a LANGE medical book

CURRENT

Diagnosis & Treatment
in Psychiatry

Edited by

Michael H. Ebert, MD
Professor of Psychiatry and Pharmacology
Chair, Department of Psychiatry
Vanderbilt University School of Medicine
Nashville, Tennessee

Peter T. Loosen, MD, PhD
Professor of Psychiatry and Medicine
Vanderbilt University School of Medicine
Chief of Psychiatry
Nashville Veterans Affairs Medical Center
Nashville, Tennessee

Barry Nurcombe, MD
Professor of Child and Adolescent Psychiatry
The University of Queensland
Director of Child and Adolescent Psychiatry
Royal Children's Hospital and District
Queensland, Australia

Professor Emeritus
Department of Psychiatry
Vanderbilt University School of Medicine
Nashville, Tennessee

Lange Medical Books/McGraw-Hill
Medical Publishing Division

New York St. Louis San Francisco Auckland Bogotá Caracas Lisbon
London Madrid Mexico City Milan Montreal New Delhi San Juan
Singapore Sydney Tokyo Toronto

McGraw-Hill

A Division of The **McGraw·Hill** Companies

Current Diagnosis & Treatment in Psychiatry

234567890 DOWDOW 09876543210

ISBN 0-8385-1462-6
ISSN 1528-1124

Notice

Medicine is an ever-changing science. As new research and clinical experience broaden our knowledge, changes in treatment and drug therapy are required. The author and the publisher of this work have checked with sources believed to be reliable in their efforts to provide information that is complete and generally in accord with the standards accepted at the time of publication. However, in view of the possibility of human error or changes in medical sciences, neither the author nor the publisher nor any other party who has been involved in the preparation or publication of this work warrants that the information contained herein is in every respect accurate or complete, and they are not responsible for any errors or omissions or for the results obtained from use of such information. Readers are encouraged to confirm the information contained herein with other sources. For example and in particular, readers are advised to check the product information sheet included in the package of each drug they plan to administer to be certain that the information contained in this book is accurate and that changes have not been made in the recommended dose or in the contraindications for administration. This recommendation is of particular importance in connection with new or infrequently used drugs.

This book was set in Times Roman by Rainbow Graphics, LLC.
The editors were Shelley Reinhardt, Isabel Nogueira, and Jeanmarie Roche.
The production supervisor was Richard C. Ruzycka.
The production service was Rainbow Graphics, LLC.
The cover designer was Elizabeth Schmitz.
The art manager was Eve Siegel.
The index was prepared by Kathy Pitcoff.

R. R. Donnelley & Sons, Inc. was printer and binder.

This book is printed on acid-free paper.

This book is dedicated to Ellen Levine Ebert, Otto Loosen, and Alison Nurcombe.

Contents

SECTION III. SYNDROMES AND THEIR TREATMENTS IN ADULT PSYCHIATRY

SECTION IV. TECHNIQUES & SETTINGS IN CHILD & ADOLESCENT PSYCHIATRY

SECTION V. SYNDROMES & THEIR TREATMENTS IN CHILD & ADOLESCENT PSYCHIATRY

Preface

Current Diagnosis & Treatment in Psychiatry reflects the current dynamic state of psychiatric knowledge. New discoveries from the basic biomedical and psychological sciences are having a major impact on psychiatric practice today. The task is to translate these new discoveries into a form useful to clinicians. This text is intended to be practical, succinct, and useful for all health care professionals who encounter and provide care for individuals with psychiatric symptoms and behavioral disturbance.

The field of psychiatry has undergone a gradual change in the last several decades. It has moved from a body of medical and psychological knowledge that was theory-bound, to an empirical approach that is more flexible with regard to reasoning about etiology. This change came about as it became apparent that developments in neurobiology, genetics, and cognitive and developmental psychology would make unanticipated inroads into our understanding of the etiology and pathogenesis of psychiatric syndromes. Furthermore, a more flexible philosophy evolved regarding the description and definition of psychiatric syndromes. Some syndromes have indistinct boundaries and shade into each other. In addition, the idea of discovering a single underlying biochemical characteristic of a psychiatric syndrome, which would in turn clarify the diagnostic description and predict treatment, was recognized as being hopelessly simplistic. Moreover, through the complexity of behavioral genetics, we now understand that those genotypes which are becoming highly significant in understanding psychopathology and developmental psychology may lead to unexpected phenotypes which do not fit our current conception of the psychiatric syndromes.

Section I of *Current Diagnosis & Treatment in Psychiatry* identifies some of the major tributaries of scientific knowledge that inform the current theory and practice of psychiatry. Sections II and IV present specialized settings and techniques for the delivery of psychiatric treatment. Sections III and V describe the syndromes of psychopathology as we understand them today and discuss current standards of treatment for each.

Current Diagnosis & Treatment in Psychiatry is written from an empirical viewpoint, with recognition that the boundaries of psychopathological syndromes may change unexpectedly with the emergence of new knowledge. Eventually, the accumulation of new knowledge will sharpen our diagnostic techniques and improve the treatment of these illnesses that have such a high impact on normal development, health, and society.

ACKNOWLEDGMENTS

We wish to thank Ellen Levine Ebert for her editorial assistance in the preparation of the text, Amy Marks for her thoughtful developmental and copy editing, Isabel Nogueira for her helpful coordination of the text, and Shelley Reinhardt for her leadership and advice throughout the process.

Michael H. Ebert, MD
Peter T. Loosen, MD, PhD
Barry Nurcombe, MD

March 2000

Authors

R. Pryor Baird, MD, PhD
Assistant Professor of Psychiatry, Vanderbilt University School of Medicine, Nashville, Tennessee
Internet: twoasprin@yahoo.com
Mood Disorders

Anna Baumgaertel, MD
Assistant Professor of Pediatrics and Developmental Pediatrician, Child Development Center, Vanderbilt University School of Medicine, Nashville, Tennessee
Internet: anna.baumgaertel@mcmail.vanderbilt.edu
Disorders Usually Presenting in Middle Childhood (6–11 Years) or Adolescence (12–18 years)

William Bernet, MD
Associate Professor of Psychiatry, Department of Psychiatry; Director, Vanderbilt Forensic Psychiatry, Vanderbilt University School of Medicine, Nashville, Tennessee
Internet: bill.bernet@mcmail.vanderbilt.edu
Psychiatry & the Law; Diagnostic Encounter; Disorders Usually Presenting in Middle Childhood (6–11 years) or Adolescence (12–18 years); Other Conditions Occurring in Childhood or Adolescence

Wade Berrettini, MD, PhD
The Karl E. Rickels Professor of Psychiatry; Director, Center for Neurobiology and Behavior, University of Pennsylvania, Philadelphia
Internet: wadeb@mail.med.upenn.edu
Psychiatric Genetics

John L. Beyer, MD
Assistant Clinical Professor, Department of Psychiatry and Behavioral Sciences, Duke University Medical Center, Durham, North Carolina
Internet: beyer001@mc.duke.edu
Mood Disorders

Tahir I. Bhatti, MD
Attending Clinical Staff, Departments of Medicine and Psychiatry, University of California, San Diego Medical Center
Internet: tsbhatt@simplyweb.net
Sleep Disorders

Leonard Bickman, PhD
Professor of Psychology, Psychiatry, and Public Policy, Vanderbilt University; Director, Center for Mental Health Policy, Nashville, Tennessee
Internet: bickmann@attglobal.net
Mental Health Services Research

Daniel G. Blazer, MD, PhD
J.P. Gibbons Professor of Psychiatry and Behavioral Sciences, Duke University School of Medicine, Durham, North Carolina
Internet: blaze001@mc.duke.edu
Psychiatric Epidemiology

George C. Bolian, MD
Associate Professor, Department of Psychiatry, Vanderbilt University School of Medicine, Nashville, Tennessee
Internet: george.bolian@mcmail.vanderbilt.edu
Emergency Psychiatry

Thomas F. Catron, PhD
Associate Professor of Psychiatry, Vanderbilt University School of Medicine; Executive Director, Vanderbilt Community Mental Health Center; Co-Director, Center for Psychotherapy Research and Policy, Vanderbilt Institute for Public Policy Studies, Nashville, Tennessee
Internet: tom.catron@vanderbilt.edu
Continuity of Care

Camellia P. Clark, MD
Clinical Instructor and Associate Physician, Department of Psychiatry, University of California, San Diego
Internet: cclark@vapop.ucsd.edu
Sleep Disorders

Kenneth A. Dodge, PhD
William McDougall Professor of Public Policy and Psychology; Director, Center for Child and Family Policy, Duke University, Durham, North Carolina
Internet: kenneth.dodge@duke.edu
Developmental Psychology

Michael H. Ebert, MD
Professor of Psychiatry and Pharmacology; Chair, Department of Psychiatry, Vanderbilt University School of

Medicine, Nashville, Tennessee
Internet: mike.ebert@mcmail.vanderbilt.edu
Psychiatric Interview; Eating Disorders

S. Hossein Fatemi, MD, PhD
Associate Professor of Psychiatry, Cell Biology, and
Neuroanatomy, Department of Psychiatry, University of
Minnesota School of Medicine, Minneapolis, Minnesota
Internet: fatem002@tc.umn.edu
Schizophrenia

Elliot M. Fielstein, PhD
Assistant Professor of Psychiatry, Vanderbilt University
School of Medicine; Clinical Neuropsychologist, Veter-
ans Affairs Medical Center, Nashville, Tennessee
Internet: elliot.m.fielstein@vanderbilt.edu
Posttraumatic Stress Disorder & Acute Stress Disorder

Robert B. Fisher, MD, MPH
Associate Professor, Department of Psychiatry and Neu-
rology, Tulane University School of Medicine; Associate
Medical Director for Adult Services, Office of Mental
Health, Louisiana State Department of Health and Hos-
pitals, New Orleans
Internet: robert_fisher73@hotmail.com
Psychiatric Epidemiology

Lee Fleisher, BS
Senior Associate and Vice Chair, Administration, De-
partment of Psychiatry, Vanderbilt University School of
Medicine, Nashville, Tennessee
Internet: lee.fleisher@mcmail.vanderbilt.edu
Continuity of Care

Charles V. Ford, MD
Professor, Department of Psychiatry and Behavioral
Neurobiology, University of Alabama School of Medi-
cine, Birmingham
Internet: cford@uabmc.edu
*Somatoform Disorders; Factitious Disorders & Malin-
gering*

Arthur M. Freeman III, MD
Professor of Psychiatry; Chair, Department of Psychia-
try, Louisiana State University School of Medicine,
Shreveport
Internet: afreem@lsumc.edu
Consultation-Liaison Psychiatry

Volney P. Gay, PhD
Professor, Departments of Religion, Psychiatry, and An-
thropology, Vanderbilt University, Nashville, Tennessee
Internet: volney.p.gay@vanderbilt.edu
Psychoanalysis

Gregory M. Gillette, MD
Assistant Professor of Psychiatry, Vanderbilt University
School of Medicine; Assistant Chief of Psychiatry, Vet-
erans Affairs Medical Center, Nashville, Tennessee
Internet: gillette.gregory@nashville.va.gov
Posttraumatic Stress Disorder & Acute Stress Disorder

J. Christian Gillin, MD
Professor of Psychiatry, University of California, San
Diego; Director, Mental Health Clinical Research Cen-
ter, University of California, San Diego, and the Veterans
Affairs San Diego Healthcare System
Internet: jgillin@ucsd.edu
Sleep Disorders

Harry E. Gwirtsman, MD
Associate Professor of Psychiatry; Director, Division of
Geriatric Psychiatry, Department of Psychiatry, Vander-
bilt University School of Medicine, Nashville, Tennessee
Internet: harry.gwirtsman@med.va.gov
*Psychiatric Interview; Mood Disorders; Eating Disor-
ders*

William A. Hewlett, MD, PhD
Associate Professor, Department of Psychiatry; Director,
Obsessive-Compulsive Disorder/Tourette Program, Van-
derbilt University School of Medicine, Nashville, Ten-
nessee
Internet: hewletw@mcmail.vanderbilt.edu
Obsessive-Compulsive Disorder

Steven D. Hollon, PhD
Professor, Departments of Psychology and Psychiatry,
Vanderbilt University, Nashville, Tennessee
Internet: steven.d.hollon@vanderbilt.edu
Behavioral & Cognitive-Behavioral Interventions

John R. Hubbard, MD, PhD
Associate Professor of Psychiatry, Vanderbilt University
School of Medicine, Nashville, Tennessee
Internet: hubbard.john_r@nashville.va.gov
Substance-Related Disorders; Personality Disorders

Joseph A. Kwentus, MD
Assistant Professor of Psychiatry, Vanderbilt University
School of Medicine, Nashville, Tennessee; Medical Di-
rector, Behavioral Sciences, Tennessee Christian Med-
ical Center, Madison
Internet: joekwentus@home.com
Delirium, Dementia, & Amnestic Syndromes

Joseph D. LaBarbera, PhD
Associate Professor of Psychiatry; Director of Psychol-
ogy, Division of Child and Adolescent Psychiatry, De-
partment of Psychiatry, Vanderbilt University School of
Medicine, Nashville, Tennessee
Internet: joseph.labarbera@mcmail.vanderbilt.edu
Diagnostic Testing

Peter T. Loosen, MD, PhD
Professor of Psychiatry and Medicine, Vanderbilt Uni-
versity School of Medicine; Chief of Psychiatry,
Nashville Veterans Affairs Medical Center, Tennessee
Internet: ptloosen@aol.com
Mood Disorders

Peter R. Martin, MD
Professor of Psychiatry and Pharmacology; Director, Division of Addiction Medicine and Vanderbilt Addiction

Center, Department of Psychiatry, Vanderbilt University School of Medicine, Nashville, Tennessee
Internet: peter.martin@mcmail.vanderbilt.edu
Substance-Related Disorders

Jonathan E. May, PhD
Adjunct Assistant Professor of Psychology, Vanderbilt University School of Medicine; Director, Psychology Training, Nashville Veterans Affairs Medical Center, Nashville, Tennessee
Internet: may.jonathan_e+@nashville.va.gov
Sexual Dysfunctions & Paraphilias

Herbert Y. Meltzer, MD
Bixler Professor of Psychiatry and Pharmacology; Director, Division of Psychopharmacology, Department of Psychiatry, Vanderbilt University School of Medicine, Nashville, Tennessee
Internet: herbert.meltzer@mcmail.vanderbilt.edu
Schizophrenia

Polly J. Moore, PhD, RPsgT
Post-Doctoral Fellow, Department of Psychiatry, University of California, San Diego, and the University of California, San Diego, Cancer Center
Internet: pmoore@ucsd.edu
Sleep Disorders

Leslie C. Morey, PhD
Professor of Psychology, Texas A&M University, College Station, Texas
Internet: icm@psyc.tamu.edu
Personality Disorders

James L. Nash, MD
Associate Professor of Psychiatry; Vice-Chairman for Graduate Medical Education, Department of Psychiatry, Vanderbilt University School of Medicine, Nashville, Tennessee
Internet: james.nash@mcmail.vanderbilt.edu
General Principles of Psychotherapeutic Management; Mood Disorders

Carol T. Nixon, MA
Program Evaluation Manager, Access Behavioral Care, Denver, Colorado
Internet: carol_nixon@coaccess.com
Mental Health Services Research

Denine A. Northrup, PhD
Research Associate, Center for Mental Health Policy, Vanderbilt University, Nashville, Tennessee
Internet: d.northrup@vanderbilt.edu
Mental Health Services Research

Barry Nurcombe, MD
Professor of Child and Adolescent Psychiatry, The University of Queensland; Director of Child and Adolescent Psychiatry, Royal Children's Hospital and District, Queensland, Australia; Professor Emeritus, Department of Psychiatry, Vanderbilt University School of Medicine, Nashville, Tennessee
Internet: i.spinks@psychiatry.uq.edu.au
Psychiatric Interview; Clinical Decision Making in Psychiatry; Dissociative Disorders; Diagnostic Encounter; Diagnostic Testing; Diagnostic Formulation, Treatment Planning, & Modes of Treatment; Disorders Usually Presenting in Infancy or Early Childhood (0–5 years); Disorders Usually Presenting in Middle Childhood (6–11 Years) or Adolescence (12–18 years); Other Conditions Occurring in Childhood or Adolescence

John I. Nurnberger Jr., MD, PhD
Joyce & Iver Small Professor of Psychiatry, Neurobiology and Medical Genetics; Director, Institute of Psychiatric Genetics and Assistant Chairman for Research, Department of Psychiatry, Indiana University School of Medicine, Indianapolis
Internet: jnurnber@iupui.edu
Psychiatric Genetics

Rudra Prakash, MD
Associate Clinical Professor, Department of Psychiatry, Vanderbilt University, Nashville, Tennessee
Emergency Psychiatry

Howard B. Roback, PhD
Professor, Departments of Psychiatry and Psychology, Vanderbilt University School of Medicine, Nashville, Tennessee
Internet: howard.roback@mcmail.vanderbilt.edu
Psychological Testing in Psychiatry

Ronald M. Salomon, MD
Assistant Professor of Psychiatry; Medical Director, Obsessive-Compulsive Disorders Clinic, Vanderbilt University School of Medicine, Nashville, Tennessee
Internet: ron.salomon@mcmail.vanderbilt.edu
Adjustment Disorders

Lucy Salomon, MD
Consultant in Psychiatry, Nantucket Cottage Hospital, Nantucket, Massachusetts
Internet: slmnlucy@nantucket.net
Adjustment Disorders

Roy Q. Sanders, MD
Attending Psychiatrist, Division of Child and Adolescent Psychiatry, Mary Imogene Bassett Hospital, Cooperstown, New York
Internet: royquincy@aol.com
Disorders Usually Presenting in Middle Childhood (6–11 years) or Adolescence (12–18 years)

Erich Seifritz, MD
Psychiatrist, Department of Psychiatry, University of Basel, Switzerland
Internet: erich.seifritz@Unibas.ch
Sleep Disorders

Samuel R. Sells III, MD
Assistant Professor, Department of Psychiatry, Vanderbilt University School of Medicine, Nashville, Tennessee
Internet: sam.sells@mcmail.vanderbilt.edu
Mood Disorders

Vernon H. Sharp, MD
Associate Clinical Professor of Psychiatry, Vanderbilt University School of Medicine, Nashville, Tennessee
Interviewing Families

Richard C. Shelton, MD
Associate Professor, Departments of Psychiatry and Pharmacology; Director, Division of Adult Psychiatry, Department of Psychiatry, Vanderbilt University School of Medicine, Nashville, Tennessee
Internet: richard.shelton@mcmail.vanderbilt.edu
General Principles of Psychopharmacologic Treatment; Other Psychotic Disorders; Mood Disorders; Anxiety Disorders

Sydney Spector, PhD
Professor, Departments of Psychiatry and Pharmacology, Vanderbilt University School of Medicine, Nashville, Tennessee
Internet: sydney.spector@mcmail.vanderbilt.edu
Neuropsychopharmacology

Wendy L. Stone, PhD
Associate Professor of Pediatrics; Director, Treatment and Research Institute for Autism Spectrum Disorders (TRIAD), Vanderbilt University School of Medicine, Nashville, Tennessee
Internet: wendy.stone@mcmail.vanderbilt.edu
Disorders Usually Presenting in Infancy or Early Childhood (0—5 years)

Fridolin Sulser, MD
Professor, Departments of Psychiatry and Pharmacology, Vanderbilt University School of Medicine, Nashville, Tennessee
Internet: fridolin.sulser@mcmail.vanderbilt.edu
Neuropharmacology

William Thomas Summerfelt, PhD
Assistant Professor, Department of Psychology, Michigan State University, East Lansing, Michigan
Internet: summerf6@msu.edu
Mental Health Services Research

John W. Thompson Jr., MD
Associate Professor, Departments of Psychiatry and Neurology; Director, Forensic Neuropsychiatry, Tulane University School of Medicine, New Orleans
Internet: jthomps3@mailhost.tcs.tulane.edu
Impulse-Control Disorder

Travis Thompson, PhD
Professor of Psychology and Psychiatry; Director, John F. Kennedy Center on Human Development, Vanderbilt University, Nashville, Tennessee
Internet: thompst@ctrvax.vanderbilt.edu
Behavioral & Cognitive-Behavioral Interventions

Michael G. Tramontana, PhD
Associate Professor of Psychiatry, Department of Psychiatry, Vanderbilt University School of Medicine, Nashville, Tennessee
Internet: michael.tramontana@mcmail.vanderbilt.edu
Diagnostic Testing; Disorders Usually Presenting in Infancy or Early Childhood (0–5 years); Disorders Usually Presenting in Middle Childhood (6–11 years) or Adolescence (12–18 years)

Larry W. Welch, EdD
Assistant Clinical Professor of Neurology, Vanderbilt University School of Medicine, Nashville, Tennessee
Internet: larry.w.welch@vanderbilt.edu
Psychological Testing in Psychiatry

James R. Westphal, MD
Professor of Clinical Psychiatry; Director of Consultation-Liaison Psychiatry, Louisiana State University Health Sciences Center, Shreveport
Internet: jwestp@lsumc.edu
Consultation-Liaison Psychiatry

Daniel K. Winstead, MD
Professor of Psychiatry and Neurology; Chair, Department of Psychiatry and Neurology, Tulane University School of Medicine, New Orleans
Internet: dan@winstead.net
Impulse-Control Disorders

Mark L. Wolraich, MD
Professor, Department of Pediatrics; Chief, Division of Child Development, Department of Pediatrics, Vanderbilt University School of Medicine, Nashville, Tennessee
Internet: mark.wolraich@mcmail.vanderbilt.edu
Disorders Usually Presenting in Infancy or Early Childhood (0–5 years) Disorders Usually Presenting in Middle Childhood (6–11 years) or Adolescence (12–18 years)

Section I.
Scientific Areas Relevant to Modern Psychiatry

Developmental Psychology

1

Kenneth A. Dodge, PhD

DEVELOPMENTAL CONCEPTS

The concept of development forms the backbone of modern behavioral science. Psychiatric practitioners and behavioral scientists are concerned primarily with change, and **developmental psychology** is the scientific study of the structure, function, and processes of systematic change across the life span. Even systems of classification of behavior (including psychiatric nosology) take into account not only contemporaneous features and formal similarities among current symptoms but also past qualities, immediate consequences, and long-term outcomes.

Whereas developmental psychology is concerned with species-typical patterns of systematic change (and central tendencies of the species), the emerging discipline of **developmental psychopathology** is concerned with individual differences and contributes greatly to our understanding of childhood disorders.

The organizing framework of developmental psychopathology is a movement toward understanding the predictors, causes, processes, courses, sequelae, and environmental symbiosis of psychiatric illnesses in order to discover empirically effective forms of treatment and prevention. This movement is girded in a developmental framework that integrates knowledge from multiple disciplines (eg, psychobiology, neuroscience, cognitive psychology, social psychology) and levels of analysis (eg, neuronal synapses, psychophysiologic responses, mental representations, motor behaviors, personality patterns). The relationship between developmental psychology and developmental psychopathology is reciprocally influential: The study of normal development gives context to the analysis of aberrations, and the study of psychopathology informs our understanding of normative development.

A developmental orientation forces a scholar to ask questions that move beyond the prevalence and incidence of disorders. Table 1–1 lists some of these questions.

THE ORTHOGENETIC PRINCIPLE

Human growth is not linear. Behavioral and psychological change is not marked merely by quantitative advances or declines. The organizational perspective on development offers a powerful theoretical framework for depicting the organism as an integrated system with hierarchically ordered subsystems and for understanding change as a progression of qualitative reorganizations within and among subsystems. The human being is a coherent integration of neural, physiologic, hormonal, affective, information-processing, mental representational, behavioral, and social subsystems. Change occurs both within these subsystems and in the relations among them.

The **orthogenetic principle** proposes that development moves from undifferentiated and diffuse organization toward greater complexity, achieved through

Table 1–1. Questions related to a developmental orientation.

How and why do some at-risk individuals become psychologically ill, whereas others do not?

How do the capacities and limitations of the human species at various life stages predispose individuals to disorder? (For example, why are females at relatively high risk for depression during adolescence?)

How are various disorders related developmentally? (For example, how does oppositional defiant disorder lead to conduct disorder, which leads to antisocial personality disorder?)

Where are the natural boundaries between normal and abnormal?

Are there critical periods, and if so, why? (For example, why is a high lead level in the blood more detrimental early in life?)

What does the concept of multifactorial causation imply for the likely success of intervention efforts?

both differentiation and consolidation within and across subsystems. The newborn infant is relatively undifferentiated in response patterns, but through development this infant achieves greater differentiation (and less stereotypy) of functioning. Each period of development is characterized by adaptational challenges resulting from environmental demands (eg, a mother who has become unwilling to breast-feed) and from emerging internal influences across subsystems (eg, growing recognition of the self as able to exert control). The challenges are best conceptualized not as mere threats to homeostasis; rather, change and the demand for adaptation define the human species, and challenges push the individual toward development. The inherent adaptational response of the species is toward mastery of new demands. The mastery motive is as yet unexplained by science, although it is paradigmatic of the human species (see "Adaptation and Competence" section later in this chapter).

Thus development is characterized by periods of disruption in the homeostasis of the organism brought on by a new challenge, followed by adaptation and consolidation until the next challenge is presented. The adaptive child uses both internal and external resources to meet a challenge. **Successful adaptation** is defined as the optimal organization of behavioral and biological systems within the context of current challenges. Adaptation requires the assimilation of past organizational structures to current demands as well as the generation of new structures equipped to meet the demands.

Consider the toddler who is confronted by an environment that becomes less indiscriminately giving (eg, a mother who needs to feed her toddler on a schedule). The toddler may respond initially with temper tantrums to indicate his or her displeasure and needs, but tantrums evolve into verbal communication as the toddler learns how to achieve desired outcomes most efficiently. Thus environmental challenge and internal chaotic responses (eg, temper tantrums) may be steps in the orthogenesis of language.

Piaget described two types of change: **assimilation,** which involves incorporation of the challenge into existing organizational structures (eg, an infant might treat all adults as the same kind of stimulus); and **accommodation,** which involves reorganization of the organism's structures to meet the demands of the environment (eg, a developing infant learns to discriminate among adults and to respond differently to different adults) (see "Organismic Theory" section later in this chapter). Accommodation is more complex than assimilation, but successful adaptation requires a balance of assimilation and accommodation.

Maladaptation, or incompetence in responding to challenge, may be characterized by the inadequate resolution of developmental challenges (as in the psychoanalytic concept of fixation). Maladaptation may be evidenced by developmental delays or lags, such as the continuing temper tantrums of an emotionally dysregulated child beyond the period when such behavior is normative. At any phase, the organism will seek some form of regulation and functioning, even if it is not advantageous for future development. Thus the child's tantrums might serve to regulate both a complex external environment of marital turmoil and an internal environment of stress. However, nonoptimal regulation will prevent or hamper the individual from coping with the next developmental challenge. Continuing the example of the dysregulated child, the repetitive pattern of anger may lead to poor peer relations, which prevent the child from acquiring new social skills through friendships.

Sometimes apparently effective responses to a particular challenge lead to maladaptation at a more general level. Consider a toddler who responds to the withdrawal of a mother's undivided attention by ignoring her. Although this pattern of response may mean calmer evenings temporarily, the toddler will be ill equipped to respond to other challenges later in development. Consistent social withdrawal may cause the child to fail to acquire skills of assertion; however, continued ignoring of the mother may lead to a phenotypically distinct response in the future (eg, depression in adolescence). Thus the orthogenetic principle calls to mind the functioning of the entire organism (not merely distinct and unrelated subsystems) and the readiness of that organism to respond to future challenges.

Horowitz FD: *Exploring Developmental Theories: Toward a Structural/Behavioral Model of Development.* Lawrence Erlbaum Assoc, 1987.

MAJOR PRINCIPLES OF ONTOGENY & PHYLOGENY

Cairns and Cairns outlined seven principles that characterize the human organism in interaction with the environment over time: conservation, coherence, bidirectionality, reciprocal interaction, novelty, within-individual variation, and dynamic systems. The first principle is that of **conservation,** or connectivity in functioning across time. Even with all the pressure to change, social and cognitive organization tends to be continuous and conservative. The constraints on the organism and the multiple determinants of behavior lead to gradual transition rather than abrupt mutation. Observers can recognize the continuity in persons across even long periods of time; that is, we know that a person remains the same "person." For Piaget, who began his career by writing scientific papers on the evolution of mollusks, this within-person continuity principle is consistent with his view that species-wide evolution is gradual. Piaget believed that development within individuals reflects development of the species (ie, ontogeny recapitulates phylogeny).

The second principle is **coherence.** Individuals function as holistic and integrated units, in spite of the multiple systems that contribute to any set of behaviors. One cannot divorce one system from another because the two systems function as a whole that is greater than its component parts. This fact is another conservative force, because an adverse effect on one part of a system tends to be offset by compensatory responses from other parts of the system. This phenomenon applies to all human biological systems and can be applied to psychological functioning.

The third principle is a corollary of the second: Influence between the organism and the environment is **bidirectional.** The person is an active agent in continuous interaction with others. Reciprocal influences are not identical; rather, at each stage of development, the person organizes the outer world through a mental representational system that mediates all experience with the world. Nevertheless, reciprocity and synchrony constrain the person, and the relative weight of these constraints varies at different points in development. At one extreme, it is possible to speak of symbiosis and total dependency of the infant on the mother; at the other extreme, behavior geneticists refer to genetic effects on environmental variables (such as the proposition that genes produce behavior that leads to the reactions that one receives from others in social exchanges).

Another corollary of the second principle is the principle of **reciprocal interaction** between subsystems within the individual. Behavioral, cognitive, emotional, neurochemical, hormonal, and morphologic factors affect each other reciprocally. Mental events have biological implications and vice versa. Even though this principle has been embraced by several areas of biology (eg, ethology, behavioral zoology), psychology and psychiatry sometimes persist in a war between biological and mental camps.

The fifth principle of ontogeny is that **novelty** arises in development. Change is not haphazard. The forces of reciprocal interaction within the individual and the environment lead not only to quantitative changes in the individual but also to the emergence of qualitatively distinct forms, such as locomotion, language, and thought. These changes represent growth rather than random events, in that previous forms typically remain and are supplemented by novel forms.

The sixth principle of phylogeny is that of **within-individual variation** in developmental rates across subsystems. Change within a subsystem occurs nonlinearly, as in language development or even physical growth. Some of this nonlinearity can be explained by species-wide phenomena, such as puberty, but much of it varies across individuals. In addition, rates of change vary within an individual across subsystems. Consider two young children, identical in age. Child A may learn to crawl before child B, but child B might catch up and learn to walk before child A. Likewise, child B might utter a recognizable word be-

fore child A, but child A might be talking in sentences before child B. This unevenness within and across individuals characterizes development and makes predictions probabilistic rather than certain. Some of the variation is attributable to environmental factors that have enduring personal effects (such as the lasting effects on cognitive achievement of early entry into formal schooling) or biological factors that have enduring psychological effects (such as the effect of early pubertal onset on social outcomes), whereas other factors may have only temporary effects (such as efforts to accelerate locomotion onset) or no effects.

Finally, according to the seventh principle, development is extremely sensitive to unique configurations of influence, such as in **dynamic systems.** Growth and change cannot be reduced to a quantitative cumulation of biological and environmental units. Also, development is not simply hierarchical, with gradual building of functions on previous ones. Rather, development often follows a sequence of organization, disorganization, and then reorganization in a different (possibly more advanced) form. In physical sciences, this principle is called **catastrophe theory,** reflecting the hypothesis that during the disorganization, events are literally random. But reorganization occurs eventually, in lawful and predictable ways. Dynamic systems models are now being used to describe the acquisition of novel functions such as locomotion and language. In theory, the same models could be used to describe individual differences in development, as in psychopathology. Even though the concept of stage-based development has lost favor because of the global nature and nonfalsifiability of some stage theories, these dynamic-system qualities have been captured in stage-based theories of change.

Cairns RB, Cairns BD: *Lifelines and Risks: Pathways of Youth in Our Time.* Cambridge University Press, 1994.

Dodge KA, Bates JE, Pettit GS: Mechanisms in the cycle of violence. Science 1990;250:1678.

AGE NORMS

A simple but powerful developmental concept that has affected psychiatric nosology is that of **age norms.** Rather than evaluating a set of behaviors or symptoms according to a theoretical, absolute, or population-wide distribution, diagnosticians increasingly use age norms to evaluate psychiatric problems. Consider the evaluation of temper tantrums. In a 2-year-old child, tantrums are normative, whereas in an adult, angry outbursts could indicate an intermittent explosive disorder or antisocial personality. More subtle examples have begun to affect the diagnosis of many disorders in the *Diagnostic and Statistical Manual of Mental Disorders,* 4th edition (DSM-IV), such as attention-deficit/hyperactivity disorder, mental retardation, and conduct disorder. With regard to major depressive episodes and dysthymic disorder, age norming has resulted in consideration of different symptoms at different ages in order to diagnose the same disorder (eg, irritability and somatization are common in prepubescent depression, whereas delusions are more common in adulthood). DSM-IV explicitly requires consideration of age, gender, and culture features in all disorders, suggesting the importance of evaluating symptoms within the context of their expression.

The importance of age norming suggests the need for empirical studies of symptoms in large epidemiologic samples and the linking of research on normative development to psychopathology. In this way, developmental psychopathology is similar to psychiatric epidemiology (see Chapter 5). Despite the increased emphasis on age norming, ambiguity pervades current practice. DSM-IV defines disorders in terms of symptoms that are quantified as "often," "recurrent," and "persistent" without operational definition. Some clinicians intuitively contextualize their use of the term "often" relative to a child's agemates (so that "often displays temper tantrums" might mean hourly for a 2-year-old child and weekly for a teenager), whereas other clinicians do not (so that "often" has the same literal meaning across all ages). The specific meaning of these terms is not clear in the context of some DSM-IV disorders. Complete age norming might imply the removal of all age differences in prevalence rates (reducing disorder merely to the statistical extremes of a distribution at an age level), whereas complete neglect of age norms implies that at certain ages a disorder is ubiquitous. To resolve these problems, developmental researchers need to learn which patterns of symptoms ought to be examined epidemiologically, and psychopathologists need to compare their observations to empirical norms.

Cairns RB, Cairns BD: *Lifelines and Risks: Pathways of Youth in Our Time.* Cambridge University Press, 1994.

DEVELOPMENTAL TRAJECTORIES

Diagnosticians must consider not only the age-normed profile of symptoms but also the developmental trajectories of those symptoms (both age-normed and individual). For example, consider three 10-year-old children who exhibit aggressive behavior. As depicted in Figure 1–1, child A has displayed a relatively high rate of aggression historically, but the trajectory is downward. Child B has displayed a constant rate of aggressive displays, and child C's aggressive displays have accelerated geometrically. Which child has a problematic profile? The diagnostician will undoubtedly want to consider not only current symptom counts (in relation to age norms) but also the developmental trajectory of these counts (and the age norm

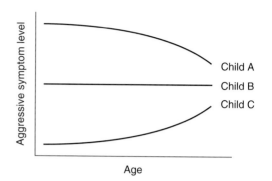

Figure 1–1. Three hypothetical developmental trajectories for aggressive behavior.

for the trajectory). Child C might be most problematic because of the age trend, unless this trend were also age normative (eg, some increase in delinquent behavior in adolescence is certainly normative). In contrast, child B's constant pattern might be problematic if the age-normed trend were a declining slope.

Some DSM-IV disorders explicitly take into account the trajectory of an individual's symptoms. For example, Rett's disorder, childhood disintegrative disorder, and dementia of the Alzheimer's type involve deviant trajectories. The diagnosis of other disorders may require trajectory information that is not yet available. This information must be based on longitudinal study of individuals and not cross-sectional data, because only longitudinal inquiry allows for the charting of growth curves within individuals over time. Population means at various ages indicate little about within-individual changes. Population-wide symptom counts might grow systematically across age even when individual trajectories are highly variable.

Costello EJ: Developments in child psychiatric epidemiology. J Am Acad Child Adolesc Psychiatry 1989;28:836.

BOUNDARY BETWEEN NORMAL & ABNORMAL

One of the tenets of developmental psychology is that a knowledge of normal development informs psychopathology partly because the boundaries between normal and abnormal are sometimes vague, diffuse, or continuous. Many disorders (eg, conduct disorder, dysthymic disorder) are defined on the basis of cutoffs in dimensional criteria rather than on qualitative distinctions that are more easily recognizable. Criteria such as "low energy" and "low self-esteem" (for dysthymic disorder) and "marked or persistent fear" (for social phobia) are matters of degree. One of the central questions is where to locate the boundary between normal and abnormal when the criteria of psychopathology are dimensional.

In some cases the boundary is arbitrary. In other cases the "true" boundary might be identified on the basis of three considerations: (1) a noncontinuous pattern of the distribution of scores, (2) a qualitatively distinct change in functioning that accompanies a quantitative difference in a score, or (3) unique etiology at the extreme of a distribution.

The first consideration is whether the population of scores is distributed normally with a single mode or bimodally with an unusually large number of cases at one extreme. A large number of cases at one extreme would suggest that a second causal agent is operating, beyond whatever agent caused the normal distribution. A second causal agent might suggest a deviant (ie, psychopathologic) process. Consider the relation between the intelligence quotient (IQ) score (a continuous measure) and mental retardation. The distribution of IQ scores in the U.S. population is not normal. Far more cases of IQs below 70 occur than would be expected by a normal distribution. Thus the distinction between normal and abnormal IQ scores is not merely one of degree.

The second consideration is whether qualitative differences in functioning occur with quantitative shifts in a criterion. For example, if a decrement of 10 IQ points from 75 to 65 makes it significantly more difficult for a child to function in a classroom than a decrement from 100 to 90, then a case can be made for locating the cutoff point near an IQ of 70.

The third consideration is the possible distinct etiology of scores at an extreme end of the distribution. A single set of causes will ordinarily lead to a normal distribution of scores. A disproportionate number of scores at an extreme often suggests a separate etiology for those scores. In the case of IQ scores, one set of forces (eg, genes, socialization) leads to a normal distribution, whereas a second set of forces (eg, Down syndrome, anoxia, lead toxicity) leads to a large number of cases at the low extreme.

American Psychiatric Association: *Diagnostic and Statistical Manual of Mental Disorders,* 4th ed. American Psychiatric Association, 1994.

MULTIPLE PATHWAYS

One vexing problem highlighted by research in developmental psychology is that some disorders involve multiple etiologic pathways. The principles of equifinality and multifinality, derived from general systems theory, hold for many disorders. **Equifinality** is the concept that the same phenomenon may result from several different pathogens. For example, infantile autism results from congenital rubella, inherited metabolic disorder, or other factors. **Multifinality** is the concept that one etiologic factor can lead to any of several psychopathologic outcomes, depending on the person and context. Early physical abuse might lead to conduct disorder or to dysthymic disorder, depending on the person's predilections and the environmental supports for various symptoms; poverty predisposes one toward conduct disorder but also substance abuse disorder.

The diversity in processes and outcomes for disorders makes the systematic study of a single disorder difficult. Unless scholars consider multiple disorders and multiple factors simultaneously, they cannot be sure whether an apparent etiologic factor is specific to that disorder. Inquiry into one disorder benefits from a conceptualization within a larger body of development of normal adjustment versus problem outcomes. The broad coverage of developmental psychology provides the grounding for inquiry into various disorders.

Rutter M: Psychosocial resilience and protective mechanisms. In: Rolf J et al (editors): *Risk and Protective Factors in the Development of Psychopathology.* Cambridge University Press, 1990.

BIOSOCIAL INTERACTIONS

Not only are multiple distinct factors implicated in the genesis of a disorder, the profile of factors often conspires to lead to psychopathologic outcomes. Empirically, this profile is the statistical interaction between factors (in contrast with the main effects of factors). Thus a causal factor might operate only when it occurs in concert with another factor. For example, the experience of parental rejection early in life is a contributing factor in the development of conduct disorder but only among that subgroup of children who also display a biologically based problem such as health difficulties at the time of birth. Likewise, health problems at birth do not inevitably lead to conduct disorder; the interaction of a biologically based predisposition with a psychosocial stressor is often required for a psychopathologic outcome.

Another example is the known effect of chronic social rejection by peers in early elementary school on the development of aggressive conduct problems. This social stressor leads to conduct problems only among that subgroup of children predisposed toward externalizing disorders prior to experiencing social rejection. Among the subgroup not predisposed, social rejection does not result in conduct problems. Of course, the experience of social rejection might well incite another disorder (such as a mood disorder), again, if a predisposition to such a disorder exists.

The importance of biosocial interactions suggests the importance of examining multiple diverse factors simultaneously, both in empirical research and clinical practice.

Garber J, Hilsman R: Cognitions, stress, and depression in children and adolescents. Child Adolesc Psychiatr Clin N Am 1992;1:129.

Lewin K: *A Dynamic Theory of Personality.* McGraw-Hill, 1935.

Plomin R et al: Nature and nurture: genetic influence on measures of the family environment. Dev Psychol 1994;30:32.

CRITICAL PERIODS & TRANSITION POINTS

A **critical period** is a point in the life span at which an individual is acutely sensitive to the effects of an external stimulus, including a pathogen. Freud argued that the first 3 years of life represent a critical period for the development of psychopathology, through concepts such as regression, fixation, and irreversibility. The concept of critical stages gained credence with studies of social behavior in animals by the ethologist Lorenz and the zoologist Scott. This concept is part of several central theories of social development, such as Bowlby's attachment theory (discussed later in this chapter). The rapid development of the nervous system in the first several years, coupled with relatively less neural plasticity in subsequent years, renders this period critical. The effects of exposure to lead and alcohol, for example, are far more dramatic when the exposure occurs in utero or in early life than later.

An alternative to the concept of a critical period is the hypothesis of gradually decreasing plasticity in functioning across the life span. As neural pathways become canalized, mental representations become more automatic and habits form. However, the notion of the primacy of early childhood has been thrown into question by empirical data that indicate greater malleability in functioning than was previously thought. Rutter, for example, suggests that a positive relationship with a parental figure is crucial to the prevention of conduct disorder and that this relationship can develop or occur at any point up to adolescence, not just during the first year of life.

Some developmental psychologists have argued for other critical periods in life, such as puberty and giving birth as critical periods for the development of major depressive disorder in women, although this assertion has been contested. Critical periods might be defined not only by biological events but also by psychosocial transitions. Developmental psychologists have increasingly recognized the crucial role of major life transitions in altering developmental course, accelerating or decelerating psychopathologic development, and representing high-risk periods for psychopathology. These **transition points** include but are not limited to entry to formal schooling, puberty and the transition to junior high school, high school graduation and entry into the world of employment, marriage, birth of children, and death of one's loved ones (particularly parents or spouse). These transitions have been associated with elevated risk for some forms of psychopathology. One task of developmental psychologists is to discover which life transitions are most crucial and how these transitions alter the course of development of some but not other forms of psychopathology.

Kandel ER, Hawkins RD: Neuronal plasticity and learning. In: Broadwell RD (volume editor): *Decade of the Brain.* Vol 1: *Neuroscience, Memory, and Language.* Library of Congress, 1995.

IMPORTANCE OF CONTEXT

One of the most important contributions of developmental psychology has been the discovery that patterns of behavior, and of process-behavior linkage, vary across contexts. In the context of U.S. society, a child who is teased by peers might find support for retaliating aggressively, whereas the same teasing experience in Japanese society might well cause shame, embarrassment, and withdrawal. Context shapes single behaviors and may also shape patterns of psychopathology.

Most theories of human behavior do not apply equally well across all contexts but are embedded within a particular context. For example, Freud's broad hypotheses must be interpreted in relation to Western culture, at a particular point in history. Indeed, his ideas about the nature of the human species changed as he saw a world war destroy the society around him. Researchers try to determine which laws of human behavior are universal and which are contextual, and they try to identify the mechanisms through which context influences behavior.

Context can be defined at many levels, from discrete situational features to broad cultural features and from internal states such as mood to external factors such as geography or time of day. Bronfenbrenner's continuum of environmental contexts forms the basis of his ecological theory (discussed later in this chapter).

Bronfenbrenner U: *The Ecology of Human Development: Experiments by Nature and Design.* Harvard University Press, 1979.

Lewin K: *A Dynamic Theory of Personality.* McGraw-Hill, 1935.

ADAPTATION & COMPETENCE

Research in developmental psychology has sometimes enabled sharper distinctions between normal and abnormal (such as when a genetic marker of a disorder is identified), but more often it has articulated the continuity between normal and abnormal. Research has suggested that disorders might be defined less by noncontextualized behavioral criteria (eg, a score on an IQ test) and more by an assessment of the individual's level of adaptation and functioning. This concept has been embraced by the term **competence,** or adaptive functioning, which is the level of performance by an individual in meeting the demands of his or her environment to the degree that would be expected given the environment and the individual's age, background, and biological potentials.

Empirical research has shown that measures of childhood social competence are important predictors of adolescent psychiatric disorders, including conduct disorder and mood disorders. Impaired social competence is a premorbid marker for the onset of schizophrenia and is a predictor of relapse.

The concurrent importance of adaptive functioning is so obvious that this concept has become part of the diagnostic criteria for some disorders. For example, a diagnosis of mental retardation requires impairment in adaptive functioning above and beyond the score on an IQ test. A diagnosis of generalized anxiety disorder requires impairment in social functioning in addition to the absolute pattern of anxiety. A diagnosis of obsessive-compulsive disorder requires marked personal distress or significant impairment in functioning. Some broad definitions of mental disorder are based on a general assessment of an impairment in adaptive functioning due to cognitive or emotional disturbance.

Asher SR, Coie JD: *Peer Rejection in Childhood.* Cambridge University Press, 1990.
Kazdin AE: *Conduct Disorders in Childhood and Adolescence.* Sage, 1995.

RISK FACTORS & VULNERABILITY

Epidemiologic and developmental researchers have introduced the notion of **risk factors** to identify variables known to predict later disorder (see Chapter 5). A risk factor is defined by its probabilistic relation to an outcome variable, without implying determinism, early onset of disorder, or inevitability of outcome. Risk factors are either markers of some other causal process or causal factors themselves. One goal of developmental research is to determine the causal status of risk markers. As noted earlier in this chapter, social competence, or level of adaptive functioning, is a broad risk factor for many disorders, but empirical research must determine whether this factor merely indicates risk that is caused by some other factor (eg, genes) or constitutes a contributing factor in itself.

Risk factors often accumulate in enhancing the likelihood of eventual disorder. For example, the probability of conduct disorder is enhanced by low socioeconomic status, harsh parenting, parental criminality, marital conflict, family size, and academic failure. The number of factors present seems to be a stronger predictor of later disorder than is the presence of any single factor, suggesting that causal

processes are heterogeneous and that risk factors cumulatively increase vulnerability to a causal process.

The concept of **vulnerability** has been applied to individuals who are characterized by a risk factor. Many empirical studies of the development of disorder use samples that are defined by a risk factor (such as offspring of alcoholics and first-time juvenile offenders); however, it is not clear that the causal and developmental factors are similar in disordered individuals who come from high-risk and low-risk populations.

Biderman J et al: Family-environment risk factors for attention-deficit hyperactivity disorder. Arch Gen Psychiatry 1995;52:464.
Rutter M: Psychosocial resilience and protective mechanisms. In: Rolf J et al (editors): *Risk and Protective Factors in the Development of Psychopathology.* Cambridge University Press, 1990.

MEDIATORS & PROCESS

Developmental psychologists study the causal process through which disorder develops. The identification of a risk factor does not necessarily imply a causal process, because (1) a risk factor might be a proxy for a causal factor and empirically related to a disorder only because of its correlation with this causal factor (the so-called third-variable problem), (2) a risk factor might occur as an outcome of a process that is related to a disorder rather than the antecedent of the disorder, or (3) a risk factor might play a causal role in a more complex, multivariate process. Therefore, developmental psychologists often attempt to understand the process through which risk factors are related to eventual disorder. The factors that are identified as intervening variables in this process are called **mediators,** which are defined as variables that account for (or partially account for) the statistical relation between a risk factor and a disorder.

Four empirical steps are required to demonstrate at least partial mediation (Figure 1–2). First, risk factor

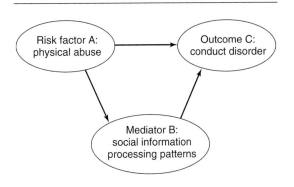

Figure 1–2. Mediation of the effect of physical abuse on the development of conduct disorder.

A must be empirically related to outcome C (ie, there must be a phenomenon to be mediated, called the **total effect**). Second, A must be related to mediator B. Third, B must be related to C. Finally, in a stepwise regression or structural equation model analysis, when B has been added to the prediction of C, the resulting relation between A and C (called the **direct effect**) must be reduced significantly from the original bivariate relation. The difference between the total effect and the direct effect is called the **indirect effect,** and it is the magnitude of the mediation of the effect of A on C by B.

An example (depicted in Figure 1–2) is the biased pattern of social information processing that often results from an early history of physical abuse. Early abuse (A) is a known risk factor for the development of conduct disorder (C) (ie, it is statistically correlated with later conduct disorder, but many abused children do not develop this disorder nor do all persons who have conduct disorder show a history of abuse). Early abuse is also correlated with the development of a social-information-processing pattern (B) of hypervigilance to threatening cues, perceiving the social world as a hostile and threatening place, and poor social-problem-solving skills. These mental factors (B) are associated statistically with later conduct disorder (C) and account for about half of the effect of early abuse (A) on later conduct disorder (C).

Baron RM, Kenny DA: The moderator-mediator variable distinction in social psychological research: conceptual, strategic, and statistical considerations. J Pers Soc Psychol 1986;51:1173.

Dodge KA: Social-cognitive mechanisms in the development of conduct disorder and depression. Annu Rev Psychol 1993;44:559.

MODERATORS & PROTECTIVE FACTORS

Rutter has enlightened scholars that the effect of a risk factor on a disorder may vary across contexts, populations, or circumstances. That is, the magnitude of an effect might be reduced (or enhanced) under different conditions. For example, the effect of early harsh discipline on the development of conduct disorder is reduced under circumstances of a warm parent-child relationship. This phenomenon is called a **moderator effect** and is defined by a significant interaction effect between a risk factor and a moderating factor in the prediction of a disorder.

Moderator variables have also been called protective, or buffering, factors. A **protective factor** protects, or buffers, the individual from the pathogenic effects of a risk factor. Intelligence and a positive relationship with a caring adult have been the most commonly studied protective factors for a variety of disorders. One remaining question is whether protective factors operate more strongly in high-risk than in low-risk groups; that is, if a variable buffers both low-risk and high-risk groups from risk, it is not clear whether that variable would be defined as a protective factor (or simply another predictor variable).

Rutter M: Psychosocial resilience and protective mechanisms. In: Rolf J et al (editors): *Risk and Protective Factors in the Development of Psychopathology.* Cambridge University Press, 1990.

INTERVENTION & PREVENTION AS EXPERIMENTS

The relation between the scientific study of behavior in developmental psychology and the application of scientific principles to psychiatry is reciprocal. Concepts from developmental psychology have been applied in psychiatric practice, but psychiatric intervention can also be viewed as a field experiment to test hypotheses about behavioral development. Systematic intervention and prevention can be viewed as experiments to test basic principles. In fact, given the complexity of human behavioral development and the ethical restraints against known iatrogenic manipulations, clinical practice may be the most powerful scientific tool available to test hypotheses from developmental psychology. Thus the relation between these disciplines is reciprocal, and communication between the disciplines must be preserved.

Dodge KA: The future of research on the treatment of conduct disorder. Dev Psychopathol 1993;5:309.

GENERAL DEVELOPMENTAL THEORIES

Seven major theories of development are listed in Table 1–2, along with key concepts and criticisms of each theory. These theories, along with their applications, are described in detail in the sections that follow.

TEMPERAMENT THEORY

Since the "human bile" theories of ancient Greeks, scholars have speculated that persons are born into the world with varying predispositions to behave in particular ways, called **traits.** Trait theorists have postulated a variety of dispositional tendencies, from Eysenck's neuroticism and extraversion to the "Big Five" traits of agreeableness, openness, extraversion, neuroticism, and conscientiousness. In developmental inquiry, temperament theory has received the greatest attention. It has been hypothesized that infants are born with biologically based temperaments that vary on a continuum from difficult to easy. This trait is ev-

Table 1–2. General developmental theories.

Theory	Key Concepts	Criticisms
Temperament theory	Traits, genetic origins of behavior	Imprecise measurement, static view of human beings
Organismic theory	Stages of development, transformational role	Empirical refutation
Attachment theory	Patterns of relationships, working models	Too much emphasis on destiny from infancy
Social learning theory	Observational learning, imitation, reinforcement	Exclusive emphasis on environmental influences and cognitive mediation
Attribution theory	Mental heuristics, causal influences	Lack of emphasis on development, too narrow
Social-information-processing theory	Mental processes during social interaction	Nonbiological
Ecological theory	Levels of systems	Vague and not falsifiable

idenced in ease of early care, including feeding, soothing, and cuddling. As children grow older, these differences are evidenced in ease of manageability (eg, the temper tantrums of 18-month-old children and the behavior difficulties of the preschool period). The trait of difficultness has been hypothesized as a risk factor for conduct disorder. Empirical studies have found significant but modest support for this hypothesis. Prospective studies indicate that infants characterized as difficult are indeed at risk for conduct problems in the early school years, but the relation is somewhat weaker (although still present) for predictions from infancy to adolescence.

A different temperament theory, proposed by Kagan, has focused on a continuum of biological inhibition as the marker variable. Some infants regularly withdraw from novel social stimuli **(inhibited pattern)** whereas others seek out social stimulation **(uninhibited pattern).** Optimal levels of inhibition may fall between these extremes. Highly inhibited infants exhibit separation anxiety from parents and are likely to grow into shy, fearful, and withdrawn children. They are thought to be at risk for panic disorder in adulthood. Most individuals demonstrate an increase in heart rate and stabilization of heart rate variability in response to a stress challenge. Individuals vary systematically in the degree to which the hypothalamus, pituitary gland, and adrenal gland (called the HPA axis) respond with glucocorticoid secretion during stress. Inhibited children have a lower threshold of sympathetic nervous system response and display a greater rise and stabilization of heart rate than uninhibited children exhibit. This pattern acts as a trait-like temperamental characteristic throughout life that may be associated with symptoms of anxiety.

Another postulate of temperament theories is that temperament elicits environmental treatment that perpetuates behavior consistent with that temperament. For example, it is hypothesized that "difficult" children elicit harsh discipline, which exacerbates difficult behavior, whereas inhibited children seek secure environments that pose minimal challenge and risk. Plomin has shown through twin and adoption studies

that environmental experiences have a heritable component; that is, inherited genes lead either to behavior patterns that elicit environmental reactions or to behaviors that seek particular environments, a phenomenon known as **niche-picking.**

Applications of the Theory

Most temperament theorists recognize the importance of both inherited and environmental sources of development, so this theory has spawned empirical research directed toward understanding how these forces interact. It may be that infants with a particular temperament will develop more favorably under certain environmental conditions than others, and the task of inquiry is to identify optimal temperament-environment matches. Researchers are examining whether temperamentally difficult infants (or highly inhibited infants) develop more favorably under conditions of environmental restraint and structure or flexibility and freedom.

Another application has been to encourage research on the process through which genetic effects may operate on human development, thus informing the age-old debate between nature and nurture influences on human behavior (see Chapter 6).

Criticisms of the Theory

One problem with research on temperament theory has been the reliance on parents for assessments of temperament. Parents may be biased or inaccurate, or they may lack a broad base of knowledge of other infants. A parent's perceptions about his or her child may be legitimate factors in the child's development, but these perceptions confound information about the child's actual behavior with the parent's construal of the behavior. More direct observational measures of behavior have been developed to assess temperament, as have measures of biological functions, including heart rate reactivity, cortisol secretions, and skin conductivity. These measures also show some stability across time and some predictive power, but the number of studies is small and the statistical effects are weak.

Another problem is the difficulty of distinguishing genetic-biological features from reactions to environmental treatment. A 6-month-old infant brings both a genetic heritage and a history of environmental experiences to current interactions. Even biological measures (eg, resting heart rate, cortisol levels) have a partial basis in past social exchanges, so that the task of sorting genetic from environmental sources in biobehavioral measures is difficult.

Gunnar MR: Psychendocrine studies of temperament and stress in early childhood. In: Bates J, Wachs T (editors): *Temperament: Individual Differences at the Interface of Biology and Behavior.* American Psychological Association Press, 1994.

ORGANISMIC THEORY

No one has had more influence in developmental psychology than Piaget. The coherence of behavior across diverse domains and the tendency for changes in abilities to occur simultaneously across domains form the basis of the organismic theory of Piaget and others such as Gesell, Werner, and Baldwin. This theory attempts to describe general features of human cognition and the systematic changes in thought across development. The organizing principle in organismic theory is **structure,** which is a closed system of transformational rules that govern thought at a particular point in development. Consider the 5-year-old girl who observes one row of nine beads placed near each other and a second row of six beads stretched across a greater distance than the first row. Even though the girl has counted the beads in each row and knows that nine is greater than six, in response to the question, "Which row has more beads?" she will answer, "The row with six beads." Moreover, the girl will see no contradiction in her answer. According to Piaget, this nonobvious phenomenon occurs because the girl's structural transformation law is to consider the whole of a stimulus, not each part separately. The child's rule structure is closed; that is, it is internally consistent and not easily altered by external contradictions.

Piaget hypothesized that infants are born with a general wiring for a crude set of transformational rules common to all sensorimotor coordination. These rules are part of the evolutionary inheritance of the human organism. Development occurs over a 12- to 15-year period in nonlinear chunks, called **stages.** Within each stage, functioning is internally consistent and stable (called an **equilibrium**). Change from one stage to the next occurs as a result of interaction between the child and the realities of the environment. When contradictory realities accumulate sufficiently, change occurs rapidly and globally. As discussed earlier in this chapter, processes of change involve assimilation and accommodation. Assimilation is the act of interpreting environmental experiences in terms that are consistent with existing rule structure (a form of generalization), whereas accommodation is the act of altering rule structures to account for environmental experience (a form of exception noting). Children engage in both assimilation and accommodation in order to maintain coherence (and the perception of consistency), until their overgeneralizations and exceptions become so contradictory that they must create higher-level, more flexible, novel structures that account for the contradictions of earlier stages. When a novel structure (ie, a new set of rules) is achieved, **equilibration** consolidates the rules until contradictions accumulate to set the scene for the next stage change. Piaget's four broad stages of cognitive development are (1) the sensorimotor period, (2) the preoperational stage, (3) the concrete-operational stage, and (4) the period of formal operations.

Applications of the Theory

Many of Piaget's concepts continue to have heuristic value even today and to provide hypotheses relevant to psychopathology. The notions of egocentrism, the invariant sequences of skill acquisition, and increasing differentiation (ie, development rather than mere change) provide hypotheses regarding the behavior of children who have conduct problems and of adolescents who are lagging developmentally. Furthermore, Piaget's discoveries of the limits of young children's abilities have inspired cognitive educational strategies.

Criticisms of the Theory

Even though Piaget's influence has been tremendous, crucial features of organismic theory have been rejected in contemporary theory. Children have repeatedly been shown to be more competent than Piaget suggested they could be at a particular age. Piaget's proposed cross-domain universality in type of thought has been shown to be false, suggesting to some scholars that the stage concept is faulty. It has been replaced by concepts of learning strategies, information-processing patterns, and the parsing of multiple components in complex task completion.

Piaget J: Piaget's theory. In: Kesson W (editor): *Handbook of Child Psychology.* Vol 1: *History, Theory, and Methods,* 4th ed. John Wiley & Sons, 1983.

ATTACHMENT THEORY

Bowlby generated a theory of attachment that has had enormous influence in contemporary developmental psychology. According to Bowlby, infants are born with innate tendencies to seek direct contact with an adult (usually the mother). In contrast to Freud's perspective that early attachment-seeking is a function of a desire for the mother's breast (and food), Bowlby argued that attachment seeking is directed toward social contact with the mother (the desire for a love relationship) and driven by fear of unknown others. By about 6–8 months of age, separation from the mother arouses distress, analogous to free-floating anxiety. The distress of a short-term separation is replaced quickly by the warmth of the reunion with the mother, but longer separations (such as occur in hospitalization or abandonment) can induce clinging, suspicion, and anxiety upon reunion. Similar effects are seen in older children until individuation occurs, at which point the child is cognitively able to hold a mental representation of the mother while she is gone, enabling the child to explore novelty.

Bowlby hypothesized that individual differences exist in patterns of parent-infant relationship quality and that the infant acquires a mental representation (or working model) of this relationship that is stored in memory and carried forward to act as a guiding filter for all future relationships. This working model of relationships generalizes to other contexts and allows future interactions to conform with the working model, thereby reinforcing the initial representation of how relationships operate. Thus the quality of the initial parent-infant relationship has primary and enduring effects on later adjustment, relationships, and parenting.

Individual differences in attachment patterns have been assessed through a laboratory procedure called the Strange Situation, devised by Ainsworth. The parent and 12-month-old child are brought to an unfamiliar room containing toys, after which a stranger enters. The parent then leaves the room for a short period, followed by a reunion. The child's behavior, especially toward the parent upon reunion, is indicative of the quality of the overall parent-child attachment. Attachment classifications are summarized in Table 1–3.

About two thirds of children fit the "secure" response pattern (type B), in which they demonstrate distress when the parent leaves and enthusiasm (or confident pleasure) upon her return. An "avoidant" response pattern (type A) involves little distress and little relief or pleasure upon reunion with the parent. A "resistant or ambivalent" response pattern (type C) involves panicky distress upon the parent's departure and emotional ambivalence upon reunion (perhaps running toward the parent to be picked up but then im-

mediately, angrily struggling to get down). Recently, scholars have identified a fourth class of response, "disorganized" (type D, empirically linked to early physical or sexual maltreatment), in which the child's behavior involves great distress and little systematic exploration or seeking of adults.

Applications of the Theory

Follow-up studies have shown that these patterns of attachment are somewhat stable over time (although not strongly correlated across relationships with different adults) and predictive of behavioral adjustment in middle childhood. Infants of types A, C, and D are all at risk for later maladjustment, although more specific patterns of outcome for each type have not been detected reliably. Developmental scholars have created methods for assessing relationship quality and working models at older ages and have related these assessments to current behavioral functioning.

Criticisms of the Theory

Critics of attachment theory suggest that the initial relationship does not determine destiny as strongly as Bowlby argued, and that any long-term predictive power is due to consistency in the environment that led to the child's initial response pattern. Attachment theory has been used to condemn the practice of early out-of-home daycare (because it interferes with the development of a secure attachment with the mother), even though most studies find little long-term effect of such care after other confounding factors (eg, economics, family stability, stress, later caregiving) are controlled. More broadly, the reversibility of the effects of early social deprivation and trauma remain controversial. The current general conclusion is that even though early experiences shape later experiences through the filter of mental representations, the plasticity of the human organism is greater than previously believed.

Ainsworth MDS et al: *Patterns of Attachment.* Lawrence Erlbaum Assoc, 1978.
Bowlby J: *Attachment and Loss.* Vol 3: *Loss, Sadness, and Depression.* Basic Books, 1980.

SOCIAL LEARNING THEORY

Bandura's social learning theory, though acknowledging the constraints of biological origins and the role of neural mediating mechanisms, emphasizes the role of the individual's experience of the environment in development. Other learning theories are based on the organism's direct performance of behaviors, whereas social learning theory posits that most learning occurs vicariously by observing and imitating models. For survival and growth, humans are designed to acquire patterns of behavior through **observational learning.** Social behavior in particular is a

Table 1–3. Attachment types and associated working models and outcomes.

Attachment Type	Working Model	Outcome
A: Avoidant	Fearful	Risk
B: Secure	Exploration with confidence	Healthy
C: Ambivalent	Panicky distress and anger	Risk
D: Disorganized	Great distress	Risk

function of one's social learning history, instigation mechanisms, and maintaining mechanisms.

Four processes govern social learning: (1) attention, which regulates exploration and perception; (2) memory, through which observed events are symbolically stored to guide future behavior; (3) motor production, through which novel behaviors are formed from the integration of constituent acts with observed actions; and (4) incentives and motivation, which regulate the performance of learned responses. Development involves biological maturation in these processes as well as the increasingly complex storage of contingencies and response repertoires in memory.

Instigation mechanisms include both biological and cognitive motivators. Internal aversive stimulation might activate behavior through its painful effect (on hunger, sex, or aggression). Cognitively based motivators are based on the organism's capacity to represent mentally future material, sensory, and social consequences. Mentally represented consequences provide the motivation for action.

Maintaining mechanisms include external reinforcement (eg, tangible rewards, social and status rewards, reduction of aversive treatment), punishment, vicarious reinforcement by observation, and self-regulatory mechanisms (eg, self-observation, self-judgment through attribution and valuation, self-applied consequences). Development in social learning theory is decidedly not stage-like and has few constraints. For example, Bandura argued that even relatively sophisticated moral thought and action are possible in young children, given relevant models and experiences.

Applications of the Theory

Social learning theory has been applied most effectively to aggressive behavior, where it has provided powerful explanations for the effects of coercive parenting, violent media presentations, and rejecting-peer interactions on the development of chronic aggressive behavior. Furthermore, it provides the basis for most current behavior-modification interventions in clinical practice.

Criticisms of the Theory

Critics dispute the primacy of cognitive mediation in understanding learning effects and the relative emphasis on environmental influences over genetic and biological influences.

Bandura A: *Social Foundations of Thought and Action: A Social Cognitive Theory.* Prentice-Hall, 1986.

ATTRIBUTION THEORY

The emphasis on cognition in social learning theory is largely consequence oriented (ie, based on individuals' cognitions about the likely outcomes of their behavior). Attribution theory is more concerned with how people understand the causes of behavior. Its origins are in the naive or common-sense psychology of Heider, who suggested that an individual's beliefs about events play a more important role in behavior than does the objective truth of events. For social interactions, an individual's beliefs about the causes of another person's behavior are more crucial than are the true causes. For example, in deciding whether to retaliate aggressively against a peer following a provocation (such as being bumped from behind), a person often uses an attribution about the peer's intention. If the peer had acted accidentally then no retaliation occurs, but if the peer had acted maliciously then retaliation may be likely. The perceiver's task in social exchanges is to decide which effects of an observed action are intentional (reflecting dispositions) and which are situational.

When judging whether another person's behavior (such as aggression) should be attributed to a dispositional rather than a situational cause, perceivers use mental heuristics, such as correspondent inference and covariation. Perceivers examine whether the person's actions are normative or unique (if unique, they may indicate a dispositional rather than situational cause). They examine the other person's behavioral consistency over time and distinctiveness across situations (if the behavior is consistent, it more likely reflects a disposition). Finally, they examine whether the action has personal hedonic relevance to the perceiver (if the action is relevant to the perceiver, perceivers tend to attribute dispositional causes).

These principles predict the kinds of causal attributions that people make about the events around them, the circumstances under which people will make errors in inference, and people's behavioral responses to events. Extensions of attribution theory have addressed differences in the causal attributions made by people about themselves versus others (actor-observer effects), the kinds of explanations that people give for their own behavior and outcomes (internal versus external attributions), and the circumstances under which people spontaneously make attributions.

Applications of the Theory

Attribution theory has been applied to problems in several domains of psychiatry and health. Studies have shown that attributions predict behavioral responses to critical events such as interpersonal losses and failure. People who attribute their failure to a lack of ability on their part are likely to give up and to continue to fail, whereas people who attribute their failure to a lack of effort are likely to intensify future efforts to succeed. People who regularly attribute their failures to global, stable, and internal causes (ie, they blame themselves) are at risk for a mood disorder and somatization disorder. People who attribute their own negative outcomes to the fault of others are likely to direct aggression toward the perceived cause of the outcome (and to develop a conduct disorder). Interventions have been developed to help people redirect attributions more accurately or more adaptively, most notably in cognitive therapies for depression.

Criticisms of the Theory

Until recently, the problem of development was relatively ignored in attribution theory. Studies only recently have begun to address topics such as the age at which attributions come to be made spontaneously, the relevance of spontaneous attribution tendencies for age differences in depression, and the experiential origins of chronic attributional tendencies.

Dodge KA: Social-cognitive mechanisms in the development of conduct disorder and depression. Annu Rev Psychol 1993;44:559.

SOCIAL-INFORMATION-PROCESSING THEORY

The comprehensive extension of social learning theory and attribution theory is to consider all of the mental processes that people use in relating to the social world. Simon's work in cognitive science forms the basis for social-information-processing theory. This theory recognizes that people come to social situations with a set of biologically determined capabilities and a database of past experiences (Figure 1–3). They receive as input a set of social cues (such as a push in the back by a peer or a failing grade in a school subject). The person's behavioral response to the cues occurs as a function of a sequence of mental processes, beginning with encoding of cues through sensation and perception. The vastness of available cues requires selective attention to cues (such as attention to peers' laughter versus one's own physical pain). Selective encoding is partially predictive of ultimate behavior. The storage of cues in memory is not veridical with objective experience. The mental representation and interpretation of the cues (possibly involving attributions about cause) is the next step of processing. A person's interpretation of a stimulus is predictive of that person's behavioral response (eg, a hostile attribution made about another's ambiguously provocative push in the back will predict a retaliatory aggressive response). Once the stimulus cues are represented, the person accesses one or more possible behavioral responses from memory. Rules of association in memory, as well as the person's response repertoire, guide this retrieval. For example, one person might follow the rule "when intentionally provoked, fight back"; whereas another person might follow the rule "when provoked, run away." Accessing a response is not the same as responding behaviorally, however, as in the case of a withheld impulse. The next step of processing is response evaluation and decision making, wherein the person (not necessarily consciously) evaluates the interpersonal, intrapersonal, instrumental, and moral consequences of accessed behavioral responses and decides on an optimal response. Clearly, evaluations that a behavior is relatively likely to lead to positive consequences are predictive of that behavioral tendency. The final step of processing involves the transformation of a mental decision into motor and verbal behavior.

Social-information-processing theory posits that people engage in these mental processes over and over in real time during social interactions and that within particular types of situations, individuals develop characteristic patterns of processing cues at each step in the model. These patterns form the basis of psychopathologic tendencies. For example, in response to provocations, one person might regularly selectively attend to certain kinds of cues (such as threats), attribute hostile intentions to others, access aggressive responses, evaluate aggressing as favorable, and enact aggression skillfully. This person is highly likely to develop conduct disorder. Likewise, in response to academic failure, another person might selectively attend to his or her own contributing mistakes, attribute the outcome to personal failure, access self-destructive responses, evaluate all other re-

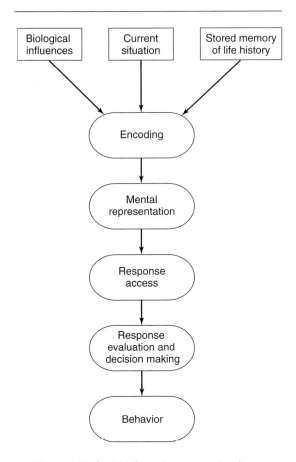

Figure 1–3. Social-information-processing theory.

sponses as leading to further failure, and enact self-destructive responses effortlessly. This person is likely to develop dysthymic disorder or major depressive disorder.

Applications of the Theory

Social-information-processing theory has been used successfully to predict the development of conduct problems in children and depressive symptoms in adolescents. Not all individuals with conduct problems display the same deviant processing patterns at all steps of the model; however, most people with conduct problems display at least one type of processing problem. Some children with conduct problems show hostile attributional tendencies, whereas others evaluate the likely outcomes of aggressing as positive. These processing differences accurately predict subtypes of conduct problems: Children with hostile attributional tendencies display problems of reactive anger control, whereas children who make positive evaluations of the outcome of aggressing display instrumental aggression and bullying.

The development of processing styles has shed light on the development of psychopathology. For example, children with early histories of physical abuse are likely to become hypervigilant to hostile cues and to display hostile attributional tendencies. These tendencies predict later aggressive-behavior problems and account for the empirical link between early physical abuse and the development of aggressive-behavior problems.

Social-information-processing theory holds the potential to distinguish among types of psychopathology. In one investigation, groups of children with depressive, aggressive, comorbid, or no symptoms were found to display unique profiles of processing patterns. The aggressive group tended to attribute hostile intentions to others, to access aggressive responses, and to evaluate the outcomes of aggressing as favorable. The depressive group, in contrast, tended to attribute hostile intentions to others as well, but they also attributed the cause of others' hostile intentions to self-blame, and they accessed self-destructive responses and evaluated aggressive responses negatively.

Social-information-processing theory has suggested interventions designed to help people construe situations differently and to act on the social world more effectively. For example, one intervention has been directed toward helping aggressive adolescents attribute interpersonal provocations in a less personalized and hostile way. This intervention has been successful in reducing the rate of aggressive behavior in these adolescents, relative to untreated control subjects.

Criticisms of the Theory

By focusing on in situ mental actions, processing theory relatively neglects enduring structural components of personality that are emphasized in psycho-analytic and Piagetian theories. Another criticism is that social-information-processing theory locates the sources of deviant behavior in the individual, in contrast to the broader social ecology.

Dodge KA: Social-cognitive mechanisms in the development of conduct disorder and depression. Annu Rev Psychol 1993;44:559.

ECOLOGICAL THEORY

Ecological theory evolved from the recognition that even though the environment has a major effect on development, many models of development have limited generalizability across contexts. Consider, for example, classic studies by Tulkin and his colleagues on the effect of mother-infant interaction patterns on the infant's development of language and mental abilities. This effect is stronger among socioeconomic middle-class families than among lower-class families. Likewise, Scarr has found that the magnitude of genetic influences on intellectual development varies according to the cultural group being studied. Greater genetic effects are observed in middle-class white groups than in lower-class African-American groups. Among lower-class families, different influences on development are operating. Findings such as these led ecological theorists such as Lewin, Bronfenbrenner, and Barker to conclude that models of development are bounded by the context in which they are framed.

Ecological theory suggests that process models of development have no universality; rather, they must be framed within the limits of a cultural and historical context. This theory must be distinguished from the radical postmodernist perspective that scientific principles have no objective basis. Ecological theorists conceptualize the environment systematically and attempt to understand how it affects development.

Bronfenbrenner has articulated an ecological model that includes developmental influences at the individual (person), person-by-environment (process), and context levels. He categorizes contextual settings into three types: microsystems, mesosystems, and exosystems. As discussed earlier in this chapter, the most proximal type is the microsystem, which includes one's immediate physical and social environment. Examples of microsystems are homes, schools, playgrounds, and work places. Each microsystem has a structure and a set of rules and norms for behavior that are fairly consistent across time. Developmental scientists study processes within each of these settings, and ecologists warn them not to overgeneralize process phenomena from one microsystem to another.

The next type is the mesosystem, which is defined as a combination of microsystems that leads to a new level of developmental influence. For example, in understanding the effects of parental versus peer influences on adolescent development, one must consider not only each of the family and peer microsystems but also the effect of the combined mesosystem, that is, the effect of the conflict between the family's values and the peer group's values on the child's development.

The final type is the exosystem, a combination of multiple mesosystems. Research on the effects of maternal employment on child development has been enhanced by an understanding of this exosystem. That is, in order to understand how maternal employment affects a child's social development, one must understand not only the family and work context but also the cultural and historical context of women's employment.

Applications of the Theory

Ecological theory has led clinicians to question the generalizability of their practices across cultural, gender, and ethnic groups. Group-specific interventions are being developed. Ecological theory has also led to policy changes in the funding of research at the federal level, in that large research studies are now required to address questions of generalizability across groups. Finally, ecological theorists have pressed clinicians to consider the possibility that interventions at a broader level might exert a powerful effect at the microsystem level.

Criticisms of the Theory

Ecological theory is not a theory in the formal sense. Rather, it is a structured framework for identifying influences at numerous levels. Thus it is not falsifiable. Its value is in alerting clinicians to factors that otherwise might be neglected.

Bronfenbrenner U: *The Ecology of Human Development: Experiments by Nature and Design.* Harvard University Press, 1979.

SYNTHESIS: DIATHESIS-STRESS MODELS & OTHER INTERACTIONIST THEORIES

It has been increasingly recognized that interactionist models of development apply to most forms of psychopathology. These models focus on the confluence of forces that must coalesce in order for a disorder to develop. The most basic of these models is the diathesis-stress model. A **diathesis** is a dispositional characteristic that predisposes an individual to disorder. The disposition may be biological (as in a genetic predisposition for schizophrenia), environmental (as in poverty), or cognitive (as in low IQ). Disorder is probabilistically related to the presence of a diathesis, but the process of development of psychopathology requires that the individual with the diathesis also be exposed to a **stressor,** which, again, might be biological or environmental. Only those individuals with both the diathesis and the stressor are likely to develop the disorder.

Consider the diathesis-stress model of major depressive disorder. According to this model, individuals who display the cognitive diathesis of self-blame for failure are at risk for the development of depression, but only if they subsequently experience a stressor that is linked to the diathesis (such as failure). Statistically, this model hypothesizes an interaction effect, and it has been supported for a variety of problems, from depression to physical illness.

Theorists have noted that individual and environmental factors interact not only in static models such as the case of major depressive disorder but also over time in transactional models. These models articulate the reciprocal influences between person and environment and the unfolding of disorder across experience. Finally, theorists have come to recognize that the unfolding occurs in nonlinear, nonuniform ways that lead to qualitative changes in the individual, as in dynamic systems (see the "Major Principles of Ontogeny and Phylogeny" section earlier in this chapter). Dynamic systems models are being borrowed from phenomena in physics to describe the development of novel behaviors in infancy (such as the onset of locomotion and language) and have the potential to be applied to the development of novel deviant behavior in psychopathology.

Garber J, Hilsman R: Cognitions, stress, and depression in children and adolescents. Child Adolesc Psychiatr Clin N Am 1992;1:129.
Hilsman R, Garber J: A test of the cognitive diathesis-stress model in children: academic stressors, attributional style, perceived competence and control. J Pers Soc Psychol 1995;69:370.

LIFE-COURSE PROSPECTIVE INQUIRY

One of the most powerful methods in developmental clinical research is that of life-course prospective inquiry, closely linked to developmental epidemiology. By identifying an important sample (either a high-risk sample or a representative sample) and then following that sample with repeated assessments across time using hypothesis-driven measures, researchers have been able to identify risk factors in the development of a disorder, moderators of that risk, and mediating processes in the etiology of the disorder. Two such longitudinal studies are described in this section as examples of ongoing research in this field.

THE DEVELOPMENT OF DEPRESSION PROJECT

The Development of Depression Project has tested the diathesis-stress model of the development of major depressive disorder in adolescents. According to

Garber, some children develop cognitive styles for attributing their failures and losses to internal, global, and stable characteristics of themselves, and they begin to have negative automatic thoughts in response to life events. Later, when confronted with failures and losses, these children are at elevated risk for developing major depressive disorder. It is the interaction of the cognitive diathesis and the life stressor, not either factor in isolation, that leads to depression. In order to rule out competing hypotheses that cognitive styles or problem life events result from, rather than lead to, depression, a research design is needed that follows children across time.

The research strategy in this study was to identify a sample of children prior to adolescence; to assess cognitive diatheses, life events, family processes, and psychopathology in this sample at that time; and then to follow the children with repeated assessments throughout adolescence in order to determine which ones develop depression following common stressors of adolescent life. The pool of subjects came from three entire cohorts of fifth-grade children in the Nashville, Tennessee, public schools. In order to ensure that the ultimate prevalence rate of major depressive disorder in the research sample was high enough to conduct statistical tests of hypotheses, written and telephone screening of 1495 families, followed by Structured Clinical Interviews for Diagnoses, was used to identify 188 offspring of parents with a life history of depression. This high-risk sample was complemented by an additional 53 low-risk offspring of parents with no psychopathology. Thus the design is not strictly epidemiologic because the community population is not representatively sampled; rather, it is a prospective high-risk sample design aimed at testing specific theoretical hypotheses of a developmental psychopathologic process.

At the first wave of assessment in sixth grade, children and parents were assessed for psychopathology, life events stressors, family processes, and most pertinent, the cognitive diathesis for depression. Analyses of the initial wave revealed that children of depressive parents demonstrated more subthreshold symptoms of depression and more negative attributional styles than did the children of nondepressed parents. Even though these findings are consistent with the hypothesized model, the critical test would come over time if initial depressive symptom levels could be controlled statistically to see whether attributional styles and life stressors interact to predict onset of depressive disorder. All children have been followed annually through 12th grade with repeated assessments using a contextual threat life events interview and structured psychiatric interviews. Analyses indicate that among those children who displayed at least some depressive symptoms, controlling for initial depressive symptom levels, the interaction of early cognitive diathesis and subsequent stressful life events significantly predicted later depressive symptom levels as determined by

psychiatric interviews. That is, only those children with a combination of initial negative automatic thoughts and subsequent stressful life events showed elevated depressive symptoms later; all other groups showed lower levels of symptoms. This is a moderator effect: The cognitive diathesis moderates (or alters) the effect of stressful life events on depressive symptoms.

How do cognitive diatheses for depression develop? Garber hypothesized that family processes might be responsible. At the initial wave of assessment, she measured parental control and lack of acceptance. Later she found that these aspects of family process predicted both cognitive diatheses and later depressive symptoms in children. Consistent with the mediation hypothesis, she also found that the child's cognitions, especially feelings of negative self-worth, mediated (or statistically accounted for) part of the effect of family interactions on the child's depressive symptoms.

This prospective study has provided empirical support for a model in which early family interactions involving psychological control and lack of acceptance lead a child to develop cognitive styles of negative self-worth, negative automatic thoughts, and negative attributions for failure. Later, in adolescence, those children who show the unique combination of experiencing stressful life events and having negative automatic thoughts about those events are most likely to develop depression. This model integrates biological (genetic risk), family process, cognitive, and ecological (stressful life events) factors in the onset and course of depression. It also suggests three points for intervention with children who are at risk for depression. First, early family interactions involving acceptance and control might be targeted through parent training. Second, the child's cognitive styles might be addressed in brief preventive cognitive therapy. Third, the child's ecology might be modified by altering the child's exposure to stressful life events (or at least the child's experience of inevitable stressful events).

Hilsman R, Garber J: A test of the cognitive diathesis-stress model in children: academic stressors, attributional style, perceived competence and control. J Pers Soc Psychol 1995;69:370.

THE CHILD DEVELOPMENT PROJECT

The Child Development Project is directed toward understanding the role of family experiences and patterns of social information processing in the development and growth of aggressive conduct problems and conduct disorder in children. The design is a developmental epidemiologic one: 585 preschool children at three geographic sites were selected randomly at kindergarten matriculation to participate in a 12-year

conconsegment

longitudinal study. The hypotheses guiding the study were based on social learning theory in developmental psychology and social-information-processing theory in cognitive science, namely, that early family experiences of physical abuse and harsh discipline would predict later serious conduct problems, and that this relation would be mediated by the child's intervening development of problematic patterns of processing social information. That is, it was hypothesized that early harsh family experiences lead a child to become hypervigilant to hostile cues, to attribute provocations to others' hostile intentions, to develop aggressive problem-solving styles, and to anticipate that aggressive strategies will result in favorable outcomes. These deviant processing patterns were hypothesized to lead to aggressive conduct problems and conduct disorder.

In-home family interviews and direct observations of family interactions provided information about the child's experience of physical abuse and harsh discipline in the first 5 years of life. About 12% of this random sample was identified as having experienced physical abuse at some time in their lives, a high rate that is consistent with Straus's national surveys of community samples. At subsequent annual assessments, video-guided interviews with each child provided measures of the child's patterns of social information processing. Finally, teacher ratings, peer nominations, direct observations, and school records provided evidence of externalizing conduct problems. The study followed this sample from preschool into high school.

Analyses indicated that the physically abused group of children had a fourfold increase in risk for clinically significant externalizing problems by middle school. This risk could not be statistically accounted for by confounding factors, such as socioeconomic status, child temperament, or exposure to other violent models. Thus it seems that the experience of harsh parenting, especially if extreme, is partially responsible for conduct problems in some children.

Consistent with the original hypotheses, the physically abused children were also at risk for problems with social information processing. Specifically, physically abused children were relatively likely to become hypervigilant to hostile cues, to develop hostile attributional biases, to access aggressive responses to social problems, and to believe that ag-

gressive behaviors lead to desired outcomes. Also consistent with hypotheses, children who demonstrated these processing patterns were likely to develop clinically significant externalizing problems in middle school and high school. Finally, the mediation hypothesis was supported, in that the child's social-information-processing patterns accounted for about half of the statistical relation between early physical abuse and later conduct problems.

CONCLUSION

Developmental psychology plays an important role in psychiatric science and practice. Concepts such as the orthogenetic principle, ontogeny, phylogeny, age-norming, and developmental trajectories can help the practicing psychiatrist to place a patient's current symptoms into developmental and ecological context. Common patterns in the development of psychopathology (eg, biosocial interactions, multiple pathway models, mediational models, and bidirectional effects) enrich the psychiatrist's understanding of the etiology of psychiatric disorders.

Even though major developmental theories (eg, temperament, attachment, social learning) have historical significance, most contemporary thinking is not directed at contrasting these theories at a macro level. Rather, it is understood that psychiatric phenomena usually involve complex interactions of factors at multiple levels. Current research is aimed at understanding how variables implicated by various theories interact to produce psychiatric disorder, rather than proving one general theory more meritorious than another.

The relation between developmental psychology and psychiatry is reciprocal. That is, knowledge gained from developmental theory and empirical findings has been useful to psychiatrists in both scientific understanding and practice, and the findings and concerns of psychiatrists have modified developmental theory and guided developmental empirical inquiry. These disciplines have been fused even more tightly in the emerging discipline of developmental psychopathology, which seeks to understand the etiology, process, and life-course of psychiatric phenomena.

2

Behavioral & Cognitive-Behavioral Interventions

Travis Thompson, PhD, & Steven D. Hollon, PhD

ROOTS OF BEHAVIORAL & COGNITIVE-BEHAVIORAL INTERVENTIONS

Although their roots can be found at the beginning of the 20th century, modern behavioral and cognitive-behavioral therapies arose during the 1950s and early 1960s when the scientific study of behavior emerged as a subject with validity in its own right. Disordered behavior was no longer taken to be purely a symptom or indicator of something else going on in the mind. Of inherent concern was its relation to past and current environmental events thought to be causally related to that behavior. Methods developed in animal laboratories began to be tested—in laboratory, institutional, clinical, and school settings—with people who had chronic mental illness or mental retardation and with predelinquent adolescents. Improvements in patient behavior and functioning were often striking. These changes took place against a backdrop of growing dissatisfaction with the prevailing notion that psychopathology typically arose from unobservable psychic causes that were assessed and treated using techniques that seemed to be based more on art than science. In addition, an accumulating literature of outcome studies revealed that much of the psychotherapy as it had been practiced until the early 1960s engendered very modest and largely unpredictable results. Thus contemporary behavior therapies emerged from three distinct psychological traditions: classical or Pavlovian conditioning, instrumental or operant conditioning, and cognitive-behavioral and rational-emotive therapies.

CLASSICAL CONDITIONING

The first major perspective within learning theory approaches is typically referred to as **classical conditioning.** This perspective dates to the first decade of the 20th century and is largely attributed to the Russian neurophysiologist Ivan Pavlov. Pavlov was interested in studying the structure of the nervous system, in particular, simple reflex arcs between external events (**stimuli**) and an organism's behavior (**response**). He chose to study salivation in dogs in response to food and developed an apparatus that held the dogs suspended in a harness while a small amount of meat powder was deposited on their tongues. He would vary the amount and timing of the delivery of the meat powder and recorded the subsequent variation in the nature and amount of salivation.

What happened next confounded his simple neurologic experiments but opened the way to revolutionary new insights regarding how organisms learn to adapt their behaviors in response to novel environments. Pavlov found that after a few trials his dogs began to salivate when strapped into the harness, well in advance of any exposure to the meat powder on a particular trial. The dogs began to salivate prior to delivery of the food. Naive dogs placed in the harness for the first time did not salivate; experienced dogs that had been through the procedure earlier began to salivate well in advance of the delivery of the food. In effect, the response came to precede the food stimulus, something that could not be explained in terms of simple reflex arcs.

Pavlov's genius lay in recognizing the importance of this complication, and he shifted his attention from the study of simple reflex arcs to those conditions necessary to support changes in behavior as a consequence of prior experience, which is, **learning.** He sounded a bell to signal the start of a trial that was followed by the delivery of meat powder and found that he could reliably train the dogs to salivate to the sound of the bell and not to respond to other aspects of the experimental situation. In effect, he introduced a particularly salient stimulus that carried all the predictive information contained in the situation (ringing the bell predicted subsequent delivery of meat powder, whereas nothing happened until the bell was sounded); and the dogs came to salivate reliably only after the bell was rung. Once the bell was established as a particularly informative stimulus, he could occasionally omit the meat powder on subsequent trials, and the dogs continued to salivate to the sound of the bell.

This simple paradigm contained the key elements of classical conditioning. The meat powder represented what Pavlov came to call the **unconditioned stimulus.** All dogs with intact nervous systems salivate in response to meat powder being deposited on their tongues, whether they have any experience with that stimulus or not. Salivation represented the **unconditioned response.** The bell (or earlier, the entire experimental apparatus) represented the **conditioned stimulus.** Dogs did not naturally salivate to the sound of a bell, but they came to do so if it was paired with the meat powder (the unconditioned stimulus). Salivation to the bell alone represented the **conditioned response,** a learned response to an originally neutral stimulus that is not found universally among all members of the species.

Early Demonstrations in Humans

J. B. Watson, one of the leading figures in American psychology, recognized the potential utility of classical conditioning as an explanation for the development of symptoms of psychopathology. Watson and a graduate student conducted a classic demonstration of how the principles of classical conditioning explicated by Pavlov could be extended to humans. In this study, Watson first showed that a 3-year-old boy called Little Albert had no particular aversion to a small white laboratory rat: He would reach for it and try to pet it, as young children are inclined to do. Watson and his assistant then placed a large gong out of sight behind Little Albert and sounded it loudly every time they brought the rat into the room. Although Little Albert had shown no initial aversion to the rat, he showed a typical startle response to the sounding of the gong (again, like most young children would). Before long, he began to become upset and burst into tears at the sight of the rat alone and would try to withdraw whenever it was brought into the room.

According to Watson, this study demonstrated that phobic reactions could be acquired purely on the basis of traumatic conditioning. Although Little Albert had previously been intrigued by the presence of the rat and showed no evidence of any fear in its presence, pairing of the rat (the conditioned stimulus) with the loud, unpredictable noise produced by the gong (the unconditioned stimulus) led him to become anxious and upset in the rat's presence (the conditioned response), just as he had naturally become upset by the sound of the gong (unconditioned response). He had not only acquired a fear response to the rat but also tried to escape from its presence or avoid exposure to it. According to Watson, Little Albert had acquired the two hallmarks of a phobia (unreasonable fear, and escape or avoidance behaviors) purely as a consequence of simple classical conditioning.

The next major study in the sequence was conducted by Mary Cover Jones in 1924. She reasoned that if classical conditioning could produce a phobic reaction in an otherwise healthy child, the same laws of learning could be used to eliminate that reaction. She also trained a young child to have a conditioned fear response to a small animal (a rabbit) and then proceeded to feed the child in the presence of the rabbit. She found that pairing of the conditioned stimulus (the rabbit) with a second, unconditioned stimulus (food)—which produced a different unconditioned response (contentment) that was incompatible with the first (anxiety)—came to override the original learning. The child began to relax in the presence of the rabbit and no longer showed the fear response that he had acquired earlier. Thus, Jones argued, she was able to provide relief via **counterconditioning.**

Despite these early demonstrations, it was several decades before behavioral principles began to be applied systematically to the treatment of psychiatric disorders. This delay resulted partly from the sense that these procedures were just too simplistic to be of practical use in the treatment of complex human problems. Required were methods based on these learning principles that could be adapted to deal with more complex problems in living. Andrew Salter provided the first such method. In a text that was somewhat ahead of its time, Salter described a series of procedures based on principles of conditioning that were suitable for addressing emotional and behavioral problems in human patients. Although that text attracted little attention when it was published in 1949, it described (in vestigial form) many of the strategies and procedures that would later be used in the clinical practice of behavior therapy.

Applications to Clinical Treatment

Joseph Wolpe provided the first coherent set of clinical procedures, based on principles of classical conditioning, that had a major impact on the field. Wolpe had studied experimental neuroses in cats. In the course of his studies, which involved shocking animals when they tried to feed and observing the results of the conflict this produced, Wolpe replicated the essential features of Jones's earlier attempt to reduce a learned fear via the process of counterconditioning. He soon extended his work to people with phobic disorders and was able to reduce his patients' distress by pairing the object of their fear with an activity that reliably produced an incompatible response. Like Salter, he experimented with the induction of anger and sexual arousal before finally settling on a set of isometric exercises developed to help reduce stress in patients with heart conditions. This procedure, called **progressive relaxation,** consists of having patients alternately tense and relax different muscle groups in a systematic fashion and can lead to a state of profound relaxation. The isometric exercises could be paired with the presumably conditioned stimulus (whatever the patient feared) in order to have the new conditioned response (relaxation) override the existing arousal and distress that patients experienced in the presence of the phobic stimulus.

Wolpe called his approach **systematic desensitization.** In addition, in progressive relaxation training a hierarchy is developed that represents successive degrees of exposure to the feared object or stimulus. For example, a patient with a fear of flying might be asked to visualize a variety of scenes that induce differing amounts of anxiety. Simply watching someone else board an airplane might induce only a minimal amount of anxiety, whereas boarding a plane oneself and flying through a thunderstorm would be expected to elicit more anxiety. Wolpe worked with the patient to develop a hierarchy of such imagined experiences and grade them on a scale from 0 to 100 in terms of how much distress they produced. He would then expose the patient to these stimuli (typically in imagination), proceeding on to the next item in the hierarchy only when the client could tolerate a particular image without experiencing distress. If the patient started to become upset while visualizing an image, Wolpe would instruct the patient to stop the image and reinitiate the relaxation exercises until the feelings of arousal had passed. In this fashion, he systematically worked the patient through the hierarchy of representations of the feared object, going only as rapidly as the patient could go without experiencing distress until the stimulus no longer elicited any anxiety.

Hundreds of studies have suggested that systematic desensitization (or its variants) is effective in the treatment of phobia and related anxiety-based disorders. Systematic desensitization has been applied widely to a host of problems and represents a safe and effective way of reducing anxious arousal in both adults and children. Major variations include substituting meditation or biofeedback for progressive relaxation as a means of producing the relaxation response (some people don't respond well to muscular isometrics) or arranging experiences in a graduated fashion. The basic approach appears to be robust to these minor modifications and is one of the few examples of a treatment intervention that is truly more effective than other interventions.

Extinction & Exposure Therapy

Despite its evident clinical utility, systematic desensitization is based on an essential misperception of the laws of classical conditioning. Classical conditioning is essentially ephemeral. Organisms stop responding to the conditioned stimulus when it is no longer paired with the unconditioned stimulus. Pavlov's dogs may have learned to salivate to the ringing of the bell, but if Pavlov kept ringing the bell after it was no longer paired with the meat powder, the dogs soon stopped salivating to its ring. This is referred to as the process of **extinction,** in which conditioned stimuli lose their capacity to elicit a response when they are presented too many times in the absence of the unconditioned stimulus.

This basic feature was considered so troublesome by early behaviorally oriented psychopathologists that they felt compelled to explain how such an ephemeral process could account for a long-lasting disorder such as a phobia (most phobias don't remit spontaneously over time). O. Hobart Mowrer solved the riddle when he postulated that phobic reactions essentially involve two learning processes: classical conditioning, to instill the anxiety response to a previously neutral stimulus; and operant conditioning, to reinforce the voluntary escape or avoidance behaviors that remove the patient from the presence of the conditioned stimulus before the anxious arousal can be extinguished. In essence, people who acquire a phobic reaction to a basically benign stimulus don't extinguish (as the laws of classical conditioning predict they should), because they don't stay in the situation long enough for classical extinction to take place.

This conclusion led some behavior theorists to suggest that although systematic desensitization was undoubtedly effective, it was unnecessarily complex and time consuming. The essential mechanism of change, they suggested, was extinction, not counterconditioning, and the only procedure needed was to expose the patient repeatedly to the feared object or situation. Of course, the therapist would also have to do something to prevent the patient from running away or otherwise terminating contact with the feared situation. Thus, according to exposure theorists, it was not necessary to ensure that patients experienced no fear in the presence of the phobic stimulus (as Wolpe claimed). Rather, all that was required was to get them into the situation and to prevent them from leaving until the anxiety had diminished on its own.

Several decades of controlled research have suggested that the extinction theorists were correct and that exposure (plus response prevention) is at least as effective as systematic desensitization and is more rapid in its effects. That does not necessarily mean that it is more useful than systematic desensitization in practice; many patients find exposure therapy very distressing and prefer the kinder, gentler alternative provided by systematic desensitization. Although exposure typically works more rapidly than does systematic desensitization (and both work more rapidly than do other nonbehavioral alternatives), it often takes as long to persuade a patient to try exposure techniques as it does to complete a full course of systematic desensitization. Nonetheless, it is now clear that exposure (with response prevention) is a sufficient condition for symptomatic change and that Wolpe was in error when he suggested that allowing a patient to experience anxiety in the presence of the phobic situation delayed the process of change. Although patients who already have acquired a conditioned fear response will undoubtedly experience distress when exposed to the object of their fears, the fact that they become anxious during the course of that exposure neither facilitates nor retards the extinction process. (This is why most behavior therapists no longer use the term "flooding" to refer to exposure therapy; although it may be descriptive of the level of anxiety induced, it is misleading in that it seems to imply that the induction of anxiety is itself curative in some way.)

Exposure plus response prevention has a clear advantage over systematic desensitization (and virtually every other type of nonbehavioral intervention) in the treatment of more complex disorders related to anxiety. It appears to be particularly helpful in the treatment of severe obsessive-compulsive disorder (OCD) and severe agoraphobia. For example, treatment for a patient who has a fear of contamination and repetitive hand-washing rituals might involve having a therapy team spend a weekend locked in the patient's home, having the patient intentionally contaminate his or her hands and food with dirt (by shutting off the water to prevent hand washing). Similarly, a patient with severe agoraphobia would be encouraged to visit settings that he or she typically avoids (eg, shopping malls or grocery stores) during the busiest times of the day and would be prevented (again by a therapy team or group) from leaving until his or her anxiety had subsided. Although systematic desensitization has had limited success with such severe disorders, the process of constructing and working through the literally dozens of hierarchies required typically makes the approach wildly impractical.

Summary

Strategies based on classical conditioning have also been used in the treatment of depression, somatoform disorders, dissociative disorders, substance abuse, sexual difficulties, medical problems, and a variety of other disorders. In general, these approaches represent some of the most effective of the therapeutic interventions. As is the case with other types of behavioral strategies, they rest on a solid foundation of basic empirical work, much of it with nonhuman animals, and on the creative adaptation of those basic principles to human populations.

Marks IM: *Fears, Phobias and Rituals.* Oxford University Press, 1987.

Masters JC et al: *Behavior Therapy: Techniques and Empirical Findings,* 3rd ed. Harcourt Brace Jovanovich, 1987.

Rachman S, Hodgson RJ: *Obsession and Compulsions.* Prentice-Hall, 1980.

Wilson GT: Behavior therapy. Pages 197–228 in: Corsini RJ, Wedding D (editors): *Current Psychotherapies,* 5th ed. FE Peacock Publishing, 1995.

Wolpe J: *Psychotherapy by Reciprocal Inhibition.* Stanford University Press, 1958.

EMERGENCE OF INSTRUMENTAL & OPERANT LEARNING THEORY

As a graduate student at Columbia University, Edward Thorndike began a series of experiments that set a new course in the study of processes underlying behavior change and learning. He placed a cat in an enclosed chamber and attached a vertical pole in the center of the compartment to a rope that passed over several pulleys. When the cat bumped against the pole, the pole would tilt, causing the rope to open the door. The cat could then leave the compartment and drink milk from a nearby bowl outside the cage. At first, the cat seemed to move about unpredictably each time it was returned to the compartment. The time required for the cat to tilt the pole grew shorter on successive repetitions of the task, and the cat's method for opening the door on each trial became progressively similar to the method used on the preceding trial. The trial-by-trial record of time to escape from what Thorndike called his "puzzle box" was the first instrumental learning curve published in a scientific journal. Eventually, each cat quickly approached the pole—seemingly purposively—and tilted it to one side, opening the door. Thorndike described this as an **instrumental conditioning** process because the pole tilting was instrumental in releasing the cat from the chamber and permitting access to a reward. Thorndike's method differed from Pavlov's classical conditioning because no specific response was elicited by a conditioned stimulus. The form of each cat's behavior that tilted the pole was idiosyncratic and variable. There was nothing fixed about the behavior, as was typical of classically conditioned behavior. Thorndike's Law of Effect described the necessary and sufficient conditions for instrumental learning to occur.

Skinner & Operant Behavior

Whereas Thorndike studied the process of behavior change, three decades later, B. F. Skinner, a graduate student at Harvard University, was interested in discovering a method for identifying the functional components of sequences of behavior. Skinner was drawn to the writings of the physiologists Charles Sherrington and Ernst Magnus. Skinner was particularly taken with Sherrington's notion of the reflex arc. Skinner believed that psychologists had gotten seriously off on the wrong track by focusing on unobservable phenomenological events, which no amount of experimentation could verify, rather than following the example of physiology in studying observable events. Skinner wondered whether Thorndike's Law of Effect might explain how a single component could be isolated from the continuously free flowing activities of an organism, so that the component could be studied scientifically, much as Sherrington had done. Using a method very similar to Thorndike's, Skinner placed a rat in an enclosed chamber, and each time the rat depressed a telegraph key protruding through the wall of the chamber, a pellet of food dropped into a receptacle near the rat. The lever-pressing methods each rat used varied: most pressed with their paws, some pushed with their muzzles, others held the telegraph key between their teeth and pulled down. All methods produced the same result—delivery of a pellet of food that the hungry rat seized and ate. Skinner said that the rat "operated" on its environment to produce reinforcing consequences, and the type of behavior was correspondingly called **operant behavior.**

In operant behavior, typically no stimulus was presented before an operant response that "caused" the behavior to occur (ie, there was no conditioned stimulus). When Skinner analyzed the sequence of the rat's activities in an operant chamber, he found that after many repetitions of the rat approaching the lever, depressing it, and hearing the device click, which had been followed by food pellet presentation, the click sound produced by the lever press began to be rewarding without food pellet presentation. If a light were illuminated above the lever (indicating periods when food would be available), alternating with periods when the light was off (indicating lever presses would not produce food), soon the rat pressed nearly exclusively when the light was illuminated. The rat's behavior continued to be variable, changing from moment to moment even when the light was illuminated, unlike a classically conditioned reflex. Skinner called the food pellet a **reinforcer** and the light that signaled that operant responding would lead to reinforcer presentation, a **discriminative stimulus.** Skinner spelled out in surprisingly accurate detail laws of operant conditioning that have stood the test of time. Immediacy, magnitude, and intermittence of reinforcement affected the pattern of behavior maintained and also determined the persistence of behavior in the absence of reinforcement.

Skinner also observed that a stimulus repeatedly paired with food presentation (eg, the "click" sound of the food pellet dispenser) came to serve as a reinforcer in its own right and would maintain considerable amounts of behavior over extended periods of time in the absence of primary reinforcement. Such previously neutral stimuli that took on reinforcing properties because of their pairing with primary reinforcers were called **conditioned reinforcers** or **secondary reinforcers.** Skinner recognized that in most developed parts of the world, relatively limited aspects of human conduct seem to be directed toward seeking food or shelter. Instead, most human conduct seems to be governed by parent or teacher approval, threat of loss of affection, or symbols of recognition from employers or peers (eg, paychecks, awards). Skinner reasoned that these reinforcers had developed their reinforcing properties (usually very early in an individual's life) from their repeated pairing with primary reinforcers. In short, they were powerful conditioned reinforcers. This observation led later educa-

tors, drug abuse counselors, psychologists, and psychiatrists working in various applied settings to develop treatment methods based on conditioned reinforcers such as social approval or concrete objects paired with other reinforcers (eg, check marks, stars, tokens, money).

Applications to Clinical Treatment

The practical utility of the operant apparatus and measurement approach was adopted quickly in experimental psychology, physiology, neurochemistry, pharmacology, and toxicology laboratories throughout the world. The methodology provided the springboard for the field of behavioral pharmacology, the study of subcortical self-stimulation, animal models of addictive behavior, and the study of psychophysics and complex human social behavior in enclosed experimental spaces. Skinner's pragmatic theory struck a popular chord with many young psychologists, special educators, and practitioners in training. In 1948, Sidney Bijou began an applied research program and experimental nursery school for children with mental retardation at the Rainier School in Washington, applying operant principles. Bijou was joined by Donald Baer, a recent graduate of the University of Chicago, and they conducted seminal research on early child operant behavior. In 1953, Ogden Lindsley and Skinner began applying operant methods to study the behavior of patients with schizophrenia at Metropolitan State Hospital in Waltham, Massachusetts.

Several major events brought the emerging field of behavior modification to the attention of psychiatry. First, Teodoro Ayllon and Nathan Azrin were granted limited funds in 1961 for an experimental program to motivate and improve the functioning of a group of severely mentally ill, mostly schizophrenic, women who were institutionalized in Illinois. The program used a token reinforcement system originally developed by Roger Kelleher, who had studied behavior of chimpanzees in laboratory settings. Tokens resembling poker chips were given to patients immediately after they completed agreed-upon therapeutic activities. Later the tokens could be exchanged for supplementary preferred activities or commodities. The changes in patient behavior were often dramatic and included markedly increased participation in therapeutic programs such as those aimed at employment, bathing, self-care, and related daily living skills.

Leonard Ullman headed a similar treatment unit in Palo Alto, California. Both programs operated on the principle that chronically mentally ill patients, primarily those with schizophrenia, had been largely unresponsive to conventional psychological therapeutic methods. Although older neuroleptic medications managed many of the florid symptoms of schizophrenia, they did little to increase the patients' positive adjustment and often produced problematic side effects. These programs demonstrated that it was possible to use laboratory-based management methods to motivate patients with chronic schizophrenia, increasing their participation in hospital therapeutic programs and decreasing the amount of disturbed behavior. Although no one claimed these methods changed the underlying disorder, they were very effective tools for improving patient compliance and management.

A less frequently cited but still important study conducted during this era was Gordon Paul and coworkers' comparison of the effectiveness of a social learning theory approach to a more traditional milieu therapy approach to managing the behavior of patients with chronic mental illnesses in an institutional setting. It is the single best study of its kind, demonstrating persuasively the effectiveness of a behavior therapy strategy for activating socially resistant patients who have schizophrenia. It also carefully documented reductions in schizophrenic disorganization and cognitive distortion; improvements in normal speech and social interactions; reductions in social isolation; and greatly reduced aggressive, assaultive, and other intolerable behavior.

The second major event was the demonstration in 1963 by Ivar Lovaas, a clinical psychologist working at UCLA, that positive reinforcement methods could be used to teach children with autism a variety of skills. Until that time, there were no known effective treatments for autism. Lovaas worked with children who were mute and with echolalic children who had autism (labeled "schizophrenic children" at that time). These children were severely mentally retarded, were self-injurious, displayed severe tantrums, and were extremely noncompliant. Lovaas used a combination of hugs and praise, edible reinforcers, and highly controversial aversive stimulation techniques to reduce self-destructive behavior. His rationale for the use of painful skin shock was that the alternative for some children was a lifetime in restraints to avoid severe self-injury. In some cases, children who, without restraints and without shock, banged their heads over 10,000 times per week, stopped head banging within 24 hours when skin shock was combined with positive reinforcement. In later years, Lovaas largely abandoned the use of aversive treatment methods, although for some researchers in the field, his name continues to be associated with this aspect of his method rather than the fact that he was the first person to develop an effective method for intervening to teach functional social, communicative, and other adaptive skills to autistic children.

The third major event that paved the way for modern behavior therapy methods was the work of Gerald Patterson and colleagues in developing a coercion model of the relationships between children with conduct disorder and their families. In the early and mid-1960s, Patterson began working with children of normal intelligence who displayed a wide array of predelinquent behavior. Some of the children displayed characteristics of attention-deficit/hyperactivity disorder, others seemed to have learning disabilities, and others were aggressive and noncompliant at home and school but exhibited no indications of other psychiatric or cognitive disability. Based on a series of laboratory and clinical studies, Patterson and his colleagues proposed that children who had conduct disorder and their families gradually learn a set of mutually coercive relationships based on interpersonal aversive stimulation and avoidance. Based on this model, he developed a behavioral treatment method drawing on basic operant methods (ie, positive social and tangible reinforcement and loss of reinforcement resulting from behavior problems, both of which were based on unambiguous and consistent contingencies). He combined these techniques with what would later be called cognitive-behavior therapy methods (ie, use of verbal self-instructions to mediate behavior changes).

Finally, in the late 1960s and early 1970s several large-scale programs were developed that applied operant behavioral principles in residential services for people with mental retardation. These early institution-based programs paved the way for subsequent community-based service and treatment programs for people with mental retardation, especially those with significant behavior problems.

Ayllon T, Azrin N: *The Token Economy: A Motivational System for Therapy and Rehabilitation.* Appleton-Century-Crofts, 1968.
Patterson GR, Gullion ME: *Living with Children; New Methods for Parents and Teachers.* Research Press, 1968.
Skinner BF: *Behavior of Organisms.* Appleton, 1938.
Skinner BF: *Science and Human Behavior.* Macmillan, 1953.

COGNITIVE & COGNITIVE-BEHAVIORAL INTERVENTIONS

One of the major changes in behavioral approaches in the past several decades has been the emergence of the cognitive and cognitive-behavioral interventions. Based largely on social learning theory, these approaches posit that organisms are not just the passive recipients of stimuli that impinge on them but instead interpret and try to make sense out of their worlds. These approaches don't reject more traditional classical and operant perspectives on learning; rather, they suggest that cognitive mediation plays a role in coloring the way those processes work in humans and other higher vertebrates.

Roots of Cognitive Therapy

The roots of cognitive therapy can be found in the early writings of the Stoic philosophers Epictetus and Marcus Aurelius, and in the later works by Benjamin Rush and Henry Maudsley, among others. It was Epictetus who, in the first century A.D., wrote that "People are disturbed not by things, but by the view which they take of them." Benjamin Rush, the father of American psychiatry, wrote in 1786 that by exercising the rational mind through practice, one gained control over otherwise unmanageable passions that he believed led to some forms of madness. A century later, Henry Maudsley reiterated the notion that it was the loss of power over the coordination of ideas and feelings that led to madness and that the wise development of control over thoughts and feelings could have a powerful effect. In more modern times, Alfred Adler's approach to dynamic psychotherapy was cognitive in nature, stressing the role of perceptions of the self and the world in determining how people went about the process of pursuing their goals in life. George Kelly is often accorded a central role in laying out the basic tenets of the approach, and Albert Bandura's influential treatise on learning theory provided a theoretical basis for incorporating observational learning in the learning process.

Modern Approaches

Modern cognitive and cognitive-behavioral approaches to psychotherapy got their impetus from two converging lines of development. One branch was developed by theorists originally trained in dynamic psychotherapy. Theorists such as Albert Ellis, the founder of rational-emotive therapy, and Aaron Beck, the founder of cognitive therapy, began their careers adhering to dynamic principles in theory and therapy but soon became disillusioned with that approach and came, over time, to focus on their patients' conscious beliefs. Both ascribe to an ABC model, which states that it is not just what happens to someone at point A (the antecedent events) that determines how the person feels and what he or she does at point C (the affective and behavioral consequences) but that it also matters how the person interprets those events at point B (the person's beliefs). For example, someone who loses a relationship and is convinced that he or she was left because he or she is unlovable is more likely to feel depressed and fail to pursue further relationships than is someone who considers his or her loss a consequence of bad luck or the product of mistakes that he or she will not repeat the next time around. Both theorists work with patients to actively examine their beliefs to be sure that they are not making situations worse than they necessarily are. Ellis typically adopts a more philosophical approach based on reason and persuasion, whereas Beck operates more like a scientist, treating his patients' beliefs as hypotheses that can be tested and encouraging his patients to use their own behaviors to test the accuracy of their beliefs.

The other major branch of cognitive-behaviorism involves theorists originally trained as behavior therapists who became increasingly interested in the role of thinking in the learning process. Bandura and Michael Mahoney represent two exemplars of this tradition, as do other theorists such as Donald Meichenbaum and G. Terence Wilson. These theorists tend to stay closer to the language and tenets of traditional behavior analysis and are somewhat less likely to talk about the role of meaning in their patients' responses to events. They are also as likely to focus on the absence of cognitive mediators (ie, covert self-statements) as on the presence of distortions. For example, Meichenbaum developed an influential approach to treatment, called self-instructional training, in which patients with impulse-control problems are trained to modulate their own behaviors via the process of verbal self-regulation.

These approaches focus on the role of information processing in determining subsequent affect and behavior. Beck, for example, has argued that distinctive errors in thinking can be found in each of the major types of psychopathology. For example, depression typically involves negative views of the self and the future; anxiety, an overdetermined sense of physical or psychological danger; eating disorders, an undue concern with shape and weight; and obsessions, an overbearing sense of responsibility for ensuring the safety of oneself and others. Efforts to produce change involve having the patient first monitor fluctuations in mood and relate those changes to the ongoing flow of automatic thoughts, subsequently using one's own behavior to test the accuracy of these beliefs. For example, a depressed patient who believes that he or she is incompetent will be asked to provide an example of something he or she should be able to do but cannot. The patient is then invited to list the steps that anyone else would have to do to carry out the task. The patient is then encouraged to carry out those steps just to determine whether he or she is as incompetent as he or she believes (typically, the patient is not).

Similarly, patients with panic disorder often misinterpret innocuous bodily sensations as signs of impending physical or psychological catastrophe, such as having a heart attack or "going crazy." The therapist provides a rationale that stresses the role of thinking in symptom formation and encourages the patient to test his or her belief in the imminence of the impending catastrophe by inducing a panic attack right in the office. As the patient experiences extreme states of arousal and panic with no subsequent consequences (ie, neither dying nor "going crazy"), he or she comes to recognize that the initial arousal was not a harbinger of impending doom (as first believed), and the patient no longer begins to panic at the occurrence of arousal. In essence, like the behavioral approaches based on classical conditioning, modern cognitive and cognitive-behavioral interventions emphasize the curative process of exposing oneself to the things one most fears as a way of dealing with irrational or unrealistic concerns.

These approaches appear to be well established in the treatment of unipolar depression, panic disorder, social phobia, generalized anxiety disorder, and bulimia. For these disorders, cognitive and cognitive-behavioral interventions appear to be at least as effective as other competing alternatives (including medications) and quite possibly more enduring. There are consistent indications that cognitive-behavioral therapy may produce long-lasting change that reduces the likelihood that symptoms will return after treatment ends. The evidence is more mixed with respect to substance abuse, marital distress, and childhood conduct disorder, although at least some indications are promising. Cognitive and cognitive-behavioral interventions are typically not thought to be particularly effective in patients who have formal thought disorder, although recent studies suggest that the interventions may reduce delusional thinking in psychotic patients who receive neuroleptic drugs.

Beck AT: *Cognitive Therapy and the Emotional Disorders.* International Universities Press, 1976.

Ellis A: *Reason and Emotion in Psychotherapy.* Lyle Stuart, 1962.

Hollon SD, Beck AT: Cognitive and cognitive-behavioral therapies. Pages 428–466 in: Bergin AE, Garfield SL (editors): *Handbook of Psychotherapy and Behavior Change,* 4th ed. John Wiley & Sons, 1994.

Marlatt GA, Gordon J: *Relapse Prevention: Maintenance Strategies in the Treatment of Addictive Behaviors.* Guilford Press, 1985.

Meichenbaum D: *Cognitive-Behavior Modification: An Integrative Approach.* Plenum Publishing Corp, 1977.

FUNDAMENTAL ASSUMPTIONS OF LEARNING THEORY–BASED THERAPIES

Several basic assumptions are common to most learning-based interventions. Perhaps most basic is that the behavior of the individual who has been referred for psychiatric treatment is of concern in its own right. Behavior is not necessarily an indication of pathology at some other level of analysis (eg, brain chemical or psychic). Moreover, pathologic behavior is often seen as the result of the demands of the environment in which the person is living, working, or going to school (or, in the case of the cognitive approaches, the person's perception of the environment). What appears to be pathologic behavior may be a best-effort adaptation to an impossible situation given the person's cognitive or personality limitations (eg, living with alcoholic parents, residing in an abusive institutional or community residential setting, interacting with people who don't use the same communication system).

Although major mental illnesses have neurochemical substrates, much of the pathologic behavior observed by psychiatrists has been learned in much the same way that more normal-appearing behavior is learned, and pathologic behavior generally follows the same scientific laws as normal behavior. Vulnerability to learning pathologic behavior is shaped by the biological substrate of inherited traits and neurochemical predispositions upon which the collective history of experiences is imposed. Individual differences in normal and pathologic behavior are attributable to dispositions created by variations in genetic makeup or differences in histories that predispose an individual to differences in motivation. Some people, by virtue of their genetic and associated neurochemical makeup, are prone to respond to a wide range of mild, negative comments by other people as though such comments are aversive and are to be avoided at all costs. Others, with different genetic makeups and correspondingly different neurochemical predispositions, may be largely impervious to similar negative reinforcers and cues. The former individuals are prone to develop avoidant behavior patterns characterized by extreme anxiety problems, whereas the latter individuals will tend to be insensitive to aversive social situations.

In the early days of behavior modification and behavior therapy treatments, targets of treatment were often circumscribed responses (eg, nail-biting, failing in school, encopresis). Since then, researchers have recognized that narrowly defined instances of pathologic behavior (ie, presenting symptoms) are usually members of larger classes of problematic responses. The treatment task is not to treat the isolated behavior (eg, arguing with parents or making self-deprecating remarks) but rather to identify factors that determine the likelihood that any member of an entire class of responses may occur. Such factors could include, for example, the child having no legitimate mechanism for determining what is going on in his or her life, combined with parental submission to a variety of unpleasant, coercive responses. Failure to properly assess the full breadth of the members composing a functional response class will tend to lead to symptom substitution. For example, successful reduction of arguing by a defiant teenager by implementing a behavioral contract limited to arguing will, in most instances, lead to emergence of other defiant behaviors (eg, staying out beyond curfew, experimenting with alcohol). The task is to identify a broader class of problem behavior, develop hypotheses concerning the purposes served by that class of behavior, and then develop an intervention plan that makes that class of behavior ineffective and unnecessary.

Most of the causes of pathologic behavior are found in the relation between the individual and the environmental antecedents and consequences of his or her actions. An individual's history creates the context within which current environmental circumstances serve as either discriminative stimuli (eg, a spouse coming home late from work) or conditioned negative reinforcers (eg, threatened disapproval). An individual's history could also establish the motivational framework that governs most of the individual's actions. As a result, assessment usually requires obtaining information from the individual or other informants about events taking place in the individual's natural environment in order to obtain valid data concerning the circumstances surrounding the pathologic behavior. The meaning of an environmental cue or a putative motivating consequence is determined contextually. Whether a social stimulus is alarming, neutral, or positive will depend on the person's history and the circumstance in which the stimulus is being experienced. Similarly, a consequence can be positive, neutral, or negative depending on the individual's history and the circumstance in which the consequence is encountered. Thus Thorndike's original Law of Effect has been contextualized. Whether this contextualization is conceptualized as residing in the cognitive domain or in the observable environment is a matter of some theoretical dispute, but the learning-based approaches emphasize the role of idiosyncratic experience in shaping the behavioral proclivities of any given individual.

Bandura A: *Principles of Behavior Modification.* Holt, Rinehart & Winston, 1969.

Craighead WE, Craighead LW, Ilardi SS: Behavior therapies in historical perspective. In: Bonger BM et al (editors): *Comprehensive Textbook of Psychotherapy: Theory and Practice.* Oxford University Press, 1995.

Kazdin AE: *History of Behavior Modification: Experimental Foundations of Contemporary Research.* University Park, 1978.

Krasner L: History of behavior modification. Pages 3–25 in: Bellack AS, Hersen M (editors): *International Handbook of Behavior Modification and Therapy,* 2nd ed. Plenum Publishing Corp, 1990.

COMBINATIONS WITH MEDICATIONS

Many of the disorders treated with behavioral or cognitive-behavioral therapy can also be treated pharmacologically, although some cannot (see Chapters 3 and 10). In some disorders, a combination of drugs and behavioral (or cognitive-behavioral) therapy is more effective than either modality alone. Despite the theoretically based concerns of advocates for each approach, one modality rarely interferes with the other, although such interference sometimes occurs. For many disorders, there are simply not adequate data to guide clinical practice; we often know that both modalities are effective in their own right but do not know whether their combination enhances treatment response.

Drugs and other somatic interventions appear to be essential to the treatment of the more severe disorders, particularly those that involve psychotic symptoms. Nonetheless, behavioral and cognitive-behavioral interventions can often play an important adjunctive role. Antipsychotic medications remain the most effective means of reducing the more florid symptoms of psychosis, and the newer, atypical antipsychotics show promise in relieving the negative symptoms of schizophrenia. Rehabilitation programs based on behavioral skills training appear to help redress impairments in psychosocial functioning in such patients and may allow the use of newer low-dose neuroleptic strategies (see Chapter 19). Lithium and the newer anticonvulsants provide the most effective means of prophylaxis in the bipolar disorders, but cognitive-behavioral therapy can enhance compliance with drug therapy (see Chapter 21).

The relative importance of pharmacotherapy is less pronounced among even the more severe, nonpsychotic disorders and quite possibly is nonexistent among the less severe disorders. Cognitive therapy appears to be about as effective as pharmacotherapy for all but the most severe nonbipolar depressions and may be more enduring in its effects (see Chapter 21). Exposure-based therapies are quite helpful in reducing compulsive rituals in OCD (see Chapter 24) and behavioral avoidance in severe agoraphobia (see Chapter 22). Such therapies are often combined with medications to treat these disorders. Cognitive-behavioral therapy appears to be at least as effective and possibly longer lasting than pharmacotherapy in the treatment of panic disorder and social phobia (see Chapter 22), and the same can be said with respect to the treatment of bulimia (see Chapter 29). Exposure-based treatment is clearly superior to pharmacotherapy (or any other form of psychotherapy) in the treatment of social phobia. There is little evidence that drugs are particularly helpful in the treatment of the personality disorders (see Chapter 33), whereas a dialectic approach to behavior therapy appears to reduce the frequency of self-destructive behavior in patients with borderline personality disorder.

In general, the more severe the psychopathologic disorder, the greater the relative efficacy of pharmacotherapy and the more purely behavioral the psychosocial intervention needs to be. Medications are often useful to control disruptive symptoms, but behavioral interventions (especially operant ones) are uniquely suited to instilling new skills or restoring those that have been lost to illness or institutionalization. Behavioral interventions based on classical conditioning models appear to be particularly helpful in reducing undesirable states of arousal and affective distress; cognitive interventions appear to reduce the likelihood of subsequent relapse by correcting erroneous beliefs and attitudes that contribute to risk. These strategies rarely interfere with one another, and it is often useful to combine them in practice to achieve multiple ends.

Klerman GL et al: Medication and psychotherapy. Pages 734–782 in: Bergin AE, Garfield SL (editors): *Handbook of Psychotherapy and Behavior Change,* 4th ed. John Wiley & Sons, 1994.

COMBINED INTERVENTIONS IN DEVELOPMENTAL DISABILITIES

Behavioral interventions can be highly effective in improving the quality of life for people who have developmental disabilities and display serious behavior problems. Sometimes behavioral methods are insufficient by themselves. Psychopharmacologic treatments can control psychopathologic symptoms and behavior in some people with mental retardation and related disabilities, much as they are effective in treating disorders (eg, major depression, bipolar disorder, anxiety disorder, schizophrenia) in non–developmentally delayed individuals.

In attempting to better understand how psychotropic drugs reduce problem behavior, it is helpful to elucidate the behavioral as well as neurochemical mechanisms of drug action. Behavioral mechanisms refer to psychological or behavioral processes altered by a drug. Neurochemical mechanisms refer to the underlying receptor-level events that are causally related to those changed behavioral processes. Some psychopathologic problems are associated so frequently with specific developmental disabilities that pharmacotherapy is often among the first treatments to be explored. Anxiety disorder, especially OCD, is commonly associated with autism and Prader-Willi syndrome. Anxiety disorder manifests itself as ritualistic, repetitive stereotypic motor responses (eg, rocking or hand-flapping) and rigidly routinized activities (eg, repeatedly lining up blocks, insisting that shoe laces be precisely the same length) that, if interrupted, provoke behavioral outbursts or tantrums. Selective serotonin reuptake inhibitors help reduce agitation, anxiety, and ritualistic behavior, including skin-picking and some self-injurious behavior associated with these problems. At times, aggression may result from an anxiety disorder. For example, a patient with autism who has severe anxiety may strike out against others who are crowding too closely, in order to keep them at a distance. Fluvoxamine reduces anxiety and the need for increased social distance, thereby diminishing the need to strike out against others to keep them at a distance. Aggression, in this example, serves as a social avoidance response that the fluvoxamine makes unnecessary. The behavioral mechanism of action is reduced anxiety and associated avoidance. The neurochemical mechanism is thought to be mediated by inhibition of serotonin reuptake with increased binding to the serotonin-2 receptors.

An individual with autism or mental retardation who strikes his or her head in intermittent bouts throughout the day may do so because head blows cause the release of β-endorphin, which binds to the μ-opiate receptor, thereby reinforcing self-injury. In this way, a self-addictive, vicious cycle is established and maintained and through years of repetition be-

comes a firmly entrenched behavioral pattern. Administration of an opiate antagonist, such as naltrexone, blocks the reinforcing effects consequent to the binding of β-endorphin to the opiate receptor. Naltrexone reduces such self-injurious behavior in approximately 40% of patients, primarily in those engaging in high-frequency, intense self-injury directed at the head and hands. Evidence indicates that elevated baseline levels of plasma β-endorphin after bouts of self-injury are predictive of a subsequent therapeutic response to naltrexone.

Repetitive self-injurious behavior, such as head banging and self-biting, can be treated effectively with complementary behavioral and pharmacologic strategies, as described in the following case example.

A 13-year-old boy with autism and severe mental retardation was nonverbal and had no communication system at baseline. An observational functional assessment of the boy's self-injurious behavior in his natural environment (a special education classroom) indicated that approximately two thirds of this behavior appeared to be motivated by the desire to obtain attention or to escape from situations he didn't like or found disturbing. Self-injury dropped 50% from baseline during the first naltrexone treatment phase. Next the patient was taught to use pictorial icons to make requests and to indicate basic needs and wants to others around him (Figure 2–1). His self-injury dropped subsequently by another 50% (a reduction of a total of 75% from baseline) when communication treatment was initiated. On follow-up 1 year later, during which time naltrexone treatment was continued, the boy's self-injurious behavior had continued to drop to nearly zero. In this case, naltrexone blocked the neurochemical reinforcing consequences of self-injury, and the communication training provided an appropriate

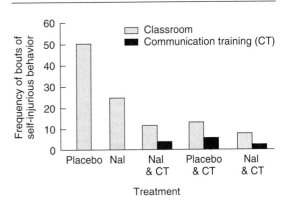

Figure 2–1. Efficacy of treatments for self-injurious behavior. Nal, naltrexone.

behavioral alternative to indicate basic needs and wants. In short, the combined treatments produced complementary, additive salutary effects.

Lutzker JR: Behavior analysis for developmental disabilities: the stages of efficacy and comparative treatments. Pages 89–106 in: Giles TR (editor): *Handbook of Effective Psychotherapy.* Plenum Publishing Corp, 1993.

Symons FJ, Fox ND, Thompson T: Functional communication training and naltrexone treatment of self-injurious behavior. JARID 1997;10:1.

Thompson T, Grabowski JG: *Behavior Modification of the Mentally Retarded,* 2nd ed. Oxford University Press, 1977.

CONCLUSION

Modern behavioral and cognitive-behavioral interventions emphasize the role of learning and adaptation to the environment both in shaping and maintaining normal life functions and in the emergence of maladaptive symptomatology. In essence, these approaches focus on behavior as important in its own right and often seek to change instances of disordered behavior via the application of clearly articulated basic principles of learning. Three basic, interrelated perspectives exist: classical conditioning, which emphasizes the learning of associations between classes of stimuli; operant conditioning, which emphasizes the learning of relations between behaviors and their consequences; and the cognitive perspective, which emphasizes the role of idiosyncratic beliefs and misconceptions in coloring each of the two earlier perspectives. There can be little doubt that the learning-based approaches have sparked a major revolution in the treatment of psychiatric disorders and that each perspective can point to a series of notable gains. These approaches can often be combined with medications for beneficial effect and should be part of the armamentarium of any well-trained clinician.

Neuropsychopharmacology

3

Sydney Spector, PhD, & Fridolin Sulser, MD

An understanding of neuropsychopharmacology provides a basis for sound therapeutics. Used as tools to probe the central nervous system (CNS), psychotropic drugs have contributed more than anything else to our understanding of the function of the brain. They have helped to establish biological psychiatry as a branch of medicine, and they have contributed to the generation of heuristic hypotheses concerning the biological basis of mental illness.

Neuropsychopharmacology reached prominence as a consequence of seminal contributions made by a number of basic scientists and astute clinical psychiatrists. Many of these contributions are acknowledged in the individual sections of this chapter. A few had such a lasting impact on the field that they deserve to be mentioned briefly at the outset. Otto Loewi and Sir Henry Hallett Dale provided the first real proof of chemical mediation of nerve impulses and established the concept of neurohumoral transmission. A corollary to the chemical transmission concept is the evolution of receptor theory, through the work of Paul Ehrlich on chemoreceptors and John Newport Langley's concept of receptive substances in the early 20th century. The impact of the receptor theory of Ehrlich and Langley was minimal during their lifetime but is now a major research area in neuropsychopharmacology. Another major milestone in our understanding of hormone and neurotransmitter function was the development of the second messenger concept in the mid-1960s by Earl Sutherland. Sutherland was the first to describe the action of a hormone (epinephrine) at a molecular level. What receptors are—how they work and how psychotropic drugs directly or indirectly interact with various receptor cascades—is a major topic to be discussed in this chapter.

The remarkable contributions of B. B. Brodie and the Brodie School have opened up the field of biochemical psychopharmacology. Discoveries made in Brodie's laboratory have paved the way for the era of cytochrome P-450 and the pivotal role of the metabolic disposition of drugs as well as the use of drugs as formidable tools to investigate brain function.

BASIC NEUROPHARMACOLOGY

Neuropharmacology is the pharmacology of the nervous system. The nervous system coordinates cellular activity, and the neuron is its basic component. The principal mechanism by which neurons communicate with one another is through the release of chemical mediators known as neurotransmitters. A chemical substance must possess several qualities before it can be classified as a neurotransmitter (Table 3–1).

A neurotransmitter has to be differentiated from another chemical messenger, namely a hormone. Hormones are secreted into the bloodstream, exert their effects throughout the body, and have a relatively long half-life. In contrast, neurotransmitters usually communicate point to point, are released by one neuron onto another neuron, and have a short half-life.

In order for a neuron to act swiftly and repeatedly it needs a synthetic mechanism to constantly replenish the neurotransmitters it releases. The synthetic apparatus is located in the cell body. After synthesis, neurotransmitters are transported down the axon to presynaptic nerve terminals where they are stored in synaptic vesicles. The presynaptic terminal is in proximity to a specialized area of the adjacent neuron referred to as the postsynaptic site. Information from the released neurotransmitter is conveyed to the adjacent neurons via the postsynaptic site. For many neu-

Table 3–1. Qualities of neurotransmitters.

The chemical is either synthesized or stored in a neuron.
It is present at the nerve terminal.
It is released following nerve stimulation.
Upon application, it mimics the effects of nerve stimulation.
Drugs that affect the receptor sites where nerve stimulation acts should also affect the action of the exogenously administered chemical.
A mechanism for inactivation of the neurotransmitter is present.

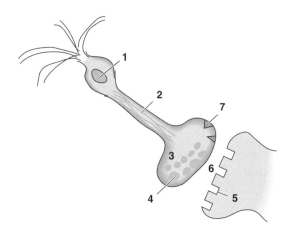

Figure 3–1. Synaptic neurotransmission sites. (1) Cell body where synthesis of the neurotransmitter occurs; (2) microtubules, involved in the transport of macromolecules between the cell body and the distal nerve terminal; (3) transport site for uptake of the precursor or neurotransmitter into presynaptic storage vesicles; (4) presynaptic storage vesicles; (5) postsynaptic neurotransmitter receptors; (6) site of transporters for the reuptake of the released neurotransmitter into the presynaptic vesicle; (7) presynaptic neurotransmitter receptors.

rotransmitters the presynaptic nerve terminal has a mechanism that rapidly replenishes released transmitter (a process referred to as **recapture**). The released neurotransmitter (or the hydrolytic product that can be reused to synthesize new transmitter substance) is taken back into the presynaptic vesicles by an active—and, in the case of some neurotransmitters, a specific—reuptake process (Figure 3–1).

The list of chemical substances classified as neurotransmitters is ever-growing. In the 1950s and 1960s norepinephrine, serotonin, dopamine, and acetylcholine were thought to be the principal neurotransmitters. Subsequent studies added the amino acids gamma amino butyric acid (GABA), glycine, glutamic acid, and aspartic acid. Several peptides satisfy criteria for classification as neurotransmitters. Furthermore, the presynaptic vesicles at the nerve terminals can contain more than one neurotransmitter, so that more than one transmitter substance is released following depolarization of the nerve ending.

CATECHOLAMINES

The **catecholamines** are molecules that contain a 3,4-dihydroxyphenyl nucleus. Norepinephrine and dopamine are neurotransmitters, whereas epinephrine, which is also a catecholamine, is classified as a hormone (Figure 3–2). Nevertheless, epinephrine is present in the CNS, and it may have a role as a neurotransmitter. Although the presence in systemic tissues of epinephrine and norepinephrine had long been known, it was not until 1948 that they were found in mammalian sympathetic nervous tissue. About the same time, researchers discovered dopamine, a catecholamine lacking a β-hydroxy group on the side chain.

Catecholamine Metabolism

The biosynthetic pathway for the catecholamines proceeds as follows: tyrosine → dopa → dopamine → norepinephrine → epinephrine (Figure 3–3). Tyrosine hydroxylase, which forms dopa from tyrosine, is the rate-limiting step in the synthesis of norepinephrine. The metabolism of dopamine and norepinephrine is shown in Figures 3–4 and 3–5.

Although the main dietary precursor of the catecholamines is tyrosine, dietary phenylalanine can be converted to tyrosine via the enzyme phenylalanine hydroxylase. The conversion of tyrosine to dopa is catalyzed by the enzyme tyrosine hydroxylase, which can also hydroxylate phenylalanine. Consequently, the conversion of phenylalanine to tyrosine occurs not only in the adrenal medulla and sympathetically innervated tissues but also in the brain. Tyrosine hydroxylase is an oxygenase that catalyzes the conversion of tyrosine to dopa, the initial step in the biosynthesis of norepinephrine. Tyrosine hydroxylase requires tetrahydropteridine as a cofactor. Because tyrosine hydroxylation is the rate-limiting step in the biosynthesis of catecholamines, it is the step to block if one wishes to halt the synthesis of norepinephrine. Tyrosine hydroxylase can be inhibited by a number of chemicals. Substrate analogues such as L-α-methyl-p-tyrosine inhibit the enzyme in vitro, and in vivo they decrease the endogenous levels of norepinephrine by

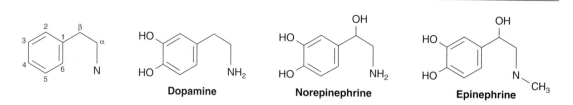

Figure 3–2. Structures of catecholamines.

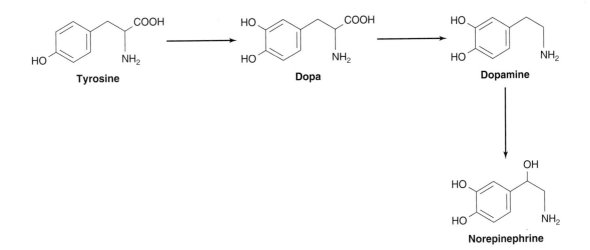

Tyrosine → **Dopa** → **Dopamine**

Norepinephrine

Figure 3–3. Biosynthesis of norepinephrine.

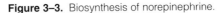

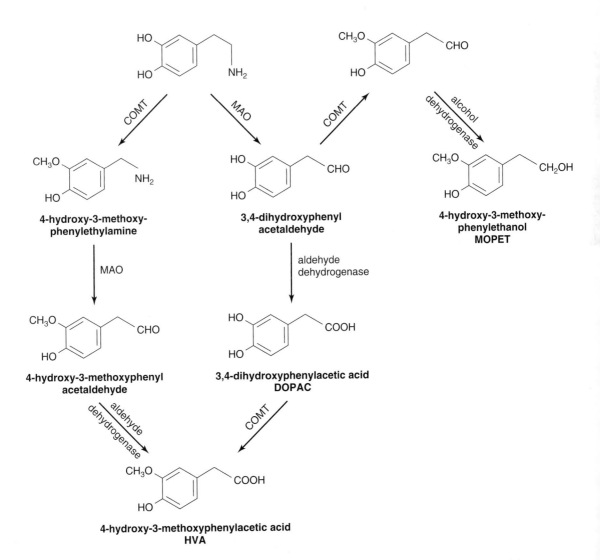

4-hydroxy-3-methoxy-phenylethylamine

3,4-dihydroxyphenyl acetaldehyde

4-hydroxy-3-methoxy-phenylethanol MOPET

4-hydroxy-3-methoxyphenyl acetaldehyde

3,4-dihydroxyphenylacetic acid DOPAC

4-hydroxy-3-methoxyphenylacetic acid HVA

Figure 3–4. Dopamine metabolism. COMT, catechol-o-methyl transferase. MAO, monoamine oxidase.

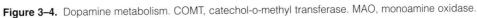

31

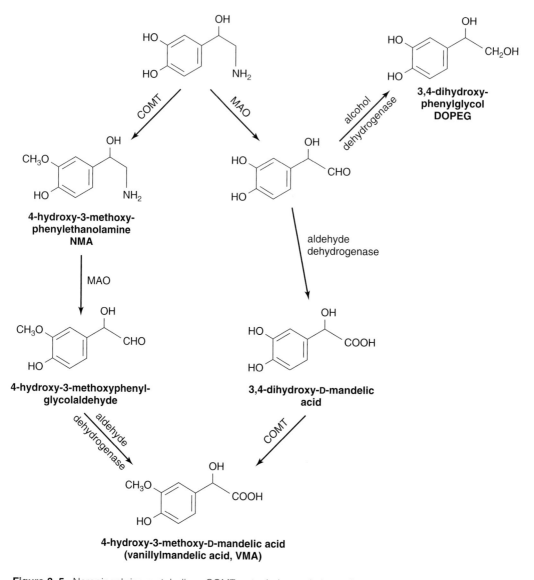

Figure 3–5. Norepinephrine metabolism. COMT, catechol-o-methyl transferase. MAO, monoamine oxidase.

competing with tyrosine. There is also a feedback regulation of catecholamine biosynthesis so that various catecholamines, such as dopa, dopamine, norepinephrine, and epinephrine, inhibit tyrosine hydroxylase by interacting with the cofactor tetrahydropteridine. The relationship between the biosynthetic pathways of catecholamine and serotonin is demonstrated by the fact that certain tryptophan derivatives can inhibit tyrosine hydroxylase. One of the most potent inhibitors of tyrosine hydroxylase is α-methyl-5-hydroxytryptophan.

The next enzyme in the biosynthetic pathway is aromatic-L-amino acid decarboxylase, otherwise known as dopa decarboxylase, which was discovered in 1938. This enzyme is not specific for the decar-

boxylation of dopa. It also decarboxylates aromatic-L-amino acids such as 5-hydroxytryptophan, phenylalanine, tryptophan, and tyrosine. Dopa decarboxylase is widely distributed in a number of mammalian organs. Pyridoxal-5-phosphate activates dopa decarboxylase and is tightly bound to the enzyme. Dopa, dopamine, and norepinephrine inhibit dopa decarboxylase by forming a Schiff's base with pyridoxal-5-phosphate. Several substances inhibit dopa decarboxylase (eg, α-methyl dopa, α-methyl-5-hydroxytryptophan, and N-m-hydroxylbenzyl-N-methyl hydrazine).

Dopamine-β-hydroxylase (DBH) is the final enzyme in the synthesis of norepinephrine. It catalyzes the conversion of dopamine to norepinephrine. DBH hydroxylates dopamine on the β carbon to form norepinephrine. The enzyme has a requirement for Cu^{++}, and ascorbic acid is necessary for the reoxidation of the Cu^{++}. Although it is referred to as dopamine-β-hydroxylase, the enzyme is not completely specific as it can also hydroxylate, on the β carbon, a number of phenylethylamines (eg, tyramine → norsynephrine [octopamine]; amphetamine → norephedrine; epinine → epinephrine; mescaline → β-hydroxy mescaline). A number of inhibitors have been found that bind the copper of DBH (eg, disulfiram, tropolone, aromatic and alkyl thioureas, fuseric acid).

Catecholamine Catabolism

Two enzymes are responsible for the catabolism of catecholamines: monoamine oxidase (MAO) and cat-echol-o-methyl transferase (COMT).

A. Monoamine Oxidase: MAO catalyzes the ox-idative deamination of amines and is a major enzyme in the metabolism of the biogenic amines (ie, norepi-nephrine, dopamine, and serotonin). MAO is found throughout the CNS. It is present in both glia and neu-rons. Studies on the subcellular distribution of the en-zyme indicate that it is principally associated with the mitochondrial fraction, although it is also present in a microsomal fraction. In the mitochondrial fraction, the enzyme is present in the outer membrane. The enzyme requires flavin adenine dinucleotide as a cofactor.

MAO exists in two forms: MAO-A, which oxida-tively deaminates serotonin, norepinephrine, and epi-nephrine; and MAO-B, which catalyzes the oxidation of benzylamine, phenylethylamine, and phenyl-ethanolamine. Tyramine and dopamine are substrates for both forms. MAO-A seems to be the predominant form in neurons.

B. Catechol-o-Methyl Transferase: COMT methy-lates the hydroxyl group meta to the side chain of cate-cholamines. The methyl donor is S-adenosylmethionine. COMT has a requirement for divalent cations such as Mg^{++}, Mn^{++}, Zn^{++}, Fe^{++}, CO^{++}, and Cd^{++}.

C. Monoamine Oxidase Inhibitors: MAO in-hibitors have antidepressant effects; however, their in-teraction with the sympathomimetic amines and tyra-mine causes many side effects. Many drugs act as antidepressants by increasing the content of the neu-rotransmitters at their respective postsynaptic recep-tors. An MAO-A inhibitor effectively increases the content of both norepinephrine and serotonin through an inhibition of their degradation.

In human brain, the major MAO is type B, for which dopamine is a good substrate. In the treatment of Parkinson's disease, L-dopa is used to replace the deficient dopamine. A large fraction of L-dopa is de-carboxylated by peripheral tissues to dopamine, and because dopamine doesn't traverse the blood-brain barrier, L-dopa is administered in combination with a peripheral decarboxylase inhibitor. A specific MAO-B inhibitor, (-) deprenyl, lacks many of the untoward side effects of other MAO inhibitors that block both A and B forms.

SEROTONIN

Serotonin Biosynthesis & Metabolism

Brain serotonin (5-HT) is synthesized in neurons that contain the enzyme tryptophan hydroxylase. Hydroxylation of tryptophan by this enzyme is the ini-tial and rate-limiting step in the synthesis of 5-HT. L-Tryptophan is converted to 5-hydroxytryptophan (5-HTP) by tryptophan hydroxylase, and 5-HTP is con-verted to 5-HT by the aromatic-L-amino acid decar-boxylase. Tryptophan hydroxylase requires oxygen and the reduced cofactor pterin (Figure 3–6).

Psychotropic drugs can influence 5-HT by (1) de-creasing the storage capacity of the serotonergic neu-ron, (2) inhibiting the synthesis of 5-HT, (3) inhib-iting the enzyme (MAO) that metabolizes 5-HT, or (4) inhibiting the reuptake transporter. Many drugs af-fect the various sites where 5-HT and norepinephrine are synthesized, stored, released, and recaptured.

PRACTICAL APPLICATIONS

Theoretical and technical advances in molecular bi-ology have provided neuropharmacology with power-ful tools to develop new psychoactive drugs. The re-ceptors of most of the neurotransmitters have been cloned and sequenced. We are now obtaining informa-tion as to where and how neurotransmitters and drugs bind to these receptors. The proteins that transport neu-rotransmitters are also being cloned and sequenced, so that psychoactive drugs can be designed to affect the transport system. We now know the genes and enzymes involved in the synthesis of neurotransmitters, and these sites too are amenable to manipulation by drugs.

Cooper JR, Bloom FE, Roth RH: *The Biochemical Basis of Neuropharmacology.* Oxford University Press, 1996.

Goodman LS, Gilman A: *The Pharmacological Basis of Therapies.* McGraw-Hill, 1996.

PSYCHOTROPIC DRUGS

All major psychotropic drugs (ie, antidepressants, antipsychotics, anxiolytics) affect directly or indirectly the various receptors that are linked via regulatory G proteins to effector systems, either enzymes or ion channels (Figure 3–7). G proteins are heterotrimers consisting of α, β, and γ subunits that are linked to spe-cific intracellular effector systems in a stimulatory (G_s) or inhibitory (G_i) manner. Effector enzymes catalyze the formation of second messengers that activate vari-ous protein kinases leading to phosphorylation and ac-tivation of pivotal proteins (**metabotropic action**). Re-ceptors linked to ion channels modify the flux of ions through the membrane (**ionotropic action**).

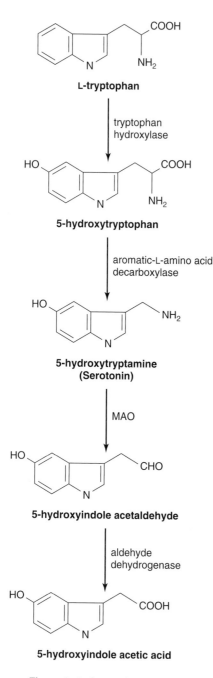

Figure 3–6. Serotonin metabolism.

antidepressants inhibit the reuptake of neurotransmitters into the presynaptic neuron. These neurotransmitters activate various receptor cascades (Figure 3–8). Norepinephrine stimulates the formation of cyclic adenosine monophosphate (cAMP) via β-adrenoceptors, whereas α-2-adrenoceptor activation by norepinephrine inhibits cAMP formation. cAMP activates protein kinase A (PKA). 5-HT receptors are linked, depending on their subtype, to adenylate cyclase (5-HT_{1A}, 5-HT_{1B}, 5-HT_{1D}, 5-HT_{1E}, 5-HT_{1F}), phospholipase C (5-HT_{2A}, 5-HT_{2B}, 5-HT_{2C}), or to ion channels (5-HT_3). Phospholipase C converts inositol 4,5-biphosphate to two second messengers: diacylglycerol (DAG) and inositol 1,4,5-tris-phosphate (IP3). DAG activates protein kinase C (PKC) and IP3 via mobilization of intracellular calcium activates calcium/calmodulin-dependent protein kinase. Thus protein phosphorylation is probably the final common pathway for signal transduction. Evidence indicates that the activation of protein kinases is an obligatory step in the sequence of events by which extracellular signals produce physiologic responses in neurons. It remains to be elucidated whether G proteins have a role in the action of antidepressants.

Studies on the mechanism of action of lithium have shown that this widely used psychotropic agent influences the synaptic availability of 5-HT and norepinephrine and has profound effects on signal transduction pathways. These findings, together with the observation that reserpine—which depletes brain 5-HT and norepinephrine—can precipitate depression, have led to the simple but heuristic hypothesis that depression results from an amine deficiency that is corrected by antidepressant drugs (eg, the catecholamine and indoleamine hypotheses of affective disorders, respectively). The well-known therapeutic delay associated with antidepressant drugs has led to modifications of these early hypotheses, involving more slowly developing adaptive processes at the level of receptors and at sites beyond the receptors.

Barden N, Reul JMHM, Holsboer F: Do antidepressants stabilize mood through actions on the hypothalamic-pituitary-adrenocortical system? Trends Neurosci 1995; 18:6.

Bourin M, Baker GB: Do G proteins have a role in antidepressant actions? Eur Neuropsychopharmacol 1996;6:49.

Budziszewska B, Siwanowicz J, Przegaliński E: The effect of chronic treatment with antidepressant drugs on the corticosteroid receptor levels in the rat hippocampus. Pol J Pharmacol 1994;46:147.

Manji HK, Potter WZ, Lenox RH: Signal transduction pathways: molecular targets for lithium's actions. Arch Gen Psychiatry 1995;52:531.

Nibuya M, Nestler EJ, Duman RS: Chronic antidepressant administration increases the expression of CREB in rat hippocampus. J Neurosci 1996;16:2365.

Rossby SP, Sulser F: Antidepressants: beyond the synapse. Pages 195–212 in: Skolnick P (editor): *Antidepressants: New Pharmacological Strategies.* Humana Press, 1997.

ANTIDEPRESSANTS

Antidepressants (eg, MAO inhibitors, tricyclic antidepressants, selective serotonin reuptake inhibitors, bupropion, venlafaxine) acutely increase the synaptic availability of norepinephrine or 5-HT or both, via different mechanisms. MAO inhibitors inhibit the metabolism of the neurotransmitters, whereas other

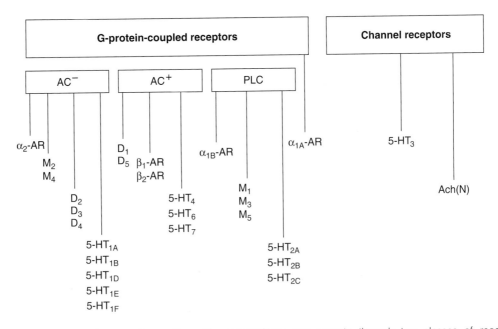

Figure 3–7. Receptors for neurotransmitters. Neurotransmitters can operate through two classes of receptors: metabotropic and ionotropic (channel) receptors. Metabotropic receptors are coupled with second messenger systems through G proteins activating phospholipase C (PLC) and activating (AC^+) or inhibiting (AC^-) adenylate cyclase. Stimulation of α_2-adrenergic (α_2-AR); M_2 and M_4 acetylcholine muscarinic; D_2, D_3, and D_4 dopaminergic; and 5-HT$_{1A}$, 5-HT$_{1B}$, 5-HT$_{1D}$, 5-HT$_{1E}$, and 5-HT$_{1F}$ serotonergic receptors inhibits adenylate cyclase and cAMP generation. Stimulation of D_1 and D_5 dopaminergic; β_1- and β_2-adrenergic (β_1-AR, β_2-AR); and 5-HT$_4$, 5-HT$_6$, and 5-HT$_7$ serotonergic receptors activate adenylate cyclase and cAMP generation. PLC is positively linked with α_{1B}-adrenergic (α_{1B}-AR); M_1, M_3, and M_5 muscarinic; and 5-HT$_{2A}$, 5-HT$_{2B}$, and 5-HT$_{2C}$ serotonergic receptors stimulating the generation of the second messengers diacylglycerol and inositol tris-phosphate. The α_{1A}-adrenergic receptor operates through a G protein–dihydropyridine–dependent calcium channel. Acetylcholine [Ach(N)] and 5-HT$_3$ can act through channel receptors as well. (Reproduced, with permission, from Nalepa I, Sulser F: Possible mechanisms for future antidepressants. In *Handbook of Experimental Pharmacology.* Springer, in press.)

Rossby SP et al: Norepinephrine-independent regulation of GRII mRNA in vivo by a tricyclic antidepressant. Brain Res 1995;687:79.

Vetulani J et al: A possible common mechanism of action of antidepressant treatments: reduction in the sensitivity of the noradrenergic cyclic AMP generating system in the rat limbic forebrain. Naunyn-Schmiedeberg's Arch Pharmacol 1976;293:109.

ANTIPSYCHOTICS

Antipsychotic drugs, or neuroleptics, are thought to exert their therapeutic action by blocking different subtypes of dopamine receptors. Neuroleptics (eg, phenothiazines, butyrophenones) display a high affinity for dopamine D_2 receptors linked in an inhibitory way via G proteins to adenylate cyclase. The rank order of antipsychotic drug affinity to the D_2 receptor parallels the rank order of clinical potency. Compared to typical antipsychotic drugs, the atypical antipsychotic clozapine exhibits about a 10-fold higher affinity for the D_4 receptor, which, like the D_2 receptor, is coupled via G_i to adenylate cyclase. Because clozapine also binds to numerous dopamine and other receptors (eg, 5-HT$_{2A}$), the question of whether D_4 receptor blockade is singly responsible for the unique therapeutic profile of clozapine (antipsychotic activity with little or no extrapyramidal side effects) remains unanswered. With the development of specific D_4 receptor antagonists, these hypotheses can be tested.

Fitzgerald LW et al: Regulation of cortical and subcortical glutamate receptor subunit expression by antipsychotic drugs. J Neurosci 1995;15:2453.

ANXIOLYTICS

Benzodiazepines, the most widely used antianxiety agents, appear to produce all of their therapeutic effects by binding to the benzodiazepine receptor. The benzodiazepine receptor is an integral binding site on the GABA$_A$ receptor channel. By allosteric modulation, benzodiazepines augment the affinity of GABA

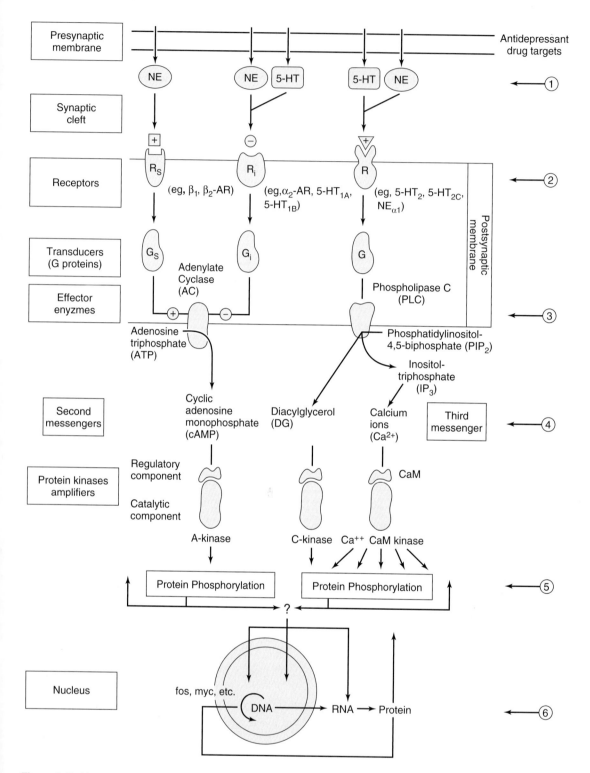

Figure 3–8. Neurotransmitter signal transduction cascades as a target for antidepressant drugs. Antidepressant drugs can influence the information flow at various levels of the signal transduction cascade: (1) change in the synaptic availability of the primary signals norepinephrine (NE) and serotonin (5-HT) (MAO inhibitors, blockade of reuptake, autoreceptor subsensitivity); (2) change in receptor number or sensitivity; (3) change in the function of G proteins; (4) change in the formation of second messengers; (5) change in the activity of protein kinases (amplifier function); (6) modification of nuclear events (eg, gene transcription). (Reproduced, with permission, from Rossby SP, Sulser F: [Historical perspective and new neurobiological aspects of the modes of action of antidepressant drugs.] ZNS J 1993;1:10 [German].)

to the GABA binding site. It remains to be seen whether buspirone (a non-benzodiazepine partial 5-HT_{1A} agonist) will be as effective as the benzodiazepines in the treatment of anxiety disorders.

Goodman LS, Gilman A: *The Pharmacological Basis of Therapies.* McGraw-Hill, 1996.

RECEPTOR ADAPTATION & RECEPTOR CROSS-TALK

The actions mediated by psychotropic drugs on receptors occur rapidly. These actions do not explain the therapeutic effect that is generally delayed for weeks after initiation of treatment. This discrepancy in the time course, particularly evident with antidepressants, has led to studies on the effect of antidepressants on more slowly developing receptor-mediated adaptive processes in brain. These studies have revealed that chronic antidepressant treatment (ie, using MAO inhibitors, tricyclic antidepressants, and electroconvulsive therapy) causes a desensitization of the β-adrenoceptor-coupled adenylate cyclase system in brain, usually associated with downregulation of the density of β-adrenoceptors. These findings have shifted the focus of research onto the mode of action of antidepressants and the pathophysiology of affective disorders, from acute presynaptic to delayed postsynaptic adaptive processes in the cascade of signal transduction. Besides causing adaptations at the β-adrenoceptor, chronic administration of antidepressants alters the density of various subtypes of 5-HT receptors (eg, $5\text{-}HT_{2A}$, $5\text{-}HT_{1A}$, and $5\text{-}HT_{1B}$).

Persistent blockade of dopamine D_2 receptors by antipsychotic drugs causes an upregulation of the density of this subtype of dopamine receptors. Upregulation of D_2 receptors has often been associated with the development of **tardive dyskinesia** (hypersensitivity to dopamine in the striatum). Clozapine, a weak D_2 blocker, does not cause upregulation of D_2 receptors and is less likely to produce tardive dyskinesia. Research into the action of antipsychotic drugs has focused on excitatory amino acids, particularly the interaction of dopamine systems with glutamate systems. After chronic (but not acute) administration, antipsychotic drugs alter the levels of expression of specific glutamate receptor subunits and extracellular levels of glutamate in specific areas of the brain. Dopamine-glutamate interactions have been implicated in the regulation of conditional, emotional, and motivational aspects of motor function in the mammalian CNS.

MECHANISMS OF REGULATION OF RECEPTOR FUNCTION

The regulation of receptor function is associated closely with the plasticity of signal transduction. The homeostasis of signal transduction is a prerequisite for emotional health. Signal transduction appears to be destabilized in patients who have emotional and cognitive disorders. Receptors are regulated at the level of their gene expression (by transcription or translation) and by posttranslational covalent modifications (eg, phosphorylation). In general, the density of receptors is upregulated in response to a decrease of their corresponding neurotransmitters and downregulated in response to an increase of the neurotransmitter. For example, β-adrenoceptor density increases after depletion of norepinephrine by reserpine and decreases after the blocking of norepinephrine reuptake by antidepressants. The phenomenon of receptor desensitization has been studied extensively in the β-adrenoceptor–G protein–coupled adenylate cyclase system. The desensitization of the β-adrenoceptor–G protein–coupled adenylate cyclase system is accomplished by receptor phosphorylation. Two types of protein kinases are involved in receptor phosphorylation: PKA, activated by cAMP; and a second messenger–independent G protein–coupled protein kinase, BARK 1. BARK 1 phosphorylates G protein–coupled receptors (such as the β-adrenoceptor), predominantly when they are occupied by agonists. BARK 1–mediated phosphorylation has also been implicated in the sequestration of β-adrenoceptors. Furthermore, the 5-HT_{2C} receptor is phosphorylated by agonist treatment, which results in desensitization of receptor signaling.

Different receptor systems "cross-talk" at different levels of their signal transduction cascade. Heteroreceptor regulation is widespread, and the interdependence of norepinephrine and 5-HT in the synaptic pharmacology of antidepressants is of particular interest. For example, supersensitivity to 5-HT and dopamine, demonstrated electrophysiologically or behaviorally following chronic administration of antidepressants or electroconvulsive therapy, is prevented by experimentally lesioning noradrenergic neurons. Furthermore, changes in cortical β-adrenoceptor density modify $5\text{-}HT_{2A}$-mediated behavior in a manner that is independent of changes in $5\text{-}HT_{2A}$ receptor number. Studies with the dual-uptake inhibitor venlafaxine have demonstrated a link between the two aminergic signal transduction pathways beyond the β-adrenoceptors. Venlafaxine failed to desensitize the β-adrenoceptor-coupled adenylate cyclase system unless 5-HT in brain was depleted. PKC, activated via $5\text{-}HT_{2A}$ or $5\text{-}HT_{2C}$ receptors, has been hypothesized to modify the PKA-mediated regulation of β-adrenoceptor sensitivity. Such counterregulation between prominent kinases on agonist-induced desensitization of β-adrenoceptors has been demonstrated in various cell lines.

Brown JR et al: Defect in nurturing in mice lacking the immediate early gene fosB. Cell 1996;86:297.

Ferguson SG et al: Role of phosphorylation in agonist-promoted β$_2$-adrenergic receptor sequestration. J Biol Chem 1995;270:24782.

Premont RT, Inglese J, Lefkowitz RJ: Protein kinases that phosphorylate activated G protein–coupled receptors. FASEB J 1995;9:175.

Westphal RS, Backstrom JR, Sanders-Bush E: Increased basal phosphorylation of the constitutively active serotonin 2C receptor accompanies agonist-mediated desensitization. Mol Pharmacol 1995;48:200.

SIGNAL TRANSDUCTION FROM SYNAPSE TO NUCLEUS

Most psychotherapeutic drugs (eg, antidepressants, antipsychotic drugs, lithium) require long-term administration to be optimally effective. Apparently, acute interaction at various steps in the agonist-receptor-mediated transduction cascades is not directly responsible for their therapeutic effects. The activation of intracellular messenger pathways and the regulation of neuronal gene expression appear to play a central role in long-term adaptive changes in neuronal function. By altering programs of gene expression, the CNS adapts to conditions that threaten the physical and psychic emotional well-being of the organism. Ultimately changes in programs of gene expression determine the intensities of incoming signals; the sensitivities of neuronal systems to those signals; and the nature, amplitude, and duration of CNS responses (ie, the plasticity of the CNS). In this way, the clinically important actions of psychotropic drugs can be viewed as the restoration of neural plasticity, a plasticity that appears to be impaired in patients with affective or cognitive disorders.

Changes in gene expression in the brain have been reported following long-term administration of antidepressants and antipsychotic drugs. Of particular interest is the role of transcription factors in the neural plasticity restored by psychotropic drugs. Transcription factors are proteins that bind to specific sequences in the promoter regions of genes and thereby increase or decrease the rate at which those genes are transcribed. Transcription factors of particular interest in neuropharmacology are steroid and thyroid hormone receptors, the CREB/ATF family and the family of immediate early gene products (eg, cFos, cJun). The regulation of transcription factors and their importation from the cytoplasm into the nucleus fine-tunes gene expression. It is of neurobiological and clinical interest that the density of glucocorticoid (GRII) receptors and their mRNA are increased following extended treatment with some antidepressants. The increase in GRII receptors following antidepressant treatment could be responsible—via feedback inhibition—for the normalization of the hyperactive hypothalamic-pituitary-adrenal axis often associated with depression. The long-term administration of several antidepressants, such as norepinephrine and 5-HT reuptake inhibitors, increases the expression of CREB in the rat hippocampus. The CREB transcription factor could be an intracellular target for antidepressants. Researchers have analyzed the expression of Fos-like transcription factors after the administration of antipsychotic drugs. Several clinically effective typical antipsychotics induce *cfos* in the striatum and nucleus accumbens, whereas clozapine increases fos levels in the prefrontal cortex and nucleus accumbens but not in the striatum. Although the target genes regulated by GRII, Fos, and CREB in brain are largely unknown, these transcription factors play a critical role in the regulation of genes and their products during long-term adaptive responses to antidepressants and other psychotropic drugs. Because most, if not all, transcription factors are phosphoproteins, phosphorylation by protein kinases and dephosphorylation by protein phosphatases play critical roles in changing transcription factor protein conformation into an active-inactive DNA-binding structure. Thus psychotropic drugs could directly or indirectly modify both transcription factor and DNA-binding activity by phosphorylation via PKA, PKC, or calcium/calmodulin-dependent protein kinases, activated via aminergic-receptor-mediated signal transduction pathways (target 5 in Figure 3–8).

CONCLUSION

The emergence of molecular neurobiology has profoundly changed the traditional focus of neuropsychopharmacologic research, shifting it toward events occurring beyond the receptors. One can now entertain the possibility that abnormal behavior patterns—affective, cognitive, and somatosensory—might be the consequence of a disarray in the temporal regulation of gene expression in response to internal (ie, neurohumoral, endocrine) and external (ie, environmental) stimuli that have rendered the individual vulnerable to psychiatric disorder. The demonstration that a nurturing defect in mice is linked to the absence of transcription factor Fos B in the preoptic area of the hypothalamus suggests that this transcription factor controls a complex behavior.

Several primary variables are involved in the effect of neuropharmacologic agents and psychotherapy: the neurotransmitters 5-HT, dopamine, norepinephrine, acetylcholine, GABA, and glutamate, acting via various subtypes of receptors; perhaps nitrous oxide and carbon monoxide; and others that are virtually unknown. Second messengers are fewer, but the number of transcription factors is enormous. It has been estimated that the human genome encodes as many as 3000 different gene-specific transcription factors. The nuclear import of these proteins is modulated in response to external stimuli whose transduction is modified by psychotropic (and other neuropharmacologic) agents. It is predicted that the nascence of molecular neuropsychopharmacology will enable the development of new, more effective psychotropic drugs and will provide the foundation for a molecular biological psychiatry.

4

Psychoanalysis

Volney P. Gay, PhD

FOUNDATIONS OF PSYCHOANALYTIC THEORY

As a form of inquiry, psychoanalysis originated in Sigmund Freud's modification of 19th-century medical consultations on what were then termed neurasthenias and other disabling psychological conditions, especially hysteria. The majority of all forms of psychiatry that claim a dynamic or cognitive orientation derive from Freud's original work and from that of his students. Although psychoanalysis began primarily as a theory of neurotic functioning and character pathology, in the past 70 years it has changed dramatically to include severe psychopathology, addictions and eating disorders, sexual abuse, and other maladies.

PSYCHOANALYTIC ASSESSMENT & DIAGNOSIS

Psychoanalysis, and dynamic psychiatry in general, face an ongoing task: How does the clinician distinguish the patient's symptoms as products of purely psychological events (eg, a headache precipitated by overt and conscious rage) from products of a purely somatic event (eg, a headache caused by caffeine withdrawal), and how does he or she distinguish both of these from mixed cases (eg, a patient who, in order to punish himself for hostile wishes, "accidentally" forgets to drink his morning coffee, realizing vaguely that he will probably have a headache later in the day)? The latter case typifies Freud's earliest discoveries regarding "parapraxes" or slips of the tongue: Sometimes careful examination of a person's associations to his or her parapraxes, to loosely associated thoughts (dreams, daydreams, free associations) and symptoms reveals unexpected connections between these manifest behaviors and latent motivations (unconscious wishes). Discovering these linkages, "making the unconscious conscious," has peculiar virtues for it can grant to patients a new measure of self-control. The precise pathways such discovery can take

are documented in thousands of published case histories. Because these linkages are often mired in personal history and personal fantasy, the psychoanalytic clinician must necessarily work ex post facto and with highly subjective, often idiosyncratic meanings. Each of these aspects makes the validation of particular interventions, assessments, and evaluating theories of pathogenesis particularly difficult. Psychoanalytic theories abound, many of them based on thousands of patient contact hours; ways to validate those theories outside the narrow confines of the analytic pair of patient and therapist are fewer. Efforts to address this problem are now under way.

Psychodynamic interviews differ significantly from medical interviews (Table 4–1). An important characteristic of psychodynamic interviews is especially noteworthy: Sudden and apparently irrational feelings in the interviewer, so-called countertransference affects, often correlate with severe forms of character pathology in the patient. Because the interviewer uses his or her own affective responses to the patient as part of the assessment process, psychoanalytic theory and training focus special attention on the clinician as part of the diagnosing instrument. The requirement that all psychoanalysts undergo their own analytic treatment, a unique demand in the field of psychiatry, derives from this clinical axiom. This "training analysis" is mandatory and remains fundamental to all forms of psychoanalytic education and training. The potential for abuse of any such training is obvious: It might simply create zealots who blindly follow their leader. However, excluding such training, or indeed rejecting the concept of countertransference, is also dangerous. To deny validity to core analytic concepts, such as unconscious process, transference and countertransference, and "character" type makes sense only if one believes that people do not have internal lives and that their private (or secret or unconscious) beliefs have no effect on their behavior. Paradoxically, the decision to minimize psychodynamic categories in the *Diagnostic and Statistical Manual of Mental Disorders,* 3rd edition, revised (DSM-III-R) has energized psychoanalytic empirical research.

Table 4–1. A comparison of medical and psychodynamic interviews.

Characteristic	Medical Interviews	Psychodynamic Interviews
Approach to signs and symptoms	Symptoms and signs are focused on immediately: Patients typically report directly and fully.	Symptoms are hidden and often sources of shame; embarrassment and dissembling are common.
Relationship to treatment	Diagnosis precedes treatment: Diagnosis is preliminary to treatment response.	Interviewing and evaluating shameful or hidden symptoms can exacerbate or ameliorate suffering: diagnosis is part of treatment.
Patient involvement	Patients are typically passive vehicles of their suffering or illness: They respond to queries but do not collaborate.	The patient must collaborate, especially by responding to open-ended questions regarding the immediate context, especially the interviewer.
Duration	History-taking ceases when a relevant diagnosis is made and treatment plans are made.	Assessment continues beyond establishing relevant DSM-IV diagnosis. The patient's and interviewer's affective responses to each other are part of assessment and diagnosis.

Psychoanalytic and psychodynamic assessment thus occurs after or in conjunction with regular medical and psychiatric assessments. In addition to knowing the patient's current medical findings, relevant medical history, and mental status, the psychoanalyst (or psychodynamic clinician) wishes to assess three features: the patient's highest and lowest personality functioning (ego strength and ego defense), the patient's past and current relationships with others (object relationships), and the patient's self state (characteristics of the self). Each of these features of the patient's life pertains to key aspects of personality functioning. Not accidentally, each also pertains to major branches of investigation in contemporary psychoanalysis. Because assessing each of these features may require an extended history, 3–4 hours of interviews may be required to make a substantial assessment. If one fails to investigate a patient's current character structure and pathology, the dangers of misdiagnosis increase dramatically. For example, narcissistic personality disorders may present with either very active or very passive forms of grandiosity. Among the criteria listed for this disorder are lack of empathy, sense of entitlement, and preoccupation with fantasies of unlimited success. Each of these concepts derives from the psychoanalysis of severe personality disorders (see Chapter 33).

Treatment planning and assessment should include a thorough and complete review of the patient's medical, sexual, family, and personal histories. Squeamishness, "politeness," and other forms of avoidance on the therapist's part (eg, the refusal to secure a complete sexual history or to ask about sexual abuse, drug or alcohol use, and other secrets the patient may wish to hide) hinder treatment from the beginning and may make it impossible in the end. To refuse to diagnose fully and properly is, in this sense, an instance of countertransference resistance, and in the absence of a proper diagnosis, it is impossible for the clinician to select the appropriate treatment.

American Psychiatric Association: *Diagnostic and Statistical Manual of Mental Disorders,* 3rd ed, revised. American Psychiatric Association, 1987.

Barron JW, Eagle MN, Wolitzky DL: *Interface of Psychoanalysis and Psychology.* American Psychological Association, 1992.

Fenichel O: *The Psychoanalytic Theory of the Neuroses.* WW Norton & Co, 1945.

Gay P: *Freud: A Life for Our Time.* WW Norton & Co, 1988.

McWilliams N: *Psychoanalytic Diagnosis: Understanding Personality Structure in the Clinical Process.* Guilford, 1994.

Miller NE et al (editors): *Psychodynamic Treatment Research: A Handbook for Clinical Practice.* Basic Books, 1993.

GENERAL CONSIDERATIONS: EGO STRENGTH & LEVELS OF DEFENSE

Ego strength refers to a classical Freudian notion that patients' psychological functioning can be assessed according to how well or how poorly they handle the entire range of stressors that affect them. **Ego defense** refers to the range of behaviors and psychological mechanisms (eg, depressive affect, anxiety, panic) that patients use to avoid psychic pain. Because psychic pain varies according to mental states such as attention, altering one's mental status through selective inattention, drug use, or dissociation decreases the severity of one's immediate pain. Some defensive maneuvers and styles, such as humor and wit, keep the ego relatively intact; others, such as splitting and dissociation, disorganize the personality in major ways and give rise to severe character pathologies.

The classic notion of ego defense found expression in Anna Freud's study in which she formalized her father's implicit concepts. Fenichel outlined the classical theory, distinguishing between successful defenses (sublimation) and pathogenic defenses (denial, projection, introjection, repression, reaction formation, undoing, isolation, and regression). E. H. Erikson's studies of personality development and character type conveyed psychoanalytic character theory to generations of educated persons even as they frustrated empirical laboratory researchers. More recently, Vaillant and his colleagues conducted extensive longitudinal and empirical studies of the concept "levels of defense" as it pertains to overall personality functioning and life-course: Subjects whom experts judged "successful" and free of major symptoms tended to manifest mature defenses, whereas those with significantly higher incidence of psychiatric illness and other measures of distress correlated with immature defenses (Table 4–2).

In addition to the theory of defense and character type, some contemporary researchers stress the value of observationally near descriptions of persons' abilities. For example, Wallerstein noted the utility of using descriptive terms (which he called capacities) that are compatible with traditional psychoanalytic theory yet are more easily agreed upon by clinicians and researchers (Table 4–3). Wallerstein and his colleagues extended this tentative list to an implicit theory of psychopathology. Those persons who cannot manifest behavior within a putative normal range are, by definition, maladapted and dysfunctional. Hyper- or hypo-functioning on any one of these scales indicates psychopathology. For example, too much self-esteem we call narcissism; if it is persistent, it figures in DSM-IV as a narcissistic personality disorder. Too little self-esteem dominates the presentation of many depressive conditions and personality disorders, especially those in cluster C, the so-called anxious, fearful group (eg, avoidant and dependent personality disorders). Deficits along the lines of sense of self as agent and sense of effectiveness and mastery dominate presentations of the schizoid and schizotypal personality disorders.

Table 4–2. Levels of defense.

Category	Defenses
Mature defenses	Anticipation Suppression Altruism Sublimation Humor Asceticism
Intermediate and neurotic defenses	Intellectualization Repression Reaction formation Displacement Externalization (including sexualization, somatization, rationalization)
Immature defenses	Passive-aggressive (masochistic character) Hypochondriasis Acting out Dissociation Projection Schizoid fantasy Blocking

Table 4–3. Ego functions.[1]

Self-esteem
Zest for life
Sense of self and
  self-coherence
Commitment to reality
Empathy
Commitment to
  standards and values
Commitment to relationships
	Reciprocity with others
	Self-disclosure and openness
	Reliance on self and others
	Trust
	Affect (emotional) tolerance
	Appropriate self-assertion
	Sexual expression
	Effectiveness and mastery

[1] Adapted, with permission, from Wallerstein J: *Forty-two Lives in Treatment: A Study of Psychoanalysis and Psychotherapy.* Guilford Press, 1986.

American Psychiatric Association: *Diagnostic and Statistical Manual of Mental Disorders,* 4th ed. American Psychiatric Association, 1994.

Benjamin L: *Interpersonal Diagnosis and Treatment of Personality Disorders.* Guilford, 1993.

Freud S: The ego and the id. In Strachey J (editor): *The Standard Edition of the Complete Psychological Works of Sigmund Freud.* Vol 19. Hogarth/Institute for Psycho-Analysis, 1923.

Langs R: Making interpretations and securing the frame: sources of danger for psychotherapists. Int J Psychoanal Psychother 1985;10:3.

Wallerstein J: *Forty-two Lives in Treatment: A Study of Psychoanalysis and Psychotherapy.* Guilford, 1986.

PERSONALITY DEVELOPMENT, OBJECT RELATIONS, & CLASSICAL THEORY

Object relations refers to the patient's current relationships to important persons, institutions, and spiritual persons, if the latter are part of the patient's lived experience. Of most immediate concern to assessment is the clinical question: What are this person's current emotional relationships to important persons? Often a patient exhibits psychiatric symptoms after a sudden change in an object relation. **Object relations theory** (ORT) refers to major European and American psychiatric and psychoanalytic groups that focus on the patient's earliest forms of intense relationship with significant others. Like Freud and Erikson before them, contemporary ORT authors have dramatically influenced scholars and thinkers not affiliated with psychiatry proper. The next several sections compare ORT with classical theory to illustrate the range of contemporary analytic thought and how it differs from Freud.

1. THEMES SHARED BY CLASSICAL THEORY & OBJECT RELATIONS THEORY

In both theories, the patient's complaints about his or her life and about the therapist are authentic complaints. The patient is an unconscious supervisor. According to Langs, a patient's disguised representations of the therapist ought to be respected as crucial elements in the process. Technique focuses upon the patient's immediate experience, the "manifest material," which reveals significant conflicts. These real conflicts are the only routes we have to reach into deeper levels of the patient's experience. Longstanding conflicts from early childhood, often preverbal, are not remembered per se. Rather they are reenacted in the transference. Because patients fear recapitulating earlier traumatic or distressing relationships, they defend themselves against recognizing their repetitious behaviors with the analyst. The concept of defense can be applied to any psychological process used to avoid repetition of childhood stressors, especially separation anxiety and fear of bodily harm (eg, castration anxiety and other forms). All persons use projection as a part of normal life. For example, when we listen to a patient we may project our past experiences onto the patient's material in order to grasp better the patient's current experience. Empathy also involves many aspects of projection. A **defense** is any psychological mechanism or operation used to prevent further insight into the source and extent of a psychological conflict. Defense is always defense against painful feelings (eg, depression, anxiety, doubt, shame).

The clinician must be able to distinguish accurate from inaccurate perceptions in order to understand how these transference experiences (and the defenses against them) recapitulate developmental stages in which similar conflicts were resolved with similar neurotic consequences (or more severe ego impairments). The universal aim of psychoanalysis is to increase the patient's freedom to speak and so discover what he or she actually feels and believes. Good technique is technique that increases the patient's freedom to speak and decreases the patient's anxiety about self-revelation. Both classical psychoanalysts and ORT analysts attempt to lay the groundwork for the "good hour." In a good hour, we see a patient work at each level of conflict: with the patient's current world of persons and struggles, with us in the transference, with us as real objects, and with us as self-objects (that is, as part of the patient's internal mechanisms of self-governance and self-control).

2. DIFFERENCES BETWEEN CLASSICAL THEORY & OBJECT RELATIONS THEORY

ORT differs from classical analysis with regard to its concept of science, intrapsychic focus, attempted reconstructions, therapeutic goals, and technique and interventions.

Concept of Science

Classical theory (including Freud's work from 1900 on and the concept of ego psychology) retained a 19th-century ideal of scientists as external observers who are to describe the forces and constraints that give rise to structure. All sciences are to be unified, sooner or later, into a single, coherent picture of the knowable universe. That which cannot be known by science in this way cannot be spoken of intelligibly. Unification also presupposes that truths in one science, such as math or physics, cannot be contradicted by claims in other sciences, especially in the less rigorous sciences such as biology and psychology. When Freud speaks of psychic energy, he does so within the constraints of the physics of his time. Hence psychic energy must obey the second law of thermodynamics and have all the tensor qualities that 19th-century scientists said were true of physical energies. Also, because physical energies are interchangeable with all forms of energy (ie, heat may be transformed into mechanical power), psychic energies are also interchangeable. Thus the psyche, too, should show similar transformations. For example, pregenital energies, genital energies, and the theory of sublimation reflect 19th-century physics.

Given this reductionistic ideal, psychic contents, such as ideas or dreams, must all be reducible in principle to states of a system that uses and binds psychic energy. In Freud's terms, because science tells us that the "really real" is only blind elements running into other blind elements, our sense that we live in a world of color, not to mention intentions, wishes, and so on, is illusory. Object relations theorists have struggled against this notion of psychological science. ORT names a widely diverse group of theoreticians, not merely the so-called English School, which uses the term "object relations" explicitly. Beginning with Carl Jung's strenuous rejection of Freud's metapsychology, all ORT authors have felt constrained by Freud's reductionistic ideals. Some, like Melanie Klein, have tried to remain true to Freud's language. Hence Klein retains the dual-instinct theory Freud promulgates in his papers on ego psychology. Yet she too found it difficult to use energic terms to account for her clinical discoveries. Instead, she created new terms that seemed closer to her patients' actual experience. A liability of wholesale rejection of Freud's reductionism is a tendency toward sentimentalism. At this extreme, empathy merges into sympathy, and tenderness replaces insight. Consequently, patients can feel that the therapists are avoiding unconscious fantasies and therefore the patient's anxiety increases. With sufficient "tenderness" patients will abandon therapy or choose some self-destructive mode to deal with their increasing sense of danger in the poorly maintained frame.

Intrapsychic Focus

Klein and other ORT authors created new terms because they worked with a class of patients—children and infants—whom Freud had not seen, and they developed their clinical explanations using their patients' categories. Freud listened to his patients; perhaps no one has ever listened better. Because he was committed to a theory of unconscious motivation, Freud refused to accept patients' conscious self-understandings as sufficient. These manifest accounts could never be the ultimate target of analytic investigation, nor could they be the ultimate authority against which we can assess psychoanalytic claims. For example, a patient's initial rage at the constraints of the "solid frame," a firmly announced set of rules for the conduct of analysis, is not, by itself, an indicator that the therapist ought to abandon ordinary rules.

In this sense, Freud was both phenomenologic and antiphenomenologic. Prior to the fully developed metapsychology of 1900, Freud adopted some of the self-descriptions hysteric patients elaborated. For this reason, Fairbairn traced the notion of "splitting" to Freud's early essays on hysteria. For example, the rule of free association not only requires the patient to speak freely about everything that passes through his or her mind but also permits the analyst to treat such data as thematically and causally related to one another. For example, in a male patient's thoughts, "Competing with boss . . . fight . . . conflict with boss . . . blood . . . death . . . lack of sexual desire for wife," one can conjecture the presence of castration anxiety and then seek clinical validation of this hypothesis. Do his recent assertive wishes to compete elicit a fixed, reflex-like pattern? Will competition yield shame around his genital functioning or elicit the fantasy that his father will try to hurt him? To remove that possibility does he deny the presence of sexual desire?

In all its forms, Freud's metapsychology is radically antiphenomenologic: The dual-instinct theory is not derived from first-order patient narratives, nor is the structural theory of mind. ORT authors rely on classical theory and elaborate on it by adopting portions of the manifest content of their patients' experience. This is most evident in the work of Fairbairn, whose ORT is "pure" because it uses only psychological terms and, then, only terms derived from first-order patient accounts. For example, sick patients often talk about feeling split or divided against themselves or about attacking themselves. It is also "pure" because Fairbairn does not seek to locate psychological theory within the grander schemata of the unified sciences, as did Freud and all who pursue biological reductionism.

Attempted Reconstructions

Classical theory contains an account of pre-oedipal experience (eg, in 1895 Freud elaborated a condensed theory of the nursing infant), but it does not contain a theory of pre-oedipal subjectivity. Freud describes the infant's behavior when frustrated and its (supposed) efforts to hallucinate the lost breast. Freud did not attempt to describe how the infant felt (thought or imagined) about that object relation. Certainly, Freud concerned himself with these issues. One can find passages in which he appears to describe infantile (preverbal) experience. But he does so always via deductive reasoning, based either on data derived from adult patients or on his metapsychological principles. When Freud reconstructs a patient's past he does so to oedipal ages, for example, "You wanted to push your mother out of the bed and have daddy to yourself." ORT authors wish to extend the range of psychoanalytic reconstructions and account for early infantile experience. Winnicott, for example, described early mother-infant interactions, using language that is, at one level, self-contradictory and unconstrained by formal, adult logic. ORT authors argue that this kind of language, full of seemingly crazy assertions, matches better the pre-oedipal child they seek to understand. Klein was explicit about this when she attempted to describe the "devouring breast" that the infant experiences.

Therapeutic Aims

Classical theory focused on neurotic patients. Only secondarily was it applied to other groups of patients. Classical theory and technique presumes the existence of a reasonable ego. No matter how much intrapsychic conflict it faces, this ego is strong enough to bring the patient to therapy and help the patient sustain the burdens of treatment. Those burdens include the rigors of analytic silence, the prohibitions against acting out, analytic neutrality, the primacy of interpretations rather than "support," and other aspects of the rigorous frame designed to induce the **transference neurosis,** the automatic repetition of the patient's earlier conflicted object relations.

ORT analysts focus on sicker groups of patients, for example, those who have schizoid, borderline, or severe personality disorders, especially those exhibiting narcissism, psychosis, or schizophrenia, or on patients who have less developed egos, especially infants and very young children. ORT authors seek to comprehend processes that precede the consolidation of the tripartite personality Freud described. Freud analyzed conflicts within a relatively consolidated personality; ORT authors analyze struggles to become a consolidated personality. When ORT analysts speak of therapeutic goals, they describe the patient's struggles to become "a person," or to "become real," or a "true self." For example, Winnicott wrote about a patient for whom dreaming replaced "living." Winnicott wished to analyze away the patient's schizoid use of dreams, not analyze the dreams themselves as representations of structural conflicts.

Technique & Intervention

Because they often work with nontraditional patient groups, ORT authors focus on nonverbal patient behaviors. Hence they may use play therapy with both children and adults, or drama, group process, patient art work, or mutually created artifacts that require a great deal of interaction with the therapist. In using these techniques, many ORT authors claim to be classical in that they retain an analytic style and regard interpretation of their patient's behavior as the ultimate agent of therapeutic effectiveness.

What fantasies and bodily sensations arise in response to this patient? Upon reflection, what sudden impulses (eg, sexual, aggressive, protective) do we experience aimed at this patient? ORT is a theory of subjectivity and intersubjectivity, of the capacity to be alone (per Winnicott) and to be sustained by others. A crucial part of ORT and object relations technique is to recognize the therapist's profound place in the patient's emotional life.

Blatt SJ, Ford RQ: *Therapeutic Change: An Object Relations Perspective.* Plenum, 1994.

Freud S: Mourning and melancholia. In Strachey J (editor): *The Standard Edition of the Complete Psychological Works of Sigmund Freud.* Vol 14. Hogarth/Institute for Psycho-Analysis, 1917.

Kernberg O: *Aggression in Personality Disorders and Perversions.* Yale University Press, 1992.

Masterson JF, Tolpin M, Sifneos PE: *Comparing Psychoanalytic Psychotherapies: Developmental, Self, and Object Relations; Self Psychology; Short-term Dynamic.* Brunner/Mazel, 1991.

A SAMPLE CONTEMPORARY DEVELOPMENTAL THEORY

Otto Kernberg represents an especially creative, contemporary current in modern American psychoanalysis. He is known both for his brilliant attempts to integrate schools of psychoanalytic theory and for his specific concepts of borderline pathology and its treatment. Linking both tasks is the notion of **integration.** In his theoretical papers Kernberg seeks to integrate classical analytic theory with other orientations that appear to be incompatible with it.

Kernberg wishes to unite three schools: (1) Freud's classic theory of the drives or set of instincts (sex and aggression), (2) the nondrive theories of British ORT, and (3) the American school of ego psychology. The concept that links these three schools together is the **internal object** and associated concepts, such as the internal object relationship.

Freud describes an internal object as that set of feelings, thoughts, images, and so on that a person associates with a particular entity (real or imagined) within a person's mind. Table 4–4 lists some sample internal objects.

Internal objects are always tied to particular feelings (ie, affects, emotions), a particular thing from one's past (whether real or imagined), and a sense of one's relationship to that thing. All three components figure into each internal object. For example, a patient may remember with strong distaste a visit to the zoo (because his mother was depressed that day and

Table 4–4. Sample internal objects.

Feelings about one's parents and representations or images of them
One's ideals (eg, about science, God, or one's nation)
Images of oneself at different ages
Fragments of childhood nightmares about "monsters" and similar fantasy creatures
Visual images, feelings, and fragments of bodily sensations evoked by discrete stimuli

seemed to avoid him), whereas another patient may remember with extreme pleasure a visit to a junkyard (because her father was happy that day and enjoyed being with her). The three components mean that each person's internal object representation of zoos and junkyard are not identical to those of anyone else. Freud asserted that we can distinguish these two responses to object loss by noting the fate of internal objects in each. In mourning, the survivor realizes that a loved one is lost, and reality testing remains intact. For example, an adult woman's mother dies. She slowly examines the internal objects linked to her dead mother and detaches herself from them by mourning. The daughter remembers her mother and feels anew the wish that she might return to her. The surviving daughter alters gradually her internal world to accommodate a change in the third component of the internal object: the linkage between representations of herself and her mother. Added to each memory of mother is the new information: "Mother is no longer with me in ordinary time and space." This requires her to use the ego function of time sense at an adult level.

In melancholia—what we would call a severe depression precipitated by object loss—the work of mourning, of slowly altering the internal object relationship, does not take place. Rather, melancholic persons attack themselves, heaping abuse on their own heads. A key feature of such attacks is the absence of feelings of shame; there is an "insistent communicativeness which finds satisfaction in self-exposure" (Freud 1917, p. 247). Freud discovered that these complaints are really "plaints" against the lost person (ie, external object). Rather than mourn the loss of the object, the melancholic person has identified with the abandoned object. "Thus the shadow of the object fell upon the ego, and the latter could henceforth be judged by a special agency, as though it were an object, the forsaken object" (Freud 1917, p. 249).

Internal object relations refers to this form of division within the mind (**ego,** or self): One part of the personality attacks or praises (loves or hates) another part. The attacking part Freud called a "special agency." Later, Freud called it the **superego.** How the superego, the agency responsible for shame and guilt, treats the ego defines one form of internal object relations. Given that older children and most adults show some form of ego and superego conflicts, we can say that most people show some degree of **splitting** of their psyches. For example, neurotic-level patients complain about guilt or shame or "feeling driven." Each utterance expresses internal conflicts (eg, "I'm my own worst enemy.").

That human beings are divided against themselves has been a staple insight of eastern and western thought for many thousands of years. Freud's insight was to study the development of such splits, both longitudinally—through the study of children and infants—and clinically—through the study of regression in deep psychotherapy. Both venues suggested that the adult patient's "divided self" stemmed from infancy.

Kernberg argued that when we examine the developmental history of splitting, we find that it begins in an archaic period—perhaps 4 months after birth—and eventually develops into adult forms of ego versus superego. During the first stage of **ego development,** intense feelings of hate toward an external object (such as the mother) and intense feelings of love toward the same object are distinctly experienced and registered separately in the infantile psyche because the ego cannot integrate introjections activated by dissimilar valences. During the next stage of ego development, to prevent the "bad" from overwhelming the "good" (eg, to prevent the "bad internal mother" from obliterating memories of the "good internal mother"), the ego, in response to anxiety, retains a split between the two internalized object relationships. During the third stage—from 4 to 12 months—a three-part psyche is present: an ego built up of positive introjections, a sense of a positive external reality intimate with the self, and a sense of a bad external reality, made up of actually dangerous objects and projected contents of the self (eg, childish notions of "monsters" who threaten to eat mommy).

Finally, these split-off parts of the psyche consolidate up to and through the oedipal period. "Bad" and "good" parts of the self are fused into a more complex sense of oneself, as are "bad" and "good" parts of the object. These fusions make possible normal psychic life, including the capacity for guilt, shame, and mourning (and the capacity to be alone, to feel that mother is with one even when she is not present). With fusion of negative and positive parts of the self comes also the dominance of a new form of defense: **repression.** Repression, when excessive, gives rise to neurotic suffering and is treated by forms of analytic psychotherapy, which aims to undo repressions and make possible new, more mature solutions to intrapsychic struggles (eg, to accept one's sexual life and one's assertiveness as elements in an adult life).

Antedating this relatively high-level form of conflict is **primitive splitting.** This form of splitting is prestructural, that is, it develops before the "structuralization" of the oedipal period (ages 3 to 5 years). When it dominates, it produces patients who manifest borderline personality disorder—what Kernberg terms borderline personality organization (BPO).

Splitting gives rise to BPO. Hence primitive defenses, such as projection, action discharge, denial, dissociation, primitive idealizations, and extreme narcissism predominate in these patients. Therapy with such patients must first deal with these primitive defenses and their structural consequences—identity diffusion and impaired reality testing—and the interpersonal chaos that accompanies BPO functioning. To treat BPO, the clinician must first confront, interpret, and undo the multiple splits that patients with BPO present. Then therapy can help the patient renew developmental processes stymied by intrapsychic and interpersonal failures. Because the patient comes to see how harmful primitive functioning has been, he or she also must mourn the time that cannot be recaptured and the love that has been lost.

Emde R: Epilogue: A beginning—research approaches and expanding horizons for psychoanalysis. J Am Psychoanal Assoc 1993;41(Suppl):411.

SELF PSYCHOLOGY

A similar use of developmental theory and observations occurs in another major contemporary school, that of self psychology. Led by Kohut, self psychologists focus their attention on the qualities and consequences of early child-parent interactions. A core technical term is **self-object,** which refers to Kohut's explication of the parent's ability to maintain a child's self-esteem. In a broader sense, the term encompasses all the ways a parent provides ego functioning for a child, not just the regulation of self-esteem. A self-object has three crucial characteristics: (1) It is a person, (2) who performs ego functions for another person, and (3) who cannot perform them for the person's self. Failures in self-object regulation between infant and adult occur because failure occurs in one or all three parts of the infant-adult interaction. For example, an infant who is grossly impaired neurologically may not be able to receive and process what would otherwise be good-enough care. When it seems possible to locate the source of self-object failure in the parent's response, and not in the child's neurologic defects, we can speak about parental failures in empathic communication. Better yet, we can speak of partial failures in empathic communication and partial failures, therefore, in ego maturation.

Observational evidence for self-object functioning derives from Demos, who expands the notion of empathic communication by distinguishing six types of infant-parent interaction. Because one can see transference events as repetitions of previous ruptures in child-parent interaction, Demos's six types pertain also to types of intervention. Relying in part on a psychoanalytic theory of affect, Demos suggests we can isolate a three-part sequence in the development of strong affects in an infant: (1) A triggering event or stimulus evokes an affect in the infant; (2) the affect (negative-like shame, or positive-like excitement) occurs; and (3) the infant responds to the affect by defense and "planning" a future response.

A well-functioning parent may recognize the triggering event, identify correctly the infant's affect state, and recognize the infant's struggle to deal with its affect. In addition, ". . . she can decide to respond to none, some, or all three components [of the infant's experience]; and her response can take a variety of forms" (Demos 1984a, p. 18). From this theorem, and an associated claim that empathy is inference about the inner state of another person, Demos generates a six-part typology (Table 4–5). Each type describes how a parent (she focuses only on mothers) interacts with the infant at a specific moment.

In type I interactions, the parent recognizes the trigger, recognizes the particular affect it arouses, and recognizes how the child attempts to cope with that affect. By acting appropriately the parent can decrease or end the child's negative affect and increase the child's positive affect. Type I interaction is the "purest" moment of empathic understanding between parent and child, but it may be neither always ideal nor always possible. Type II interaction, in which the parent cannot immediately reduce negative affect but can prolong positive affect, is a feature of much parenting (eg, a visit to the dentist).

Like other analytic theorists, Demos suggests that parents who are less attuned to their child's inner world, and who either misinterpret or ignore the process that produces negative affect in their children, produce the sickest children. Type V and type VI interactions generate the most severe deprivations. As Mahler found in her classic studies, children of alcoholic parents, or of parents prone to psychotic states or severe altered states of consciousness, have numerous experiences of type V and type VI interactions.

Self-object failures occur along this spectrum of parental oversight and include hostility and, in extreme cases, rage. Naturally, if an infant cannot perceive the good-enough parent because of organic or

physical limitations, he or she will experience type V or type VI interactions. Conversely, some children can extract from type V or type VI interactions enough emotional supplies to make ego maturation possible.

How does a parent's type V or VI response inhibit ego maturation? How do these accurate moments of empathic interaction enhance ego maturation? Demos's careful study of child-parent interactions yields valuable clues to the interpersonal mechanisms by which specific ego functions, or ego capacities, are deformed by parental response. In brief, because types IV, V, and VI increase the child's negative affect and decrease the child's positive affects associated with a particular challenge, these types of interactions squelch adaptive forms of problem solving. The squelching may be specific to particular kinds of behavior (eg, sexuality), may relate to intensity levels (eg, of noise), or may be references to interactions with other people ("Act this way in these circumstances") and other parameters. In each case, the child's developing sense of mastery in specific areas is hampered.

For example, Demos discusses a particular 15-month-old girl throwing a ball back to an older child. Because the girl's throw was not "good enough," the mother refused to acknowledge the little girl's efforts and her enthusiasm. "By the third and fourth repetitions of this sequence, the child's expression had become sober; she was no longer clapping" (Demos 1984a, p. 28). One can imagine that a steady diet of such "instruction" would create a woman whose ego functions such as self-esteem, zest for life, and sense of effectiveness and mastery were compromised.

Further, as a consequence of these compromises and failures, all tied to negative affects such as shame and guilt, we would tend to find that behavioral extremes, such as perfectionism and grandiosity, would mark the adult woman's efforts in her adult spheres. Current empirical studies of the inner world have attempted to bridge the conceptual gap that has separated clinical psychoanalysis from laboratory studies of self-representation and self-schemata.

Table 4–5. Six types of interaction and their effect on emotional learning.[1]

Parent Interaction Type	Recognize Trigger	Recognize Affect	Recognize Child's Plan	Negative Affect	Positive Affect
I	Yes	Yes	Yes	Ends	Increases
II	Yes	Yes	Yes	Persists	Persists
III	Yes	Yes	Yes	Persists	Decreases
IV	Yes	Yes	Yes	Persists	Increases
V	Sometimes	Sometimes	Sometimes	Increases	Decreases
VI	No	No	No	Increases	Decreases

[1] "Yes" indicates correct recognition of the child's affective state, "sometimes" indicates partial failure to recognize the child's state, and "no" indicates failure to recognize the child's state.

Demos V: A perspective from infant research on affect and self-esteem. In: Ablon S, Mack J (editors): *The Development and Sustenance of Self-esteem.* International Universities Press, 1984a.

Demos V: Empathy and affect: reflections on infant experience. In: Lichtenberg et al (editors): *Empathy.* Analytic Press, 1984b.

Kohut H: *How Does Analysis Cure?* Goldberg A, Stepansky P (editors). University of Chicago Press, 1984.

Kohut H: *The Kohut Seminars on Self Psychology and Psychotherapy with Adolescents and Young Adults.* Elson M (editor). WW Norton & Co, 1987.

Stolorow R, Atwood G: *Contexts of Being: The Intersubjective Foundations of Psychological Life.* Analytic Press, 1992.

PSYCHOANALYTIC THEORY APPLIED

PSYCHOLOGICAL TESTING

All psychological tests that claim to be projective derive ultimately from psychoanalysis through either Freud or his pupils, such as Jung. For example, Rorschach, originator of the famous inkblot test that bears his name, was influenced by Jung. The Rorschach Inkblot Test, Thematic Apperception Test (TAT), Draw-a-Person Test, and hundreds of other instruments all presume validity of the psychoanalytic concepts of internal psychic conflict and ego defense, especially projection and displacement (see Chapter 12). Thirty years ago projective testing fell into disrepute and seemed on the verge of collapse, but some contemporary research psychoanalysts have sought to place the Rorschach on rigorous, objective footings.

The validity and utility of projective tests are of central concern to contemporary research because Rorschach findings are often part of the test battery used to evaluate the effectiveness of particular therapies. For example, to investigate Freud's claim that sicker patients get less benefit from psychotherapy than do healthier patients, Luborsky et al used a battery of tests that included the Barron Ego Strength Scale (derived from ego psychology), the TAT, and the Rorschach Prognostic Rating Scale. Each of these tests derives wholly or mainly from psychoanalysis. To avoid circularity, research psychologists have attempted to validate projective instruments before using them to evaluate the effectiveness of psychoanalytic treatment. For example, Blatt and Riggs examined outcomes on 90 patients undergoing intensive, long-term psychotherapy. They too used the TAT, the Rorschach, and the human figure drawings test for both pretreatment and posttreatment evaluations. In a manner typical of such research, they also used contemporary theory (ORT) to reevaluate standard Rorschach protocols. Indeed, they claim that

their data support a new clinical distinction between anaclitic and introjective types of psychopathology: Anaclitic patients (those whose defenses are primarily avoidant) do better with psychotherapy, whereas introjective patients (those whose defenses are counteractive and focused on self-cohesion) do better with psychoanalysis.

CHARACTER PATHOLOGY

Psychoanalysis, having the advantage of seniority, has named and given substance to most of the major terms and concepts used to designate character pathology, or what in DSM-IV is termed personality disorder. In addition to drive theory (S. Freud), ego psychology (A. Freud), ORT, and self psychology, McWilliams (1994) notes the utility of other bodies of theory from classical authors such as Jung, Otto Rank, and Alfred Adler. Unlike the laboratory sciences, psychoanalysis and dynamic psychology cannot afford to dismiss the contributions of texts and traditions that preceded them by dozens or even hundreds of years. The great novelists, poets, and playwrights of our own and other cultures have seen deeply and wisely into human character in ways most clinicians cannot match, nor often fathom. The best trained research clinician, of any school and of any theoretical persuasion, has much to learn from Shakespeare, Goethe, and Chekhov.

Yet to remain plausible and contribute to the medical sciences as progressive enterprises, psychoanalysis must also find ways to exclude competing theories. Given the range of psychoanalytic theory and the complexity of its subject matter (the human mind in conflict), psychoanalysis needs a critical, research-based way to decide between competing theories. Happily this need is addressed in new empirical studies.

Erikson EH: *Gandhi's Truth.* WW Norton & Co, 1969.

Gabbard G: *Psychodynamic Psychiatry in Clinical Practice.* American Psychiatric Press, 1990.

Gedo JE: *The Biology of Clinical Encounters: Psychoanalysis as a Science of Mind.* Analytic Press, 1991.

Kernberg O et al: *Psychodynamic Psychotherapy of Borderline Patients.* Basic Books, 1989.

Winnicott DW: *Playing and Reality.* Tavistock, 1971.

Wollheim R. *The Mind and Its Depths.* Harvard University Press, 1993.

PSYCHOANALYTIC CLINICAL FINDINGS

Psychoanalytic technique, especially the sustained empathic investigation of the patient's lived experience, aims to foster ego-syntonic regression, which permits the patient to observe psychological processes that would otherwise go unnoticed. In this sense the psychoanalytic situation, like the telescope in astronomy, permits the observer to record new facts about human behavior. These newly discovered facts constitute the core clinical findings of psychoanalysis. Chief among these findings are (1) the decentering of consciousness, (2) the massive complexity of desire and self-experience, and (3) the ubiquity of transference events. The decentering of consciousness refers to the psychoanalytic aim of enlarging the scope of patients' conscious awareness of their motivations and thoughts. Freud called this his Copernican revolution, because it revealed that human beings are not always masters of their own psyche, just as the earth is not at the center of the solar system. Second, central to psychoanalytic theory and practice is the attempt to follow the contours of a patient's multiple desires (sexual, aggressive, narcissistic, and altruistic). In many important ways, contemporary research has refined classical theory about childhood fantasies about love.

The third finding—that transference events occur in most (some would say all) relationships—pertains to the core features of psychoanalytic technique. Minimally, it means that we construe contemporary relationships according to patterns we have established in previous relationships and that we do so unconsciously. Psychoanalytic research into infancy and childhood, severe character pathology, and even schizophrenia has added to this finding sustained insights into what constitutes "normal" character.

Given the intensity of most forms of psychotherapy, the patient quickly comes to experience the therapist as a transference figure (or figures—some benign, others malignant) and so distorts the new relationship. This distortion may be mild or severe (from momentary conscious slips to complete delusional beliefs). In all instances, such distortion impinges on the therapist and elicits in the therapist a large range of psychic discomfort (from fear of the unknown, to anxiety about seeing the "insides" of another, to homosexual panic and other forms of dread). Hence all therapists will experience "neurotic-like" moments with all patients. With adequate training and adequate safeguards, these moments (almost always countertransference issues) do not dominate the dyadic relationship. For experienced therapists working well within the therapeutic relationship, these neurotic moments act as signal events. For example, a disturbing sexual thought or sudden aggressive wish toward a patient elicits self-analysis, not action.

To lay the foundation for adequate protection of the therapist and the patient from overt errors and distortions generated by the therapist's neurosis, therapists should undertake their own psychotherapy. The experience of patienthood for psychotherapists is vital for a number of reasons. First, it helps stabilize one's own psychological states and so deepens one's relationship to the therapeutic profession. In this sense, psychotherapy is a transformational experience. Second, being a patient permits one to understand directly the kinds of feelings and profound anxieties that one's patients undergo. Third, one's own therapy helps develop the "analytic instrument," the use of one's own inner experience, to grasp empathically the feeling state of another person.

To say that therapists who wish to understand dynamic psychotherapy must become patients first would seem to place dynamic theory within the realm of religiosity and not science. Although one may argue that the analytic setting (or similar psychotherapeutic setting) fosters an especially well-developed form of unconscious processes, one does not want to say that the former creates the latter. For this reason, Freud began his general lectures on psychoanalysis with a lengthy description of ordinary behaviors, parapraxes, to which everyone can give ready credence; then dreams, which most people recognize; and finally neurotic symptoms, which only a few people are willing to ascribe to themselves. In each step of his argument, Freud tried to show how what began as a narrow theory of special psychological states, the neuroses, became a general theory of behavior. Freud's dominant concern was to found a general theory of all human behavior. He classified neurotic and even psychotic behaviors as subsets of nonneurotic behaviors. Basic psychoanalytic theorems will appear clearer and more persuasive when generated within an analytic situation, but they are observable in principle outside that relationship as well. (By analogy, the stars shine during the daytime, but only a total eclipse will reveal this truth.)

Understanding Past Behaviors

One could say humanists attempt to understand, social scientists attempt to explain, and natural scientists attempt to predict the behavior of complex systems. To the degree that psychodynamic theorems are advanced post facto they easily fall into the first kind of proposition: they are attempts to bring order and pattern to behavior that has occurred in the past. Post facto reasoning is not illegitimate, but it sometimes falls into post hoc ergo propter hoc claims [after that; therefore, because of that] that are not valid. That the rain fell after a rain dance was performed does not prove the efficacy of rain dances.

Motives as Explanations

We can distinguish hermeneutic reconstruction from explanation. (Of course, one usually finds both hermeneutics and explanations tied up together in a single account.) **Hermeneutics** is the attempt to find a coherent pattern post facto. Explanations for this pattern—why one finds a particular behavior and not another—typically require one to assign motives to the actors on the scene. To explain is to offer an analysis of motives: for example, John Hinckley, Jr., shot President Reagan because he wanted to be famous. At this level, finding the motives for behavior, one finds an important dynamic issue: One may have multiple reasons for doing something. Freud's initial discoveries about the meaning of parapraxes fall within this category. One can often discover a dual set of motives: one public and overt, the other private and hidden (or repressed). Freud's discovery of such dual structures (an unconscious wish and its conscious counterpart) has entered popular culture, never to be removed. An unfortunate aspect of this success has been an understandable urge to confuse psychoanalytic technique with precisely the discovery of such hidden motives. With adequate cleverness one can impute to others some base motive that often is a portion of that person's thinking. Although early psychoanalytic authors offered shorthand definitions of analysis as the uncovering of repressed motives, it would be a mistake to assume that such uncovering constitutes the core of technique. Rather, the main task of technique is the fostering of the transference, which is the reenactment of the patient's idiosyncratic and all too human conceptions and fantasies of why he or she suffers and how that suffering will be overcome.

A CONFLUENCE OF EMPIRICAL FINDINGS

Thanks to the advent of videotaping, entire analyses, some of them more than a thousand hours long, are available for study. To evaluate this massive amount of material, researchers need organizing hypotheses and principles. Rigorous outcome studies in psychotherapy have been conducted for more than 30 years. These studies enable research analysts to refine clinical generalizations into much more precise concepts subject to empirical examination. Initial evidence suggests that the patient-analyst mix is much more important than earlier thought; that the term "unconscious" is too narrow and should be refined with new evidence about "nonconscious" events, especially data derived from the clinical neurosciences; and that early fears that rigorous and objective empirical work would contaminate the analytic process are unfounded. This last discovery is particularly important, for it gives to analytic clinicians additional criteria with which to distinguish useful from less useful theories, and it gives to psychodynamic psychiatry a renewed grounding in empirical studies that preserve the nuances of the analytic encounter.

Complications & Negative Outcomes

Psychoanalysis as therapy is the examination of a person's interior life in the context of an intense transference-countertransference matrix. Although Freud claimed therapeutic value for such investigation, he realized quickly that it was not appropriate for every patient nor for every condition. Yet even when psychoanalysis is not pertinent as therapy, the analytic investigation of severe psychopathology has given to western thought an important vocabulary for understanding human interior experience. Given Freud's insight that psychoanalysis is not for everyone, issues of complications and negative outcome are extremely important. For example, if we learn that specific forms of medication, or medication and focal psychotherapy, or focal-behavioral therapy, or long-term psychodynamic-cognitive therapy are best for specific conditions, then ethically one must prescribe those interventions for those maladies, at least until they fail. The problem is that there are no consistent findings that demarcate clearly the virtues of one form of therapy from another for specific diagnostic categories. Hence, although behaviorists have been particularly industrious in arguing for the superiority of strictly behavioral techniques, meta-analytic reviews of their findings and effects of different psychotherapies yield little consistent evidence for those claims.

Complications of psychoanalytic treatment include missed diagnosis, heroic efforts with unsuitable patients, and according to new research, errors in treatment modality. In a larger sense of complications, some of the most important advances in psychoanalysis derive from abject failures. For example, Freud abandoned the seduction theory of hysteria when he found that not all of his patients' stories were true. Although a noisy debate has raged over the degree to which Freud thereby excluded discovering actual abuse, it is typically psychoanalytic that he revised his theory in light of his findings. So, too, when his famous patient "Dora" quit her treatment abruptly, Freud had to assess both his theory and his technique: From that failure came his dramatic discovery of transference repetition and, later, countertransference resistances. In a similar way, Kohut's formulations on the theory of narcissism derived from his failures with narcissistic patients, some of whom he saw for a second analysis.

Efficacy & Outcome Studies

Given the complexity and richness of psychoanalytic theory, the many hundreds of hours over which psychoanalytic treatment occurs, the many patient variables (eg, diagnostic category, motivation, age, education), and the many therapist variables (eg, empathic ability, training, innate skills, negative countertransference), assessing the efficacy of psychoanalysis has long been a challenging and important task. The most naturalistic form of study is the sustained case history. This remains the dominant tradition: Novel theories find their first expression in case books.

The more rigorous scientific tests of efficacy are intergroup comparison and longitudinal studies, which can evaluate predicted outcomes. The latter has been a particular forte of psychoanalytic research. The most systematic and complete study, begun in 1945 at the

Menninger Clinic, lasted for more than 30 years and devoted hundreds of pages of tests, reviews, interviews, physical examinations, and recordings to each of the 42 patients. Bachrach et al evaluated a large effort conducted at Columbia University, where researchers studied 700 patients receiving psychoanalysis and 885 patients receiving psychotherapy between 1945 and 1971. Still other efforts to systematically evaluate predictive values of analytic therapy took place at the Boston Psychoanalytic Institute, the New York Psychoanalytic Institute, and other institutions.

Treatment improvements lie in the 60% to 90% range when they are calculated using standard measures. Although this improvement is impressive, important issues remain. Bachrach et al noted five: (1) patients suitable for psychoanalysis derive considerable benefit from it, (2) assessment should be done after a suitable termination phase because analyzability (the capacity to carry out introspection, free association, and so on) does not predict reliably positive outcome, (3) initial consultations do not predict analyzability and treatment outcomes, (4) suitability for analysis remains ambiguous and requires much more study, and (5) the studies vary in the soundness of their design. The cost-effectiveness of psychoanalysis and intensive psychoanalytic psychotherapy compared to other modalities is a serious issue for third-party payers. Researchers have found that intensive outpatient psychotherapy is highly valuable and decreases subsequent hospitalization for all illnesses, not just psychiatric ones. Others have reported that overall treatment costs decreased when psychoanalysis was used. Similar findings have appeared in large-scale studies that compare cost-benefit structure of psychotherapy and psychoanalysis compared to hospital treatment or no treatment. Thanks to many decades of analysis of children, researchers have conducted retrospective studies comparing treatment outcomes in children seen in intensive analytic sessions with those seen in less intense therapy and found that analytic treatment was more effective.

Within psychiatry, the biopsychosocial model of disease describes three major sources of constraint and, roughly speaking, causation. The traditional tripartite model of disease production is attractive in its eclecticism, but it does not help clinicians and researchers organize treatment along priority lines. A rule of thumb that seems to be emerging now is to assess patients sequentially: beginning with biological, then psychological, and then psychosocial perspectives. For example, many psychiatrist-psychoanalysts treat psychiatric disorders with medication, especially for panic and depression, and analysis or intensive psychotherapy. Given this approach, issues of diagnosis and assessment loom even larger, especially for the psychiatrist-psychoanalyst.

[An open-door review of outcome studies in psychoanalysis. Report prepared by the Research Committee of the International Psychoanalytic Association. Editor and Chair: Peter Fonagy.] http://www.ipa.org.uk/research/complete.htm

Luborsky L: The benefits to the clinician of psychotherapy research: A clinician-researcher's view. In: Talley PF, Strupp HH, Butler SF (editors): *Psychotherapy Research and Practice: Bridging the Gap.* Basic Books, 1994.

Luborsky L et al: Psychological health-sickness (PHS) as a predictor of outcomes in dynamic and other psychotherapies. J Consult Clin Psychol 1993;61:542.

Weiss J: *How Psychotherapy Works.* Guilford Press, 1993.

CONCLUSION

Until the late 1980s, becoming a psychoanalyst in the United States meant doing postdoctoral work, primarily post-MD, in an approved institute of the American Psychoanalytic Association. Of the 3000 or so certified analysts, the majority were psychiatrists or other physicians who had completed 4–5 years of additional course work, undertaken a personal analysis, and passed written and oral assessments of their capacities as clinicians and therapists. In addition to the 29 institutes of the American Psychoanalytic Association, nonmedical institutes exist, some of them run by psychologists and other non-psychiatrists. With the death of Freud and the passing of the generation of psychiatrist-psychoanalysts who knew him personally, and with the rise of biological and laboratory methods in psychiatric research, American psychoanalysis confronts new demands.

The relevance of a patient's internal world (defined as "unconscious ideas," personal schemata, self-representations, ego states, core conflicts, and so on) to the patient's overt behavior, including psychopathology, is indisputable. How best to conceive of that world, how to modify it toward health, and how to assess the various and competing theories that make up contemporary psychoanalysis and its points of view is an exciting and major research task for the future. One task will be comparative psychoanalysis. Also, thanks to new research instruments generated primarily by psychologists investigating psychotherapy effectiveness, we can look forward to sophisticated studies that can distinguish the most effective treatments for given diagnostic categories and for use with particular types of patient-therapist interactions.

In the political battles of the 1950s and 1960s, between strict behaviorists who denied the relevance or even existence of an inner world and Freudians who championed such a belief, little exchange took place. Both sides tended to caricaturize the other and rained polemics down upon the other camp. The simultaneous rise of cognitive-behavioral-developmental research efforts and a focus on cognitive aspects of the inner world in contemporary psychoanalysis suggests a confluence of two heretofore independent research traditions.

Researchers long ago answered the extreme skepticism of the placebo argument: We can show systematically that treatment enhances patients' positive outcomes along most lines of interest. Indeed, some forms of intensive psychotherapy, such as cognitive-behavioral therapy, are more effective than antidepressant medication alone for treating some forms of depression. In its best moments, psychoanalysis has added immeasurably to our grasp of human self-understanding. That it was oversold and idealized for many years should not require now the reverse error of denigration and abandonment.

We know that some people are expert and highly effective clinicians whose talents and efforts cannot be duplicated with medication alone. We know that some patients, recalcitrant to all other forms of treatment, blossom with some therapists, overcoming lifelong disability and impairment. The question remaining before us is how, precisely, all these wonderful things occur.

Psychiatric Epidemiology

5

Robert B. Fisher, MD, MPH, & Dan G. Blazer, MD, PhD

THE BIOPSYCHOSOCIAL MODEL & THE WEB OF CAUSATION

The late George Engel promulgated a theoretical model, based on general systems theory, of the etiology of mental disease. Research had demonstrated, and indeed continues to demonstrate, that unitary explanations are not adequate to explain disease etiology or thus indicate appropriate prevention and treatment strategies. Engel suggested an interrelatedness among biological, psychological, and social factors. Biological factors included anatomic and molecular factors and those factors related to gender, age, ethnicity, and genetics. Psychological factors related to the individual's personality. According to Engel's theory, social factors included family, society, culture, and environment; other authors would include religious and spiritual as well as economic factors in this group. Engel also believed that the physician's contribution, through a psychosocial presence, to this "collaborative pathway to health" was often inseparable from that brought by the patient.

CONCEPT OF THE "CASE"

Epidemiologists, for better or for worse, typically allocate people to being either a "case" or a "non-case." *Diagnostic and Statistical Manual of Mental Disorders,* 4th edition (DSM-IV) and other psychiatric diagnostic systems do virtually the same thing. For example, either an individual meets criteria for a diagnosis of major depressive disorder or he or she does not. To identify a case, one must have criteria for identifying cases, but these criteria may vary from one nomenclature to another. For example, the criteria for a case in DSM-IV differ from those in DSM-III in some circumstances.

The use of the concept of a case in epidemiology makes it easier for practicing clinicians to interpret the types of studies performed by epidemiologists, although by arbitrarily assigning an individual to a category of either "case" or "non-case," one loses considerable data. Several early epidemiologic studies were cognizant of this dilemma and attempted to assign patients to groups based on how well they met the predetermined criteria for each group; these researchers recognized that the ability of clinicians to assign individuals as either cases or non-cases was not perfect and was more applicable to a probability function than to a simple yes or no decision. Similarly, the use of symptom rating scales, such as the Hamilton Depression Rating Scale, does not require that an individual be assigned to a case or non-case category but rather permits the assessment of depressive psychopathology as a continuum.

American Psychiatric Association: *Diagnostic and Statistical Manual of Mental Disorders,* 4th ed. American Psychiatric Association, 1994.

OTHER EPIDEMIOLOGIC CONCEPTS

To discern the relationship(s) between what has been described as the **web of causation,** and to determine relevant patterns, the clinical investigator must study not only the impaired individual but also persons within the context of their community. The concept of a web of causation is that specific relationships, such as the relationship between social stressors and a mental disorder, may be connected through a variety of intervening variables that interrelate in a way best illustrated by a web consisting of nodes (etiologic factors) and strings (interrelationships of these etiologic factors). **Epidemiology** here is defined as a ". . . method of reasoning about disease that deals with biological inferences derived from observations of discrete phenomena in population groups." Epidemiology allows more exact determinations as to the contribution(s) that biological, psychological, sociodemographic, and cultural differences may contribute to the **prevalence** and **incidence** of mental disorders. Table 5–1 defines these and other key terms used in epidemiology.

According to Morris, epidemiology has several vital uses: (1) in the study of the historical health of

Table 5–1. Key terms in epidemiology.

Prevalence: The frequency of a given disorder in a population at a particular point of time (ie, it is the ratio of the number of cases of a disorder in the population divided by the number of persons in the population). Although community surveys take time to complete (usually 3 months to 1 year), it is assumed that the results of such studies estimate the frequency of a disorder within a population (usually given as a percentage) on a given day. In some cases, prevalence is measured not as the frequency on a given day but as the frequency of all cases of the disorder that are present during some interval of time, such as 1 month or 1 year.

Denominator: In the prevalence ratio, the denominator is the number of persons in the population. This number becomes important because the prevalence may vary depending on the population from which cases are selected. For example, the denominator may be all persons in a community, all females in a community, all persons attending a clinic, all persons 65 years of age or older attending a clinic, or all African Americans in the community. For each denominator, prevalence may vary.

Incidence: The likelihood, over a period of time (usually 1 year), that an individual who is free from a given disorder will develop it. For example, if 1000 persons are free of a disorder on January 1 and 100 develop the disorder during the next 12 months, then the incidence of that disorder is 10%. In most cases, incidence is much lower than prevalence, and, naturally, because incidence reflects a rate, the collection of data at two or more points in time is necessary to determine incidence.

Risk: The likelihood that an individual will experience a psychiatric disorder. In this sense, risk is basically a measure of incidence.

Risk factor: Any factor that may increase the likelihood that a person will develop a psychiatric disorder. For example, it is known that female gender, younger age, lower socioeconomic status, and being divorced are risk factors for developing major depression. A risk factor may not necessarily be causal.

Risk profile: The array of risk factors associated with a specific disorder.

Relative risk: The increased (or decreased) risk for developing a disorder among persons with a risk factor, compared to persons without a risk factor.

Comorbidity: The presence of at least two distinct disorders in the same individual, each with its own etiology, presentation, and course.

communities and the estimation of morbidity for different disorders, (2) in the assessment of the efficiency of health programs and services, (3) in the determination of individuals at **risk** of acquiring a disease or disability in all their various presentations, (4) in the identification of syndromes as the unified collection of related signs and symptoms, and (5) to assist in ". . . the search for the causes of health and disease." Proper epidemiologic studies can promote sound health policy, enable more rational health care planning, and facilitate cost-effective prevention and treatment. An essential component of all these uses is the determination of valid **denominators** to compare the characteristics of populations with and without disease.

The study of **comorbidity** required advanced statistical methods, available only relatively recently for the study of disease in populations. Epidemiology and statistics have become vital partners in the development of approaches to delineate and disentangle the interrelatedness of psychiatric disorders, or the web of causation.

Lilienfeld DE: Definitions of epidemiology. Am J Epidemiol 1978;107:87.

MacMahon B, Pugh TF, Ipsen J: *Epidemiological Methods.* Little, Brown, 1960.

Morris JN: *Uses of Epidemiology.* Williams & Wilkins, 1964.

HISTORICAL PERSPECTIVE

FIRST-GENERATION STUDIES

The earliest formal psychiatric epidemiologic studies were undertaken during the first part of the 20th century. They were generally of limited scale, relied on institutional records, and used small groups of informants for their data. These were "convenience" studies in which, instead of initiating the surveys themselves, epidemiologists assembled health data from those persons who had already received treatment for a medical problem or had committed suicide. A notable exception was Brugger's study in Thuringia, in which he attempted to use census tracts to identify mental illness in a defined population. Ferris and Dunham's relatively large pre–World War II study examined the geographic distribution of patients with mental disorders in mental hospitals in the Chicago area. They found that manic-depressive illness was distributed equally throughout the geographic area, whereas schizophrenia clustered in the lower socioeconomic areas.

SECOND-GENERATION STUDIES: THE STIRLING COUNTY & MIDTOWN MANHATTAN STUDIES

In comparison to pre–World War II investigations, the studies that followed World War II took advantage of the considerable health information gathered on the military forces during the war. This was the beginning of the "community survey" era of epidemiology. Postwar studies—such as the Stirling County (Nova Scotia) Study and the Midtown Manhattan Study (which are discussed in this chapter) and the Baltimore Study of mental illness in an urban population—were second-generation studies that attempted to determine prevalence rates of mental illness by interviewing community residents using nonpsychiatrist clinical interviewers. The postwar studies examined general health as well as psychiatric disorders and tended to gather and interpret rates of symptom presentation in groups rather than assess the presence of discrete cases. The gathering of often-isolated symptoms, or the finding of psychopathology or emotional illness using the data collection system of the World War II era, was not helpful to health planners or policymakers.

Contributing to the ascension of psychiatric epidemiologic research during the early postwar period was the realization that the increase in mortality and morbidity associated with chronic disease (including that of mental disorders) was more important than was the mortality and morbidity associated with acute, generally infectious, disorders. Difficulty with case identification in the community continued to preclude the determination of prevalence rates for specific clinical disorders.

The initial paradigms for these newer studies were often quite different. The Stirling County Study attempted to determine rates for qualitatively different disorders as well as for overall impairment. The Midtown Manhattan Study assumed that mental disorders were on a continuum and—reflecting the thinking at that time (that mental illness differed in degree and not kind)—that all clinical manifestations of illness could be evaluated in terms of functional impairment. The overall prevalence of psychiatric impairment from both of these studies was approximately 20%. Dohrenwend and colleagues reviewed most of the major European studies and, despite some individual study differences, found a prevalence rate of psychiatric disorder of 16–25%, quite similar to the North American studies. Leighton and colleagues demonstrated in Stirling County that the mental illness of the individual could be influenced, for benefit or detriment, by the attributes of the community, thus ushering in an emphasis, during the late 1950s and early 1960s, on social psychiatry. During this period, Hollingshead and Redlich studied a population of individuals receiving psychiatric treatment in the New Haven, Connecticut, area and found that socioeconomic class was an important correlate of both the presence of a psychiatric disorder and the kind of treatment provided.

Leighton DC et al: *The Character of Danger: Psychiatric Symptoms in Selected Communities.* Basic Books, 1963.

Pasamanick B et al: A survey of mental disease in an urban population. Am J Public Health 1956;47:923.

Strole L et al: *Mental Health in the Metropolis: the Midtown Manhattan Study.* McGraw-Hill, 1962.

THIRD-GENERATION STUDIES

Third-generation epidemiologic studies were based on more advanced epidemiologic and statistical techniques and on a move toward scientific or evidence-based medicine. These studies began with the important development of operational criteria for mental disorders. Newer methodological techniques helped address the increasing need for more exact rates of specific disorders for specific persons in specific settings. Indeed, effective treatment has been shown to be related directly to accurate and thus specific assessment and diagnosis. Similarly, appropriate mental health policy planning for the unique health needs of persons with various psychiatric disorders depends greatly on an accurate and precise definition of boundaries between disorders. Further, research into the etiology and thus effective treatment and, it is hoped, eventual prevention of psychiatric disorders must derive from the specificity of operational criteria. Otherwise, the blurring that has occurred between symptom patterns can lead only to similar blurring in the assessment of treatment and prevention effectiveness.

The Present State Examination (PSE), designed as an instrument that demonstrated diagnostic reliability when used cross-nationally, was used by the World Health Organization in the early 1970s in its study of schizophrenia in a number of countries. About this same time, Feighner and colleagues published diagnostic criteria for 14 major psychiatric illnesses. These criteria both provided a framework for the comparison of data gathered by different research groups and facilitated communication among investigators. This work was followed by the development of the Research Diagnostic Criteria by Spitzer and his colleagues, which led to the American Psychiatric Association's DSM-III. DSM-III was a clear departure from its predecessors in that the specificity and boundaries that demarcated a foundation of this evolving instrument led to specific case and non-case determinations. Many etiologic assumptions in DSM-II that were not demonstrated by empirical research were abandoned in DSM-III. Although interview instruments have been derived from each of these criteria sets, the Diagnostic Interview Schedule (DIS), associated with the development of DSM-III, was the first instrument designed for use by (trained) lay interviewers in community-based epidemiologic studies, a decision based on cost-benefit considerations. The DIS became the preferred instrument for use in most large epidemiologic studies during the 1980s, such as the Epidemiologic Catchment Area (ECA) study (see next section).

American Psychiatric Association: *Diagnostic and Statistical Manual of Mental Disorders,* 3rd ed. American Psychiatric Association, 1980.

Spitzer R, Endicott J, Robins E: Research Diagnostic Criteria. Arch Gen Psychiatry 1978;35:773.

THE NIMH ENVIRONMENTAL CATCHMENT AREA STUDY

The National Institute of Mental Health's ECA study was the most comprehensive and sophisticated epidemiologic study accomplished in its time in the United States. When it was undertaken between 1980 and 1984, its purpose was to provide the best estimates, for the United States, of the prevalence of alcohol and drug abuse and other mental disorders, based on a formalized criteria set (DSM-III) rather than global impairment. Unlike previous studies, this investigation included not only data from institutional and community samples but also longitudinal data and information on disease severity. ECA investigators explored the specific demographic, biological, psychosocial, and environmental factors that might influence the presence and the severity of a mental disorder (ie, the biopsychosocial model). The study not only allowed investigators to follow-up on possible clinical change but also assessed the service utilization of both mental health and general health services. The ECA study has assisted greatly in the planning for future health care service needs—including physical resources, financing, personnel, and educational requirements. The ECA study also confirmed the capability of DSM-III criteria to discriminate among mental disorders and generally helped sharpen the nosology of mental illness.

Although the methodology of the ECA study was a great improvement on previous work, the use of DSM-III as the basis for case identification tended to emphasize reliability rather than validity. DSM-III diagnostic criteria, in contrast to DSM-II criteria, were intended to enhance diagnostic reliability, which, although necessary, is insufficient to establish diagnostic validity. Further, because lay interviewers were utilized in the ECA study, in-depth, qualitative data could not be collected.

Compared to previous surveys, the ECA study found lower rates of virtually all disorders, except for severe cognitive impairment in younger age groups. Women exhibited higher rates of mental disorders than did men, although there were important differences in the rates for specific disorders. Men had higher rates of substance abuse and antisocial personality disorder, and women had significantly higher rates for anxiety-based, affective, and somatization disorders. Men and women exhibited similar rates for schizophrenia and manic episodes. The ECA study showed that individuals with comorbid conditions were more likely to receive treatment than were those with a single disorder; yet, less than one third of persons with mental illness, a substance abuse disorder, or both received any treatment. An important methodological finding was that, in comparison to international studies (after adjusting for differences in diagnostic categories and time frames), disease rates based on the DIS were found to be essentially compatible with previous epidemiologic studies based on the PSE.

THE NATIONAL COMORBIDITY STUDY

The National Comorbidity Study (NCS) was the first attempt in the United States to estimate the prevalence of specific psychiatric disorders, with and without comorbid substance abuse, in a national population sample. The NCS was designed to further the findings of the ECA study, but in contrast to the ECA study (which was drawn from local and institutional groups), the NCS had a national focus. The NCS sought risk factors as well as prevalence and incidence rates, in contrast to the ECA study, which focused only on the latter. Table 5–2 provides comparison data from the two studies. With its national focus, the NCS made possible regional comparisons, including rural and urban differences, and it was possible to establish, on a national basis, more precise investigations into unmet mental illness treatment needs. Furthermore, the NCS was referenced to the DSM-IIIR rather than DSM-III and also contained some questions that would allow comparison to the future DSM-IV and the *International Classification of Diseases,* 10th edition (ICD-10). The NCS found a higher prevalence of mental disorders in the U.S. population, and this prevalence was aggregated in approximately one sixth of the population (ie, in individuals who had three or more comorbid disorders).

In the NCS, risk profiles were constructed for depression alone and when found in association with other psychiatric disorders: 4.9% of persons studied were found to have current major depression (ie, within the last 30 days). The lifetime prevalence of depression was 17.1%. Multiple studies, often using quite different instruments, have found reasonably uniform results on depression: a point prevalence of about 3%, a 6-month to 1-year prevalence of about 6%, and a lifetime prevalence of approximately 16%.

Risk factors for both current and lifetime depression were as follows: being female; having a lower level of education; and being separated, widowed, or divorced. The rates for all time frames and the demographic distributions were higher than those found in the ECA study. The fact that a different method of case identification was used probably explains most of the difference in prevalence between the NCS and the ECA study. The sample from the NCS was younger, and younger persons are known to have a higher prevalence of major depression. The NCS also suggested that although "pure" depression may have a strong biogenetic contribution, comorbid depression may be more environmentally determined. Furthermore, as in the ECA study and other international investigations, more recent birth cohorts were found to be at increased risk for major depression.

Table 5–2. Comparison data from the NCS and ECA study.[1]

Disorder	Prevalence Rates (%, Standard Error)	
	NCS (12 months)	ECA Study (1 month)
Any disorder	29.5 (1.0)	15.4 (0.4)
Any disorder except cognitive impairment, substance abuse disorder, and antisocial personality	N/A	11.2 (0.3)
Substance abuse disorders	11.3 (0.5)	3.8 (0.2)
Alcohol abuse and dependence	7.2 (0.5), dependence only	2.8 (0.2)
Drug abuse and dependence	2.8 (0.3), dependence only	1.3 (0.1)
Schizophrenia/schizophreniform disorders	0.5 (0.1)	0.7 (0.1)
Schizophrenia	N/A	0.6 (0.1)
Schizophreniform disorders	N/A	0.1 (0.0)
Affective (mood) disorders	11.3 (0.7)	5.1 (0.2)
Manic episode	1.3 (0.2)	0.4 (0.1)
Major depressive episode	10.3 (0.6)	2.2 (0.2)
Dysthymia	2.5 (0.2)	3.3 (0.2)
Anxiety disorders	17.2 (0.7)	7.3 (0.3)
Phobia	7.9 (0.4), social phobia	6.2 (0.2)
Panic	2.3 (0.3)	0.5 (0.1)
Obsessive-compulsive disorder	N/A	1.3 (0.1)
Antisocial personality disorder	3.5 (0.3)	0.5 (0.1)
Cognitive impairment		1.3 (0.1)

[1] ECA study data are from Regier DA et al 1988; NCS data are from Kessler RC et al 1994. N/A, not available.

Many explanations have been offered for the striking finding of high estimates of childhood depression and the unexpectedly low estimates of depression in the elderly: methodological limitations including the bias found in diagnostic instruments for the assessment of psychopathology in both children and the elderly, differential morbidity, faulty sampling, response-biased memory, institutionalization, and selective migration. Some or all of these explanations may play a role.

Continued investigation of the NCS data, building on the findings of the Medical Outcome Study (which showed that depressive symptoms themselves were a significant risk factor for other diseases—see next section), found that major and minor depression were not distinct entities but were actually on a continuum. Further, and also using the NCS data, the lifetime prevalence of major and minor depression associated with seasonal affective disorder (SAD) was found to be much lower (1%) than that found in previous studies. This was probably because the instrument used more accurately reflected DSM-IIIR criteria for SAD. Another study, using the NCS data, found a significant lifetime association between panic disorder and

depression in patients who first present with panic disorder and a less powerful but statistically valid association for those who first present with depression. An investigation from Germany, using the revised version of the Composite International Diagnosis Interview on a community sample of adolescents and young adults, found that agoraphobia and panic disorder had "marked differences in symptomatology, course, and associated impairments" and were not necessarily linked, a finding at odds with some earlier studies. If confirmed, this study, which used a more sophisticated epidemiologic design than was available in much earlier studies, will demonstrate a more precise separation between several disorders previously considered to be closely related. This finding may lead to a more definitive basis for both prevention and treatment strategies.

More narrowly focused epidemiologic studies have contributed to increased understanding of psychiatric disorders associated with social conditions. Through a population survey, Breslau and colleagues demonstrated that posttraumatic stress disorder occurred in 9.2% of the population following exposure to trauma. Not only was this prevalence lower than that reported previously, but the most common trauma experienced was the unexpected death of a loved one, not the usually reported combat, rape, or other serious physical assault. Bassuk and colleagues investigated the prevalence of mental illness and substance abuse disorders among homeless and low-income-housed mothers, compared to the prevalence of these disorders among all women in the NCS, and found the prevalence of trauma-related disorders among poor women to be significantly higher than that found among women in the general population.

Bassuk EL et al: Prevalence of mental health and substance use disorders among homeless and low-income housed mothers. Am J Psychiatry 1998;155:1561.

Blazer DG, Kessler RC, Swartz M: Epidemiology of recurrent major and minor depression with a seasonal pattern. The National Comorbidity Survey. Br J Psychiatry 1998;172:164.

Breslau N et al: Trauma and post traumatic stress disorder in the community: The 1996 Detroit Area Survey of Trauma. Arch Gen Psychiatry 1998;55:626.

Kessler RC et al: Lifetime and 12-month prevalence of DSM-III-R psychiatric disorders in the United States. Results from the National Comorbidity Study. Arch Gen Psychiatry 1994;51:8.

Kessler RC et al: Prevalence, correlates, and course of minor depression and major depression in the National Comorbidity Survey. J Affect Disord 1997;45:19.

Kessler RC et al: Lifetime panic-depression comorbidity in the National Comorbidity Survey. Arch Gen Psychiatry 1998;55:801.

Regier DA et al: One-month prevalence of mental disorders in the United States. Arch Gen Psychiatry 1988;45:977.

Regier DA et al: One-month prevalence of mental disorders in the United States and sociodemographic characteristics: the Epidemiologic Catchment Area study. Acta Psychiatr Scand 1993;88:35.

Wittchen HU, Reed V, Kessler RC: The relationship of agoraphobia and panic in a community sample of adolescents and young adults. Arch Gen Psychiatry 1998;55:1017.

RURAL-URBAN DIFFERENCES & THE SOCIAL DRIFT HYPOTHESIS

Another important finding of most epidemiologic studies is that the prevalence of some mental disorders, particularly schizophrenia, has been found to be higher in urban and industrialized areas than in rural areas. A number of explanations for this finding have been suggested: social migration (the downward drift of persons and families experiencing schizophrenia to lower socioeconomic levels), inbreeding among the mentally ill, and the greater availability in urban areas of services for the chronically mentally ill. These differences may also reflect the comparative integration and stability of rural areas. Leighton and colleagues, in their study of rural Nova Scotia, found that depres-

sion (and other psychiatric disorders) were more common for all ages in "disintegrated" communities. Given the recent emphasis on the genetic basis of many psychiatric disorders, more research must be done on the degree of possible inheritance of these disorders in populations, and on the social drift hypothesis, before firm conclusions can be reached.

RELIGION & MENTAL HEALTH

Although limited investigation has suggested an association between religion (or spiritual) health and general health (including mental health), the nature and degree of this association is not clear. Several authors have found an increase in depression among larger and generally older Protestant denominations. The specific religious creeds involved; the internalization of these creeds by the members of the organization; the psychological, social, and behavioral characteristics demanded of these beliefs; and the adherence of the believers to these demands have yet to be elucidated.

MENTAL DISORDER, PHYSICAL HEALTH, & SOCIAL FUNCTIONING

A survey of the point prevalence of schizophrenia within three regions of Scotland was undertaken in 1996, replicating a similar survey conducted in 1981. In comparison to the 1981 study, the patients studied in 1996 had both more positive and negative symptoms and more nonschizophrenic symptoms. Some of the symptoms encountered involved physical health.

An increasing number of epidemiologic studies have demonstrated that depression is a serious illness in its own right and that depressive disorder, and depressive symptoms without a formal depressive disorder being present, can have a serious impact on the general physical health of an individual. The Medical Outcome Study looked carefully at this association by evaluating processes and outcomes of care for patients with the chronic conditions of hypertension, diabetes, coronary heart disease, and depression. Patients with either a current depressive disorder or depressive symptoms in the absence of a disorder tended to have worse physical health, poorer social role functioning, worse perceived current health, and (perceived) greater bodily pain than did patients without a chronic depressive condition. Further, the poor functioning associated with depression or depressive symptoms was equal or worse than that associated with eight major medical conditions, and the effects of depressive symptoms and chronic medical conditions were addictive. For example, the combination of advanced coronary artery disease and depressive symptoms was associated with roughly twice the reduction in social functioning than was found with either condition alone. These authors and subsequent studies concluded that it was important to correctly assess and treat depression in all health care settings in order to improve overall patient outcome, reduce patient and family suffering, and reduce societal costs. The Medical Outcome Study was one of the first to directly compare the social and occupational costs of physical and psychiatric disorders, emphasizing that psychiatric disorders are a major public health concern. More recent research has extended these findings.

Spitzer and colleagues found that depression, anxiety, somatoform disorders, and eating disorders were associated with considerable impairment in health-related quality of life scales. As in the Medical Outcome Study, impairment was found in patients with subclinical symptoms and in those with clinically diagnosable disorders. Mental disorders appeared to contribute to overall impairment to a greater degree than did medical conditions.

From 1982 to 1996, the comorbidity of physical and psychiatric disorders was studied in an unselected 1966 northern Finland birth cohort. In comparison to individuals without a psychiatric diagnosis, psychiatric patients were found to have been hospitalized more frequently for injuries, poisonings, or indefinite symptoms. Men were more commonly hospitalized with a variety of gastrointestinal and circulatory disturbances; women with a comorbid psychiatric disorder were more commonly hospitalized with respiratory disorders, vertebral column disorders, gynecologic disorders, or induced abortions. Epilepsy, nervous and sensory organ disorders in general, and inflammatory disorders of the bowels were more common in patients with schizophrenia as compared to those without the disease. The National Treatment Outcome Research Study, the first large-scale prospective, multisite treatment outcome study of drug users in the United Kingdom, found an extensive range of psychological and physical health problems among this population. Studies looking at the comorbid features of physical and psychological health have consistently demonstrated a high correlation, and these findings have given leaders in the health, social service, and criminal justice systems impetus to plan integrated approaches to this vulnerable, and at least dually afflicted, population.

Gossop M et al: Substance use, health, and social problems of service users at 54 drug treatment agencies. Intake data from the National Treatment Outcome Research Study. Br J Psychiatry 1998;173:166.

Kelly C et al: Nithsdale Schizophrenia Surveys. 17: Fifteen year review. Br J Psychiatry 1998;172:513.

Makikyro T et al: Comorbidity of hospital-treated psychiatric and physical disorders with special reference to schizophrenia: a 28 year follow-up of the 1966 Northern Finland General Population Birth Cohort. Public Health 1998;112:221.

Spitzer RL et al: Health-related quality of life in primary care patients with mental disorders. J Am Med Assoc 1995;274:1511.

Wells KB et al: The functioning and well-being of depressed patients. J Am Med Assoc 1989;262:914.

CONCLUSION: EPIDEMIOLOGY, ETIOLOGY, & PUBLIC HEALTH

Epidemiology places psychiatric disorders in a broad context, which is not always apparent with individual patients. This comprehensiveness is the basis of the biopsychosocial model. Goldberg suggests a version of this model that considers three kinds of factors: those that promote vulnerability (or indeed resilience), those that "release" symptoms at a particular time, and those that determine how long a particular disorder will last. Koopman adds that there is now a shift to studying complex systems that create patterns of disease. Such studies are conducted by the comprehensive monitoring of individuals as individuals and when they interact with others and their environment.

Research by Kendler and colleagues, investigating the risk factors for depression among twins, is among the first of an increasing number of epidemiologic studies based on an integrated biopsychosocial approach. Henderson extends this approach along the causal continuum in a slightly different way, noting that "the concept of populations having different frequency distributions of morbidity, not just different prevalence rates for clinical cases, carries with it the implication that some factor or factors are pushing up the over-all distribution in some groups, but not in others." He suggests that there may be some instrumental "force" in the environment that promotes disease. According to Susser and Susser, epidemiology historically offered the paradigm of the "black box," in which exposure was related directly to outcome, without much interest (and thus investigation) into contributing factors or pathogenesis. Moving toward a more fundamental, comprehensive, and integrative goal, these authors would suggest the alternative paradigm of "eco-epidemiology" or the study of "causal pathways at the societal level and with pathogenesis and causality at the molecular level." Among the lessons that may be drawn then are (1) that intervention by those in health policy and practice must involve a population-based strategy rather than a singular focus on afflicted or vulnerable individuals, (2) that the web of causation is multidimensional, and (3) that theory and practice are interdependent.

Korkeila and colleagues investigated factors predicting readmission to a psychiatric hospital during the early 1990s in Finland. Frequently admitted patients were found to be an identifiable group with three defining characteristics: previous admissions, long length of stays, and a diagnosis of psychosis or personality disorder. This study was particularly important because it reconfirmed earlier work that showed that, in this era of an emphasis on community care, there may be a small group of patients who, with the current treatment strategies available, may always need frequent or longer hospital treatment.

Another important lesson was carefully drawn by Vander Stoep and Link, who emphasized the importance of using valid data in the formation of health policy. They revisited Edward Jarvis's landmark study on the prevalence of mental illness in Massachusetts in the early 19th century. In examining social class, ethnicity, and insanity, Jarvis, wrongly interpreting his data, concluded that immigrants born in Ireland had a higher prevalence of insanity in each social stratum than did those from other ethnic groups. Jarvis then formulated elaborate theories to explain his findings, and his work had a major impact on the formation and direction of health policy of that day. A later reanalysis of the data showed that, to the contrary, the prevalence of mental illness was much lower in the foreign born than in those persons born in the United States.

Public health prevention and treatment strategies drawn from any research must be carefully and critically constructed. This will not be easy. Intervention with individuals and even populations of individuals may be both more difficult and less effective when the real ". . . target is a social entity with its own laws and dynamics." To begin to address these issues of profound complexity and increasing topical relevance, many authors have strongly supported the reintegration of population-driven epidemiology into public health. Adding support and some urgency to this drive has been the advent of managed care, which has created information needs that only more sophisticated epidemiologic investigations can address. Questions on specific treatments for specific patient populations in specific settings; the effectiveness of various forms of health care, including management and finance strategies; and the relentless quest for ways to improve quality while simultaneously attending to related costs will all require methodologically sound investigations.

Goldberg D: A biosocial model for common mental disorders. Psychiatr Scand 1994;90:66.

Henderson AS: The present state of psychiatric epidemiology. Aust N Zeal J Psychiatry 1996;30:9.

Kendler KS et al: The prediction of major depression in women: towards an integrated etiologic model. Am J Psychiatry 1993;150:1139.

Koopman J: Comment: emerging objectives and methods in epidemiology. Am J Public Health 1996;86:630.

Korkeila JA et al: Frequently hospitalized psychiatric patients: a study of predictive factors. Soc Psychiatry Psychiatr Epidemiol 1998;33:528.

Susser M, Susser F: Choosing a future for epidemiology. I. Eras and paradigms. Am J Public Health 1996;86:668.

Susser M, Susser F. Choosing a future for epidemiology. II. From black box to Chinese boxes and eco-epidemiology. Am J Public Health 1996;86:674.

Vander Stoep A, Link B: Social class, ethnicity and mental illness: the importance of being more than earnest. Am J Public Health 1998;88:1396.

Psychiatric Genetics[*]

6

John I. Nurnberger, Jr., MD, PhD, & Wade Berrettini, MD, PhD

METHODS IN PSYCHIATRIC GENETICS

A scientific revolution has occurred in the field of genetics, with the advent of molecular biological techniques. Using these techniques, researchers have located genes, in specific regions of chromosomes, for many neuropsychiatric diseases: Huntington's disease (chromosome 4), Friedreich's ataxia (chromosome 9), neurofibromatosis (chromosome 17), and familial Alzheimer's disease (chromosomes 1, 14, 19, and 21). After strong evidence for inheritance of a disorder has been found through family, twin, and adoption studies, the tools of molecular biology can be used to locate the relevant gene(s) and designate the precise abnormality.

POPULATION GENETICS OF PSYCHIATRIC DISORDERS

Three types of population genetic studies—family, twin, and adoption studies—are conducted to ascertain whether a particular human phenomenon is genetically influenced.

Family Studies

Family studies can answer three critical questions concerning the inheritance of a human phenomenon: First, is the phenomenon found more frequently among the blood relatives of an affected individual compared to relatives of control subjects? That is, are relatives of an affected subject at increased risk for the disorder compared to relatives of control subjects? Second, what other phenomena (possibly genetically related) are also found more frequently among relatives of an affected individual? That is, what other disorders may share a common genetic vulnerability with the phenomenon in question? Third, can a specific mode of inheritance be discerned?

A family study should be differentiated from a family history study in which the relatives are not examined directly but information from the **proband** (ie, the initially ascertained patient) or other persons

is used to establish the presence or absence of the illness. The reliability of the family history method is obviously not as high as the family study method. The discrepancy in reliability is a function of the phenomenon under study, but for psychiatric diseases, the discrepancy is usually great enough to render the family history method undesirable. A family study typically begins with a proband whose relatives are then studied. Prevalence rates in relatives are generally corrected for age (the resulting rate is referred to as the **morbid risk** or **lifetime risk**).

Gershon ES et al: A family study of schizoaffective, bipolar I, bipolar II, unipolar, and normal control probands. Arch Gen Psychiatry 1982;39:1157.

Nurnberger JI Jr. et al: Diagnostic interview for genetic studies: rationale, unique features, and training. Arch Gen Psychiatry 1994;51:849.

Weissman MM et al: Family genetic studies of psychiatric disorders: developing technologies. Arch Gen Psychiatry 1986;43:1104.

Twin Studies

Twin studies are based on the fact that monozygotic (MZ), or identical, twins represent a natural experiment in which two individuals have the exact same genes. This is in contrast to dizygotic (DZ), or fraternal, twins, who share 50% of their genes and are no more genetically similar than any pair of siblings. A phenomenon that is under genetic control should be more concordant (ie, similar) in MZ twins than in DZ twins. By comparing the **concordance rate** (how often the second member of a twin pair demonstrates the phenomenon in question when the first member has it) for MZ and DZ twin pairs, investigators can obtain evidence for the genetic determination of a phenomenon. Concordance may be reported as **pairwise** (each pair of twins is counted once) or **probandwise** (each affected subject is considered together with his or her co-twin). If twin pairs are identified through affected subjects, the probandwise method may be more correct.

---

[*] Some of this material also appears in Nurnberger JI Jr., Berrettini WH: *Psychiatric Genetics.* Chapman & Hall, 1998. Reprinted, with permission.

Nurnberger JI Jr., Goldin LR, Gershon ES: Genetics of psychiatric disorders. Pages 459–492 in: Winokur G, Clayton PJ (editors): *The Medical Basis of Psychiatry,* 2nd ed. WB Saunders, 1994.

Adoption Studies

Adoption studies represent the strongest test of inheritance of a disorder within the field of population genetics. In the most straightforward type of adoption study, a group of affected subjects who have been adopted is identified. Similarly, a control group of unaffected, adopted subjects is identified. The risk for the disorder is then evaluated in four groups of relatives: the adoptive and biological relatives of affected adoptees and the adoptive and biological relatives of control adoptees. If the disorder is heritable, one should find an increased risk among the biological relatives of affected subjects, compared to the other three groups of relatives. One can also compare risk for illness in adopted-away children of ill parents to risk for illness in adopted-away children of well parents.

Kety SS, Wender PH, Rosenthal D: Genetic relationships within the schizophrenia spectrum: evidence from adoption studies. Pages 213–223 in: Spitzer RL, Klein DF (editors): *Critical Issues in Psychiatric Diagnosis.* Raven, 1978.

High-Risk Studies

Biochemical studies of individuals with psychiatric diseases are always confounded by disease effects: For example, are biochemical differences between affected individuals and control subjects related to the cause of the disorder, or are they related to the effects of the disorder (or its treatment)? When investigating possible biochemical differences for a genetic disease, researchers can address this difficult issue by studying a group of individuals (usually adolescents or young adults) who are at high risk to develop the disorder under study (usually because they have parents or other relatives with the disorder). The high-risk group may then be followed over time to assess whether the biochemical abnormalities observed are predictive of the disease.

Schuckit MA, Smith TL: An 8-year follow-up of 450 sons of alcoholics and controls. Arch Gen Psychiatry 1996; 53:202.

GENETIC ANALYSIS METHODS

Specific methods of formal analysis have been developed to assess the way in which a condition is inherited and to determine the location of the gene(s) involved.

Segregation Analysis

Segregation analysis is used to determine whether the pattern of illness in families is consistent with a specific mode of transmission. In 1971, Elston and Stewart developed a general model for single-gene inheritance that allowed researchers to estimate the likelihood that a particular mode of transmission could explain a given set of pedigrees (ie, families in which individuals are defined as ill, not ill, or illness status unknown). Computer-generated segregation analysis can now be used to detect not only single major locus inheritance but also polygenic inheritance and multifactorial inheritance (ie, in which both environmental and inherited factors are important in pathogenesis). However, four confounding variables, characteristic of many psychiatric illnesses, reduce the power of segregation analysis to confirm or exclude a particular mode of inheritance: (1) variable penetrance (some individuals with the genetic predisposition will not manifest the disease), (2) phenocopies (some individuals without the genetic predisposition will manifest symptoms of the disease), (3) genetic heterogeneity (more than one type of genetic cause can produce the same syndrome), and (4) uncertainty regarding the diagnostic boundaries of a syndrome.

Although segregation analysis is a powerful tool for delineating data from family studies for many disorders, it has been less useful in psychiatry thus far.

Elston RC, Stewart J: A general model for the analysis of pedigree data. Hum Hered 1971;21:523.

Linkage Analysis

At any given genetic locus, each individual carries two copies (alleles) of the DNA sequence that defines that locus. One of these alleles is inherited from the mother, and the other is inherited from the father. These alleles will be transmitted with equal probability (ie, $\frac{1}{2}$), one of the two alleles to each offspring. If two genetic loci are close to each other on a chromosome, their alleles tend to be inherited together (not independently) and are known as linked loci. During meiosis, crossing-over (also known as recombination) can occur between homologous chromosomes, thus accounting for the observation that alleles of linked loci are not always inherited together.

The rate at which crossing over occurs between two linked loci is directly proportional to the distance on the chromosome between them. The genetic distance between two linked loci is defined in terms of the percentage of recombination between the two loci (this value is known as theta [θ]). Loci that are far apart on a chromosome will have a 50% chance of being inherited together and are not linked. Thus the maximum value for θ is 0.5, and the minimum value is 0. Linkage analysis is a method for estimating θ for two or more loci.

The probability that two loci are linked is the probability that $\theta < 0.5$. The probability that the two loci are not linked is the probability that $\theta = 0.5$. Thus a LOD (logarithm-of-the-odds ratio) score is defined:

$$\text{LOD score} = \log_{10} \frac{P(\theta) < 0.5}{P(\theta) = 0.5}$$

In practice, probabilities are calculated for values of θ varying between 0 and 0.5, and the value of θ that gives the highest probability is assumed to be correct for the numerator. Given the distribution of the marker alleles and the disease phenotype in question among members of the sampled pedigrees, one can calculate the probabilities in the preceding equation and arrive at a LOD score. Although it is possible to perform such calculations by hand, LOD scores are usually calculated using computer programs. Because a LOD score is a log value, scores from different families can be summed. A LOD score of 1.0 indicates that linkage is 10 times more likely than is nonlinkage. For simple genetic conditions, a LOD score of 3 or greater is evidence for linkage, and a score of -2 or less is sufficient to exclude linkage for the sample studied. For disorders with more complex forms of inheritance (including most psychiatric disorders), a higher positive LOD score may be required to be confident of linkage.

LOD score analysis requires the estimation of genetic parameters such as gene frequency in affected and unaffected subjects. Such estimates are difficult to determine in a complex disease. Alternative statistical methods are available that assess allele sharing among affected persons without requiring parameter estimation. The best known of these methods is the affected sib pair method.

Kong A, Cox NJL: Allele-sharing methods: LOD scores and accurate linkage tests. Am J Hum Genet 1997;61:1179.

Lander E, Kruglyak L: Genetic dissection of complex traits: guidelines for interpreting and reporting linkage results. Nat Genet 1995;11:241.

Ott J: *Analysis of Human Genetic Linkage.* Johns Hopkins University Press, 1985.

Reich T et al: Genome-wide search for genes affecting the risk for alcohol dependence. Am J Med Genet 1998;81:207.

Suarez BK et al: Problems of replicating linkage claims in psychiatry. Pages 23–46 in: Gershon ES, Cloninger CR (editors): *Genetic Approaches to Mental Disorders.* American Psychiatric Press, 1994.

Association Studies

Not all clinical genetic investigations of disease utilize families. In association studies the investigator compares allele frequencies for a given locus in two populations, one of which is composed of unrelated individuals who have a disease and the other of which (the control population) is usually composed of ethnically similar, unrelated persons who do not have the disease. If a particular allele commonly predisposes individuals to the disease in question, then that allele should occur more frequently in the disease population than in the control population.

There are pitfalls to an association study, however. The locus chosen for study must predispose individuals to illness (or be extremely close to a predisposing locus—this is known as linkage disequilibrium). Thus loci chosen for association studies are often known as candidate genes. False-positive results can easily oc-

cur if the two populations are not matched carefully for ethnic background. A preferable strategy is to also sample DNA from the parents of affected individuals, in which case the nontransmitted alleles are used as a control (known as the haplotype relative risk method).

Kidd KK et al: DRD2 haplotypes containing the TaqI A1 allele: implications for alcoholism research. Alcohol Clin Exp Res 1996;20:697.

Nielsen DA et al: A tryptophan hydroxylase gene marker for suicidality and alcoholism. Arch Gen Psychiatry 1998;55:593.

Spielman RS, Ewens WJ: The TDT and other family-based tests for linkage disequilibrium and association. Am J Hum Genet 1996;59:983.

MOLECULAR GENETIC METHODS

Advances in our understanding of the human genome have allowed the development of new and powerful techniques for gene localization. The first commonly employed technique using DNA markers involved detection of restriction fragment length polymorphisms (RFLPs). Restriction enzymes are proteins of bacterial origin that have the enzymatic capacity to cleave double-stranded DNA wherever a particular linear sequence of base pairs is found in the DNA exposed to the enzyme. The sequence of base pairs may be four, six, or even eight pairs in length, but each restriction enzyme (over 100 different restriction enzymes have been isolated) is highly specific for a particular sequence of base pairs and, given the proper incubation conditions, will cut DNA only at the appropriate sequence of base pairs. This sequence is termed the recognition site for the enzyme. If human genomic DNA is cut by one of these restriction enzymes, more than one million fragments of various sizes may result. A restriction enzyme can be used to reveal a polymorphism (DNA variant) if digestion of an individual's DNA results in fragments that differ in size from those usually obtained in a specific region of DNA. Table 6–1 lists the steps involved in this technique.

A variant of the RFLP polymorphism is known as the variable number of tandem repeat (VNTR) polymorphism. In these VNTR polymorphisms (also known as minisatellites), the variation in length of the DNA fragment comes from differences in the number of a tandemly repeated specific DNA sequence that is found between two adjacent restriction fragment sites. In the example diagrammed at the end of this section, consider that each box, |—|, represents a 200-base-pair repeated DNA sequence that has no recognition site for the restriction enzyme BamHI within the repeated sequence. Thus when the diagrammed sequence is cut with BamHI, one fragment will contain 800 base pairs and the other will contain 1000 base pairs, a difference easily detectable with the RFLP techniques described in Table 6–1.

Table 6–1. Steps involved in the detection of polymorphisms.

1. Isolation of intact DNA from blood, cultured cells, or tissue.
2. Cleavage of the DNA with one or more restriction enzymes, which cut the DNA into specific fragments of varying size.
3. Separation of the fragments by size using gel electrophoresis.
4. Separating the double-stranded DNA fragments into single strands, a process known as denaturation.
5. Transfer of the single-stranded fragments from the gel to a nylon membrane, a procedure known as a Southern transfer.
6. Incubation of the nylon membrane in a solution containing a radiolabeled single-stranded DNA fragment (known as a probe) which binds to homologous single-stranded DNA fragments on the membrane to form stable double-stranded fragments of DNA.
7. Detection of the various genomic DNA fragments which bind the probe, a process accomplished by exposing the nylon membrane to an X-ray film (a process known as autoradiography).

Unfortunately, VNTRs have a tendency in the human genome to cluster at the ends of chromosomes, and sets of VNTR markers have been difficult to find in the middle of chromosomes. This difficulty in finding evenly spaced VNTR markers throughout the human genome has spurred the development of simple sequence repeat (SSR) markers, also known as microsatellites.

SSR markers represent a group of polymorphisms that resemble the VNTR markers in that the polymorphism is based on a variable number of a tandemly repeated sequence. However, in the case of SSR markers, the tandemly repeated sequence is not unique and usually consists of two to five nucleotides. The repeated sequence is often $-(CA)_n-$, $-(AG)_n-$, or $-(AAAT)_n-$, although other SSR sequences have been described. The region containing the SSR is amplified by using a thermostable DNA polymerase in a polymerase chain reaction (PCR).

Chromosome workshop summaries from the 1998 World Congress on Psychiatric Genetics. Am J Med Genet 1999;88 (whole issue).

Collins FC et al: New goals for the US Human Genome Project: 1998–2003. Science 1998;282:682.

Petronis A, Kennedy JL: Unstable genes—unstable mind? Am J Psychiatr 1995;152:164.

Shuler GD et al: A gene map of the human genome. Science 1996;274:540.

Strachan T, Read AP: *Human Molecular Genetics.* Wiley-Liss, 1996.

GENETIC STUDIES OF SPECIFIC PSYCHIATRIC DISORDERS

The following sections describe the application of the methods described in the preceding sections to particular syndromes in psychiatry.

AFFECTIVE DISORDERS

Population Genetics

A. Family Studies: Family studies of affective disorders have continually demonstrated aggregation of illness in relatives (Table 6–2). In a study at the National Institute of Mental Health, 25% of relatives of bipolar probands were found to have bipolar disorder or unipolar illness (depression) themselves, compared to 20% of relatives of unipolar probands and 7% of relatives of control subjects. In the same study, 40% of the relatives of schizoaffective probands demonstrated affective illness at some point in their lives. These data demonstrate increased risk in relatives of patients; they also show that the various forms of affective illness appear to be related in a hierarchical way. Relatives of schizoaffective probands may have schizoaffective illness themselves but are more likely to have bipolar or unipolar illness. Relatives of bipolar probands have either bipolar or (more likely) unipolar illness.

If pedigrees of patients with affective disorders are considered as a group, it has generally not been possible to fit single-gene models to them. Some data have supported multifactorial models. These models imply multiple factors: genetic, environmental, or both. An alternative explanation is heterogeneity. In other words, single major genes are important in at least some families, but it is not the same gene in each family.

Age at onset may be useful in dividing affective illness into more genetically homogeneous subgroups. Relatives of early-onset probands seem to be at increased risk of illness.

A birth cohort effect has been observed in recent family studies: There is an increasing incidence of affective illness among persons born more recently. The cohort effect appears to be true for schizoaffective, bipolar, and unipolar illness. The cohort effect is also true among relatives, who are at greater risk than the general population; that is, we are now seeing an increased manifestation of illness among vulnerable persons or (if vulnerability is a single locus defect) greater penetrance. A series of neuropsychiatric conditions has been shown to be related to expansion of short repeated sequences within genes as they are passed from one generation to the next (eg, expanded trinonucleotide repeats). This type of gene expansion may be associated with anticipation (increased severity or earlier onset in younger generations). Anticipation might cause an apparent cohort effect.

B. Twin Studies: Twin studies show consistent evidence for heritability (Table 6–3). On average, MZ

Table 6–2. Lifetime prevalence of affective illness in first-degree relatives of patients and control subjects.[1]

Reference	Number at Risk[2]	Morbid Risk (%)	
		Bipolar	Unipolar
Bipolar Probands			
Perris 1966	627	10.2	0.5
Winokur and Clayton 1967	167	10.2	20.4
Goetzl et al 1974	212	2.8	13.7
Helzer and Winokur 1974	151	4.6	10.6
Mendlewicz and Rainer 1974	606	17.7	22.4
James and Chapman 1975	239	6.4	13.2
Gershon et al 1975	341	3.8	8.7
Smeraldi et al 1977	172	5.8	7.1
Johnson and Leeman 1977	126	15.5	19.8
Pettersen 1977	472	3.6	7.2
Angst et al 1979, 1980	401	2.5	7.0
Taylor et al 1980	601	4.8	4.2
Gershon et al 1981b, 1982	598 (572)	8.0	14.9
Unipolar Probands			
Perris 1966	684	0.3	6.4
Gershon et al 1975	96	2.1	14.2
Smeraldi et al 1977	185	0.6	8.0
Angst et al 1979, 1980	766	0.1	5.9
Taylor et al 1980	96	4.1	8.3
Weissman et al 1984	Severe: 242 (234)	2.1	17.5
Weissman et al 1984	Mild: 414 (396)	3.4	16.7
Gershon et al 1981b, 1982	138 (133)	2.9	16.6
Normal Probands			
Gershon et al 1975b	518 (411)	0.2	0.7
Weissman et al 1984	442 (427)	1.9	5.6
Gershon et al 1981b, 1992	217 (208)	0.5	5.8

[1] Full references are found in Nurnberger et al 1994.
[2] Number at risk (corrected for age) for bipolar illness appears first in "number at risk" column; in parentheses is the number at risk for unipolar illness (when this value is available separately).

twin pairs show concordance 65% of the time, and DZ twin pairs show concordance 14% of the time.

C. Adoption Studies: Several adoption studies have focused on affective illness. The results have been generally consistent with genetic hypotheses. In one study, the risk for affective disorder in the biological relatives of bipolar probands was 31% as opposed to 2% in the relatives of control probands. The risk in biological relatives of adopted bipolar probands was similar to the risk in relatives of bipolar probands who were not adopted away (26%). Adoptive relatives did not show increased risk. Adoption studies that used a broader class of affective probands showed evidence for genetic factors but also possible

environmental influences. In some of these studies, adoptive relatives of affective probands had a greater tendency to develop affective illness themselves, compared to the adoptive relatives of control subjects. These data suggest that genetic factors are more prominent in bipolar illness than in other forms of affective illness.

Genetically Related Disorders

A. Bipolar II Disorder: Most investigators have found that bipolar II disorder is genetically related to bipolar I disorder and unipolar illness. Some evidence from recent family studies indicates a specific increase of bipolar II disorder in relatives of bipolar II

Table 6–3. Concordance rates for affective illness in monozygotic and dizygotic twins.[1,2]

Reference	Monozygotic Twins		Dizygotic Twins	
	Concordant Pairs/ Total Pairs	Concordance (%)	Concordant Pairs/ Total Pairs	Concordance (%)
Luxenberger (1930)	3/4	75.0	0/13	0.0
Rosanoff et al (1935)	16/23	69.6	11/67	16.4
Slater (1953)	4/7	57.1	4/17	23.5
Kallman (1954)	25/27	92.6	13/55	23.6
Harvald and Hauge (1965)	10/15	66.7	2/40	5.0
Allen et al (1974)	5/15	33.3	0/34	0.0
Bertelsen (1979)	32/55	58.3	9/52	17.3
Totals	95/146	65.0	39/278	14.0

[1] Data not corrected for age. Diagnoses include both bipolar and unipolar illness.
[2] Full references are found in Nurnberger et al 1994.

probands. Bipolar II disorder tends to be a stable life-time diagnosis (ie, patients do not frequently convert to bipolar I disorder).

B. Bipolar Disorder with Rapid Cycling: Bipolar disorder with rapid cycling has been the subject of great theoretical and clinical interest. The diagnosis is given to patients with four or more episodes of mania or depression per year; individual patients have been described who have regular cycles of 48 hours. The disorder is relatively resistant to lithium prophylaxis. A link with thyroid pathology has been proposed. Bipolar disorder with rapid cycling appears to arise from factors that are separable from genetic vulnerability to bipolar illness and that do not lead to aggregation within families.

C. Unipolar Mania: The diagnosis of unipolar mania describes patients with bipolar I disorder who have no history of major depression. They tend to be male, are responsive to lithium, and on further history or follow up are usually found to have at least subclinical depressions. This group is not distinguishable from other bipolar I patients on the basis of family pattern of illness.

D. Cyclothymic Disorder: Cyclothymic disorder, which involves repetitive high and low mood swings that generally do not require clinical attention, is probably genetically related to bipolar disorder.

E. Schizoaffective Disorder: Patients with psychotic symptoms, intermittently or chronically, between mood episodes may share genetic vulnerability factors for schizophrenia and affective illness. Schizoaffective disorder (bipolar type) appears to be more closely related to mood disorder, whereas schizoaffective disorder (depressed type) may be more closely related to schizophrenia.

F. Schizophrenia: Some studies have found an increased prevalence of depression in relatives of schizophrenic patients. Bipolar illness has generally not been found, nor is schizophrenia more prevalent in relatives of bipolar probands than in control subjects. Evidence indicates that there may be some common genetic factors in bipolar disorder and schizophrenia (discussed later in this chapter).

G. Eating Disorders: Family studies of anorexia and bulimia have generally found an increased prevalence of affective illness in relatives of patients with these disorders. The risk of affective disorders in relatives of anorexic patients may be similar to that in relatives of bipolar probands.

H. Attention-Deficit/Hyperactivity Disorder (ADHD): The relatives of children with ADHD are more likely to have depression than are control subjects. The opposite has not been demonstrated (ie, bipolar and unipolar probands have not been reported to have increased risk of ADHD in their offspring).

I. Alcoholism: Alcoholism is probably genetically distinct from bipolar illness, but overlapping vulnerability traits may exist. Winokur assembled evidence that unipolar depressive patients with alcoholic or sociopathic relatives (depressive spectrum disorder) are distinct from those without. Alcoholism appears to be comorbid with unipolar and bipolar disorders. Some evidence indicates that alcoholism with comorbid affective disorder may aggregate within families.

Linkage Studies

Linkage studies in affective disorder have been both newsworthy and controversial (Table 6–4). One study reported linkage to markers on the short arm of chromosome 11 in a large Amish family; however, a number of investigators failed to find similar results. Failure to replicate a linkage finding in a separate family is not necessarily a disconfirmation. It may simply indicate heterogeneity. X-chromosome linkage has been reported by some investigators and a meta-analysis suggests a gene of partial effect at Xq26.

Researchers have reported a linkage between bipolar illness and markers on chromosome 18p near the cen-

Table 6–4. Putative linkages for affective disorders.[1]

Chromosomal Location	Reference
18p	Berrettini et al 1993 Stine et al 1995
21q	Straub et al 1994 Detera-Wadleigh et al 1996
Xq26	Pekkarinen et al 1995
11p15	Egeland et al 1987 Kelsoe et al 1991 Gurling et al 1995
5q	Coon et al 1993
4p	Blackwood et al 1996
18q	Freimer et al 1996 Stine et al 1995
Other (including 10p, 12q)	Craddock et al 1994 Ewald et al 1995 Ginns et al 1996 NIMH Genetics Initiative 1997

[1] Full references are found in Nurnberger and Berrettini 1998.

tromere. This finding is supported by data from several other investigators, although there is also evidence for an 18q locus. Another study reported linkage to markers on chromosome 21. This observation has been partially replicated by several other researchers. Loci on 4p and 12q have also been reported. Some findings appear to be common to bipolar disorder and schizophrenia. The 13p32 region has a confirmed schizophrenia susceptibility locus, and there is a statistically robust report of linkage at this locus in bipolar disorder.

Velocardiofacial syndrome (VCFS) is characterized by conotruncal cardiac defects, facial dysmorphology, cleft palate, and learning disabilities. The majority of patients have an interstitial deletion on chromosome 22q11. In addition to physical abnormalities, a variety of psychiatric illnesses have been reported in patients with VCFS, including schizophrenia, bipolar disorder, and ADHD. The psychiatric manifestations of VCFS could be due to disruption of a gene within 22q11. There are several reports of bipolar disorder and schizophrenia linkage to the 22q11–13 region.

Potential Biological Vulnerability Markers

The quest for the physiologic basis of genetic vulnerability to mood disorder has led in many different directions. Most putative biological vulnerability markers have not passed the tests of heritability and association with illness within pedigrees. A discussion of some of the more notable work in this area follows:

A. Lithium Transport: The lithium erythrocyte-plasma ratio may be higher in some cases of familial bipolar disorder.

B. Cholinergic REM Induction: Sleep disturbance is common in depression; one of the most con-

sistent observations is the shortening of rapid eye movement (REM) latency. REM may be induced in volunteer subjects by an injection of a small dose of physostigmine or arecoline during sleep. A series of studies showed that bipolar patients are more sensitive than are control subjects to the REM-inducing effects of arecoline, even when the patients are euthymic and are not taking medication. Further studies have shown that sensitivity to REM induction may be heritable and that it associates with affective disorder within pedigrees. These studies suggest the possibility of central muscarinic cholinergic supersensitivity in brainstem areas in bipolar illness. Methodologic issues require resolution, and the precise neurochemical and anatomic interpretation of these studies remains to be elucidated.

C. Melatonin Suppression: Some studies have found that, in comparison to control subjects, patients with bipolar disorder, and their offspring, are more sensitive to light suppression of melatonin secretion by the pineal gland. This observation may be found more consistently in bipolar I disorder.

Summary & Empirical Data for Genetic Counseling

Molecular genetic studies hold great promise for families with affective disorder, particularly bipolar disorder. The availability of DNA markers would make genetic counseling for these disorders much more precise. Such counseling has already begun for families with Huntington's disease. At present, however, the field has not reached the point at which such markers are clinically useful for affective disorder. This is also the case for etiologic markers. Consequently genetic counseling must be based on empirical risk figures.

The lifetime risk for severe affective disorder is about 8% (about 5–6% for unipolar disorder and 2–3% for bipolar I and bipolar II disorders). Risk is increased to about 20% in first-degree relatives of unipolar patients and to 25% in first-degree relatives of bipolar patients. Risk appears to be 40% in relatives of schizoaffective patients. The risk to offspring of two affectively ill parents is more than 50%. Overall risk figures appear to be rising in recent years, more so in relatives of patients than in the general population.

Freimer NB et al: Genetic mapping using haplotype, association and linkage methods suggests a locus for severe bipolar disorder. Nat Genet 1996;12:436.

Ginns EI et al: A genome-wide search for chromosomal loci linked to bipolar affective disorder in the Old Order Amish. Nat Genet 1996;12:431.

Klerman GL et al: Birth-cohort trends in rates of major depressive disorder among relatives of patients with affective disorder. Arch Gen Psychiatry 1985;42:689.

NIMH Genetics Initiative Bipolar Group; Nurnberger JI Jr. (chair): Genomic survey of bipolar illness in the NIMH genetics initiative pedigrees: a preliminary report. Am J Med Genet 1997;74:227.

ALCOHOLISM

Population Genetics

A. Family Studies: A review of 39 studies on families of 6251 alcoholic subjects and 4083 nonalcoholic subjects reported a 27.0% prevalence of alcoholism in fathers of alcoholic subjects and a 4.9% prevalence in mothers; 30.8% of the alcoholic subjects had at least one alcoholic parent. The same preponderance of alcoholism was not seen in the parents of comparison groups of patients with other psychiatric disorders. The nonpsychiatric control subjects included in the same review showed a 5.2% prevalence of alcoholism in fathers and a 1.2% prevalence in mothers. A recent multicenter study confirmed familial aggregation of alcoholism, with more severe forms showing greater familiality.

B. Twin Studies: Twin studies tend to show heritability of drinking behavior and heritability of alcoholism. Heritability of alcohol consumption is about 40%, at least in males (ie, twin studies show that about 40% of the variance between members of a twin pair is due to genetic factors).

Twin studies of alcoholism itself have generally shown heritability. In a total of 205 twin pairs, in which at least one was alcoholic, probandwise concordance was 54.2% in MZ twins and 31.5% in DZ twins ($P < .01$). Concordance rates in MZ twins increased with the severity of the disturbance. Heritability appears to vary from 40% to 90%, and the more serious forms of alcoholism are more heritable.

In a population-based study of female twin pairs from the Virginia twin registry, personal interviews were completed on 1033 of 1176 pairs. MZ concordance varied from 26% to 47% (as the definition of alcoholism varied from narrow to broad); DZ concordance ranged from 12% to 32%. Calculated heritability was 50–61%. This observation suggests substantial genetic influence in alcoholism in women in the populations studied.

C. Adoption Studies: One study compared 55 adopted-away male children with an alcoholic parent to 78 adoptees without an alcoholic parent. The groups were matched by age, sex, and age at adoption. The principal finding was that 18% of the proband group were alcoholic compared to 5% of the control subjects ($P < .02$). Adopted-away sons with an alcoholic parent were also compared to sons whose alcoholic parent raised them. There was no difference in rates of alcoholism.

One investigation studied 2324 adoptees born in Stockholm between 1930 and 1949. Male adoptees whose fathers abused alcohol (excluding those who were also sociopathic) were more likely to be alcoholic themselves (39.4% vs 13.6%, $P < .01$) compared to adoptees without an alcoholic (or sociopathic) father. Cloninger postulated a familial distinction between types of alcoholism: milieu-limited (type I) and male-limited (type II). Individuals with type I alcoholism usually have onset after age 25, manifest problems with loss of control, and have a great deal of guilt and fear

about alcohol use. Individuals with type II alcoholism have onset before age 25, are unable to abstain from alcohol, and have fights and arrests when drinking but less frequently show loss of control and guilt and fear about alcohol use. The Stockholm adoption data were reanalyzed using these specific categories. This analysis showed that the prevalence of type I alcoholism was increased significantly only among those adoptees with both genetic and environmental risk factors (ie, alcoholism in both biological and adoptive parents). Type I was the most common type of alcoholism and was present in 4.3% of the control subjects with no risk factors. Type II alcoholism was present in 1.9% of the control subjects and in 16.9–17.9% of adoptees with genetic risk factors; the presence or absence of environmental risk factors (alcoholism in adoptive parents) did not appear to make a difference.

Genetically Related Disorders

In some family studies, an increased prevalence of depression has been reported in the female relatives of alcoholic individuals, roughly comparable to the increased prevalence of alcoholism in male relatives. Some forms of illness may result from shared vulnerability factors. Recent studies suggest that alcoholism with comorbid affective illness may itself run in families. Adopted-away daughters of parents with type II alcoholism manifest no increase in alcoholism but show an increased prevalence of somatization disorder.

Some sociopathic alcoholic individuals may transmit both alcoholism and sociopathy as part of the same syndrome. However, it is not clear that a single genetic predisposing factor may be manifest as either alcoholism or sociopathy.

Various behavioral disorders (eg, ADHD, oppositional defiant disorder, conduct disorder, substance use disorders) are more common in offspring of alcoholic parents.

Linkage Studies

No linkages are confirmed in alcoholism at this time. A multicenter study of alcoholic families recently reported loci for vulnerability on chromosomes 1, 7, and 2, with a possible protective locus on chromosome 4.

Association Studies

An association between alcoholism and an allele at the D_2 receptor locus has been reported. This finding has caused much controversy. It has been very difficult to separate the effects of ethnicity from those of alcoholism. A family-based control study that took ethnicity into account was not encouraging.

Potential Biological Vulnerability Markers

The search for a potential biological trait marker of alcoholism has focused on (1) enzymes of alcohol metabolism and other enzymes, (2) electroencephalogram (EEG) and evoked potentials before and after alcohol consumption, and (3) behavioral and neuroendocrine responses to alcohol.

Alcohol is metabolized primarily in the liver by the enzymes alcohol dehydrogenase (ADH) and aldehyde dehydrogenase (ALDH). Four isozymes of ALDH are known. Three are found in the cytoplasm and one (ALDH$_2$) in the mitochondria. ALDH$_2$ is probably responsible for most acetaldehyde metabolism in vivo. The ALDH$_2$ enzyme is lacking in about 50% of Japanese subjects tested and apparently in other Asian groups. Such individuals are subject to a so-called flushing reaction caused by alcohol (similar to a reaction seen in patients receiving disulfiram treatment for alcoholism). The rate of alcoholism is significantly lower in those individuals who lack ALDH$_2$.

Monoamine oxidase (MAO), a primary catabolic enzyme for dopamine, norepinephrine, and serotonin (among other substrates), has been found in lower levels in alcoholic subjects in comparison to control subjects. Perhaps most interesting are several reports suggesting that a low MAO level is related only to type II alcoholism. However, recent data suggest that the effect of cigarette smoking in lowering MAO levels may explain many of the findings in studies of alcoholism.

A poorly synchronized resting EEG (ie, decreased time of alpha rhythm) may be related to a predisposition for alcoholism. The change in alpha rhythm following alcohol consumption was found to be more concordant in MZ twins than in DZ twins (as are many other EEG parameters). A relationship was noted between the resting EEG of the unselected twins and drinking behavior (less alpha in the twins who were heavier drinkers). In subsequent studies, relatives of alcoholic individuals with poorly synchronized resting EEGs demonstrated the same characteristic themselves. A change in alpha rhythm following alcohol consumption has also been found to differentiate young adult subjects at high risk for alcoholism from control subjects.

Measurements of event-related potentials (ERPs) have shown smaller P300 waves following visual stimuli in 7- to 13-year-old sons of alcoholic parents compared to sons of control subjects; the age range studied lessens the likelihood of previous alcohol exposure. Similar findings using an auditory stimulus have been reported in older groups, both before and after alcohol administration. Other researchers have found a significant increase in P300 latency in adolescent and adult relatives of alcoholic individuals compared to control subjects. The EEG/ERP area remains one of the more promising in the field of pathophysiologic markers for alcoholism.

A study of behavioral and neuroendocrine responses to alcohol infusion in a series of high-risk populations found that sons of alcoholic parents displayed less subjective intoxication than did sons of control subjects. A follow-up study showed that decreased subjective intoxication is correlated with later development of alcoholism.

Summary

Hereditary factors appear to operate in normal drinking behavior and in individual vulnerability to alcohol abuse. The flushing reaction to acetaldehyde is a clear instance of a pharmacogenetic variant that influences human behavior. Alcoholism runs in families and is manifest in men more often than in women. The familial preponderance is related primarily to genetic factors, and the differentiation by gender is primarily the result of sociocultural factors. There may be two distinct types of alcoholism with different patterns of inheritance: type I (or milieu-limited) and type II (or male-limited). Type II alcoholism is more severe and more likely to be influenced strongly by major gene effects. Genetic markers for the vulnerability to alcoholism have yet to be verified. Of most interest are studies suggesting EEG/ERP differences in those at risk and studies showing decreased responsiveness to alcohol in those at risk. The neurochemical investigation of animal models of alcoholism is showing links to the serotonin system, as are recent genetic studies. Genetic linkages to areas on chromosomes 1, 2, 4, and 7 and elsewhere are being explored in ongoing studies.

Begleiter H, Kissen B (editors): *The Genetics of Alcoholism.* Oxford University Press, 1995.

Begleiter H et al: Quantitative trait loci analysis of human event-related brain potentials: P3 voltage. Electroencephalogr Clin Neurophysiol 1998;108:244.

Cloninger C: Neurogenetic adaptive mechanisms in alcoholism. Science 1987;236:410.

Cotton NS: The familial incidence of alcoholism. J Stud Alcohol 1979;40:89.

Kendler KS et al: A population-based twin study of alcoholism in women. JAMA 1992;268:1877.

Merikangas K, Gelernter C: Comorbidity for alcoholism and depression. Psychiatr Clin North Am 1990;13:613.

ALZHEIMER'S DISEASE

Population Genetics

Genetic etiologies for some forms of Alzheimer's disease have been found, and specific genes that influence vulnerability have been identified (Table 6–5). A review of epidemiologic studies, however, is remarkable in that it does not show high heritability of the disorder. This observation is partly attributable to multiple environmental and genetic etiologic factors. It is also related to the variable age at onset for the condition. Early-onset causes are more likely to be heritable and may be determined by single genes. Late-onset cases are more likely to be multifactorial. Important genetic factors in late-onset cases may be obscured by the fact that mortality from other causes decreases familial aggregation.

Table 6–5. Genes implicated in Alzheimer's disease.

Chromosomal Location	Clinical Correlate	Frequency	Gene Name	Reference
21q	Early onset	Rare	APP	Goate et al 1991
1	Early onset	Rare	Presenilin II	Levy-Lahad et al 1995
19	Late onset	Common	ApoE	Strittmatter et al 1993
14	Early onset	Rare	Presenilin I	Schellenberg et al 1992

A. Family Studies: Most of the relatives of late-onset Alzheimer's probands will have died of other causes before passing the age of risk. For example, in one study, 60% of 125 autopsy-confirmed Alzheimer's probands did not have an affected first-degree relative. However, the risk to siblings of probands (with an affected parent) whose age at onset was less than 70 years is close to 50%. The risk to first-degree relatives at age 90 has been estimated to be 40%. Another study reported that first-degree relatives of demented subjects with amnesia, apraxia, and aphasia have a corrected lifetime risk of close to 50% for Alzheimer's disease at age 90, compared to 7% for relatives of control subjects (ie, demented subjects without agraphia).

B. Twin Studies: A total of 81 twin pairs, in which at least one member was affected by Alzheimer's disease, have been reported in the literature. In these pairs, the MZ concordance rate (approximately 45%) is not different from the DZ concordance rate (approximately 35%).

Linkage Studies

One study reported linkage of familial Alzheimer's disease to RFLP markers on chromosome 21. The peak LOD score of 4.25 suggested a causative gene near these markers. Subsequently, several studies identified isolated, rare cases of familial Alzheimer's disease in which a point mutation in the gene for amyloid precursor protein was found in ill pedigree members. These studies suggest that abnormalities in this gene are sufficient to cause the disease. Amyloid is a proteinaceous material that accumulates in the extracellular space of the brain in persons with Alzheimer's disease. Another cause of early-onset familial Alzheimer's disease is a gene on chromosome 14. Other familial cases are linked to a gene on chromosome 1. The genes on chromosomes 1 and 14 both code for proteins called presenilins. These proteins appear to be highly homologous; they may metabolize any bound precursor protein.

Many families with late-onset Alzheimer's disease show linkage to a region of chromosome 19 that codes for apolipoprotein E (ApoE), which is also implicated in cardiovascular illness. One copy of the E4 allele will increase an individual's risk fourfold compared to individuals with the more common form, E2. Two copies of E4 increase risk by a factor of 12. It is not yet clear whether E4 is a risk factor for all ethnic groups or just for certain populations. The molecular mechanisms for the Alzheimer's disease vulnerability genes are the subject of intense investigation. There is reason to suspect that all of the causative genes may have an effect on accumulation of amyloid.

Breitner JCS, Folstein MF: Familial Alzheimer dementia: a prevalent disorder with specific clinical features. Psychol Med 1984;14:63.

Goate A et al: Segregation of a missense mutation in the amyloid precursor protein gene with familial Alzheimer's disease. Nature 1991;349:704.

ANTISOCIAL PERSONALITY DISORDER

Population Genetics

A. Family Studies: According to one family study of 223 male criminals, 80% were found to have a diagnosis of antisocial personality disorder (ASPD). Of the first-degree male relatives who were interviewed, 16% also received this diagnosis, whereas only 2% of female relatives were so diagnosed. In comparison, 3% of male control subjects and 1% of female control subjects had ASPD. Increased rates of alcoholism and drug abuse were also found among the relatives in this study.

A family study of 66 female felons and 228 of their first-degree relatives revealed increased rates of ASPD (18%), alcoholism (29%), drug abuse (3%), and hysteria (31%); all of the hysteria occurred in female relatives. Predictably, the male relatives had a threefold increase in ASPD (31%) compared to the female relatives (11%). The increased risk for ASPD among first-degree relatives of female felons (31%), compared to the risk in relatives of male felons (16%), may be related to a greater genetic loading in the families of the female felons.

B. Twin Studies: In a Danish twin study, 32.6% of MZ twins were concordant for criminal behavior, compared to 13.8% of DZ twins ($P < .001$).

C. Adoption Studies: Adoption studies in the 1970s reported that the adopted-away offspring of biological parents with ASPD had a higher risk for ASPD than did control adoptees. Outcome was unrelated to the length of time the adoptees remained with their biological mothers. In a study of 57 adoptee ASPD probands and 57 control probands, ASPD was found among 3.9% of biological relatives of adoptees with ASPD, compared to 1.4% of biological relatives of control adoptees, a highly significant difference. Of the biological fathers of probands, 9.3% received a diagnosis of ASPD, compared to 1.8% of the biological fathers of control adoptees.

A larger study, using adoption and criminal registries, reported that when neither the biological nor the adoptive parents had a criminal record, 13.5% of adoptees had a criminal record. If only the adoptive parents had a criminal record, the adoptee criminality rate rose to only 14.7%. If only the biological parents had a criminal record, the adoptee rate was 20%. And when both sets of parents had criminal records, the adoptee rate was 24.5%. The risk for conviction in a male adoptee increased as a function of the number of parental convictions.

These findings were confirmed in a study of criminality among a cohort of adoptees from Stockholm. The study reported that both genetic and environmental influences were detectable in the risk for ASPD. Of adoptees with a background of predisposing environmental factors, 6.7% were criminals, compared to 2.9% of male adoptees with nonpredisposing environmental and genetic backgrounds. When the genetic background, but not the environment, was predisposing, 12.1% of male adoptees were criminal, compared to 2.9% of control male adoptees. When both the genetic background and environment were judged to be predisposing, 40.0% of male adoptees were criminal. These results are consistent with the additive effects of genetic and environmental influences. Specific environmental influences implicated were multiple foster homes (for men) and extensive institutional care (for women).

Potential Biological Vulnerability Markers

Several reports have suggested that the prevalence of XYY males among the populations in prisons and in penal or mental institutions is higher than in the general population. The XYY karyotype is associated with slightly lower than normal intelligence, tall stature, and cystic acne. This karyotype is found in approximately 0.1% of male newborns but was noted in about 2% of males in penal and mental institutions. In a survey of all tall Danish men from a birth cohort, 12 out of 4139 (0.29%) had the XYY karyotype. Five of the twelve had a criminal record, involving primarily petty crimes. Lower than average intelligence may partially account for the excess of criminal activity among XYY males. This karyotype does not seem to be associated with a predisposition to impulsive violence.

A variant of the tryptophan hydroxylase gene (which codes for the synthetic enzyme for serotonin) has been associated with low 5-hydroxyindoleacetic acid (5-HIAA) in cerebrospinal fluid and with suicide attempts in violent criminal offenders. This finding

deserves follow up using family-based association methods. Low 5-HIAA has been associated with impulsivity and violence in experimental colonies of rhesus monkeys and in humans.

A Dutch family was reported with lowered MAO-A activity caused by a point mutation on the eighth exon of the MAO-A gene. The males with this mutation (both MAO genes are on the X chromosome) had committed impulsive aggressive acts, arson, attempted rape, or exhibitionism. It seems likely that other familial monoamine defects may be associated with aggressive behavior.

Summary

Family, twin, and adoption studies of ASPD demonstrate that the disorder has a heritable component. This component probably includes genes that increase several characteristics associated with ASPD, including impulsivity and substance abuse. The existence of a specific genetic susceptibility to criminal acts is less certain.

Brunner HG et al: Abnormal behavior associated with a point mutation in the structural gene for monoamine oxidase A. Science 1993;262:578.
Cloninger CR, Guze SB: Psychiatric illnesses in the families of female criminals: a study of 288 first-degree relatives. Br J Psychiatry 1973;3:697.

ANXIETY DISORDERS

Population Genetics

A. Family Studies: Family studies provide evidence that some anxiety disorders may be transmitted separately from one another. This is best established for panic disorder and least so for generalized anxiety disorder (GAD). Observations on the increased familial risk for anxiety disorders have been recorded in the literature for over 100 years. Family studies of panic disorder are often complicated by comorbidity with social phobia and GAD. One family study of pure panic disorder probands found a significantly higher risk for panic among first-degree relatives compared to relatives of controls. There was also a fivefold increase in risk for any anxiety disorder. Similarly, an increased risk for agoraphobia (11.6%) has been reported for the relatives of agoraphobic probands, compared to 1.9% for relatives of panic disorder probands and 1.5% for relatives of control probands. A study of simple phobia found an increased risk for simple phobia (31%) among relatives of probands with that diagnosis (but no other anxiety disorder) compared to relatives of control probands (11%). A family history study of social phobia demonstrated that relatives of phobic probands were at increased risk for this disorder (6.6%), compared to relatives of panic disorder probands (0.4%) or relatives of control probands (2.2%).

Distinctly separate genetic transmission is not well established for GAD. A family study found that relatives of GAD probands had a greater risk of GAD than relatives of control probands, but this risk was not greater than the risk for relatives of panic disorder probands. Conversely, a separate study reported similar risks for GAD among relatives of panic disorder probands and relatives of probands with GAD. Thus although some evidence suggests familial transmission of GAD, the transmission may not be specific.

B. Twin Studies: In a Norwegian sample, the concordance of all anxiety disorders for MZ twins (34.4%) was significantly greater than that for DZ twins (17.0%).

C. Linkage Studies: A study of 26 families with multiple cases of panic disorder included 77 persons with definite or probable panic disorder. Screening of the entire genome for linkage is now in progress in this and other samples. No definite linkage findings have been reported, but current interest centers on chromosome 7.

Fyer AJ et al: Familial transmission of simple phobias and fears. Arch Gen Psychiatry 1990;47:252.

ATTENTION-DEFICIT/HYPERACTIVITY DISORDER

Population Genetics

Early family studies of ADHD noted alcoholism and sociopathy in male relatives of children with ADHD and hysteria in female relatives. This same constellation was not manifest in the adoptive parents of adopted children with ADHD.

Recent family studies suggest that ASPD aggregates in the relatives of children with ADHD, but only when the probands have had conduct disorder or oppositional defiant disorder. One study found increased rates of affective illness in relatives of the ADHD probands as well. ADHD itself was also more common in relatives, and ADHD and antisocial behavior tended to occur together.

A report on the association between minor physical anomalies and ADHD found a relationship consistent with a genetic latent trait model (ie, an underlying autosomal dominant gene producing ADHD, physical anomalies, or both). Other findings include a report of mutations in the gene for the thyroid hormone receptor in one group of subjects with ADHD and a family-based association study implicating a gene for the dopamine transporter.

Biederman J et al: A family study of patients with attention deficit disorder and normal controls. J Psychiatr Res 1987;20:263.

AUTISTIC DISORDER

Population Genetics

The pooled frequency of autistic disorder in siblings of autistic probands is about 3%, which is 50–100 times the frequency in the general population. A twin study reported an MZ concordance of 36% and a DZ concordance of 0%. When the phenotype was extended to include language and cognitive abnormalities, concordance rates rose to 82% and 10%. This sample of twins, though carefully selected, was small ($N = 21$), but the essential conclusions regarding heritability were borne out in later studies.

Genetically Related Disorders

What is perhaps most striking about the known genetics of autistic disorder is the association of multiple single-gene disorders with the syndrome. The most clearly documented of these disorders is the fragile X syndrome; perhaps 8% of autistic subjects have the cytogenetic fragile X, and 16% of males with fragile X syndrome are autistic. However, studies in a series of families did not provide evidence for a major role of fragile X mutations in autistic disorder in general. There are also probable associations with tuberous sclerosis, neurofibromatosis, and phenylketonuria. Thus a variety of single-gene abnormalities may serve as the first step in the pathophysiology of autistic syndrome. Although these abnormalities account for only a fraction of the total number of cases of autistic disorder, they may provide important biochemical and anatomic clues.

Rutter M et al: Genetic factors in child psychiatric disorders. II. Empirical findings. J Child Psychol Psychiatry 1990;31:39.

DRUG ABUSE

Population Genetics

A. Family Studies: Considerable comorbidity has been reported for alcoholism and other Axis I disorders in individuals who abuse drugs, and a relationship has been found between the type of comorbid disorder (eg, alcoholism or affective disorder) in probands and the rate of that same disorder in relatives. Relatives of opiate-dependent probands are at significantly increased risk for substance abuse, alcoholism, antisocial personality disorder, and major depression, compared to control subjects.

B. Twin Studies: A study from a sample of 32 MZ twins raised apart found significant heritability for drug abuse or dependence, with a probandwise concordance rate of 36%. Concordance in this range suggests a combination of genetic and environmental effects.

C. Adoption Studies: Of 443 adoptees included in an adoption study of drug abuse, half were selected for psychopathology in biological parents and the other half were matched for age and sex. The parents were not examined directly, but information from adoption records was available. Of the adoptees, 40 manifested drug abuse of one kind or another. Antisocial behavior in a biological relative predicted drug abuse in the adoptee, and alcohol problems also predicted drug abuse. Possible environmental factors included divorce and significant psychiatric pathology in the adoptive parents.

Candidate Gene Studies

Variants of the sigma (σ) opiate receptor gene are being studied in a mouse model and in humans who abuse opiates. Initial results are promising.

Berrettini WH et al: Quantitative trait loci mapping of three loci controlling morphine preference using inbred mouse strains. Nat Genet 1994;7:3.

Cadoret RJ et al: An adoption study of genetic and environmental factors in drug abuse. Arch Gen Psychiatry 1986;43:1131.

Rounsaville BJ et al: Psychiatric disorders in relatives of probands with opiate addiction. Arch Gen Psychiatry 1991;48:33.

EATING DISORDERS

Population Genetics

A. Family Studies: The risk of eating disorders in relatives of anorexic patients is higher than that found in control subjects (Table 6–6). Affective illness is also increased in relatives. Even if probands without a major affective illness are considered as a separate group, an excess of affective illness is observed in relatives compared to relatives of control subjects. In one study, 40 bulimic probands were compared to 24 control subjects. Relatives of bulimic probands had a 27.9% risk of major affective illness compared to 8.8% in relatives of control subjects. In comparison, the risk of major affective illness in relatives of bulimic probands without major affective illness was lower (19.1%), but this risk is still higher than for relatives of controls. The same study found that 11.8% of relatives of bulimic probands had an eating disorder, compared to 3.5% of relatives of controls. In the study of bulimia, relatives of probands also showed an excess of alcoholism and ASPD in comparison to relatives of controls.

B. Twin Studies: One study reported pairwise concordance of 56% in MZ twins and 5% in DZ twins (71% and 10% with probandwise figures) (Table 6–7). Family history assessment (including additional informant data from parents) showed that 4.9% of female first-degree relatives and 1.16% of female second-degree relatives had had anorexia at some point in their lives, a risk considerably higher than the reported population prevalence. The MZ co-twins were much more similar in body dissatisfaction, drive to thinness, weight loss, length of amenorrhea, and minimum body mass index.

The heritability of the body mass index (weight in kilograms/height in meters squared) has been calculated as 0.77 at age 20 and 0.84 at age 45. A special sample of MZ twins raised apart ($N = 93$) was ascertained as part of the Swedish Adoption/Twin Study of Aging. The correlation for body mass index in that group was 0.70 for males and 0.66 for females. For MZ twins raised apart, the intrapair correlation coefficient may be considered a direct estimate of heritability.

C. Adoption Studies: Adoption studies of obesity in Denmark showed a significant correlation between body mass index of adoptees and that of their biological parents but not that of their adoptive parents. Genetic effects are less clear in the very obese, suggesting that environmental factors operate to determine the degree of obesity.

Table 6–6. Family studies of eating disorders.[1]

Study	Morbid Risk Among First-degree Relatives	
Anorexia Nervosa	**Anorexia Probands (N)**	**Control Subjects (N)**
Gershon et al 1983	2.0% (99)	0% (265)
Strober et al 1990	4.1% (387)	0% (703)
Bulimia	**Anorexia Probands (N)**	**Control Subjects (N)**
Gershon et al 1983	4.4% (99)	1.3% (265)
Strober et al 1990	2.6% (387)	1.1% (703)
Bulimia	**Bulimia Probands (N)**	**Control Subjects (N)**
Kassett et al 1989	2.0% (185)	0% (265)
Strober et al 1990	4.1% (387)	0% (703)

[1] Full references are found in Nurnberger and Berrettini 1998.

Table 6–7. Twin studies of anorexia nervosa.[1]

Reference	Concordance	
	MZ	**DZ**
Garfinkel and Garner 1982	10/27 (38%)	0/9 (0%)
Holland et al 1988	11/25 (56%)	1/20 (5%)
Fichter and Noegel 1990	5/6 (83%)	4/15 (27%)

[1] Full references are found in Nurnberger and Berrettini 1998.
[2] Population-based sample of unselected female twins.

Linkage Studies

No linkage studies of eating disorders have been reported, but a large collaborative effort is in progress to accumulate data on sibling pairs with bulimia.

MENTAL RETARDATION

Mental retardation is defined by subnormal scores on standardized testing. Intelligence quotient (IQ) cutoffs of 90, 70, and 50 are commonly considered to be the boundaries for mild, moderate, and severe mental retardation.

Population Genetics

Twin studies performed 40–60 years ago showed an MZ twin concordance of 100% ($N = 83$) and a DZ twin concordance of 55% ($N = 10$). These studies would undoubtedly be performed today with separation according to specific etiologies. Adoption studies have not been performed.

The recurrence of risk (ie, the risk to siblings of an affected child) for mental retardation has been estimated at 9.5–23%, depending on severity of the disorder and the mother's reproductive history. For mothers who have already had more than one retarded child, the risk is 25–50% for siblings.

Specific Etiologic Causes

Many medical syndromes are manifest as mental retardation, such as specific errors of metabolism and chromosomal anomalies. It is estimated that 4% of human conceptions are chromosomally abnormal but that 85–90% of these are selectively eliminated as spontaneous abortions. Of live births, 6% may have a genetic or developmental abnormality of some type, including 0.5% surviving with a chromosomal abnormality, 4% with another developmental anomaly, and 1.5% with a single-gene disorder of some type. Single-gene causes of mental retardation include dominant diseases (eg, tuberous sclerosis, neurofibromatosis, Sturge-Weber syndrome, Hippel-Lindau disease, and craniosynostosis), recessive diseases (Hurler's syndrome, Hunter's syndrome, galactosemia, G-6 phosphodehydrogenase deficiency, and familial hypoglycemia), and several recessive aminoacidurias and lipid-related disorders. Many more are listed in McKusick's compendium *Mendelian Inheritance in Man*.

If we consider disorders that cause mental retardation according to their frequency in the population, we may see the following: (1) Down syndrome accounts for mental retardation in 1.5 persons per 1000 and is the most common single cause of the condition. The prevalence of Down syndrome varies greatly and is determined primarily by maternal age. (2) Familial microcephaly is present in about 1 out of 40,000 births but may account for a significant proportion of mental retardation because of effects in heterozygotes. (3) Fragile X syndrome accounts for about 0.5 out of 1000 births, and other X chromosome syndromes account for another 1 out of 1000 births. (4) All metabolic causes together are responsible for 1 out of 1000 births, and chromosomal abnormalities account for 3 out of 1000 births. We discuss Down syndrome and fragile X syndrome here.

A. Down Syndrome: Down syndrome is caused by a triplication of genetic material on a portion of chromosome 21. The area is presently being localized precisely using molecular techniques combined with cytogenetics. Sections of 21q22.2 and 21q22.3 are likely involved, although some research implicates 21q21. The areas implicated include genes for amyloid and superoxide dismutase. The ETS-2 protooncogene is also near this area, and its presence may be related to an increased incidence of leukemia in persons with Down syndrome and their relatives. Human 21q21–22.3 is homologous to portions of mouse chromosome 16. A mouse model of Down syndrome has been developed based on a laboratory-generated translocation involving this area.

The reasons for triplication, or nondisjunction, in Down syndrome are not entirely clear. The likely etiologic factors are environmental rather than genetic, and vulnerability for the condition does not seem to be inherited. A small proportion of patients with Down syndrome have a translocation rather than a triplication.

As noted previously, the clearest correlate is maternal age; yet it has been known for some years that the origin of the nondisjunction may be paternal instead of maternal. Serum markers (eg, decreased α-fetoprotein and estriol and increased human chorionic gonadotropin) may be able to contribute to prenatal determination and may aid in the selection of women for referral to amniocentesis.

It has been reported that an association exists between Alzheimer's disease and Down syndrome within certain families, but this does not seem to be generally true.

B. Fragile X Syndrome: Fragile X syndrome is named after a cytogenetic observation in which cultured cells from some patients show chromosomal breakage under appropriate conditions. Human chromosomes actually have multiple fragile sites. Fragile X syndrome (breakage at Xq27.3) is merely the best known. The syndrome itself was originally described by Martin and Bell, who described a large pedigree with mental retardation segregating in an X-linked recessive pattern.

Fragile X syndrome is the most common form of X-linked mental retardation and is, in general, the most common heritable form (Down syndrome is genetic but not inherited). It is estimated that 1 out of 850 persons carry the defect. Of those, 4 out of 5 males will express the clinical phenotype, compared to 1 out of 3 females (thus some homozygotes are nonpenetrant and some heterozygotes are penetrant). Tests are now available to determine carrier status in nonpenetrant individuals; the error rate should now be 5% or less with available probes and new polymorphisms that are being developed at a rapid rate. The precise genetic error in the Xq27.3 region is now known to be a triplet repeat of variable length. More repeats (associated with greater severity of illness) occur as the gene is passed to succeeding generations. When the number of repeats exceeds a threshold, clinical manifestations are seen.

Most female heterozygotes do not have mental retardation; however, schizotypal features have been demonstrated in about one third of a sample of carriers, and a weaker association was found with chronic or intermittent affective disorders. Several studies have suggested a connection with autistic disorder. One study described a family in which fragile X syndrome segregated with bipolar affective disorder; data were consistent with linkage to the Xq27 area.

Sutherland GR, Richards RI: *Dynamic Mutations.* American Scientist 1994;82:157.

OBSESSIVE-COMPULSIVE DISORDER

Population Genetics

A. Family Studies: One study evaluated 145 first-degree relatives of 46 children with obsessive-compulsive disorder (OCD). The investigators found that of the 90 parents evaluated in person, 15 (17%) received a diagnosis of OCD, compared to 1.5% of the parents of 34 children with conduct disorder who served as a control group. This 17% rate is also significantly higher than the prevalence rate of 2% in the general population. Fathers were three times as likely as mothers to receive a diagnosis of OCD. Of the 56 siblings evaluated personally, three (5%) met criteria for OCD. When data were corrected for age, the morbid risk was 35% in siblings. This result should be viewed with caution because of the magnitude of the age correction for siblings. The probands all had severe childhood-onset OCD and were referred to the

investigators for treatment protocols. It is possible that childhood-onset OCD represents a more severe form of the illness. Nevertheless, this carefully conducted family study reveals an increased risk for OCD among the first-degree relatives of OCD probands.

B. Twin Studies: There are no large twin studies of OCD. A review of reported series noted that 63% of MZ pairs were concordant. However, assignment of diagnosis and zygosity has been questioned in some of these cases. There is general agreement on 13 concordant MZ twin pairs and 7 discordant MZ twin pairs. There are several unquestioned reports of discordant MZ twin pairs for OCD, implicating some nongenetic factors in incidence or age at onset.

Genetically Related Disorders

When OCD occurs in the familial context of Tourette's syndrome, the OCD may be considered part of the spectrum of Tourette's syndrome. However, most OCD occurs in individuals who have no first-degree relatives affected by Tourette's syndrome. Occasionally, an individual destined to develop Tourette's syndrome will present with symptoms of OCD, and the motor tics appear subsequently. These patients are often diagnosed as having OCD until the motor tics develop.

Summary

There is limited evidence from family, twin, and adoption studies regarding the inheritance of OCD. Although OCD may be familial, there is insufficient data from twin studies and no data from adoption studies. Several avenues of research suggest a serotonergic abnormality in OCD patients.

Nurnberger JI, Jr., Berrettini W: *Psychiatric Genetics.* Chapman & Hall, 1998.

SCHIZOPHRENIA

Population Genetics

A. Family Studies: Pooled family study data from Europe show an age-corrected morbid risk for schizophrenia of 5.6% in parents, 10.1% in siblings, and 12.8% in children. It is thought that the lower rate in parents is related to a relative decrease in fertility among schizophrenic patients. Because general population figures for morbid risk for schizophrenia are around 1%, all classes of first-degree relatives have a clear increase in prevalence. The risk for offspring of two schizophrenic parents is difficult to estimate because of the small number of cases but probably runs between 35% and 45% (in the pooled data it is 46.3%). Among second-degree relatives (eg, uncles, aunts, nephews, nieces, grandchildren), half-siblings, and cousins, the risk ranges from 2% to 4%.

Close relatives of schizophrenic patients are at about a 5- to 10-fold excess risk for the illness, and the risk diminishes in more distant relatives. An additional group of first-degree relatives appear to develop related or so-called spectrum disorders; however, the majority of close relatives of schizophrenic patients are psychiatrically normal.

It is hard to make a strong case for genetic determination of the classical subtypes of schizophrenia (Kraepelin's hebephrenic, catatonic, and paranoid forms). Although there is significant concordance in MZ twins for subtype, this does not hold true in family studies.

Are schizophrenia and affective disorders truly distinct? Evidence of an overlap in genetic liability was found in a large family study that used lifetime diagnoses and separately examined relatives of control probands and probands who had schizophrenia, chronic schizoaffective disorder, acute schizoaffective disorder, bipolar affective disorder, or unipolar depression. An increase in unipolar disorder was found in all groups of relatives. Relatives of schizoaffective probands (both chronic and acute) showed both an excess of affective disorders and an excess of chronic psychoses, compared to relatives of control subjects. However, bipolar probands did not show an excess of schizophrenic relatives, nor did schizophrenic probands show an excess of bipolar relatives. The most parsimonious explanation of these data is that a "middle" group of disorders (ie, the schizoaffective disorders) is genetically related to both schizophrenia and affective illness and that it may not be possible to completely separate the groups using clinical criteria.

With regard to mode of transmission, results generally favor a multifactorial rather than a single-locus model.

B. Twin Studies: Twin studies of schizophrenia are summarized in Table 6–8. Several points may be made with reference to these data. First, in each study, MZ twin concordance is greater than DZ twin concordance, an observation that is consistent with genetic hypotheses. Second, the heritability of broadly defined schizophrenia is greater than the heritability of strictly defined schizophrenia. This is consistent with a spectrum concept (ie, some individuals with the genetic loading for schizophrenia manifest a somewhat different condition). Third, the amount of discordance is considerable; even with a broad definition of illness, the total discordance in the twins is 51%.

A series of nine monozygotic twins with schizophrenia who were raised apart from infancy has been reported. Three were regarded as completely concordant, and three were partially concordant. A twin study paradigm has also been used to generate data regarding environmental effects in schizophrenia. Examining age at onset in the Maudsley Hospital twin series, one study found that there was a high incidence of illness in the second of a pair of twins within 2 years of onset of the illness in the first twin. Further categorizing the group on the basis of whether the twins lived together or lived apart, the investigator found the higher incidence to be primarily in those living together. That is, twins living together show

Table 6–8. Twin studies of schizophrenia.[1,2]

Reference	Strictly Defined Schizophrenia				Broadly Defined Schizophrenia				
	MZ Concordance[3]		Same-Sex DZ Concordance[3]		Heritability	MZ Concordance[3]		DZ Concordance[3]		Heritability
Luxenberger 1928	10/17	59%	0/13	0%	.59	13/17	76%	0/13	0%	.76
Rosanoff et al 1934	18/41	44%	5/53	9%	.38	25/41	61%	7/53	13%	.55
Essen Möller 1941	1/7	14%	2/24	8%	.06	5/7	71%	4/24	17%	.65
Kallman 1946						120/174	69%	34/296	11%	.65
Slater 1953						23/37	65%	8/58	14%	.59
Inouye 1963						33/55	60%	2/11	18%	.51
Tienari 1975	3/20	15%	3/42	7.5%	.08					
Kringlen 1966	14/50	28%	6/94	6%	.24	19/50	38%	13/94	14%	.28
Fischer et al 1969	5/21	24%	4/41	10%	.16	10/21	48%	8/41	19%	.36
Gottesman and Shields 1972	8/20	40%	3/31	10%	.33	11/22	50%	3/33	9%	.45
Kendler and Robinette 1983						30/164	18%	9/268	3%	.15
Totals	59/176	33%	23/298	8%	.27	289/588	49%	78/891	9%	.44

[1,2] If multiple publications have resulted from the same data, only the most definitive is included. Full references are found in Nurnberger et al 1994.
[3] Pairwise concordance figures, in general following the interpretation of Fischer et al 1969.

concordance in age at onset, whereas twins living apart do not. This is an intriguing finding that suggests an environmental factor.

C. Adoption Studies: A series of large, systematic studies were based on adoption and psychiatric hospitalization registries in Denmark. In later studies in the series, subjects were interviewed directly. In all studies, adoptees were separated from their biological parents at an early age and adopted by nonrelatives. More schizophrenia and schizophrenia spectrum disorders were present in the biological relatives of schizophrenic adoptees than in the biological relatives of psychiatrically normal adoptees. The prevalences of psychiatric illnesses in adoptive relatives of the two groups were small and comparable.

The frequency of schizophrenia spectrum disorders is higher in adopted-away offspring of schizophrenic parents than in adopted-away offspring of normal parents. These studies have been criticized for the methods used to select subjects, the validity of the diagnoses, and the validity of comparisons. However, further independent analysis of the data has confirmed the essential results: Biological relatives of schizophrenic patients who have not shared the same environment have a significantly higher prevalence of schizophrenia and schizophrenic spectrum disorders than do biological relatives of comparable control groups.

Up to 30% of first-degree relatives of schizophrenic patients have associated disorders. The particular diagnostic categories that seem to be implicated are schizotypal personality disorder, paranoid personality disorder, and schizoid personality disorder. Older studies used the term borderline schizophrenia to include some individuals who had these personality disorders. Other researchers have argued for a separate entity characterized by paranoid delusions only (eg, simple delusional disorder) with inheritance independent of schizophrenia and affective disorder.

Linkage Studies

Reports have implicated loci on chromosomes 22q, 6p and 6q, 8p, 13q, and 10p (Table 6–9). The evidence is strongest for a locus on chromosome 6p. No specific genes have yet been confirmed.

Potential Biological Vulnerability Markers

Certain psychophysiologic abnormalities appear to be genetic vulnerability indicators for schizophrenia. For instance, a deficit in smooth pursuit eye movements (SPEMs) is observed in schizophrenic patients and their relatives. However, there is not a clear differentiation between ill relatives and well relatives: Many well relatives exhibit the SPEM abnormality. Holzman and colleagues formulated what they call the latent trait model to describe the relationship. In this model, a single gene variant may manifest as schizophrenia in some individuals and eye movement dysfunction in others. Family studies are consistent with dominant inheritance. SPEM abnormalities are also observed in some patients who have schizotypal personality disorder.

There are many reports of attentional deficit measures in schizophrenia. Results on the continuous performance test distinguished high-risk offspring of schizophrenic patients from age- and sex-matched control subjects. These young people have now passed through the period of greatest risk for onset of schizophrenia, and about 20% have become psychotically ill.

Auditory evoked potential measures also seem to differentiate high-risk offspring from control subjects. A defect in auditory gating has been described in schizophrenia that may be related to a gene on chromosome 15 that codes for a subunit of the nicotinic cholinergic receptor.

Summary

The heritability of broadly defined schizophrenia approaches 50%. Related disorders appear to include schizotypal and paranoid personality disorders. Psychophysiologic abnormalities are particularly promising as vulnerability markers. Linkage analysis implicates genes on chromosome 6 (perhaps on both 6p and 6q), 8p, and 5q. Additional areas (10p, 13q, 18p, 22q) may be implicated in both schizophrenia and bipolar disorder.

Baron M et al: A family study of schizophrenia and normal control probands: Implications for the spectrum concept of schizophrenia. Am J Psychiatry 1985;142:447.

Gershon ES et al: A controlled family study of chronic psychoses. Arch Gen Psychiatry 1988;45:328.

Gottesman II, Shields JS: *Schizophrenia: The Epigenetic Puzzle.* Cambridge: Cambridge University Press, 1982.

Holzman PS et al: A single dominant gene can account for eye tracking dysfunctions and schizophrenia in offspring of discordant twins. Arch Gen Psychiatry 1988;45:641.

SOMATIZATION DISORDER

Population Genetics

A. Family Studies: A family history study evaluated first-degree relatives of 49 probands with somati-

Table 6–9. Putative linkages for schizophrenia.[1]

Chromosomal Location	Reference
6p	Straub et al 1995
22q	Pulver et al 1994a,b
8p	Pulver et al 1995
Other (13q, 10p, 5q)	

[1] Full references are found in Nurnberger and Berrettini 1998.

zation disorder. The control groups comprised first-degree relatives of probands with other somatoform disorders and affective disorder. The risk for a complicated medical history was 8.0% in the first-degree relatives of the somatization disorder probands, compared to 2.3% and 2.5% in the control groups ($P < .01$).

A family study of somatization disorder reported a significantly increased risk for the disorder among first-degree female relatives of somatization disorder probands (6.7%), compared to female relatives of control probands (2.4%). The study also reported an increased risk for antisocial personality disorder among the male (18.8%) and female (8.6%) relatives of the somatization disorder probands, compared to the risk in male (10.5%) and female (2.6%) relatives of control probands.

B. Twin Studies: Twin studies have evaluated 14 MZ twin pairs and 21 DZ twin pairs in which one member had a somatoform disorder (including somatization disorder, conversion disorder, psychogenic pain disorder, and hypochondriasis). Of the MZ twin pairs, 29% were concordant for some type of somatoform disorder, compared to 10% of DZ twin pairs (not a significant difference in this small sample).

C. Adoption Studies: An analysis of a large Swedish adoption cohort identified a set of discriminant function variables that distinguished female adoptees with repeated brief sick leaves for somatic complaints and psychiatric disability (so-called somatizers) from other female adoptees. In a subsequent analysis, these somatizers were divided into two groups: high-frequency somatizers (those who had a high rate of psychiatric, abdominal, or back complaints) and diversiform somatizers (those who had a lower frequency of complaints but with multiple and highly variable symptoms). Of the high-frequency somatizers, 30% had histories of alcohol abuse or criminality (based on the national registries for these behaviors). Their male biological relatives were at increased risk for violent criminal behavior and alcohol abuse. For both types of somatizers, a cross-fostering analysis provided evidence for both congenital and postnatal influences on the development of the disorder.

These studies suggest a familial connection between some types of somatoform disorders and alcoholism and criminality.

Bohman M et al: An adoption study of somatoform disorders. Arch Gen Psychiatr 1984;41:872.

TOURETTE'S SYNDROME

Population Genetics
A. Twin Studies: One study evaluated 43 pairs of same-sex twins, including 30 MZ pairs and 13 DZ pairs. MZ twin concordance was 77% for any tics, compared to 23% for DZ twins. For Tourette's syndrome per se, the MZ twin concordance was 53%, compared to the DZ twin concordance of 8%. These differences are significant.

B. Adoption Studies: One adoption study found that among biological relatives of 38 Tourette's probands, 8.3% had Tourette's syndrome, 16.3% had chronic tics, and 9.5% had OCD. These risks are all significantly greater than the risks for the relatives of control subjects.

Although one study reported that the transmission of Tourette's syndrome and chronic tics was consistent with a single-locus model, other studies have been unable to differentiate between a single-locus model and polygenic models.

Linkage Studies
A collaborative effort to use systematic genomic screening to find genes causing Tourette's syndrome has been under way for several years. It is expected that a reproducible linkage will be found, although large samples may be needed.

GENETIC COUNSELING

Empirical data for genetic counseling are summarized in Table 6–10. Some illnesses have fairly narrow age-at-onset distributions in the general population. For example, first episodes of bipolar illness almost always occur before age 50. Fully 50% of bipolar individuals develop an initial episode (either depressive or manic) before age 25. Age at onset should be considered in a general way when assessing risk. For example, an unaffected 40-year-old son of a parent with bipolar disorder has already passed through most of the age at risk; thus his risk of developing bipolar disorder is substantially less than 9%. An estimate of approximately 2% would be more accurate in this case.

Risk estimates should be provided in a psychotherapeutic context. That is, the particular question and its meaning for the individual should be explored carefully. A pedigree diagram should be constructed. Empirical risk information should be provided (at this point no specific biological tests are indicated in the great majority of cases). Finally, the subject's response to the information provided should be explored, with support and further counseling offered as appropriate.

Nurnberger JI Jr., Goldin LR, Gershon ES: Genetics of psychiatric disorders. Pages 459–492 in: Winokur G, Clayton PJ (editors): *The Medical Basis of Psychiatry,* 2nd ed. WB Saunders, 1994.

Quaid KA et al: Issues in genetic testing for susceptibility to alcoholism. The lessons from Alzheimer disease and Huntington disease. Alcohol Clin Exp Res 1996;20:1430.

Table 6–10. Family study data for genetic counseling.

Family History[1]	Unselected General Population Risk	Increased Risk for Offspring
Unipolar disorder (UP)	6%	2-fold (16%) for UP 4-fold (4%) for BP
Bipolar disorder (BP)	1%	9-fold (9%) for BP 2-fold (16%) for UP
Schizophrenia (SZ)	1%	10-fold (10%) for SZ 2-fold (15%) for UP
Alcoholism	5% males, 1% females	5-fold (27% for males, 5% for females)
Panic disorder	0.5%	12-fold (6%)
Tourette's syndrome	0.25%	100-fold (25%)
Alzheimer's disease	3%	5-fold (15%) at age 75
Attention-deficit/hyperactivity disorder	3%	5-fold (15%)
Anorexia nervosa	0.5%	10-fold (5%)

[1] These data assume that only one parent is affected.

CONCLUSION

Major psychiatric disorders are substantially heritable; however, with few exceptions their inheritance patterns are complex and suggest multiple genes. As a result, linkage studies have been difficult to carry out, although multiple studies are implicating certain chromosomal areas (including some common areas for bipolar disorder and schizophrenia). Identification of specific genes is expected to proceed over the upcoming decade and should enable the development of more specifically targeted strategies for treatment and prevention of psychiatric disorders.

7 Mental Health Services Research

Carol T. Nixon, MA, Denine A. Northrup, PhD,
William Thomas Summerfelt, PhD, & Leonard Bickman, PhD

WHAT IS MENTAL HEALTH SERVICES RESEARCH?

Although mental health services research is not easily defined, it "consists mainly of those studies examining the effectiveness of the health care system in the prevention, diagnosis, and treatment of individuals with or at risk of mental disorders" (Kelleher and Long 1994, p. 133). **Effectiveness** should be defined broadly, allowing examination of issues such as service access, utilization, cost, and quality in addition to issues of service impact (ie, outcome evaluation) but deemphasizing specific disorders or conditions. The classic delineation of areas within services research distinguishes between clinical (or process) and systems (or structural) research. **Clinical health services research** is relatively more narrow in focus and includes, for example, investigation of the outcome of specific interventions and the relationship between clinicians and patients. **Systems research** is typically broader, encompassing organizational and financial factors that affect the delivery or quality of health care.

The National Institute of Mental Health (NIMH, 1990) identified five major areas of investigation in mental health services research: (1) **Epidemiology** focuses on the individual, family, and cultural characteristics of those seeking mental health services; (2) **assessment** emphasizes the best means of assessing disorders or functioning; (3) **treatment** examines the methods to assess effectiveness, treatment intensity and modality, setting, and specified target population; (4) **rehabilitation and habilitation** explores the methods of examining the effect of rehabilitation services for social skills, independent living, or vocational rehabilitation; and (5) **outcome** focuses on estimating the impact of mental health services on clinical symptoms, social and vocational functioning, family and patient well-being, and public welfare.

Mental health services delivered in naturalistic settings require not only effective psychiatric and medical treatment but also a variety of social, educational, voca-

tional, and housing services. Many people have recognized the importance of interagency collaboration to plan and implement multifaceted treatment. In turn, mental health services research must be interdisciplinary in nature, drawing on individuals with backgrounds in psychology, psychiatry, epidemiology, statistics, biostatistics, economics, sociology, political science, and the law. Because of the necessity of interorganizational relationships and coordination for optimal functioning of the mental health system, mental health services research also must rely on research that focuses on the process of providing mental health services to patients and their families. It is necessary to understand the treatment process and interorganizational interactions to appropriately interpret any outcome that results.

Mental health services research is still in its infancy. Seemingly basic issues are still being examined. How much do systems of care cost? How can costs be controlled? Which models of care lead to the best outcome? How can quality be defined, assessed, and maintained? With the complexity of all the features that contribute to an integrated, coordinated mental health service system, and in light of system reform and managed care, multidisciplinary teams of researchers are best equipped to examine the process and effects in all the substantive areas (eg, economic, organizational, psychological).

Kelleher K, Long N: Barriers and new directions in mental health services research in the primary care setting. J Clin Child Psychol 1994;23:133.
National Institute of Mental Health: *National plan for research on child and adolescent mental disorders.* Rockville, MD: National Institute of Health, 1990.

FUNCTIONS OF MENTAL HEALTH SERVICES RESEARCH

The ultimate goal of mental health services research is to influence policy and programmatic decision-making in order to improve mental health services. The evaluation of programs, services, and systems provides a relatively objective means of choosing among alternative programs or services competing for limited resources and informing decisions that will affect public policy. Services research may provide information about the services that are being delivered as compared to those intended, how services are being utilized and by whom, the extent to which services are effective, and the costs of services. In addition, evaluation encourages accountability, cost-consciousness, and responsiveness to those in need of and utilizing services. Further, services research can synthesize what is already known, unearth false assumptions, debunk myths, develop new information, and explain the implications of this information for future decision-making. Moreover, it may be unethical to continue to provide untested, perhaps invalid, services to children and their families in the name of treatment.

In order to make such an impact, it is necessary to build a knowledge base about what is currently known in the field. It is then possible to identify and focus on the gaps in the existing research. To overcome some of the limitations of existing research, multidisciplinary research using multiple methods and innovative methodologies and analytic strategies have been used. For instance, drawing on the perspectives of all stakeholders in the process of evaluation increases the relevance of research findings for practice in the field. Further, analytic strategies such as meta-analysis have been used to synthesize the existing research.

The link between clinical practice and services research must be captured to provide balance in the representation of the variety of stakeholders in the professional community. Clinicians and services researchers jointly can examine patient selection processes; effectiveness of complex interventions; and the effect of financial and organizational factors on selection of treatment settings, choice of treatment, intensity of care, and the provider mix.

In addition to enhancing clinical practice, mental health services research also can inform public policy. With the proliferation of managed care in the health services, services research that examines the impact of managed care on service delivery and the associated outcome will help to guide public policy. The mental health services system is constrained by external stakeholders such as health insurance companies, entitlement programs, and social welfare legislation. Mental health services research informs public policy by examining the effect of these external constraints on the individual-, service-, system-level outcome.

Finally, one of the major functions of mental health services research is disseminating the findings and informing the community as a whole. In order to make services research as useful as possible, researchers must carefully report evaluation results, even though potentially unpopular, and thoroughly note the constraints and limitations of any study as well as the generalizability of the findings. Chelimsky (1995) emphasized two types of credibility, relating both to substance and to presentation, that are necessary for effective dissemination. Three critical means of enhancing substantive credibility include conducting a thorough literature review, critiquing the methodology, and anticipating potential attacks on the evaluation findings. Regarding credibility of presentation, Chelimsky suggested that even an ideal study can be misrepresented if it is presented in a careless fashion. Finally, services research findings must be communicated appropriately to a diverse audience including patients and their families, policy makers, clinicians, funding agencies, insurers, and the public at large.

Chelimsky E: Preamble: new dimensions in evaluation. In Picciotto R, Rist RC (editors): *Evaluating Country Development Policies and Programs: New Approaches for a New Agenda.* Jossey-Bass, 1995.

CHILD VERSUS ADULT RESEARCH

Services research is often dichotomized into child versus adult mental health issues. This child-adult split has been characterized as just one of many categories in services research (eg, psychology versus psychiatry, community versus inpatient). Child mental health and adult mental health research offer qualitatively different challenges to researchers. Some researchers have asserted that mental health policy regarding children is arguably more important nationally than adult policy. However, research, theory, knowledge, and legislation in children's mental health services has lagged far behind that in the adult field. In contrast, as the average age of the U.S. population continues to climb, issues facing the elderly will demand attention. The key is the realization that research in these areas is qualitatively different and that findings in one area may not generalize to another. However, as discussed in the "Implications for Future Research" section of this chapter, now is the time for researchers, clinicians, and advocates to develop mutual respect for one another and collaboratively advocate for parity in resources allocated to mental health issues.

RELEVANCE TO PSYCHIATRY

As psychiatry develops a more biomedical emphasis, it will be important to retain a comprehensive perspective in the treatment of mental disorders while concurrently researching the biological etiology of such disorders. There has been a shift away from simplistic causal theories to multidimensional causality across all types of psychiatric research. The interplay among genetic predisposition, brain processes, and psychosocial events has been represented in complex conceptions of etiology and perpetuation of various disorders.

In mental health services reform efforts for children and adolescents, the emphasis on the Child and Adolescent Service System Program (CASSP), which, among other principles, recommends serving patients in the least restrictive environment possible, has led to reliance on community-based resources (CASSP is discussed in further detail in the next section). In the future, the practice of psychiatry will have to be more in partnership with community-based agencies. The success of mental health services provided within the community context will require professional leadership, interagency communication and cooperation, and a supportive community environment.

Most important, with the current rhetoric regarding improved outcome and cost control, all disciplines will have to demonstrate that the services provided under their leadership are cost-effective and competitive. Research data will be required to substantiate claims of effectiveness. Status, tradition, and prestige will be less significant than competency in determining who will provide what types of services.

HISTORY OF SERVICES RESEARCH

Mental health services research has been slow to evolve; however, much of the current thinking in the field has stemmed from ideas formed decades ago. Mental health services, since the beginning of the 20th century, have been influenced more by federal initiatives than by individuals. From the 1930s through the 1960s, the mental health field did not focus on its relationship with other agencies (eg, schools, juvenile courts), nor did it seem to be concerned with social problems influenced by poverty. In essence, mental health services were isolated from other agencies dealing with those in need.

The National Mental Health Act in 1946 was critical in the creation of the National Institute of Mental Health. This legislation promoted a social model of mental disorders and encouraged community-based treatment as opposed to institutionally based treatment. With the Joint Commission on Mental Illness and Health in the 1950s recommending the establishment of community mental health centers (CMHCs), the late 1950s witnessed a deinstitutionalization movement, although there were few resources to support deinstitutionalized individuals. In the 1960s welfare reforms and other social programs further promoted deinstitutionalization. Medicaid and Medicare encouraged a reduction in psychiatric hospital beds and at the same time stimulated placement in alternative settings such as nursing homes. In recent decades,

there has been some growth in insurance coverage for treatment of chronic mental health disorders, which has further encouraged care in community settings. Recently the emphasis on managed mental health care has influenced mental health services in many ways (discussed later in this chapter).

In the 1960s the community mental health movement flourished. The rapid expansion of federal support of CMHCs dramatically improved the living conditions for individuals with mental disorders. However, it was not until 1965 that any national initiatives paid attention to mental health services for children. Amendments to the Social Security Act that year mandated that a program be created to examine the "resources, methods, and practices for diagnosing or preventing emotional illness in children and of treating, caring for, and rehabilitating children with emotional illnesses" (Joint Commission, 1969, p. 2, as cited in Meyers 1985). In 1969 the Joint Commission on Mental Health of Children produced an 800-page report called *Crisis in Children's Mental Health: Challenge for the 1970's.* The report detailed the number of children in need of services and those who were at risk. It also emphasized the role of early intervention and prevention.

A decade later, little had been done in response to the *Crisis in Children's Mental Health* report. For this reason, President Carter's Commission on Mental Health identified children and adolescents as an underserved population with available resources unable to meet the needs. The Mental Health Systems Act passed into law in 1981 recommended an increase in funding for all mental health services, particularly for individuals with severe psychiatric disorders. The Act was intended to promote the design of a coordinated national plan for comprehensive services, quite a breakthrough for mental health. However, as often happens in the political arena, things went awry, and when President Reagan came into office, the law was repealed.

In the children's field, however, the Children's Defense Fund's report, *Unclaimed Children,* was influential in highlighting, once again, the disparity between the number of children in need and those actually receiving services (Knitzer, 1982). The report identified fragmentation of the service system as a major problem, and 4 years later, the Congressional Office of Technology Assessment produced a report that documented the gap between the number of children in need of treatment and those who received treatment. This unmet need influenced the call for more coordinated systems of care so that children and families could access a wide range of community-based services.

CASSP was developed by NIMH to support state and local systems of care for children and adolescents with serious emotional problems and their families. CASSP also developed principles to be followed in the creation of systems of care for children. Some of these principles include that services should be family focused, children should be served in the least restrictive environment possible, services should be appropriate to the child and family's needs, and the services should be community based.

In an effort to better coordinate mental health services, Stroul and Friedman (1986) developed a system-of-care conceptual model to provide a framework for communities trying to develop a service delivery system. The model's seven dimensions of service include mental health services, social services, educational services, health services, vocational services, recreational services, and operational services. The goal for the system is to provide all the services necessary to meet the comprehensive needs of children and their families.

In addition, a variety of innovative community services have been developed both for adults and children. Included among these new services are intensive home-based services, therapeutic foster care, individualized wrap-around services, and crisis services as well as developments in prevention and early intervention. Many of these services have focused on the risk factors for mental illness.

More recently, some large-scale evaluations in the field have been undertaken. For example, the Fort Bragg Evaluation Project compared mental health outcome between children served in a system with a full continuum of care and those served in a more fragmented service system restricted primarily to inpatient and outpatient services. The Robert Wood Johnson Foundation funded the national Mental Health Services Program for Youth to demonstrate the feasibility of coordinated systems that integrate services across a community's service agencies. Other projects evaluating children's mental health services have emerged across the country, from the National Adolescent and Child Treatment Study in Florida, to the evaluation of California's system of care. A major multisite initiative to develop interagency systems of care for children with serious emotional disturbance has been led by the Center for Mental Health Services (CMHS) of the Substance Abuse and Mental Health Services Administration. Since beginning in 1992, CMHS has awarded millions of dollars matched by dozens of project sites. CMHS funded 13 new projects in 1998 and 20 projects in 1999 at an annual cost of over $70 million.

In the adult field, two major epidemiologic studies of the prevalence of mental illness have been conducted. Between 1980 and 1985, the Epidemiologic Catchment Area (ECA) study surveyed respondents older than 18 years of age about their need for, use of, and access to mental health services. The second study, the National Comorbidity Survey (NCS), was conducted between 1990 and 1992. More recent studies in adult mental health services research include investigations focusing on outcomes of mental health services, particularly for capitated (ie, fixed) systems.

Bickman L, Noser K, Summerfelt WT: Long term effects of a system of care on children and adolescents. J Behav Health Serv Res 1999;26:185.

Bickman L, Summerfelt WT, Bryant D: The quality of services at the Fort Bragg Demonstration. J Ment Health Admin 1995;23:30.

Kessler RC et al: Lifetime and 12-month prevalence of DSM-III-R psychiatric disorders in the United States: results from the National Comorbidity Study. Arch Gen Psychiatry 1994;51:8.

Knitzer J: *Unclaimed Children.* Children's Defense Fund, 1982.

Mechanic D: Evolution of mental health services and areas for change. Pages 3–13 in: Mechanic D (editor): *Improving Mental Health Services: What the Social Sciences Can Tell Us. New Directions for Mental Health Services.* No. 36. Jossey-Bass, 1987.

Meyers JC: Federal efforts to improve mental health services for children: breaking a cycle of failure. J Clin Child Psychol 1985;14:182.

Regler DA et al: The de-facto U.S. mental and addictive disorders service system: Epidemiologic Catchment Area prospective 1-year prevalence rate of disorders and services. Arch Gen Psychiatry 1993;50:85.

Rog DJ: Child and adolescent mental health services: Evaluation challenges. Pages 5–16 in: Bickman L, Rog DJ (editors): *Evaluating Mental Health Service for Children.* Jossey-Bass, 1992.

Stroul BA, Friedman RM: *A system of care for severely emotionally disturbed children and youth.* Georgetown University Child Development Center, CASSP Technical Assistance Center, 1986.

CURRENT ISSUES & FINDINGS IN MENTAL HEALTH SERVICES RESEARCH

Although not an exhaustive review of current issues, this section discusses some of the salient issues in mental health services research. Current issues include management, use, accessibility, cost, effectiveness, and quality of mental health services.

Bloom R et al: Mental health costs and outcomes under alternative capitation systems in Colorado: Early results. Journal of Mental Health Policy and Economics 1998;1:3.

DeLeon PH, VandenBos GR, Bulatao EQ: Managed mental health care: A history of the federal policy initiative. Professional Psychology, Research and Practice 1991;22:15.

Dickey B, Azeni H: Impact of managed care on mental health services. Health Aff (Millwood) 1992;11:197.

MANAGED CARE

Although earlier events contributing to the rise of managed care can be singled out, the passage of the Health Maintenance Organization (HMO) Act in 1973 led to the rapid growth of managed health care systems, particularly HMOs. One of the primary aims of managed mental health care has been the containment of costs due in large part to high inpatient utilization rates, much of which is asserted to be inappropriately restrictive and costly. Another primary goal of managed care is to increase access to needed care, particularly for those who are underinsured. By law, HMOs were to provide eight basic services, including emergency and outpatient crisis intervention services and treatment and referral for substance abuse in addition to general health services: consultation and referral, emergency health, diagnostic laboratory and radiologic, home health, and preventive health services.

Managed mental health care, or **behavioral health care,** generally refers to the third-party oversight of the cost and quality of mental health services. Providers and insurers define a specific target population and benefits package aimed at providing integrated, comprehensive, and coordinated care, often at a capitated rate. Although managed care is now the primary model for the majority of those privately insured, development in the public sector has been much slower. However, state mental health authorities more frequently are increasing controls on expenditures, restructuring the financing and delivery of health care under Medicaid, and opting to contract out for managed mental health care services. Between 1991 and 1995, Medicaid managed care increased threefold, from covering 9.5% of enrollees to a total of 32.1% in 45 states.

Managed mental health care may be provided by a number of mechanisms: (1) "carve-out" programs, whereby a specialty behavioral group contracts with a net-work of individual clinicians, sets up its own clinic, or does a combination of these things; (2) employee-assistance programs; (3) integrated delivery systems (ie, a "carve-in" system), in which individual treatment facilities expand to take on mental health care; (4) HMOs, in which a primary care physician serves as a gatekeeper to additional, more specialized services; and (5) Medicaid carve-out experiments, whereby CMHCs collaborate with managed care companies. Managing mental health care typically entails many of the following elements: prepayment of care; prior authorization; utilization review or case management; preferred providers; negotiated rates; practice guidelines; or the development of comprehensive managed mental health programs for employers, insurers, or HMOs.

The HMO Act expanded mental health coverage, and the prepayment mechanism allowed more flexibility in service delivery than traditional indemnity plans. However, in the 1980s, indemnity plans expanded their mental health benefit packages. Criticism of HMOs subsequently arose, contributing to the rise of carve-out programs. Traditional indemnity insurance is generally more restrictive than managed care approaches, limiting reimbursement to specific diagnoses and particular treatment processes and settings, whereas prepayment options tend to encourage more flexibility and innovation such as the use of paraprofessionals in service delivery.

Health care reform has not been without concern. The 1973 mandate for mental health services was imprecise, leaving considerable flexibility and latitude to administrative decision-making regarding the nature and extent of services provided by HMOs. There has been a general lack of awareness about services delivered within HMOs, particularly regarding the delivery of mental health services. Further, several legal and ethical issues have been raised in relation to managed mental health care.

Research Findings

Little research has addressed the effects of health care reform, particularly in publicly funded populations. As states increasingly incorporate a managed care model in service delivery, research is needed that examines the impact of such broad-based reform on the quality of care received by individuals with severe emotional disturbance and by other vulnerable populations. The original focus of the HMO movement was the delivery of high-quality, accessible services at an affordable cost, but emphasis has shifted to containing costs, providing investment opportunities, and extracting profits. Although the emphasis of managed care has diverged from its original focus, the effects of managed care that have been debated are those original issues—quality, access, and cost.

Capitation alone does not appear to result in reductions in access, adequacy, and appropriateness of services for seriously emotionally disturbed individuals. Studies of access to general health and mental health services have demonstrated equal or superior access for managed care as compared to fee-for-service arrangements for both publicly funded and privately insured populations. However, managed care appears to limit access to specialists, including mental health specialists. Client, family, and system outcomes need to be maintained to see whether system and financing changes negatively affect quality of mental health services and outcomes.

Some research has reported that managed mental health care has been successful in achieving its goal of reducing inpatient hospitalization for both publicly funded and privately insured populations. An evaluation of a prepaid plan, carve-out approach implemented in Utah also has demonstrated reduced utilization of inpatient care. The Fort Bragg Demonstration Project resulted in significant shifts from inpatient to less restrictive outpatient mental health care with no decrements in mental health outcomes. Efforts in New York to develop a community-based, family-centered system of care cut inpatient utilization rates for children with serious emotional disturbance.

Further, managed care has been shown to reduce costs of mental health as well as general health care. Results from an evaluation of Massachusetts' carve-out approach yielded reduced costs, as did Utah's approach. A Government Accounting Office (1993) review of several states' managed Medicare approaches found reductions in cost. Additional evidence of cost savings has been collected by an evaluation of service system change in California. However, not all results have been positive.

There is general agreement that managed care has the potential to reduce and contain costs of care. Although some positive evidence indicates better access for managed health and mental health care, and scant results in general health care indicate comparable or improved quality in managed care, debate and suspicion regarding these assertions continues. For example, Miller (1996) claimed that evidence indicates the quality of outpatient mental health care suffers under managed care because of efforts to reduce costs by denying needed services and providing inadequate treatment (eg, by cutting long-term treatment for individuals with moderate to severe illness that may benefit from such treatment). Moreover, surveys of clinicians indicate that many are frustrated and dissatisfied with managed behavioral health care and that they feel that it negatively affects the quality of delivered care.

The uncertainty of the impact of managed care approaches on access to and quality of care is especially true in the public sector, where fewer evaluations have been conducted than for managed care approaches in the private sector. Investigations that have been conducted have demonstrated some success as well as areas of concern. For example, the evaluation of the Massachusetts approach highlighted that although costs were reduced, readmission rates and lengths of stays were higher, specifically for children and adolescents.

Clearly, more research is needed in order to examine how broad-based system reform affects the utilization, access, cost, quality, and outcome of mental health care. Attention should be given to conducting implementation studies to determine the nature and extent of reform efforts before impact assessments are conducted; to evaluating services and systems using a systems perspective; and to collecting both process and outcome data. In studies of publicly funded populations, additional investigation must be aimed at vulnerable populations such as children and adolescents. Although variability exists across state models of care (thereby making inferences more difficult), the differences in findings between studies of publicly funded and privately insured populations needs further investigation.

Finally, in prelude to the remainder of this chapter, the changing structure of the health care system can be expected to influence utilization, access, and cost, but there is strong doubt that system change alone can influence the effectiveness of mental health services.

Attkisson CC et al: Effectiveness of the California System of care model for children and youth with severe emotional disorder. In Nixon CT, Northrup DA (Eds): *Evaluating Mental Health Services: How Do Programs for Children "Work" in the Real World?* Sage, 1997.

Bickman L: A managed continuum of care: More is not better. Am Psychol 1996;51:689.

Callahan JJ et al: Mental health/substance abuse treatment in managed care: the Massachusetts Medicaid experience. Health Aff (Millwood) 1995;14:173.

Christianson et al: Utah's prepaid mental health plan: The first year. Health Affairs 1995;14:160.

Hoagwood K et al: Introduction to the special edition: efficacy and effectiveness studies of child and adolescent psychotherapy. J Consult Clin Psychol 1995;63:683.

Leff HS et al: The effects of capitation on service access, adequacy, and appropriateness. Admin Policy Ment Health 1994;21:141.

Mechanic D, Schlesinger M, McAlpine DD: Management of mental health and substance abuse services: state of the art and early results. Milbank Q 1995;73:19.

Miller JJ: Managed care is harmful to outpatient mental health services: A call for accountability. Professional Psychology: Research and Practice 1996;27:349.

Summerfelt WT, Foster EM, Saunders RC: Mental health services in a children's mental health managed care demonstration. J Ment Health Admin 1996;23:80.

UTILIZATION

Introduction

It has been estimated that 12–22% of children and adolescents have a diagnosable mental disorder, and some researchers suggest an increase in prevalence over recent years. The ECA study and the NCS estimated that 30% of adults will have a diagnosable mental illness in any given year and that as many as one out of every two adults will experience one or more disorders in their lifetime. Findings suggest that mental illness is widespread, often chronic, and highly comorbid; however, it is estimated that only a small proportion of those in need of services receive them. Studies of service utilization aim to describe what types of services are used, by whom, in what amount, and in what context.

Research Findings

Research has demonstrated substantial unmet mental health service needs. The Great Smoky Mountains Study of Youth (GSMS), a population-based community survey of youth, found that 20.3% of the surveyed youth had a diagnosable mental disorder, although this result did not include those adolescents with substantial impairment but no diagnosis. Generally, less than one third of those in need of services received them, and specifically, only 40% of adolescents with severe emotional disorder received services. Findings from the ECA study and the NCS illustrate an even gloomier picture for adults in terms of unmet mental health needs. According to these two studies, 70% to 79% (respectively by study) of adults with a disorder in the past 12 months reported that they had not received services. Barriers to service utilization that contribute to unmet needs are considered later in this chapter, in the section titled "Access."

Utilization research also has examined the service sectors, or settings in which services are obtained (eg, juvenile justice, education, child welfare, specialty mental health, and general medical care settings). Although not drawing from a nationally representative sample, the GSMS found that of the 19% of adolescents who received services in one or more than one sector, approximately 18% utilized services in specialty mental health settings, 85% in education settings, 11% in primary care, 2.5% in child welfare, and 7.6% in juvenile justice settings. Children with serious emotional disturbance tended to be served in multiple sectors, including specialty mental health settings, underscoring the importance of coordination across multiple sectors. A sad footnote to these findings is the relative dearth of research in settings outside specialty mental health, particularly in educational settings.

In contrast, research on adult utilization has demonstrated relatively more mental health service use in the general medical sector as compared to child and adolescent utilization findings. Nonpsychiatric physicians provide close to half of all mental health services. In fact, the trend is growing, attributed partially to increasing partnerships between primary care physicians and mental health professionals. Finally, in addition to general medical settings, the importance of informal voluntary support networks (eg, self-help groups, friends, relatives), which provide a significant proportion of services, is beginning to be acknowledged.

Utilization research also has investigated demographic variables as they relate to service use. Service utilization has been linked to education, marital status, race, distress, and insurance coverage. Additionally, education, income, and insurance coverage have predicted the length of outpatient treatment. Because of the importance of demographics, utilization research should incorporate a minimum standard data set including these variables.

System reform efforts of states and communities is ongoing. For example, CASSP principles that aim at improving access, limiting barriers, providing a continuum of care, and increasing coordination among service sectors motivate reform efforts for providing mental health services to children, adolescents, and their families. These and other broad-based reform efforts, such as state Medicaid reform, can be expected to change patterns of mental health service utilization. Utilization and de facto policy are influenced by insurance mechanisms that often undermine intended or de jure policy. Thus further research is needed to inform public policy and planning because inasmuch as aims of reform better address unmet mental health needs, they may increase service utilization. It is likely that these efforts will put further strain on limited financial and human resources.

Burns BJ, Friedman RM: Examining the research base for child mental health services and policy. J Ment Health Admin 1990;17:87.

Burns BJ et al: Children's mental health service use across service sectors. Health Aff (Millwood) 1995;14:147.

Fisher AJ et al: Correlates of unmet need for mental health services by children and adolescents. Psychol Med 1997;27:1145.

ACCESS

Introduction

Although there may be substantial disagreement about the way in which care is delivered, there is more agreement that everyone, regardless of financial status, should be entitled to some health care. Access to general health care as a public policy objective has been debated since the early 1900s. The enactment of Medicare and Medicaid in the mid-1960s greatly expanded health insurance coverage for certain populations. Limited federal initiatives addressed the provision of mental health services and indirectly improved access to mental health care. Such initiatives included the HMO Act and the Community Mental Health Center Act, amended in 1971 to specifically mandate the provision of mental health services for children and adolescents. Additionally, among the goals of managed care is to improve access to health and mental health care.

The findings reported in the "Utilization" section indicate that a substantial proportion of those individuals with a diagnosis or functional impairment do not report receiving mental health services. This discrepancy may be due to **individual barriers** such as personal economics, attitudes and beliefs, knowledge about services, family history of mental health problems, family support, stigma, or perceived need for services. Howard et al (1996) illustrated the potential pathway to mental health services by distinguishing between (1) intrapersonal decisions about the presence of a mental health problem and what to do about it and (2) interpersonal and external behaviors needed in order to overcome treatment barriers and enter into services. Further, the failure to receive services could be due to **system barriers,** such as inadequate transportation, limited service hours, unavailability of appropriate services, poor coordination of services, unhelpful staff, and restrictive eligibility criteria.

Access to mental health services for children and adolescents is more complicated. Parents often serve as additional gatekeepers by making decisions about the initiation or termination of services. A child's receipt of services depends not only on the child's willingness but also in part on the parent's perceived need for and ability to obtain services. Access can be increased by utilizing standardized screening for emotional, behavior, and substance abuse in children and adolescents, particularly those at high risk, such as children in foster care. For example, Halfon et al (1995) reported that only about 41% of foster parents of children demonstrating emotional, behavior, or developmental problems reported or were aware of the problems. Because children depend almost solely on their parents or primary caregivers to seek needed services, when access to needed services is not facilitated through alternative routes (eg, screening in primary care, schools, courts), children and adolescents will remain underserved.

Research Findings

Research has indicated that individual barriers to service utilization are more problematic than are system barriers. In the ECA study, 80% of the participants were very receptive to mental health services, but 83% perceived at least one barrier to receiving those services. Child and adolescent perceptions of services were critical as two of the most frequently perceived barriers to services. Both were related to the child's refusal to seek services. However, parents who previously had sought services reported more barriers than did those who had not recently used services. In contrast, families who subsequently had utilized school-based services reported fewer barriers. Ultimately, parent-reported barriers to access have been linked to lower utilization of services.

Issues of access have been particularly salient with the rapid growth of managed care and health care reform in general. A substantial body of literature claims positive findings. For example, the Fort Bragg Evaluation Project found that a continuum of care in North Carolina greatly increased access to mental health services for children and adolescents compared to more traditional services at the two control sites. In fact, access at the demonstration site increased more than threefold over a 5-year period, whereas access remained stable at the control sites.

Although some research has suggested fairly good availability of psychological services, particularly in larger HMOs, service utilization patterns and treatment patterns are likely to be influenced by capitation. For example, Glied (1997) found that women receiving mental health care within an HMO were more likely to see a primary care provider than a specialist. Moreover, when compared to fee-for-service providers, HMO providers were more likely to prescribe medication and less likely to recommend psychotherapy.

Concerns about inappropriate barriers to mental health services delivered within HMOs and managed behavioral health care have been raised partly because of the model of care in which the primary care physician is a gatekeeper. Usually, the approval of the patient's primary care physician is required for mental health services even though general practitioners and pediatricians often, and unfortunately, are not well-trained in mental health issues. Although roughly half of existing HMOs, for example, have some self-referral mechanism, patients often are not aware of these or how to access services. Problems limiting access include delays in scheduling nonemergency services, caps or limits on mental health coverage, patient copayments, and procedural difficulties in applying for psychological services.

Research has implied that managed behavioral health care may indeed enable better access to services, at least initially. However, mechanisms of managed care affect mainly system barriers to care, which may not be as important as individual barriers in determining access and service utilization.

Glied S: The treatment of women with mental health disorders under HMO and fee-for-service insurance. Women and Health 1997:26:1.
Halfon N, Mendonca A, Berkowitz G: Health status of children in foster care: the experience of the center for the vulnerable child. Arch Pediatr Adolesc Med 1995; 149:386.
Howard KI et al: Patterns of mental health service utilization. Arch Gen Psychiatry 1996;53:696.

COST

Introduction

Research regarding the costs of mental health services is linked directly to service utilization. Programs designed to alter utilization patterns are typically designed so that costs of services can be reduced while maintaining quality of services. This endeavor intrinsically examines the efficiency of services or delivery systems (ie, how costs relate to benefits). The estimation of costs and benefits depends on the accounting perspective chosen. These perspectives include buyers (ie, individual patients), insurers (ie, insurance companies, Medicaid, Medicare), and society at large. For example, from the patients' perspective, only resources that the individual pays out for treatment should be included in a tabulation of cost. These resources include out-of-pocket payments, lost wages due to treatment participation, and travel expenses. From the insurers' perspective, only direct reimbursements for services or expenditures should be included. From a societal perspective, all of the resources mentioned above would be included as well as communal costs such as the lost productivity of family members or the ultimate costs of not providing treatment to those in need.

Hence, when examining the costs, one's accounting perspective will determine the goods or services included as costs. Typically, in the analysis of social programs, it is difficult to identify and estimate costs from a societal perspective. Moreover, cost analyses seldom are conducted for the benefit of individual patients or families but rather for the agencies delivering services. This is especially true of publicly funded programs, where the cost to families is rather low. In light of these multiple perspectives, researchers have defined costs in two ways: the cost of mental illness and the cost of mental health treatment. The cost of treatment reflects a combination of the patient and insurer perspectives and considers only monies spent for mental health care. It includes costs of direct services (eg, the cost of an inpatient hospital stay or outpatient session) and indirect services (eg, family travel costs, missing work). The cost of mental illness reflects the societal perspective and considers the costs to society when an individual has a mental illness. These costs include lost productivity, the consumption of public resources, and the destruction of community property. Although both types of cost analyses are complex, cost of illness studies are much more difficult to conduct than are cost of treatment studies. As a result, cost of illness studies are rare and very expensive to execute.

Most studies on the costs of mental health services report the aggregate costs of mental illness, but they leave important questions unanswered. The primary problem is that because the estimates are pieced together from different data sources, there is no complete picture of the costs of mental illness for any given person. For example, in the children's field, juvenile justice costs are derived from one source and costs of inpatient psychiatric care from another. These different costs are combined only at the aggregate level.

These cost considerations have several important implications. First, aggregate estimates do not allow one to look at how total costs vary across individuals of different ages, diagnoses, or family background. Second, aggregate estimates do not allow one to look at the relationships among the different types of costs. For instance, one cannot examine the relationship between the direct and indirect costs of mental illness and how that relationship varies across settings. The receipt of mental health services may reduce costs in other areas; thus the costs of mental health services would actually be much lower than the direct expenditures associated with them. A narrow focus on the direct costs can produce a vastly different picture about the costs of mental health services and may lead to very different public policy options. Third, the fact that aggregate estimates are not based on a single sample of individuals further obscures information about the variation that exists across individuals. Costs may vary substantially over the course of an illness, and different interventions may produce different cost trajectories over time; however, yearly aggregate cost estimates will obscure these observations. If mental health services represent an investment in children, spending now may reduce costs later. In contrast, foregoing current expenditures may only shift costs into the future, where they will be borne by other members of society. The best information will be provided with data that follows individuals over time and offers information on diagnoses, family environment, and other characteristics.

Research Findings

The increase in the cost of health care from the 1970s has been astronomical. Health care costs rose from $90 billion in 1973 to $735 billion in 1991, and it is predicted that health care expenditures will total $1.5 trillion in the year 2000. Mental health and substance abuse treatment costs have risen at a rate exceeding those for any other insured conditions.

A broader understanding of the full costs of mental illness includes consideration of direct and indirect costs, including mortality and morbidity, beyond specialty mental health services alone. Family members of those with mental illness bear still other costs, for example, limiting a parent's ability to maintain an income.

Given the national environment of managed care, most current cost analyses concern the effects of financing of mental health services. A key determinant of who bears the costs of mental illness is the financial arrangement through which a family pays for mental health services. Unfortunately, there are gaps in our knowledge about the ways in which mental health services for children are financed and about the effect of financing on service utilization. Children and adolescents covered under more generous private insurance are reportedly more likely to use services and to use more services than are children and adolescents with less generous coverage. This was evident in the Fort Bragg Demonstration Project, in which access, utilization, and costs of services rose dramatically with the implementation of a no-copayment financing structure.

These studies, however, are rather limited. They have examined only families with private insurance and thus provide no means of comparing service utilization in uninsured families or in families with Medicaid. In addition, because prior studies do not examine services in all settings, they offer a narrow view of how families respond to financial incentives. These questions involve difficult methodological problems, most deriving from the fact that individuals are not assigned to insurance randomly. Because there is self-selection (ie, people choose insurance), factors other than insurance may determine their behavior.

Managed care is promoted as a powerful tool to increase cost-effectiveness, preventive care, and service quality. However, little research has examined the impact of managed care on actual costs, and the studies that have been undertaken have provided inconsistent findings. Whereas some researchers have reported little to no reductions in costs associated with managed care strategies, several evaluations have found evidence of cost savings as a result of incorporating a managed care approach. For instance, the California System of Care Model Evaluation Research Project, a longitudinal study initiated in 1989, sought, among other goals, to reduce California's group home utilization rate. Researchers (Attkinson et al, 1997) found that time-series analyses of data provided evidence of real cost savings attributable to the System of Care implementation for the demonstration counties in comparison to aggregate state expenditures. Another study (Goldman et al, 1998) found that an introduction of managed mental health care with a carve-out model resulted in a decrease in costs of over 40% that was maintained over a 6-year follow-up period. The cost reductions were not attributed to reductions in access. Rather, lower costs were associated with fewer outpatient sessions per patient, lower inpatient utilization, reduced inpatient lengths-of-stay, and lower costs per unit of service. Researchers also found evidence in Colorado of cost savings for managed care. Preliminary findings indicated decreased costs and probability of outpatient use under capitation as compared to fee-for-service. The researchers found no adverse changes in patient outcomes. Although inconsistent results have been observed, many researchers believe that managed care has the potential to reduce and contain health care costs.

Frank RG, McGuire TG: A review of studies of the impact of insurance on the demand and utilization of specialty mental health services. Health Serv Res 1986;21:241.
Goldman W, McCulloch J, Sturm R: Cost and use of mental health services before and after managed care. Health Aff (Millwood) 1998;17:40.

EFFECTIVENESS

Introduction

In the mental health services research field, a basic distinction has developed between the **efficacy** of an intervention and its **effectiveness.** Studies of the efficacy of an intervention examine the relationship between intervention processes and outcome under tightly controlled or optimal conditions. The investigator usually has substantial control over sample selection, the intervention, its delivery mechanisms, and the environmental setting. For example, randomized clinical trials (RCTs), often conducted within a university-based laboratory, are typically efficacy studies. In contrast, studies of effectiveness examine the impact of interventions in naturalistic settings or under average conditions of use. The researcher loses much of the control over factors such as sample selection, fidelity of services delivery, and choice of clinicians. Studies of effectiveness usually are conducted in real-world clinical settings (ie, schools, general medical settings, CMHCs, or HMOs).

One of the critical differences between the two types of studies is the trade-off between internal and external validity. **Internal validity** is the extent to which a causal linkage can be drawn between the intervention and the desired outcomes by ruling out alternative explanations of the observed effect (eg, maturation). The tighter the control held by the experimenter, the more likely he or she will be to rule out other explanations of observed change other than the studied intervention. **External validity** refers to the likelihood that the results observed in one investigation would be repeated, or would generalize, to other settings, samples, or times. Real-world delivery

of interventions tends to include heterogeneity in the patient population, the services, and the environmental context in which they are delivered. According to Cronbach et al (1980), evaluation has placed too high an emphasis on internal validity. Furthermore, threats to external validity always are present, and attempts to control them lead to the evaluation of the intervention in an artificial setting, nothing like the setting for which the intervention was intended.

As mentioned earlier in this chapter, effectiveness research is the ultimate goal of services research, although both types of research are ultimately important. The following five-phase model (Haywood et al, 1995) serves as a basic, yet ideal, framework for conducting research: (1) hypothesis development; (2) methods/instrumentation development and refinement; (3) controlled intervention trials such as RCTs; (4) defined population studies in which subgroups of the population are studied; and (5) demonstration and implementation studies that examine the transfer of efficacious interventions to more applied settings. Studies that follow this model are studies of effectiveness.

Research Findings

A plethora of efficacy studies of psychological treatments and services (primarily psychotherapy) have been carried out in both the adult and the children's mental health fields. Many of the individual studies have failed to demonstrate significant effects because of a number of possible causes (including methodological problems or the possibility that the treatment simply was not effective); however, meta-analytic reviews have produced "stark, dramatic patterns of evidence for the general efficacy of such treatment" (Lipsey and Wilson 1993, p. 1182). Several meta-analyses have indicated that children and adolescents who receive some form of mental health intervention function better than those in control conditions. Lipsey and Wilson concluded that "well developed psychological, educational, and behavioral treatments generally have meaningful effects on the intended outcome variables" (1993, p. 1199). Lambert and Bergin (1994) concluded that psychotherapy was effective for adults, more so than placebo interventions, and that gains were maintained for extended periods. Finally, many psychopharmacologic studies have demonstrated efficacy under controlled conditions.

Efficacy research of psychological interventions compares favorably to similar research in general health care. In 1985, the Office of Technology Assessment estimated that only 10–20% of medical practices had demonstrated medical efficacy by RCTs. Moreover, treatment effect sizes for psychological interventions are generally as large as many found in general health care.

Relative to the number of efficacy studies, few studies have examined the effectiveness of mental health interventions or services, particularly in regard to children. More investigations of this type are greatly needed. The effectiveness research that has been conducted has focused primarily on system-level variables (eg, administrative and financing structures, service coordination, access, utilization) with little investigation of clinical outcome and specific mental health treatments. According to Henggeler et al (1994, p. 230)

> the dearth of clinical outcome data in the services research literature raises the frightening possibility that evidence of increased access and variety of services may be construed as a proxy for quality and effectiveness of clinical services rendered.

The majority of studies that have examined the effectiveness of mental health services have not demonstrated a general link between the intervention studied and improved clinical outcome for children or for adults. For example, the Fort Bragg Evaluation Project found that children in a continuum of care had increased access to the appropriate services compared to children at the control sites who received traditional inpatient and outpatient services only. Both the experimental and control groups improved but equally as much: The clinical and family outcomes did not differ between the two groups. The findings of the Fort Bragg study were replicated in a randomized effectiveness study of publicly funded children and adolescents. A multisite Robert Wood Johnson Foundation project did not find a relationship between system changes and clinical outcome for the seriously mentally ill adults who were served. However, other researchers have obtained promising results demonstrating the potential effectiveness and cost impact of assertive community treatment for adults with severe emotional illness and multisystemic therapy for adolescents with serious emotional disturbance.

The 39 studies included in Speer and Newman's (1996) review of outcome evaluations of community support services for adults with persistent and severe mental illness varied tremendously in research designs, patient groups, and outcome measures. According to the reviewers, "the findings of these studies should in no way be interpreted as reflecting the effectiveness of community-based mental health services in general" (p. 123). However, approximately half of the studies had positive or mixed findings (ie, positive findings on at least one measure, no or negative results on others). Seven studies reported no-difference effects, and four reported negative effects for the intervention. The authors asserted that (1) many of the studies had inadequate power to detect treatment effects due to insufficient sample sizes, and (2) many suffered from follow-up patient attrition that can bias outcome evaluation results, but (3) research design weakness did not seem to play a part in null findings. The reviewers emphasized the critical need

for clinicians to collect outcome measures in order to develop knowledge regarding intervention effectiveness that will contribute to policy-making decisions in the future.

Some researchers have proposed potential explanations that might account for the differences in findings between efficacy and effectiveness studies. Similarly, several other researchers have discussed possible methodological reasons for failing to detect a statistically significant impact of services. One possible reason for the difference in clinical findings between efficacy and effectiveness studies is the yet untested belief that practitioners are not using treatments that have been found to be effective. Because of this strong possibility, professional societies are developing treatment guidelines that reflect the findings from these efficacy studies. However, it remains to be determined whether these techniques can be transferred to the real world and whether practitioners will adopt them.

More attention needs to be devoted to conducting well-designed effectiveness studies that have methodological advantages rather than obstacles to overcome (eg, small sample sizes, poor theoretical framework, inappropriate instrumentation) in order to bridge the gap between positive efficacy and null effectiveness findings. Research is needed that examines the components or specific processes within an intervention in order to determine those that are the most effective and under what circumstances.

Bickman L: Designing outcome evaluations for children's mental health services: improving internal validity. New Directions for Program Evaluation 1992;54:57.

Cronbach LJ et al: *Toward Reform of Program Evaluation.* Jossey-Bass, 1980.

Henggeler SW et al: The contribution of treatment outcome research to the reform of children's mental health services: multisystemic therapy as an example. J Ment Health Admin 1994;21:229.

Lambert MJ, Bergin AE: The effectiveness of psychotherapy. Pages 143–189 in: Bergin AE, Garfield SL (editors): *Handbook of Psychotherapy and Behavior Change,* 4th ed. John Wiley & Sons, 1994.

Lipsey MW, Wilson DB: The efficacy of psychological, educational, and behavioral treatment: Confirmation from meta-analysis. Am Psychol 1993;48:1181

Padgett DK et al: Ethnic differences in use of inpatient mental health services by blacks, whites, and Hispanics in a national insured population. Health Serv Res 1994; 29:135.

Speer DC, Newman FL: Mental health services outcome evaluation. Clinical Psychology: Science and Practice 1996;3:105.

Weisz JR et al: Effectiveness of psychotherapy with children and adolescents: a meta-analysis for clinicians. J Consult Clin Psychol 1987;55:542.

Weisz JR et al: The lab versus the clinics: effects of child and adolescent psychotherapy. Am Psychol 1992; 47:1578.

Weisz JR et al: Bridging the gap between laboratory and clinic in child and adolescent psychotherapy. J Consult Clin Psychol 1995;63:688.

QUALITY

Introduction

The quality of health and mental health care has received renewed attention since the mid-1980s. There has been increasing emphasis on accountability and routine monitoring of access to and the quality of health and mental health care delivered by clinicians and health plans. Many of the factors discussed earlier in this chapter—skyrocketing costs, changes in reimbursement strategies, including capitation and prospective payment systems, and recent health care reform efforts—have contributed to a renewed surge of concern about the quality of services.

The focus on quality of care is not new. Early emphasis on quality, beginning as early as the 1900s, was primarily self-imposed by professional organizations in regard to the education of physicians or hospital performance. More recently, emphasis on quality has buttressed the marketing of hospital services as well as the development and dissemination of practice guidelines in order to shape physician behavior. Current efforts have focused on making information about quality of health care more user friendly and accessible to patients. This latest trend emphasizes influencing the quality of services through market competition rather than by externally imposed standards and criteria (eg, practice guidelines, external peer or utilization review).

The advent and growth of managed mental health care has caused concern about the resulting quality of services, particularly if reduction in health care costs is a prime focus. Although most of the evidence for equal or improved quality in managed care versus fee-for-service care comes from general health care, there is reason to hypothesize that managed care will lead to better quality in mental health services. For example, managed care organizations usually offer a fuller array of services—including case management and wrap-around services—that could theoretically lead to benefits such as increased continuity of care. Further, it has been predicted that the cost of mental health services will eventually level off, thereby forcing managed care companies to compete on the quality of services alone. However, others have expressed much concern about the quality of managed mental health services.

Currently, several related, more specific issues have sparked the attention of researchers. These issues include: (1) the definition and conceptualization of quality, (2) stakeholder evaluation of quality, and (3) the validation of indicators of quality.

Definition & Conceptualization of Quality

The manner in which quality is defined has always been a source of debate. Yet the definition of quality is critical in that it leads directly to the assessment of and efforts to improve quality of care. Both the conceptualization and the measurement of quality should be clinically relevant as well as useful for stakeholders including patients, policy makers, researchers, and program evaluators.

Numerous definitions of quality have been offered. Much of the discussion of quality in the field today revolves around Donabedian's tripartite model of quality—structure, process, and outcome—as well as his distinction between technical and interpersonal care. Similar in many respects to definitions offered by others, Menninger (1977, p. 476) defined quality as:

> the goodness of fit between the problem requiring therapeutic attention; the desired outcome (the goal or purpose of treatment); the treatment used, as sensed or experienced by the patient, as judged by the physician and his colleagues, and as verified by outcome studies.

Definitions of quality generally portray it as consisting of multiple domains or components. Most definitions emphasize quality in terms of outcome. That is, the criterion for determining quality is the extent to which care improves desired outcomes. Moreover, many definitions address process, although indirectly. Process is the "black box," so to speak, detailing the components of a specific intervention or service.

Typically, the inconsistencies between various definitions of quality arise primarily as a result of differences in level of concern (eg, patient-level versus systems-level) and perspective (eg, patient, clinician, insurer). Additionally, definitions of quality may be invoked for a variety of purposes (eg, research, evaluation of program effectiveness, accountability to funding agencies, internal process reviews) and thus may emphasize different aspects of structure, process, and outcome.

Stakeholder Evaluation of Quality

With the increasing push to control the quality of health services through market competition, more recent research has focused on assessing quality of care from the viewpoint of different stakeholders, particularly consumers of health services, rather than from the traditional clinician viewpoint. Stakeholders should be broadly defined to include all those whose lives are affected by programs, services, and the evaluation of those services. Thus individuals who have a stake in mental health services include (but are not limited to) the following: (1) policymakers, at federal, state, and local levels; (2) practitioners, acknowledging differences among professionals in educational training and contact with patients; (3) administrators, including managed care professionals, upper-level managers at care facilities, and purchasers; and (4) patients, again including and acknowledging potential differences in perceptions among patients, their family members, and members of the general public who are not currently receiving services. Following the lead of researchers in evaluation and systems theorists, the best picture of quality may be gleaned from the input of multiple stakeholders, each experiencing different parts of the service system. Input from multiple stakeholders in the evaluation of quality increases the chance that the ultimate goal of improving the quality of care will be realized by increasing the validity, fairness, range, and responsiveness of the information upon which program decisions are based.

Research typically has not included all relevant stakeholders in the study of quality of care and thus has not incorporated a true systems framework. The vast majority of efforts examine only one or two perspectives simultaneously, usually the views of patients and physicians, and exclude other groups such as policy makers, purchasers, administrators, and the general public (ie, non–service users). Most research has addressed quality of health and mental health care indirectly by exploring stakeholders' views of physician or clinic performance or by investigating patient satisfaction.

Recent research has explored patients' desire for, understanding of, and use of disseminated information on quality. In 1994, a multistakeholder conference including patients, families, clinicians, managed care representatives, and insurers among others was convened by the National Alliance for the Mentally Ill (NAMI), John Hopkins University, and NIMH. More theoretically based work is beginning to appear in the literature. This work promotes a multiperspective view of service quality, but much work remains to be done. The Fort Bragg Evaluation Project used a formalized brainstorming technique, called concept mapping, to allow various stakeholder groups to define the key elements of quality in that mental health service delivery system. Key elements were given operational definitions and measured by various stakeholders as part of the assessment of the quality of services delivered within the program.

Validation of Indications/ Indicators of Quality

In the history of quality assessment, most research has focused on the process of care, particularly the technical rather than interpersonal aspects of care. The pendulum has recently swung heavily toward outcome while generally remaining focused on technical aspects of care. Quality improvement techniques have included peer review, accreditation, patient-oriented report cards, and practice standards or guidelines. However, the indicators of quality have not, for the most part, been validated empirically. In other words, traditional research methodology has not been used to demonstrate the necessary linkages between structural or process indicators of quality and desired outcomes, thus demonstrating criterion-related validity. Furthermore, assessments of quality often have inadequate content validity because too few indicators have been used to cover the construct of quality. For example, mortality or readmission rates are taken to

represent quality, even though these measures are quite limited and represent only a small piece of the quality picture. The field is in dire need of more research aimed at establishing the reliability and validity of indicators thought to measure quality of care.

Donabedian A: *Explorations in Quality Assessment and Monitoring: The Definition of Quality and Approaches to Its Assessment.* Michigan Health Administration, 1980.

Menninger KW: What is quality care? Am J Orthopsychiatry 1977;47:476.

Nash D: Quality and utilization management: the cutting edge for 2000. Presentation at the American Managed Care and Review Associations Quality and Utilization Management Conference, Nashville, TN, October 1995.

Salzer MS et al: Validating quality indicators: quality as a relationship between, structure, and outcome. Evaluation Review 1997;21:292.

IMPLICATIONS FOR FUTURE RESEARCH

Mental health services research is still in its infancy. Much work is yet to be done, particularly in light of health care reforms expected to have a substantial effect on many of the issues discussed in this chapter.

POLICY & SERVICE DELIVERY ISSUES

Current goals of community service delivery (eg, treatment in the least restrictive environment, continuity of care, provision of a continuum of care) tend to be inconsistent with current financing and reimbursement practices. Third-party payers have been resistant to reimbursement for ambulatory services and often have placed arbitrary limits on outpatient reimbursement. Attention to the deficiencies in current research, including a scarcity of community-based effectiveness studies, may help to bring parity in resources to mental health services and research. Financing and reimbursement, however, are only part of the dilemma. Implementing systems of care requires strong leadership and increased interagency communication and coordination.

In light of figures indicating substantial unmet needs, limited access to mental health services, and the need to control costs while maintaining quality of care, the use of paraprofessionals and nonprofessionals in service delivery has received renewed attention. Interventions offering promise of effectiveness, such as assertive community treatment and multisystemic therapy, are typically delivered by nondoctoral-level mental health providers. Even as the states are assuming a more prominent role in the financing of CMHCs and mental health care in general, the employment and patient-care responsibility of psychiatrists in CMHCs has decreased. The recruitment and training of additional service providers for innovative service delivery, with psychiatrists and psychologists serving as expert consultants, directors, or supervisors, may be an effective method of addressing unmet mental health needs. Although most research has revealed bias in the views of some professionals in their opinions of self-help groups or service delivery by non-professionals, there is growing emphasis and involvement of consumers and family members in service delivery and in service evaluation efforts. For instance, family members are more often being employed in care coordination and patient advocacy roles at provider sites. Further, evaluators are more often hiring consumers and family members to collect patient data or to cofacilitate focus groups.

The process of defining current policies in health and mental health is largely political, reflecting the agglomerations of advocacy strength and professional coordination; thus more emphasis should be placed on building a strong constituency across professions and interests as well as with consumer and family advocacy groups. This is particularly true in the new age of managed health care that is driven in large part by profit.

Because mental health services remain primarily supported by categorical funding streams, interagency coordination continues to be a system-level problem with potential negative consequences at the patient and family levels. States and local governments need to incorporate, into managed care contracts, incentives for interagency coordination, and agencies need to forge interagency agreements.

SERVICES RESEARCH ISSUES

Current Limitations

Several factors limit evaluation and thus its contributions to service delivery and effective policy. First, there is a paucity of longitudinal funding that allows sufficient start-up time for the development, implementation, and stabilization of the interventions, services, and systems being studied. Research agencies, among others, often underestimate the amount of time needed to realize significant improvement in outcome; thus research projects may be of insufficient duration.

Second, although the array of funding mechanisms is broadening, fundamental biases exist in the way proposals for extramural funding are reviewed. For example, with the current shift to results-based accountability, there are pressures to avoid efforts that pose measurement difficulties and do not promise quick results. Also, research agencies often prefer traditional scientific research methods, emphasizing, for example, strong internal validity and low risk of false-positive errors, contrary to the views of Cronbach et al

discussed earlier in this chapter. The result is cookie-cutter evaluations with little innovative or informative value.

Third, partly because of some of these pressures, researchers falter and fail to conduct research informed by the problems of applied research documented in the literature. Too often, warnings described in the scientific literature are overlooked because funding allows too little time or too few resources. In order to further the field, researchers must be innovative and creative by drawing from a broader range of methodologies and increasing stakeholder involvement in the research process in order to overcome the problems discussed in this chapter and elsewhere.

Research Needs

The construction of a solid base of knowledge regarding the effectiveness of interventions provided in the community will promote parity in economic resource allocations for mental health services. It is incumbent on the mental health field to support outcome evaluations that examine what works best for whom and under what circumstances. For instance, researchers must establish the conditions under which patients need and can benefit from longer-term interventions. In order to overcome the shortcomings of traditional mental health services, clinicians and researchers must collaborate to develop interventions and services that address the multidimensional nature of mental illness within patients' natural environments. Research is needed to inform public policy regarding alternative modes of treatment, the training of alternative service providers and paraprofessionals, the relative effectiveness of various treatment modalities (and combinations of treatment), and the impact of social helping networks. Research synthesis methods (eg, meta-analyses) have grown since the late 1980s or so and provide a critical tool for assessing the effectiveness of psychological interventions. Unfortunately, funding for such efforts often is inadequate.

Micro-level examinations of interventions (eg, RCTs) must be united with macro-level (or service system) research drawing on a systems framework that addresses how the separate components of the service system fit together most effectively. Some researchers have pointed to the lack of research on traditional clinical interventions and have advocated for the use of RCTs in order to investigate the effectiveness of services. Research on specific interventions is needed to address potential interaction effects and to broaden the picture of which specific components within the "black box" are related to outcome. However, the establishment of intervention efficacy, as we have already seen, is no guarantee of its effectiveness in community-based settings or within the context of a system of care. Thus controlled studies of interventions in natural settings are critically needed. Real-world contexts often involve barriers to access and treatment, such as a politicized environment, competition between professionals, poor communication, and professional ignorance. In order to accomplish these goals, there must be better cooperation among researchers, practitioners, and managed care companies. Managed care companies should take responsibility for supporting research and development rather than the federal government being solely responsible for funding research in this field.

Some evaluators have referred to many micro-level efforts as self-defeating and have emphasized the need to test the impact of the entire system. Such research is consistent with systems thinking, according to which the service system will have a synergy of its own, not defined or understood by the parts taken alone. Chelimsky has questioned how we can expect such findings to have a large impact on public policy when the fundamental link between an intervention and its putative effect has not been established. Rather than arguing the relative merits of research focusing on different levels of services, the limitations of each type of research should be acknowledged. Micro-level studies can inform authorities in the development and implementation of programs and system-reform ef-

forts, and macro-level systems research can address the effectiveness of system-level reform.

CONCLUSION

Mental health services research is a new and growing area in mental health. Services research addresses questions that are significant to all stakeholders, including patients, clinicians, and policy makers: What are the best ways to assure access to services? How can we best describe the treatments that patients receive? Which treatments are most effective with which types of patients? What are the best ways to affect clinician practices? These are all questions posed by services researchers. In this chapter we have noted that we do not know the answers to these questions. We have also described the political and methodologic difficulties encountered in trying to answer them. If we are to achieve any real progress in serving those who need services, then we need to answer these and similar questions with well-designed research.

Section II.
Techniques & Settings

Psychiatric Interview*

8

Barry Nurcombe, MD, Harry E. Gwirtsman, MD, & Michael H. Ebert, MD

Human behavior is multifaceted and complex. When it becomes dysfunctional because of environmental stressors or brain disease it can be mysterious and frustrating to the inexperienced clinician who must master the tasks of diagnosis and management. This is especially true of neurobehavioral disorders, which involve organically related changes in cognitive or emotional behavior that appear to fall between the boundaries of psychiatry and neurology. The clinician needs to be able to appreciate and assess the signs and symptoms of these neurobehavioral disorders with the same discernment as the more traditional physical syndromes, such as myocardial infarction or common infections.

In this chapter we discuss the psychiatric history and the mental status examination (MSE), in the context of conducting an effective psychiatric interview. We explain the steps of the interview process and describe techniques that the clinician must master in order to elicit in an orderly and complete fashion information relevant to the psychiatric history. We describe the components of the psychiatric history and the MSE in our discussion of the specific interview stage during which they would normally be obtained.

What can be achieved at the initial psychiatric interview? The outcome depends on the situation in which it is conducted and what the physician and the patient are seeking. For example, a brisk, focused interview in an emergency room contrasts with the more extensive survey appropriate to an outpatient clinic. These types of interview differ from what is possible at the bedside of a patient who is severely ill in a medical or surgical ward. Despite these observations, fundamental issues can be addressed to varying degree in any clinical situation, as illustrated in Table 8–1. We

return to these issues in our discussion of the elements of the psychiatric history.

STAGES OF THE PSYCHIATRIC INTERVIEW

INCEPTION

If the interviewer works in a clinic, at the opening of the psychiatric interview he or she goes to the waiting room, introduces himself or herself to the patient, accompanies the patient to the interview room, and shows him or her to a seat. After taking identifying data from the patient, the interviewer can tell the patient what he or she already knows. This approach avoids unnecessary mysteries and clears the way for action. Consider the following example:

Psychiatrist: Your parents came to see me yesterday. They told me they're worried because your schoolwork has fallen off, although you've always been a good student; you've dropped most of your friends; and you seem to have become depressed. Last week they found one of your assignments in which you spoke about suicide. They think you may need help for an emotional problem.

Table 8–1. Issues to be addressed in the psychiatric interview.

Chronology of events and development of symptoms; subjective concerns of the patient; and concerns of patient's family, friends, neighbors, or employers
Insight, judgment, and motivation for treatment
Precipitation of illness and relevant stressors
Predisposition and family history of psychiatric illness
Presentation
Previous psychiatric illness and behavioral problems
Previous psychiatric treatment and/or mental health intervention

* Some of this material also appears in Nurcombe B, Gallagher RM: *The Clinical Process in Psychiatry: Diagnosis and Management Planning.* Cambridge University Press, 1986. Reprinted with the permission of Cambridge University Press.

Patient (a 16-year-old boy): So?
Psychiatrist: So they asked you to see a psychiatrist. I get the impression you're not too happy about that.
Patient: No.
Psychiatrist: Maybe we can start by you telling me how you feel about it.

Interviews are not always conducted in an office; they may be transacted beside a patient's bed, or between pieces of equipment in the examination room of an emergency clinic, or even while driving a car. Wherever they occur they include a pattern to the beginning, a certain formality. The interviewer introduces himself or herself, says why he or she is there, and invites the patient to respond by telling his or her story. If the patient doesn't want to do so, the interviewer helps the patient to explain why.

RECONNAISSANCE

The interviewer helps the patient tell his or her story as spontaneously as possible. He or she listens and does not interrupt any more than is necessary to keep the story flowing. The interviewer does not rush the reconnaissance nor try to direct it prematurely. If all the interviewer does is ask questions, all he or she will get is answers. Open-ended probes should be used as much as possible. The more leading the probe, the less valid the response, unless the issue in question is a simple, unequivocal one. The facilitating techniques we describe later in this chapter are particularly appropriate for the reconnaissance stage.

DETAILED INQUIRY

After the patient has finished his or her story, the interviewer seeks further information about the present illness, past illness, medical history, early environment, education, and other relevant matters from the psychiatric history. A full detailed inquiry will take several interviews, but a scanning of the features most important for a provisional diagnosis can be completed within an hour.

Table 8–2 lists the content of the psychiatric history. The order suggested in the table should not be followed blindly. The interviewer should be prepared to deal with topics in whatever sequence is natural. Some areas will be emphasized and others pursued in less detail, as different cases demand.

Detailed inquiry involves questioning, but the questions are kept as open ended as possible at the outset. They move from general to specific as more detail is required. Compare the following questions:

- How are things in your marriage?
- How are things between you and your wife?
- How do you and your wife get on?

Table 8–2. Content of the psychiatric history.

Identifying data
Presenting problem
History of present illness
History of past psychiatric illnesses
Medical history
History of drug or alcohol intake or of antisocial behavior
Early development and childhood environment
Educational history
Vocational history
Family history
Sexual history
Marital history
Characteristic coping mechanisms, values, ideals, aspirations

- Is your marriage a happy one?
- Do you love your wife?

This approach is similar to the way a surgeon approaches a guarded section of a painful abdomen: from the outside in. Direct questions provoke circumscribed responses and are most appropriate to issues of fact (eg, What year were you married?).

Some issues are left to a later time after a therapeutic alliance has developed. Unless the patient presents his or her sexual life as a problem at the outset, an exploration of this area is usually postponed.

1. TRANSITIONS

The interviewer never moves abruptly from one topic to another. Change should be signaled. For example, the psychiatrist could say, "Okay. I'd like to go on from there to something else. Could you tell me about the jobs you've had? What did you do after you left school?"

2. ROUTINE VERSUS DISCRETIONARY INQUIRY

Part of the detailed inquiry is routine, including questions obligatory for patients of a given age, in a specific clinical situation, or as part of a minimum database. The components of a routine inquiry should be defined in each clinical setting. The rest of the detailed inquiry is largely discretionary and involves the eliciting of evidence supporting or refuting the diagnostic hypotheses generated after reconnaissance.

3. ELEMENTS OF THE PSYCHIATRIC HISTORY

We now discuss the components of the psychiatric history, which are shown in Table 8–1. Each issue addressed in Table 8–1 must be addressed and the information related to one of the categories shown in Table 8–2.

The Present Illness

It is important to delineate the present illness, the episode for which the patient is seeking help. In some patients it is difficult to draw the line between the present episode and a much longer pattern of pathologic behavior or chronic illness resulting from external circumstances. A successful psychiatric history serves as a guide for diagnosis, intervention, and treatment. To this end, it is useful to define the present episode with its precipitants and then determine whether the present episode constitutes a discrete psychiatric illness or is an episode of a more chronic psychiatric illness that can then be documented chronologically.

Some patients may present a variety of subjective concerns. Others may have a more focused complaint and identify specific issues as problems. Whatever the problem(s) for which the patient or his or her associates seek help, the clinician attempts to delineate them; to understand how the patient experiences them; and to ascertain their duration, onset, development, and persistence.

Precipitation of Illness & Relevant Stressors

If the problems had an onset, the interviewer attempts to determine whether the patient experienced physical or psychosocial stress at that time. The mere coincidence of stress and the onset of pathologic behavior does not substantiate a causal association; causation may remain speculative in some cases. It is supported, however, if the patient previously had a breakdown when exposed to a similar stress or if the patient's account of the stress indicates its personal significance.

Some stressors have universal impact. Others are highly idiosyncratic, and painstaking work may be required before they are unraveled in psychotherapy. In some cases it is an open question whether an event was a precipitant, the result of a disorder in its early stages, or mere coincidence.

Previous Psychiatric Illness & Behavioral Problems

The interviewer considers the following questions in evaluating the patient for previous psychiatric illness and behavioral problems: Has the patient had any problems of a similar nature in the past? What precipitated them, if anything? Has the patient had any other emotional disorders or physical symptoms related to tension? Has the patient had, or does he or she have, physical or neurologic disease that could contribute to the present problem? Does the patient have, or has he or she had, personal habits (eg, substance abuse) that could cause, precipitate, or complicate the present problem?

Previous Psychiatric Treatment & Mental Health Intervention

The interviewer should be aware of any therapeutic interventions that occurred before the current evaluation. This includes formal psychiatric treatment (or treatment by another mental health professional), emergency evaluations, hospitalizations, or mental health treatment rendered by a primary care physician. The clinician who carried out the treatment and the treating facility should be identified, as should the approximate date(s) and duration of treatment. The patient's response to each pharmacologic agent and associated side effects should be documented. Type, duration, and results of psychotherapy should be identified. The interviewer will need to amplify and verify some of this information by requesting records from previous treating professionals and facilities, with appropriate written consent from the patient.

Predisposition & Potentials

The interviewer considers the following questions in evaluating the patient for predisposition to and family history of psychiatric illness: What kind of person was the patient before he or she became ill? What biopsychosocial strengths and weaknesses predisposed the patient to breakdown? These questions require a comprehensive evaluation, and it is unrealistic to expect all of this information to be elaborated in a single interview. Important pieces of the jigsaw puzzle are usually lying around, if the interviewer keeps his or her eyes and ears open. The interviewer can ask the following additional questions: What personal and environmental strengths, resources, and liabilities are apparent at the present time? What has the patient got going for him or her now? What holds the patient back? What hurdles does he or she face? This too requires a full inventory of the patient's physical, intellectual, emotional, and social assets and deficiencies. This inventory is crucial to the design of an individualized plan of management.

Presentation

The interviewer considers the following questions in evaluating the patient's current presentation for treatment: Why does the patient seek help now? Is the patient being seen at the onset of a disorder or later, either when a relatively defined pattern of symptoms has developed or after the patient has recovered partially but remains troubled by residual difficulties? Did the patient come of his or her own accord, or was he or she persuaded to do so? Did others bring in the patient for treatment? Why?

Insight, Judgment, & Motivation for Treatment

The interviewer considers the following questions in evaluating the patient's insight, judgment, and motivation for treatment: Does the patient think he or she is unwell? Does the patient think he or she has been referred inappropriately? The patient may be correct. If the patient recognizes his or her own disturbance, does he or she have any idea of its nature or cause? How realistic are these notions?

What kind of help does the patient seek, if any? Is this in line with what is advisable, appropriate, or feasible? Is the patient troubled by doubts concerning his or her problem and the kind of treatment he or she will receive? Fears of craziness or of exotic psychiatric treatments are likely to be inflamed by deep-seated anxieties about helplessness and victimization. These fears are often aggravated by images derived from family or cultural values, including those depicted in the media. It is better that such concerns be expressed as soon as possible and corrected when they are the result of misinformation.

4. MENTAL STATUS EXAMINATION: CONTEXT, PURPOSE, & FORMAT

The MSE is a set of systematic observations and assessments undertaken by a diagnostician during the clinical interview. Properly conducted, the MSE provides a detailed and systematic description of the patient at that time, information essential to the consolidation of those patterns of clues and inferences that are required for the generation of diagnostic hypotheses. The MSE, guided by the hypothetico-deductive approach to diagnosis, is an essential part of the subsequent inquiry plan. In this section we offer a comprehensive description of the components of the MSE. In regard to a particular patient—and in accordance with the clinical context, background information, and psychiatric history—the interviewer will apply the MSE tactically, pursuing brief, comprehensive, or discretionary lines of inquiry, as warranted.

The Need for Standardization

Because the MSE, like the psychiatric history, should involve routine and discretionary lines of inquiry according to the diagnostic hypotheses being entertained, it should not be standardized as a whole. Instead the separate observations and assessments that compose the MSE should be standardized. The techniques of eliciting data should be formalized, the phenomena in question clearly defined, and the weight to be placed on each phenomenon clarified.

Reliability

The **reliability** of a test refers to the likelihood (usually expressed as a correlation) that similar results will be obtained on retesting (**test-retest reliability**) or that similar results will be obtained by different observers (**interrater reliability**). Test-retest reliability applies to relatively stable characteristics such as the use of language; it is not to be expected in characteristics (eg, mood) that are changeable and often linked to a current situation.

When psychiatrists test for the patient's abstracting ability, for example, by asking the patient to explain proverbs in his or her own words, how certain can the psychiatrist be that the clinical test is a true measure of the ability in question? In other words, what is the **validity** of the test? Over the years a set of informal mental state assessments has accumulated, but in some instances their validity is questionable. When we describe any clinical test in this chapter, we will consider its validity along with the mental faculties required for adequate performance on the test.

Types of Mental Status Examinations

A. Brief Screening Mental Status Examination: When a patient has been referred to an ambulatory clinic for a situational or personality problem, and none of the indications for a comprehensive screening examination pertain (see next section), a brief, informal screen is sufficient. The brief screening MSE is completed during the inception, reconnaissance, and detailed inquiry stages of the psychiatric interview. In particular, the interviewer notes the patient's general appearance, motor behavior, quality of speech, relationship to the interviewer, and mood. From the patient's demeanor, conversation, and history, the interviewer makes inferences about consciousness, orientation, attention, grasp, memory, fund of information, general intellectual level, language competence, and thought process. Abnormal thought content is not investigated unless clinical clues indicate the need for such discretionary inquiry (eg, into hallucinations, obsessions, depersonalization). Physiologic function (eg, sleep, appetite, libido, menstrual cycle, energy level) and insight should always be assessed.

B. Comprehensive Screening Mental Status Examination: The interviewer should be alerted to the need for a comprehensive screening MSE whenever there is a reasonable possibility that the patient has psychosis or primary or secondary brain dysfunction. Table 8–3 summarizes the settings and clues that mandate a comprehensive MSE. If the clinician has any doubts, the comprehensive screen should be completed.

Components of the Mental Status Examination

Table 8–4 summarizes the areas to be covered in the MSE. The following sections describe these areas in more detail:

A. Appearance & Behavior: From the moment the interviewer first greets the patient, he or she will be aware of the patient's appearance. The interviewer should try to describe it in detail before drawing inferences from it. What is the patient's physique and habitus? Is there evidence of weight loss or gain? Does the patient have any conspicuous marks or disfigurement? The interviewer should describe the patient's face and hair. Does the patient look ill? What is the expression of the eyes and mouth? Does the patient appear to be in touch with the surroundings? Is the patient clean and neat, or does he or she exhibit

Table 8–3. Indications for a comprehensive screening mental status examination.

The patient is seen in a hospital emergency room or crisis clinic; is being managed on a nonpsychiatric ward and has been referred for consultation; or is being admitted to a psychiatric unit.
The patient is over age 40 years.
The patient has a history of psychiatric disorder, substance abuse, organic brain disorder, or physical disorder that could affect brain function.
The patient's personal habits, memory, concentration, or grasp have deteriorated recently.
The patient or other informant presents clinical clues that suggest current mood disorder, psychosis, or organic brain dysfunction (eg, persistent or intermittent depression, withdrawal, elation, overactivity, bizarre ideation, hallucinations, delusions, ideas of influence and reference, headaches, loss of memory and grasp, disorientation, disordered language, headaches, seizures, motor weakness, tremor, or sensory loss).
Physical examination indicates or suggests brain dysfunction.
In forensic referrals, when mental competence or legal insanity are in question.

deficiencies in personal hygiene revealed by poor grooming of the skin, hair, or nails? How is the patient dressed? Is the patient's clothing neat? Is it appropriate or peculiar? After the interviewer describes these characteristics, he or she determines whether an inference may be made about the kind of "statement" the patient is attempting to make with his or her attire.

The interviewer notes general overactivity or underactivity; abnormalities of posture; gross incoordination; or impairment of large muscle function. What is the patient's gait like and how does he or she sit? The interviewer notes any abnormalities of finer movement and posture, such as tremor, tics, or fidgeting.

Stereotypies are organized, repetitive movements or speech or perseverative postures. They are usually associated with schizophrenia, particularly the catatonic type. A striking variant of postural stereotypy is **waxy flexibility,** in which the patient will remain indefinitely in a position into which the interviewer places him or her (eg, standing on one leg). Other disorders of movement associated with catatonia include a stiff expressionless face; facial grimacing or contortions; stiff, awkward, or stilted body movement; and unusual mannerisms of expressive movement or speech. The latter should not be confused with the gracelessness of someone who is socially anxious. The interviewer also notes whether the patient exhibits any rituals such as a need to touch objects repetitively, as in obsessive-compulsive disorder, or any habits such as nail biting, thumb sucking, lip licking, yawning, or scratching.

The interviewer attends to the accent, pitch, tone, and tempo of the patient's speech, paying particular attention to unusually high or low pitch and abnormal tone, as in the high-pitched "squawking" monotone sometimes encountered in children with early infantile autism.

In mutism, which may occur in advanced brain disorder, severe melancholia, catatonia, or conversion disorder or in the elective mutism of negativistic children, the patient is unable or unwilling to utter anything. In conversion disorder, mutism is less common than is aphonia, in which the patient is able to speak only in a hoarse whisper.

B. Relationship to the Interviewer: The interviewer should infer the quality of the patient's relationship by how he or she behaves and by what he or she says. The relationship may be constant, it may vary with the topic being discussed, or it may be influenced by other factors. These factors may remain obscure if they are unexpressed (eg, when the patient is privately amused by an auditory hallucination). The interviewer should note whether this is the case.

Affective states are difficult to assess, aside from noting whether they are inconstant or are influenced by obscure factors. The interviewer draws on a number of behavioral clues to assess the quality of the patient's relationship and mood. As a rule, the more inferential the judgment, the more unreliable the conclusion. Interviewers may differ in their inferences concerning a patient's affect, especially when it is unstable, ambiguous, complex, or shielded by interpersonal caution.

The interviewer's behavior will inevitably affect the ebb and flow of the patient's feelings. The patient may be responding appropriately to the interviewer's friendly approach (or rudeness, for that matter). He or she will also be responding to highly idiosyncratic internal predispositions. For example, a patient may harbor mingled anxiety and deference for somebody he or she perceives as a threatening authority figure who must be placated.

Given the fallibility of inference, the interviewer is well advised to stick closely to observations and be able to cite them. This skill requires training. The beginner may be overly impressed by brilliant intuitive leaps; the expert heeds intuition but realizes how unreliable it is. The beginner grasps for, and holds firmly to, an infer-

Table 8–4. Sections of the mental status examination.

A. Appearance and behavior
B. Relationship to the interviewer
C. Affect and mood
D. Cognition and memory
E. Language
F. Disorders of thought
G. Physiologic function
H. Insight and judgment

ence, sometimes in spite of contrary evidence. The expert makes the inference, cites the clues on which it is based, can offer alternative explanations, and discards the inference for a better one if the evidence indicates it.

The quality of the patient's eye contact is of great importance in gauging affective states. Negativistic patients, especially those with catatonia, may avert their gaze from the interviewer. Children with early infantile autism characteristically demonstrate eccentricities of eye contact, for example, staring "through" the interviewer or averting their gaze from him or her. A delirious patient, whose sensorium is impaired, may stare into space, as may a melancholic or schizophrenic patient whose thoughts are dominated by ruminations or preoccupations. Intermittent staring is a feature of different forms of epilepsy. The interviewer notes whether the patient's attention can be captured, albeit briefly. If not, the interviewer should suspect an organic brain disorder.

Some patients stare at the interviewer intently. He or she should distinguish the wide eyes of awe and fear from the narrowed slits of hypervigilant suspiciousness. Other patients make hesitant eye contact, particularly when they are embarrassed about what they are saying. Not all patients with shifty gaze are liars, and some prevaricators have learned to deliver their lines without batting an eyelash.

The impact of the eyes on interpersonal relations cannot be overestimated. The configuration of supraorbital, circumorbital, and facial musculature; eyelids; palpebral fissure; gaze; depth of ocular focus; pupil size; and conjunctival moisture combine to produce a range of social signals of great significance for interpersonal dominance, competition, attraction, hostility or avoidance, the initiation and punctuation of conversation, and the feedback one requires to know how another has responded to what one has said.

Eyes and face are combined with body posture and movement in a gestalt. The face provides the clues to remoteness, bewilderment, and perplexity, whereas the whole body is involved in tenseness (eg, clenched fists, sweaty palms, stiff back, leaning forward), restlessness, preoccupation, boredom, and sadness.

The patient may be uncommunicative or, in the extreme, quite mute. In contrast, he or she may be friendly and communicative, even loquacious or garrulous. Patients convey antagonism by hectoring; by being uncooperative, impertinent, or condescending; or even by making direct threats, criticizing, or verbally abusing the interviewer. In contrast, by tone of conversation and demeanor, the patient can convey respect, deference, anxiety to please, or ingratiation. The interviewer notes and describes the following attitudes in the patient: shyness, fear, suspiciousness, cautiousness, assertiveness, indifference, passivity, clowning, interest in the interviewer, clinging, coyness, seductiveness, or invasiveness.

C. Affect & Mood: **Affect** refers to a feeling or emotion, experienced typically in response to an ex-

ternal event or a thought. The patient's relationship to the interviewer is a particular manifestation of affect. Affects are usually associated with feelings about the self or others who are of personal significance to the individual. Less often an affect is experienced alone, as though adrift from its reference point. Affect is the conscious component of a monitoring system that signals whether the individual is on track toward a personal goal; whether he or she is obstructed, frustrated, or prevented from achieving the goal; or whether he or she has already attained it. Compare, for example, the anticipatory pleasure at preparing to meet someone beloved; the anxiety and fear at seeing the beloved with a serious rival; the rage and despair of loss; and the exaltation of reunion. Similar, though more complex, affects may attend mountain climbing, solving mathematical puzzles, or giving birth. Whatever the goal, its remoteness, proximity, loss, repudiation, attainment, or inaccessibility are all accompanied by self-monitoring affect.

In contrast to an affect, which may be momentary, **mood** refers to an inner state that persists for some time, with a disposition to exhibit a particular emotion or affect. For example, a mood of depression may not prevent an individual from deriving momentary amusement from a joke; however, the expression of gloom, sadness, or desolation prevails. Affects and mood are inferred from the patient's demeanor and spontaneous conversation. A general query such as "How are you feeling, now?" or "How have your spirits been?" can be helpful. The interviewer should try to avoid leading questions such as "Do you feel depressed?"

Demeanor and affect usually coincide, but sometimes they do not. For example, a stiff smile can mask anxiety or depression. If the interviewer suspects this to be the case, he or she can offer an indicating or clarifying interpretation to help the patient recover suppressed emotion, such as "I notice that even though you speak of sad things, you are smiling" or "It's hard to smile when you feel bad inside."

The interviewer describes in the mental status report the general qualities of the patient's emotional expression. Particular morbid affects or moods are noted. For example, is the patient **affectively flat,** that is, emotionally dull, monotonous, and lacking in resonance? This presentation is characteristic of chronic schizophrenia and dementia. Is the patient **emotionally constricted,** with a narrow range of affect, as in obsessional or schizoid personality? Does the patient exhibit **inappropriate or incongruous affect,** in that it is not in keeping with the topic of conversation?

Does the patient show evidence of **lability,** suddenly changing from neutral to excited or from one emotional pole to the other? Lability is often associated with emotional intemperateness, an abrupt unreflective expression of heightened emotion (eg, excited anticipation, affection, irritation).

The interviewer notes the presence of **histrionic affect,** the blatant but rather shallow expression of emotion often observed in those who exaggerate their feelings in order to avoid being ignored and who need to capture, or who fear to lose, the center of the interpersonal stage. Histrionic affect is often encountered in people with histrionic, narcissistic, or borderline personality disorder.

Morbid euphoria, a sense of well-being expressed in inexorable good spirits, is encountered in hypomania or mania and less commonly in schizophrenia and organic brain disorder. Frontal lobe dysfunction, characteristic of neurosyphilis and disseminated sclerosis and after lobotomy, may be associated with fatuous joking and lack of foresight. Silliness is sometimes encountered in histrionic or immature people overwhelmed by the enormity of a difficult situation. Morbid silliness is also characteristic of some disorganized schizophrenic patients.

As it becomes exaggerated, euphoria merges into elation and excitement; although the manic patient commonly also exhibits irritation if obstructed or thwarted. An extreme and transcendent exaltation of mood may be observed in the ecstatic states that are rarely associated with acute schizophreniform or schizophrenic disorders and epilepsy.

Apathy, a pervasive lack of interest and drive (also known as **anergia**), may be observed in patients with preschizophrenic, schizophrenic, depressive, and organic brain disorders. The apathetic patient has little or no enthusiasm for work, social interaction, or recreation. Anergia is usually associated with a decrease in sexual activity. **Anhedonia,** a subjective sense that nothing is pleasurable, is commonly associated with anergia and is observed in preschizophrenic, schizophrenic, and melancholic patients. **Excessive fatigue,** which may be manifested as hypersomnia, is associated with many disorders such as organic brain disorder, schizophrenia, anxiety disorders, depressive disorders, and somatization disorder.

When applied to an affect or mood, **depression** refers to a pervasive sense of sadness. Depression is often related to a life event involving loss, rejection, defeat, or disappointment. It may be associated with tearfulness and anger about the event. In more severe depression or melancholia, the patient feels emotionally deadened or empty, the world stale and unprofitable, and the future hopeless. The patient is preoccupied with dark forebodings and may be agitated by persistent self-recrimination about past misdeeds. Diminished concentration and a slowing of thinking and movement characteristically accompany depressed affect and gloomy ruminations. In some patients agitated depression is associated with psychomotor restlessness. Severe depression has important somatic features, including characteristic posture and facies, headache, irritability, precordial heaviness, gastrointestinal slowing, anorexia, weight loss, loss of sexual interest, and insomnia. Depression typically has a diurnal variation: dysphoria, hopelessness, and agitation are worse in the morning, and the patient brightens up by evening.

The interviewer will readily recognize **open anger** and **irritability.** These feelings may be quite understandable in the context of the patient's circumstances. Morbid anger, however, is defined by pervasiveness, frequency, disproportionate quality, impulsiveness, and uncontrollability. Morbid anger is associated with organic brain disorder, usually in the form of catastrophic reactions to frustration, especially when the patient can no longer complete a familiar or easy task. Abnormal anger is also associated with some forms of epilepsy; personality disorders of the aggressive, antisocial, borderline, or paranoid type; attention-deficit and disruptive behavior disorders of childhood; drunkenness; paranoid disorders; hypomania or mania; and intermittent or isolated explosive disorders.

Controlled hostility may be expressed as sullenness, uncooperativeness, superiority, or mockery. It can be helpful to invite the patient to express anger or resentment directly and to define its origin. This is particularly the case with adolescents. When working with adolescents, the interviewer might consider saying, "Whenever I ask you a question, you close up. Something about being here is making you pretty uptight. Can you tell me what it is?"

Anxiety and **fear** refer to the subjective apprehension of impending danger, together with widespread manifestations of autonomic discharge (eg, dilated pupils; cold, sweaty palms; tachycardia; tachypnea; nausea; bowel hurry; urinary urgency). Fear has an object: the need to defend oneself against uncertain odds (eg, a charging bull, a near accident in an automobile). Anxiety is associated with the threat to an essential value, for example, being attached to someone beloved, not being a coward, being successful, or being highly regarded. Direct action (ie, fight or flight) can eliminate fear, whereas the adaptive solution to anxiety is likely to require planning and persistence. Anxiety and fear are biologically advantageous because they signal the need for constructive responses.

In morbid anxiety, affect is cast adrift from its moorings, either to float free or fasten on a substitute, phobic object or situation (eg, heights, a particular animal, elevators, enclosed spaces, being fat). Morbid anxiety appears disproportionate or eccentric and is recognized as pathologic by the patient and others. Many of the disorders of thought content (described later in this chapter) can be regarded as unconsciously determined, pathologic mechanisms that detach anxiety from its object or block and divert it at its origin.

D. Cognition & Memory: Table 8–5 lists the cognitive functions that can be assessed in a MSE. We describe them in more detail in the following sections:

1. Level of consciousness & awareness— The psychiatrist may be asked to consult on a comatose or stuporous patient, if a nonorganic cause is hypothesized. **Coma** is a state of nonawareness from

Table 8–5. Cognitive functions.

Level of consciousness and awareness
Orientation, attention, and concentration
Memory
Information
Comprehension
Conceptualization and abstraction

which the patient cannot be aroused. Diminished awareness is called semicoma or **stupor,** in which case the subject is temporarily rousable (eg, by pain or noise) but reverts to stupor when the stimulus ceases. In stupor, eye movements become purposeful when the painful stimulus is applied, and wincing or pupillary constriction may occur, but the patient remains akinetic and mute. Stupor and coma occur in primary neuronal dysfunction (eg, Alzheimer's disease), secondary neuronal dysfunction (eg, metabolic encephalopathy), supratentorial lesions (eg, infarction, hemorrhage, tumor), subtentorial lesions (eg, infarction, hemorrhage, tumor, abscess), and psychiatric disorder (eg, dissociative disorder, depression, and catatonia).

Psychogenic coma is suggested by normal vital and neurologic signs, resistance to opening the eyes, normal pupillary reactions, and staring (rather than wandering) eyes. Swallowing, corneal, and gag reflexes are usually intact, and electroencephalography and oculovestibular reflexes are normal. Intravenous barbiturate may increase verbalization in psychogenic stupor. It depresses awareness further in organic conditions.

Torpor denotes a lowering of consciousness short of stupor. Awareness is narrowed and restricted, and apathy, perseveration, and psychomotor retardation are observed, but the more dramatic phenomena of delirium (ie, illusions, hallucinations, agitation, and so on) are lacking. Torpor is associated with severe infection and multi-infarct dementia.

In **twilight or dreamy states,** restricted awareness is manifested as disorientation for time and place, with reduced attention and short-term memory. In addition, the patient may have the sense of being in a dream.

Delirium is a common condition in medical and surgical wards. It is caused by a diffuse cerebral dysfunction of acute or subacute onset and fluctuant or reversible course. After prodromal restlessness and insomnia, delirium typically presents with obtundation, emotional lability, and visual illusions. The clinical features tend to worsen at night (so-called sundowning), with insomnia, agitation, hallucinations, and delusions. So-called quiet deliria are common, with little more to note than clouding of consciousness, mild disorientation for time and place, and reduced concentration. Restlessness, tremor, asterixis (irregular, asymmetrical jerking of the extremities), myoclonus, and disturbance of autonomic function

are also common. Patients vary in their psychological reactions to delirium: depressive, paranoid, schizophreniform, anxious, and somatoform responses may be encountered. Patients may be fearfully or combatively hypervigilant, or torpid and apathetic.

Visual illusions, which are characteristic of delirium, involve the patient misinterpreting the moving shadows, curtains, and surrounding bedroom furniture. Physical sensations may also be misperceived. For example, the patient may mistake abdominal pain for the knives of malefactors and tinnitus for radio waves. If poorly systemized delusional beliefs arise, the patient may act on them, seeking escape or defense. Visual hallucinations are more common than auditory hallucinations in delirium. Visual hallucinations are sometimes playful (eg, animals romping), sometimes personal (eg, the face of a dead relative), or sometimes horrible or threatening (eg, dismembered bodies, accidents). They are most evident at night and can be provoked when the eyes are closed, especially when the orbits are pressed. Affect is usually labile in delirium, but persistent blunting, anxiety, suspiciousness, hostility, depression, or euphoria may be encountered and is usually congruent with the prevailing illusions or hallucinations.

Delirious patients may exhibit wandering attention and concentration; their thinking may become disconnected or incoherent and their memory impaired. These patients sometimes confabulate, linking memories out of correct sequence. Subtle restriction of consciousness often occurs during acute anxiety and results in vagueness or amnesia for traumatic experiences. Sometimes the amnesia is accentuated. The patient may wander off in a daze, turning up in an emergency room unaware of his or her name or address. This is known as **dissociative fugue state** and should be differentiated from epilepsy or postictal conditions.

2. Orientation, attention, & concentration— Disorders of orientation are most often involved when the sensorium is clouded, as in torpor, obtundation, dreamy states, delirium, or fugue. Orientation is usually lost in the following order: time, place, person. Disorientation for time and place usually indicates organic brain disorder. Disorientation for personal identity is rare and is associated with psychogenic or postictal fugue states, other dissociative disorders, and agnosia (loss of the ability to recognize sensory inputs). The interviewer assesses the patient's orientation by asking him or her for the information listed in Table 8–6. The reliability of the clinical assessment of orientation is high, but its predictive validity is uncertain.

Attention is involved when a patient is alerted by a significant stimulus and sustains interest in it. Concentration refers to the capacity to maintain mental effort despite distraction. An inattentive patient ignores the interviewer's questions, for example, or soon loses interest in them. The distractible patient is diverted

Table 8–6. Clinical tests of orientation.

Time
Hour
Day
Date
Month
Year
Place
Building
City
State
Person
Name
Address and telephone number
Age
Occupation
Marital status

from mental work by incidental sights, sounds, and ideas.

Table 8–7 describes simple clinical tests for attention and concentration. These tests have high reliability but little validity. Primarily they test the ability to concentrate. A patient's ability to answer arithmetic questions requires not only concentration but also intelligence and education. Errors are common and are related to psychiatric disturbance, socioeconomic status, intelligence, and the patient's ability to cope with an interview situation. The procedure helps to identify organic brain disorder but has little diagnostic specificity.

3. Memory—Memory has several stages. Information must first be registered and comprehended. It is then held in short-term storage. If the material is to be retained beyond immediate recall, a more durable memory trace is formed. Memory traces in long-term storage will decay, consolidate, or become simplified and schematized, partly as a result of subsequent experience. Long-term memories are retrieved or recalled from storage by tagging a pattern of sensory phenomena and matching it with long-term memory schemata.

In clinical practice, abnormal memory is manifest as **amnesia** (memory loss) or **dysmnesia** (distortion of memory). Psychogenic amnesia occurs in several forms. During and after severe anxiety, memory is likely to be defective. Some people have the ability to repress unwelcome anxiety-laden ideas; their memory is thereby rendered patchy or selective. In dissociative disorders, such as psychogenic amnesia and fugue,

Table 8–7. Clinical tests of attention and concentration.

Subtract sevens or threes, serially, from 100.
Reverse the days of the week or months of the year.
Spell simple words backwards (eg, *world*).
Repeat digits (two, three, four, or more) forward and backward.
Perform mental arithmetic (Number of nickels in $1.35? Interest on $200 at 4% for 18 months?).

the patient usually loses memory for a circumscribed period of time during which profoundly disturbing events took place. Less commonly the amnesia is generalized (ie, total) or subsequent (ie, amnesia for everything after a particular time).

In addition to displaying generalized amnesia, patients in a psychogenic fugue state may travel a distance from home and assume a new identity. Often it is unclear in such cases whether unwitting self-deception or conscious imposture are involved.

Organic amnesia occurs in acute, subacute, and chronic forms. After acute head trauma, **retrograde amnesia** (loss of memory of past events) is likely to occur as a result of a disruption of short-term memory. The extent of **anterograde amnesia** (inability to form new memories) after head trauma is an index of the severity of brain injury. Amnesia also occurs in association with alcoholism (ie, blackouts) and after acute intoxication, delirium, or epileptic seizures.

Subacute amnesia (the amnestic syndrome) occurs after Wernicke's encephalopathy, a disease caused by thiamine deficiency and encountered most commonly in alcoholic patients. Wernicke's encephalopathy is characterized by conjugate gaze ophthalmoplegia, nystagmus, ataxia, and delirium. After the delirium clears, most patients experience a residual Korsakoff's syndrome with disorganized memory in an otherwise clear sensorium. Patients with Korsakoff's syndrome have difficulty recalling events from before the onset of the encephalopathy. They also experience severe impairment of the ability to lay down new memories after the encephalopathy. The retrograde amnesia affects the patient's ability to remember the precise order in which events occurred. The anterograde amnesia, however, tends to be even more marked; the most severely affected patients, for example, are unable to store new information. As a consequence, these patients are often disoriented for place and time and may confabulate to fill the memory gaps. Thus the characteristic pattern of Korsakoff's syndrome is of amnesia, disorientation, confabulation, a facile lack of concern, and a tendency to get stuck in the one groove of thought. Chronic amnesia, as in dementing illnesses, extends back for years. Recent memory is lost before remote memory.

Disorders of recognition include déjà vu, déjà vécu, and psychotic misidentification. **Déjà vu** and **déjà vécu** are common and normal, particularly in adolescents. They involve the sudden uncanny feeling that one has experienced the present situation, or heard precisely the same current conversation, on a previous occasion. These phenomena are associated with anxiety and less commonly with temporal lobe epilepsy. **Psychotic misidentification** may occur in schizophrenia. These patients describe familiar people as strangers or claim to recognize people they never met. Patients with Capgras's syndrome regard familiar individuals (such as family members) as doubles, or impersonators of themselves.

Disorders of recall include retrospective falsification and confabulation. All people indulge at times in **retrospective falsification,** embellishing the past to present a more appealing, tragic, or amusing impression. Histrionic people sometimes invent such an extensive and impressive past that they are drawn into imposture. Depressive individuals find sin, failure, and occasion for self-recrimination in their unexceptional lives. After recovery from psychosis, patients often repress their memories of illness and retain only bland or vague reminiscences of the acute disorder. It is inadvisable to ask them to recall their experiences in detail.

A **confabulation** is a false memory that the patient believes is true. Confabulations may be quite detailed, but they are often inconsistent and fanciful. Confabulations commonly fill memory gaps, especially in the amnestic syndrome. Some schizophrenic patients confabulate, spinning complicated fantasies about telekinesis, extrasensory perception, nuclear radiation, and the like. It is difficult to draw the line between confabulation and deception in the hysterical impostor or the dramatic abnormal illness behavior of the patient with Munchausen's syndrome.

Table 8–8 lists the clinical tests for immediate, recent, and remote memory. These tests have good test-retest and interrater reliability. Their validity is affected by intelligence and age and by emotional states such as depression and to a lesser extent anxiety. The most useful tests for detecting organic lesions appear to be orientation, delayed recall, sentence repetition, and general information.

4. Information—The patient's fund of general knowledge depends on education and current interest in contemporary affairs. Table 8–9 provides a clinical test of information. Organicity is suggested if the patient makes 12 or more mistakes (≥60%) on this test. If administration is standardized, reliability is high. The test is quite useful as an estimate of organicity, although it does not assess a unitary cognitive function.

Table 8–9. Clinical test of information.

Name the last four presidents, starting with the current president.
Name the mayor, state governor, and state senators.
Name four large United States cities.
Discuss four important current events.
For what are these people famous: George Washington, Christopher Columbus, William Shakespeare, Albert Einstein?

5. Comprehension—A patient's comprehension is evaluated by his or her grasp of the importance of the immediate situation. For example, does the patient know why he or she is where he or she is? Does the patient appreciate that he or she is ill or in need of treatment? Does the patient understand the purpose of the examination?

There are no tests for comprehension. It is evaluated as the interview proceeds. Although comprehension is often disturbed in delirium and dementia, for example, there is no evidence that this disturbance contributes anything to the diagnosis of organicity beyond what is provided by other tests of the sensorium (ie, orientation, concentration, memory).

6. Conceptualization & abstraction—Simple levels of conceptualization are assessed by testing the patient's capacity to discern the similarities and differences between sets of individual words. The patient's capacity to abstract is tested by asking the patient to discern the meaning of well-known metaphorical statements (Table 8–10). The tests listed in Table 8–10 have poor reliability and validity. They are affected by intelligence, educational level, culture, and age and have little discriminating power. The tests do not effectively detect organicity. Research has shown that clinicians using these tests could not distinguish between manic patients, schizophrenic patients, and creative writers. They are of most use when

Table 8–8. Clinical tests of memory.

Testing immediate recall
Repeat digits forward and backward. (Present digits at 1-second intervals. The average adult performance is up to six forward and four backward.)
Repeat three unrelated words (eg, *apple, table, grass*) immediately.
Repeat three three-part words (eg, *33 Park Avenue, brown mahogany table, 12 red roses*).
Testing recent memory
Repeat the three one-part phrases after 1, 3, and 5 minutes.
Repeat the three three-part phrases after 1, 3, and 5 minutes.
Recall events in the recent past (eg, a chronological account of the present illness, the last meal, an account of how the patient got to the office, the names of the physicians and nurses who are caring for the patient in the hospital).
Repeat this sentence: *One thing a country must have to become rich and great is a large, secure supply of wood.*
Recount the following story with as many details as possible:
   William Stern/ a 63-year-old/ state representative/ from Walton County,/ Utah,/ was planning his reelection campaign/ when he began experiencing chest pain./ He entered Logan Memorial Hospital/ for three days of medical tests./ A harmless virus was diagnosed/ and he, his wife,/ Sandra,/ and their two sons,/ Rick and Tommy,/ hit the campaign trail again. (The average patient should be able to reproduce 8 of the 15 separate ideas in this paragraph. Less adequate performance suggests defective recall of information that requires hierarchical analysis, short-term memory storage, and sequential recall.)
Testing remote memory
Recall parents' names, date and place of birth, graduation dates, age and year of marriage, and occupational history.

Table 8–10. Clinical tests of conceptualization and abstraction.

1. How are the following pairs similar or alike?
   a child and a dwarf
   a tree and a bush
   a river and a canal
   a dishwasher and a stove
2. How are the following pairs different?
   a lie and a mistake
   idleness and laziness
   poverty and misery
   character and reputation
3. What is the meaning of the following proverbs? (Ask the patient if he or she has heard them before.)
   "A rolling stone gathers no moss."
   "People who live in glass houses should not throw stones."
   "Strike while the iron is hot."

they tap unmistakable formal psychotic thought disorder. Consider the following examples:

> A young man with disorganized and accelerated thinking responds thus to the proverb "People in glass houses should not throw stones": "Oh yeah. My California uncle passed the shotgun out the windows and started firing!"
>
> To the proverb "A rolling stone gathers no moss," he answers, "Put a few pebbles in your mouth when you're hiking. You'll go a few more miles."

> Another young patient, who has the delusion that he is Christ, responds to the glass houses proverb as follows: "Those who know that it has been seen what they have done—and believe me it has all been seen—Let him who is without sin cast the first stone. Okay? That's what I believe it means."

> The same patient responds to the rolling stone proverb in this way: "If you can continue to move and always move and always follow yourself and no one else, you'll never have the evil one within yourself."

Unfortunately the sample of thinking provoked by these tests is usually so small, and its pathology so equivocal, that these tests are of dubious virtue.

E. Language: Language is a system of communication that is also used as a tool of thought. Language facilitates thinking by the way semantics hierarchically organizes ideas and concepts and by the way in which syntax indicates the relationship between those ideas and concepts.

Language competence is assessed from the patient's speech during the psychiatric interview. Any history of spoken or written language difficulty, or any observation of clumsy articulation, disordered rhythm, and difficulty in the understanding or choice of words, should be noted and investigated further. **Language comprehension** is tested by asking the patient to point to single objects, and then to point to a number of objects in a particular sequence. The inter-

viewer may also ask the patient to perform a series of actions in an arbitrary sequence (eg, "Touch your nose with your right index finger, then point that finger at me, then put it behind your back."). **Language expression** is evaluated by asking the patient to repeat words, phrases, and sentences and to name correctly a number of objects. Expression and comprehension are evaluated by asking the patient to read a passage aloud and to answer questions about it. Asking the patient to take dictation tests graphic language. Any errors and slowness in performance should be noted. The following sections describe some common disorders of language.

1. Aphasia—Aphasia is a dysfunction in the patient's ability to express himself or herself. The three most common forms of aphasia are all manifest as difficulty in repeating words or phrases. In **Broca's aphasia,** comprehension is relatively intact but expression dysfluent, sparse, telegraphic, and full of circumlocution. In **Wernicke's aphasia,** comprehension is affected. Expression, though fluent, rambles, lacks meaning, and is full of errors to which the patient seems oblivious. In **conduction aphasia,** comprehension is intact, expression is fluent but full of errors and pauses, and repetition is difficult; however, reading is relatively intact.

2. Muteness—Muteness is seldom found in neurologic disease, except in the acute phase, in seizure disorder, or in advanced cerebral degeneration. The aphasic patient is never mute. Muteness is much more commonly a sign of melancholia, stupor, catatonic stupor, somatoform disorder, dissociation or negativism in children (ie, elective mutism).

3. Schizophrenic language—The psychiatrist's main diagnostic problem is to differentiate schizophrenic language from the "jargon" of Wernicke's aphasia. Schizophrenic patients tend to be heedlessly bizarre in thought content; aphasic patients are more aware of their errors and are more likely to use substitutions to overcome their language defects. The confused speech of schizophrenic patients is known as **word salad.** It may be so chaotic as to be barely comprehensible.

4. Paralogia—Paralogia, or talking past the point, occurs when the patient gives answers that are erroneous but that reveal knowledge of what should be the correct answer. For example, the interviewer may ask, "How many legs has a cow?" and the patient responds, "Five." Talking past the point occurs in Ganser syndrome (also called the syndrome of approximate answers). It is most likely to be observed in patients for whom hospitalization for insanity is preferable to incarceration for crime.

5. Neologisms—Neologisms are new words coined by the patient. They are often condensations of ideas that attempt to capture the ineffable. Neologisms are most common in schizophrenia; they must be distinguished from aphasic paraphasia, and circumlocution, to which the patient resorts in order to overcome expressive difficulty. Sometimes a neologism reveals that the patient has been "derailed" by the sound or sense of an associated word or idea. At other times, neologisms are a response to hallucinations or a defense (in a private code) against the intrusion by the interviewer upon the patient's privacy.

F. Disorders of Thought: Pathology of thought may be found in the process, in the form, or in the content of thinking. The process and form of thinking may be disordered in terms of tempo, fluency (including continuity and control), logical organization, and intent. Normal thinking is characterized by reasonable, but not excessive speed, and a smooth and continuous flow from one idea to the next. Normal thinking has clear goal-direction, organization, and consensual logic in the links between, and the sequence of, its constituent ideas.

In psychological illness, particularly the turmoil associated with psychoses such as schizophrenia and mania, any or all of the above characteristics may be disorganized. Pathologic thinking can be sluggish, headlong, disconnected, meandering, halting, and prone to lose its track, wander off at tangents, or follow an illogical line.

Abnormal thinking can be experienced by the thinker as invading, inserted, or controlled by alien forces. It can also be sensed as leaking, stolen, lost, or broadcast from the mind into the outside world. Finally, the psychotic thinker, oblivious to the need to make sense, may lose contact with the audience or use language as a mocking camouflage.

1. Abnormalities of thought process & form—

a. Tempo. Thinking is accelerated in **flight of ideas,** which may reach such a pitch that goal direction is lost and the connection between ideas is governed not by sense but by sound or idiosyncratic verbal or conceptual associations. Alliteration, assonance, rhyme **(clang associations),** and punning may determine the torrent of ideas that is distracted readily by internal or environmental stimuli. Flight of ideas is usually associated with **pressured speech** and may be experienced by the patient as racing thoughts. Flight of ideas is characteristic of mania, but it may occur also in excited schizophrenic patients, especially those in acute catatonia. In hypomania the flight of ideas is less marked, the tempo being accelerated but the associations less disorganized.

The tempo of thinking may be slowed in **retardation of thought,** especially in major depression. The patient often complains of fuzziness, woolliness, and poor concentration. Response time to questions is increased. There are long silences during which the patient may lose the thread of the conversation. In the extreme, retardation of thought becomes mutism or even stupor.

b. Fluency. In **circumstantiality,** although the goal direction of thinking is retained, associations meander into fruitless, overly detailed, or barely relevant byways. The listener may feel impelled to hurry the speaker along. Circumstantiality is said to be characteristic of some epileptic patients whose peculiar combination of pedantry, perseveration, religiosity, and cliché lend their thinking a so-called viscous quality.

Perseveration refers to a tendency to persist with a point or theme, even after it has been dealt with exhaustively or the listener has tried to change the subject. It is also observed, for example, when a child fixedly repeats one aspect of a drawing, leaving multiple lines or dwelling on the shading in an exaggerated manner.

c. Continuity. In **thought blocking,** the patient's speech is interrupted abruptly by silences that last for from less than a second to much longer, even a minute or more. During the pause the patient's eyes often flicker, particularly if he or she is listening to an auditory hallucination; sometimes the patient becomes blank mentally. Blocking is often precipitated by questions or ideas that have personal significance, particularly if their import is threatening. Blocking is an uncommon but striking sign. It tends to be identified far too often, the observer mistaking the retarded thinking of a depressed or preoccupied patient for the sudden roadblock of the true phenomenon. It is almost pathognomonic of schizophrenia but must be differentiated from the absences of petit mal epilepsy, the hesitation caused by anxiety, and the peculiar mental fixity of amphetamine intoxication.

During the period of blocking, intermediate associations may be lost, and the patient recommences on an apparently different track **(tangential thinking).** This can give rise to a phenomenon known as the **knight's move in thought:** The listener can sometimes intuit how the patient got from A to E and realizes that the unspoken intermediate associations (B, C, and D) were quite indirect. On other occasions, the patient's thinking appears subject to **derailing** (jumping the track to proceed on a quite different subject), particularly when a sore point has been touched on. Patients are often aware of disturbances in the continuity of their thinking and will describe how their thoughts become paralyzed, interrupted, or jumbled.

d. Control. Akin to the subjective phenomena described in the previous section is the patient's sense that speed, direction, form, or content of thought are out of control. Complaints such as "confused," "racing thoughts," "unable to concentrate," "scatterbrained," "jumbled," and "going crazy" often reflect the subjective perception of pathologically accelerated, dysfluent, or discontinuous thinking.

Sometimes schizophrenic patients report that their thinking is controlled by external forces or people, often by means of radio waves or other transmissions. Thinking may be perceived as directed by the external agency, or particular thoughts experienced as having been implanted by it. This is known as **thought insertion** or **thought alienation.**

In **thought deprivation** or **thought broadcasting,** the patient senses that ideas are leaking out of the mind, being stolen by others, or being broadcast via radio or television. The perception that the television picks up and repeats one's thoughts may lead to a grandiose or persecutory delusional misinterpretation.

e. Logical organization. Psychotic thinking may reflect a deterioration in the capacity to think formally or logically. Commonly the schizophrenic patient uses a private logic, with overpersonalized concrete symbols. Within this logical framework, conceptual boundaries are blurred, and the thinking patterns are metaphorical and idiosyncratic, almost as if they emerged directly from a dream-state. Thus, to the observer, when such thoughts are expressed, they appear on the surface to be diffuse or bizarre, and lack clarity. However, it is possible to interpret their meaning in the context of the patient's personal situation, and the issues that he or she is struggling with.

f. Intent of communication. The conventional purpose of discourse is to communicate, but the clinician may be misled by the intentions of a schizophrenic patient. The schizophrenic patient may attempt to remain private or to deride the clinician, subtly, by conversing in an obscure, remote, supercilious, attacking, caricatured, or farcical manner.

2. Abnormalities of thought content—Several disorders are virtually defined by the presence of abnormalities of thought content. In many instances the patient will complain of these phenomena (eg, a phobia of heights); in other cases the patient appears to have accepted an eccentric idea (eg, the delusion of being a reincarnation of Christ) and to be acting accordingly. Abnormal thought may be divided into the following categories: abnormal perceptions, abnormal convictions, abnormal preoccupations and impulses, and abnormalities in the sense of self.

a. Abnormal perceptions. Perception is physical sensation given meaning, the integration of sensory stimuli to form an image or impression, in a manner or configuration influenced by past experience. Perception may be increased or decreased in intensity. **Heightened perception** occurs in delirium, mania, after hallucinogens, and in the rare ecstatic states that occur as part of acute schizophrenia or "transported" hysterical trances. **Dulled perception** occurs in depression and organic delirium.

In **derealization,** the external world seems different, changed, vague, unreal, or distant. This symptom is common in adolescence, in association with **depersonalization.** It is also associated with anxiety or dissociative disorders, depression, schizophrenia, organic brain disorder, and after hallucinogen use. In **synesthesia,** the subject perceives color in response, for example, to music. It is a common psychedelic experience.

Time may be experienced as accelerated under the influence of hallucinogens, in mania, or during an epileptic aura. Time may seem slowed or stopped in depression or epilepsy. In some conditions, time seems to lack continuity and the subject feels uninvolved in the temporal stream. This is particularly likely to be encountered in depersonalization, amnestic syndromes, depression, schizophrenia, or toxic-confusional states.

An **illusion** is sensory stimulation given a false interpretation, that is, a false perception. Illusions are most likely to occur when the mind is under the sway of an emotionally determined ideational "set" (eg, vigilance for an intruder), when sensory clarity is reduced (eg, at night), or when both sets of circumstances are operating (as when a frightened elderly patient has both eyes bandaged following ophthalmic surgery). Illusions are common in delirium and may be visual (eg, fluttering curtains seen as intruders), auditory (eg, a slamming door interpreted as the report of a pistol), tactile (eg, skin sensations thought to be caused by vermin), gustatory (eg, poison detected in the taste of food), kinesthetic (eg, flying), or visceral (eg, abdominal pain thought to be caused by ground glass). Illusions may also occur in hysteria, depression, and schizophrenia, particularly when perception is subordinated to a delusional idea (eg, of guilt or persecution) or an emotion of great force (eg, abandonment or erotic yearning).

A **hallucination** is a false perception that occurs in the waking state in the absence of a sensory stimulus. It is not merely a sensory distortion or misinterpretation, and it carries a subjective sense of conviction. A true hallucination appears to the subject to be substantial and to occur in external objective space. In contrast, a mental image is insubstantial and experienced within internal subjective space. Deafness, tinnitus, or blindness, usually in association with dementia or delirium, may determine the modality of hallucinations.

Sensory deprivation experiments have produced visual and auditory hallucinosis in many subjects. Hallucinosis and delirium following cataract operation probably acts by the same mechanism, especially in association with dementia. Diencephalic and cortical disease may be associated with hallucinations (usually visual). Tumors of the olfactory or basal temporal regions may cause olfactory hallucinosis, for example, as an aura. Hallucinations, especially visual (though sometimes vestibular and kinesthetic), are common in the delirium caused by toxins (eg, drugs, hallucinogens, alcohol, toxins), fever, cerebrovascular disease, and central degenerative disorders. Hallucinations may also be a prominent feature of the uncommon schizophrenia-like psychosis associated with epilepsy. Aside from these medical circumstances, hallucinations are common and normal, especially in some people, when falling asleep (hypnagogic) or waking (hypnopompic). Severe sleep deprivation can cause hypnagogic hallucinosis.

Hallucinations can be auditory, visual, olfactory or gustatory, tactile, or somatic. In form, they may be amorphous, elementary, or complex. They may be experienced as emanating from inner or outer space and, if from outside, from near or far. Hallucinations may be unsystematized, appearing to have no link to life circumstances, or systematized and part of a causally interconnected delusional world.

Auditory hallucinations may be inchoate (eg, humming, rushing water, inaudible murmurs), fragmentary (eg, words or phrases such as "fag," "get him," or "beastly") or complex. Typically the schizophrenic patient locates complex hallucinations in inner or outer space, as a voice or voices speaking to or about him or her. The voice may be soothing, mocking, disparaging, or noncommittal. Sometimes the voice echoes the patient's thoughts or comments neutrally on his or her actions. Sometimes the voice orders the patient to perform actions, or puts thoughts into his or her head, a notion verging on thought insertion. The voice may be perceived as coming from the radio or television, from outside the window, or even from a distant place. In alcoholic hallucinosis, typically, a conspiracy of threatening whisperers plan to injure the patient, provoking the patient to defend himself or herself or to take flight.

Visual hallucinations vary from elemental flashes of light or color, as in disorders of the visual pathways and cortex, to well-formed scenes of people, animals, insects, and things. In delirium, insects or other small objects may be seen moving on the bed or in the surroundings. Lilliputian hallucinations, of little people on the bed, for example, occur in delirium and other organic brain syndromes. Complex audiovisual hallucinations may occur in temporal lobe epilepsy. In general, visual hallucinosis suggests acute brain disorder rather than functional psychosis and tends to occur in a setting of confusion or obtundation. Sometimes, however, a schizophrenic patient will report visual hallucinations (eg, trips in flying saucers) aligned with his or her prevailing delusions. The visual hallucinations of hysteria or dissociative disorder have a pseudo-hallucinatory quality and sometimes represent a traumatic event, as when a war veteran relives a battle incident.

Olfactory and gustatory hallucinations (eg, burning rubber, steak and onions) may occur in epilepsy. Schizophrenic patients may perceive gas being pumped into their bedrooms by persecutors or may think they taste poisonous substances in their food. Melancholic patients may be conscious of the stench of corruption rising from their unworthy bodies or may complain of the changed, metallic, tasteless quality of their meals.

Tactile hallucinations are characteristic of cocaine and amphetamine intoxication, the patient being distracted by the sensation of insects crawling on the skin. Schizophrenic patients may detect the effect on the skin of radioactivity beamed at them from a hostile source.

Somatic hallucinations occur in schizophrenia, whereby genital, visceral, intracerebral, or kinesthetic sensations are often referred to the influence of persecutors or machines. The melancholic patient may have the sense of having no stomach, with food dropping from the throat into a void.

In schizophrenia, or under the influence of hallucinogens, the patient may have the uncanny sense that somebody, a presence, is behind him or her. This can occur in states of extreme fear, but it may become a central feature of schizophrenia, in the guise of the doppelgänger or Horla, a hallucinatory double of the self who always lurks just behind the periphery of vision.

b. Abnormal convictions. A **delusion** is a false belief that is not susceptible to argument and that is inconsistent with the subject's sociocultural background. Bordering on delusion is the **overvalued idea,** a notion that may be eccentric rather than false but that becomes a governing force in the patient's life.

It is not always easy to draw the line between an eccentric individual, somebody who holds unfamiliar views that are nevertheless consistent with a different sociocultural system, and a deluded person. Indeed, some people drift across the misty boundaries between these categories. An active delusion, however, is rigid, unshakable, and self-evident. It dominates the subject's life, subordinating all other matters. It is private, idiosyncratic, ego-centered, and inconsistent with the common experience of people from the same background. A delusion, therefore, isolates the subject from others and alienates them from him or her.

Severe sensory deprivation, or exhaustion and physical privation, may lead to delusional misinterpretation, often associated with wish-fulfilling hallucinations. A delusion can act as a transcendental escape from an existential wasteland. This is the ground from which cosmic, messianic, and redemptive delusions grow.

As for the content of delusions, the commonest are of persecution, jealousy, love, grandeur, disease, poverty, and guilt. **Delusions of persecution** are most frequently encountered in schizophreniform disorders or schizophrenia, paranoid disorders, organic mental disorder (especially alcoholic hallucinosis, amphetamine delirium or delusional disorder, other hallucinogenic syndromes, epilepsy, and all forms of delirium) and, less commonly, in melancholia or during transitory psychotic breaks in the life-course of borderline personality. The patient may perceive others as talking conspiratorially about him or her (delusions of reference) or spying on him or her. External agencies (eg, communists, FBI, freemasons) are regarded as acting in concert and disconcerting the subject with radiation, poisonous gases, radio and television, intruders, assassins, and so on. The patient often alludes to the use of tape recorders, cameras, and other surveillance paraphernalia. Delusions of poisoning, particularly by the spouse, are sometimes encountered.

Delusions of jealousy occur in the same syndromes as delusions of persecution but are especially likely in association with alcoholism in men. In that case, delusions of marital infidelity (possibly related to alcoholic impotence) are characteristic, and the patient closely scrutinizes his wife and her belongings for evidence of adultery.

Delusions of grandeur occur in mania, schizophrenia, paranoid disorders, and organic delusional syndromes (eg, neurosyphilis). In mania and organic grandiosity, the patient's megalomania (eg, of being God, the governor, the Virgin Mary, Napoleon) are in line with his or her general high spirits. In schizophrenia and paranoid disorders, an inflated sense of importance may be reinforced by auditory hallucinations and the grandiosity of a delusional explanation for ideas of persecution: Why else would important agencies (eg, the FBI, the Vatican, the PLO) be persecuting the patient?

Erotic delusions (erotomania) are more common in female schizophrenic or paranoid patients. A lonely person develops a crush on another, often a celebrity or prominent citizen. Fantasies evolve into delusions, and the subject bombards the other person with telephone calls and messages. The failure of the loved one to reciprocate is put down to conspiratorial forces that stand in the way of destiny. In schizophrenia, the patient may receive erotic hallucinations from the beloved.

Somatic delusions, usually of disease or ill health, occur in many psychiatric disorders. Schizophrenic patients may have bizarre complaints, possibly in an attempt to explain somatic hallucinatory experiences, for example, of blood running backward in the head, of radiation being trained on the genitals by an outside agency, or of objects placed inside the body by malevolent forces. In melancholia, the patient may have delusions of being dead (no blood in the body), of the internal organs rotting away, or of the brain being destroyed by syphilis, in retribution for an unpardonable sin. The boundary between hypochondriasis, disease phobia, and disease conviction on the one hand and somatic delusions on the other may be difficult to define.

Melancholic patients are prone to **delusions of poverty** and **delusions of nihilism.** The future is hopeless, the present desolate, the patient destitute and abandoned to a bleak fate. Depressive patients may also complain of inordinate guilt, the most extreme punishments being meted out to them for unremarkable, ancient transgressions.

c. Abnormal preoccupations & impulses. A **phobia** is a morbid and irrationally exaggerated dread that focuses on a particular object, situation, or act (see Chapter 22). Phobias differ from generalized anxiety in their focused quality; although a diffuse anxiety state sometimes precedes a phobic disorder. The patient is aware of the exaggerated, irrational nature of a phobia and regards it as symptomatic. The patient often tries to avoid the phobic situation or is compelled to perform actions (such as hand washing) in order to eradicate the object of the fear, or atone for tabooed action.

An **obsession** is a persistent idea, desire, image, phrase, or fragment of music that cuts into the stream of conscious thinking. The patient recognizes the alien nature of the obsession and attempts to resist it, without success. The obsession often presses the subject to perform compulsive acts, to relieve anxiety. The key characteristics of obsessions are their persistent, irresistible, imperative nature; their ego-alien quality; and their repetitiousness. Obsessional symptoms have been reported after encephalitis. They occur in the premonitory phase of schizophrenia or as part of a major depression (eg, the patient may experience persistent ruminations that old tax returns were in error and that ruin will result). Obsessive-compulsive symptoms are most characteristic of the anxiety disorder that bears the same name (see Chapter 24).

Impulsions differ from compulsions in that the former are less likely to be resisted, and they are episodic rather than repetitious, although the distinction may be blurred at times. Impulsions tend to occur in externalizing personalities, whereas compulsions are more typical of inhibited, constricted people. Impulsions cause difficulty for others and may lead to legal entanglements. Impulsive acts often spring from an emotional setting of anger, anxiety, frustration, rejection, sadness, or humiliation, particularly when the subject is disinhibited by alcohol. Common impulsions include violent assault, fast driving, excessive drinking or eating, gambling, sexual assault, sexual exhibitionism, shoplifting, stealing, and fire-setting. Sudden, episodic, if not explosive, onset is the hallmark of these phenomena. The subject does not or cannot exercise inhibition or self-control. Feeling short circuits thought, leading to action without reflection.

d. Abnormalities of the sense of self. The normal person has a sense of selfhood composed of the following elements: a sense of existing and being involved in one's own body and activity; a sense of personal continuity in time between past, present, and future; a sense of personal integrity; and a sense of distinction between self and outside world. In psychiatric disorders, any or several of these phenomena may be disturbed. For example, the individual may feel uninvolved in his or her own body or actions, like a spectator looking at another person (as in depersonalization); the individual's sense of temporal continuity may be dislocated, with the past and future seeming remote and the present but a series of disconnected scenes; the individual's ego may feel as though it is falling apart, shedding, fragmented, or split in two; or the difference between the self and other persons or objects may have become blurred.

The sense of depersonalization, often associated with derealization, occurs in adolescence, epilepsy, dissociative disorders, schizophrenia, and depression. Adolescents in severe emotional turmoil sometimes develop a sense of discontinuity, disintegration, and dedifferentiation. These symptoms are very common after ingestion of hallucinogens (and may be reexperienced as flashbacks) and in reactive psychosis, schizophreniform disorder, or schizophrenic disorders.

G. Physiologic Function: Sleep disturbances are often encountered in psychiatric practice. Sleep deprivation may precipitate or accentuate psychiatric disorder. Sleep disturbance may be a prodrome, a symptom, or a sequel of psychiatric disorder. Many psychopharmacologic agents also affect sleep. See Chapter 30 for more on sleep disorders.

Appetite may be increased in depression (especially dysthymic personality) and after psychotropic drug medication. Eating binges (not necessarily determined by increased appetite) may occur in bulimia nervosa as a condition separate from, in alternation with, or following, anorexia nervosa (see Chapter 29).

Anorexia and weight loss can occur in almost any stress condition but are particularly likely in major depression, paranoid schizophrenia, somatoform disorders, alcoholism or drug addiction, and, of course, anorexia nervosa. A comprehensive physical screening investigation is always required when anorexia and weight loss are present.

Sexual desire may be increased in mania, in some forms of acute schizophrenia, and in narcissistic or borderline personality under stress. Sexual behavior may be disinhibited after alcohol or drug ingestion, in delirium, or in organic dementia. Sexual desire is decreased by any debilitating disorder, by anxiety, worry, tiredness, age, poor nutrition, and lack of affection for the partner. It is usually reduced by depression, schizophrenia, alcoholism, substance abuse, and by neuroleptic, antihypertensive, and antidepressant medication.

Absent, irregular, infrequent and scanty menstrual periods may occur in psychiatric disorder, particularly in depression, anorexia nervosa, anxiety disorders, schizophrenia, and substance abuse. Any condition that reduces total body fat to below 14%, in the female, produces anovulation and amenorrhea. Dysmenorrhea, dyspareunia, vaginismus, and other pelvic complaints are common in somatoform disorders, and in abnormal illness behavior generally, but a discretionary physical screen is required before a stress-related condition is diagnosed. See Chapter 28 for a more complete discussion of sexual dysfunctions.

Any or all body systems may be accelerated in the hyperdynamic states of anxiety, delirium, mania, and catatonic excitement or slowed in the general hypomotility of depression, organic dementia, and hypothyroidism. The patient's level of energy, or fatigue, may also be affected by disorders with accelerated or sluggish mental processes. Anergia, weakness, or obscure bodily discomfort are encountered frequently in somatoform disorders.

H. Insight & Judgment:

1. Insight—The patient's attitude or insight into the illness has several aspects. For example, does the patient recognize that he or she has a problem? Does he or she identify the problem as personal and psychological in nature? Does he or she understand the nature and cause of the illness? Does he or she want help and, if so, what kind of help?

The hypomanic patient has no problem. He or she feels very well (eg, high-spirited, amusing, energetic, expansive, and optimistic). The manic or schizophrenic patient may view the problem as external (ie, other people or agencies are stupidly obstructive or malevolent). Many patients with externalizing personality disorders (eg, borderline, antisocial, narcissistic) blame others for their predicament.

Sophisticated patients, particularly those who have undergone previous treatment, may have considerable knowledge of the formal diagnosis and the theoretical or actual causes of their disorder. Indeed, sometimes this causes problems in treatment: Other mental health professionals who develop psychiatric illness are notoriously difficult to manage for this reason.

The patient may be aware of having a problem but want no help, or he or she may want help of a particular sort or from a particular kind of clinician. Whenever this is reasonable and feasible, it should be arranged. The patient's desires should be respected as much as possible in the negotiation phase of the clinical process.

2. Judgment—The interviewer can ask the patient one of the following questions to test judgment: What would you do if you found a stamped, addressed envelope in the street? Why are there laws? Why should promises be kept? Good judgment requires intact orientation, concentration, and memory. There is no evidence that a finding of poor judgment adds anything to diagnosis beyond that provided by the detection of deficits in the lower-order functions, such as accomplishing household chores, maintaining personal hygiene, or selecting appropriate attire.

TERMINATION

A psychiatric interview may last 15 minutes or go on for much longer. The usual time is about 50 minutes: long enough for a rapid survey but not so long as to exhaust the patient. The interviewer can signal the approach of the conclusion by saying, for example, "Our time is almost finished, and there are a few things we need to discuss . . ."

A concluding summary of the material points of the interview can be very helpful. It allows the patient to correct or modify misinterpretations and leads naturally into the interviewer's plan for what happens next—another interview, for example, or special investigations.

PRACTICAL MATTERS

LABORATORY TESTING

Psychiatrists must increasingly rely on laboratory testing to confirm their diagnostic impressions, to detect medical or neurologic illness that may underlie or coexist with neuropsychiatric symptoms, and to ensure the safe and maximally effective use of certain psychotropic medications. Clinicians should understand the relevance of any laboratory test to the clinical problem presented by the patient and be ready to use the information obtained to enhance the findings of the psychiatric history and MSE. Table 8–11 summarizes the common laboratory tests the interviewer considers ordering in certain classes of psychiatric disorders, although it is by no means an exhaustive

Table 8–11. Selected laboratory tests useful in supporting the diagnosis of psychiatric illnesses.[1]

Laboratory Test(s)	Major Psychiatric Illness					
	Alcohol & Substance Dependence	Anxiety Disorders (eg, panic disorder)	Cognitive Disorders (ie, dementia, delirium)	Eating Disorders	Mood Disorders	Psychosis
Amylase				X		
Calcium			X	X		
Carotid ultrasound			X			
Cerebrospinal fluid			X			
Complete blood count	X		X	X		
Computed tomography scan			X		X	X
Cortisol					X	X
Creatine phosphokinase		X				
Electroencephalograph			X			
Electrolytes[2]	X	X	X	X		
Erythrocyte sedimentation rate			X			
Glucose		X	X		X	X
Human immunodeficiency virus antibody			X		X	X
Liver functions[3]	X		X			X
Magnesium	X					
Magnetic resonance imaging			X			
Myoglobin						X
Porphobilinogen						X
Prolactin						X
Psychotropic drug monitoring		X	X		X	X
Renal functions[4]			X		X	
Urinalysis			X			
Urinary catecholamines		X				
Urine drug screen	X					
Venereal Disease Research Laboratory			X			X
Vitamin B$_{12}$		X	X			X

[1] Adapted, with permission, from Rosse RB, Deutsch LH, Deutsch SI: Medical assessment and laboratory testing in psychiatry. Pages 601–618 in: Kaplan HI, Sadock BJ (editors): *Comprehensive Textbook of Psychiatry,* 6th ed. Williams & Wilkins, 1995.
[2] Electrolytes = sodium, potassium, chloride, bicarbonate.
[3] Liver functions = alanine aminotransferase, aspartate aminotransferase, bilirubin, glutamyl transaminase, alkaline phosphatase.
[4] Renal functions = blood urea nitrogen, creatinine.

listing. It can be used as a guideline for determining which test might be germane to a patient when considering a particular psychiatric diagnosis.

FACILITATING THE INTERVIEW

If an interview is to achieve its purpose (ie, to gather information), the interviewer must develop an atmosphere favoring the expression of ideas, feelings, and attitudes. The patient must develop a sense of trust and confidence in the interviewer, in order to be as spontaneous as possible. He or she will thereby see the interview as encouraging participation and collaboration toward a therapeutic end, through free expression and self-exploration.

What can the interviewer do to promote trust, spontaneity, and free expression? The interviewer must accept the patient, without moral judgment. If he or she cannot do so, it is better to be honest about it and refer the patient to another physician. Anybody can help somebody, but nobody can help everybody. If a patient angers, repels, or frightens the interviewer, and the feeling persists, the interviewer should seek help from a colleague.

The interview is facilitated if the interviewer understands the patient and conveys this understanding by facial expression, intonation, and well-timed reflections of the content and emotion behind the patient's story. The deepest affective understanding is empathy, that is, feeling with, or sharing the feelings of, the patient. It contrasts with sympathy, which is a feeling for the patient.

The open-ended style of questioning we described earlier in this chapter as being most appropriate to reconnaissance and detailed inquiry helps to convey the spirit of collaboration, free expression, and self-exploration. An atmosphere of trust is fostered if the interviewer is relaxed and receptive, not preoccupied, rushed, abrupt, or irritable. Interviewers will likely adapt to their own purposes the techniques of others that have impressed them.

INTERVIEW SETTING

A skilled interviewer can be effective walking along a corridor, playing catch, or sitting by the side of a bed. Nevertheless, offices are preferable to closets, and chairs are an improvement over packing boxes. If the interviewer has the opportunity, he or she should arrange the interview room to take advantage of its size, proportions, furnishings, and design.

The fundamental principles are simple. The room should be large enough to fit the patient, a desk, chairs, and other equipment, without crowding the interviewer. It is desirable, though not always possible, to have enough room and seating to accommodate the patient and four others, particularly if the interviewer

plans to see families as well as individuals. The arrangement of the desk and chairs should allow entry and egress, but the interviewer should not sit between the patient and the door. He or she should try not to interview people from across a desk. Harsh lighting should be avoided. The patient should not be blinded by glare shining directly from a window or a lamp. The chairs should be comfortable, and the interviewer should not tower over the patient. The interviewer should not leave the patient stranded in the middle of the room; people feel less exposed with something solid behind them. The interviewer should not sit too close (ie, knee to knee) or too far away. He or she should be near enough to make arm contact by leaning forward.

INTERVIEW TECHNIQUES

The interviewer should encourage free expression during the reconnaissance and detailed inquiry stages of the psychiatric interview. He or she does so by the setting provided, the atmosphere created, and the interview techniques used. The interviewer should be at ease with these techniques, and they should be used naturally, without flamboyance or stiltedness. If a particular technique does not suit the interviewer, he or she should not use it; an alternative should be found that conveys the same spirit and has a similar purpose.

The following are examples of useful techniques: attentive listening, subtle vocal and nonvocal encouragement, support and reassurance, the reflection of feeling, gentle indication, and judicious paraphrasing.

Having invited the patient to tell his or her story, the interviewer waits and listens. He or she does not stare but meets the patient's gaze from time to time to indicate he or she is following. The interviewer's intent but relaxed posture indicates involvement. If the interviewer takes notes, they are brief and unobtrusive.

While the flow of associations proceeds, the interviewer need do little but maintain relaxed concentration, signaled by posture, eye contact, and subtle nonvocal or vocal encouragement. A nod or an "uh-huh" or "mm-mm" at strategic points may be all that is needed. Sometimes, when the flow seems to waver or slow, it is very effective to pick up and repeat a significant phrase or the last word the patient has said. But the interviewer should not be mechanical and should not do something unless it feels natural.

The interviewer needs to be alert to the patient's reactions, particularly to changes in voice intonation and speech tempo, tensing of facial muscles, alterations of skin color, and moistening of conjunctivae, which herald a flush of anxiety or anger or a sudden feeling of sadness.

How does the interviewer handle silences? If the patient is thinking fruitfully, all the interviewer need do is wait. Similarly, if the patient has broken down in tears, it may be better to wait calmly until the patient can continue. If the silence occurs when the patient has lost track of or has confused feelings about the topic, the interviewer can facilitate associations with a subtle oral reflection, picking up a key word, phrase, or idea from the recent conversation and repeating it gently, sometimes with a questioning intonation. Oral reflection is also useful to help circumstantial patients get back on track.

The reflection of feeling is a variant of the technique of oral reflection. The interviewer picks up and echoes feelings explicit or implicit in what has been said but that have been expressed incompletely up to that point.

TRANSFERENCE & COUNTERTRANSFERENCE

Transference refers to the unreasonable displacement of attitudes and feelings that originated in childhood to people in the here and now. This phenomenon is particularly likely to affect the doctor-patient relationship when patients are made vulnerable by fear, anxiety, guilt, despair, and hope.

Note the term "unreasonable" in the definition. The patient who is angered by overt rudeness is not displaying transference. However, if the patient is angered because the interviewer has a mustache or wears pearls, it is apparent that something is being added to an objectively neutral situation.

The patient may unconsciously regard the physician as a parent or a sibling, casting him or her in a caring or antagonistic role. Some examples of the commonest roles are of nurturing mother, demanding mother, protective father, punitive father, and rivalrous sibling. Sometimes older patients will relate to the physician as though they themselves were parents, reversing the roles.

How can the interviewer recognize transference? When the patient is exceptionally deferential, hanging onto the interviewer's opinions, singing his or her praises to others, or is easily slighted by a brief or delayed appointment, the interviewer may suspect a positive transference. When the patient is unexpectedly hostile, suspicious, or competitive, and there is no reasonable explanation for such antagonism, a negative transference is likely.

It is not difficult to imagine how a positive transference can become eroticized, with the patient falling in love with an idealized parental figure. Most of these infatuations are transitory, like the crushes of adolescence. If the interviewer recognizes them and responds in a professional manner, they will go no further. Occasionally, however, unscheduled visits, notes, telephone calls, or seductive dress indicate that the matter is more serious. The interviewer may need to consult a psychiatric colleague to decide how to proceed. The interviewer should not respond impulsively, out of fear or affront, lest a vulnerable patient be hurt.

Transference has its counterpart in a physician's **countertransference,** which occurs when a physician irrationally transfers to a patient his or her attitudes and feelings derived from childhood experiences. Psychiatric interviewers must be alert for countertransference. They should suspect it whenever they have powerful feelings of affection, protectiveness, fear, frustration, irritation, hatred, or erotic excitement toward a patient; when they very much look forward to the next appointment; or when they cannot tolerate a particular patient. If the interviewer recognizes these feelings, they will be much less likely to respond impulsively with rejection, flight, or self-indulgence. Once again, the interviewer should seek the help of a colleague or group of colleagues if he or she is unsure how to proceed in the patient's best interests.

There is no need to be embarrassed by transference or countertransference. Experienced clinicians know that these emotional displacements are ubiquitous and inescapable. They are most likely to be problematic when the interviewer is overworked, preoccupied, or rendered emotionally vulnerable by the vicissitudes of his or her personal life. The interviewer must look after himself or herself physically and emotionally and should do the best he or she can to ensure a fulfilling life outside of medicine itself.

CONCLUSION

The purpose of the psychiatric interview is to obtain information from the patient about the presenting problem and its precipitation and about previous disorders, predisposition, biopsychosocial strengths and limitations, reason for the current presentation, insight, and desire for help. The psychiatric history covers topics that range from identifying data to coping mechanisms. The four stages of the interview—inception, reconnaissance, detailed inquiry, and termination—are adapted to different topics.

In the inception stage, the interviewer makes introductions, gets the patient or family seated, takes identifying information, and summarizes what he knows. The quality of the interview is enhanced if the interviewer creates an atmosphere of trust, spontaneity, and expressiveness by his or her acceptance, empathic understanding, open-ended style, and natural manner. The decor, lighting, furnishings, and arrangement of the room can also promote (or subvert) the desired atmosphere.

During the reconnaissance stage, the interviewer helps the patient describe the presenting problem and its precipitation and development.

During the detailed inquiry, routine and discretionary, the interviewer explores past illness; early development and environment; later educational, occupational, social, and marital history; interests, values, and aspirations; habitual coping style; family history; and mental status.

During the interview, the clinician fosters free expression and association by being attentive and by using certain techniques such as vocal and nonvocal encouragement, support and reassurance, reflection of ideas or feelings, indication of inconsistencies, and paraphrasing.

The clinician will seldom, if ever, need to turn over every stone and pebble in this chapter. What is required is a set of criteria to decide whether comprehensive or brief discretionary screening MSE is indicated.

At termination, the interviewer summarizes the interview and negotiates with the patient over what the next step should be.

Colby KM: *A Primer for Psychotherapists.* Ronald Press, 1951.

McKinnon RA, Michaels R: *The Psychiatric Interview in Clinical Practice.* WB Saunders, 1971.

Nicholi AM: *The Harvard Guide to Modern Psychiatry.* Belknap Press of Harvard University Press, 1978.

Scheiber SC: The psychiatric interview, psychiatric history, and mental status examination. Pages 187–220 in: Hales RA, Yudofsky SC, Talbott JA (editors): *The American Psychiatric Press Textbook of Psychiatry,* 2nd ed. American Psychiatric Press, 1994.

Siegman AW: Review of interview research. Pages 481–530 in: Balis et al (editors): *The Behavioral and Social Sciences and the Practice of Medicine.* Butterworth, 1978.

Strauss G: The psychiatric interview, history, and mental status examination. Pages 521–530 in: Kaplan HI, Sadock BJ (editors): *Comprehensive Textbook of Psychiatry,* 6th ed. Williams & Wilkins, 1995.

Strub RL, Black FW: *The Mental Status Examination in Neurology.* FA Davis, 1993.

Rosse RB, Deutsch LH, Deutsch SI: Medical assessment and laboratory testing in psychiatry. Pages 601–618 in: Kaplan HI, Sadock BJ (editors): *Comprehensive Textbook of Psychiatry,* 6th ed. Williams & Wilkins, 1995.

Clinical Decision Making in Psychiatry

9

Barry Nurcombe, MD

PURPOSE OF CLINICAL REASONING

It is through clinical reasoning that clinicians collect, weigh, and combine the information required to reach diagnosis; decide which treatment is required; monitor treatment effectiveness; and change their plans if treatment does not work. The study of clinical reasoning, therefore, concerns the intellectual processes that underlie diagnosis and the planning and implementation of treatment.

Diagnosis has three purposes: to aid research, to summarize information, and to guide treatment. For clinicians, the chief purpose of diagnosis is to summarize information in such a way as to guide treatment. In one approach to diagnosis, the clinician matches a pattern of clinical phenomena elicited from the patient against the idealized patterns of disease entities and chooses the diagnosis that best fits. In another approach, the clinician attempts to understand the particular environmental, biological, psychological, and existential factors that have both led to the current problem and perpetuated it. The first approach, therefore, seeks commonality and lends itself to generic treatment planning. The second approach stresses uniqueness and the adaptation of treatment to the individual. In good clinical practice the two approaches are complementary.

CLINICAL REASONING & ACTUARIAL PREDICTION

Diagnosis and treatment are risky ventures. They are fraught with the possibility of error that can have serious consequences. How can error be minimized? On the one hand are the clinicians who, having elicited information that is generally both incomplete and inferential, diagnose patients and use subjective probabilities to predict outcome. On the other hand are the psychological actuaries who regard natural clinical reasoning as so flawed as to be virtually obsolete and who seek to replace it with reliable statistical formulas.

A considerable amount of research has been conducted into the fallacies and biases that can lead clinicians astray. Such research has had little effect on clinical practice for several reasons. Actuarial experiments sometimes seem artificial, irrelevant, or even rigged (against the clinician). Clinicians are prone to concede that others may make a particular mistake but that they are unlikely to do so. Indeed, clinicians often have a degree of self-confidence that enables them to survive in an uncertain world, and they are not likely to accept their defects unless they see a practical remedy. Finally, clinicians may fear that, if tampered with, their mysterious diagnostic skills will evaporate and that they will be replaced by computing machines.

RESEARCH INTO CLINICAL REASONING

There are three types of research into clinical reasoning: clinical judgment, decision theory, and process tracing. **Clinical judgment research** attempts to identify the criteria used by clinicians in making decisions. **Decision theory** explores the flaws and biases that deflect accurate clinical judgment. **Process tracing** elucidates the progressive steps of naturalistic reasoning. The first two types are statistical and prescriptive, the third is normative.

CLINICAL JUDGMENT & DECISION THEORY

According to the "lens" model of clinical judgment, each patient exhibits a set of symptoms, signs, or criteria that the clinician weighs and combines to reach a decision (eg, whether the patient is at risk for suicide or whether he or she should be hospitalized). Researchers attempt to "capture the policy" of the expert decision maker in order to construct mathematical models that replicate clinical judgment.

Given the fuzzy nature of clinical data, medical decisions have to be probabilistic. Accordingly, decision theorists base their research on Bayes' theorem. This theorem states that $P(D/F)$ (the probability that a diagnosis is present given a clinical finding) is a function of $P(F/D)$ (the probability that a finding will be associated with that diagnosis), $P(D)$ (the probability of the diagnosis in that population), and $P(F)$ (the probability of the finding in that population). Thus

$$P(D/F) = \frac{P(F/D) \times P(D)}{P(F)}$$

The intuitive clinician gauges $P(F/D)$ from theoretical knowledge and experience. However, $P(F/D)$ must be combined with the local base-rates for both the disease and the finding, base-rates that are often either unknown or ignored by the clinician. Unfamiliarity with Bayes' theorem and other biases can introduce several errors into clinical reasoning (Table 9–1).

Decision theory has been applied most often to convergent problems, for example, whether or not to hospitalize a patient. The better choice should be the one that has the highest expected utility. **Expected utility** is the product of the probability of an outcome and its subjective utility (eg, how highly the patient or physician values that outcome). Consider the following case:

A 14-year-old girl is evaluated in a pediatric hospital ward after she has taken an overdose of 50 acetaminophen tablets. She has made one previous suicide attempt. The recent suicide attempt occurred after she was rejected by a boyfriend. The patient is emotionally labile and clinically depressed. She is hostile to her mother and refuses to agree to a "no-suicide contract." The consequences of hospitalizing the patient versus not hospitalizing her but referring her for outpatient treatment can be represented in Figure 9–1.

Action	Outcome	Probability	Utility
Hospitalizing	Death	0	0
	No change or worse	.3	0
	Lost to treatment	.1	0
	Improved	.6	100
Not Hospitalizing	Death	.01	0
	No change or worse	.4	0
	Lost to treatment	.3	0
	Improved	.2	100

Expected utility of hospitalizing =
  $(0 \times 0) + (.3 \times 0) + (.1 \times 0) + (.6 \times 100) = 60$

Expected utility of not hospitalizing =
  $(.01 \times 0) + (.4 \times 0) + (.3 \times 0) + (.2 \times 100) = 20$

Figure 9–1. Expected utility estimation.

The clinician is expected to opt for the choice that leads to the greater expected utility.

Clinical decisions are often more complex than can be represented by a simple decision tree of the type shown in Figure 9–1. Multiple branching yes-no decision trees have been constructed to aid diagnostic decision making (eg, Appendix A in *Diagnostic and Statistical Manual of Mental Disorders,* 4th edition [DSM-IV]) and to encode expert treatment decisions. Utility and probability are also important considerations when cost-benefit analyses are undertaken, for example, concerning the desirability of mass screening procedures.

Table 9–1. Common errors in clinical reasoning.

If a set of clinical findings (F) matches a textbook syndrome (D), clinicians are apt to diagnose it without sufficiently taking $P(D)$ and $P(F)$ into account.

Clinicians must often rely on their subjective estimations of $P(D)$ and $P(F)$. They tend to be overconfident concerning the accuracy of these estimations.

Clinicians may overestimate $P(D)$ as a result of recent experience (eg, reading a journal article). Thus, exotic disorders may be overdiagnosed.

Clinicians are conservative. Despite corrective feedback, they are slow to correct their subjective base-rates.

Clinicians are prone to rely too much on confirmatory data, whereas negative evidence is more powerful.

Early preference for a particular diagnostic hypothesis may be hard to dislodge and can deflect the subsequent collection or evaluation of evidence.

Research has shown that clinicians do not always follow the expected utility model. For example, decision making may be biased by the readiness with which a particular outcome can be remembered, particularly if it has had an emotional impact on the clinician (eg, a patient's recent suicide). Decision making is also affected by the way problems are presented. For example, a treatment that saves 800 lives out of 1000 may be preferred to one that sacrifices 200 out of 1000 (although the two situations are equivalent in risk). Furthermore, the probability of an outcome can sometimes affect the subjective estimation of its utility, whereas theoretically the two should be independent.

American Psychiatric Association: *Diagnostic and Statistical Manual of Mental Disorders,* 4th ed. American Psychiatric Association, 1994.

Schwartz S, Griffin T: *Medical Thinking.* Springer Verlag, 1986.

Weinstein MC et al: *Clinical Decision Analysis.* WB Saunders, 1980.

PROCESS TRACING

Comparing experts and novices, researchers have traced the steps of naturalistic reasoning in areas such as chess, physics, mathematics, neurology, family practice, internal medicine, radiology, and psychiatry. A chess expert, for example, has built up from experience the memory of perhaps 50,000 chessboard patterns. Each pattern is associated with possible moves. Rapid pattern matching dynamically linked to good choice of next move explains the capacity of the chess expert to play and defeat many novices simultaneously. Thus pattern recognition is linked to strategic option choice. The expertise of the diagnostician is similar: The recognition of an incomplete clinical pattern that matches, in part, the memory of a diagnostic syndrome is linked to tactical choices for eliciting, evaluating, and integrating further evidence to solve the diagnostic puzzle.

Clinical reasoning is a species of "bounded rationality" in which the clinician converts an open problem (ie, a problem with no clear endpoint) into a series of closed problems (each with a hypothesized endpoint). In other words, the open problem is reframed as an array of closed problems that organize the search for evidence. Furthermore, diagnosis is not a static endpoint but rather a dynamic way station on the road to treatment. The decision pathway toward diagnosis is shown in Table 9–2 and is described in more detail in the sections that follow.

Eliciting & Perceiving Salient Cues

Even before the patient is seen, the clinician may have gathered cues, for example, from the referring agent. As the patient enters the office, before the interview begins, the clinician scans the patient's eyes, face,

Table 9–2. Decision pathway toward diagnosis.

1. Communicate and elicit pertinent data.
2. Perceive salient cues.
3. Evaluate the significance of salient cues.
4. Make clinical inferences.
5. Assemble significant cues and clinical inferences as a clinical pattern.
6. On the basis of the pattern, generate an array of categorical and dynamic diagnostic hypotheses.
7. Design an inquiry plan and search for both disconfirmatory and confirmatory evidence.
8. On the basis of new evidence, progressively revise, rule out, or rule in the diagnostic hypotheses.
9. Reach a diagnostic conclusion.

skin, clothes, gait, coordination, posture, and voice in order to perceive salient cues (eg, "pale, elderly, frail, shabbily dressed, worried-looking woman using a walking stick, favoring her left leg"). The clinician must be alert to pertinent cues, distinguishing them from the immense amount of noise in the perceptual field. Initially, the net is cast widely so as to maximize the chance of correctly recognizing salient cues, perhaps at the expense of perceiving data that turn out to be irrelevant. As the diagnostic process proceeds, however, the gathering of evidence becomes more focused.

The patient sits down and the interview begins. The clinician's demeanor, receptiveness, and empathic communication encourage the patient to tell her story. More cues are elicited from the patient's spontaneous account of herself.

Evaluating Cues & Making Inferences

Out of the enormous amount of noise, the experienced clinician knows what to look for. Freckles, for example, are less likely to be pertinent than are blue lips (although, in certain circumstances, freckles could be relevant). Blue lips, however, must be evaluated before they are regarded as significant (ie, abnormal). Has the patient been eating berries, or is the blueness circulatory in origin? If the blueness is circulatory in origin—that is, cyanotic (a clinical inference)—is it central or peripheral in origin?

If a patient says that people are talking about him, the clinician must decide whether this complaint is based on reality, whether it is an exaggeration of reality, or whether it is based on a false conviction (ie, a delusion). The experienced clinician makes tentative inferences, at first, which he or she is prepared to revise if subsequent information does not bear them out.

Assembling Cues & Inferences as a Clinical Pattern

Soon after the clinical encounter has begun, the clinician has begun to form cues and inferences into tentative patterns that form the gist of clinical reasoning, for example: (1) potentially lethal suicide attempt; (2) angry, depressed, disheveled adolescent girl lying in a hospital bed; (3) uncooperative and dismissive toward the examiner; (4) said to have made one previous suicide attempt (the time and lethality of which are uncertain at this point).

The efficiency and accuracy of pattern discernment distinguishes the expert from the novice, as does the efficiency with which the expert matches clinical patterns, incomplete though they may be, against his or her memory of diagnostic syndromes.

Generating Categorical & Dynamic Hypotheses

The pattern prompts hypotheses, and hypotheses organize the subsequent clinical inquiry. The capacity of working memory limits the array of hypotheses to between four and six. The array of hypotheses may be linear or hierarchical (see Figures 9–2 and 9–3 for examples). Hypothetical reasoning prevents premature closure on one diagnosis and spares short-term memory by dividing the information derived from cues and inferences into strategic units, from each of which a systematic search for evidence can be planned. Hypotheses are open to revision in the light of new information derived from the inquiry process.

The diagnostic hypotheses generated are usually a mixture of categorical and dynamic types. **Categorical hypotheses** are expressed in the familiar terms of DSM-IV or a similar taxonomy. **Dynamic hypotheses** (eg, "vulnerability to rejection related to abandonment by father") operate in parallel with categorical hypotheses and are not exclusive of them.

Designing an Inquiry Plan & Searching for Evidence

The inquiry plan (ie, history; mental status examination; physical examination; laboratory testing; special investigations; and information from collateral sources, past records, and consultations) has two aspects: **standard** and **discretionary.** Clinicians standardize their data collection (eg, past medical history, mental status examination), casting the net widely to gather important cues and evidence in people from

particular age, ethnic, or social groups. For example, questions about substance abuse, physical and sexual abuse, suicidal ideation, and antisocial behavior are virtually obligatory for adolescent patients. Similarly, certain urine and blood chemistry and hematologic tests may be part of a standard screen for hospitalized patients. For the most part, however, the inquiry plan is discretionary. It is designed to elicit information relevant to the array of diagnostic hypotheses.

Revising, Deleting, or Accepting Hypotheses

Modifications of the standard history, mental status examination, and physical examination are determined by the diagnostic hypotheses. For example, if lead poisoning is hypothesized (eg, as a cause of childhood hyperactivity), the clinician will inquire about the child's physical environment (eg, exposure to old paint, batteries, or tetraethyl lead), examine the child's teeth and gums, and test the child's blood and urine. The inquiry plan yields data that complete the clinical pattern from which the preliminary hypotheses were derived and allows the clinician to refine hypotheses or to disconfirm them.

Reaching a Diagnostic Conclusion

When enough evidence has been gathered, the clinician weighs and summarizes the evidence supporting or refuting hypotheses that have not already been rejected. Sometimes, a single diagnosis is insufficient, and two or more diagnoses are required to account for a heterogeneous pattern of clinical features. Next, the clinician expands the diagnosis, combining dynamic and categorical diagnoses in a diagnostic formulation (see Chapter 36).

Dowe J, Elstein A: *Professional Judgment.* Cambridge University Press, 1988.
Elstein AS, Shulman LS, Sprafka SA: *Medical Problem Solving.* Harvard University Press, 1978.

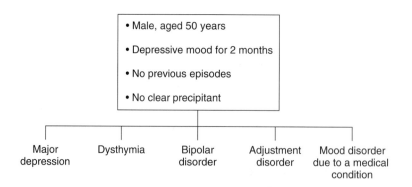

Figure 9–2. Example of a linear array of hypotheses.

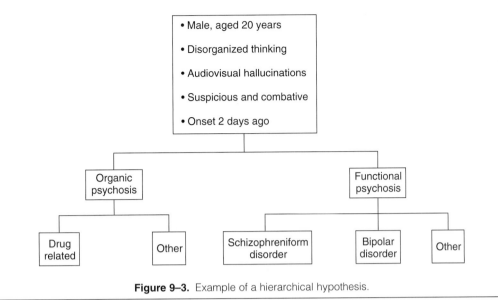

Figure 9–3. Example of a hierarchical hypothesis.

THE STRATEGY OF CLINICAL REASONING

Diagnostic reasoning is a feed-forward, feedback hypothetico-deductive process involving cue recognition, clinical inference, hypothesis testing, inquiry, planning, the search for evidence, the reaching of a diagnostic conclusion, and diagnostic formulation. In order to support the complexity of this process, the diagnostician must do several things (Table 9–3).

Nurcombe B, Gallagher RM: *The Clinical Process in Psychiatry.* Cambridge University Press, 1986.

FLAWS

Flexible and efficient though diagnostic reasoning may be, it is subject to a number of errors that are a consequence of the fact that the human computer has

Table 9–3. The strategy of diagnostic reasoning.

Tolerate uncertainty, avoid premature closure, and consider alternatives.
Separate cue from inference; be able to refer inferences to the salient cues from which they were derived.
Be aware of personal reactions to the patient.
Be alert for fresh evidence, particularly evidence that demands a revision or deletion of a hypothesis or diagnosis.
Value negative evidence above positive evidence.
Be prepared to commit to a diagnosis when enough evidence has been gathered.

inherent capacity limitations and is vulnerable to interference by intrinsic and extrinsic factors.

The diagnostician's judgment can be clouded by fatigue or illness. Clinical judgment can also be biased when the clinician has an emotional reaction to the patient based, for example, on unresolved conflict from his or her own childhood experience (ie, countertransference).

As mentioned earlier in this chapter, no more than four to six diagnostic hypotheses can be juggled at one time because the capacity of short-term memory is limited. This limitation is even more evident in the case of dynamic hypotheses, in which case the clinician will often be satisfied with a single hypothesis, failing to consider alternatives.

The human computer is more impressed by information and hypotheses that appear early in the diagnostic encounter and is relatively less efficient at accounting for later data, especially if the data run counter to first impressions. However, the expert clinician is able to adjust initial hypotheses in response to new information and to drop them when they no longer fit. Expert radiologists, for example, know where to look, what to see, and how to frame an anomalous pattern conceptually. They then engage in "top-down, bottom-up" recursive thinking, testing their initial flexible hypotheses against the details of the radiologic film and progressively adjusting or discarding their hypotheses in accordance with the evidence.

In the same way, the expert psychiatrist quickly discerns significant cues, makes tentative inferences, and assembles a dynamic pattern that allows efficient hypothesis generation. From these hypotheses, he or she begins recursive hypothesis testing, seeking both standard and discretionary data. Table 9–4 lists the chief potential flaws in this process.

Table 9–4. Potential flaws in diagnostic reasoning.

Only a limited number of hypotheses can be dealt with.
Subjective probabilities may be inaccurate (eg, because of recent vivid experience).
Clinicians may lack a systematic inquiry plan.
Clinicians may fail to test all hypotheses in an impartial manner.
Clinicians may fail to refine or discard hypotheses in accordance with the evidence.
Clinicians may rely on a natural inclination to prefer confirmatory to disconfirmatory evidence.
Clinicians may be reluctant to commit to a diagnostic conclusion.

CONCLUSION

Even after training, experience, and self-reflection, the clinician's reasoning is not perfectible. How can it be improved? No contemporary computer can match the skill of the expert clinician in recognizing and weighing cues and inferences, and assembling efficient patterns. However, computers excel at storing information, generating extensive arrays of hypotheses, calculating Bayesian probabilities, avoiding judgment biases, and ensuring that inquiry plans will be systematic. In the future, when base-rate probabilities are better understood, computers will become indispensable to accurate diagnosis and treatment planning. Self-report questionnaires, structured interviews, and search protocols could also enhance the reliability and comprehensiveness of data collection.

Although computers, questionnaires, standard interviews, and inquiry protocols can supplement the human computer, they cannot, as yet, replace it. Whether they will ever be able to do so is conjectural. Until then, they should be regarded as potential aids to the clinical decision maker, not rivals.

General Principles of Psychopharmacologic Treatment

10

Richard C. Shelton, MD

Most psychiatric disorders remain without well-established biological substrates; however, standardized diagnostic nosology has gained acceptance, primarily in the form of the *Diagnostic and Statistical Manual of Mental Disorders,* 4th edition. As with other areas of medicine, there is no substitute for a careful diagnostic evaluation using externally validated diagnostic criteria. Whenever possible, the diagnostic evaluation should draw on a comprehensive database that includes family members, previous or concurrent providers, and other sources of information, and the evaluation should focus on longitudinal data.

PHARMACOKINETICS & PHARMACODYNAMICS

An understanding of the basic pharmacokinetics and pharmacodynamics of psychotropic drugs is required for their safe and effective utilization. With the exception of lithium (which is an element), most psychotropic drugs are lipophilic polycyclic amines. These drugs interact with neurotransmitter-binding sites, which confers their psychotropic effects. For example, most antidepressants act by allosteric binding to catecholamine- or indolamine-uptake binding sites (or with the monoaminergic catalytic enzyme monoamine oxidase), which enhances the synaptic availability of monoamines such as norepinephrine and serotonin. These effects can produce direct antidepressant actions but also may produce side effects such as nausea or nervousness. These drugs also interact with muscarinic cholinergic–binding sites, producing significant side effects such as dry mouth, blurred vision, and constipation, and with histamine-binding sites, producing drowsiness and weight gain. The relative profile of receptor binding affinities will allow the clinician to predict both the beneficial effects and side effects of specific drugs.

Most psychotropic drugs are fairly rapidly and completely absorbed from oral and intramuscular sites and, because of their relatively high lipid solubility, readily cross the blood-brain barrier. Intramuscular administration yields rapid absorption and distribution and bypasses first-pass hepatic metabolism. Therefore, plasma levels are achieved much more rapidly. Intramuscular delivery of antipsychotic drugs (eg, haloperidol) or antianxiety agents (eg, lorazepam) are reserved primarily for the acute management of agitated and psychotic patients. An exception to this is the use of haloperidol or fluphenazine decanoate. These drugs are provided in oil suspension for long-term treatment of psychotic conditions. They require injection every 2–4 weeks and are given to patients who have problems with treatment compliance.

Most psychotropic drugs have high levels of protein (eg, α_1 acid glycoproteins) binding. Notable exceptions include lithium and venlafaxine. Therefore, drug interactions could occur at the level of protein binding, in which case these drugs will displace (and be displaced by) other drugs with significant binding. This can result in unexpected toxicities; therefore, clinicians should take a careful drug history whenever they plan to prescribe a new drug to a patient.

With the exception of lithium, all psychotropic drugs are metabolized, at least in part, via cytochrome enzymes. After one or more metabolic steps, water-soluble products (eg, glucuronides) are formed and eliminated via the kidney. Certain psychopharmacologic agents may induce or inhibit metabolism by cytochrome P-450 (CYP) enzymes. For example, carbamazepine can induce CYP 3A4, 2B1, and 2B2 enzymes, whereas certain serotonin selective reuptake inhibitor (SSRI) antidepressants may inhibit metabolism via CYP 2D6 and, possibly, 3A4 mechanisms. These metabolic interactions must be considered when drugs are coadministered.

Most psychotropic drugs produce widely varying plasma levels, and monitoring may be helpful. However, plasma-level ranges are established only with certain tricyclic antidepressants (eg, imipramine, desipramine, nortriptyline), with antipsychotics such as haloperidol and clozapine, and with lithium. Because of the narrow therapeutic index, plasma-level monitoring of lithium is part of accepted practice. With other drugs, where there are no established plasma level–response relationships, plasma-level monitoring can be used to check compliance or when severe side effects suggest supratherapeutic levels. In addition, plasma levels may clarify a situation in which one drug may be increasing or decreasing the level of another. For example, an SSRI such as paroxetine may elevate plasma levels of other drugs that are metabolized by CYP 2D6 (eg, haloperidol). Unexpected side effects could occur that would be clarified by a plasma-level measurement.

Mavroidis ML et al: Plasma haloperidol levels and clinical response: confounding variables. Psychopharmacol Bull 1985;21:62.

Nemeroff CB, DeVane CL, Pollock BG: Newer antidepressants and the cytochrome P450 system. Am J Psychiatry 1996;153:311.

Preskorn SH: Clinically relevant pharmacology of selective serotonin reuptake inhibitors: an overview with emphasis on pharmacokinetics and effects on oxidative drug metabolism. Clin Pharmacokinetics 1997;32(Suppl 1):1.

Preskorn SH, Dorey RC, Jerkovich GS: Therapeutic drug monitoring of tricyclic antidepressants. Clin Chem 1988;34:822.

PHARMACOKINETICS IN SPECIAL POPULATIONS

Pharmacokinetics change significantly depending on the population. For example, children have a higher relative percentage of hepatic mass and a greater-than-expected elimination of drugs by first-pass metabolism. The elderly often have relatively reduced hepatic clearance and protein binding, which increases the relative plasma levels of psychotropic drugs. Dosage adjustments must be made for differences in kinetics, and these adjustments should be based on research data, when available.

Pregnancy poses its own set of problems. Women of reproductive potential are exposed regularly to psychotropic drugs, raising the possibility of birth defects or spontaneous abortion should pregnancy occur. All women of reproductive potential should be counseled about pregnancy and drug exposure (ie, to avoid pregnancy or to inform the physician before becoming pregnant). Lithium, anticonvulsant mood-stabilizing agents (eg, carbamazepine or divalproex), and benzodiazepines have been associated with increased rates of specific birth defects and, generally, should be avoided. The effects of antidepressants and antipsychotics are less clear. Drugs should be withdrawn if possible; however, drug withdrawal is sometimes impossible. A risk-benefit analysis should be undertaken in which the potential risks of drug exposure are weighed against the hazards of no drug therapy. Because the first trimester is the most important period of organogenesis, efforts should be made to avoid drug exposure during this period. Another consideration is that drugs could be withdrawn prior to delivery and reinstated afterward. This will help prevent untoward reactions such as excessive sedation or withdrawal in the newborn.

Nursing mothers usually should avoid taking psychopharmacologic agents because most drugs are excreted into breast milk. Although the excreted amount is small, the absolute short-term and long-term risks are unknown.

Altshuler LL et al: Pharmacologic management of psychiatric illness during pregnancy: dilemmas and guidelines. Am J Psychiatry 1996;153:592.

Ambrosini PJ: Pharmacotherapy in child and adolescent major depressive disorder. Pages 1247–1254 in: Meltzer HY (editor): Psychopharmacology: The Third Generation of Progress. Raven, 1987.

Catterson ML, Preskorn SH, Martin RL: Pharmacodynamic and pharmacokinetic considerations in geriatric psychopharmacology. Psychiatr Clin North Am 1997;20:205.

Simeon JG: Pediatric psychopharmacology. Can J Psychiatry 1989;34:122.

Stowe ZN et al: Sertraline and desmethylsertraline in human breast milk and nursing infants. Am J Psychiatry 1997; 154:1255.

Vitiello B: Treatment algorithms in child psychopharmacology research. J Child Adolesc Psychopharmacol 1997; 7:3.

PRINCIPLES OF PSYCHOPHARMACOLOGIC MANAGEMENT

Although psychopharmacology often is thought of as a technical discipline, clinical practice involves establishing and maintaining an effective working relationship with a patient—the therapeutic alliance. This process requires the therapist and the patient to establish mutually acceptable goals and to agree on a plan to achieve these objectives. This is especially important in psychiatry because the beneficial effect of a drug may be delayed and because some patients may not have insight into their problem. The challenge of psychopharmacologic management is to maintain an effective working relationship with patients in the face of such obstacles.

The effective pharmacotherapist will maintain a broad biopsychosocial view of the patient's problem and will plan accordingly. Medications will help to address identified symptoms, but patients exhibit a wide array of problems, including psychosocial stressors (eg, family and work issues) and more purely psychological factors that put the patient at risk for further problems. Pharmacotherapy, therefore, shares significant elements with psychotherapy. The pharmacotherapist must establish rapport and a working relationship with the patient, based on the expertise of the therapist and on mutual trust. The patient will depend on the therapist's ability to perform a risk-benefit analysis and to provide an adequate rationale for all elements of treatment. A therapeutic trial of medication may then be undertaken; however, this process of education and negotiation with the patient is an ongoing part of treatment.

Analyzing Risks & Benefits

The risk-benefit analysis considers many factors. The most basic of these factors is the presence of any medical or psychiatric contraindications to the use of a particular drug, including the potential for drug interactions. For example, although bupropion is an effective antidepressant, it generally is not given to patients who have a history of seizure disorder or a current psychotic condition because the drug has the potential to aggravate these problems. However, bupropion may be an especially good choice for patients who are impotent. Alternatively, the pharmacotherapist may determine that medications are not required at all, preferring a course of individual or family therapy. The risk-benefit analysis involves the process of maximizing the potential benefit while minimizing the possible harm of pharmacotherapy.

Managing Nonresponse

Lack of complete response to a given treatment is common. The management of nonresponse should begin before treatment is initiated. The clinician should inform the patient of the possibility of nonresponse and the steps that might be taken in such a circumstance. Patients must be warned of the possible delay in response and of the importance of continuing compliance in face of incomplete improvement. If the response to treatment is inadequate, the clinician should review the treatment plan with the patient and explain to him or her the rationale for each next step. This review should always include the instillation of realistic hope. Suicidal potential must be evaluated as well.

Managing Side Effects

The review, documentation, and management of side effects is an important part of pharmacologic treatment. The clinician should warn patients of the possibility of side effects and should review with them a range of common side effects. A general rule of thumb is that any side effect that occurs in 5% or more of patients in clinical trials should be discussed. However, the clinician should address any serious adverse experience, even those that might be rare, and should warn the patient that other unusual effects may

occur. For example, although hypothyroidism is an uncommon outcome of lithium treatment, patients should be warned of this possibility. The clinician should review and document side effects with each patient and undertake a plan to manage unacceptable effects. Most side effects will improve with time, but noncompliance may be the price of ongoing serious problems. Each patient has his or her own tolerance for side effects, and the patient's tolerance must be considered. For example, sexual side effects of drugs may be completely unimportant for some patients (especially those with no current sexual partner) but critical for others. Further, sexual side effects may be unimportant in one phase of treatment and monumental in others (eg, when a new relationship is established).

Laboratory evaluations may be required to determine if certain serious reactions have occurred (eg, hepatotoxicity or nephrotoxicity). Certain drugs require regular plasma-level monitoring to provide the patient with a margin of safety. Biweekly white blood counts are an absolute requirement for clozapine therapy, and annual or biannual thyroid-stimulating hormone and creatinine tests may be performed for patients on lithium. Proper medication management requires regularly scheduled laboratory evaluations for many patients.

Addressing Concurrent Alcohol or Drug Use

Another safety issue is the concurrent use of alcohol or drugs of abuse. The clinician must take a careful drug and alcohol history; however, ongoing evaluation of the patient's drug and alcohol use also is required. In most cases, modest alcohol use is allowed while a patient is taking psychotropic drugs; however, patients must be warned of potential drug interactions with alcohol with a potentiation of the sedative effects of both the prescribed medication and the alcohol.

Evaluating Response

The clinician should target specific symptoms as indicators of response to treatment. In the case of psychosis, the presence and severity of hallucinations, delusions, or agitation can be effective indicators of early response; however, a more comprehensive view of the patient's condition is required for longer-term management. This involves an ongoing evaluation of a variety of symptomatic domains, including cognitive and mood symptoms and social impairments. As a result, symptoms such as occupational impairment may be important indicators of the effectiveness of pharmacotherapy. Whatever the condition, the goal of pharmacotherapy is to minimize or eliminate symptoms and to return the patient to his or her maximal level of functioning. To this end, the clinician should review and document in each patient the change in a broad range of symptoms.

CONCLUSION

Psychopharmacotherapy ultimately represents a human endeavor in which the challenge to the clinician is the competent synthesis of the scientific basis of pharmacology with the psychosocial skills of the psychiatrist. The most successful pharmacotherapists have a thorough knowledge about the nature of psy-chiatric disorders, the mechanisms of drug action, and the applications of drug therapies, but they also have remarkable interpersonal skills in the management of patients. This integrative skill set in many ways defines competent contemporary psychiatry.

Janicak PG et al: General principles. Pages 1–28 in: *Principles and Practice of Psychopharmacotherapy*. Williams & Wilkins, 1993.

Marder SR: Facilitating compliance with antipsychotic medication. J Clin Psychiatry 1998;59(Suppl 3):21.

General Principles
of Psychotherapeutic Management

11

James L. Nash, MD

Many medical and perhaps most psychiatric conditions cannot be eradicated totally. The affected individual must often learn to manage a protracted or chronic condition. The scope of medical, surgical, and psychiatric intervention is therefore appropriately not limited to acute pathologic states in which a definitive therapy is applied and the person is restored to perfect function. Humans are subject to a multitude of adverse influences, both external and internal. Whether these adverse influences are from bad luck, bad genes, bad environment, or simply the effects of aging, suffering is inherent in the human condition, and the individual must learn to manage personal suffering. It is appropriate that physicians provide others with assistance in the management of suffering.

Psychotherapeutic treatment is an important weapon in the armamentarium of the physician and a necessary component of the management strategy of many and diverse forms of human suffering. It is both common knowledge and the finding of considerable research that human suffering is eased by the ministrations of another caring human being. For example, children learn to comfort themselves via the comforting presence of their mothers, participation in therapy groups may enhance the immune response of patients who have malignant melanoma, and patients who have schizophrenia and who receive psychotherapy in addition to psychopharmacologic agents spend less time hospitalized.

Physicians need to learn the principles of psychotherapeutic management of human suffering in the interest of easing their patients' pain and transferring to them an improved ability to self-manage. It is not clear that a particular type of psychiatric disorder (eg, depression) should necessarily be treated with a particular type of psychotherapy (eg, interpersonal psychotherapy). Individual human suffering is so unique, and the life circumstances of any individual so varied, that psychotherapy must perforce be custom designed, at least in part. It is therefore more important to learn to conduct a coherent and useful psychotherapeutic experience for a patient than to learn one narrowly defined therapeutic style and expect all patients to fit its procrustean bed.

This chapter is also concerned with another form of management: that of the physician's career and life. Coexisting with the many blessings and pleasures that derive from the privilege of knowing other humans so intimately and from the position of power and influence that physicians hold in their patients' lives, is a real and multifaceted peril. Physicians are subject not only to the same suffering that afflicts all people but also to the various forms of exquisite and potentially devastating suffering that can follow when mischief infects the physician-patient bond. In order for physicians to lead long, happy, productive professional lives, they must learn not only to manage their patients' care but also to manage their relationships with their patients. By the attentive acquisition of the principles of professional life management, physicians can largely avoid a chronic state of fear of their patients. Physicians' fear of patients derives from two related sources: (1) The patient will cross some boundary and render the physician uncertain how to behave. This leads the physician to an inability to be natural. (2) The patient will commit some act of aggression against the physician (eg, sue him or her) because of some dissatisfaction. Fear of patients is learned in residency training and must be unlearned in order for the physician to have a comfortable professional life. Fearful physicians cannot be creative, convey hope, or model joy in living. By doing three things the physician can come to enjoy life and the practice of the Art to which Hippocrates referred: (1) by understanding the nature of human vulnerability, both one's own and that of the patient; (2) by understanding the mechanisms whereby patients construct their experience of the physician and vice versa; and (3) by learning to apply the concepts of empathy, transference, and boundaries.

DEFINITION OF PSYCHOTHERAPY

Psychotherapy can be defined in general terms as the use of verbal means to influence beneficially another person's mental and emotional state. Such a definition does not concern itself with training of the therapist and does not distinguish the activities of a well-intentioned friend from those of a paid professional. Psychotherapy will be understood here to refer to a process wherein an individual (ie, the patient) participates in a structured encounter or series of encounters with another person who—by dint of training, licensure, certification, and ethical proscription—is qualified to influence the mental state of another. There is no fundamental difference between the patient and the therapist other than the training of the therapist for the role. This point is made to emphasize that a psychotherapist is not superior to the patient. The patient may be inclined to think so, but the therapist must avoid this prejudice. Nevertheless, the difference inherent in the training and preparation for the role is crucial.

QUALIFICATIONS OF A PSYCHOTHERAPIST

Personal Traits

Although training is the chief distinguishing feature of a psychotherapist, it alone cannot make a good psychotherapist out of every individual. The potential psychotherapist is an individual who is fascinated by the human condition and is not consciously exploitative, significantly emotionally handicapped, or impulsive. Intelligence is important, but more important are thoughtfulness and sensitivity. Some individuals may be said (semifacetiously) to be "too normal" to be psychotherapists. By this, it is meant that some energetic and optimistic people become quickly impatient with others' foibles. Other individuals have no diagnosable psychiatric conditions but do have strongly developed personality traits (eg, pessimism, narcissism) or cognitive styles (eg, suspicious, histrionic) that deter the patient. Some individuals represent a potential danger, both to themselves and to the patient, if allowed to assume the psychotherapist's role. This group includes the charismatic leader and (in contrast) the emotionally needy or love-starved individual. These individuals have powerful personal agendas that overshadow the patient's needs.

Training

Psychoanalytic institutes have, over decades, evolved a tripartite structure of training that can be criticized on various grounds but that is in principle fundamentally sound and provides a prototypical

model. Ideally, a psychotherapist has first passed through some sort of screening to assess personal attributes as outlined in the preceding section. Other qualifications are generally specified (eg, a particular terminal degree), but these requirements are usually in the interest of turf definition and are arbitrary. Having satisfied a training body that one is of reasonable character and is trainable, the student therapist then enters a course of theoretical study, supervised practice, and personal therapy experience. The length and content of such a training program varies considerably in practice. Some training programs emphasize theory; others emphasize the acquisition of specific skills and attitudes. The length of a training program (some months to many years) is a function of the ideals and scope of the learned method (ie, a skill to be acquired or an identity to be forged). Mechanisms are in place to weed out candidates who do not pass muster and to graduate those who have achieved competence. Graduates are eligible to present their work to a national oversight organization that qualifies training programs, sets standards for the profession, admits new graduates into the profession, and requires its members to be accountable to its standards.

There are many such programs in the United States, although most are dedicated to teaching a specific psychotherapeutic discipline. Within these disciplines, the student is expected to master a particular body of theoretical knowledge. This knowledge, in conjunction with the student's personal therapy experience, is intended to provide a framework for understanding another's experience and for structuring therapeutic interventions while avoiding self-serving exploitation of the patient. In practice, a great deal of psychotherapy undoubtedly is practiced by individuals who have had less training than the ideal version outlined here. A typical psychiatric residency training program, for instance, does not require its graduates to have had a personal psychotherapy experience. Some therapists practice various forms of psychotherapy with little training and in an unregulated way.

Robertson MH: *Psychotherapy Education and Training: An Integrative Perspective.* International Universities Press, 1995.
Rogers CR, Dymond R: *Psychotherapy and Personality Change.* University of Chicago Press, 1954.

MAJOR FORMS OF PSYCHOTHERAPY

There may be hundreds of forms of psychotherapy; however, considerable overlap exists among the legitimate forms because the general principles on which they are based are mostly agreed upon. The different forms of psychotherapy place special emphasis on one or another general principle. Whether a given therapy is significantly different from another, or more the brainchild of its originator, is often a matter of debate.

Four major forms of psychotherapy result from the different ways workers conceptualize the nature and development of psychic distress: dynamic, experiential-humanistic, cognitive-behavioral, and eclectic or integrated.

Dynamic Psychotherapies

The dynamic psychotherapies are based on the belief that much of human behavior, especially that which is troublesome to the individual, is motivated by psychological forces outside of the individual's awareness. One is compelled therefore to maintain self-defeating perspectives, and repeat ultimately unsuccessful and maladaptive behaviors, for unknown (ie, unconscious) reasons. Defense mechanisms operate to stabilize the individual's emotional state, but the price paid for this stabilization may be high. The development of these problematic behaviors, personality traits, affect states, and other symptoms is generally understood to have occurred because of some unfortunate mix between the individual's inherent traits (eg, intelligence, temperament) and the caregiving surround into which he or she has been thrust. In the dynamic therapies, improvement is measured by improved function in various realms of the person's life and by results from the new understandings gained in the context of a therapeutic relationship with the therapist. Traditionally, the dynamic therapies have been seen to exist along a somewhat artificial continuum with support at one end and insight at the other. Developments over the past 20 years have placed increased emphasis on the quality of the therapist-patient relationship as a central factor in a beneficial therapy experience.

Experiential-Humanistic Psychotherapies

The experiential-humanistic models of psychotherapy attempt to eliminate the objectivist perspectives seen as inherent in psychodynamic models and replace them with perspectivalist attitudes. That is, the individual's lived experience is viewed as the most, or only, important consideration. No attempt is made to decode the patient's distorted vision of the therapist in order to reconstruct an infantile experience, presumed to be repressed but inferred by the therapist based on knowledge of the universal phases of development. These therapy approaches take the patient's experience, including the patient's experience of the therapist, at face value. Psychopathology is viewed as resulting from the failure of caregivers to provide the empathic responsiveness necessary for the development of a self-structure that organizes experiences in the most adaptive way. The therapist will play a wider array of roles than in the more classically dynamic approaches, determined by the patient's needs and characteristics. Therapeutic effects derive from the formation of a personal narrative that, in the atmosphere of a new self-object experience (ie, patient with therapist in a safe, gratifying, and development-enhancing relationship), allows for a reordering of the processing of personal experience.

Cognitive-Behavioral Psychotherapies

Cognitive-behavioral models of psychotherapy view psychopathology as the result of faulty thinking (ie, cognitions) based on illogical beliefs. Various forms of mental illness (eg, anxiety, inhibitions, depression) result from the powerful influence of these cognitions, for which there is understood to be little or no rational basis. Little time is spent attempting to explain the etiology of these beliefs, and the concept of a dynamic unconscious is seen as unnecessary. The patient's unsubstantiated beliefs (eg, "others would be better off if I were dead") are challenged, with more adaptive beliefs implicitly or explicitly suggested and supported. The patient is thereby persuaded to discard irrational perspectives on the world (eg, "no one will want you if you are not perfect") and replace them with more realistic, validated beliefs. Although other psychotherapies frequently include cognitive elements, the behavioral components of cognitive-behavioral therapy (eg, flooding, blocking) involve action interventions that carry these methods into a clearly different realm (see Chapter 2).

Eclectic or Integrated Psychotherapies

In the practice of psychotherapy, most patients and clients receive a therapy that is an amalgam of the dynamic, experiential-humanistic, and cognitive-behavioral perspectives. This results less from the inherent difficulty in staying within the confines of a particular method and more from the failure of each of the methods to account for the multifaceted presentation of human psychopathology. Unless he or she is immune to the possibility of reductionism, views therapy as a tour de force, or simply elects to ignore certain material, the therapist will not fail to recognize that the typical patient presents clinical material best handled by first one and then another perspective.

It would be ludicrous to attempt to paint a picture of a typical psychotherapy patient. The following case is presented to illustrate the typical complexity of the clinical picture that confronts the psychotherapist, and the usefulness of being familiar with a range of theoretical perspectives and techniques:

The patient was an early-middle-aged mother of two healthy children. She was an intelligent, sensitive, and kind woman who had been married for 15 years to a hard-working man who she felt did not understand her. Indeed, he was frustrated by her manifest pessimism, her guilt, and her inability to enjoy the many fruits of their hard work. She was chronically depressed, anxious, phobic, and compulsive. She was also hypochondriacal, sexually unresponsive, and indecisive. Her father died when she was 12 years old—a critical time in a girl's life. She had been sexually abused by her older brother, and her sister had committed suicide. As the eldest girl in the family, she had been assigned domestic responsibilities inappropriate to her age following her father's death. The first-born brother's presence, however, stood between her and a sense of specialness. She grew up embittered and thinking that she was not, and never would be, "good enough." Her sense of self was defined by her failures. Her successes were discounted as aberrations.

Although the patient might have benefited from pharmacotherapy, she said that she did not wish to take medication. She wanted a psychotherapy experience that would help her learn to enjoy her life more and unlock what she experienced as untapped potential. She feared that she might be contaminating her children's world views, and she felt she was being unfair to her husband and restricting their life together. She saw her problem as chronic and severe and worried that she might one day follow her sister's suicidal path, an act that, for her family's sake, she desperately wanted to avoid.

In planning a psychotherapy for this patient, the therapist was struck by the myriad symptoms she exhibited, noting that all were in the "neurotic" sphere. She did not abuse substances and had no psychotic thought content. She seemed to experience both irrational thoughts and personal isolation. Her low self-esteem was related to chronic abusive experiences, and her guilty fears and inhibitions suggested unconscious themes of an oedipal nature. The pervasiveness of the patient's suffering and the history of her personal losses suggested that short-term work would not be effective and might even be damaging. A purely cognitive approach seemed inappropriate given the patient's overwhelming symptomatology: It would not address her many interpersonal needs. An open-ended and eclectic therapy seemed indicated.

Gabbard GO: *Psychodynamic Psychiatry in Clinical Practice: The DSM-IV Edition.* American Psychiatric Press, 1994.

Gill MM: *Psychoanalysis in Transition: A Personal View.* Analytic Press, 1994.

Stolorow RD, Atwood GE, Brandchaft B: *The Inter-subjective Perspective.* Jason Aronson, 1994.

EXPECTATIONS OF A PSYCHOTHERAPY

Patients approach psychotherapy with a mixture of hopes and expectations, many of which are conscious and some of which are unconscious. Some of the patient's goals are reasonable and some are not. Patients do not intend to be unreasonable; their demands are a function of their neediness and their lack of information. Therapists have knowledge, acquired through training and experience, of what is and is not attainable from psychotherapy. The therapist's ambitions and goals for the therapy may not, however, coincide with the patient's. More mature and experienced therapists become increasingly confident in the usefulness of a psychotherapy experience, while simultaneously becoming impressed with the unpredictable and nonspecific nature of the benefit. They understand the importance of allowing the patient to use therapy in a uniquely personal and creative way.

Therapists themselves are not immune to influences that induce them to place unreasonable expectations on therapy. Chief among these influences are pressures to move more quickly, more efficiently, and more definitively. The therapist may unwittingly accept the demand to become a magician whose aims are accomplished by special power, not hard work. Some therapists feel apologetic for their limitations, ashamed of their imperfections, and guilty about their fees. These vulnerabilities, which signal a need for supervision or personal treatment, may combine with the patient's unreasonable demands to create an "unholy alliance" in which goals are implied but never stated, boundaries are fluid, and roles are not defined.

Patients and therapists should agree explicitly on the goals of the work they are performing mutually. If goals are not made explicit, they will likely become idiosyncratic and unmeasurable as well as unreasonable and probably unattainable. Goals can be changed; indeed, it is good practice to compare notes from time to time, especially in a longer treatment, in order to assure that patient and therapist are still on the same track. In any event, one goal should always be to provide the patient with a positive experience. The therapist may be the first significant other in the patient's life who has not wished to exploit the patient, or who has genuinely wished to hear and understand the patient. Such quite general influences may nevertheless be profoundly salutary. It is not necessary for change to be a goal, and setting change as a goal may doom the treatment to failure and thus to its being seen as a negative event in the patient's life. Humans, most especially neurotic ones, are resistant to change. Neurosis is understood to describe the mind in conflict with itself over two opposing wishes—those that are reasonable and those that are unreasonable (Table 11–1)—and suffering is experienced as the result of the conflict. Most humans will, regrettably, tend to continue to suffer rather than let go of one or the other wish. A positive experience with the therapist will likely have a continuing effect on the patient long after the treatment is ended, and changes will likely occur, albeit out of sight of the therapist.

Table 11–1. Patients in (or entering) psychotherapy.

Reasonable wishes
To achieve more mature development (eg, decrease emotional investment in parents and increase independence of function, decrease self-absorption and increase awareness of needs of others)
To restructure ways of organizing experience, including changing cognitive style and irrational beliefs
To decrease fear of one's own thoughts and feelings with less reliance on immature coping mechanisms
To increase communication skills in situations in which former limitations were the result of past untoward experiences leading to pathologic character structures
Unreasonable wishes
To become completely well-adjusted; mythically perfect; free of irrational, embarrassing, or shameful thoughts or feelings
To be changed without active effort
To have one's past erased, or be transformed in the present, for example, to become the therapist's child

THE PSYCHOTHERAPEUTIC PROCESS

PATIENT SELECTION & THERAPY PLANNING

What principles should guide the therapist in deciding whom and how to treat? Many individuals may be recognized as needing therapy, in the sense that their loved ones or personal acquaintances recognize them as suffering or causing others to suffer. Needing therapy in this sense is not the same as having the potential to use a psychotherapy experience. The process of assessing the likelihood that a prospective patient can benefit from psychotherapy of any type begins with the first encounter (often via the telephone) and should continue until therapist and patient are ready to close the evaluation phase and begin the treatment.

The first level of screening involves the question of need for hospitalization or the likelihood that hospitalization will be necessary in the near future. Although many of the principles discussed here are applicable to inpatients, psychotherapy is not feasible in the face of active psychosis or immediate suicide threat. Similarly, a patient who is in the throes of active substance abuse or who is currently involved in a legal proceeding should be referred to a specialized help provider.

The telephone call may be used to screen out patients who might become involved in an encounter with a therapist that will be frustrating and essentially a waste of the patient's time and money. The patient should be asked how he or she came to call the particular therapist, in the interest of assessing what the patient likely knows about how the therapist works, and should be told what fees will be charged. The therapist should consider the following questions: Does there seem to be a beginning goodness-of-fit in that the referral makes sense? What is the nature of the complaint? Is the problem within the competence or interest range of the therapist? Does the prospective patient indicate a degree of reflectiveness, or is

there the sound of demandingness? Does the patient "hear" the therapist during the phone call? The patient may well be asked to pay for the about-to-be-scheduled evaluation session at the time of the service. This serves as a useful screen for motivation and ensures that the therapist will be compensated for the time spent, even if the patient elects not to return. Obviously, this strategy applies only in a fee-for-service setting.

An initial phone call need not be lengthy, but it can be useful, and the patient should not be scheduled for a first visit unless the therapist feels a sense of enthusiasm about working with the patient. The patient may also have some questions for the therapist, which should neither threaten nor offend the therapist.

Occasionally, the patient will ask the therapist a question that will indicate that referral to a colleague, or simply a refusal, is the best strategy. Although some questions may need to be answered, others may seem so provocative or challenging that they alarm the therapist. It is better not to begin working with a patient in the first place than to have to refer the patient to another therapist after treatment has begun.

FIRST SESSION: EVALUATING THE PATIENT

The prospective patient is told that one session will be scheduled for an evaluation of the problem. At the end of that hour, the therapist and patient will compare notes and discuss options. Treatment has at this point not been offered and no such contract has been entered into. A first psychiatric session will generally be a mixture of medical interviewing, with a focus on the symptom picture and the patient's mental status, and open-ended interviewing, wherein the patient is given an opportunity not only to be heard but also to demonstrate ease with carrying the conversation. Given a reasonably cooperative patient, the first session should yield three things: (1) an Axis I diagnosis, if any; (2) a sense of goodness-of-fit between patient and therapist; and (3) an ever-growing sense in the therapist of "getting it," that is, of the patient's story beginning to make sense according to the therapist's understanding of the nature and development of psychopathology.

If the therapist is to plan a psychotherapy experience for the patient (either as primary treatment or as an adjunct to other interventions), an understanding of what is "wrong" with the patient must be developed. This extends beyond a clinical diagnosis and addresses the question of how psychotherapy will be designed to enable the patient to do a needed body of psychological work. The straightforward and succinct statement that forms in the therapist's mind is a basic version of the elaborate psychodynamic formulations from the heyday of psychoanalysis. It becomes the skeleton on which the flesh of the therapy will be hung. In the absence of the therapist's ability to explain to an observer (or to the patient) what he or she proposes to do and why or, better yet, what the therapist and patient will do together and why, it is likely that a kind of "chronic undifferentiated psychotherapy" will be undertaken. Such an enterprise will be unfocused. It may be pleasant, but it will lack thrust.

It bodes well for psychotherapy when the prospective patient engages the therapist in a personal way. Psychotherapeutic work in the realm of what has traditionally been referred to as the transference adds immediacy and zest to the treatment. Psychotherapy can be done without working with the patient's experience of the therapist, but such treatments are more sterile, intellectual, and distant. However, some patients cannot work effectively in this manner. Patients with narcissistic personality disorder, especially, need a considerable period of time before they feel comfortable revealing what to them represent humiliating notions about the therapist. The therapist cannot force transference into the foreground, but it can be a powerful tool when the patient will allow its use.

As the time allotted for the first evaluation session draws to a close, a number of complex and interlocking issues come to the forefront. If the evaluator is a psychiatrist, then four decisions must be made: (1) Is hospitalization indicated? If so, the whole psychotherapy matter will probably be tabled. The administrative details of getting the patient hospitalized become the focus of attention. (2) Is a different immediate intervention demanded by the patient's condition? If the therapist is required immediately to assume the role of active change agent (eg, by prescribing psychotropic medication), certain other roles will be made less easily established in the future. (3) How comfortable does the therapist feel about having "gotten it?" Generally, the patient will want to feel that the time has been well spent and that the therapist is forming a clear understanding of the patient's situation. The patient does not, however, want to experience the therapist as having decided too quickly about diagnosis and treatment. This will lead the patient to be suspicious of the therapist from the beginning. (4) Does the therapist feel that a therapeutic fit is likely to happen and is worth pursuing, or should this session be the last? Referral for whatever reason is best done at the time of the first visit.

A recommendation of no treatment should remain a possibility in the therapist's mind. If, however, the therapist is beginning to understand the patient and imagine a potential contract for a therapy, it is appropriate near the end of the first hour for the therapist to share with the patient reflections on the interview so far. This preliminary interpretive statement, which should be followed by the patient's invited response, will set the stage for an agreed-upon second evaluative session that explores areas that both parties feel are important but for which no time is left. In most cases the therapist can reassure the patient that things should be clear, both for therapist and patient, by the end of a second interview, and that a recommendation for treatment will be discussed at that time. The second interview should be scheduled sooner rather than later, preferably within less than 1 week. Patients who have made the decision to seek help generally have delayed for some time but, having begun the process, hope that it will move swiftly.

SECOND SESSION: PROCESS & CONTRACT

A second evaluation hour is necessary for several reasons. The therapist may not be ready to present the patient with a therapy recommendation because the formulation is incomplete, or he or she may not want to rush the patient or may want to test the patient's reaction to the first session. Will the patient be able to share thoughts and reactions to the first hour? Will the patient feel better already, more hopeful of an improved future? Will there be evidence of self-reflection that generates fresh associations?

The therapist may begin the second session with a statement that it will be useful to explore further a number of areas, but first, what were the patient's thoughts and reactions to the first hour? Such early alliance building demonstrates that much of the responsibility for the treatment rests with the patient. The patient will often tell the therapist that he or she feels better or will report that new information has been recalled. An exploration of this material generally will enable the therapist to call attention to areas noted after the first session that need exploration (with the upcoming therapy recommendation clearly in mind). If left unexplored, these areas may erupt later as major obstacles (eg, substance abuse, legal trouble, experience with other therapists).

The therapist is also considering further the nature of the problem and the type of treatment to be recommended. This will inevitably result in a compromise between what is ideal and what is feasible. The therapist needs to know the patient's capacity to fund therapy, ability to conform to the therapist's work schedule and office hours, and ways of handling separations. The therapist is also assessing how easily the patient talks, and about what. Patients who wish to discuss situational issues may need more time between sessions to allow events to occur. Patients who have strong reactions to the therapy encounters may have difficulty waiting for the next session. Patients who live some distance from the therapist's office, or who must exert considerable effort to get back and forth, will have trouble sustaining their initial enthusiasm. How much is the patient suffering? How motivated does the patient seem to be to initiate change? How stable and supportive is the patient's social support network? Does the patient have the ways and means to effect change?

By the midway point of the second session, an experienced therapist will generally feel comfortable with an extraordinary amount of important information. A less experienced therapist may wish to obtain supervision at this point, but the seasoned therapist will have assessed and decided upon three key issues: (1) whether or not to prescribe medication; (2) whether tests (eg, psychological, chemical, neuropsychological) are needed; and (3) what type of psychotherapy to recommend and at what frequency.

These issues are matters of the utmost importance to the patient's life and to other lives that psychotherapy will affect. The therapist is now poised to make recommendations that will have such an impact on the patient as to be remembered possibly for the rest of the patient's life. The patient may need help in sorting through the most salient implications. If third-party payment will be used, does the patient understand that confidentiality cannot be complete and that the future may bring difficult questions regarding history of treatment? Does the patient plan to make significant life decisions that could affect the course and outcome of the treatment? What are the dynamic forces at work between the patient and most significant other over the need for and possible result of therapy? The need for informed consent is great in the case of the potential psychotherapy patient, who may have little appreciation of what is about to be undertaken.

The therapist will then tell the patient precisely what is being recommended and why. Three areas must be covered: (1) the name of the psychotherapy, its rationale, its frequency, its anticipated length, and its cost; (2) the hoped-for outcome of the treatment, couched in terms that express optimism for realistic and attainable goals, and the likelihood of that outcome; and (3) alternative treatments, their anticipated length and costs, and their risks and likely outcome.

A schedule for visits will be negotiated, and a clear description will be provided of procedures regarding payment of the bill, appointment cancellation and lateness on the part of the patient or the therapist, and vacations. A standard written policy statement may be used. If third-party payment or certification procedures (eg, health maintenance organizations [HMOs]) will be a part of the picture, these procedures, including the provision of a diagnosis, should be outlined clearly. The therapist should explain to the patient the diagnosis and should tell the patient what is expected of him or her during the treatment and what can be expected of the therapist. Some issues may be addressed only when they arise and become integrated into the context of the treatment. These issues include details such as telephone calls, chance meetings outside the office, and what names will be used.

By the end of the second session, the therapist and the patient may look forward with optimism and anticipation to the beginning of a psychotherapeutic endeavor between an informed patient and a therapist who knows where things are headed. The framework of treatment has been carefully built. Both parties know what to expect. Therapy is off to a good start.

BEGINNING OF PSYCHOTHERAPY

It can be said justifiably that therapy has been underway since its conception as a thought in the patient's mind, and certainly since the patient's first encounter with the therapist. Nevertheless, the therapist has made a point of separating evaluation from treatment, because of the wish not to enter into a formal medico-legal contractual responsibility for the patient's ongoing welfare (ie, beyond handling any immediate needs the patient may have) until he or she is confident that the treatment is manageable. The treatment phase has now been launched, and the therapist becomes concerned with those phenomena that characterize the opening phase.

Whatever goals for the treatment enterprise the patient and therapist have agreed upon, the therapist knows that there is one overarching goal: to provide the patient with an experience that will enable some measure of healing to occur. The therapist cannot will the patient into mental health, and the patient may find that personal resistances to change are too great to overcome. The therapist is confident, however, that careful attention to the application of considered strategies and tactics, informed by a detailed understanding of the nature of the patient's psychopathology against the background of his or her unique developmental experiences, and delivered with skill and sensitivity, will, over time, create a healthy atmosphere that the patient will use to the best possible advantage. To this end, the therapist considers the various or predominant role(s) to be played and the basic interventions to be undertaken. Staying in role, and consistently and effectively intervening over time, the therapist will have a corrective effect. The therapist has the emotional well-being and personal attributes to make this possible.

Whatever the nature of the therapy, the opening phase is understood to involve two parts. First, the patient passes through the stages of engagement into the therapy process. The signs of the patient becoming "in therapy" will vary according to the structure of the particular therapy being used. In psychodynamic therapy, for instance, patients might be said to be "in therapy" when they begin to attach emotional importance to the therapist as a real person or to the nature of the intersubjective experience of patient and therapist. In therapy designed along more educational or supportive lines, the patient may report having been reflecting on the last session and provide additional thoughts about it. In some cases, the engagement will be revealed in a dream or in an unconscious but undeniable act of resistance.

After engagement has occurred, the second part of the opening phase plays out, with the unfolding and illumination before the eyes of the patient and the therapist of the nature of the problem. The way the problem is conceptualized is intensely personal. It is worked out between the patient and the therapist in language to which they will refer by mutual agreement. This language is a derivative of the blending of the therapist's methods of organizing the experience of the therapy with the patient's organization of the experience. The words used to describe the nature of the problem will reveal the predominant theoretical orientation of the therapist merging with the narrative that the patient is constructing. Once the problem has been defined, the opening phase is over.

MIDDLE PHASE OF PSYCHOTHERAPY

Before the middle phase of psychotherapy can begin, the alliance between patient and therapist must be established firmly and the core conflictual issue identified and agreed upon. The process of working through begins. The patient is confronted repeatedly with manifestations of problematic ways of organizing experiences and relating to others. In some therapies, this process occurs in the cauldron of the transference-countertransference. In other therapies in which the patient is unable to work with transference material, working through takes place once-removed, by examining relationships outside the therapy, both current and past. This confrontation has variable effects on the patient. There may be moments of new understanding and growth. There may be periods of flight away from the process via resistance maneuvers and regressive detours. The therapist's role is to "follow the red thread" of the patient's unconscious and automatic attitudes and behaviors and—through a mixture of empathic responsiveness, probing, clarifying, confronting, and interpreting—"hold the patient's nose to the grindstone" of the work of the treatment.

Many difficulties are encountered during the middle phase; some are inevitable and some are incidental to therapist error. All the desirable personal attributes and all the therapeutic competence that the therapist can muster will not ensure a smooth middle

phase. Empathic failures by the therapist will lead to failures to intervene and to mismatches between patient need and therapist role selection. The therapist will lose sight of the patient's experience, and the patient's feelings will be hurt. A number of middle-phase problems are typical and are mentioned individually in the sections that follow.

A. Acting Out: The term "acting out" is used in different ways, but it is generally understood to refer to behavior that discharges the affects generated by the therapy process. A variety of behavior is seen, involving both conscious and unconscious motivations. Individuals who are prone to impulsiveness or destructive behavior make relatively problematic psychotherapy subjects. The most flagrant behavior, such as substance abuse, suicide attempts, and middle-of-the-night phone calls, may be so difficult to manage as to make therapy impossible. If the therapist lacks the ability to bring administrative control to bear in order to preserve the treatment, he or she can be placed in the untenable position of being responsible for the patient's irresponsible acts.

Less dramatic forms of acting out must be recognized by the therapist, who should then confront the patient and bring the affects and associated thoughts into the therapy. The patient may quote the therapist to another person and arouse ire, especially if the other person is paying the bill. The patient may fail to pay the bill, miss sessions, cancel appointments, or be late; or the patient may make serious life decisions abruptly, especially regarding love relationships. The mutual analysis of these behaviors nearly always leads to an improved alliance and forward motion. Failure to confront the behavior retards or disrupts therapy.

The patient may demonstrate ego-syntonic acting out, in which he or she enacts unconscious themes through behavior that causes no harm. For example, the patient may come early for the appointment (the attendant hope being to see the therapist's other patients), or the patient may watch the clock so as not to overstay (the unconscious fear is of feeling dismissed). It is sometimes useful in therapy to look the gift horse in the mouth.

B. Acting In: Novice therapists are frequently troubled when patients do things in their presence that throw them off balance, disorient, or even frighten them. Many of these behaviors merely need to be experienced once in order to know how to handle them next time. Some behaviors may prompt the therapist to seek personal treatment.

A patient may put the therapist off balance by exhibiting overly familiar behavior. For example, a patient calls the therapist by her first name or asks to be called by his first name; a patient brings the therapist a small gift; or a patient asks personal questions about the therapist's life. The smooth management of these personal moments requires self-awareness, compassion, flexibility, and objectivity. It also requires factual knowledge of the nature of boundaries, boundary violations, and medical ethics, as well as theoretical knowledge of the nature of psychopathology and of the science of psychotherapy. Beginning therapists need regular forums in which they can process such events. In general, it is best to err on the side of awkward, stiff refusal than on the side of boundaryless permissiveness. One's technique will become smoother with time.

Some behaviors by the patient are more provocative and troublesome. For example, a patient asks for hugs or other personal contact or asks for a gift from the therapist; a patient wears revealing clothing or directly propositions the therapist; or a patient requests out-of-the-office contact. In such situations, the therapist should begin with gentle limit setting accompanied by sensible explanations. One does not say "I'd like to, but the ethics of my profession won't let me." One says, "Therapy is conducted through talk, not through action." Occasionally a patient will persist, despite firm but gentle limit setting. The therapist then confronts the patient with his or her seeming inability to take no for an answer and invites an exploration.

A common behavior on the border between acting out and acting in involves encounters between the patient and the therapist's office personnel. The patient may pump the secretary for personal information about the therapist. The patient may attempt to befriend or even romance the office staff. These situations are easily dealt with when the staff is knowledgeable and well-trained. Considerable trouble can result, however, when the office person has no understanding of the nature of a patient-therapist relationship or, even worse, harbors resentment toward the therapist-boss. Beginning therapists must take nothing for granted in the hiring and training of office personnel. Such individuals represent the therapist to the public, for better or for worse.

C. Stalemate: The term "stalemate" covers a variety of conditions, the essence of which is that the patient becomes dissatisfied with the therapy, makes no progress, and threatens to quit. This phenomenon has traditionally been seen from an objectivist perspective and understood as a manifestation of resistance (eg, negative therapeutic reaction). More contemporary views of the therapy process interpret these states as commentaries on the nature of the relationship between the two parties. Active interpretation is usually required to restore the alliance and the therapy, and generally some degree of therapist self-disclosure involving the immediate interaction calls to the patient's attention the failure to get something from the therapist that the patient very much wants. It is not, of course, the gratification of these wishes that is the purpose of the therapy but rather their identification. Awareness and acknowledgment that the therapist plays an active role in the creation of the "analytic third" is necessary to uncover and illuminate these states of depletion in the patient.

D. Third-Party Interferences: Threatened spouses and parents are joined by third-party payers of all varieties in placing pressures on the very existence of psychotherapy. For example, an angry wife may request equal time to "set the record straight"; a jealous husband may knock on the door during a therapy hour; or an HMO may need more information before a claim for benefits can be processed. Sensitivity, flexibility, and strength are required of the therapist in order to protect the patient's confidentiality and preserve the life of the therapy.

E. Other Negative Effects: Many complications are possible in psychotherapy. Constant pressure against the frame of a therapy is created by necessary restrictions. It is not easy to avoid boundary violations, but the task is made easier if the therapist has a knowledge of behaviors that are considered to be boundary violations. Experience shows that it is folly to expect the patient to understand and control these matters. It is the therapist's responsibility.

The vulnerabilities of the psychotherapist are all too real, and patients can present many attractions to a therapist. The therapist is of course in danger of participating in boundary violations but is also vulnerable to painful affect states tied to the rigors and restrictions of the work. Commonly experienced signs of untoward therapist stress include excessive fatigue at the end of the day; depression, depletion, and having nothing left for life outside the office; inability to take time off (called "dance of the hours"); or loss of objectivity and intemperate identification with the patient.

Rarely, the therapist will realize that a serious mistake has been made in the original conceptualization of the therapy and that the therapy should not be allowed to continue. It is better to interrupt treatment than to persist in the face of an untenable situation. The therapist may, for example, realize that the patient has been misdiagnosed and that significant antisocial elements are present. The patient may become engaged in behavior that runs counter to the contract or that the therapist finds intolerable (eg, an HIV-positive patient who continues to expose unknowing partners). Consultation with a colleague may show the therapist the way out of the dilemma. If not, the only path may be to make alternative arrangements with careful consideration of the therapist's legal and ethical responsibilities.

In a gratifyingly high percentage of cases, when the patient-therapist fit has been a good one and the alliance has held together, the patient achieves most of the contracted-for goals. The patient is easier to be with, both for the therapist and significant others. The patient reports that life is better. Symptoms melt away, and characteristic ways of organizing experiences become less rigid and stereotyped. Relationships with other people improve. The patient begins to talk about life without the therapy, and the therapist begins to think that a successful ending for the therapy is in view. The middle phase is finished.

TERMINATION OF PSYCHOTHERAPY

The ending of a psychotherapy can occur under a variety of circumstances, some very satisfying for both parties, and some painful or traumatic, especially for the patient.

Termination by Mutual Agreement: Satisfied

In this situation, circumstances are optimal. The therapist and the patient are in agreement that the therapy should end because the work has gone well and the desired effect has occurred. If the therapy has been open ended, the classic phases of termination will be seen, as always, colored by the particular patient's circumstances. The therapist will have begun to muse that termination has become a consideration, seeing that the patient is functioning well, both within and outside the therapy hour: There is no acting out, the original symptoms are no longer problematic, and the patient is being affirmed by the environment. When the patient raises the issue, it feels congruent to the therapist. It is discussed, and a mutually agreeable ending date is set. During the ensuing phase (brief or extended, according to agreement), a resurgence of symptomatology is typical, and the pain of loss of a relationship is experienced by both parties. The therapist knows the pain must be worked through by the patient and does not collude in any defensive maneuvers of the patient. The therapy ends on a bittersweet note, with recognition that good work was done and each party has devoted appreciated effort; but the work is over, and the patient is ready to move on. The therapeutic relationship is left intact. The therapist does not cross previously respected boundaries. The patient may well never return, but if the need arises, there would be no barriers.

Termination by Mutual Agreement: Elements of Dissatisfaction

More typical than the previously described ideal situation is one in which the patient and therapist agree to the ending of the therapy, but one or both feel a degree of dissatisfaction with what has been accomplished and would prefer to continue. The therapy may have been time limited from the beginning, either because the therapist conceptualized a time-limited treatment as optimal or because the patient had limited resources. Artificial limits may have been set by a managed care organization. Nevertheless, one or both parties may wish the treatment could go on. The patient and the therapist may agree that a hoped-for

goal for the treatment will not be realized. These endings are painful to a degree, but they are not traumatic. The limitations of the experience are acknowledged, but there is a sharing in appreciation of the good work. The pain of separation is experienced, but there is no recrimination or bitterness.

Interruption of Psychotherapy: Disagreement

When one or both parties disagree with the ending of psychotherapy, the word "interruption" is a more descriptive designation than is "termination." The treatment is ending over the objections of one or both participants. For example, the patient announces the intention not to return, the patient is told that the therapist is leaving (eg, relocating for a career move, rotating off residency service), or the financial support for the treatment is withdrawn unexpectedly. In these situations, psychological trauma will be experienced, generally more acutely by the patient, although losing a therapy case can be a staggering blow to a therapist's self-esteem. In any case, the nature of the felt trauma will be a function of the reason for the interruption and the psychological structure of the injured party.

When the patient leaves the therapist, it is important that the therapist remain in role. Although shocked, insulted, or frightened, the therapist must help the patient deal with the emotions surrounding the decision. Any impulse to counter with threats or dire predictions must be stifled, perhaps to be worked through in an ad hoc personal therapy encounter. Because of the chronic nature of psychopathology, there is a good chance that the patient who interrupts therapy will seek therapy elsewhere, sooner or later. Therapists should always endeavor to make any encounter with a patient as therapeutic as possible.

When the therapist leaves the patient, the scene is ripe for damage to be inflicted on the patient, although the degree of damage can be controlled by sensitive and thoughtful management of the situation. To do so, the therapist must transcend the narcissistic investment in the reason for the interruption. The excitement one is feeling over an upcoming relocation or graduation or new baby will not be shared by the patient, informed or otherwise. The patient will feel variously bereft, abandoned, devalued, jealous, envious, or a plethora of other feelings determined by circumstances and character structure. The patient must be allowed to explore these states and express the attached affects. The therapist must remain in role, acknowledging nondefensively as many of the facts as is consistent with his or her established way of working. The patient's pain is not underestimated, and the patient's individuality is respected within reason as a schedule for the interruption is worked out.

In announcing the interruption, the therapist has two decisions to make: (1) when to announce it and (2) whether transfer to another therapist is indicated.

Patients need adequate time to process an interruption, but announcing the interruption too soon may cause the remaining time to be a "lame duck" period in which little is accomplished. Likewise, the patient may be soothed to know that therapy will continue, but the new therapist will immediately assume great importance in the patient's mind even if never met, and this will distract the patient from dealing with feelings about the interruption.

In some cases, it will be obvious that further treatment will be needed, and the therapist will offer help in locating a replacement therapist. In these cases, the therapist can leave the interruption announcement until relatively late in the sequence, perhaps with only several sessions remaining. Other patients may not need a replacement therapist. The patient may be near enough to a termination that the work can be truncated. The patient may feel that transfer to a new therapist is not worth the trouble involved. The patient may wish to find further therapy in the future but wants to take a break from the process after the interruption. The therapist will profit from avoiding a premature and unilateral decision to recommend continued treatment. Such a recommendation may be more defensive against the therapist's guilt over leaving than it is sensitive to the patient's individuality. In such situations, where there is a good chance that the patient's therapy experience will end with the interruption, the therapist must give the patient more time. The therapist must assess the patient's record of dealing with separations. Some patients may need 6 months or more, and various tapering schedules and other modifications of the usual ways of working may be useful. Therapist inflexibility is usually experienced as damaging.

The management of an interruption or a termination requires sensitivity and skill. Having had the experience of being in therapy oneself adds immeasurably to the therapist's ability to be sensitive to the importance one attains in the eyes of the patient.

Gutheil TG, Gabbard GO: The concept of boundaries in clinical practice: theoretical and risk-management dimensions. Am J Psychiatry 1993;150:188.

Ogden TH: *Subjects of Analysis.* Jason Aronson, 1994.

Strupp H, Binder J: *Psychotherapy in a New Key: A Guide to Time-Limited Psychotherapy.* Basic Books, 1984.

CONCURRENT TREATMENTS

Individual psychotherapy as the sole therapeutic agent is the best treatment for many of the patients who present themselves to mental health professionals. Individuals with common personality disorders such as narcissistic personality and borderline personality, and those troubled by what may be called disorders of the spirit, are frequently best managed in the containing acceptance of an individual therapy. Such patients may seek psychotherapy from psychologists, social workers, and pastoral counselors, reasoning not only that such professionals are uniquely qualified to help them but also that psychiatrists will be either too expensive or disinterested in their problems. Although this recent historical development is unfortunate for the field of psychiatry, it is hoped that the recognition that psychiatry is in danger of "losing its soul" will spur the field to reclaim its place in the psychotherapy tradition.

Many patients, especially those encountered by psychiatrists, need more than individual therapy to manage their conditions. Depression seems to have replaced narcissism as the illness of our time, and combined psychotherapy and pharmacotherapy for mood disorders has become commonplace. In addition, a new recognition of the important role of supportive psychotherapy in the care of the seriously mentally ill has led to more collaboration between psychiatrists and non-psychiatrist psychotherapists. Debates about whether psychotherapy can withstand the resistances set in motion by combined use of medication, and about whether the therapist should have a psychopharmacologist handle the medication, have been replaced by concerns over the impact of contemporary agents (eg, fluoxetine) on the core of personality structure. Amidst this sea of change, however, it is easy to trivialize truths about the patient-therapist relationship. Fortunately the concept of dynamic pharmacotherapy has provided a framework within which to consider the positive and negative effects of combining psychotherapy and medication.

It is now well-established that problems with medication compliance in patients who have chronic illnesses such as bipolar disorder and schizophrenia are common and costly realities in psychopharmacology. The sensitive application of psychotherapy by the psychopharmacologist makes for more successful pharmacotherapy. In contrast, therapists may be concerned that their psychotherapeutic zeal could bias them against potentially helpful biologic agents. This may lead them paradoxically to recommend medication too quickly. In many clinical situations the determination of the need for a psychopharmacologic agent is far from clear-cut. In these situations many patients do not want to take medication; they want the physician's time, person, and perceptual, conceptual, and executive skills. Many patients do not like the way medication affects them and fear that the doctor will lose interest in talking to them. Psychotherapists, including psychiatrists, commonly see patients who have been dissatisfied with their experience with a physician who seemed too quick to prescribe medication in lieu of engaging them in even a brief psychotherapy. Psychiatric treatment is clearly more satisfying to all concerned when the physician has the time and the freedom to prepare a truly customized treatment plan.

Psychiatrists are regularly called upon to perform medication evaluations for patients in psychotherapy with a non-psychiatrist. Such collaborations can be very satisfying when the psychiatrist knows the psychotherapist and understands and trusts the psychotherapy. If this mutual knowledge and trust is not in place, there is too much room for divisive splitting to occur. The patient's treatment will suffer, and such an arrangement is not recommended.

CONCLUSION

In undertaking to learn the basic principles of psychotherapeutic management, contemporary beginning psychiatric residents and medical students considering psychiatry as a career are inclined to question whether the effort is worthwhile. They are intrigued by the ideas and the history of the field, but they are overwhelmed by what seems both vast in scope and mysterious and impenetrable in concept. They question whether they will be "allowed" (by managed care organizations) to perform psychotherapy. They question whether they or their patients will be able to afford to spend an hour (or any significant portion thereof) together. Trainees at this level may be reminded that psychiatry as practiced in the emergency room of a city hospital at 3:00 A.M., although necessary, represents only a small portion of the influence they can bring to bear on the toll taken by mental illness in our time. Advanced psychiatric residents quickly rediscover the lost soul of psychiatry and clamor for seminars and supervision in psychotherapy. They have learned again what was almost forgotten, what was almost buried under the avalanche of medical school facts and early residency sleepless nights. They rediscover the central role of relatedness in the definition of emotional well-being, and they learn to appreciate the pernicious impact of its loss in the manifestations of emotional despair. The road to the recovery of human relatedness is through the process of relatedness, and many times this requires a therapist. The quality of human life, whether that of the professional or that of the patient, is a function of relatedness. No amount of bottom-line accounting can alter that truth.

Psychological Testing in Psychiatry

12

Howard B. Roback, PhD, & Larry Welch, EdD

PSYCHOLOGICAL TESTING IN THE PSYCHIATRIC CONTEXT

Psychological testing in the psychiatric context generally refers to measurements made for the purpose of helping delineate and classify a patient's psychopathology. Personality testing is also used to address specific clinical issues such as the patient's need for hospitalization, personality factors complicating Axis I symptoms, the possible presence of malingering, identification of major therapeutic issues, the patient's potential for suicide, his or her primary defense mechanisms and coping style, and the most appropriate discharge options. Questions a psychiatrist might ask in a neuropsychological referral are typically related to the role of possible central nervous system dysfunction in a patient's pathology and its impact on daily functioning. For example, does a patient have dementia or pseudodementia, is a patient's behavioral or emotional dyscontrol the result of personality factors or impaired central nervous system mechanisms that modulate such reactions, and what is the extent of organic damage and associated cognitive impairment? In addition to clarifying the diagnosis and assisting in treatment planning, psychological testing can play an important role in outcome assessment by helping to document the effectiveness of the treatment provided to a given patient. In today's health care environment, the demonstration of treatment effectiveness to insurance companies, managed care corporations, and patient-consumers is becoming increasingly important.

Maruish ME (editor): *The Use of Psychological Testing for Treatment Planning and Outcome Assessment.* Lawrence Erlbaum Assoc, 1994.

PERSONALITY ASSESSMENT

Interest in personality assessment predates the scientific advances in psychological testing. Throughout the ages, people have evaluated their own conduct and the actions of others for the purpose of understanding and predicting behavior. Scientific personality testing has its origins in the study of individual differences through psychological measurement.

MEASUREMENT CONCEPTS

Measurement concepts provide the foundation for evaluating the utility of all psychological tests. What follows is a brief outline of the important concepts of standardization, validity, and reliability.

Standardization
Standardization refers to the uniform administration and scoring of a test instrument. This is necessary in order to meaningfully interpret differences in test scores between individuals. To ensure this uniformity, the test constructor provides the psychologist with a manual of detailed instructions for administering and scoring the test. Another important component of a standardized test is the establishment of norms. That is, the instrument is administered to a large representative sample of the type of persons for whom it has been designed (eg, English-speaking adults with at least a third-grade reading level). The sample used to establish the norms is known as the **standardization sample.** Norms establish comparison scores and the degree of score deviation from the mean.

Validity
Validity is the most important criterion for a test. It refers to the degree to which a test actually measures what it claims to be measuring. For example, does the

Medical College Admission Test (MCAT) score actually predict medical student performance as measured by relevant external criteria, such as grades, faculty evaluations, and successful completion of training? When the test measure agrees adequately with such external criteria, the measure is said to have **criterion validity.** Another type of validity, **content validity,** involves a systematic analysis of the individual items comprising the test in order to determine how well the items sample the behavior domain under study. For example, a measure of depression should consist of items that sample all major aspects (eg, cognitive, physiologic, and behavioral) of the construct with respect to their relative importance. This type of validity information should also be included in the test manual.

Reliability

Reliability refers to consistency of measurement or repeatability of scores. Two major types of reliability are test-retest reliability and internal consistency. For example, if a medical school applicant scores in the 98th percentile on the MCAT on Saturday and in the 60th percentile on Monday using the same test version, or an equivalent form, the measure is said to be nonreliable because little confidence can be put in either score. Various methods are available for determining the reliability of a test score. **Test-retest reliability** refers to administering the identical test on a second occasion (eg, within 2 weeks). One then correlates the two scores for the same individual. The higher the correlation, the less likely that scores are influenced heavily by chance fluctuations, such as uncontrolled testing conditions or changes in the test-taker (eg, through illness). Reliability information about a test should also be reported in the test manual. Test-retest changes that occur over longer periods of time are likely not random. However, a major disadvantage of the retest method is that the first testing will likely influence the person's responses in the second testing (termed **practice effects**). It is possible to determine a test's internal consistency from a single administration of the measure. **Internal consistency** refers to how well items of a single scale intercorrelate, thus demonstrating that items are measuring the same construct. **Split-half reliability** refers to dividing a single test into equivalent halves (eg, odd and even items) for each individual. The person's scores are then correlated. The difficulties with the split-half method is that the correlation between halves may vary according to how items are divided (eg, odd-even, random), and the resulting correlation gives the reliability of only half of the test. The challenge for the test constructor is to develop a stable and internally consistent measure of the construct under investigation. If the test does not reliably measure the trait under evaluation, then it is unclear whether differences in scores are due to the trait being measured or the unreliability of the test instrument. That is, a test that is not reliable is not valid.

Anastasi A: *Psychological Testing,* 6th ed. Macmillan, 1988.
Sattler J: *Assessment of Children,* 3rd ed. Jerome M Sattler, 1988.

CONTEMPORARY PERSONALITY TESTING

Contemporary personality tests are typically described as being either objective or projective in type. Simply stated, **objective personality tests** are usually structured paper-and-pencil self-report instruments whose items are answered in a standard format (eg, true-false). These tests are scored in a quantitative manner, and resulting numerical scores are subjected to statistical analyses. Typically, a profile is generated that contrasts the patient's scores with those of the normative sample. Normative data are provided in the test manual, as are reliability and validity information. In **projective personality testing,** the individual is provided unstructured test stimuli (eg, inkblots, incomplete sentences, pictures of human figures) and required to give meaning to them. The theoretical assumption is that the patient's responses reflect primarily a projection of the individual's inner needs, motivations, defenses, and drives. That is, tests are intended to elicit a projection of "unconscious" material from the subject's inner life. There are objective scoring systems for some projective tests, such as the Exner Comprehensive Scoring System, one of the most sophisticated and widely used for the Rorschach. However, some clinicians prefer to make psychodynamic interpretations from the thematic content of the patient's Rorschach responses, arguing that they are achieving a much richer understanding of the patient than that provided through more sterile numerical analysis of the person. Proponents of objective personality inventories often criticize their counterparts who favor projective testing for not meeting higher standards of validity, reliability, and standardization. Many clinicians, however, utilize a test battery of both objective and projective tests when performing a psychological workup on a patient. Such a strategy will likely result in a more comprehensive evaluation of a patient and provide more confidence in replicated findings from different types of test stimuli. Although intelligence testing is frequently a part of such a test battery, our discussion of it will appear in the neuropsychological assessment section of this chapter.

The number of personality tests available to the clinician is enormous. We discuss here six measures (three objective and three projective) commonly used in the mental health field. These tests provide a comprehensive assessment of personality functioning rather than an assessment of the severity of specific symptoms (eg, depression). The latter tests, such as the Beck Depression Inventory, are used frequently in treatment effectiveness research; however, such tests are seldom used to make a clinical diagnosis. General comments about the applications and advantages and limitations of objective and projective personality tests follow each section.

1. OBJECTIVE PERSONALITY TESTS

Minnesota Multiphasic Personality Inventory

The Minnesota Multiphasic Personality Inventory (MMPI) is the most frequently used personality inventory in clinical practice. In the 1930s, psychiatrists and psychologists had to rely almost exclusively on interview procedures to assist them in making clinical decisions. Starke Hathaway and Charley McKinley, a psychologist-psychiatrist collaborative team at the University of Minnesota, published the MMPI in 1943. It proved a successful attempt to develop an empirically based objective personality inventory. This 566-item true-false test was designed to yield 10 clinical subscales: Hypochondriasis, Depression, Hysteria, Psychopathic Deviate, Masculinity-Femininity, Paranoia, Psychasthenia, Schizophrenia, Hypomania, and Social Introversion. For ease of communication, each scale has an associated number. For example, Hypochondriasis = 1, Depression = 2, and so forth. Psychologists typically refer to these numbers when discussing an MMPI profile among themselves, as many scale names are clinically outdated (eg, Psychasthenia). In addition, there are four validity scales (Q, K, L, F), which essentially measure the respondent's test-taking attitude (eg, defensiveness, exaggeration of symptoms). Sets of items selected for inclusion in the test's final version differentiated a specific clinical sample (eg, depressed patients) from the normal subjects who comprised the standardization group.

The MMPI was revised in 1989 as the MMPI-2, which consists of 567 self-descriptive statements. In the revision, several original items were reworded or deleted, and statements focusing on suicide, substance abuse, and related matters were added. The revised version also includes a standardization sample that is more representative of the U.S. population (based on census data).

Interpretation of both versions of the MMPI is based primarily on a profile analysis consisting of the two or three highest scale elevations. On the MMPI, raw scores are translated into T-scores (ie, standardized scores with a mean of 50 and standard deviation of 10), and the latter are coded onto the profile sheet. On the MMPI-2, scales with T-scores above 65 are considered clinically significant. Abnormally low scores are also interpretable. Numerous books are available to help the clinician interpret specific code types. The basic profile form of the MMPI-2 is shown in Figure 12–1. The patient's profile suggests a major depression with psychotic features (elevated Depres-

sion and Schizophrenia scales) in an individual who is overly dependent and self-centered (elevated Hysteria scale). In both clinical and research settings, many psychologists continue to use the original MMPI version because of the vast amount of research conducted with it.

Millon Clinical Multiaxial Inventory-II

The Millon Clinical Multiaxial Inventory-II (MCMI-II) was developed by Theodore Millon, a professor of psychology at the University of Miami. It consists of 175 true-false test items. The items are self-references (eg, "I often have difficulty making decisions without seeking help from others"), much like the MMPI, but the MCMI-II items are grouped into 25 subscales. The 22 clinical scales were developed in accordance with constructs or syndromes derived from personality theory and to correspond with *Diagnostic and Statistical Manual of Mental Disorders,* 3rd edition, revised (DSM-III-R) criteria. The Axis II scales include Schizoid, Avoidant, Dependent, Histrionic, Narcissistic, Antisocial, Aggressive/Sadistic, Compulsive, Passive-Aggressive, and Self-Defeating. Scales for severe personality pathology include Schizotypal, Borderline, and Paranoid. Clinical syndromes (Axis I) include Anxiety; Bipolar, Manic; Alcohol Dependence; and Major Depression. Each scale has an associated number or letter. For example, Schizoid = 1, Paranoid = P, and so forth. The interpretation of the MCMI-II is complex and requires a sophisticated understanding of the scales and theoretical underpinnings of the overall instrument. At the time that this chapter was being prepared, the MCMI-III had been published with modifications for correspondence with the *Diagnostic and Statistical Manual of Mental Disorders,* 4th edition (DSM-IV) psychiatric classification system. The sample MCMI-II profile form shown in Figure 12–2 is consistent with major depression (elevated CC scale) and associated agitation (elevated A scale). The patient also appears to have histrionic personality features (elevated scale 3) and the presence of borderline traits (elevated scale C).

Personality Assessment Inventory

The Personality Assessment Inventory (PAI) was constructed in 1991 by Leslie Morey, a professor of psychology at Vanderbilt University. The test consists of 344 items answered on a four-point Likert-type format: totally false, slightly true, mainly true, and very true. In addition to the 11 clinical scales (diagnosis), there are 5 treatment consideration scales (prognosis), 2 interpersonal scales (social support), and 4 validity scales. The clinical scales are Somatic Complaints, Anxiety, Anxiety-Related Disorders, Depression, Mania, Paranoia, Schizophrenia, Borderline Features, Antisocial Features, Alcohol Features, and Drug Features. An important feature of the PAI scales is that

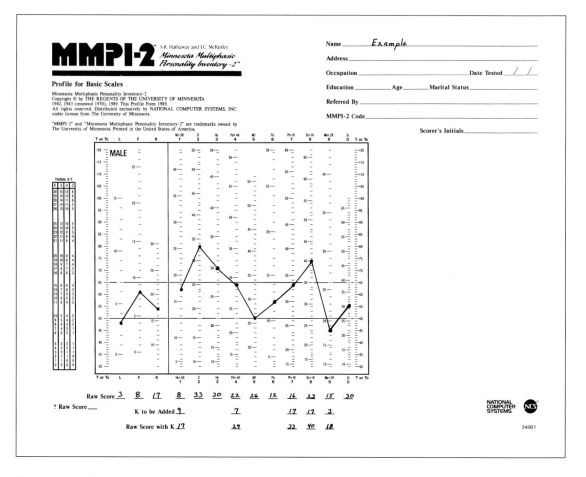

Figure 12–1. Minnesota Multiphasic Personality Inventory-2 (MMPI-2) Profile for Basic Scales. Copyright © 1989 the Regents of the University of Minnesota. All rights reserved. "MMPI-2" and "Minnesota Multiphasic Personality Inventory-2" are trademarks owned by the University of Minnesota. Reproduced by permission of University of Minnesota Press.

they are further divided into subscales that reflect specific components (eg, cognitive, affective, and physiologic symptoms). For example, a patient's specific manifestation of anxiety may be in excessive worry and concern (ie, cognitive) rather than trembling hands (eg, physiologic). The treatment scales (Suicidal Ideation, Treatment Rejection, Nonsupport, Stress, Aggression) also provide the clinician with pertinent information for treatment planning, an especially useful feature of this test. The PAI profile shown in Figure 12–3 suggests a severely depressed person with suicidal ideation (elevated Depression and Suicide scales).

Applications of Objective Personality Tests

The MMPI, MCMI, and PAI are three important objective personality inventories for diagnostic classification and treatment planning. The MMPI is used primarily for an assessment that focuses on Axis I is-

sues and the MCMI and PAI for an evaluation of Axis II traits or character pathology. Sometimes the Axis II problem is the focus of psychotherapy, whereas the Axis I problem is treated by medication.

Advantages & Limitations of Objective Personality Tests

There are several advantages to using objective personality measures. They are relatively simple to administer, and many are capable of being scored and interpreted by computer. Test manuals provide standardization and psychometric information (eg, validity and reliability data) for the user. The three measures discussed here have satisfactory reliability and validity for the purposes they were intended. For example, compared to the standardization sample, a person with a T-score of 70 on the PAI Anxiety scale would be two standard deviations above the mean score for that scale. This score would be significantly higher than the anxiety scores of normal adults.

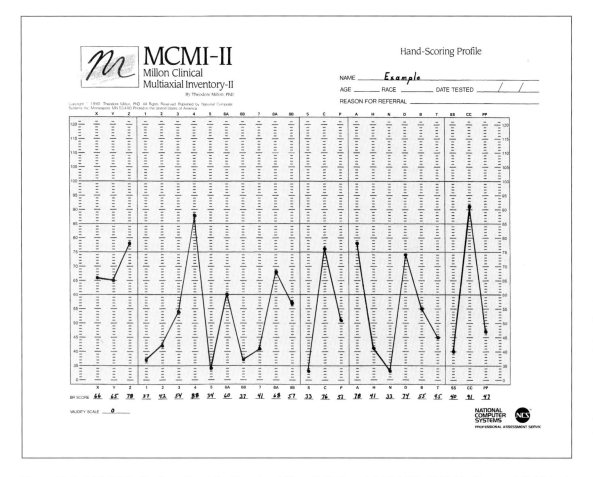

Figure 12–2. MCMI-II Profile Face Sheet, by Theodore Millon, PhD. Copyright © 1990. All Rights Reserved. Published by National Computer Systems, Inc., Minneapolis, MN 55440. Portions reproduced by permission of NCS.

Objective personality instruments also have some limitations. They are primarily behavioral in content and may provide inadequate information about the respondent's underlying motives or psychodynamics. For example, two patients may produce identical profiles indicating that they feel depressed and anxious. In one case the symptoms may be the result of acute situational stress (eg, financial reversals), whereas in the other case, the symptoms may be long-standing and result from childhood trauma. Further, the forced choice method (eg, true-false) prevents the two patients from elaborating or qualifying their responses. Thus the four-point PAI scale has an advantage here.

2. PROJECTIVE PERSONALITY TESTS

As noted earlier, projective personality tests are unstructured tests that are designed to elicit responses that provide information on the respondent's inner life, including unconscious motivations, wishes, and conflicts. In theory, the manner in which the patient organizes and perceives the ambiguous test stimuli reveals something about his or her distinctive personality. Three of the projective tests that have stood the test of time are the Rorschach Inkblot Test, the Thematic Apperception Test (TAT), and the Sentence Completion Test (SCT).

Rorschach Inkblot Test

The Rorschach Inkblot Test was the creative effort of a Swiss psychiatrist, Hermann Rorschach, who published the test in 1921. Out of several hundred inkblot configurations, he selected 10 cards because of the variety of responses they elicited. Five of the bilaterally symmetrical inkblots are achromatic, two have additional spots of red, and three combine several colors (Figure 12–4).

During the test administration, the examiner asks the patient what each card looks like (ie, "What might this be?"). The examiner then records the patient's responses verbatim, the time it takes to generate re-

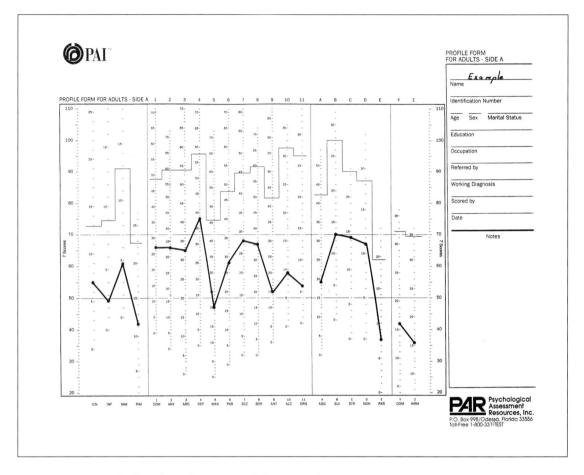

Figure 12–3. PAI Profile Face Sheet (manual, p. 25). Reproduced by special permission of the Publisher, Psychological Assessment Resources, Inc., 16204 North Florida Avenue, Lutz, Florida 33549, from the Personality Assessment Inventory by Leslie Morey, PhD, Copyright © 1991 by PAR, Inc. Further reproduction is prohibited without permission of PAR, Inc.

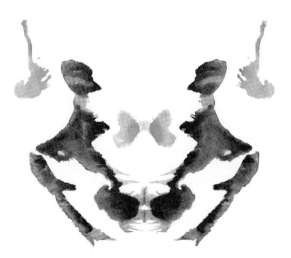

Figure 12–4. Rorschach Test Plate 1, by Rorschach H. Copyright © Verlag Hans Huber AG, Bern, Switzerland, 1921, 1948, 1994. Reproduced by permission.

sponses, and any nonverbal reactions. After the responses are compiled, the examiner asks the patient to go through the cards again. This is referred to as the **inquiry phase.** The examiner is attempting to identify the factors influencing the response—what parts of the blot are used and what features made the blot look a certain way (eg, color, movement, texture, shading, and form). All of these factors are interpretable. For example, perception of movement (eg, the percept of a bird in flight) is considered to relate to the richness of an individual's fantasy life. The form determinant (eg, how closely the response corresponds with the selected area of the inkblot) is believed to indicate an individual's reasoning powers and reality testing. Persons with good psychological equilibrium tend to have refined and differentiated perceptions, whereas the perceptions of psychologically impaired persons generally fit poorly with the form of the blot associated with their response. Color responses are believed to reflect the emotional life of the respondent. For example, pure color responses (ie, the blot color itself stimulates the respondent's associative process) are considered to reflect an individual with poorly integrated emotional reactions. Location choice (eg, the area of the blot where the respondent associates his or her response) is also considered to reflect something about one's personality. For example, an emphasis on very small details is considered to reflect an individual who has a very critical attitude or is overly concerned with trivialities.

Responses are analyzed in terms of the number that fall into various categories (eg, movement, form, location), the normative frequency of these categories for different clinical groups, and the relationships among determinants (ie, ratios such as percentage of conventional form). Psychodynamically oriented examiners also interpret the content of responses in terms of symbolic meaning (eg, perception of an island may reflect a sense of isolation). When interpreted within the respondent's specific experiences, the latter analyses are considered to reveal a great deal about an individual's unique personality style.

A number of Rorschach scoring and interpreting systems have been developed since its inception. Irving Weiner and John Exner have attempted to put contemporary Rorschach assessment on a psychometrically sound basis. For instance, the Exner Comprehensive Scoring System emphasizes structural rather than thematic content of responses. This complex scoring system involves categorizing responses in an objective manner into ratios, percentages, and other indices. Interpretations are primarily data based rather than theoretically based. The Exner system has been well received by the current generation of Rorschach testers whose graduate training has emphasized the importance of psychometric standards in assessment.

Thematic Apperception Test

The TAT was developed in 1943 by Harvard psychologist Henry Murray. The test consists of 29 pictures and 1 blank card. The cards have recognizable human figures (Figure 12–5), and the patient is asked to make up a story of what is happening in the scene. In addition, the subject is asked to tell what led up to the situation, what the people are thinking and feeling, and how the situation will end. There is significant variability in the scoring of TAT responses. Some examiners prefer a more intuitive approach to understanding the psychodynamic implications of a story; others favor a more complex scoring system (eg, Murray's drive system analysis). In the former case, the psychologist attempts to identify significant emotions and attitudes projected onto the cards. Each card is intended to elicit information about a specific type of relationship (eg, child-mother, child-father) or an important psychological area (eg, sexuality). Themes that recur with unusual frequency are judged to reflect prominent psychological needs. As on the Rorschach, the examiner records the verbatim responses of the

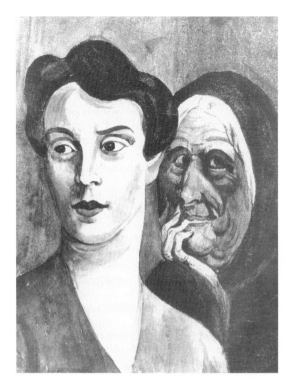

Figure 12–5. Card 12F from Thematic Apperception Test. Reprinted by permission of the publishers from Henry A. Murray, THEMATIC APPERCEPTION TEST, Cambridge, Mass.: Harvard University Press, Copyright © 1943 by the President and Fellows of Harvard College, © 1971 by Henry A. Murray.

examinee for later analysis. Because of its familiar content, TAT stimuli are less ambiguous than are Rorschach cards.

Sentence Completion Tests

Like the Rorschach and the TAT, sentence completion tests are used frequently in personality assessment. They generally consist of a number of incomplete sentences (eg, I feel guilty when . . .) that are completed by the patient. They are intended to provide information about the respondent's interpersonal attitudes and relationships, personality style, and other issues that are important to the examiner. The referral questions will help determine which one of several different published sentence completion test versions is used in a given case. Many psychologists would agree that the SCT is more likely a semiprojective test because the items are more transparent than are the Rorschach inkblots and the TAT cards. As psychologists who have reviewed these instruments have pointed out, incomplete sentences arc among the least researched of projective methods. They appear to persist because, like a slot machine, there is an intermittent payoff in their usage. It may be that some patients are more comfortable communicating information to the clinician in a written form than they are in the face-to-face conversational context.

Application of Projective Personality Tests

Psychodynamically oriented psychologists use the Rorschach as part of a test battery for evaluating clinical issues such as the degree of a patient's cognitive-perceptual pathology. For example, to evaluate whether a patient has a low-grade thought disorder, the psychologist may examine the Rorschach protocol in terms of idiosyncratic responses with a distorted form level. Further, persons with a thought disorder often emit three types of pathologic responses: (1) **confabulated whole responses** (using a single detail as a basis for an entire response, for example, "This looks like a whisker, so the rest of the card is a cat's face."); (2) **fabulized combinations** (making one incongruous concept out of two percepts in close physical proximity, for example, "This looks like a bridge and this looks like legs, so this area is a bridge with legs."); and (3) **contaminated responses** (seeing two different things at the same blot area and then fusing them together, for example, "This is a dog. It's a bug. No, it's a dog-bug."). In these responses, the patient is demonstrating inadequate conceptual boundaries, as well as confusion in thought, perception, and reasoning. The Rorschach is also useful for generating hypotheses about the individual's personality style; however, psychologists often look for collateral support for their inferences about personality style in the patient's objective personality data, interview statements, and case history. The TAT and the SCT are used primarily to generate hypotheses about an individual's family and social relationships, areas of conflict, and related Axis II issues.

Advantages & Limitations of Projective Personality Tests

A great deal of controversy surrounds projective personality tests. Many clinicians find the instruments described here as highly useful for diagnostic purposes and for evaluating personality functioning. However, results of studies examining the psychometric properties of these tests are generally discouraging, perhaps with the exception of the Exner Comprehensive Scoring System for the Rorschach Inkblot Test. Nonetheless, a sizable number of clinicians continue to argue that projective personality tests should not be subject to standard psychometric evaluation and that such attempts are damaging to the potential richness of these methods for understanding an individual's distinctive personality. It is highly unlikely that these differences will be resolved anytime soon.

American Psychiatric Association: *Diagnostic and Statistical Manual of Mental Disorders,* 4th ed. American Psychiatric Association, 1994.

Phares E: *Clinical Psychology,* 4th ed. Brooks/Cole, 1992.

Maruish ME: *The Use of Psychological Testing for Treatment Planning and Outcome Assessment.* Lawrence Erlbaum Assoc, 1994.

CLINICAL DECISION MAKING IN PERSONALITY ASSESSMENT

Following the gathering of test data, the psychologist analyzes the materials for purposes of clinical decision making and prediction. If testing included both objective and projective measures, then the examiner performs two functions—one being that of the psychometrist who minimizes subjective interpretation and the other that of the psychodynamic clinician who relies heavily on clinical interpretation. The objective of such a dual role is to use both sets of tools as a means of cross-validating test findings. For example, if a patient scores two deviations above the mean on the MMPI Schizophrenia scale, the clinician anticipates bizarre responses (eg, contaminated responses) on the Rorschach. If the assumption is correct, then there is increasing support for the presence of a psychotic adjustment. If not, then an alternative explanation is sought. TAT responses may inform us of how the patient's impaired cognitive-perceptual processes may be manifesting themselves in the interpersonal sphere. For example, on the TAT "family card," the patient may perceive the pregnant female figure as a "cheating wife carrying the baby of the man with whom she is having an affair."

After analyzing the data, the psychologist communicates the findings, resulting clinical impressions, and any treatment recommendations to the referring psychiatrist in the form of a psychological test report. The report is crafted to communicate a meaningful picture of the patient in a format most useful for the referring physician. For example, a psychodynamically oriented psychiatrist generally prefers a report that helps him or her better understand the patient from that perspective. A psychiatrist whose practice is primarily medication focused may prefer a report that focuses on specific symptoms, suggested by objective testing, that the psychiatrist can address pharmacologically. The psychiatrist may ask that a patient be retested after treatment to assess quantitatively the effectiveness of his or her intervention. With the psychiatrist's approval, the psychologist will review test findings with the patient. However, psychotherapy-oriented psychiatrists often prefer to have the patients discover on their own in therapy the insights provided in the report. That is, they want the patient to be psychologically ready to confront the information.

An example of a psychological test report follows. A pretest interview was conducted with the patient, as it is with all testing cases. The goals of the interview are to establish rapport, gain clinically useful information, and address any concerns that the patient may have about the evaluation.

The patient is the 19-year-old son of a hard-driving and successful attorney living in a medium-sized southeastern city. The patient's father was very concerned about his son's suspension from an Ivy League college for academic reasons. According to the father, the patient appeared depressed, withdrawn, and somewhat uncommunicative since his return home. He sought only minimal contact with long-time friends attending a local college. The patient's inability to hold down a job as a salesman in a small store owned by a family friend was embarrassing to the patient's parents. His father consulted with a physician-friend who recommended that the patient be referred to a psychiatrist for a formal evaluation.

Tests Administered: Minnesota Multiphasic Personality Inventory (MMPI), Wechsler Adult Intelligence Scale-Revised (WAIS-R), Personality Assessment Inventory (PAI), Thematic Apperception Test (TAT), Suicide Probability Scale (SPS), Sentence Completion Test (SCT), Rorschach Inkblot Test

Background: The patient, a 19-year-old single male, was referred by his psychiatrist for psychological evaluation. The focus of this assessment was to explore whether the patient's recent emotional, academic, occupational, and social dysfunction are related to individual or family dynamic issues or are a manifestation of some other more malignant underlying pathology.

Interview: The patient reported that he was suspended by his university for academic failure after one semester but hoped to reenroll this coming fall. He noted that, despite experiencing no academic difficulties in high school, "a lot of stuff happened at [college]." He specified that motivational difficulties (inability to get out of bed) and increasing alcohol abuse contributed to his academic troubles. He denied the use of other illicit substances. He added that he initially was comfortable with the move away from home and family to a new city and college dorm life. However, he then became progressively more isolated, socially disconnected, and lonely. The patient claimed, "Even in a room full of people I would feel left out." He further qualified that such a situation did not always distress him, as he sometimes preferred to remain aloof, withdrawn, and to "wallow in my misery." He claimed that his pattern of isolation was long-standing. He admitted to periods of depressed mood of varying severity, during which his preference for isolation was enhanced. The patient endorsed passive thoughts of suicide in the past but denied urges to act on impulses for self-harm or elaboration of a plan to do so.

The patient revealed a number of idiosyncrasies centering around social interaction. For example, he admitted to often pretending that one of his friends or acquaintances is riding in the car with him, or sitting in his bedroom with him, and he will rehearse how he would act if the person were really present. He acknowledged that such fantasy is much less threatening than social reality, as it "gives me an idea of what I'd be like in front of others and helps me boost my self-image."

He mentioned that his deflated self-image and low self-esteem have troubled him throughout his life. He claimed that he continually worries "if I'm good enough" and that he will "mess up." The patient stated that his parents, especially his father, often reacted to his mistakes with "a lot of yelling and shouting, and making me feel guilty." He described his relationship with his parents and only sister to be much like his social experiences, characterized by a lack of connectedness and belongingness. In reference to his father, the patient said, "I have no real connection, I guess; I don't identify with him and don't even really talk to him." However, the patient added that his father had "smoothed out" after having a heart attack a few years earlier, resulting in him being more talkative than volatile. Still, the patient denied the growth of a close emotional bond with his father.

The patient was employed by a local sporting goods store after being dismissed from college, but he was fired because of "disagreements with the boss." He stated that he is not presently in a romantic relationship but has been in the past. Interestingly, he described past sexual experiences as "emotionally confusing," adding, "I want more than just a squeeze toy, I want someone I can talk to."

Test Findings:

Intelligence: The patient achieved an estimated Full Scale intelligence quotient (IQ) score of 105 on selected subtests of the WAIS-R, which places him in the average range of intellectual functioning. His Verbal Scale IQ score of 107 and Performance scale IQ score of 102 are also within the average range. Although the patient's Verbal-Performance IQ score discrepancy (5 points) is not diagnostically significant, his inter- and intratest scatter suggests the likelihood of a disruption in cognitive functioning. This is further indicated by the pattern of WAIS-R subtests on which he performs best (Vocabulary, Information) and worst (Comprehension, Similarities, and Digit Symbol). Based on these findings, one would anticipate that academically he performed best on courses depending on long-term memory (eg, history) and poorest on those requiring complex abstraction and new learning. His social judgment is also likely poor. Finally, it appears that his cognitive inconsistency has resulted in lower-than-expected IQ scores.

Personality: On objective testing (MMPI, PAI), the patient's profiles consistently suggest someone making a "plea for help" in the midst of intense psychological turmoil. His PAI profile is remarkable for symptoms of depression, anxiety, and a possible thought disturbance. Individuals with similar profiles often experience feelings of hopelessness, worthlessness, and personal failure. Their affective distress is often accompanied by a backdrop characterized by social isolation and detachment. They typically have few interpersonal relationships that could be described as deep, close, and supportive. These individuals experience great ambivalence between urges to fulfill unmet needs for affiliation and belongingness and the threatening anxiety they feel related to intimate involvement. His MMPI profile is invalid because of excessive endorsement of pathologic items. That is, he overstated his symptoms to an unusual degree.

The patient's scores on both the Suicide Probability Scale (SPS) and PAI Suicidal Ideation scale indicate that he is experiencing intense and recurrent thoughts related to suicide. He should be considered at serious risk for self-harm.

Projective test results also suggest that the patient is experiencing substantial psychological turmoil at this time. Numerous responses on the Rorschach reflect inner disharmony, intense anger, and a possibly burgeoning paranoid cognitive process. A review of his Rorschach protocol reveals descriptors such as "frightening" and "menacing" to card 3 (see Figure 12–4) and "mad," "angry," "being attacked," "decaying," and "about to collapse" to other cards. These projections lead to speculation that the patient is externalizing the emotions and sense of deterioration that he is experiencing internally. The lack of human content perceived on the Rorschach suggests that the patient has likely established a wall between himself and others and is experiencing significant social isolation.

The patient's TAT scenarios provide rich themes of disruptive relations with each parent figure. The patient described a card depicting a father-son interaction as "two ships passing in the night as the father has no awareness or insight into the son's emotional needs." To the family card, he referred to the figures as immersed in their own activities while the son is left to feel "lonely, depressed, and unneeded." He responded to the mother-son card with a scenario in which the child is confused as to what he needs to do to gain his parents' approval or positive attention. Of concern, the patient responded with an upbeat theme of contentment to a TAT card that often generates depressive and sometimes suicidal scenarios.

On the SCT, the patient also provided prominent themes of detachment from parental figures, loneliness, rumination, and social isolation. Most alarming is "Sometimes . . . I think about my own funeral." After the four SCT stems "I am," the patient responds: "lost," "worried," "alone," and "exhausted."

Clinical Impressions: Although the patient denied suicidal ideation or impulses on interview, test results (SPS, PAI, TAT, SCT) consistently suggest that he may be experiencing severe and recurrent thoughts related to self-harm at this time. Close monitoring of the patient in this regard is indicated, with consideration of future hospitalization if warranted. His tendency for isolation and excessive rumination, his apparent perplexity and apprehension about his own functioning, his lack of perceived support, and his age all combine to make him a worrisome patient.

The patient's overall personality test data (including Rorschach perceptions of "decay" and things "collapsing") likely reflect on the patient's own subjective experience of decline. The patient appears preoccupied with his symptoms and failures to the extent that he has lost all interest in others. So apprehensive is this morbid self-concern that the patient appears to be exhibiting profound passivity and social lethargy and, for all practical purposes, appears to be approaching virtual immobility. The patient reported spending much of his day in his room, withdrawn from peer or substantial familial interaction. We would also anticipate that he is moving in the direction of the bottom of the mood cycle with recurring self-annihilative thought content.

On the SPS he responded that he feels he cannot be happy no matter where he is and that the world is not worth continuing to live in. His morbidly depressed feeling tone may reflect grieving over loss of functioning or a component of a possible schizoaffective disorder. We suspect that the patient was able to function academically in a highly structured high school environment but was also perceived as "odd" by teachers and peers. However, the transition to a less-structured college situation may have highlighted how poor his adjustment actually was. Further complicating the situation are his family dynamics, which leave him feeling even further disconnected and unsupported. A major concern in this case is that the patient may be developing a chronic pattern of apathy, dysfunction, severe social disruption, and peculiarity. That is, an evolving schizophrenic or schizoaffective disorder cannot be ruled out.

In addition to pharmacologic management of his cognitive and affective disturbances, some important practical issues will need to be addressed. The patient reported that he anticipates returning to college in the fall. It is difficult at this point to envision that being anything other than another failure experience. He will likely have significant difficulty in attention, persistent concentration, and processing of complex intellectual tasks. If his condition is stabilized by medication, a less severe transition might be considered. For instance, living at home and taking a significantly reduced college course load at a less academically stressful local institution might be worth a try. However, even that might prove a stretch.

An alternative would be referral to a vocational rehabilitation service that could evaluate and direct the patient to an appropriate training or work situation that would be low pressure and highly structured. The patient would likely confront serious difficulties if he tried on his own to enter a competitive work environment. However, with his family background, if he chose the latter option, a job such as a clerk in a hospital medical records' division might be a consideration. Perhaps this option would be more attractive to him and his high-achieving family than would blue collar work. Further, it would entail relatively limited public contact.

NEUROPSYCHOLOGICAL ASSESSMENT

Neuropsychological assessment refers to the application of standardized measurement techniques to determine the relationship between brain impairment and its behavioral concomitants. Interest in cases that focus on the interface between psychiatry and neurology provided the impetus for the modern clinical development of neuropsychology as an important subspecialty within clinical psychology.

The practice of contemporary neuropsychological assessment in the psychiatric setting is indicated when a complex set of symptoms and referral questions dictates the need for more than clinical interview or mental status examination alone.

A 57-year-old mail carrier was referred by his psychiatrist for neuropsychological testing 10 months after a car accident. The patient sustained a closed head injury with a brief loss of consciousness. Although neuroimaging tests were negative, the patient complained of various post-concussive symptoms including headache, dizziness, neck and back pain, attention and memory problems, and increased emotional lability. A

change in personality ensued, in which the patient was described by his family as more withdrawn and irritable. He had a history of narcotic abuse, which escalated after the onset of post-traumatic pain. He also reported past treatment for alcohol dependence. During his psychiatric interview, the patient reported neurovegetative signs of depression. His symptoms have prevented him from returning to his mail route, and he is seeking disability.

The patient's mental status examination prior to his neuropsychological referral was inconclusive regarding the etiology for his lingering memory complaints, pain, and personality changes. Neuropsychological testing documented normal new-learning and problem-solving ability and indicated that all of the patient's cognitive functions had returned to baseline. Thus the result of neuropsychological examination suggested that psychological factors were primary in the case. After receiving supportive counseling and medication for depression, the patient was able to return to his previous work activity.

The preceding case example demonstrates the contribution that careful neuropsychological evaluation may have in untangling the multiple factors that can affect a patient's functioning. In-depth, standardized, quantifiable, and individualized testing can often be a critical factor in differential diagnosis and appropriate treatment. Moreover, formal testing makes it easier to track disease progression and recovery of function than does mental status examination.

Carefully planned neuropsychological testing requires the establishment of a referral relationship between the psychiatrist and psychologist. In the latter context, the psychiatrist learns how to best frame the referral questions. The following are three of the more common referral questions addressed by neuropsychological testing: (1) Are the patient's symptoms the result of psychiatric, neurologic, or combined etiologies; (2) when is the best time to refer a patient; and (3) can the patient resume normal activity such as living alone, driving, or working?

Symptom Etiology

Once used to help identify focal brain lesions, the role of neuropsychology in diagnosis has diminished somewhat with the advent of advanced neuroradiologic techniques. However, neuroimaging may provide equivocal results in many instances (eg, mild head injury, neurotoxic exposure, early dementia). Magnetic resonance imaging (MRI) techniques may detect gross structural damage but not changes at the molecular or cell level, which can also affect function. Under such circumstances, neuropsychological testing may provide a more sensitive measure of brain function.

For example, neuropsychological testing is useful in distinguishing between early dementia and those symptoms of depression that mimic cognitive impairment. Because these conditions may be present simultaneously, sorting out the relative contribution of each can help indicate appropriate treatment. Depressed elderly patients perform differently on neuropsychological tests than do patients with genuine or irreversible cognitive deficits, although the deficits may be indistinguishable on mental status examination. In-depth neuropsychological testing can lead to a better perspective of the patient's effort and level of energy, frequency of giving up on more difficult items, attempts to minimize deficiencies, and patterns of strengths and weaknesses.

Timing for Referral

Referral for assessment of patients in the acute recovery process from stroke or traumatic brain injury can assist with treatment planning regardless of whether diagnosis is an issue. However, within the first few days or weeks of recovery from acute compromise in ability, as occurs with head injury or stroke, a comprehensive evaluation may not be appropriate for two reasons. First, data may not be reliable because of disruption of attentional mechanisms and, therefore, may not reflect the patient's true capacities at the time of testing. Second, until the patient has stabilized and begun to reach a plateau of recovery, limited predictive value can be gathered from testing. For example, the prognostic value of testing a patient at 3 weeks after cessation of drinking will more accurately predict long-term recovery than will similar testing done at 3 days. In degenerative illnesses (eg, dementia), repeated longitudinal evaluations are essential for accurate diagnosis and tracking of symptom progression. Differential diagnosis is sometimes not possible without follow-up testing, in which case the first evaluation serves as a baseline.

In variable or ongoing illness, such as multiple sclerosis or epilepsy, timing is also essential in that the referring psychiatrist must have an idea of whether a recent exacerbation has occurred. Also, fatigue, anxiety, and performance inconsistencies due to recent seizures, motivational problems, and lack of tolerance in brain-compromised patients must be considered in the referral process. These issues are critical because results will have varying prognostic value depending on the point at which the patient is evaluated.

Resumption of Normal Activities

Another important set of referral questions addresses the patient's level of residual functional capacity after recovery. Normal resumption of activities of daily living, socialization, and performance in work-like settings may not be possible depending on age, course of illness, severity of injury, and the presence of concomitant psychiatric illness. These are functional questions that may be best answered by a combination of assessment techniques, including administering formalized tests (see next section), observing the patient in demanding environments, interviewing the family, and taking a complete history of illness.

Neuropsychological testing is most predictive of functional limitations when used in the context of the patient's premorbid abilities (ie, educational and occupational background). For example, after receiving a left frontal head injury, a law student may expect to encounter difficulty in classes that tap verbal reasoning, whereas a factory worker might be just as debilitated from a comparable right-hemisphere lesion.

APPROACHES TO ASSESSMENT: FIXED VERSUS FLEXIBLE BATTERIES

In deciding how to address specific referral questions, the psychologist must determine which tests can best describe the patient's current level of function and predict further recovery or decline. The **fixed-battery approach** has the advantage of a standardized set of tests administered to all patients, thus making comparison of performances more accessible; however, it may result in unnecessary testing. The more recent trend has been to individualize the battery. The **flexible-battery approach** (also called the hypothesis-driven approach) uses the referral question and patient characteristics to determine which tests to administer. Most neuropsychologists use a combined approach to testing, with a basic core of tests administered to all patients and variations depending on the particular patient and referral question.

The Fixed Battery

A. Halstead-Reitan Neuropsychological Test Battery: The Halstead-Reitan Neuropsychological Test Battery (HRNTB) is the most widely used fixed battery. It originated from the work of Ward Halstead, who in 1947 at the University of Chicago published his observations of several hundred case studies of patients who had frontal lobe damage. By using 10 scores, Halstead blindly distinguished patients with confirmed brain lesions from control subjects. Ralph Reitan, a student of Halstead's, modified the battery in 1955 to identify lateralizing features of patient performances such as motor deficits expected in subtle stroke, the effect of temporal lobe epilepsy on memory, and the loss of abstraction ability associated with frontal damage. Reitan also modified the original battery to include tests that would accurately measure aphasia and variations of normal aging. The battery often had limited utility other than in merely determining the presence of organicity before other techniques (eg, neuroimaging) were available to do so. From continued use of the battery over the decades, 3 of the original 10 scores were dropped because of questionable validity.

Currently, the Halstead Impairment Index is the most widely accepted global measure of brain dysfunction in neuropsychology. Most normal subjects are able to pass 60–100% of the tests included in the Index. Patients who have moderate impairments may be within the normal range on only 30–60% of the tests, and those with severe dysfunction on less than 30%. The Index includes seven scores within the following five subtests:

1. Category Test—The Category Test is an abstract reasoning task consisting of 180 items. The patient is required to use mental flexibility and problem solving to form concepts with minimal feedback from the examiner other than correctness. Most normal individuals are able to complete this task with fewer than 50 errors.

2. Tactual Performance Test—The Tactual Performance Test contributes to the Index three scores (total time to completion, number of items remembered correctly, and number of items placed in correct location). The patient is blindfolded, then asked, in each of three trials, to place 10 blocks into their proper spaces, using their dominant, nondominant, and both hands, a task usually requiring 15 minutes or less for normal subjects. The second and third scores derived from the test (following removal of the blindfold) are the memory and location components. The patient is asked to draw the shapes and remember them in their correct location on the board in relation to the other blocks. This complex task is sensitive to difficulty in adaptation by the brain-injured patient.

3. Finger Tapping Test—Finger tapping is a test of fine motor speed. Five consecutive 10-second trials are obtained with the dominant and nondominant index fingers. Although this test is age dependent, most young adults are expected to average at least 50 taps per 10 seconds with their dominant hand. This task has been especially useful in detecting subtle lateralizing motor damage.

4. Rhythm Test—The Rhythm Test originated from the Seashore Measures of Musical Talent test, in which the patient is asked to differentiate between 30 pairs of rhythmic patterns. These pairs are presented in rapid succession on a tape recorder, and the patient must distinguish whether they are the same or different. Most normal subjects are able to do so for 25 or more of the 30 pairs.

5. Speech Sounds Perception Test—The Speech Sounds Perception Test involves 60 spoken nonsense words that are administered by audiotape. The patient is required to underline the corresponding printed response on an answer sheet, measuring verbal discrimination and sustained attention.

B. General Neuropsychological Deficit Scale: In addition to the seven scores provided by five Index subtests, other subtests from the HRNTB are used to represent patients' performances on the General Neuropsychological Deficit Scale (GNDS). Subtests used to contribute to this scale, in addition to those in the Index, include the Lateral Dominance Examination, Grip Strength, the Sensory-Perceptual Examination, Tactile Form Recognition, the Trail Making Test Parts A and B, and the Aphasia Screening Test. The GNDS, much like the Impairment Index, provides a global impairment rating but takes into account 42 variables, thus increasing reliability.

C. Luria-Nebraska Neuropsychological Battery: Another popular fixed battery is the Luria-Nebraska Neuropsychological Battery (LNNB). Based on work by the Russian neurologist and neuropsychologist A. R. Luria, it was first translated to English by A. L. Christensen of the University of Copenhagen. It was later modified with original and new items by psychologist C. G. Golden at the University of Nebraska. In its most recent and widely used form, this battery has been criticized for lack of adequate subjects in original standardization samples, sparse item selection, and limited generalizability of test findings to certain populations. Despite these validity and reliability issues, the LNNB has had considerable success because of its ease of interpretation and brevity relative to the HRNTB.

The LNNB consists of 11 clinical scales and 269 individual items. Commonly used research scales number over 50. The clinical portion includes the following scales: Motor Function (51 items that test motor speed, construction, coordination, and laterality), Rhythm (nonverbal auditory perception), Tactile Perception, Visual (perception, orientation, and spatial reasoning), Receptive Speech, Expressive Speech, Writing, Reading, Arithmetic, Memory, and Intellectual Processes. A proposed short form for elderly patients has correctly distinguished in validity studies Alzheimer's disease from depression.

Hartlage LC, Asken MJ, Hornsby JL: *Essentials of Neuropsychological Assessment.* Springer-Verlag, 1987.

Reitan R, Wolfson D: *The Halstead-Reitan Neuropsychological Test Battery: Theory and Clinical Application.* Neuropsychology Press, 1993.

The Flexible Battery

Advocates of a flexible neuropsychological test battery are likely to select particular instruments depending on information being requested and the patient's particular features. Major contributors to this approach are Boston University School of Medicine psychologist Edith Kaplan and University of Oregon psychologist Muriel Lezak, each of whom has emphasized the advantages of hypothesis testing in patients of undetermined diagnosis. At any stage of the examination process, the psychologist may choose a different course of testing based on the patient's performance. Depending on the patient's history and the referral question, the clinician may select all cognitive areas described in the sections that follow or may choose to focus on particular areas of investigation. For example, although the patient described in the case study at the beginning of this section was screened in all cognitive areas, much of the examination involved tasks related to learning and retaining new information, retrieval of old knowledge, and assessing whether challenges disrupt learning (eg, distractions to attention). This particular emphasis was made in order to delineate psychiatric from truly organic causes of his memory complaints. The following sections highlight the generally accepted cognitive domains in a flexible battery.

A. Attention & Concentration: After assuring an adequate level of consciousness, assessment of attention provides fundamental information as to whether evaluation of other cognitive domains, such as intelligence, memory, or language, will be valid. Further, because the ability to focus and maintain attention is highly sensitive to many acute and ongoing conditions (eg, alcohol withdrawal, certain medications, metabolic encephalopathy), a stable, chronic process may be affected less than will a recent or changing one. At the most basic level, this domain measures the patient's ability to attend to incoming information without being distracted. Examples of simple attentional tasks include digit repetition or visual tapping span, requiring forward or backward sequencing of auditory or visual stimuli. Sustained attention, known as vigilance or continuous performance, is a more complex level of attention. Signaling when hearing a target word or letter in a long sequence, or searching for visual targets on a computer screen, are examples of vigilance. Figure 12–6 represents the attempt of a right parietal stroke patient to complete a sustained visual attention task, the Mesulam Visual Cancellation Task, revealing neglect in the left visual field. The patient resumed driving after her stroke, but she likely contributed to an accident when she pulled into traffic and was struck by a car she did not see on the left side.

Similar lateralized inattention may occur in other modalities (eg, tactile) when patients have focal le-

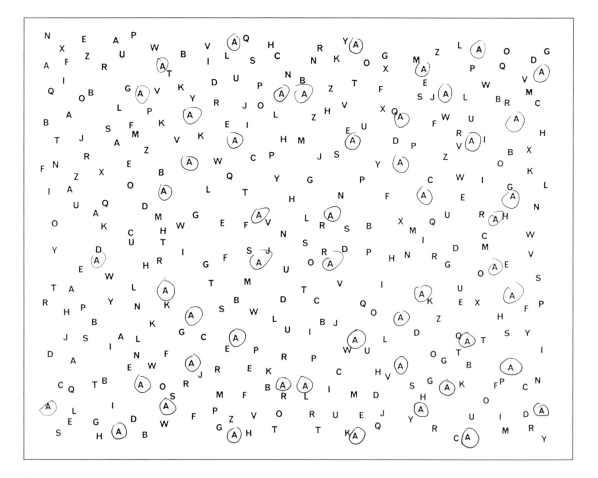

Figure 12–6. The Visual Cancellation Task from Mesulam (1986) showing neglect of target letters (A's) on extreme left. Reproduced by permission of F.A. Davis Co.

sions. More global deficits may emerge in the examination of patients who are delirious (eg, as a result of alcohol withdrawal or metabolic encephalopathy). The major limitation of tasks that measure only global attentional problems is lack of specificity: Without additional data, they may not distinguish a neurologic condition from a psychiatric disorder.

B. Learning & Memory: Compromise of memory is the most common patient complaint and referral question for neuropsychological testing. Milder memory problems, and particular learning parameters such as visual memory, may not be readily apparent on screening tasks from the mental status examination. Because memory is not a static or unitary process, careful assessment can help to characterize variations in performance, which can have diagnostic value. Recent memory versus long-term memory is the most common dichotomy and refers to recent information of up to about 4 hours as opposed to transitional phases for longer storage. Patients who have anterograde amnesia, or faulty learning of new material or events after the onset of their disorder, have more difficulty consolidating this learning into longer storage. Retrograde amnesia, or the inability to retrieve remote memories, is less prominent in organic memory loss, especially if the onset is sudden, as in head injury. However, certain chronic conditions and disease processes, such as Korsakoff's syndrome and Alzheimer's disease, may produce a more dense retrograde amnesia. Memory is often evaluated in the mental status examination by assessing orientation, current events, and recall of words or objects. Although screening is sometimes adequate to determine the presence of a gross learning disorder, full neuropsychological evaluation can detect whether the difficulty is with encoding, storage, or retrieval mechanisms, and whether the impairment is associated more with one modality than another (eg, verbal or visual).

The most widely used global memory test is the Wechsler Memory Scale (WMS), developed by David Wechsler, and its 1987 revision, the WMS-R, both of which yield memory quotients similar to IQ scores (expected mean is 100; standard deviation is 15). The WMS-R is composed of nine subtests: Orientation and Information, Mental Control (recitation of the alphabet, counting backwards, and serial three additions), Figural Memory (recognition recall of abstract designs), Logical Memory (recall of stories), Visual Paired Associates (association between designs and colors), Verbal Paired Associates (association between word pairs), Digit Span, Visual Memory Span (tapping), and Visual Reproduction (spontaneous recall of designs). Thirty-minute delayed recall is gathered for stories, visual designs, and word lists. Scores are derived through age comparisons. Performances on tests such as the WMS-R provide evidence of the patient's ability to engage in visual and verbal memory, immediate and delayed recall, spontaneous recall and recognition, and one-trial versus multi-trial learn-

ing. The third edition of the Wechsler memory series, published in 1999 with updated norms and some subtest revisions, retained the basic format of reporting verbal, visual, and general learning and recall capacity.

C. Language: Testing for aphasia is a necessary part of diagnosis and treatment planning in some developmental and learning disabilities, progressive disorders (eg, dementia, tumor), or recovery from an acute injury such as stroke or head injury. Impairment of language on a gross level is often more noticeable because of the frequent need for clear communication. However, subtle language deficits can go undetected in informal conversation and occasionally in more formal assessment. At the very least, language screening should include tasks to measure quality of spontaneous speech, naming, comprehension, repetition, reading, writing, calculation, and left-right orientation. Naming, the most sensitive element of most underlying language disturbances, is often measured through confrontational naming tasks such as the Boston Naming Test, a 60-item test of picture identification. Well-studied aphasia screening batteries include the Boston Diagnostic Aphasia Examination, the Western Aphasia Battery, and the Reitan-Indiana Aphasia Screening Test. If the neuropsychological assessment confirms the presence of aphasia, a speech evaluation may be required for more detailed treatment.

D. Intelligence: Intelligence has been defined as the ability to adapt effectively to one's environment. Psychometric intelligence is regarded as one's comparable ability to perform on a test of intelligence. The Wechsler tests, including the Wechsler Adult Intelligence Scale-Revised (WAIS-R), are the most widely used measures of intellectual functioning. The WAIS-R yields Verbal, Performance, and Full scale IQs (expected mean is 100; standard deviation is 15) based on age ranges from 16 to 74 years. The WAIS-R is divided into 11 subtests, 6 of which make up the Verbal Scale. General fund of knowledge is assessed on the Information subtest, whereas expressive word knowledge is tapped by the Vocabulary subtest. The Arithmetic subtest measures the patient's ability to compute numerical problems mentally. Digit Span assesses the patient's ability to complete number repetitions forward and backward, thus tapping simple auditory focusing. The patient's social judgment and reasoning are evaluated on the Comprehension subtest, on which interpretation of proverbs is also required. On the Similarities subtest, the patient is asked to explain how opposite or unrelated objects (eg, an orange and a peach) are alike in some obvious or abstract way (eg, both fruits).

The Performance Scale contains five subtests, all of which are timed and involve visual and, in most cases, motoric interaction with test materials. The Picture Completion subtest is a visual analysis task in which the patient indicates the essential missing parts of pictures (eg, a handle on a car door). The Picture Arrangement subtest requires the patient to create a logical sequence for cartoon-like cards that tell a story. On the Block Design subtest, a nonverbal test of abstraction, the patient must use colored blocks to replicate in three dimensions a two-dimensional construction shown on a card. The Object Assembly subtest requires the patient to place jigsaw puzzle pieces together to form familiar objects. Finally, the Digit Symbol subtest requires the patient to match numbers to symbols, measuring speed of visual processing. A newer edition of this instrument (WAIS-III) is available with updated norms and three new subtests (Matrix Reasoning, Letter-Number Sequencing, and Symbol Search).

Estimation of the patient's premorbid intellectual level arises frequently in the referral question, particularly when a suspected change in function has occurred in a patient who has psychiatric disturbance (eg, schizophrenia) or neurologic disturbance (eg, suspected dementia). Demographic data are useful in this regard as are procedures (eg, measures of long-term memory) that are usually preserved in the earlier stages of organic disturbances such as dementia.

E. Executive Functioning: Executive functioning refers to those areas of cognition and personality subserved by the frontal lobes in interaction with other brain regions. The frontal lobes themselves comprise one third of the human cortex, and interactions with more posterior brain regions require whole brain integrity. Neuropsychological functioning under the rubric of executive tasks includes abstraction, problem solving, set generation and sequencing, ability to maintain or terminate behaviors, and ability to plan and organize. These functions are mediated by the frontal lobes. Personality characteristics having to do with judgment, social appropriateness, inhibition versus impulsivity, and motivation are also at least partially related to frontal activity. The best example of an organically driven personality change is that of Phineas Gage, a railroad worker in the 1880s, who sustained a traumatic injury to the frontal lobes when a tamping iron was blown through his head. This formerly docile, responsible worker became irascible, foul mouthed, and disinhibited. As his reckless and menacing behavior continued, his coworkers described him as "no longer Gage."

Specific tasks that are frequently used to study the integrity of the frontal systems include the Wisconsin Card Sorting Test. This procedure provides an index of how well the examinee can formulate hypotheses and solve problems. Cards are matched by principles that are not stated directly, and the patient must shift cognitive sets as the rules for sorting change without forewarning. Other good measures of executive functioning include Controlled Oral Word Fluency, which requires verbal set generation (eg, words beginning with certain letters), the Category Test (concept formation), and the Trail Making Test (measuring visual shifting and sequencing).

F. Visuospatial Functioning: Visuospatial functioning measures both the patient's ability to function within his or her environment with regard to recognition of objects and his or her construction and perception of spatial relations. Such abilities are important in daily activities that require the patient to recognize faces and remember geographic location and spatial orientation and in procedural learning tasks such as driving a car. Because patients with progressive neurologic disorders such as Alzheimer's disease or right hemisphere strokes are particularly susceptible to deficits in this area, careful testing will be able to determine whether the patient is likely to encounter problems in getting lost or living independently. Figure copying, clock drawing, visual organization of parts to whole, facial recognition, and map orientation are samples of tasks used to assess this domain.

Lezak MD: *Neuropsychological Assessment,* 3rd ed. Oxford University Press, 1995.
Mesulam M: *Principles of Behavioral Neurology.* FA Davis Co, 1986.
Tranel D: Neuropsychological assessment. Psychiatr Clin N Am 1992;15:283.

CLINICAL DECISION MAKING IN NEUROPSYCHOLOGICAL ASSESSMENT

Valid and reliable interpretation of neuropsychological test scores must be based on consideration of several factors in addition to the patient's test performances. Conclusions about particular test findings, and how they are conveyed to the referring psychiatrist, will differ markedly depending on several patient variables. First, scores must be related to the educational and occupational background of the patient. Accordingly, if the patient had a third-grade education and experience only in factory work before retirement, then low scores on a given test might not be interpreted as a decline from previous levels. Similarly, if low test scores were gathered in the context of a recent mental status change in someone who has a college degree and previous professional work, then a reasonable conclusion is that poor performance represents a decline.

Before a psychiatrist can be assured of a diagnosis of a particular disorder (eg, dementia), a host of alternative diagnoses must be ruled out. Depression, delirium caused by physical illness or medication effects, a recent but recovering brain insult (eg, closed head injury), and recent seizures are only a few possible explanations for transiently deficient test scores. In cases of documented brain compromise from treatable conditions, the psychiatrist may wish to begin appropriate therapy (eg, treatment of depression in pseudodementia). If cognitive recovery is less than expected, follow-up neuropsychological examination or referral for further neurodiagnostic procedures may be warranted.

The neuropsychological evaluation may provide the only means for detecting alteration or recovery in brain function in more subtle disorders. Additionally, an estimate of the patient's capacity to return to normal work and social activities will be addressed most effectively in an open dialogue with the referring psychiatrist. The following case example illustrates the need for such close communication.

A 23-year-old single female was seen in psychotherapy for depression, which was thought to be a reaction secondary to an unwanted pregnancy. Although distinct neurovegetative signs were absent, the patient's family noticed that she was socially withdrawn and had lost interest in usual activities. She had difficulty initiating behavior and spent most of her day appearing "bored," according to her concerned family. She spent most of her time sitting motionless in front of the television. Although she did not exhibit improvement from psychotherapy, sessions were continued. The patient's development of severe headaches was thought to be related to depression. When she developed a slight right facial droop, language abnormalities, and a right hemiparesis, she was referred for organic workup, including neuropsychological testing. Examination revealed an expressive aphasia, slowness in initiating activ-

ity, poor planning ability, decreased judgment, and a marked visual neglect on the right visual field. This finding coincided with her clock drawing (Figure 12–7A), which showed obvious right-sided neglect due to the frontal mass shown on MRI (Figure 12–7B). On surgical removal, the mass was found to be a rare meningioma.

CONCLUSION

This chapter has attempted to provide the reader with an introduction to adult personality and neuropsychological testing in psychiatry. The importance of immediately delineating a diagnosis and instituting treatment lends psychological testing great value. Psychological testing provides clinicians with greater diagnostic confidence than interview data alone. For instance, the clinician can relate test patterns to normative data for different diagnostic groups (both inpatient and outpatient). This capability enables the psychologist to arrive at increased accuracy in correctly classifying an individual's psychiatric disorder.

Psychological testing referrals from medical specialties other than psychiatry are becoming much more commonplace. Internists and orthopedists typically refer for psychological testing patients with pain complaints for which no organic basis can be de-

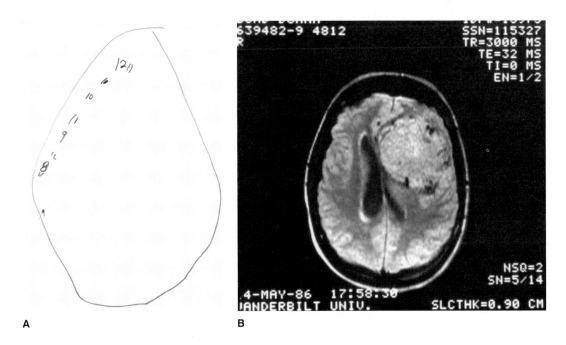

A   **B**

Figure 12–7A. Clock drawing showing neglect of right side. **B.** MRI showing left front parietal tumor.

tected, or for which the complaints are far in excess of what one would anticipate from physical findings. Transplant surgeons want information about an individual's cognitive ability to follow a complex medical regimen and how personality factors may affect treatment compliance. Other referrals may come from neurologists and neurosurgeons wanting help in differentiating the relative contributions of neurologic and psychological factors in a patient's behavioral symptoms.

Contemporary personality and neuropsychological techniques are linked closely to advances in statistical methodology. The increasing partnership between quantitative psychology and psychological assessment holds promise for improving our understanding and measurement of complex human behavior.

Emergency Psychiatry

13

George C. Bolian, MD, & Rudra Prakash, MD

Emergency psychiatry is a set of circumstances under which clinical psychiatry is sometimes practiced. It is best regarded as a subset of emergency medicine. Its four distinguishing features within that domain are (1) enhanced verbal communication and acute behavioral observation, (2) enhanced psychosocial and cultural awareness, (3) widespread collaboration with nonmedical personnel, and (4) increased time expenditure.

GOALS OF EMERGENCY PSYCHIATRY

The goals of emergency psychiatric care are identical to those of medical-surgical care: (1) triage; (2) expeditious, pertinent assessment; (3) accurate diagnosis; (4) initiation of treatment, when appropriate; and (5) disposition.

Triage

In triage, the clinician must first distinguish between situations that constitute a genuine emergency and those that, although perceived as such by the patient or others, can safely await later assessment. This distinction has assumed added significance in an era of managed reimbursement. Next, the clinician must correctly identify, among a variety of emergency situations, those that reflect a dominant need for psychiatric evaluation as a first step. It is here that the experience and skill of the triage person is crucial because so many patients may have combined medical-psychiatric complaints. Finally, the clinician must assure the safety and comfort of emergency psychiatric patients at least until they can be evaluated by a psychiatrist or other appropriate mental health professional.

Although initial triage is most commonly undertaken by nursing or other personnel, the psychiatrist must assume an active role in the training and supervision of those persons and in the formulation of standards and clinical criteria applied during the triage "sorting"

function. Triage is only as effective as the quality of the standards and the accuracy of their application.

Assessment

Assessment of psychiatric patients under emergency circumstances is essentially no different from competent assessment in general, except for time constraints and the resultant need to quickly focus the evaluation on the pertinent aspect(s) of the case. The examiner assembles as much data as possible before addressing the patient directly. For example, if information suggests that the patient may be dangerous to others, appropriate security arrangements should be made. However, the initial moments of the direct encounter with the patient are probably the most revealing. It is then that the examiner gets an initial overall impression of the patient's appearance, style and appropriateness of dress; openness or suspiciousness; weeping or smiling; menacing gestures; furtive glances; seductive poses; agitated pacing; somnolent dozing; and so forth. Equally revealing are whether or not the patient greets the examiner conventionally and his or her speech and language (eg, accent, thought sequencing, neologisms, indication of probable intellectual level, use of profanity). At that moment, the examiner is well advised to heed the admonition of many emergency room clinicians: "Don't just do something . . . stand there" (and assimilate what is before you). Although the examiner's task is to focus on the most pertinent details, only the inexperienced examiner will assume that what the patient (or spouse, parent, police officer, and so on) identifies first is necessarily the central problem. For example, a parent may report that his or her teenage daughter is sullen, depressed, has spoken of suicide, and refuses to attend school; the problem may be that she is secretly pregnant and fearful that she is HIV positive. Despite the common pressure to proceed expeditiously, the assessment phase is no time to short-circuit thoroughness in either medical or psychiatric evaluations. Taking into account the incidence and prevalence of various behaviors, the clinician must include in the assessment the patient's history, physical examination, and mental status examination as well as appropriate laboratory, radiologic, and other ancillary studies.

Diagnosis

The pressures of the emergency setting do not allow the detailed diagnosis possible in inpatient hospitalization. However, the emergency evaluation must move the clinical process in the right direction. Table 13–1 lists four sequential questions that must be considered in making a differential diagnosis.

Treatment Intervention

Treatment intervention, when appropriate as an emergency procedure, will usually follow the diagnostic assessment. However, sometimes the clinician must intervene before gathering all the diagnostic information. This is particularly true when the patient must be physically restrained if he or she presents an obvious and imminent danger to self or others. In most circumstances, emergency intervention will fall into one or more of three categories: medication, crisis intervention, and education.

A. Medication: Rapid treatment with a neuroleptic such as haloperidol is sometimes useful for treating acute psychotic states. Similarly, the prompt use of benzodiazepines may be appropriate treatment for agitation associated with sedative withdrawal. Clinical judgment, on a case-by-case basis, is required to determine whether a patient should be given an initial dose of medication prior to outpatient follow-up care. Some factors to consider are the patient's compliance, issues of safety, and the amount of time before outpatient follow-up care will begin. A patient should not be given more than a few days' supply of medication at any one time.

B. Crisis Intervention: Psychological strategies based on a biopsychosocial understanding of the situation can often deescalate a crisis. Such techniques include ventilation, identification of alternatives, clarification of interpersonal roles, interpretation of meaning, or simply empathic listening. Environmental modification can sometimes eliminate the need for hospitalization (eg, providing respite care or emergency placement of a child).

C. Education: Often overlooked is the opportunity for preventive education in the emergency setting. Family members, significant others, and even other caretakers will sometimes benefit greatly from clarification of the situation in a way that can avert unwarranted guilt or confusion. The patient may avoid a sense of alienation, shame, and hopelessness by better understanding the diagnosed illness, its prevalence, and its prognosis.

Disposition

Disposition of a psychiatric emergency depends on the resources that are realistically available. In general, at least four issues must be considered: (1) initial level of care, (2) timing of initial follow-up care, (3) interval provisions, and (4) communication with the patient and subsequent caretakers.

1. Initial level of care—As the most restrictive and expensive alternative, 24-hour inpatient care should be used only after careful consideration of several factors. Commonly accepted criteria for such care include mental illness associated with imminent danger to self or others, grave impairment of function to a degree that prohibits self-preservation in the most supportive environment available, and diagnostic uncertainty that could result in a lethal outcome. Less restrictive alternatives include 23-hour observation, partial hospitalization, or intensive or routine outpatient follow-up care. The objective is to provide the least restrictive level of care that meets the patient's clinical needs. Managed reimbursement is a factor, but it should not unduly influence sound clinical decision-making.

2. Timing of initial follow-up care—If the patient is admitted to the hospital, it should be established that all services required immediately are available. If the patient is not admitted, the disposition should include determination of the clinically permissible time interval before a less restrictive level of care is available. For example, a situation that requires urgent outpatient follow-up care should not be scheduled 2 or 3 weeks later.

3. Interval provisions—If time will elapse before follow-up care, the patient and relevant others should be informed of what to do if the need for emergency care recurs. In most cases the clinician who provided the initial emergency assessment is best prepared to handle any such interval recurrence.

4. Communication with the patient & subsequent caretakers—A breakdown in communication often frustrates the patient and leads to criticism of the health delivery system. The precise disposition plan should be made clear to the patient (and, when appropriate, to the family or significant others). An oppor-

Table 13–1. Differential evaluation.

1. Is the disordered affect, thought, or behavior the product of detectable pathophysiology, especially that associated with alcoholism or other substance-induced toxicity?
2. If not, is the disordered affect, thought, or behavior of psychotic quality, especially that associated with schizophrenia or manic states?
3. If not, is the disordered affect, thought, or behavior compatible with some other formal diagnostic entity, especially anxiety states, depression, or personality disorder?
4. If not, is the disordered affect, thought, or behavior contrived to obtain an advantage or to avoid an undesirable consequence (eg, incarceration)?

tunity to raise questions, seek clarification of details, better understand the clinical rationale, and so on should be a routine part of this process. Equally important is timely communication with other professional caretakers who are to provide subsequent treatment. This communication should provide enough detail for other clinicians to assume an active stance immediately and to prevent the patient from having to repeat large volumes of information. Quality care gives the patient a reassuring sense of continuity from emergency onset to final resolution.

SPECIAL SITUATIONS

The variety of human predicaments that may constitute a psychiatric emergency for any given individual is virtually endless. Three general conditions deserve mention: suicide, homicide and other violence, and epidemic emotional expression.

Suicide

Suicide accounts for 30,000 deaths each year in the United States. The number of attempted suicides is many times larger. Many individuals who committed suicide saw a physician or other health care personnel shortly before their deaths, often (it appears in retrospect) in an effort to signal their distress. Perhaps the single most important element in the assessment of suicidal risk is constant awareness of the possibility that it exists. The patient may make no direct reference to self-destruction unless asked. He or she may exhibit vague somatic symptoms, anxiety, or depression. His or her mood may seem devoid of hope, and he or she may mention some recent life crisis or a family history of suicide. Although no definitive list of risk factors exists, several factors should be considered (Table 13–2).

Table 13–2. Suicide risk factors.

Age (especially adolescents and older adults)
Marital status (suicide is more common among single, widowed, or divorced adults)
Sex (females attempt suicide more often than do males, but males succeed more often than do females)
Economic status (unemployment or economic reverses increase risk)
History of prior attempt
Family history of suicide
Recent separation or loss
Presence of a plan and available means to accomplish it
Lethality of an attempt (more lethal attempts increase risk)
Diagnosis (especially major depression, schizophrenia, alcoholism or other substance dependence, and borderline personality disorder)
Specific symptoms (especially command hallucinations, delusional thinking, and profound hopelessness)
Lack of social support

Table 13–3. Homicide and other violence: clinical and epidemiologic factors.

Age (violent individuals tend to be young)
Sex (males predominate)
Criminality (some individuals violate social rules without significant psychological impairment)
History (physical or sexual abuse as a child, fire setting, or cruelty to animals)
Proposed victim is a family member or close associate
Environmental influence (violent subcultures beget violence)
Diagnosis (especially manic states, schizophrenia, alcoholism or other substance dependence, conduct disorder, antisocial personality disorder, and intermittent explosive disorder)
Specific symptoms (especially command hallucinations, agitation, and hostile suspiciousness)

Homicide & Other Violence

Homicide and other social violence are important social problems in the United States as we enter the 21st century. Their relationship to bona fide mental illness is a complex clinical and legal issue. Although the clinician who is called upon to make an emergency assessment must be aware of the legal ramifications (see Chapter 15), he or she is best advised to approach the task with the admonition that justice is served best by thorough, objective, accurate assessment and documentation. As with self-directed aggression, many clinical and epidemiologic factors need to be considered (Table 13–3).

Epidemic Emotional Expression

Epidemic emotional expression, although not an emergency in the more traditional sense, is an increasingly common psychosocial problem. It reflects the growing interdependence of a larger population coupled with the ready accessibility that some individuals have to technologically sophisticated instruments of destruction. Two general patterns exist: the response to the sudden, unexpected, and violent death of one individual; and the response to multiple, simultaneous violent deaths.

A. Response to the Death of One Individual: The sudden, unexpected, and violent death of one individual can sometimes trigger a nearly overwhelming emotional response in a large number of others. The dimensions of this phenomenon vary, from the effect of an adolescent's suicide on his or her classmates, to the effect of a president's assassination on an entire nation. When the size of the group permits it, early direct intervention can be therapeutic and prevent longer-term morbidity. Because the most common dynamic reflects some form of identification with the individual who died, the strategies listed in Table 13–4 may be helpful.

B. Response to Multiple Deaths: Multiple, simultaneous violent deaths can also ignite profound group response. The dynamics have less to do with identification with any one individual than with sheer

Table 13–4. Common strategies for dealing with epidemic emotional expression.

Empathic listening
Encouragement of ventilation
Nurturance of preexisting group bonds
Participation in culturally prescribed rituals (eg, burial rites, eulogies, wakes)
Rededication to the positive principles represented by or associated with the person who died
Alertness for the emergence of any bona fide psychopathology in response to the event

horror at the dimension of the event. Examples include a lone gunman who enters a school and shoots several innocent children in a matter of seconds, an airplane crash with no survivors, and the explosive demolition of a huge office building at a time of peak occupancy. Formal intervention in such circumstances is usually limited to specific survivors (eg, family members). Most of the public perception of, and reaction to, such tragic circumstances is influenced heavily by the media. This area deserves more careful psychological investigation.

MAJOR CLINICAL SYNDROMES

Patients with a variety of clinical syndromes may present in a health care setting for emergency psychiatric treatment (Table 13–5). The following sections discuss the disorders most commonly requiring emergency treatment.

Table 13–5. Clinical syndromes that may present as psychiatric emergencies.[1]

Syndrome	Assessment	Dispositions
Geriatric syndromes	Review of systems Laboratory tests Look for delirium, delirium with dementia, depression, and psychosis	Inpatient care Collaboration with medical team High-potency neuroleptics (eg, haloperidol, 0.5–1 mg orally or intramuscularly) for agitation
Substance abuse	Look for intoxication or withdrawal	Quiet environment Inpatient care for neuropsychiatric signs Lorazepam (1–2 mg intramuscularly or orally) or haloperidol (5 mg orally or 2 mg intramuscularly) for agitation
Psychosis	New onset versus exacerbation? Rule out substance abuse and medical illness Evaluate for compliance, dangerousness, and ADL	Inpatient care for new-onset psychosis, dangerousness, or severely impaired ADL Collaboration with outpatient team
Depression	Evaluate for suicidal risk, comorbidities, current stressors, and substance abuse	Inpatient care for suicidal risk, agitation, or substance abuse Collaborate with outpatient team
Mania	Evaluate for dangerousness and substance abuse	Inpatient care for psychosis, dangerousness, or substance abuse Lorazepam (1–2 mg intramuscularly) or haloperidol (1–5 mg intramuscularly) for agitation
Catatonia	Two subtypes: withdrawn and excited Look for schizophrenia, mood disorders, and medical disorders (eg, using amobarbital, 500 mg, 50 mg/min intravenously)	Inpatient care Lorazepam (1–2 mg, intramuscularly or intravenously)
Acute anxiety states	Types include panic disorder, acute stress disorder, posttraumatic stress disorder, conversion states, dissociative states Evaluate for ADL	Inpatient care if ADL markedly impaired Lorazepam (1–2 mg orally or intramuscularly)
Personality disorders	Evaluate for substance abuse, legal history, relationships, "micropsychotic" episodes, mood changes, aggression, and comorbidities	Interdisciplinary treatment Focus on "here and now" issues
Neuroleptic malignant syndrome	Look for sudden onset, autonomic changes, neuromuscular changes, elevated CPK, and leukocytosis	Medical emergency Inpatient care: stop neuroleptic and provide supportive treatment (rehydration, antipyretic) Dantrolene (2–3 mg/kg) or bromocriptine (2.5–10 mg three times daily)

[1] ADL, activities of daily living; CPK, creatine phosphokinase.

GERIATRIC CONDITIONS

Assessment

A geriatric patient with a psychiatric emergency almost always poses an assessment challenge. Coexisting medical disorders and medical treatments often influence psychiatric presentation. Therefore, a thorough review of systems, a complete physical examination, and appropriate laboratory tests are imperative in this age group. A medically oriented evaluative approach may be more effective than a traditional psychiatric one. The clinician must ask short and simple questions in a straightforward manner and repeat them as necessary. He or she should speak clearly and slowly to geriatric patients. Due respect should be given to such patients by addressing them properly, usually formally. Further, the clinician should always consider a collateral source of history within the framework of confidentiality.

Common geriatric emergencies include delirium, delirium with dementia, depression, and psychosis. Delirium is a medical emergency that has a potentially fatal outcome if not treated in time. Physical symptoms, generally related to a hyperadrenergic state, and acute cognitive and perceptual changes are hallmarks of delirium. Fluctuating consciousness, extreme attentional deficits, memory disturbance, disorganized thinking, and hallucinations are to be expected in some combination. The onset is acute and the course turbulent. Delirium may be comorbid with a preexisting dementia. As soon as the clinician suspects delirium, he or she should initiate a thorough evaluation of etiology. Adverse drug interactions or an anticholinergic syndrome are present in some cases.

Intoxication secondary to an unintentional overdose (related to cognitive impairment) may also be associated with delirium. Depressed elderly patients may exhibit somatic symptoms and pseudodementia and may underreport their suicidality. Suicidal risk is high. Depression may be related to a general medical condition and medication. Depression and psychosis may also be part of a dementing illness. Aggression is sometimes associated with psychosis. The etiology of such cognitive and behavioral change is often unclear.

Disposition

Because of the likely fragility of a geriatric emergency patient's mental or medical status, geriatric disorders are best treated on an inpatient basis and in collaboration with a medical team. The utmost care should be taken before referring such a patient to outpatient care. A high-potency neuroleptic (eg, haloperidol) is a safer tool for the management of agitation than is a benzodiazepine. Low-potency neuroleptics (eg, thioridazine or chlorpromazine) are likely to be associated with strong anticholinergic side effects, thereby precipitating delirium.

ALCOHOL ABUSE

Assessment

Alcohol-related presentations are among the most common psychiatric emergencies. They are associated with the following disorders: intoxication, withdrawal, intoxication delirium, withdrawal delirium, psychotic disorders with delusions or hallucinations, mood disorders, and anxiety disorders.

The clinical picture of intoxication generally depends on the patient's blood alcohol level (BAL), but BAL cannot be used exclusively. Pathologic intoxication, for example, is characterized by excessive behavioral reaction to an insufficient amount of alcohol. The concept is rather controversial. In most jurisdictions, an individual with a BAL of .1 or greater is considered legally to be intoxicated. If a patient is intoxicated, the clinician must ascertain whether another chemical in addition to ethanol is related to the clinical presentation. A toxicology screen is essential. An intoxicated state is characterized by a combination of markedly maladaptive behavior or psychological changes and physical changes (eg, slurred speech, ataxia, nystagmus, stupor, coma) that appear during or after alcohol ingestion.

Alcohol withdrawal appears within several hours to a few days after cessation of or reduction in heavy and extended alcohol use. It is characterized by a hyperadrenergic state, agitation, insomnia, gastrointestinal symptoms, hallucinations, hand tremors, and seizures. Both intoxication and withdrawal may be associated with delirium. Psychotic, mood, and anxiety disorders may be related to alcohol use. A thorough medical evaluation is warranted to exclude physical conditions that resemble intoxication or withdrawal.

Disposition

Coma must be managed as a medical emergency. A belligerent, drunk patient should be moved to a quiet environment. Lorazepam or haloperidol should be effective in managing agitation. Physical restraints or higher dosages of lorazepam or haloperidol may be used, as needed.

A common and complex question is, When can a patient with alcohol intoxication or withdrawal be discharged from the emergency room? The clinician must consider carefully whether the following conditions are present: ataxia; significant psychosis; cognitive or mood impairment; suicidal, homicidal, or aggressive behavior; or coexisting medical conditions. A patient who exhibits any of these problems may be better served in an inpatient setting. It is wise and safe, if feasible, to discharge a patient to the custody of family or friends. Appropriate referral may include an outpatient detoxification or rehabilitation program, partial hospitalization, intensive or routine outpatient treatment, and Alcoholics Anonymous.

OTHER DRUGS OF ABUSE

Assessment

Clinical history, specific physical examination findings, and a drug screen may offer evidence of other drugs of abuse (Table 13–6).

Disposition

The management of intoxication or withdrawal depends on the specific type of drug. Associated physical and psychiatric symptoms must be factored into the immediate treatment plan. Violence, blatant psychosis, or overt mood symptoms, in association with suicidal behavior, warrant immediate inpatient care. Chemical restraints (eg, lorazepam or haloperidol), seclusion, or physical restraints may be needed to manage violent behavior. Methadone or clonidine is specifically indicated in opioid withdrawal. The principles of outpatient referral are the same as for alcohol.

PSYCHOSIS

Assessment

A psychotic state may occur either as a completely new event or as the exacerbation or reactivation of chronic psychosis (see Chapters 19 and 20). The distinction is important because new-onset psychosis frequently warrants hospitalization, whereas the chronic condition often can be managed readily in cooperation with an outpatient team. Substance abuse and medical illness should be considered among the possible causes. Assessment should consider the patient's compliance with prior treatment recommendations; the severity of impairment in activities of daily living; the patient's dangerousness to self and others; the presence of delusions, command auditory hallucinations, or thought disorder; and the presence of judgment or insight impairment.

Disposition

First-time acute psychotic conditions generally require hospitalization. Impaired judgment in the presence of dangerous behavior may warrant involuntary hospitalization. Marked agitation often requires physical restraint or psychopharmacologic intervention (eg, lorazepam). Determination of the most appropriate and least restrictive level of care should include consideration of 23-hour observation, partial hospitalization, full 24-hour admission, and respite care. When outpatient follow-up care will suffice, attention must be given to appropriate inclusion of family members, case managers, and other caretakers. Initiation or adjustment of neuroleptic medication may be indicated after necessary laboratory studies are completed. Disposition instructions should be precise, preferably written, and followed by telephone contact to ensure compliance.

DEPRESSION

Assessment

By far the most common psychiatric emergency, a depressed patient typically presents with melancholic features and suicidal ideation or behavior (see Chapter 21 and the discussion on suicide earlier in this chapter). In addition to identifying current stressors and probing for a history of depression, the clinician must pay close attention to comorbid conditions such as medical illness, psychosis, substance abuse, anxiety, and personality disorders.

Disposition

Potentially lethal suicidal behavior associated with a mood of hopelessness and worthlessness generally warrants 24-hour inpatient care, although the availability of a vigorous, reliable support system may allow a less restrictive alternative to be considered. The judgment of an experienced clinician who has examined the patient should prevail over opinions of managed care utilization reviewers. Patients who exhibit significant depression, coexistent with substance abuse, should be referred to a dual-diagnosis program when available. Referral for outpatient follow-up care requires forethought about many factors such as safety, availability of supportive monitoring, time interval to next visit, access to help in the event of recurrent emergency, and

Table 13–6. Evidence of other drugs of abuse.

Drug	Physical Findings	Psychiatric Findings
Amphetamines	Increased blood pressure, mydriasis	Euphoria, hypervigilance
Cannabis	Tachycardia	Anxiety, social withdrawal
Cocaine	Increased temperature, tachycardia, tremor	Euphoria, hypervigilance
Hallucinogens	Mydriasis, tachycardia, tremor	Anxiety, paranoia
Inhalants	Nystagmus, arrhythmia	Belligerence, apathy
Opioids	Miosis in intoxication, mydriasis in withdrawal	Agitation, dysphoria
Phencyclidine	Nystagmus, increased blood pressure, arrhythmia	Labile mood, amnesia
Sedative-hypnotics	Decreased respiration, tremor	Aggression, mood lability

advisability of medication use. The clinician should not automatically give the patient antidepressant medication, but the judicious provision of a small quantity of a serotonergic antidepressant as one component of a biopsychosocial plan is warranted. The clinician must communicate promptly with follow-up caretakers.

MANIA

Assessment

The cardinal features of mania are ignitability, expansiveness, and elevation of mood (see Chapter 21). Other frequently associated findings include grandiosity, pressured speech, flight of ideas, insomnia, increased psychomotor activity, social or economic indiscretion, and poor concentration. The manic patient generally does not initiate the search for help, but rather the people around him can no longer tolerate his or her talkativeness, grandiosity, irresponsible behavior, and so on. The patient who offers a self-diagnosis of bipolar disorder should be evaluated carefully for comorbid conditions such as chemical dependence or cluster B personality traits. Cocaine, amphetamines, phencyclidine, and various hallucinogens can precipitate or aggravate a manic state. Cluster B traits, or borderline, histrionic, or narcissistic disorders, may underlie a manic state. For example, the mood swings of borderline personality disorder must be differentiated from cyclothymia and rapid cycling bipolar disorder.

Disposition

A clear-cut manic episode, especially if associated with psychotic symptoms, usually warrants inpatient care. A dual-diagnosis program should be considered when mania is associated with chemical abuse or dependence. Recognition of any associated personality disorder is particularly important if the clinician is to avoid resistance and the misperception of treatment, followed by the unnecessary trial-and-error use of several different psychopharmacologic agents. Proper treatment of such comorbid conditions requires intervention other than the use of mood-stabilizing drugs. In the emergency room, a typical agitated patient with mania warrants immediate intervention. As in the case of acute psychosis, pharmacotherapy (eg, lorazepam) with or without physical restraint may be required. Haloperidol can be used as an alternative or adjunctively. The primary goal is to contain the patient's agitation immediately so that he or she may be transferred safely to an inpatient setting.

CATATONIA

Assessment

Catatonia is characterized by either excitement or withdrawal. The excited type is characterized by extreme purposeless motor activity; the withdrawn type is characterized by negativism, mutism, rigidity, posturing, waxy flexibility, and stupor. Catatonia is no longer synonymous with schizophrenia, even though a significant subpopulation of catatonic patients have schizophrenia. Other etiologies to consider are mood disorders, especially depression and "organic" states (eg, encephalitis, neurotoxicities). Catatonia is an emergency situation that requires immediate inpatient care, because dehydration and stupor are major complications. If the patient has a medical illness underlying catatonia, there is additional risk of medical complications. Neuroleptic malignant syndrome (described later in this chapter) merits exclusion. Amobarbital may help distinguish diverse etiologies.

Disposition

Inpatient care must be delivered immediately. A thorough medical workup is generally indicated. Lorazepam can bring about quick improvement. Specific treatment depends on etiology.

ACUTE ANXIETY STATES

Assessment

Panic attack, acute stress disorder, adjustment disorder, posttraumatic stress disorder, conversion disorder, and dissociative states may lead patients to visit the emergency room (see Chapters 22, 23, and 25). Psychophysiologic symptoms of intense anxiety; sudden attacks, with or without recurrence; and agoraphobia characterize panic attack and panic disorder. Acute stress reactions involve intense anxiety following exposure to a major stressor. Symptoms include flashbacks, nightmares, numbing, reliving experiences, preoccupation with trauma, and phobic avoidance.

Adjustment disorder (see Chapter 32) occurs when a commonly encountered stressor leads to an excessive reaction characterized by anxiety. A sudden loss of physical function (eg, paralysis, mutism) without physical basis is the hallmark of conversion hysteria (see Chapter 25). The unconscious nature of this illness distinguishes it from malingering (see Chapter 26), which involves the intentional fabrication of symptoms for obvious gain. Amnesia without an organic basis, fugue state, and multiple personality disorder are different forms of dissociative states (see Chapters 17 and 25). Depersonalization is occasionally a patient's chief complaint in the emergency room. Common comorbidities are chemical abuse or dependence, generalized or other anxiety disorders, cluster B and cluster C personality traits or disorders, mood disorders, eating disorders, and medical illnesses. A thorough medical evaluation is often warranted, especially when panic and conversion states are present.

Disposition

A marked restriction of activities of daily living, acute stress disorder, posttraumatic stress disorder, and multiple personality disorder may require inpatient care. Depersonalization and impaired reality testing (eg, hallucinations) are sometimes present in acute or posttraumatic stress reactions and generally warrant hospitalization. However, most anxiety disorders can be managed on an outpatient basis with a balanced combination of pharmacotherapy and psychosocial interventions. Panic and other acute anxiety states respond favorably and quickly to a benzodiazepine such as lorazepam.

PERSONALITY DISORDERS

Assessment

Patients with personality disorders per se do not present routinely in the emergency room. Almost invariably, a crisis associated with these disorders leads to a visit to the emergency room. Suicidal or homicidal behavior, aggression in general, "micropsychotic episodes," drug-abuse-related complications (eg, arrest, infidelity), dissociation, impulsive behavior (eg, spending sprees), and discordant relationships often lead to one or another form of crisis (see Chapter 33). Cluster B personality disorders and the borderline personality subtype form the bulk of emergency psychiatric presentations related to personality disorders. Common comorbidities include anxiety disorders, mood disorders, substance abuse, eating disorders, somatoform disorders, and medical illnesses such as migraine, temporomandibular joint dysfunction, pain syndromes, carpal tunnel syndrome, irritable bowel syndrome, and fibromyalgias.

Disposition

Delineation of acute changes in the patient's mental status and assessment of the effect of these changes on the patient's level of functioning will determine the proper approach to triage. A "here and now" approach is nowhere more important than in this clinical situation. The managed care industry is keeping a close watch on overutilization of inpatient care by patients who have severe personality disorders. Strong teamwork and a broad-based yet unified multidisciplinary therapeutic approach—for example, a variable combination of pharmacotherapy and individual, group, family, and marital psychotherapies—is more effective than one treatment alone.

OTHER EMERGENT CONDITIONS

Neuroleptic malignant syndrome (NMS) is a serious and potentially lethal symptom-complex. In NMS, two sets of symptoms appear very rapidly in response to neuroleptic treatment. Autonomic symptoms include tachycardia, labile hypertension, hyperthermia, and tachypnea; neuromuscular symptoms involve muscle rigidity. Elevated creatinine phosphokinase level and leukocytosis are common findings. A triad of rigidity, elevated temperature, and hypertension appearing for the first time following neuroleptic intervention must arouse the clinician's suspicion that NMS is present. Neuroleptic medication must be stopped at once. The prescription of dantrolene or bromocriptine, together with aggressive supportive treatment (eg, rehydration, antipyretic medication), must be implemented in an intensive care facility. A common clinical error is to increase the dosage of the neuroleptic drug.

Rape and domestic violence may lead to acute anxiety states (eg, acute or posttraumatic stress disorder) or brief reactive psychosis. Adjustment disorder can also follow such trauma.

Acute grief reactions may occur in the presence of anxiety, depression, or somatic complaints. Management should include treatment of the coexisting psychiatric syndrome, if abnormal grief reaction is present, and facilitation of the mourning process. Pharmacotherapy should be used sparingly.

CONCLUSION

As in other fields of medical practice, sudden and unanticipated psychiatric situations occur and can be life threatening. The first duty of a well-prepared clinician is to recognize which of those situations is more critical than others and then to identify correctly the pertinent problem(s) and to intervene appropriately. Central considerations include whether the patient presents an imminent danger to self or others and whether grave psychological or behavioral impairment prevents the patient from caring for himself or herself. Common interventions include safety precautions, astute observation, sensitive inquiry, attentive listening, alertness to unsuspected medical or surgical conditions, judicious use of psychopharmacologic agents, and referral to the most appropriate and least restrictive level of follow-up care. Not to be overlooked is the admonition that psychiatric emergency care should always be provided in a manner that respects the basic dignity of the patient, no matter how disturbed or disruptive he or she may be.

Hillard JR: *Manual of Clinical Emergency Psychiatry.* American Psychiatric Press, 1990.

Hyman SE: *Manual of Psychiatric Emergencies,* 2nd ed. Little, Brown, 1988.

Kleespies PM: *Emergencies in Mental Health Practice: Evaluation and Management.* Guilford Press, 1998.

Slaby AE: *Handbook of Psychiatric Emergencies,* 4th ed. Appleton & Lange, 1994.

Consultation-Liaison Psychiatry

14

James R. Westphal, MD, & Arthur M. Freeman III, MD

Consultation-liaison (C-L) psychiatry involves the study of the psychosocial aspects of medical care and the detection and treatment of psychiatric disorders in the medically ill. The original definition of liaison psychiatry was any psychiatric activity—clinical, educational, or research—performed in a general hospital rather than an asylum. As C-L psychiatry matured and expanded, the term "consultation" came to mean clinical activities with identified patients formally requested by physicians usually through written consultation requests. These activities are usually billed to individual patients on a fee-for-service basis. The term "liaison" referred to activities of psychiatrists on medical and surgical services, such as regular attendance on rounds, multidisciplinary patient care conferences, and supportive group staff meetings. These services are considered general and are not billed to individual patients. Liaison activities could be considered the forerunner of contemporary quality improvement in health care.

As medical techniques (eg, renal hemodialysis and organ transplantation) advanced, consultation psychiatrists focused on the distress these new techniques created in patients. Assessment of psychiatric morbidity associated with medical procedures and their overall effect on quality of life became part of the C-L clinical evaluation in the 1950s. During the 1960s, psychiatric consultations in the general hospital became more pragmatic and focused on relief of patients' presenting symptoms, using eclectic combinations of medication and brief psychotherapies.

C-L psychiatrists became sensitive to the often detrimental effects of the hospital environment on the psychological well-being of patients. Particular emphasis is given to syndromes arising in intensive care units. As medical care became more specialized, some patients were lost between numerous specialists, alienated by overemphasis on one organ or disease, or sandwiched between specialty-oriented "turf" conflicts. To understand this new dimension, C-L psychiatrists added systems theory to their formulations.

C-L psychiatrists also became interested in the diagnostic distinctions between the depressive syndromes often exhibited by medical patients and the presumed organically induced syndromes of delirium and dementia. The three diagnostic *d*'s (depression, delirium, and dementia) then became central to the differential diagnoses offered by C-L psychiatrists.

Increasingly, the C-L psychiatrist has been asked to play a role in medical ethics. Psychiatrists are often called on in issues related to death or dying, such as deciding whether to extend the life of the patient. The concepts of patient choice and quality of life have become important components in the debate. Psychiatrists have called on a range of professionals to help as they have not wished to make moral judgments alone. Clergy, lawyers, medical ethicists, and health economists among others have been drawn into discussions and decisions relating to life and death.

C-L psychiatry currently draws from law, religion, ethics, health economics, systems analysis, neurobiology, pharmacology, communication arts, psychology, and medicine. As C-L psychiatry continues to evolve, new fields of knowledge will be applied to the continuing challenge of understanding the psychosocial aspects of medical care. The study of C-L psychiatry can be lifelong, but the first steps involve learning the basic skills of identifying, diagnosing, discussing, and treating psychiatric and chemical dependency problems in medical patients. These skills are the foundation of effective physician-patient communication and of patient management.

Billings EG, McNary WS, Rees MH: Financial importance of general hospital psychiatry to hospital administrator. Hospitals 1937;11:40.

Sutherland A: Psychological impact of cancer and cancer surgery. Cancer 1952;5:857.

BASIC SKILLS OF CONSULTATION-LIAISON PSYCHIATRY

The basic skills of C-L psychiatry are case finding, diagnosis, intervention, treatment, and communication. **Case finding** is commonly defined as identifying patients that are likely to have a psychiatric disorder or chemical dependency. **Diagnosis** can be defined in two phases. The first is information gathering from the patient, family, significant others, health care team members, medical records, and testing. The second phase applies diagnostic criteria to the information in the formulation of a diagnosis. **Intervention** can be defined as discussing the diagnosis and treatment alternatives with the patient up to the point when the patient accepts treatment. **Treatment** is defined as treating the patient's illness in the medical setting (outpatient or inpatient) or referring the patient for psychiatric care in a setting different from that in which the medical care is provided.

Communication with patients, family members, and other members of the health care team is a highly valued and integrating skill of C-L psychiatrists. Effective physician communication is associated with enhanced patient satisfaction, improved treatment compliance, better patient outcome and fewer malpractice suits. For example, the ability of family practice residents to detect and treat psychiatric disorders in their patients is associated with generally superior communication skills. The study and practice of C-L psychiatry will enhance the physician's ability to address the psychosocial aspects of medical care and improve his or her ability to communicate with and manage patients. These abilities are important components of physician performance, regardless of specialty.

Effective communication starts with the information-gathering aspect of diagnosis and continues to flow through the other phases. A C-L psychiatry consultation is not complete until the patient, relevant family or significant others, and relevant members of the health care team understand the diagnosis and treatment plan (within the bounds of confidentiality) sufficiently to coordinate their efforts. This is usually accomplished through face-to-face or telephone communication, not through written notes. Communication and the expansion of the physician-patient dyad into an integrated and coordinated treatment team are important skills for any physician. Physicians who collaborate with peers and consultants are better problem solvers and are regarded as more effective by the medical community.

CASE FINDING

The identification of patients who would benefit from psychiatric treatment or consultation has not been standardized or performed adequately by physicians. Psychiatric disorders are recognized in only 1.5–3.0% of hospitalized patients who have them. Psychiatric and chemical dependency disorders are misdiagnosed or untreated in 50–75% of the primary care patients who have them. Taking a systems perspective, if the majority of psychiatric disorders are not identified in the patients who have them, no mat-

Table 14–1. CAGE questionnaire.[1]

Have you ever felt you should cut down on your drinking?
Have people annoyed you by criticizing your drinking?
Have you felt bad or guilty about your drinking?
Have you ever had a drink first thing in the morning to steady your nerves or get rid of a hangover (eye-opener)?

[1] Reproduced, with permission, from Ewing JA: Detecting alcoholism: the CAGE questionnaire. JAMA 1984;252:1905.

ter how effective the diagnostic and treatment phases are, the system itself will fail. The clinician's detection skills of case finding are also critical in assessing the patient's communication abilities and needs, which in turn enhance effective physician-patient communication.

Approaches to Case Finding

Case finding can be accomplished by (1) unstructured interviewing during the medical history portion of the physical examination or during an outpatient visit, (2) structured interviewing (ie, a specific set of interview questions with an interview protocol), or (3) self-report questionnaires, either computerized or using paper and pencil. Because psychiatric and chemical dependency disorders are missed in the majority of medical patients who have them, this section focuses on the structured interview and self-report instruments that can be applied systematically to screen and identify psychiatric disorders in large populations of medical patients.

A. Structured Interview: The CAGE is a set of four structured interview questions that identify possible alcohol dependence or abuse (Table 14–1). These questions have also been adapted to include drug abuse or dependence, CAGE-AID (Table 14–2). To be effective, this instrument must be administered at the initial evaluation and during periodic reassessment of every patient that a physician evaluates and manages. Uniform administration of this type of case-finding instrument allows the physician to develop enough experience in applying and scoring the instrument. Uniform administration also circumvents physician bias (conscious or unconscious) and dis-

Table 14–2. CAGE-AID questionnaire.[1]

Have you ever felt you should cut down on your drinking or drug use?
Have people annoyed you by criticizing your drinking or drug use?
Have you felt bad or guilty about your drinking or drug use?
Have you ever had a drink first thing in the morning to steady your nerves or get rid of a hangover or to get the day started?

[1] Reproduced, with permission, from Brown RL: Identification and office management of alcohol and drug disorders. In: Fleming MF, Barry KL (editors): *Addictive Disorders*. Mosby Yearbook, 1992.

comfort in questioning patients about possibly stigmatizing disorders.

B. Self-Report Instruments: Many psychiatric disorders are associated with self-administered symptom-rating scales that can be used for case finding. The 21-question Beck Depression Scale is an example of a self-administered symptom-rating scale for a single disorder (ie, depression). Figure 14–1 shows sample Beck Depression Scale questions. When the Beck Depression Scale is used as a case-finding instrument, patients fill out the questionnaire according to the severity of their depressive symptoms, and the physician or an assistant scores it. If the patient scores higher than a predefined level, he or she is identified

---

BECK INVENTORY

Name _____ Date _____

On this questionnaire are groups of statements. Please read each group of statements carefully. Then pick out the one statement in each group which best describes the way you have been feeling the *PAST WEEK, INCLUDING TODAY!* Circle the number beside the statement you picked. If several statements in the group seem to apply equally well, circle each one. *Be sure to read all the statements in each group before making your choice.*

1   0   I do not feel sad.
     1   I feel sad.
     2   I am sad all the time and I can't snap out of it.
     3   I am so sad or unhappy that I can't stand it.

2   0   I am not particularly discouraged about the future.
     1   I feel discouraged about the future.
     2   I feel I have nothing to look forward to.
     3   I feel that the future is hopeless and that things cannot improve.

3   0   I do not feel like a failure.
     1   I feel I have failed more than the average person.
     2   As I look back on my life, all I can see is a lot of failures.
     3   I feel I am a complete failure as a person.

4   0   I get as much satisfaction out of things as I used to.
     1   I don't enjoy things the way I used to.
     2   I don't get real satisfaction out of anything anymore.
     3   I am dissatisfied or bored with everything.

5   0   I don't feel particularly guilty.
     1   I feel guilty a good part of the time.
     2   I feel quite guilty most of the time.
     3   I feel guilty all of the time.

6   0   I don't feel I am being punished.
     1   I feel I may be punished.
     2   I expect to be punished.
     3   I feel I am being punished.

7   0   I don't feel disappointed in myself.
     1   I am disappointed in myself.
     2   I am disgusted with myself.
     3   I hate myself.

8   0   I don't feel I am any worse than anybody else.
     1   I am critical of myself for my weaknesses or mistakes.
     2   I blame myself all the time for my faults.
     3   I blame myself for everything bad that happens.

9   0   I don't have thoughts of killing myself.
     1   I have thoughts of killing myself, but I would not carry them out.
     2   I would like to kill myself.
     3   I would kill myself if I had the chance.

Figure 14–1. Representative portion of Beck Depression Scale.

for further investigation into the possibility of depression.

An example of a multidisorder case-finding questionnaire used in a similar manner is the 60-question Medical Inpatient Screening Test. This questionnaire is designed to be followed by a psychiatric consultation when it identifies a possible psychiatric diagnosis. A limitation of this instrument is its lack of questions covering chemical dependency. This type of case-finding instrument accurately identifies patients who have psychiatric problems. As with structured interview questions, self-report instruments need to be administered systematically to populations of patients in order to be reliable and precise.

C. PRIME-MD Self-Report and Physician-Administered Evaluation: Another approach to case finding is the PRIME-MD system, which uses a 1-page self-report instrument (Figure 14–2) together with a physician-administered 12-page evaluation instrument that prompts the physician concerning mood, anxiety, somatoform, and alcohol abuse disorders. The physician administers a particular section of the evaluation if the patient responds to specific case-finding questions (in this example, questions 23 through 26) that trigger the administration of that section. The PRIME-MD system is similar to the Medical Inpatient Screening Test, but it adds a focused physician-structured interview instead of a psychiatric consultation.

D. Cognitive Case-Finding Instruments: Cognitive assessment is essential to case finding of dementia and delirium, the general assessment of the patient's communication ability, and the evaluation of the cognitive basis of functional behavior. The Standardized Mini-Mental State Exam (SMMSE) is a 20-question examination that takes approximately 5 minutes to administer (Figure 14–3). This examination provides a single score, ranging from 0 to 30, as an estimate of general cognitive function. A more sophisticated cognitive case-finding instrument is the Neurobehavioral Cognitive Status Exam (NBCSE). This examination evaluates 10 areas of cognitive functioning: orientation, attention, language comprehension, language repetition, naming, constructional ability, memory, calculations, similarities, and judgment. Each area is scored and a profile developed. Changes in cognitive status over time can be monitored and specific problem areas identified. Figure 14–4 illustrates a profile of a patient with hepatic encephalopathy and the profile's change with treatment. The NBCSE instrument, although more sophisticated, takes the same amount of time to administer as the SMMSE because of its screen and metric test construction. The screen questions are difficult. If the patient performs the screening question correctly, the metric section, a series of questions ranging from easy to difficult, is skipped. If the patient does not perform the screening question correctly, the metric section is administered. The severity of the specific deficit is quantified by the metric section. In patients who are cognitively intact, the NBCSE involves 17 questions, a brief interview, shorter than the SMMSE. If the patient has cognitive deficits, the interview will be prolonged, but the results will identify and quantify the specific cognitive deficits.

The SMMSE and the NBCSE generally test the posterior cortical area associated with specific cognitive abilities. The frontal cortex, which has been relatively less studied, is involved in executive abilities or organizing specific cognitive abilities into chains of tasks involved in functional activities such as cooking or grooming. The current emphasis on functional outcome has led to the development of clinically oriented tests of frontal lobe functions. Frontal lobe functioning has not been evaluated systematically in the classic mental status examination. The Trail Making Test is a case-finding instrument for frontal lobe or executive dysfunction, and the Executive Interview, a bedside assessment, assesses the cognitive basis of many functional activities.

Cognitive deficits are important not only in the diagnosis of cognitive disorders but also in the evaluation of the patient's communication abilities and in his or her ability to comply with medical treatment. Patients with cognitive deficits are less likely to understand, remember, and follow medical regimens. They may need more intensive patient education and follow-up care than patients who are not cognitively impaired. For example, a patient identified by any of the cognitive examinations as impaired may need written rather than verbal instructions and, possibly, family monitoring and assistance to ensure compliance with medical regimens. For physicians in any specialty who wish to improve compliance, a brief investment in assessing cognitive status and adapting management to fit the patient's cognitive strengths and weaknesses will be well rewarded.

E. Literacy Assessment: Many physicians provide written instructions to their patients. An assessment of the patient's literacy level is important for evaluating the patient's ability to understand written instructions, especially instructions written at advanced reading levels. In addition, knowledge of a patient's reading level is often more accurate than is the highest grade level attended for determining the appropriate level of language and concepts with which to communicate. Often patients are too embarrassed to inform their physicians directly of their illiteracy. Unrecognized illiteracy can be mistaken as patient noncompliance. A literacy assessment such as the REALM (Figure 14–5) will enable the physician to adjust communication to the patient's reading level. The REALM takes less than 5 minutes to administer and is a brief investment in effective physician-patient communication.

Use of Case-Finding Instruments by Physicians

The use of case-finding instruments in routine evaluation of medical patients requires time on the

PATIENT QUESTIONNAIRE

NAME: _____ SEX: ☐ Male ☐ Female AGE: _____ TODAY'S DATE: _____

MARITAL STATUS
☐ Married
☐ Widowed
☐ Separated
☐ Divorced
☐ Never married

YOUR BACKGROUND
☐ Black (not Hispanic)
☐ Hispanic
☐ White (not Hispanic)
☐ Asian
☐ Other Describe: _____

HOW FAR YOU WENT IN SCHOOL
☐ 8th grade or less
☐ Some high school
☐ High school graduate or equivalency (GED)
☐ Some college or associate degree
☐ Completed college

INSTRUCTIONS: This questionnaire will help your doctor better understand problems that you may have. Your doctor may ask you more questions about some of these items. Please make sure to check a box for <u>every</u> item.

During the *PAST MONTH*, have you *OFTEN* been bothered by...						During the *PAST MONTH*...		
	YES	NO		YES	NO		YES	NO
1. stomach pain	☐	☐	12. constipation, loose bowels, or diarrhea	☐	☐	22. have you had an anxiety attack (suddenly feeling fear or panic)	☐	☐
2. back pain	☐	☐	13. nausea, gas, or indigestion	☐	☐			
3. pain in your arms, legs, or joints (knees, hips, etc)	☐	☐	14. feeling tired or having low energy	☐	☐	23. have you thought you should cut down on your drinking of alcohol	☐	☐
4. menstrual pain or problems	☐	☐	15. trouble sleeping	☐	☐	24. has anyone complained about your drinking	☐	☐
5. pain or problems during sexual intercourse	☐	☐	16. the thought that you have a serious undiagnosed disease	☐	☐	25. have you felt guilty or upset about your drinking	☐	☐
6. headaches	☐	☐	17. your eating being out of control	☐	☐	26. was there ever a single day in which you had five or more drinks of beer, wine, or liquor	☐	☐
7. chest pain	☐	☐	18. little interest or pleasure in doing things	☐	☐			
8. dizziness	☐	☐	19. feeling down, depressed, or hopeless	☐	☐	Overall, would you say your health is:		
9. fainting spells	☐	☐				Excellent	☐	
10. feeling your heart pound or race	☐	☐	20. "nerves" or feeling anxious or on edge	☐	☐	Very good	☐	
						Good	☐	
11. shortness of breath	☐	☐	21. worrying about a lot of different things	☐	☐	Fair	☐	
						Poor	☐	

RTI113X93C © 1993, Pfizer Inc   Printed in USA/May 1993

Figure 14–2. PRIME-MD patient form.

part of the physician, ancillary personnel, and the patient. For example, the average amount of time spent by physicians using the PRIME-MD system is about 8 minutes per patient. Ease of use is an impor- tant operational criterion if case-finding systems are used systematically. Self-report case-finding sys- tems are the most cost-effective. Any of the struc- tured methods, if used systematically, will increase

STANDARDIZED MINI-MENTAL STATE EXAMINATION (SMMSE)

INTRODUCTION: Prior to the initiation of this questionnaire, assess the patients ability to see and hear. Attempt to make the environment non-distracting and establish a cooperative rapport with your patient.

SUPPLIES: A wristwatch, pencil, eraser, 2 blank sheets of paper. A sheet of paper with " **CLOSE YOUR EYES**" in large capital print. A sheet of paper containing (2) five sided figures intersecting to create a four sided figure:

DIRECTIONS: Ask each question a maximum of 3 times. Do not prompt or correct answers. If asked, "What did you say?" repeat the question. If asked, "Why?" say you will explain later and continue.

SCORING: Scores for each question are provided in the chart. No response = 0, Incorrect = 0: Total = 30 points

QUESTIONS	INSTRUCTIONS	TIME	SCORE
What year is this?	Ask each question a maximum of 3 times	10 seconds	1
What season is this?	"	"	1
What month of the year is this?	"	"	1
What is today's date?	"	"	1
What Day of the week is this?	"	"	1
What Country are we in?	"	"	1
What Province/State/County?	"	"	1
What City/Town are we in?	"	"	1
What is the name of this Hospital/Building?	"	"	1
What floor of the building are we on	"	"	1
Repeat these three items: BALL CAR MAN	Remember these, I will ask them again. Repeat until learned or a maximum of 5 times	20 seconds 1 point ea.	3
Spell the word: WORLD	Now spell it backwards. Score 0 if help is needed	30 seconds	5
What were the 3 objects I asked you to remember?	Order of response does not matter	10 seconds 1 point ea.	3
What is this called?	Show the wristwatch. Accept watch or wristwatch, not clock or time	10 seconds	1
What is this called?	Show the pencil. Accept pencil only		1
Repeat this phrase: NO IF'S, AND'S OR BUT'S	Must be exact	10 seconds	1
Read the words on this page and then do what it says: CLOSE YOUR EYES	If subject reads and does not close eyes repeat the instructions up to 3 times. Score only if subject closes eyes.	10 seconds	1
Take this paper in your (Right/Left) hand, Fold the paper in half and put it on the floor	Give the paper to the subjects non-dominant hand. One point for each step	30 seconds	3
Write a complete sentence on this paper	Give the subject a pencil and paper. The sentence should make sense. Ignore spelling	30 seconds	1
Copy this design:	Provide a copy of the design. Allow multiple tries. Must draw a 4-sided figure between the two 5-sided figures	Max. time 1 minute	1

Figure 14–3. SMMSE. (Reprinted, with permission.)

the yield. That is, they will identify more medical patients who have psychiatric disorders than will current practices.

The most significant issue in case finding is the setting of thresholds to determine which patients need psychiatric evaluation and intervention. For example, some studies have suggested that depressive symp-toms, even at subsyndromal levels, affect the patient's ability to function in everyday life. If the treatment of subsyndromal depressive symptoms is found effective in improving patient functioning, subsyndromal levels of depressive symptoms will also need to be identified, which will require the current case-finding thresholds to be lowered.

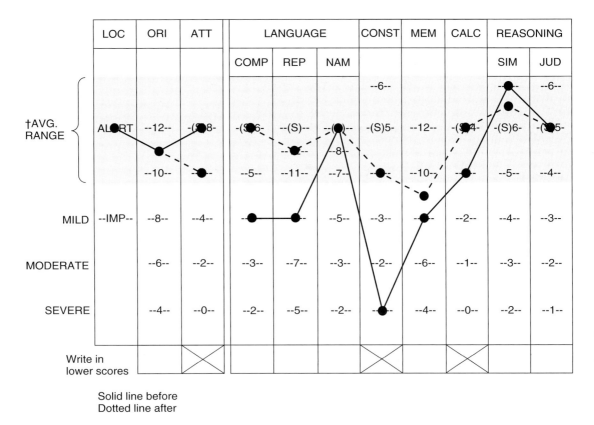

Figure 14–4. NBCSE cognitive profile of patient with hepatic failure and response to treatment. (Reprinted, with permission, from Neurobehavioral Group: *Manual for the Behavioral Cognitive Status Examination,* Figure 6.)

Davis TC et al: Rapid estimate of adult literacy in medicine: a shortened screening instrument. Fam Med 1993; 25:391.

Levenson JL, Hamer RM, Rossiter LF: A randomized controlled study of psychiatric consultation guided by screening in general medical inpatients. Psychiatry 1992;149:631.

Mayfield D, McLeod G, Hall P: The CAGE questionnaire: validation of a new alcoholism screening instrument. Am J Psychol 1974;131:1121.

McDowell I, Newell C (editors): *Measuring Health: A Guide to Rating Scales and Questionnaires,* 2nd ed. Oxford University Press, 1996.

DIAGNOSIS

Once case finding has identified patients likely to have a psychiatric diagnosis, the causation, consistency, severity, and duration of the symptoms and their effect on the patient's ability to function must be evaluated. Often sources of information beyond the patient are needed in order to collect enough information for a diagnostic formulation. Information can be obtained from collateral interviews with family or significant others, chart review, and other health care providers (especially the nursing staff if the patient is an inpatient). By expanding information gathering to other members of the patient's social network, the physician sets the foundation for effective communication and participation during the intervention and treatment phases.

The introduction of a psychiatric diagnostic manual for primary care physicians marked a significant step for C-L psychiatry. *Diagnostic and Statistical Manual: Primary Care Version* (DSM-PC) organizes the criteria sets developed for *Diagnostic and Statistical Manual of Mental Disorders,* 4th edition (DSM-IV) into algorithms for the primary care physician. The basic diagnostic categories and criteria in DSM-PC and DSM-IV are identical, but the methods used by the physician to apply the diagnostic criteria are different in the two systems. DSM-IV is not used widely in primary care because it is perceived as cumbersome and impractical. The use of psychiatric casefinding instruments combined with the simplified diagnostic approach of DSM-PC and the use of combined case-finding and diagnostic systems such as PRIME-MD hold the promise of improving case detection and diagnostic accuracy.

**RAPID ESTIMATE OF ADULT LITERACY IN MEDICINE
(REALM)©**

Terry Davis, PhD • Michael Crouch, MD • Sandy Long, PhD

Reading
Level _____

Patient Name/
Subject # _____ Date of Birth _____

Grade
Completed _____

Date _____ Clinic _____ Examiner _____

List 1		List 2		List 3	
fat	_____	fatigue	_____	allergic	_____
flu	_____	pelvic	_____	menstrual	_____
pill	_____	jaundice	_____	testicle	_____
dose	_____	infection	_____	colitis	_____
eye	_____	exercise	_____	emergency	_____
stress	_____	behavior	_____	medication	_____
smear	_____	prescription	_____	occupation	_____
nerves	_____	notify	_____	sexually	_____
germs	_____	gallbladder	_____	alcoholism	_____
meals	_____	calories	_____	irritation	_____
disease	_____	depression	_____	constipation	_____
cancer	_____	miscarriage	_____	gonorrhea	_____
caffeine	_____	pregnancy	_____	inflammatory	_____
attack	_____	arthritis	_____	diabetes	_____
kidney	_____	nutrition	_____	hepatitis	_____
hormones	_____	menopause	_____	antibiotics	_____
herpes	_____	appendix	_____	diagnosis	_____
seizure	_____	abnormal	_____	potassium	_____
bowel	_____	syphilis	_____	anemia	_____
asthma	_____	hemorrhoids	_____	obesity	_____
rectal	_____	nausea	_____	osteoporosis	_____
incest	_____	directed	_____	impetigo	_____

SCORE

List 1 _____

List 2 _____

List 3 _____

Raw
Score _____

Figure 14–5. Representative section from the REALM. (This material is the property of the author, Terry C. Davis, who may be contacted for full copies of the REALM.)

American Psychiatric Association: *Diagnostic and Statistical Manual of Mental Disorders,* 4th ed. American Psychiatric Association, 1994.

Pincus HA et al: Bridging the gap between psychiatry and primary care: the DSM-IV-PC. Psychosomatics 1995; 36:328.

Spitzer RL et al: Utility of a new procedure for diagnosing mental disorders in primary care: the PRIME-MD 1000 study. JAMA 1994;272:1749.

INTERVENTION

Intervention is the step between diagnosis and the patient's acceptance of treatment. Communication skills are crucial in the link between identifying and diagnosing a disorder and engaging the patient in constructive efforts to treat the disorder. Intervention can also be conceptualized as the preparation of the patient for psychiatric or chemical dependency treatment. This phase is one of the more challenging areas for effective physician-patient communication, because patients usually perceive the diagnosis of a psychiatric or chemical dependency disorder as threatening to their self-esteem. The communication model we present here is also applicable to circumstances in which physicians inform patients of other threatening diagnoses or events, for example, informing a patient that he or she has a life-threatening medical disease such as AIDS or cancer.

Patients may require several discussions before they are able to accept the diagnosis and engage in treatment. Some physicians are unrealistic about the ability of their patients to respond effectively to diagnosis of a psychiatric or chemical dependency disorder. Physicians who are effective communicators expect to discuss chemical dependence and psychiatric treatment many times before patients take action. Persistence is the key to effective communication. Physicians who seek collateral information from families and significant others in the diagnostic phase usually are more effective in interventions. Family members are more likely to support a physician's intervention if they feel that the physician has considered their concerns and information.

The skills necessary for effective brief interventions can be summarized by the acronym FRAMES (see Table 14–3). When discussing a psychiatric or chemical dependency disorder, brief individualized **feed-**back of the patient's risk, emphasis on the patient's **responsibility,** specific **advice** on the change recommended, a **menu** of alternatives, **empathy,** and a positive view of the patient's (**self**) ability to change and the treatment's efficacy are the important components. Dialog boxes 1 and 2 offer brief examples of these concepts.

Dialog Box 1: Alcohol-dependent male hospitalized with pancreatitis

Mr. A, if you continue to drink, you risk another episode of pancreatitis *(feedback).* I would suggest that you stop drinking completely *(advice).* In my experience with patients, I know it's very difficult to stop drinking alone *(empathy).* I recommend attending Alcoholics Anonymous. You can call this telephone number to obtain a meeting schedule, or I could also recommend inpatient treatment at our local hospital or the outpatient program at the nearby clinic *(menu).* It's your decision *(responsibility).* I know that both inpatient treatment and Alcoholics Anonymous work *(self-efficacy).*

Dialog Box 2: Female outpatient worked up for weight loss by primary care physician

Ms. B, I think your sleep problems, weight loss, crying spells, and difficulty working are caused by depression. Without treatment, you could continue to have these symptoms or feel worse for up to a year. You could also become suicidal without treatment *(feedback).* I suggest treatment *(advice).* I can prescribe an antidepressant or you can go to the mental health center or to our local psychiatrist *(menu).* It's your choice *(responsibility).* I know treatment works in the majority of patients *(self-efficacy),* and I'd like to help you *(empathy).*

The style of intervention should be empathic or caring rather than confrontational or accusatory, optimistic rather than pessimistic, and it should place the responsibility for change on the patient, rather than the physician, health care system, family, or others.

Intervention is also needed when a patient is referred for psychiatric consultation. Simple statements such as those in dialog boxes 3 and 4 will make consultation a more effective process for the patient, the consulting psychiatrist, and the referring physician. Intervention using the same communication skills and attitudes prepares the patient for psychiatric consultation and will increase the chance of a successful referral.

Dialog Box 3: Male alcoholic inpatient with hepatitis

Mr. C, I think your drinking is causing your liver disease *(feedback),* and you need to stop drinking before your liver becomes worse *(advice).* I'd like you to talk with Dr. X to discuss what you can do about your drinking *(responsibility).* I've asked him to see you today. I think he can help you with your problem *(empathy and self-efficacy).*

Table 14–3. FRAMES acronym.

F	=	Feedback on the patient's risk or impairment
R	=	Responsibility for change belongs to the patient
A	=	Advice to change should be specific and nonambiguous
M	=	Menu of alternative strategies
E	=	Empathetic rather than confrontational counseling style
S	=	Self-efficacy: a positive view of patient's ability to change and the treatment's efficacy

Dialog Box 4: Female inpatient with angina and depressive symptoms

> Ms. D, I think your problems with insomnia, crying spells, and fatigue may be caused by depression *(feedback)* rather than your heart. I'd like you to talk with Dr. Y *(advice)*, who's an expert in this area to see if we can help you with these symptoms *(empathy)*. I've arranged for her to come by and see you today. There's a good chance that you will feel better *(self-efficacy)* if you are depressed and follow through with treatment. I'd like to see you feeling better and doing more in your life *(empathy)*.

Intervention requires communication skills, positive attitude, persistence, and practice, but the rewards of successful treatment of psychiatric and chemical dependency disorders in terms of patient satisfaction, improved patient health and functioning, and increased professional satisfaction are worth the effort.

Stern TA, Herman JB, Slavin PL (editors): *The MGH Guide to Psychiatry in Primary Care.* McGraw-Hill, 1998.

TREATMENT

The site of psychiatric treatment and the use of psychiatric consultants is currently a matter of preference, the patient's acuteness, risk factors, and availability of local resources. Some physicians use their own training and experience to work with their patients who have chemical dependency or psychiatric disorders; others work with their own patients using psychiatric recommendations, either formal or informal; and still others refer their medical patients who have psychiatric disorders to mental health and chemical dependency treatment sites or have C-L psychiatrists evaluate and recommend treatment for patients during patient hospitalizations for medical and surgical conditions.

C-L psychiatrists usually use biological and psychotherapeutic treatments that have demonstrated efficacy. However, some researchers suggest that ambulatory medical patients who have depressive symptoms may have a disorder with different etiology, severity, and duration than the patients studied in depression treatment research. Until research determines whether specific populations of the medically ill with psychiatric disorders have definably different treatment responses, the most conservative treatment choice is application of proven psychiatric treatments.

COMMUNICATION

The C-L psychiatrist has the primary task of facilitating information flow between the patient and others regarding issues that either enhance or impede the overall care of the patient. The presence of so many different participants and stakeholders in the individual's care makes the job of integration and clarification essential. Facilitating and integrating this information is an essential; otherwise, fragmentation and chaos will triumph over rational care. If the significant people in the patient's life have been involved in the information-gathering phase of diagnosis and intervention, it is natural to integrate them into the treatment team. Using a systems model, the C-L psychiatrist will at times devote significant effort to working with members of the health care team who are involved with a particular patient. The ultimate goal is to harmonize elements of the treatment team toward effective care of the current identified patient and, ideally, those patients who follow with similar sorts of distress.

Brown RL: Identification and office management of alcohol and drug disorders. In: Fleming MF, Barry KL (editors): *Addictive Disorders.* Mosby Yearbook, 1992.
Rundell JR, Wise MG (editors): *Textbook of Consultation-Liaison Psychiatry.* American Psychiatric Press, 1996.

COMMON CONSULTATIONS

C-L psychiatry is based on the biopsychosocial model, which attempts to understand a patient's behavior as an interaction of biological factors (eg, physical trauma, infectious agents, nutritional status); psychological factors (eg, personality traits, motivation, previous experience, intelligence); and social factors (eg, current influences from parents, spouse, children, employment, church, and community). Current application of the biopsychosocial model in many patients adds a complex health care system to the social influences. Often patients have multiple complex interactions—with specialists, primary care physicians, gate keepers, benefit managers, and clerical staff—that influence their behavior. Efficient information-gathering skills are necessary in the review of medical and psychiatric records, interview of patient caregivers (eg, nurses, ancillary personnel, physicians), and interview of collateral sources (eg, family and significant others). Also needed are skills in diverse psychiatric treatments such as brief individual psychotherapies, psychopharmacology, brief marital and family interventions, systems interventions, and educational interventions for patient, family, and health care providers. The "difficult patient" is the area in which the most diverse skills are required.

CONSULTATIONS WITH DIFFICULT PATIENTS

Most difficult-to-manage patients have personality disorders or somatoform disorders.

Patients With Personality Disorders

The personality disorders described by DSM-IV often overlap (see Chapter 33). Patients often qualify for more than one personality disorder diagnosis. Unrecognized personality disorder is thought to be a significant factor in treatment resistance. Approximately 10% of the community can be diagnosed as having one or more personality disorder. The percentage of the population diagnosed as having a personality disorder increases significantly in various health care populations to highs of 48% in a behavioral medicine clinic and 67% in hospitalized chronic psychiatric patients.

Cloninger's three-dimensional concept of character postulates three character dimensions: self-directedness, cooperativeness, and self-transcendence. In this system, low self-directedness and low cooperativeness are common to all personality disorders. The Tridimensional Personality Questionnaire, a 100-item self-report inventory, diagnoses personality disorder according to this theoretical model.

Personality disorders may be easier to learn about and to assess according to the two-step process illustrated by Figure 14–6. The first step determines the presence or absence of personality disorder by assessing for the common factors of low cooperativeness and low self-directedness. The second step is to determine the DSM-IV personality disorder cluster: aloof, dramatic, or anxious. For most patient management issues in general health care, the diagnosis of personality disorder and its cluster is sufficient. For example, in HIV-infected populations, the diagnosis of personality disorder predicts Axis I disorders and impaired functioning. Furthermore, the presence of personality disorder can predict morbidity and mortality in cardiac transplantation patients.

A. Patients With Cluster B Personality Disorders: Some of the most difficult patients are in the cluster B personality disorder group, and patients with borderline personality disorder represent one of the greatest treatment challenges. Both pharmacotherapy and psychotherapy are exceedingly difficult with these patients. In addition to their low self-directedness, low cooperativeness, and erratic and dramatic emotions, patients with borderline personality disorder tend to split individuals and groups into all-good or all-bad categories. One moment they idolize the physician, and in the next they demonize him, projecting their negative feelings onto others. They are emotionally quite labile and fragile, and they tend to make frequent suicidal threats or gestures.

The best approach to these patients is through firmness, consistency, and management of the physician's own rage and feelings of humiliation in dealing with these patients. Support of these patients' strengths is essential. Minimization of the intensity and frequency of the destructive cycles in a borderline patient's emotional life can sometimes occur through an ongoing

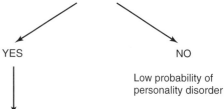

1. Does the patient have a personality disorder?

   A. Does the patient exhibit low self-directedness? Is the patient unable to accept personal responsibility, set goals, and retain a positive outlook when challenged?

   AND

   B. Does the patient exhibit low cooperativeness? Is the patient intolerant of others, revengeful, unhelpful to others, and socially disinterested?

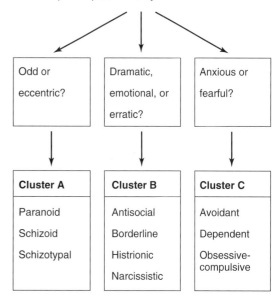

Figure 14–6. Algorithm for diagnosing personality disorder in general medical settings.

helpful, clarifying relationship. On medical wards, the physician must explain to staff about the dynamics of these patients and how the staff must avoid being split or accepting the projected abuse. Anxiolytics, antidepressants, mood stabilizers, and neuroleptics can be useful on an intermittent basis.

Patients who have antisocial personality disorder can be especially difficult because they typically attempt to hide their adverse traits. These patients are often clever, charming, and manipulative and, initially, may seem to be self-directed and cooperative. Many physicians have expressed unwillingness to deal with such patients. A firm, unyielding approach is generally required. The physician must make clear to these patients that he or she is aware of, and will not tolerate, their manipulation and conscious undermining of the treatment regimen. The more an antisocial patient can see value from adhering to a treatment plan, the better the results will be. If treatment is presented as an arbitrary rule, results are likely to be sabotaged. Unfortunately, antisocial patients are notorious at undermining the best-designed therapeutic regimens.

B. Patients With Cluster A Personality Disorders: Patients with the cluster A personality disorders—paranoid, schizoid, and schizotypal—often present in medical settings. In addition to the core traits of low self-directedness and low cooperativeness, these patients are typically distant, aloof, and suspicious, which makes it difficult for them to comply with medical treatment. The principal issue with these patients is the preservation of their personal psychological boundaries. Medical staff must avoid being overly intrusive. Respect for the distance these patients require is necessary; at the same time, the clinician should gently attempt to engage them in a collaborative treatment process. Often patients in this personality cluster, particularly those with paranoid traits, respond best when they are prepared for medical interventions, when these interventions occur slowly, and when frequent feedback is given to and sought from the patient. Success can be achieved if attention is given to boundaries and the timing of interaction.

Patients With Problems Dealing With Medical Systems

Medicine has been fragmented by specialization. This has been the result of the rapid pace of biomedical research, the establishment of subspecialty boards, and until recently, the economic principle that specialization was good for the physician's income. Unfortunately, numerous patients have been lost in the shuffle between high-powered subspecialists. Many patients who are "lost" in the health care system, or who are the focus of specialty conflicts, have personality disorders. An appreciation of the core issues of personality disorder (ie, low self-directedness and low cooperativeness) explains why these patients develop problems in a fragmented health system. The core personality traits of passivity and decreased ability to cooperate lead to the patient's inability to follow through on recommendations and to seek appropriate care if not given guidance. The health professional's reaction to these patients is usually to "turf" the patient to another provider, to treat the patient in such a manner that he or she is unwilling to come back, or to make less than a full effort to follow up on these patients.

An economic and consumer protest has led to the renascence of the importance of the primary care physician. The primary care physician is seen as the guarantor of a strong doctor-patient relationship and of a continuity of care that integrates the disparate elements of that care. The C-L psychiatrist often plays a role similar to that of the primary care physician while continuing to serve as a psychiatric subspecialist. To the extent that the C-L psychiatrist can work with designated primary care physicians and enhance their role, the same objectives will be achieved. Optimal medical care for most patients requires a blend of primary care and specialty care. An important role for the C-L psychiatrist may be to fine-tune the balance between these two components.

Patients With Somatoform Disorders

Patients who have somatoform disorders (see Chapter 25) can be difficult to manage in health care settings. These patients typically present with physical complaints that suggest a general medical condition but that have a psychological origin. The most dramatic of these patients have somatization disorder (formerly called hysteria or Briquet's syndrome), which begins before age 30, is chronic, and is associated with multiple symptoms related to pain, the gastrointestinal tract, sexuality, and the nervous system. Conversion disorder also involves symptoms that affect voluntary motor or sensory function. Hypochondriasis is encountered in patients who as a result of their misinterpretation of bodily symptoms think that they have a serious disease.

As a group, patients with these disorders respond poorly to traditional psychotherapy. These patients require respectful treatment. Some patients are willing to examine the psychological origin of their problems. To the extent that a supportive and consistent doctor-patient relationship is established, some attenuation of distress may be achieved. These patients are often incapable of introspection or the use of psychological concepts. Anxiety and depression in these patients can be treated, in part, with medications. Supportive group therapy can also be helpful for some patients.

Pain Patients

A particularly difficult group of patients includes those who have somatization or personality disorders as well as chronic pain. Acute and chronic pain are often undertreated by physicians. The Agency for Health Care Policy and Research practice guidelines for acute pain management estimate that half of the 20 million surgical operations performed in the United States in 1989 provided adequate pain relief. Chronic pain affects 78–80 million people in the United States and has been estimated to cost the United States $16 billion per year. A C-L psychiatry referral for chronic pain patients usually indicates that the referring physician considers that psychiatric disorder or chemical dependency are likely, that the physician has difficulties in managing the patient, or that the physician can find no "organic" cause for the pain.

All psychiatric diagnoses in patients with pain behavior need to fit the standard DSM-IV diagnostic criteria. Even though an organic etiology for pain cannot be determined, it does not mean that the patient has a psychiatric disorder. The most likely Axis I psychiatric diagnoses in these patients are depression, anxiety, or somatoform disorders. In addition, chemical dependency disorders may be encountered in patients with chronic pain.

The most important distinction is between the physical sensation of pain and the patient's affective response to the physical sensation. Many pain patients develop behavior that becomes a dominant part of their lives. Suffering, that is, a negative behavioral reaction to the pain, dominates their subjective experience. These patients often somatize, and their pain is very difficult to treat with psychiatric methods. Some success has been obtained from specific behaviorally oriented pain programs for chronic pain patients. C-L psychiatrists need to know the local referral resources for chronic pain treatment.

Assisting With Countertransference in Difficult Patients

Difficult patients elicit strong reactions (usually defined as **countertransference**) from physicians and other caregivers. An important role in the management of the difficult patient is for the C-L psychiatrist to help dampen the disruptive effects these patients have on the treatment setting. Education in the form of psychiatric diagnostic clarification and clear practical treatment approaches will often be helpful. The C-L psychiatrist can help the staff by accepting their negative feelings, lessening the intensity of these feelings by identifying the origin and the mechanisms being used by patients to create emotional reactions in the staff. Liaison psychiatry can generalize this ability for treatment staff members so that they can apply it to other patients.

A 17-year-old black male with sickle cell disorder was an inpatient for treatment of sickle cell crisis. Pediatrics sought a C-L consultation to evaluate the patient for depression and drug-seeking behavior. He was admitted approximately every 2–3 months for sickle cell crisis with little outpatient follow-up care. When the C-L psychiatrist interviewed the nursing staff, some nurses spontaneously described the patient's behavior of screaming and loud crying that disrupted most of the unit with both open and indirect hostility. However, several other staff members were quite sympathetic to the patient.

On examination, the patient was a short, frail adolescent who appeared younger than his stated age and who huddled in a fetal position in his hos-

pital bed. He was crying quietly. His speech was slow and sparse but organized. The patient denied all current psychiatric symptoms and described a normal life outside the hospital. His only spontaneous speech were pleas to stop the interview, because of the pain he was experiencing, and requests for medication. The C-L team was able to confirm the patient's history with brief interviews of an older sister and a girlfriend. They reported that the patient was an active, popular, high school student with a social life and involvement in extracurricular activities and who did not complain of depression or seek medication when not in sickle cell crisis. A discussion with the resident staff found one physician who had seen the patient as an outpatient and again confirmed the patient's history. The family also stated that the patient's exaggerated response to pain occurred only while he was hospitalized and that they did not tolerate screaming and disruption at home. The family said that they had moved to their current home when the university hospital where the patient was previously treated, and where the behavior developed, refused to admit him when he was in sickle cell crisis.

The C-L team diagnosed the patient as exhibiting a learned behavior to the inpatient setting and acute pain. They met with the nursing and house staffs to design a behavioral plan for the patient's pain, reinforcing mature behavior and ignoring inappropriate behavior. In addition, the C-L team offered to meet with the pediatric nursing staff to discuss behavioral management for all pediatric pain patients. Many issues in managing pediatric pain patients were explored and discussed. The nursing staff decided to design pain management protocols for all pediatric units.

Carr DB et al: Acute Pain Management: Operative or Medical Procedures and Trauma. Clinical Practice Guideline No. 1. AHCPR Publication No. 92–0032. U.S. Department of Health and Human Services, 1992.

Cloninger CR, Svrakic DM, Przybeck TR: A psychobiological model of temperament and character. Arch Gen Psychiatr 1993;50:975.

Oldham JM: Personality disorders. JAMA 1994;272:1770.

Weiner RS (executive editor): *Pain Management: A Practical Guide for Clincians,* 5th ed. Vol 1. CRC Press, 1998.

CONSULTATION WITH PATIENTS WHO REQUIRE COGNITIVE ASSESSMENT

C-L psychiatry consultations often are needed for patients who require cognitive assessment. This group includes patients with postoperative delirium, patients whose competence to make medical decisions is questioned, and medically ill patients who have acute psychiatric symptoms.

Consultation With Patients Who Have Delirium, Especially Postoperative

Delirium occurs more often than suspected in postoperative patients. Up to 13% of general medical inpatients have been found to have delirium. The cardinal signs of delirium are loss of short-term memory, disturbance in consciousness, and a change in cognition that cannot be accounted for by dementia. Delirium is caused by a general medical condition, substance intoxication or withdrawal, use of a medication, toxin exposure, or a combination of these causes. The patient cannot focus attention and may be distracted easily. Short-term memory impairment, disorientation, language disturbance, or perceptual disturbance may occur. Usually delirium develops over a short period of time and is caused by infection; metabolic disorder; electrolyte imbalance; hepatic or renal disease; B_{12}, folate, or thiamine deficiency; neurologic syndromes; and postoperative states. Without systematic evaluation of cognitive functioning, delirium is missed in many patients, especially if they are not agitated.

Important practical measures help in the management of these patients. Because darkness may be quite frightening to them and may further disrupt their fragmented sleep-wake cycle, a nightlight is imperative. Frequent orientation and reassurance by staff is helpful. Clocks and calendars and other orienting instruments can be very helpful. Overstimulation should be avoided. Low doses of high potency neuroleptics such as haloperidol at bedtime may be useful in treating acute delirium. Fortunately, these states are usually transient and usually remit with the correction of the underlying medical problem.

Consultation With Patients Whose Competence Must Be Assessed

The assessment of patient's competency to consent to medical treatment is a variant of the cognitive capacity examination. Because the legal requirements for consent to medical treatment vary from state to state and can change with legal precedents, it is always advisable to have access to a local attorney who understands the state's medical competency laws (see Chapter 15). However, C-L psychiatrists are often consulted to give an opinion on medical competency. Several factors are important in the determination: the patient's ability to make the decision voluntarily, to understand the illness and its prognosis, and to understand the risk and benefits of treatment (and of refusal of treatment). These abilities usually depend on the patient's general cognitive ability. Up to 79% of patients referred for medical evaluation of competency issues have undetected delirium or dementia.

A well-documented general mental status examination, standardized cognitive status examinations, such as the SMMSE or NBCSE, and documentation of the patient's specific competency abilities are required for this evaluation. In the general mental status examination, particular attention should be paid to eliciting potential delusions about the illness or treatment. Once the patient's cognitive status and general mental status have been examined, his or her understanding of the illness, risks of treatment, and risks of refusal of treatment are assessed. If the patient understands and can verbalize these issues, then in most jurisdictions he or she is considered to be competent to consent to medical treatment. The patient's competence to consent to medical treatment may vary over short time spans in accordance with the temporal variation of delirium. The examination for medical competency must be dated and timed, and the examinations need to be repeated in order to demonstrate the stability of the findings. An important emerging area of competency evaluation is the assessment of frontal lobe executive function, because frontal lobe dysfunction may prevent patients with adequate knowledge from applying that knowledge to themselves or their situation.

Henneman PL, Mendoza R, Lewis RJ: Prospective evaluation of emergency department medical clearance. Ann Emerg Med 1994;24:4.

Kiernan RJ et al: The Neurobehavioral Cognitive Status Examination: a brief but differentiated approach to cognitive assessment. Ann Intern Med 1987;107:481.

CONSULTATION WITH MEDICALLY ILL PATIENTS WHO HAVE ACUTE PSYCHIATRIC SYMPTOMS

The majority of acute psychiatric symptoms of recent onset, and without previous psychiatric history, have organic causes. The most effective assessment protocol includes a medical history; physical examination; serum sodium, potassium, chloride, carbon dioxide, glucose, creatinine, and urea nitrogen; serum calcium; serum creatinine phosphokinase (if myoglobinuria is present); urine alcohol and drug screens; computed tomography scan; and lumbar puncture (if patient is febrile). In hospitalized patients who have no psychiatric history and who develop acute psychiatric symptoms, the first priority is medical evaluation (including a careful cognitive status examination) organized to rule out medical causes, especially of delirium.

If no medical cause is found, psychiatric evaluation should consider acute reactive psychosis and affective disorder in the differential diagnosis. Treatment of psychotic symptoms in the medical patient on the general hospital unit is very similar to the treatment of acute delirium. The patient needs to be observed regularly. A sitter, either a professional or a family member, is usually acceptable to the patient. Sometimes restraints are necessary, but they must be used in accordance with hospital policy and procedures. If the medical condition for which the patient is being treated has stabilized, and the patient continues to have acute psychiatric symptoms not of organic origin, transfer to a psychiatric unit should be considered.

The general surgery service asked the C-L service to conduct a competency evaluation on a 63-year-old nursing home resident who had been diagnosed as having chronic schizophrenia and acute renal failure. She had been a state hospital resident for 20 years before transfer to a local nursing home 2 years earlier. The patient had consented to the placement of a vascular shunt in her arm so that hemodialysis could be started. Surgery had been scheduled several times, but the patient refused to have an intravenous drip started on the day of surgery and surgery had been canceled. At this point, the surgeons were concerned that the patient was not competent.

The patient was obese and appeared older than her stated age. She had sparse, slow speech, which was organized. Her affect was blunted. She denied hallucination or delusions. The patient's daughter confirmed that her mother did not express any delusions about her illness or her treatment. The patient could verbalize what her medical problems were and the need for treatment. Her SMMSE score was 22/30. The NBCSE revealed defects in similarities and constructional ability. The Executive Interview revealed significant executive dysfunction. The patient could not understand that the painful intravenous puncture was a necessary step in the treatment of her renal failure. After consultation, the hospital attorney advised that a majority of her local family (five adult children) was required to give consent. A meeting with the family by the C-L team found that only the daughter who had attended the initial examination and was the primary caretaker was willing to give consent. The C-L team guided a brief family exploration of the issues, but found that the family members were all firm in their respective opinions. A further session with the daughter who supported surgery was scheduled to explore her feelings and explain her legal options.

Royall DR, Mahurin RK, Gray KF: Bedside assessment of executive cognitive impairment: The Executive Interview. J Am Geriatr Soc 1992;40:1221.

CONSULTATION WITH MEDICALLY ILL PATIENTS WHO HAVE DEPRESSIVE SYMPTOMS

The assessment of affective symptoms in the medically ill has a long and controversial history. Perhaps the most frequent and practical work done by the C-L psychiatrist is in the diagnosis of depression in the medically ill. Such work is often difficult because medical illnesses can have symptoms that mimic depression and because the drugs used to treat medical illnesses can cause depression. Yet another complication is that the clinician must determine whether the depression is a reaction to the illness or is organically caused. The diagnosis of depression as a syndrome without respect to causality and with more emphasis on the psychological or cognitive symptoms of depression has been helpful in this regard. The Endicott criteria for the diagnosis of depression in patients with cancer are an example of this type of approach (Table 14–4). The Endicott criteria substitute the cognitive symptoms of depression for vegetative symptoms that may be associated with the patient's physical disease.

Depression is the psychiatric disorder most commonly treated by nonpsychiatrists. Several problems are related to this trend: Nonpsychiatrists tend to prescribe inadequate dosages of antidepressants, terminate the medication prematurely if the patient does not respond immediately, and terminate the continuation phase (after the therapeutic effect occurs) prematurely. All of these problem areas can be remedied.

A 48-year-old single, female college professor was admitted to a tertiary care hospital for an autologous bone marrow transplant. She had been physically healthy until the diagnosis of metastatic breast cancer approximately 4 months before her admission. She had no history of chemical dependency or previous psychiatric treatment. She received chemotherapy and a radical mastectomy within 2 weeks of the initial diagnosis. The metastatic breast cancer did not respond to chemotherapy, and the patient was referred for

Table 14–4. Endicott criteria for depression in patients with cancer.

A. Dysphoric mood or loss of interest
B. At least four of the following present at least 2 weeks (if medical condition is likely to affect a specific symptom, substitute according to items below)
  1. Poor appetite or weight loss[1]
  2. Insomnia or hypersomnia[1]
  3. Psychomotor agitation or retardation
  4. Loss of interest or pleasure
  5. Loss of energy or fatigue[1]
  6. Feelings of worthlessness, self-reproach, or guilt
  7. Difficulty thinking or concentrating[1]
  8. Thought of death or suicide
C. Mood-incongruent delusions or hallucinations and bizarre behavior not dominant when affective syndromes absent
D. Not superimposed on schizophrenia, schizophreniform, or paranoid disorder
E. Not due to organic mental disorder or uncomplicated bereavement

[1] Substitution items: (1) fearful or depressed appearance; (2) social withdrawal or decreased talkativeness; (5) brooding, self-pity, or pessimism; (7) mood not reactive (ie, cannot be cheered up, doesn't smile, no reaction to good news)

evaluation for bone marrow transplantation. She reported that, since the diagnosis of breast cancer, 4 months earlier, she had experienced periodic depression and anxiety. She described crying episodes, depressed mood, initial insomnia, and agitation lasting 3–4 days at a time with normal mood and neurovegetative functioning between episodes. She denied weight loss and anhedonia. She disclosed persistent feelings of hopelessness, helplessness, and worthlessness. She denied suicidal thoughts.

The C-L service was consulted because the patient was agitated and crying throughout her first day in the hospital. The bone marrow team was concerned about the patient's ability to tolerate the stress of transplantation and isolation in the clean room and consulted the C-L psychiatry service. The patient scored 26/30 on the SMMSE. The NBCSE was completely normal except for mild deficits in attention and constructional ability. All routine admission blood work was within normal limits, and a magnetic resonance imaging scan performed 1 month earlier was normal.

The patient's symptoms and history fit the DSM-IV classification of a mood disorder due to metastatic breast cancer. The treatment literature on this diagnosis is minimal. The patient was started on trazodone 50 mg at bedtime, and the dose was increased rapidly to 150 mg at bedtime over 1 week. The patient's sleep, anxiety, and mood symptoms stabilized. She received brief cognitive therapy approximately three times per week for 15- to 20-minute sessions. The therapy focused on how the patient's thinking could affect her emotional and physical condition. She tolerated the transplant well. At discharge, the psychotropic medication was stopped at her request, and she was referred to her local physician.

Endicott J: Measurement of depression in patients with cancer. Cancer 1984;53:2243.

SPECIAL TOPICS IN CONSULTATION-LIAISON PSYCHIATRY

Disfiguring Conditions

Disfiguring conditions and injuries are a special area of interest in C-L psychiatry. Extensive scarring, the loss of a limb, and a malformation such as a cleft palate are all conditions that disfigure a patient's physical appearance. What are the psychosocial consequences of such disfigurement? Although it is intuitively obvious that a developmental anomaly affecting physical attractiveness could cause social and sexual dysfunction, the results of limited studies in this area are surprising. Cleft palate is the most stud-ied disfiguring condition. Results of studies on children born with this defect demonstrate minimal effect on normal development and little behavioral or personality pathology in these children.

Studies of burn patients demonstrate similar results. Most psychiatric disorders in patients with severe burns are transient, and only a minority of such patients have depressive disorders. The long-term effects of disfiguring burns were usually limited to decreased socializing in men and decreased sexual satisfaction in women. Surprisingly, self-esteem was not impaired in the majority of burn patients. Family and hospital staff may have a tendency to overpathologize burn patients' psychological reactions to their injuries. Studies of development in burned children also demonstrate minimal personality pathology as a result of burns. The majority of patients exhibit resilience to the psychosocial effect of disfiguring conditions.

Transplantation Psychiatry

Because of the significant expense of solid organ transplants and the problem of treatment noncompliance as the major factor in late transplant morbidity and mortality, C-L psychiatrists are often consulted about decisions relating to selection for transplantation. Far more patients meet criteria for solid organ transplantation than there are donor organs available, especially in heart and liver transplantation. C-L psychiatrists have learned that psychopathology does not represent an absolute contraindication to transplantation. Judgments in this area are exceedingly complex and are determined by laws of supply and demand and by unconscious bias as much as by a rational evaluation based on the clinical examination. The problem with this area of C-L psychiatry is the difficulty in predicting which patients can best utilize the gift-of-life extension. Research on psychosocial risk factors and treatment to ameliorate the risk factors are active areas of current research.

Anderson BJ, Robin RR (editors): *Practical Psychology for Diabetes Clincians: How to Deal with the Key Behavioral Issues Faced by Patients and Health Care Teams.* American Diabetes Association, 1996.

THE FUTURE OF CONSULTATION-LIAISON PSYCHIATRY

C-L psychiatry diversified and flourished in general hospitals in the latter half of the 20th century, but its future lies in its adaptation to managed care and its integration with primary care. The role of C-L psychiatry in primary care is ill defined and problematic. Currently, more patients with psychiatric diagnoses are treated by primary care physicians than by all mental health providers combined. As economic forces shift the majority of medical care into outpatient primary care settings and away from specialist care in tertiary hospitals, the role of the C-L psychiatrist will become even more important.

Models for psychiatric participation in primary care include the shifted outpatient model, the selected consultation model, and the liaison attachment model. The shifted outpatient model is represented by traditional psychiatric outpatient practice located in a primary care setting. It is the most prevalent form of collaboration in Great Britain. The selected consultation model involves a formal association between a psychiatrist or psychiatric interdisciplinary group and a primary care practice where primary care patients are seen by a psychiatrist in the psychiatric setting and feedback is given to the primary care physician. The liaison attachment model links a psychiatric team and a primary care team involving not only the treatment of primary care patients but also education and support.

Interesting preliminary findings have emerged from early studies of these models. Psychiatric patients seem to prefer the shifted outpatient model. Their compliance as measured by outpatient clinic attendance is higher and hospital admissions of patients in this model are lower. The liaison attachment model study showed mixed results in terms of patient outcome with significantly increased costs. More pilot programs with cost-benefit outcome studies are needed to develop effective collaborative services in the primary care setting.

It is useful to take a future-oriented view of C-L psychiatry. Much has been done of value in the past; however, there has been very little measurement of its effectiveness. Some studies have looked at process, that is, the percentage of consultations followed carefully by consultees. Only a few studies examine the effect of a liaison psychiatrist on positive outcome (eg, reduced length of hospital stay in patients with hip fractures). Additional studies are required that examine not only symptom reduction and length of stay but also functional outcomes such as self care, school, family and social participation, and return to work.

As managed care dominates U.S. health care, significant questions arise. Establishing the value of traditional inpatient C-L psychiatric services in terms of decreasing other health care services and improving patient satisfaction and quality of life will be an area of active research. An example of a cost-effective C-L psychiatry service is screening for and treatment of delirium in hip replacement surgery patients. More studies of specific C-L psychiatry interventions are needed to delineate the cost-effective services. Key questions include the following: In primary care, which of the three models is cost-effective? How can the quality of psychiatric services provided by primary care physicians be assessed and improved? Are C-L psychiatric services cost-effective in primary care? Are innovative models necessary for primary care? The future holds many challenges.

Blount A (editor): *Integrated Primary Care: The Future of Medical and Mental Health Collaboration.* WW Norton & Co, 1998.

CONCLUSION

Whatever the future course of C-L psychiatry, it will continue to address and study the important psychosocial issues associated with medical care and to model effective physician-patient communication skills. Liaison psychiatry was one forerunner of quality improvement. To improve patient functional outcomes and quality of life, physicians of all specialties will need to be able to address the psychosocial aspects of their medical care.

15

Psychiatry & the Law

William Bernet, MD

Forensic psychiatry is the medical subspecialty, recognized by the American Psychiatric Association since 1991, in which psychiatric expertise is applied to legal issues. The American Board of Psychiatry and Neurology started in 1994 to examine individuals for "added qualifications in forensic psychiatry," and there are about 30 1-year fellowship programs in forensic psychiatry.

There are four divisions of forensic psychiatry. The first pertains to the legal aspects of general psychiatric practice, such as the civil commitment of involuntary patients, the doctrine of informed consent, the requirement to protect third parties from dangerous patients, and matters of privilege and confidentiality.

The second division of forensic psychiatry covers the assessment of mental disability. This includes the evaluation of individuals who have been injured on the job; the assessment of a plaintiff who claims that he or she was injured and is now seeking compensation from a defendant; and the assessment of the competency of individuals to perform specific acts such as making a will.

The most colorful aspect of forensic psychiatry deals with individuals who have been arrested. This division includes the evaluation of competency to stand trial, the assessment of criminal responsibility, evaluations that relate to sentencing, and the treatment of incarcerated individuals.

The fourth division of forensic psychiatry is forensic child psychiatry, which includes child custody evaluations, the evaluation of children who may have been abused, and consultation regarding minors who are involved with juvenile court.

Appelbaum PS, Gutheil TG: *Clinical Handbook of Psychiatry and the Law,* 2nd ed. Williams & Wilkins, 1991.

Melton GB et al: *Psychological Evaluations for the Courts,* 2nd ed. Guilford Press, 1998.

Rosner R: *Principles and Practice of Forensic Psychiatry.* Chapman & Hall, 1994.

Simon R: *Clinical Psychiatry and the Law.* American Psychiatric Press, 1992.

LEGAL ASPECTS OF PSYCHIATRIC PRACTICE

PROFESSIONAL LIABILITY

Psychiatrists are less likely than other physicians to be sued for professional negligence. However, we live in a litigious society—most psychiatrists will be the subject of at least one professional liability claim during the course of their professional careers.

In a case of professional liability or malpractice, a patient (the plaintiff) sues the psychiatrist (the defendant). In order to prevail legally, the plaintiff must prove each of four elements: (1) The psychiatrist had a duty of care to the patient, (2) there was a breach of the duty to the patient, (3) the patient was injured, and (4) the negligent care was the proximate cause of the patient's injury. That is, if it were not for the negligent act, the injury would not have occurred. At a trial, the plaintiff will attempt to prove each of the four elements by a preponderance of the evidence. Both the plaintiff and the defendant may ask expert witnesses to testify.

Psychiatrists are at risk of being sued in several clinical situations. For example, a psychiatrist may be held responsible when a patient commits suicide, if the suicide was foreseeable, and if the psychiatrist failed to take a proper history from the patient or from other individuals or if he or she failed to take appropriate precautions. A psychiatrist may be liable for negligent psychopharmacology if a patient sustains injury as a result of (1) failure to obtain an adequate history, (2) use of a drug that is not efficacious or not indicated, (3) use of the wrong dosage of medication, or (4) failure to recognize or treat side effects. A particular concern is the occurrence of tardive dyskinesia (a serious side effect caused by certain psychotropic medications), especially if the patient and family members were not warned of the risk and if the psychiatrist did not monitor the patient properly for side effects. A lawsuit may arise out of the use of electroconvulsive therapy if its use was inappropriate or if informed consent was not obtained.

Psychiatrists have been sued for engaging in sexual conduct with a patient or with the spouse of a patient. Because it has been clearly stated by professional organizations that sexual activity with patients is a breach of the psychiatric standard of care, the major issue in these cases is to prove that the sexual activity occurred. In some cases patients have made false allegations of sexual conduct against psychiatrists. Even if the sexual activity never occurred, the psychiatrist may have mishandled the case through boundary violations that created the foundation for the false allegations (ie, through negligent management of the transference).

INFORMED CONSENT

Informed consent refers to the continuing process through which a patient understands and agrees to the evaluation and treatment proposed by the physician and mental health professional. Although informed consent is a concept that all psychiatrists claim to endorse, many practitioners do not understand what the concept means or give only lip service to its implementation. A patient, of course, must be competent to give informed consent.

There are four components to informed consent: (1) understanding the situation, (2) considering the consequences of the decision, (3) having adequate information, and (4) giving consent voluntarily. "Understanding the situation" means, for instance, that the patient knows he or she has a particular illness and that the patient is discussing his or her care with the doctor. "Considering the consequences of the decision" means that the patient knows the possible outcomes, which might be continuing illness, disability, or recovery. Considering the outcomes also means that the patient is capable of weighing the risks and benefits of the proposed treatment. "Having adequate information" means that the patient knows the facts needed in order to make the decision. In general, the legal standard is for the physician to relate as much detail as a reasonable person would want to know. Ordinarily this means telling the patient the purpose of the treatment, the possible consequences of providing or withholding the treatment, and alternative treatments that should be considered. The last requirement is that the patient must be "giving consent voluntarily." That is, the patient should not be coerced or offered inducements by the physician, by other members of the treatment team, or by family members.

Informed consent is more than just a signature on a form. As treatment progresses, there should be a continuing dialogue regarding the nature of the treatment and its possible side effects. In some circumstances, such as starting a psychotic patient on neuroleptic medication, the patient will be able to discuss these topics coherently only after treatment has begun. In some cases informed consent should involve a discussion with close family members as well as the patient. When a chronically suicidal patient is being discharged from the hospital, for instance, it is useful for the immediate family to understand both the pros and cons of the discharge and to understand that all parties (ie, patient, family, and psychiatrist) share and accept the inherent risks.

CIVIL COMMITMENT

In some circumstances, psychiatric patients are hospitalized involuntarily. The legal bases for involuntary or civil commitment are the principle of *parens patriae* (ie, the government may act as "father of the country" to protect individuals who are unable to take care of themselves) and the police power of the state (ie, the government has the authority to protect society from dangerous individuals). Psychiatrists participate in this process by evaluating patients as to whether they meet criteria for civil commitment. Although the specific procedures vary from state to state, the criteria for involuntary commitment generally include all of the following: (1) The patient has a serious psychiatric disorder, such as a psychosis or bipolar disorder; (2) there is significant risk that the patient will harm himself or others; and (3) hospitalization is the least restrictive alternative. In some jurisdictions, civil commitment is hard to justify (requiring an overt act rather than mere risk of danger) or less difficult to justify (allowing civil commitment if the patient is not likely to take care of basic personal needs).

THE RIGHTS OF PATIENTS

On many occasions, hospitalized psychiatric patients and institutionalized mentally retarded persons have been railroaded, warehoused, and abused. As a result, state and federal courts and legislators have declared that patients have specific rights. For example, the right to treatment means that civilly committed mental patients have a right to individualized treatment. Likewise, patients also have the right to refuse treatment. That is, a patient who is civilly committed may still be competent to decide whether to agree to use psychotropic medication. If the psychiatrist proposes to use medication even though the patient refuses, he or she should follow the appropriate local procedures. Such procedures may include referring the question to a treatment review committee or asking the court to appoint a guardian for the patient.

In some jurisdictions, psychiatric patients have the following rights: to receive visitors; to send uncensored mail; to receive uncensored mail from attorneys and physicians, although other mail may be examined before being delivered; to confidentiality; to have medical records available to authorized individuals; and to a written statement outlining these rights. An important patient right is that seclusion and mechanical restraint will not be used unless required for the patient's medical or treatment needs. Seclusion and restraint may not be used for punishment or for the convenience of staff.

CONFIDENTIALITY

Psychiatric patients have a right to be assured that information that they have related in therapy will not be revealed to other individuals. The American Medical Association has promulgated ethical principles for many years. These principles include the importance of confidentiality. The American Psychiatric Association has published both general principles and detailed guidelines regarding patient confidentiality. Federal law and federal regulations protect the confidentiality of patients treated in alcohol and substance abuse programs. In some states, the medical licensing act or a separate statute defines the physician's obligation to maintain patient confidentiality.

The issue of confidentiality in clinical practice is complex. In some situations, confidentiality should be given great importance; but in other situations, it is therapeutically important to share information with other clinicians or with family members. For example, the treatment of chronically ill patients may require continuing collaboration with family members. The sharing of clinical information is almost always done with the patient's knowledge and consent. In treating a minor, the importance of confidentiality will depend on the patient's age and developmental level, his or her psychopathology, his or her relationship with the parents, and the specific topic in question. For example, most therapists would maintain confidentiality regarding an adolescent's sexual activities and occasional drug usage that might be considered normal youthful experimentation. However, therapists would want parents to become aware of extreme sexual promiscuity, pregnancy, serious delinquent behavior, and serious substance abuse. The concept of confidentiality is not absolute.

Table 15–1 lists some of the many exceptions to confidentiality in clinical and forensic practice. Clinicians have a strong impulse to discuss case material with colleagues, and these conversations sometimes occur in elevators, cafeterias, and other public places where they can be overheard by strangers. This urge to discuss cases occurs because clinical material is both extremely interesting (so the therapist wants to tell about it in order to show off in some way) and extremely anxiety provoking (so the therapist wants to find reassurance by sharing the case with a colleague). If a psychiatrist is concerned or puzzled about a clinical issue, he or she should confer in a formal setting with a consultant or a supervisor.

Table 15–1. Exceptions to confidentiality.

If the patient is suicidal or homicidal, protective steps may have to be taken that breach confidentiality.

Child abuse must be reported to protective services.

If the plaintiff in a lawsuit has made his or her medical or psychiatric condition an issue, the defendant has the right to know about and to obtain the records of the plaintiff's evaluation and treatment.

A court may order a physician to disclose confidential information.

The results of a court-ordered pretrial evaluation may be available to the defense attorney, the prosecuting attorney, and the judge.

The results of a disability evaluation will be available to the attorney or agency that requested the evaluation.

The clinician should be aware that any written record may later be read by the patient or by many other people. The wise psychiatrist will protect himself or herself from future chagrin by always keeping this in mind when he dictates an evaluation or writes a progress note. Prospective patients should know the limits of confidentiality. One way that therapists can ensure patient understanding of such limits is to provide them with an office brochure that explains that the therapist values confidentiality very highly but that particular exceptions to confidentiality exist.

The right to confidentiality continues after a patient's death, but it must be balanced against the family's right to certain information. After a patient's suicide, for instance, it may be appropriate for the patient's therapist to meet with immediate family members and for all of them (ie, including the therapist) to try to make sense of what happened. That meeting might involve the therapist's sharing certain kinds of information with the family, but it need not involve extensive or detailed revelations.

PRIVILEGE

The concept of privilege is a specific aspect of confidentiality that may arise in a judicial setting. A person has the right of testimonial privilege when he or she has the right to refuse to testify or to prevent another person from testifying about specific information. For instance, a woman may claim privilege and refuse to testify about conversations she had with her attorney, because such discussions are considered private under the concept of attorney-client privilege. Likewise, a man may claim that his therapy is covered by physician-patient privilege and prevent the psychiatrist from testifying about him. The man may waive the right to physician-patient privilege and allow his psychiatrist to testify. In fact, the psychiatrist needs to realize that it is up to the patient, not the psychiatrist, to make that decision. In other words, the psychiatrist should ordinarily go ahead and testify, if the patient has waived his right to privilege.

PROTECTION OF THIRD PARTIES

Occasionally, a patient may reveal that he or she has murderous feelings toward a specific other person. The psychiatrist should assess, of course, the cause and the seriousness of these feelings. In addition, the psychiatrist should devise a treatment plan to protect the other person (ie, the third party). Ideally, the psychiatrist and patient should cooperate in devising a safety plan. For example, a psychiatrist was treating a patient who had chronic schizophrenia and who expressed thoughts of hurting his parents. The psychiatrist and the patient agreed to a joint telephone call to the parents to inform them of the danger; an adjustment in the patient's medication; and a written statement that the patient would not visit the parents until the crisis was resolved.

If the psychiatrist and patient cannot agree on a safety plan or if it is clinically inappropriate to attempt such an agreement, the psychiatrist must take steps unilaterally to protect the third party. For example, an acutely paranoid man has told his psychiatrist that he intends to take revenge against his former boss. The psychiatrist protects both the patient and the boss by arranging for an involuntary commitment.

Warning a potential victim is usually done with the patient's knowledge, if not with his or her permission. But this is not always possible. For example, an extremely angry and jealous man, who has been threatening his wife, has eloped from a supposedly secure inpatient program. It is no longer possible to discuss the issue therapeutically, but the psychiatrist immediately notifies the wife and also the police.

State legislatures have adopted a variety of laws and local courts have held a variety of opinions, so psychiatrists should become familiar with the local standards. There may be contradictory practices as a person moves from one state to another. Some states have laws that protect mental health professionals from liability if they disclose in good faith confidential information to the patient's intended victim.

American Psychiatric Association: *Opinions of the Ethics Committee on the Principles of Medical Ethics with Annotations Especially Applicable to Psychiatry*. American Psychiatric Press, 1995.
Simon RI, Sadoff RL: *Psychiatric Malpractice: Cases and Comments for Clinicians*. American Psychiatric Press, 1992.

ASSESSMENT OF MENTAL DISABILITY

There are several circumstances in which psychiatrists evaluate clients to determine the degree of disability, if any, that is present. These circumstances include claims under workers' compensation programs; personal injury lawsuits; and evaluations to determine mental competence to perform specific acts.

DISABILITY & WORKERS' COMPENSATION

The Social Security Administration provides financial benefits for individuals who are not able to work at any occupation for at least 12 months because of a serious physical condition or psychiatric illness. The federal government, through the Veteran's Administration, provides benefits to veterans who are partially or fully disabled because of a service-related condition. Individual states administer workers' compensation programs that provide defined and limited compensation to individuals who were injured during the course of their employment. Finally, some people have individual or group disability insurance policies and apply for benefits from the insurance company.

Clients who are seeking disability benefits or workers' compensation should be evaluated in a thorough and systematic manner. The clinician should carefully read the referral information, because the agency or company may be asking the evaluator to address very specific questions. In some cases the cause or the date of onset of the illness may be very important. In other cases the issue may be whether the client can currently engage in a particular occupation.

In addition to a thorough interview, a psychiatric disability evaluation may include the following: psychological testing, neuropsychological assessment, review of medical and psychiatric records, review of military and employment records, and interviews with family members and other informants. The evaluator should actively consider the possibility of malingering or exaggeration of symptoms. The American Medical Association has published guidelines for the assessment of physical and mental disability.

PERSONAL INJURY

Personal injury litigation is part of a large domain called tort law, the law of civil wrongs. A person who injures another can be arrested and tried (under criminal law) or sued (under tort law). A successful tort action requires proof of the four elements mentioned previously: (1) A duty was owed to the plaintiff by the defendant, (2) the duty was breached, (3) an injury occurred, and (4) the breach of duty caused the injury.

Courts allow plaintiffs to be compensated for both physical and psychological injuries. If a person was severely injured physically, it is easy to see how he or she may have sustained psychological damage as well. In some circumstances courts will allow compensation for psychological injury even when no physical injury occurred at all. This may happen when the plaintiff was so close to the incident (within the "zone of danger") that he or she could have been physically injured or when the plaintiff was not in the zone of danger but observed a close relative being injured.

Psychiatrists become involved in these cases by evaluating whether a plaintiff has been psychologically injured and whether the injury was the result of the negligent act by the defendant. The evaluator should interview the client carefully and collect information from other sources, in order to compare the person's psychological and social functioning before and after the alleged trauma. Several psychiatric conditions may follow a serious trauma: posttraumatic stress disorder, generalized anxiety disorder, phobias, panic disorder, adjustment disorder, dysthymia, and major depression. The evaluator should clarify whether the condition antedated the alleged trauma, whether there were other psychological stressors that could have caused the symptoms, and whether there was a direct relationship between the alleged injury and the psychiatric disorder.

COMPETENCE

In psychiatry, competence refers to a person's mental capacity to perform or accomplish a particular task. Although the details of the competency evaluation will depend on the circumstances of the case, the general principles are the same:

The individual must understand what is happening. For example, an elderly woman who is making a will must understand that she is meeting with her attorney and they are drawing up a document.

The individual must understand the consequences of the proposed action. For example, the woman who is drafting her will must realize that her children will not receive anything if she puts her entire estate in a trust fund for her cats.

The individual must have adequate information. That is, the elderly woman who is preparing her will must know both the extent of her property and who the potential heirs would be.

The individual must not be under coercion. For example, the elderly woman must not be unduly influenced to leave a large bequest to her nurse, psychic, or chauffeur.

The evaluation of competence occurs in a variety of clinical situations, both in general medical and psychiatric practice, as well as in forensic settings (Table 15–2).

American Medical Association: *Guides to the Evaluation of Permanent Impairment.* American Medical Association, 1993.

Rogers R (editor): *Clinical Assessment of Malingering and Deception,* 2nd ed. Guilford Press, 1997.

Table 15–2. Circumstances in which competency is an issue.

In criminal law
  to waive Miranda rights
  to stand trial
  to testify
  to be executed
In civil law
  to write a will
  to make a contract
  to vote or hold office
  to manage one's own funds
  to care for a child
In medical practice
  to consent to surgery or electroconvulsive therapy
  to refuse surgery or electroconvulsive therapy

INDIVIDUALS WHO HAVE BEEN ARRESTED

Forensic psychiatrists sometimes evaluate individuals who have been arrested and are awaiting trial. Usually, it is the defense attorney who is concerned about the defendant's mental competency to go to trial and his or her state of mind at the time of the alleged offense.

COMPETENCY TO STAND TRIAL

In order to be competent to stand trial, the defendant must understand the charges that have been brought against him or her and the nature of the legal proceedings. For example, the defendant needs to understand the roles of the defense attorney, prosecuting attorney, and judge. The defendant must be aware of the possible outcome of the legal proceedings (eg, release to the community, prison, capital punishment). Finally, the defendant must be able to cooperate with his or her attorney, disclose to the attorney the facts regarding the case, and testify relevantly.

If the defendant is found not competent to stand trial, the court will arrange for psychiatric treatment in the jail or at a state psychiatric facility. In some cases a defendant becomes competent following psychotropic medication or psychoeducational intervention. A person who is permanently incompetent, such as a severely retarded individual, may never go to trial. He or she may simply be released or, if dangerous to self or others, civilly committed.

CRIMINAL RESPONSIBILITY

A person who has committed a crime is not held responsible for his or her behavior if he or she was legally insane at the time the crime was committed. In this sense, "insanity" is a legal term that implies a severe mental disorder or a significant degree of mental retardation. The courts have applied several standards to define criminal insanity. The most common are the M'Naghten rule and the American Law Institute (ALI) test.

The M'Naghten rule provides for only a cognitive test for the insanity defense. That is, the person is held not responsible for a crime if "the party accused was labouring [sic] under such a defect of reason, from disease of the mind, as not to know the nature and quality of the act he was doing; or, if he did know it, that he did not know he was doing what was wrong."

The ALI test provides for both a cognitive and a volitional test. That is, a defendant would not be responsible for criminal conduct "if at the time of such conduct as a result of mental disease or defect he lacks substantial capacity to appreciate the criminality of his conduct or to conform his conduct to the requirements of the law." Jurisdictions that use the ALI test usually include the proviso that "mental disease or defect" does not include any disorder that is manifested simply by antisocial conduct.

If a judge or jury finds a defendant not guilty by reason of insanity, the person does not go to prison. He or she does not go home, either. Usually the disposition is to a secure inpatient facility to determine if the person can be civilly committed to either hospital or outpatient treatment. Some states have provided an alternative outcome, in that the defendant can be found guilty but mentally ill. That is, the defendant had a mental illness at the time of the alleged offense, but it was not severe enough to acquit him or her. The defendant found guilty but mentally ill goes to prison, where treatment presumably is available.

PRISON PSYCHIATRY

Our jails and prisons have much higher proportions of mentally ill and mentally retarded individuals than are found in the general population. Forensic psychiatrists provide treatment to these individuals, who may have serious conditions manifested by chronic depression, violent and aggressive behavior, and overt psychosis.

Perlin ML: *The Jurisprudence of the Insanity Defense.* Carolina Academic, 1998.
Wettstein RM: *Treatment of Offenders with Mental Disorders.* Guilford Press, 1998.

FORENSIC CHILD PSYCHIATRY

The interface between child psychiatry and the law is a very young discipline. The forensic child psychiatrist is likely to be consulted regarding child custody disputes, on the question of physical or sexual abuse, and with regard to minors involved in the juvenile justice system.

CHILD CUSTODY EVALUATION

When parents divorce and disagree regarding the custody of the child, mental health professionals sometimes evaluate the family and make recommendations to the court. Since the 1920s, lawmakers and courts have emphasized "the best interests of the child," which implies that the needs of the child override the rights of either parent. The American Academy of Child and Adolescent Psychiatry has developed practice parameters for child custody evaluations.

In conducting these evaluations, it is best to have access to all members of the family, including both parents. In some circumstances the psychiatrist may conduct a one-sided evaluation by interviewing only one parent and the child. In such a case the psychiatrist may make only limited observations and recommendations, such as commenting on the psychiatric condition of one parent and his or her relationship with the child. Usually the psychiatrist would not be able to make any recommendations regarding custody because he or she had no way of evaluating the relative parental adequacy of the mother and father.

Typically, the psychiatrist has an initial conference with both parents together; meets with each parent individually in order to complete a psychiatric evaluation and to assess each person's parenting attitudes and skills; and meets twice with the child, so that each parent can bring the child for an appointment at least once. The psychiatrist should collect information from outside sources, such as grandparents, nannies, the pediatrician, and teachers. It is important to speak to previous and current psychotherapists of the child and of the parents.

Decisions regarding custody are guided by the best interests of the child, but there are no standard guidelines for what specific factors should be taken into consideration and what weight should be given to each factor. The following factors are generally considered important: parental attitudes and parenting skills; which parent has been more involved with day-to-day child rearing activities; continuity of placement, in that it is usually presumed preferable to maintain the status quo unless there is good reason to change it; the physical health of the parents; the mental health of the parents (the psychiatric diagnosis is less important than the person's parenting skills in the present and the future); substance abuse; the relative merits of the two households (eg, whether the parent has remarried); allegations of physical or sexual abuse; the child's attachment to the parents; and the child's preference, if he or she articulates a definite preference for reasons that seem valid.

CHILD MALTREATMENT

Psychiatrists in private practice, as well as those employed by courts or other agencies, see children who are alleged to have been psychologically, physically, or sexually abused. The purpose of the evaluation may be to assist the court in determining what happened to the child, to make recommendations regarding placement or treatment, or to offer an opinion on the termination of parental rights. The evaluation of a child who is alleged to have been maltreated is described in Chapter 39.

JUVENILE JUSTICE

Forensic child psychiatrists may consult with the juvenile justice system to evaluate a juvenile's competency to go to trial and his or her state at the time of the alleged offense, if an insanity defense is being considered. Psychiatrists can also assist the court in determining if a juvenile, who has been accused of committing an unusually serious offense, should be tried as an adult.

American Academy of Child and Adolescent Psychiatry: Practice parameters for psychiatric custody evaluations. J Am Acad Child Adolesc Psychiatr 1997;36(10 Suppl):57S.

Grisso T: *Forensic Evaluation of Juveniles.* Professional Resource Exchange, 1998.

Nurcombe B, Partlett DJ: *Child Mental Health and the Law.* Free Press, 1994.

Schetky DH, Benedek EP (editors): *Clinical Handbook of Child Psychiatry and the Law.* Williams & Wilkins, 1992.

THE PSYCHIATRIST IN COURT

THE WRITTEN REPORT

The report should be carefully written. It will be read by several people, and the reader will tend to attach great significance to particular sentences or phrases. Probably the best approach is to make the report detailed enough for the reader to understand fully the procedure that was followed and the basis for the conclusions and recommendations but not to include every scintilla of data. Table 15–3 offers an outline of a typical forensic report.

ROLE DEFINITION

There are many times when the psychiatrist must keep straight in his or her own mind, and for others, both who is the client and what precisely is the psychiatrist's role in the current situation. The client may be the person the psychiatrist is examining or it may be somebody else. The psychiatrist may have the role of therapist or simply that of an evaluator. In forensic work, any confusion regarding the psychiatrist's role will be magnified and highlighted by the legal process and will compromise his or her work, whether the psychiatrist is intending to be a therapist, an evaluator, a consultant, or an administrator.

THE PROBLEM OF BIAS

Psychiatrists and other mental health professionals may not realize how easily and how often they become biased in their work with patients and families. Despite all that is known about unconscious processes (such as countertransference) and conscious motivations (such as greed and the desire for popularity and fame), it is common for therapists to base their conclusions on preconceived assumptions rather than on the data that have been presented. Bias may be more prevalent in forensic cases, because the evaluator is exposed to anger, threats, deceit, tragedy, innuendo, and various forms of hypocrisy, flattery, and inducement. It is extremely important for the psychiatrist to be aware of his or her own motivations, as well as the agendas of the other professionals involved in the case.

Bias is a distorting glass, through which the evaluator views the situation. For example, an evaluator who is a very strong believer in law and order may always interpret the facts to support criminal responsi-

Table 15–3. Outline for typical forensic report.

I. **Identifying information:** for example, names and birth dates
II. **Referral information:** a brief chronology of the situation and a statement about the circumstances of the referral and the specific purpose of the evaluation
III. **Procedure for this evaluation:** an explanation of the various meetings held, the psychological tests administered, and the outside information collected (it may be appropriate to state specifically that the client gave informed consent for the evaluation)
IV. **Observations:** a systematic presentation of the data collected during the evaluation
V. **Conclusions:** a list of specific statements that the psychiatrist believes are supported by his or her data
VI. **Recommendations:** these should follow logically from the conclusions
VII. **Appendices:** associated information (eg, psychological test results)
VIII. **Qualifications of the evaluator:** may be a curriculum vitae

bility rather than a finding of not guilty by reason of insanity. Also, the psychiatrist who enters a case with a particular bias is likely to change a situation despite a belief that he or she is studying it objectively. For example, an evaluator who is predisposed to find child abuse may interview children in such a suggestive manner that the children start to allege abusive acts that did not occur.

Several safeguards against bias are available. The psychiatrist should try to be aware of his or her own conscious and unconscious motivations. It may be helpful if the psychiatrist says something like this to himself or herself: "My job is not to win this case. My task is to collect accurate and pertinent data and to organize it in a way that is scientifically and medically valid." Another safeguard against bias is for the psychiatrist to carefully indicate in the written report the reasons for his or her conclusions, so that the court will truly understand the basis for the opinion.

Some forensic psychiatrists misuse their expertise by manipulating the court into believing something that may not be true. Sometimes, unscrupulous psychiatrists and other mental health professionals use obfuscating jargon in order to cloak their shaky reasoning with a false air of certainty.

DEGREES OF CERTAINTY

An important aspect of legal decisions is the standard of proof or the level of certainty that must be established in order for a particular decision or verdict to be reached. There are several levels of certainty.

The least exacting level of certainty to achieve is **probable cause.** In the practice of criminal law probable cause would be defined as cause sufficient to lead a reasonable man to suspect the person arrested had committed a crime. In psychiatric practice, that may be a sufficient level of certainty to report a suspected instance of child abuse.

In civil cases the side that prevails is the one that establishes a **fair preponderance of the evidence.** This can be expressed roughly as being 51% certain.

In some cases that involve psychiatric evidence, the level of certainty is **clear and convincing proof,** which is proof necessary to persuade by a substantial margin, which is more than a bare preponderance. In most states civil commitment, paternity suits, and legal insanity must be proven to a degree that is clear and convincing. In most circumstances the proof that child abuse has occurred or that parental rights should be severed must be clear and convincing.

Criminal cases require proof that is **beyond a reasonable doubt,** which means proof that is beyond question. To convict a specific person of child abuse would require proof beyond a reasonable doubt.

One of the most puzzling terms in forensic psychiatry is **reasonable degree of medical certainty.** When a physician testifies in court, he or she is frequently asked if his or her opinions are given with a reasonable degree of medical certainty. Unfortunately, there is no specific meaning for that term. At one time or another, physicians have taken it to mean about the same as "beyond a reasonable doubt," the same as "clear and convincing," and even the same degree of certainty as "preponderance of the evidence." It has

Table 15–4. Important cases in forensic psychiatry.

Addington v. Texas, 441 U.S. 418 (1979). The U.S. Supreme Court found that the standard of proof for civil commitment is "clear and convincing evidence."

Ake v. Oklahoma, 470 U.S. 68 (1985). The U.S. Supreme Court said that an indigent defendant, who raised the question of insanity, had the right to have a court-appointed psychiatrist perform an evaluation and assist the defense in preparation of an insanity defense.

Dillon v. Legg, 441 P.2d 912 (1968). The Supreme Court of California found that a person could be awarded damages for psychological injury that was caused by witnessing the physical injury of a close relative.

Dusky v. United States, 362 U.S. 402 (1960). The U.S. Supreme Court defined the test for competency to stand trial: whether the defendant "has sufficient present ability to consult with his lawyer with a reasonable degree of rational understanding—and whether he has a rational as well as a factual understanding of the proceedings against him."

In re Gault, 387 U.S.1 (1967). The U.S. Supreme Court defined the due process rights of a juvenile who has been arrested: written and timely notice of the charges, protection against self-incrimination, defense counsel, and right to cross-examination.

Landeros v. Flood, 551 P.2d 389 (1976). The Supreme Court of California established the standard of care for diagnosing the battered child syndrome, which was "whether a reasonably prudent physician examining this plaintiff . . . would have been led to suspect she was a victim of the battered child syndrome . . . and would have promptly reported his findings to appropriate authorities. . . . "

Rennie v. Klein, 720 F.2d 266 (1983). The Third Circuit Court of Appeals found that civilly committed patients have a constitutional right to refuse treatment.

Tarasoff v. Regents of the University of California, 551 P.2d 334 (1976). The Supreme Court of California found that the therapist of a dangerous patient "bears a duty to exercise reasonable care to protect the foreseeable victim of that danger."

Wyatt v. Aderholt, 503 F.2d 1305 (1974). The Fifth Circuit Court of Appeals said that civilly committed patients "unquestionably have a constitutional right to receive such individual treatment as will give each of them a realistic opportunity to be cured or to improve his or her mental condition."

been proposed that reasonable medical certainty is a level of certainty equivalent to that which a physician uses when making a diagnosis and starting treatment. The implication is that the degree of certainty depends on the clinical situation. For example, the diagnosis of syphilis is accomplished with almost 100% certainty, because there is a reliable laboratory test for that purpose. The determination that a patient has posttraumatic stress disorder as a result of a specific event is made with considerably less certainty.

Gutheil TG: *The Psychiatrist in Court: A Survival Guide.* American Psychiatric Press, 1998.

Rappeport J: Reasonable medical certainty. Bull Am Acad Psychiatry Law 1985;13:5.

Ziskin J, Faust D: *Coping with Psychiatric and Psychological Testimony.* Law and Psychology Press, 1995.

CONCLUSION

Forensic psychiatry is an unusual medical specialty because of the diverse clinical situations and the broad scope of practice that it encompasses. For instance, a forensic evaluation might involve a very young child (regarding child maltreatment), a very old person (regarding competency to make a will), or anybody in between. The forensic practitioner must be familiar not only with the clinical literature but also with the applicable law and important legal precedents. Several important legal cases have influenced both the practice of law and the practice of psychiatry (Table 15–4).

In addition, it is challenging to apply psychiatric expertise to legal situations—both through written reports and oral testimony—in a manner that is even handed and unbiased. Finally, forensic psychiatrists experience a wealth of human relationships and a variety of roles. They may consult with clients in the office, in the hospital, in jail, on death row, and in the corporate board room. After conducting an evaluation, they frequently take on the role of teacher or lecturer, as they explain their findings to family members, attorneys, and perhaps a judge and jury. This diversity within forensic psychiatry gives this medical specialty its own blend of suspense, accomplishment, and satisfaction.

Continuity of Care

Thomas F. Catron, PhD, & Lee Fleisher, BS

A **continuum of care in mental health services** refers to a range of services of different levels of intensity designed to meet the mental health needs of individual patients or target populations. Until recently, the range was limited to inpatient, residential, and outpatient treatment. However, a variety of economic and ideologic pressures have prompted the development of expanded services. The first attempts to expand the continuum of care developed out of the community mental health movement. Coincident with pressures to deinstitutionalize the chronic mentally ill, the Community Mental Health Centers Act was passed in 1963 to establish a range of community-based services and prevention efforts. This act was never fully implemented or realized, but it laid the groundwork for expanding the scope of available services and putting an increased emphasis on providing services in community-based settings.

A second major focus on the development of a continuum of care came from the National Institute of Mental Health Child and Adolescent Service System Program (CASSP). This program, begun in 1984, went beyond defining a continuum of mental health services for youth with serious emotional disturbances. The program defined a system of care that included mental health, social, educational, health, vocational, and recreational services. Moreover, the program defined a set of operational services including case management, advocacy, transportation, and legal services. At the core of this model, and perhaps its greatest contributions, were its aim to achieve continuity of care through aggressive case management and interagency cooperation, as well as its emphasis on the provision of services in the least restrictive setting and on an individual's movement through the system in accordance with changing treatment needs. Table 16–1 shows the range of services defined by CASSP that comprise a comprehensive system of care for children and youth who have severe emotional problems.

Most recently, the rapid growth of managed care in the mental health field has brought several new elements into the arena of continuum of care. The most significant of these elements are the emphasis on the relationship between costs and benefits, the shift of control from providers to insurers, and the creation of formal practice guidelines in an attempt to determine the appropriate level of care for the individual patient.

MENTAL HEALTH SERVICE PROGRAMS

Typically, in a continuum of care in mental health services, the endpoints in the range of treatment programs are residential and nonresidential services that vary by intensity and restrictiveness. Figure 16–1 represents such a continuum.

As Figure 16–1 demonstrates, various programs have evolved to fill the gap between the traditional inpatient and outpatient services. Several nonresidential programs provide a significant intensity of service, sometimes close to that of inpatient services. For example, day treatment (or partial hospitalization) typically offers the same intensity of treatment as an inpatient hospitalization, without the overnight stay. Some school-based interventions can vary the level of intensity to meet the needs of the individual patient. At the same time, residential services such as independent living programs or therapeutic foster care do not provide treatment per se. The mental health services programs listed in Table 16–1 are described in more detail in the sections that follow.

NONRESIDENTIAL SERVICES

The main purpose of nonresidential programs is to provide services to individuals who are maintained in their natural community setting (eg, home or school).

Table 16–1. A system of care for seriously emotionally disturbed children and youth.

Mental Health Services

- Nonresidential services
  - Prevention
  - Early identification and intervention
  - Assessment
  - Outpatient treatment (clinic-, home-, and school-based treatment)
  - Vocational and rehabilitation services
  - Day treatment, partial hospitalization, and intensive outpatient treatment
  - Emergency and crisis services
- Residential services
  - Therapeutic foster care
  - Therapeutic group care
  - Therapeutic camp services
  - Independent living services
  - Residential treatment
  - Crisis residential services
  - Hospitalization

Social Services

- Protective services
- Financial assistance
- Home aid services
- Respite care
- Shelter services
- Foster care
- Adoption

Health Services

- Health education and prevention
- Screening and assessment
- Primary, acute, and long-term care

Educational Services

- Assessment and planning
- Resource rooms
- Special education
- Special schools
- Home-bound instruction
- Residential schools
- Alternative programs

Vocational Services

- Career education
- Vocational assessment
- Job survival skills training
- Work experiences
- Job finding
- Placement and retention services
- Supported employment

Recreational Services

- After-school programs
- Summer camps
- Special projects

Operational Services

- Case management
- Self-help and support groups
- Advocacy
- Transportation
- Legal services
- Volunteer programs

Less (low) — INTENSITY — More (high)

RESTRICTIVENESS: Less (low) → More (high)

Prevention

Early Identification and Intervention

Outpatient — **Foster Care**

Intensive Outpatient (IOP) — **Independent Living**

Vocational Rehabilitation — **Group Care**

Day Treatment/Partial Hospitalization

Emergency Services — **Residential Treatment (RTC)**

Hospitalization

Figure 16–1. The level of intensity and restrictiveness of programs comprising a continuum of care in mental health services.

Furthermore, the level of services has been expanded to provide a varying degree of intensity of treatment for the purpose of preventing mental disorders, avoiding hospitalization, or providing an appropriate step-down or transition program.

PREVENTION SERVICES

Prevention services aim to reduce the incidence of mental health problems. Preventative programs are directed at populations at risk for mental health disorders. These programs address three types of prevention: (1) fostering mental health competencies (eg, problem-solving skills, coping skills, social skills), (2) improving natural support systems, and (3) promoting system changes in order to foster environments that avert situations that could lead to maladaptation. The prevention of mental health problems could reduce the incidence of disorders in later life. Some examples of prevention programs include the tactile or kinesthetic stimulation program to improve the physical and mental development of preterm infants, assertiveness training to promote better adaptation for young children, alcohol and drug education programs for adolescents, and depression prevention programs for adults.

Assessment

A competent assessment of the patient's functioning and psychopathology is needed so that the clinician can understand the nature and extent of the patient's disorder. Assessment can be conducted using observation, psychometrics, and interviewing techniques with a variety of informants (eg, patient, parent, teacher). Observation allows the clinician to note behavior in a variety of naturalistic settings and activities and in structured events in the clinic. Psychometrics can provide normative information regarding the patient's functioning in areas of intelligence, behavior, and adaptive functioning. Some psychometrics such as intelligence and personality measures require administration and interpretation by a licensed psychologist, whereas other psychometrics can be administered and scored by any clinician. Many assessment devices can be administered or scored using a computer. Assessments are often used to establish treatment goals, techniques, and setting with the patient.

Early Identification & Intervention

The rationale for early identification and intervention is that if problems can be addressed early, they might be treated more effectively. These efforts are often referred to as **secondary prevention.** Examples of early identification and intervention can be found in school systems where screening for mental health problems might be used to identify those children ex-hibiting initial indicators of disorders and to initiate appropriate services. Early intervention services can be clinic, home, or school based and can provide linkages to multiple agencies.

Outpatient Treatment

Individual, group, and family therapy may occur in a variety of outpatient settings including private offices, community mental health centers, schools, public health offices, and hospital-based outpatient clinics. Typically, patients are seen for therapy one or more times per week (sometimes less frequently). Outpatient therapy is usually the first approach to addressing psychiatric problems because it is flexible and relatively inexpensive. Sometimes outpatient services are provided in conjunction with other forms of treatment (eg, therapeutic foster care or independent living). Outpatient therapy can be offered in a variety of modes (eg, psychopharmacologic, psychodynamic, behavioral, cognitive-behavioral, or family systems treatment).

Recently, there has been an effort to adapt research-based psychotherapies to clinic settings in order to enhance the effectiveness of outpatient treatments. Empirically derived treatments have been implemented using manual-based treatment procedures in order to assure treatment integrity and improve treatment efficacy.

The provision of outpatient services outside the clinic setting is often used with special populations to improve access or address specific treatment issues. Home-based services offer the opportunity to work with individuals and families in their home environments. In some instances, crisis care can be provided in the home to prevent hospitalization. In addition, some home-based treatment techniques are effective for adolescents with severe conduct disorders. The school setting offers a unique platform from which mental health services can be provided. School-based services can increase the accessibility of mental health services to children who might otherwise be unserved.

Day Treatment, Partial Hospitalization, & Intensive Outpatient Treatment

If the patient cannot function in normal daily routines and functions, partial hospitalization may be recommended. Services offered in partial hospitalization programs typically resemble those of an inpatient program (eg, individual, group, and family therapy; pharmacotherapy; activity therapy; and recreation). Many psychiatric hospitals now offer this service as an alternative to (or a step up to or down from) inpatient care. Partial programs typically last 4–8 hours per day. Partial programs for children and adolescents include academic instruction as part of daily activities. Day school programs are often confused with day treatment programs. Although day schools offer a therapeutic milieu via highly structured classrooms, the objectives remain educational rather than psychiatric. Day schools are often used for children and adolescents who have serious emotional and behavioral problems and who cannot function in regular classrooms.

Outpatient services occur with varying frequency in order to increase intensity, and the length of each treatment session is 60 minutes or less. Intensive outpatient (IOP) services occur with varying frequency (1–7 times per week) and typically last no more than 3 hours per visit. IOP offers an opportunity to provide a relatively intense level of treatment without disrupting other functions or routines in which the patient must participate (eg, school, work, or family care). IOP often includes a high degree of structure and a variety of treatment modalities (eg, experiential, group, and individual therapy).

Emergency & Crisis Services

Sometimes an individual in crisis requires close supervision and monitoring for an extended period of time. This can be accomplished in a hospital-based service (often called a 23-hour admission) or independent crisis unit. Once the crisis has passed the individual is referred to an appropriate level of treatment. Other forms of crisis intervention (eg, emergency room visits, crisis hotlines) are available.

RESIDENTIAL SERVICES

Residential mental health services are provided in facilities, such as hospitals, group homes, schools, or foster homes, that house the patient. Continua of care are designed to minimize the utilization of costly residential services. Indeed, the average length of stay for children, adolescents, and adults in inpatient programs has declined drastically over the last decade. However, as there will always be a need for residential services, it is unlikely that these programs will be eliminated. The common thread amongst all residential facilities is that patients are admitted because they cannot be managed in their natural setting and require constant supervision and maintenance.

Therapeutic Foster Care

Residential programs that use foster parents have some advantages over other residential facilities. Foster parents are trained to work with emotionally disturbed children. Therapeutic foster care is much less expensive than are other residential programs. The patient is exposed to a home-like environment and has access to the foster family's natural support system as well as to other community services (eg, outpatient services, social services). A low staff-to-patient ratio allows clinical staff to work closely with the foster parents and patient. Although therapeutic foster care is typically used for children, some adult-oriented programs exist.

Therapeutic Group Care

Therapeutic group homes typically serve 5–10 patients per setting. Usually the setting consists of homes found in local communities and staffed by trained professionals. Mental health services can be provided by group home staff (if appropriately trained) or through community resources. Secure group homes provide a high degree of supervision. All services may be located at the facility. Open group homes allow for a greater degree of flexibility and movement. For example, children may attend the neighborhood school, or adults may continue employment.

Therapeutic Camp Services

Therapeutic camps differ from other residential treatment programs in that they tend to use more basic living accommodations and treatment themes. For example, wilderness-type therapeutic camps might be located in a wooded area, and living quarters might be tents or handcrafted cabins. The focus of the wilderness camp is to impress on the patient the importance of mutual effort and collaboration for survival purposes. Other camp services might use a regimented form of daily routines of very basic exercises (including physical exercise and strenuous physical labor). Such camps might appear similar to military boot camps.

Independent Living Services

Independent living skills are often an extension of group home or residential placement. Although some of the requisite skills may be taught in other placements, independent living placements are typically apartments or similar residences occupied by one to three individuals. Supervision is provided, but there is usually no resident staff to monitor the patient. The focus of these programs is independence through the development of financial, medical, housing, transportation, social, and daily living management skills.

Residential Treatment

Often confusion occurs in distinguishing between residential treatment centers (RTC) and other residential programs. RTCs are mental health facilities that provide 24-hour treatment and care to patients, under the age of 18 years, who have a diagnosable psychiatric illness. Although similar to psychiatric hospitals, RTCs do not usually have the same licensure or accreditation requirements as psychiatric hospitals. RTCs also offer more intensive treatment than do foster care, group homes, or independent living centers. Many of the elements of inpatient treatment are available at the RTC facility. RTCs, like group homes, have different degrees of security and restrictiveness. Some RTCs are organized around a large facility or campus. Wilderness camps are becoming popular for children and adolescents. RTCs are often used for long-term treatment.

Crisis Residential Services

Crisis residential services provide a 24-hour placement. These services may include diagnostic/evaluation and acute/intensive treatment services. Some crisis shelters provide placements for battered women or adolescents who are in need of respite.

Hospitalization

Hospitalization represents the most expensive and restrictive form of treatment. Until recently, hospitalization was the only treatment alternative to outpatient services. Currently, psychiatric hospitalization is used primarily for disturbances of high anxiety (eg, psychotic deterioration, violent behavior, refusal to eat or drink, or active suicidal ideation). Following comprehensive evaluation and multidisciplinary treatment, the aim is stabilization and discharge to a less intensive level of care. Inpatient facilities are rarely used today for long-term treatment.

Psychiatric hospitals can be organized into generic or specialized treatment units. **Generic units** accept patients on the basis of broad characteristics such as age and provide diagnosis and treatment for a variety of disorders. **Specialized units** accept patients on the basis of a particular psychiatric problem (eg, eating disorders) and related conditions (eg, emotional trauma) and might also group patients according to age and gender. Inpatient units are very structured and provide a full range of intensive services: psychopharmacology, psychotherapy (eg, individual, group, family), and activity therapy. Each unit typically has a group room, a recreation room, a nurse's station, a close observation room, and staff offices. Inpatient units provide around-the-clock medical coverage and very close monitoring of suicidal, homicidal, assaultive, or psychotic patients.

VOCATIONAL & REHABILITATION SERVICE PROGRAMS

For patients who require highly structured, psychoeducational resources, vocational and rehabilitation services offer an alternative to institutional care. Through these programs, chronic mentally ill patients can be taught daily living and vocational skills to help them attain gainful employment and, in some cases, independence. These programs help the individual adjust to mental illness and develop requisite social and vocational skills. Most programs operate on a daily basis and have individualized objectives. Once the objectives are achieved, the patient is assisted in gaining employment or independence and is provided ongoing support.

CONCLUSION

A continuum of care in mental health offers a range of coordinated services in which to provide patients with the most appropriate level of care, from both a financial and an ideologic point of view. Highly specialized continua may be developed to meet the needs of distinct patient groups. For any continuum to effectively meet the needs of a given patient or patient population, it must provide a broad range of services that differ in intensity, setting, and function. Processes must be in place that ensure access to the full range of services, coordination among services, and efficient movement among appropriate levels of care. The various components of the continuum described here represent the most commonly used or developing programs. Clinical innovation will undoubtedly generate additional components. Although research on the clinical efficacy and cost-effectiveness of services is in its infancy, there will continue to be pressures to decrease utilization of residential services in favor of less costly and less restrictive, nonresidential services.

The challenge to successful implementation of a continuum of care is to provide effective treatment within the various program components and to improve the continuity of care for patients. Unfortunately the different components of the continuum may not be organized in such a manner as to allow the primary clinician to work with the patient throughout all components. Multiple providers can interfere with therapeutic progress. However, with creative strategizing and multiagency collaboration, such problems can be overcome.

Bachrach LL: Continuity of care for chronic mental patients: a conceptual analysis. Am J Psychiatr 1981; 138:1449.

Bachrach LL: Continuity of care and approaches to case management for long-term mentally ill patients. Hosp Community Psychiatry 1993;44:465.

England MJ, Cole RF: Building systems of care for youth with serious mental illness. Hosp Community Psychiatry 1992;43:630.

Lefkovitz PM: The continuum of care in a general hospital setting. Gen Hosp Psychiatry 1995;17:260.

National Association of Psychiatric Health Systems: *The Mental Health Continuum of Care.* National Association of Psychiatric Health Systems, 1993.

Stroul BA, Friedman RM: *A System of Care for Severely Emotionally Disturbed Children and Youth.* CASSP Technical Assistance Center, Georgetown University Child Development Center, 1986.

Stroul BA, Friedman RM: Principles for a system of care. Children Today 1988;17:11.

Stroul BA, Friedman RM: Putting principles into practice. Children Today 1988;17:15.

Section III.
Syndromes and Their Treatments in Adult Psychiatry

Delirium, Dementia, & Amnestic Syndromes

17

Joseph A. Kwentus, MD

In everyday practice, psychiatrists serve as members of medical teams in providing treatment to patients who have delirium, dementia, or other cognitive disorders. More often, psychiatrists see these patients in hospitals, nursing homes, and other institutional settings. A psychiatrist may be the attending physician but usually acts as a consultant to a primary care physician. Psychiatrists help primary care physicians understand the degree to which medical illness contributes to psychiatric symptoms or confusion. Proper treatment of the medical problem may lead to substantial improvement in psychiatric symptoms. Psychotropic medication may be helpful in the management of the patient's illness. Psychiatrists must consider medical diagnoses, treatments, drug interactions, and side effects when they prescribe psychotropics as part of their role on the medical team.

Patients who have cognitive disorders are not usually able to give a reliable history, and the history obtained from third parties usually does not totally reveal the diagnosis. The psychiatrist must rely heavily on data obtained from laboratory tests, electroencephalogram (EEG) findings, and brain imaging. The medical model provides the most appropriate understanding of patient care in cases of delirium and dementia because the medical model stresses a biological etiology for the patient's symptoms. This approach helps the physician establish crucial links between the patient's medical pathology and the psychiatric symptoms. Once links have been established, the psychiatrist can recommend drug therapy and psychotherapy integrated in a comprehensive medical treatment plan.

Delirious patients and patients with the behavioral complications of dementia often require complicated therapeutic regimens. In some older patients, treatment is not well tolerated and may produce cognitive changes. This is particularly true when patients are receiving treatment for medical disorders. The clinician should understand the behavioral side effects of medical therapies. The removal of drugs that cause confusion corrects cognitive deficits in these patients. Psy-

chiatrists may attempt to treat agitation or hallucinations by adding psychotropics. In some cases psychotropics may worsen the patient's condition. Psychiatrists must be prepared to analyze the possibility of multiple drug interactions before launching into psychopharmacotherapy.

Physicians who treat cognitive disorders need to cross the traditional boundaries between psychiatry and neurology. More often than not, older patients have multiple disorders. Delirium, dementia, and affective disorder often coexist. It is the psychiatrist's job to treat depression and other correctable disorders. Simultaneously, the psychiatrist must determine the existence of dementia and establish a prognosis so that patients are not treated inappropriately.

The physician must educate the patient and the family about the nature of the specific illness and the rationale for treatment. Disease processes that cause cognitive deficits may be very complex. Families are often exceedingly anxious because they expect to be forced to accept change in a meaningful relationship. They demand answers. Serious social and financial hardships add to a sense of dread about the future. Most families benefit from a thorough explanation of the patient's condition. Ultimately, the physician must be prepared to explain the contribution made by various disease processes. The physician must know how to deliver bad news so that family members can take proper steps to prepare for the future. In the process, families have a reasonable expectation that the physician will respect the dignity of the patient who experiences cognitive deficits. Whenever possible, the psychiatrist must try to help the family salvage hope and meaning.

THE AGING BRAIN

Although organic mental disorders occur at any age, they are more common in older patients. As the number of elderly people increases, clinicians will more frequently encounter patients who have these disorders. The diagnosis of cognitive disorders is more complex in older patients because physical problems interact with emotional and social troubles in a significant way. This interaction is rendered more complicated because normal aging also brings about distinct cognitive change. The psychiatrist must be familiar with the cognitive changes associated with normal aging before determining the impact of a neurologic illness or a psychiatric disorder. Assessment of these patients requires meticulous attention to the mental status examination. If physicians are not thorough in the cognitive assessment of their geriatric patients, they may miss significant deficits, some of which may be treatable.

Anatomy

Delirium, dementia, and amnestic disorders can develop at any age, but cognitive disorders are more likely to afflict older people than younger people. As a person ages, his or her brain becomes more vulnerable to a variety of insults. The brain's weight and volume attain their maxima by the time the individual is in his or her early teens, but the brain loses both weight and volume as it ages. Gradual shrinkage of the brain has begun by the time that most people reach their 60s. By the 10th decade, the ratio of the brain to the skull cavity has fallen from 93% to 80%. When cortical neurons decrease in number, the cortical ribbon also begins to thin. Large neurons decrease in number whereas the number of small neurons increases.

Normal aging affects the frontal and temporal lobes more than the parietal lobe. The limbic system, the substantia nigra, and the locus coeruleus all exhibit a sizable loss of neurons. Despite the loss of neurons, the aged brain continues to undergo dynamic remodeling. In normal older people, dendrites in the hippocampal regions continue to show plasticity. When dendritic arborization fails, mental powers decline.

The relationship between cognitive functions and the morphologic changes that occur as the brain ages is incompletely understood. The volume of the cerebral ventricles increases with age, but the range of ventricular size is greater in old age than in youth. Increases in the size of ventricles, sulci, and subarachnoid spaces are observed easily with modern imaging techniques.

On a microscopic level, lipofuscin granules collect in neurons of aging brains. Fibrous astrocytes increase in size and number. The hippocampus exhibits granulovacuolar changes. Senile plaques and neurofibrillary tangles may occur in the brains of normal older individuals. The number of plaques and tangles in normal brains is usually less than the number observed in the brains of patients with Alzheimer's disease. The overlap can be difficult to discriminate even after an autopsy. However, some brains of people who have normal cognition have the same number of plaques or tangles as in people who have mild Alzheimer's symptoms. Small infarcts are observed in the brains of many normal older people.

Physiology & Neurotransmitters

Aging brains have a diminished capacity to respond to metabolic stress. The brain's demand for glucose decreases. EEG activity slows. Blood flow declines, and oxygen use diminishes. Glucose metabolism is crucial because it contributes to the synthesis of the neurotransmitters acetylcholine, glutamate, aspartate, gamma amino butyric acid (GABA), and glycine. Effects of slight abnormalities in glucose metabolism are obvious even in the resting state. The senile brain shows impaired transmitter synthesis and reduced transmitter levels.

Acetylcholine has been studied because of its role in memory. Older people exhibit a decrease in the synthesizing enzyme for acetylcholine, choline acetyl transferase. Uptake of circulating choline into the brain decreases with age. Deficits of acetylcholine in the hippocampus may account for age-related decline in short-term memory. In Alzheimer's disease, damage to the ascending cholinergic system plays an important role in the loss of memory and in other cognitive deficits.

Decrease in catecholamines is linked more closely to affective changes than to cognitive changes in older people. There is an age-related loss of noradrenergic cell bodies from the locus coeruleus, but concentrations of noradrenaline appear to remain normal in target areas. In contrast, monoamine oxidase increases whereas tyrosine hydroxylase decreases. Research also suggests reduced serotonergic innervation in the neocortex.

Loss of dopaminergic innervation of the neostriatum is a prominent age-related change that corresponds with the age-related loss of dopaminergic cell bodies from the substantia nigra. Age-related decreases in basal ganglia dopamine make older patients more sensitive to the side effects of neuroleptics. Dopaminergic innervation of the neocortex and the neostriatum are not affected.

Studies of the brains of older patients have revealed a decrease in norepinephrine, serotonin, acetylcholine, and dopamine receptors. A decrease in β-receptor density results in reduced cyclic adenosine monophosphate and decreased adaptability to the external environment. Brain receptors sensitive to hormones such as glucocorticoids, estrogens, and androgens diminish. In contrast, older patients exhibit an increase in benzodiazepine-GABA receptor inhibitory activity and an increased sensitivity to benzodiazepines.

The capacity of mitochondria declines with age. Mitochondrial oxidants may be the chief source of the mitochondrial lesions that accumulate with age. The brain becomes susceptible to injury by free radicals that damage mitochondrial DNA, proteases, and membranes. Free radicals are likely to be a major contributor to cellular and tissue aging.

Cognitive Performance

Changes in cognitive performance related to aging vary greatly. Information processing, particularly verbal speed and working memory, show the most pronounced changes. Older people who possess highly developed cognitive abilities can mask memory defects for a time. After age 70, brain functions and capabilities decline rapidly. Cognitive decline related to aging produces impaired memory, diminished capacity for complex ideas, mental rigidity, cautious responses, and behavioral slowing. Slowing of responses is the most consistent cognitive change. As a result, it takes longer to provide professional services to older people.

Physicians who spend sufficient time testing mental status in older individuals are more likely to obtain accurate results than are physicians who rush through the examination. Given enough time, older people will complete the following tasks accurately: (1) random digits forward, (2) untimed serial arithmetic problems, (3) simple vigilance tests, (4) basic orientation, and (5) immediate memory. Unfamiliar stimuli, complex tasks, and time demands cause trouble for the older person. When older patients are asked to reorganize material (eg, repeating digits backward), they often become anxious. Immediate memory continues to be normal in most patients, but if the memory task calls for split attention or reorganization, older people will have a harder time. Whenever the items to be remembered exceed primary memory capability, seniors show a decrement in memory acquisition and retrieval. Seniors have more difficulty remembering names and objects when they are not in a familiar routine. They do poorly on memory tasks that involve speed, unfamiliar material, or free recall. Although older people have a hard time organizing information, their memory performance improves if they control the rate of presentation. Practice also improves performance. Cognition does not operate in isolation from personality or social relationships. Because learning and memories occur within a range of contexts, a more useful test is one that emphasizes real-life memory.

Seniors usually perceive themselves as less effective than when they were younger, a perception that affects performance. The memory complaints of older adults are often related to low self-confidence or other personality variables. As a result, when seniors experience an increase in self-esteem and motivation their objective performance also improves. Similarly, lack of confidence reduces cognitive expectations even further.

Bartus RT et al: The cholinergic hypothesis of geriatric memory dysfunction. Science 1982;217:408.

Hultsch DF, Dixon RA: Learning and memory in aging. Pages 258–274 in Birren JE, Schaie KW (editors): The *Handbook of the Psychology of Aging.* Academic Press, 1990.

McCartney JR: Physician's assessment of cognitive capacity. Failure to meet the needs of the elderly. Arch Intern Med 1986;146:177.

DELIRIUM

DSM-IV Diagnostic Criteria

Delirium Due to General Medical Condition

A. Disturbance of consciousness (ie, reduced clarity of awareness of the environment) with reduced ability to focus, sustain, or shift attention.
B. A change in cognition (such as memory deficit, disorientation, language disturbance) or the development of a perceptual disturbance that is not better accounted for by a preexisting, established, or evolving dementia.
C. The disturbance develops over a short period of time (usually hours to days) and tends to fluctuate during the course of the day.
D. There is evidence from the history, physical examination, or laboratory findings that the disturbance is caused by the direct physiological consequences of a general medical condition.

Substance Intoxication Delirium

A–C. Same as above
D. There is evidence from the history, physical examination, or laboratory findings of either (1) or (2):
　(1) the symptoms of Criteria A and B developed during substance intoxication
　(2) medication use is etiologically related to the disturbance

Substance Withdrawal Delirium

A–C. Same as above
D. There is evidence from the history, physical examination, or laboratory findings that the symptoms of Criteria A and B developed during, or shortly after, a withdrawal syndrome.

General Considerations

A. Major Etiologic Theories: A variety of conditions lead to delirium. These conditions can be categorized into four major groups: (1) systemic disease secondarily affecting the brain, (2) primary intracranial disease, (3) exogenous toxic agents, and (4) withdrawal from substances of abuse. The *Diagnostic and Statistical Manual of Mental Disorders,* 4th edition (DSM-IV) classifies delirium according to the presumed etiology. If delirium is due to a systemic medical condition or to primary intracranial disease, then the medical cause is listed in the Axis I diagnosis. Substance-induced delirium and substance withdrawal delirium are classified separately. Substance-induced delirium includes delirium caused by toxins and by drugs of abuse. If the etiology is not found, the diagnosis is delirium not otherwise specified. In most clinical situations, delirium is caused by multiple factors.

1. Systemic disease—Delirium can be caused by any type of systemic disease. When a medical condition causes delirium, the primary disease has caused either failure in cerebral blood flow or failure in cerebral metabolism. Cardiac conditions cause delirium by decreasing cerebral perfusion. Patients who have experienced cardiac arrest, cardiogenic shock, hypertension, or heart failure are at risk of delirium. Endocrine and metabolic disturbances affect metabolism. Hyponatremia and hypoglycemia may be the most prevalent causes in this category.

Central nervous system (CNS) causes of delirium include vasculitis, stroke, and seizure. Paraneoplastic phenomena in the brain (eg, limbic encephalitis) may cause altered mental status in cancer patients.

Nutritional status also contributes to delirium; the most notable example is vitamin B_1 deficiency in alcoholic patients. Infections may affect the nervous system directly but more often cause delirium indirectly through toxins. In elderly patients who have generalized sepsis, altered mental status may precede both fever and leukocytosis. Mental status change may be the only manifestation of infection. In at least half the cases, the cause of delirium is multifactorial. Urinary tract infection, low serum albumin, elevated white blood cell count, and proteinuria are among the most significant risk factors. Other risk factors include hyponatremia, hypernatremia, severity of illness, dementia, fever, hypothermia, psychoactive drug use, and azotemia.

No matter what systemic illness causes delirium, the clinical consequences are stereotypical. The diverse insults that cause delirium seem to act by the same metabolic and cellular final pathways. A cascade of pathology in central neurotransmitter systems destabilizes cerebral function. Ultimately, dysfunctional second messenger systems may provide the cellular mechanism of metabolic delirium.

2. Primary intracranial disease—Delirium is a symptom complex that arises from so-called brain failure, which can be caused by lesions in crucial brain centers. Vascular pathology is more likely to cause confusional states if lesions are present in the basal nuclei and thalamus. Right temporoparietal, prefrontal, and ventromedial strokes also predispose to delirium. Lesions in the right inferior parietal lobule also seem to predispose to delirium. In traumatic brain injury, deeper brain lesions are associated with longer periods of delirium. Anteromedial thalamic lesions can also cause a confusional state.

3. Exogenous toxic agents—Delirium due to substances may occur as the result of substance abuse or as an undesirable effect of medical therapies. Patients with delirium may exhibit symptoms suggesting pathology in specific neurotransmitter systems. Delirium that occurs when substance abusers overdose is the best example of a neurotransmitter-specific delirium.

Stimulants act through dopamine and other catecholamine pathways. Stimulant overdoses can cause confusion, seizures, dyskinesia, and psychomotor agitation; however, the most common presentation is that of an agitated paranoid state. Patients with stimulant-induced delirium can be dangerous, to which the saying "speed kills" attests. People who abuse stimulants are involved in violent acts more often than are those who abuse other substances. The dopamine excess observed in stimulant-induced delirium may provide a model to understand delirium in other general medical conditions. The effectiveness of dopa-blocking agents such as haloperidol in the treatment of delirium suggests that excess dopamine relative to acetylcholine may produce delirium in general medical conditions and in stimulant-induced delirium.

D-Lysergic acid diethylamide (LSD) causes a different form of delirium through its action at serotonin receptors. This hallucinogen causes intensification of perceptions, depersonalization, derealization, illusions, hallucinations, and incoordination. Patients with delirium due to medical conditions may also experience illusions and hallucinations. Serotonin systems also may be affected in these patients. Under certain circumstances patients who are taking selective serotonin reuptake inhibitor (SSRI) antidepressants develop the serotonin syndrome, of which delirium can be a prominent feature.

Disruption of pathways served by NMDA receptors induces patients who are intoxicated with phencyclidine to display yet another symptom complex. Phencyclidine overdose is well recognized because of its tendency to produce assaultive behavior, agitation, diminished responsiveness to pain, ataxia, dysarthria, altered body image, and nystagmus. The NMDA receptor is also involved in the biological effects of alcoholism, such as intoxication and delirium tremens. Ethanol-induced upregulation of NMDA receptors may underlie withdrawal seizures. The NMDA receptor also mediates some of the more damaging effects of ischemia during a stroke. Stimulation of NMDA receptors can lead to permanent brain damage. For this reason, conditions that lead to NMDA stimulation should be treated promptly.

Action at brain GABA receptors causes some manifestations of sedative or alcohol overdoses. Sedative intoxication causes slurred speech, incoordination, unsteady gait, nystagmus, and impairment in attention or memory. Some manifestations of hepatic encephalopathy may be the result of excessive stimulation of GABA receptors. Delirium tremens occurs when insufficient stimulation of GABA receptors results from withdrawal from benzodiazepines or alcohol. Treatment with benzodiazepines improves delirium tremens.

Drugs that have anticholinergic properties are very likely to contribute to delirium. In hospitalized patients, symptoms of delirium occur when serum anticholinergic activity is elevated. Total serum anticholinergic activity also helps predict which patients in intensive care units become confused. Symptoms of anticholinergic delirium include agitation, pupil dilation, dry skin, urinary retention, and memory impairment.

Physicians must be cautious when prescribing psychoactive drugs to seniors. One of the most common causes of delirium is iatrogenic. Common agents such as digoxin may induce cognitive dysfunction in older people even when digoxin serum concentrations are therapeutic. In the intensive care unit, antiarrhythmic agents such as lidocaine or mexiletine may cause confusion. Among the narcotics, meperidine is particularly likely to cause confusion and hallucinations. Benzodiazepines, other narcotics, and antihistamines are also frequent contributors to delirium. In psychiatric patients, tricyclic antidepressants (TCAs) and low-potency neuroleptics are frequent contributors. The list of other drugs that may induce confusion is extensive.

The misuse of psychoactive drugs causes as many as 20% of psychogeriatric admissions. The odds of an adverse cognitive response increase as the number of drugs taken rises. Adverse drug reactions are a source of excess morbidity in elderly patients. A high index of suspicion, drug-free trials, and careful monitoring of drug therapy reduce this problem. Occasionally a specific antidote is available for a drug-induced delirium. Physostigmine may reverse anticholinergic delirium and is sometimes useful in treating TCA overdoses. Narcotic-induced delirium can be reversed with naloxone. Flumazenil is an imidazobenzodiazepine that antagonizes the effects of benzodiazepine agonists by competitive interaction at the cerebral receptor. Naloxone and flumazenil have short half-lives and may have to be readministered.

B. Epidemiology: The prevalence of delirium in general hospital patients is 10–30%. Up to 50% of surgical patients become delirious in the postoperative period. Delirium accompanies the terminal stages of many illnesses. It occurs in 25–40% of patients who have cancer and in up to 85% of patients with advanced cancer. Close to 80% of terminal patients will become delirious before they die.

Distinguishing delirium from depression in this population is important because physicians can treat both conditions and improve quality of life for the terminally ill. Many patients today make living wills or assign loved ones a durable power of attorney for health care. By explaining the causes and treatment of delirium to family members, the physician empowers them to decide what is best for the patient.

Age is the most widely identified risk factor for delirium. Patients with dementia are at high risk for delirium. Forty-one percent of dementia patients have delirium on admission to the hospital. Twenty-five percent of patients who are admitted to the hospital with delirium will ultimately be diagnosed as having dementia. The incidence of delirium in nursing homes is also quite high. Because the onset of delirium is more insidious in seniors than in young people, there is an even higher probability that delirium will be overlooked in nursing homes. Illnesses such as unrecognized urinary tract infection may cause delirium. More serious, life-threatening illnesses can also present with delirium. Hospital staff must be trained to recognize delirium at an early stage so that they can identify and promptly treat the primary medical condition. Common causes of delirium in older people include hypoxia, hypoperfusion of the brain, hypoglycemia, hypertensive encephalopathy, intracranial hemorrhage, CNS infection, and toxic-confusional states. Even when delirium is recognized and treated promptly, it predicts future cognitive decline. Many elderly patients who have been delirious never fully recover.

Erkinjuntii T et al: Dementia among medical inpatients. Arch Intern Med 1986;146:1923.

Francis J, Martin D, Kapoor WN: A prospective study of delirium in hospitalized elderly. J Am Med Assoc 1990;263:1097.

Gibson GE et al: The cellular basis of delirium and its relevance to age-related disorders including Alzheimer's disease. Int Psychogeriatr 1991;3:373.

Gleckman R, Hibert D: Afebrile bacteremia. A phenomena in geriatric patients. J Am Med Assoc 1982;248:1478.

Lipowski AJ: Delirium (acute confusional states). J Am Med Assoc 1987;258:1789.

Mach JR Jr. et al: Serum anticholinergic activity in hospitalized older persons with delirium: a preliminary study [see comments]. J Am Geriatr Soc 1995;43:491.

Mesulam MM et al: Acute confusional states with right middle cerebral artery infarction. J Neurol Neurosurg Psychiatry 1976;39:84.

Clinical Findings

A. Basic Evaluation: Although the evaluation of delirium entails the analysis of very straightforward data, physicians often miss the diagnosis. The physician must obtain a careful history, perform a relevant physical examination, conduct a mental status examination, and review the patient's medications and laboratory tests. Physicians who do not conduct a careful physical examination may overlook asterixis, tremors, psychomotor retardation, and other motor manifestations of delirium. An organized mental status examination is the cornerstone of the assessment. The clinician who makes assumptions about the patient's cognitive status will make mistakes. This is particularly true in patients who are apathetic. After the physician has assessed the patient's mental status, he or she should carefully review laboratory data and the patient's medications.

B. Signs & Symptoms: Delirium is associated with the acute failure of the brain. The essential feature of acute brain failure is an alteration in attention associated with disturbed consciousness and cognition. One of the most disconcerting clinical characteristics of delirium is its fluctuating course. Symptoms are ever-changing. The patient's mental status varies from time to time. Cognitive deficits appear suddenly and disappear just as quickly. Patients may be apathetic at one moment yet a short time later be restless, anxious, or irritable. Other patients become agitated and begin hallucinating without apparent change in the underlying medical condition. Waxing and waning of symptoms and perceptual disturbances may reflect the fact that the nondominant cortex is involved.

Common features of delirium include sleep disturbance and decreased consciousness. Delirium may first present as **sundowning** with daytime drowsiness and nighttime insomnia with confusion. As the patient becomes more ill, disorientation and inattention dominate the clinical picture. Nonetheless, consciousness does not always follow the course of the underlying illness. When the patient's sleep is disturbed and his or her affect is labile, delirium usually lasts longer. This cluster of delirious symptoms points to involvement of the brainstem's reticular activating system and ascending pathways. Symptoms usually resolve quickly when the underlying problem is treated, but some degree of confusion can last as long as 1 month after the medical condition has resolved.

C. Psychological Testing: The Mini-Mental Status Exam (MMSE) is often used to quantify cognitive impairment, but only certain items on the MMSE are useful for evaluating delirium. Delirious patients have the most difficulty with calculation, orientation, and memory. Their higher cortical functions and language are usually preserved. The MMSE may be normal in as many as one third of patients with clinical delirium. More specific delirium scales can be helpful. The Confusion Assessment Method is a rapid test designed to be administered by trained non-psychiatrists. The Delirium Rating Scale is a 10-item scale for assessment of delirium severity. One study found that patients whose delirious episode improved within 1 week had much lower Delirium Rating Scale scores at the time of psychiatric consultation than did patients whose delirium lasted more than 1 week. The Trail Making Test (Parts A and B) and clock drawing tests are psychomotor tasks that are sensitive and easy to administer. Unfortunately, these tests measure specific cognitive functions that may not be impaired in some delirious patients. For the busy clinician, the MMSE is the most practical tool; however, clock drawing tests also provide a lot of information in a short amount of time.

D. Laboratory Findings: The delirious patient's vital signs are often abnormal. Common tests that often reveal the etiology of the delirium include complete blood count, sedimentation rate, electrolytes, blood urea nitrogen, glucose, liver function tests, toxic screen, electrocardiogram (ECG), chest X ray, urine analysis, and others. Blood gases or appropriate cultures may be helpful in more complex cases. A computed tomography (CT) scan is sometimes necessary to diagnose structural damage. Prompt lumbar puncture will confirm the diagnosis of suspected intrathecal infection.

Imaging studies are needed when the neurologic examination suggests a focal process or when initial screening tests have not revealed a treatable cause of the delirium. Even in delirious patients without neurologic disorder, CT scans often reveal ventricular dilatation and cortical atrophy. Low attenuation areas are seen in the CT scans of delirious patients. The right-hemisphere association cortex is often involved when some patients who are not paralyzed become delirious, suggesting a predisposing role for structural brain disease in the elderly with delirium. Subarachnoid hemorrhage, subdural hematoma, or right-hemisphere stroke cause early mental status changes. Structural neurologic injury is sometimes the sole reason for delirium.

The EEG is useful in the evaluation of delirium when all other studies have been unrevealing. Generalized slowing is the typical pattern. A normal EEG supports a nonorganic etiology but does not rule out delirium. Confusion and clouding of consciousness correlate partially with EEG slowing. In mild delirium, the dominant posterior rhythm is slowed. In more severe cases, theta and delta rhythms are present throughout all head regions. Quantitative methods of EEG analysis supplement visual assessment in difficult cases. The severity of EEG slowing is correlated with the severity and duration of delirium and with the length of hospital stay. In more severe cases of metabolic or toxic delirium, triphasic waves replace diffuse symmetrical slowing. The appearance of periodic lateralized epileptiform discharges suggests a structural etiology. Rarely, the EEG reveals nonconvulsive status epilepticus as the cause of the delirium. In sedative or alcohol withdrawal, the EEG may show low-voltage fast activity.

Differential Diagnosis

Distinguishing delirium from dementia can be difficult because many clinical findings on mental status examination are similar. According to DSM-IV, the most common differential diagnoses are as follows: whether the patient has dementia rather than delirium; whether he or she has a delirium alone; or whether the patient has a delirium superimposed on preexisting dementia. Regardless, the clinical history is the most important tool in the diagnosis. Delirium is an acute illness. Dementia is longstanding. Physical examination and mental status are also important. Tremor, asterixis, restlessness, and other motor abnormalities are more common in delirium than dementia. Cortical disorders such as dysphasia (language impairment) or apraxia (motor impairment) are not as common in delirium as in dementia. Clinicians should remember, however, that the two conditions often coexist.

Patients who are delirious frequently have altered perceptions. As a result, delirium is sometimes mistaken for a psychosis. It is usually possible to separate delirium from a psychosis because signs of cognitive dysfunction are more common in delirium than in psychotic disorders. The EEG is normal in psychoses. When the laboratory evidence does not support a medical illness, the clinician should consider the possibility of a psychiatric cause. When a psychiatric illness causes symptoms of delirium, patients are said to have a **pseudodelirium.** A history of past psychiatric illness may help clarify whether a patient has delirium or a psychiatric illness with pseudodelirium (eg, a dissociative fugue or trauma state).

In some clinical situations, the boundaries are blurred between delirium and other psychiatric illness. Psychiatric illness causes certain populations to become prone to physical disease. As a result, delirium can be surprisingly prevalent in psychiatric patients. Delirium and depression often coexist in seniors because depressed older patients are prone to become dehydrated and malnourished. Psychiatric patients may misuse prescribed drugs or abuse street drugs. Psychiatrists must be alert for delirium in all psychiatric patients.

Treatment

The correct treatment of delirium entails a search for the underlying causes and an attempt to treat the acute symptoms. Close nursing supervision to protect the patient is essential. Staff should remove all dangerous objects. Brief visits from a familiar person and a supportive environment with television, radio, a calendar, and proper lighting help orient the patient. The physician should review the patient's medications for unnecessary drugs and stop them; he or she should also monitor the patient's electrolyte balance, hydration, and nutrition.

A. Handling Treatment Resistance: When delirious patients become agitated, they may resist treatment, threaten staff, or place themselves in danger. Of equal importance, these patients have elevated circulating catecholamines, which causes an increase in heart rate, blood pressure, and ventilation. Hospital personnel must protect patient rights and apply the least restrictive intervention when dealing with an agitated patient (see Chapter 15). The use of mechanical restraints increases morbidity, especially if the restraints are applied for more than 4 days. A sitter, although expensive, can sometimes obviate the need for physical restraint. Specially designed beds can also reduce the need for restraints. The Health Care Financing Administration has recently introduced strict guidelines for the use of restraints in psychiatric settings.

When other methods fail to control agitated patients, chemical sedation is usually more effective and less dangerous than physical restraint. According to the practice parameters of the Society of Critical Care Medicine, haloperidol is the preferred agent for the treatment of delirium in the critically ill adult. Haloperidol and other high-potency neuroleptics are less likely to produce adverse reactions than are low-potency agents. In emergencies, haloperidol should be administered intravenously for a painless, rapid, and reliable onset of action that occurs in about 11 minutes. The dose regimen can be adjusted every 30 minutes until the patient is under control. For mildly agitated patients, 1–2 mg may suffice. Severely agitated patients may do better with an initial dose of 4 mg. Every 30 minutes the dose is doubled until the patient's behavior is contained. About 80% of patients will respond to less than 20 mg per day of intravenous haloperidol. Although intravenous haloperidol is safe, significant Q-T interval prolongation and torsades de pointes (an atypical rapid ventricular tachycardia) are possible complications of high-dose intravenous haloperidol therapy. Hypotension may occur rarely. Acute dystonic reactions occur in fewer than 1% of patients.

B. Treating Comorbid Anxiety: Patients admitted to the intensive care unit are often anxious and in pain, conditions that make delirium worse. Anxiety and delirium may be difficult to distinguish from one another. The interplay between confusion and anxiety may cause patients to become agitated when they are encouraged to engage in stressful activities such as weaning from mechanical ventilation. Benzodiazepines, if carefully monitored, can help in these situations. If benzodiazepines are given intravenously, they can cause respiratory depression or hypotension; however, this class of drugs can be easily titrated when monitoring is appropriate. As a result, benzodiazepines are effective in the treatment of delirium in many patients. Neuroleptic agents such as haloperidol may act synergistically with benzodiazepines, resulting in control of agitation. The patient's level of consciousness and respiratory drive are usually maintained but should be monitored. Once sedation has been achieved, intermittent administration of a neuroleptic agent in combination with a benzodiazepine can usually maintain control.

C. Managing Side Effects: Physicians need to be aware of the side effects of benzodiazepines. Even when these medications are used as hypnotics, they may cause a decrease in the patient's MMSE score. A variety of factors, including reduction in hepatic metabolism, modify the pharmacokinetics of many benzodiazepines in elderly patients. Lorazepam and oxazepam may be less affected by hepatic factors and are therefore preferred. Midazolam has been used as an intravenous infusion in intensive care settings because it is safe and has a short half-life.

Barbiturates are highly effective sedatives, but they depress the respiratory and cardiovascular systems.

Given the efficacy of benzodiazepines, barbiturates should probably be reserved for agitated patients who have special indications for these drugs. Etomidate and propofol should be avoided for long-term use in agitated patients because of potentially serious side effects.

D. Managing Pain: Pain relief is important. Opiates are the cornerstone of analgesia, but they may also contribute to delirium. In acute settings, opiates with short half-lives are the most efficacious. The Society of Critical Care Medicine recommends morphine; however, the total daily dosage must be monitored carefully in situations in which as-needed dosing is permitted. Naloxone can reverse the effects of a morphine overdose, but the clinician must be aware of the 20 minute half-life of this antagonist. Morphine is contraindicated in patients who have renal failure. Meperidine has been associated with hallucinations and should not be given to delirious patients.

E. Special Considerations: The determination of the effective dosage of sedatives and analgesics in patients who have multiple organ system insufficiency requires careful planning and monitoring. Because the liver and kidney eliminate these drugs, organ system failure usually affects their distributive volume and clearance. The physician must assess the patient's creatinine clearance and liver function. Malnourished patients may have reduced plasma binding. By reducing the size and frequency of doses, the physician can avoid toxic effects. In life-threatening delirium, consultation with the anesthesia service is recommended, and therapeutic paralysis with muscle relaxants and anesthetic agents can be considered.

Prognosis & Course of Illness

Patients who are delirious have longer hospital stays than do lucid patients. About half of all patients with acute organic brain syndrome improve if they receive proper treatment. Of the remainder, half will die and half will prove to have early signs of dementia. The severity of the underlying illness determines whether the delirious person will live or die, and patients with the poorest cognitive status on admission have the poorest long-term outcome. Ideal management requires awareness of the causes of delirium and active preventive efforts. Exceptionally elderly patients and patients with sensory impairment are at highest risk. The alert physician who recognizes systemic illness early and avoids complicated drug regimens can help prevent delirium.

Adams R, Victor M: Delirium and other acute confusional states. In: *Principles of Neurology,* 6th ed. McGraw-Hill, 1996.

Ayd FJ: Intravenous haloperidol-lorazepam therapy for delirium. Drug Ther Newslett 1984;19:33.

Bowen BC et al: MR signal abnormalities in memory disorder and dementia. Am J Roentgenol 1990;154:1285.

Frye MA et al: Continuous droperidol infusion for management of agitated delirium in an intensive care unit. Psychosomatics 1995;36:301.

Inouye SK: The dilemma of delirium: clinical and research controversies regarding diagnosis and evaluation of delirium in hospitalized elderly medical patients. Am J Med 1994;97:278.

Koponen H et al: EEG spectral analysis in delirium. J Nerv Neurosurg Psychiatry 1989;52:980.

Ross CA et al: Delirium: phenomenologic and etiologic subtypes. Int Psychogeriatr 1991;3:135.

Trzepacz PT, Dew MA: Further analyses of the Delirium Rating Scale. Gen Hosp Psychiatry 1995;17:75.

DEMENTIA

General Considerations

Slow evolution of multiple cognitive deficits characterizes dementia. Usually dementia patients have some degree of memory impairment; however, dementia has many presentations. Personality disturbance or impaired information processing may reflect the early stages of a dementing process. Sometimes the clinical syndrome suggests the underlying pathology. Just as often, the presentation may reflect a variety of possible pathologies. DSM-IV categorizes dementias according to presumed etiology, but this categorization will undoubtedly continue to undergo substantial revision because of the explosion of knowledge derived from dementia research. In this chapter, DSM-IV criteria are included wherever possible (see "DSM-IV Diagnostic Criteria" sections, where applicable); however, in some cases alternative classifications better express the growing field of knowledge (see "Essentials of Diagnosis" sections, where applicable).

Evaluation

Clinical diagnosis is ultimately an attempt to deduce the neuropathologic basis of the patient's problem. Most dementias are associated with destruction of large parts of the brain. The autopsy shows whether the damage is the result of degenerative disease, vascular disease, infection, inflammation, tumors, hydrocephalus, or traumatic brain injury. Multiple causes for dementia are often apparent at an autopsy. Because the autopsy comes too late to help the patient or the family, the clinician must be knowledgeable about the pathology that is most likely to be associated with a given clinical presentation.

Clinical diagnosis is based on the patient's history and mental status and on laboratory examination. Several basic tests are recommended in the evaluation of dementia. These include complete blood count with differential, electrolytes, liver function tests, blood urea nitrogen, creatinine, protein, albumin, glucose, vitamin B_{12}, syphilis serology, urine analysis, and thyroid function tests. Optional tests include sedimentation rate, blood gases, folate, HIV screen, heavy metals screen, PET (positron emission tomography) scan, SPECT (single photon emission computed tomography) scan, magnetic resonance imaging (MRI), genetic testing (for apolipoprotein E), cerebrospinal fluid (CSF) tau, and neural thread protein.

Structural brain imaging is sometimes helpful in the initial evaluation of dementia; however, brain imaging is not a routine part of the clinical examination of the dementia patient. Although CT and MRI scans exclude focal disorders in dementia, clinical examination and mental status examination may serve the same practical purpose. Imaging in dementing conditions should be performed only if questions about the patient's presentation suggest that an imaging test is necessary for diagnostic clarification. CT scans rarely add clinical information. MRI is much more useful in distinguishing conditions such as the vascular dementias or normal pressure hydrocephalus.

EEG was previously used more commonly in the evaluation of dementia; however, EEG slowing is difficult to interpret. Intermittent slowing is not related to MRI change or to decline in neuropsychological function. Runs of intermittent slowing increase in frequency with advancing age, but such episodes are brief and infrequent. Focal slow waves sometimes occur in temporal and frontal areas without significance. When any of these changes become prominent, pathology is usually present. Older people in good health may have an average occipital frequency that is a full cycle slower than young adults; however, they do not show EEG dominant frequencies below 8 hertz.

Rarely, dementia evaluation leads to definitive treatment, especially when the dementia has toxic or metabolic etiologies. More commonly the physician establishes a plausible explanation of the clinical findings and suggests palliative care. Because families come to physicians for a diagnosis and a prognosis, the physician's explanation should include statements about what is likely to happen to the patient. The family needs an interpretation of the observed behavior and suggestions about ways to deal with it. The physician gives the family some understanding of what is happening and helps them in planning for future decline in the patient's status. The psychiatrist often manages the troubling behavior that occurs toward the end of many dementing illnesses. The psychiatrist also recognizes the needs of the caregiver and makes suitable suggestions to help the caregiver relinquish part of the burden.

CLINICAL SYNDROMES

DEGENERATIVE DEMENTIAS

Alzheimer's disease, frontal lobe dementias (ie, Pick's disease), and diffuse Lewy body disease are primary degenerative processes occurring within the CNS. These syndromes are progressive and probably represent final common pathways for many different factors. Other degenerative dementias are associated with specific brain diseases such as Huntington's disease or progressive supranuclear palsy.

1. DEMENTIA OF THE ALZHEIMER'S TYPE

Essentials of Diagnosis

The most widely applied criteria for the clinical definition of Alzheimer's disease are those of the National Institute of Neurological and Communicative Disorders and Stroke and those of the Alzheimer's Disease and Related Disorders Association. The diagnosis of probable Alzheimer's disease requires the presence of dementia established by clinical examination, documented by standardized mental status assessment, and confirmed by neuropsychological tests. These tests must demonstrate deficits in two or more areas of cognition, with progressive worsening of memory and other cognitive functions in the absence of delirium. The onset must be between ages 40 and 90 years, and there must be no other brain disease that could account for the clinical observations. Supportive features include family history, specific progressive deficits in cognitive functions, and laboratory data such as PET or SPECT scans.

General Considerations

Alzheimer's disease is the most common form of dementia, accounting for over half of all dementias. Oddly enough, just 25 years ago, many textbooks considered Alzheimer's disease to be rare. Before 1975, a computer search of the medical literature identified fewer than 50 papers that addressed Alzheimer's disease as a key word. By contrast, a recent search revealed 12,718 citations.

Although memory problems dominate the early stages of the disorder, Alzheimer's disease affects cognition, mood, and behavior. Cognitive impairment affects daily life because patients are unable to perform normal everyday tasks. Behavioral manifestations of the disease such as temper outbursts, screaming, agitation, and severe personality changes are more troubling than the cognitive difficulties. No two patients with Alzheimer's disease are exactly alike when it comes to the behavioral manifestations of the disorder. Only recently has this aspect of the disease received substantial attention.

A. Major Etiologic Theories: In general, Alzheimer's disease represents an imbalance between neuronal injury and repair. Factors contributing to injury may include free radical formation, vascular insufficiency, inflammation, head trauma, hypoglycemia, and aggregated β-amyloid protein. Factors contributing to ineffective repair may include the presence of the apolipoprotein E (ApoE) E4 gene, altered synthesis of amyloid precursor protein, hypothyroidism, and estrogen deficit. Some researchers hypothesize that β-amyloid causes chronic inflammation. Others give a more primary role to neurofibrillary tangles. Ultimately, the deficit of key neurotransmitters, such as acetylcholine, produces cognitive symptoms.

Plaques and tangles identify the illness at the microscopic level. Amyloid plaques occur in vast numbers in severe cases. Amyloid plaques were first recognized in 1892. PAS or Congo Red stains identify these structures. β-Amyloid protein, which is concentrated in senile plaques, has been linked to Alzheimer's disease. The β-amyloid protein appears early in the brain in Alzheimer's disease. Some studies suggest that β-amyloid is toxic to mature neurons in the brains of Alzheimer's patients. Neurons in these areas begin to develop neurofibrillary tangles. Amyloid plaques and neurofibrillary tangles gradually accumulate in the frontal, temporal, and parietal lobes. The density of plaques determines postmortem diagnosis. The number of neurons and synapses is reduced. This is particularly true of acetylcholine-cholinergic-containing neurons in the basal nucleus of Meynert, which project to wide areas of the cerebral cortex. PET studies demonstrate a reduction in acetyl-cholinesterase and decreased binding of cholinergic ligands. Hirano bodies and granulovacuolar degeneration occur in the hippocampus and represent further degeneration.

Neocortical neurofibrillary tangles are extremely rare in normal individuals; however, neuropil threads and neurofibrillary tangles appear at the onset of dementia. These intracytoplasmic filaments displace the nucleus and the cellular organelles. Neurofibrillary tangles contain an abnormally phosphorylated protein named tau. The abnormal phosphorylation of tau protein probably causes defective construction of microtubules and neurofilaments. The neurofibrillary tangles in brains affected by Alzheimer's disease abnormally reexpress Alz-50, a protein antigen commonly found in fetal brain neurons. Neural thread protein is present in the long axonal processes that emerge from the nerve cell body and is found in association with neurofibrillary tangles. This protein may be involved in neural repair and regeneration. Neural thread protein can be identified in the CSF of patients with Alzheimer's disease and is the basis of the AD7C test for Alzheimer's disease.

Neurons bearing neurofibrillary tangles often project to brain regions that are rich in senile plaques containing β-amyloid. These plaques are found in areas innervated by cholinergic neurons. Cholinergic neurons in the hippocampus and the basal nucleus of Meynert degenerate early in Alzheimer's disease, causing impairment of cortical and hippocampal neurotransmission and cognitive difficulty. The affected cortical areas become anatomically disconnected. One of the earliest areas to be disconnected is the hippocampus, which explains why memory disorder is one of the early manifestations of Alzheimer's dis-

ease. As time goes on, there is a loss of communication between other cortical zones and subsequent loss of higher cognitive abilities.

These basal forebrain cholinergic projections not only mediate cognitive function but also mediate brain responses to emotionally relevant stimuli. In the late stages of Alzheimer's disease, a wide range of behavioral changes occur, including psychosis, agitation, depression, anxiety, sleep disturbance, appetite change, and altered sexual behavior. These changes are mediated by cholinergic degeneration and by degeneration in other neural systems. Serotonergic neurons and noradrenergic neurons degenerate as the disease progresses. Degeneration of these systems also contributes to some of the later cognitive and behavioral manifestations of the disorder. Because dopaminergic neurons are relatively immune to degeneration in Alzheimer's disease, the performance of well-learned motor behaviors is preserved well into the late stages of the disease.

B. Epidemiology: Alzheimer's disease is the most common type of progressive dementia. This degenerative disease reaches 20% prevalence in 80 year olds and afflicts as many as four million Americans. It is projected to affect eight million by the year 2040. The disease affects women more often than men. The economic impact of Alzheimer's disease has been estimated at approximately $58 billion annually.

C. Genetics: Alzheimer's disease has demonstrated genetic diversity. Chromosome 21 has been implicated for many years because it is well known that patients with Down syndrome are very likely to develop the histologic features of Alzheimer's disease. Genetic mutations usually cause familial early-onset Alzheimer's disease. These mutations are inherited in an autosomal dominant mode. Several mutations of the amyloid precursor protein gene on chromosome 21 have been described. These mutations increase the production of an abnormal amyloid that has been associated with neurotoxicity. Another form of early-onset disease has been localized to a variety of defects on chromosome 14. These mutations are associated with presenilin 1 and account for the majority of familial Alzheimer's cases. A mutation on chromosome 1 is associated with presenilin 2. Both of these mutations also cause increased production of amyloid.

The ApoE E4 allele is associated with the risk of late-onset familial and sporadic forms of Alzheimer's disease. ApoE, a plasma protein involved in the transport of cholesterol, is encoded by a gene on chromosome 19. Disease risk increases in proportion to the number of ApoE E4 alleles. The population that is positive for ApoE E4 has a lower age at onset. The ApoE E2 allele may offer some protection. Although patients with the ApoE E4 allele may be more likely to have Alzheimer's disease, a full diagnostic evaluation including imaging, laboratory tests, and neuropsychological evaluation is still indicated when the clinical situation warrants. It is premature to regard ApoE testing as a screening tool for Alzheimer's disease.

Clinical Findings

A. Signs & Symptoms: A subjective sense of memory loss appears first, followed by loss of memory detail and temporal relationships. All areas of memory function deteriorate including encoding, retrieval, and consolidation. Patients forget landmarks in their lives less often than other events. Agnosia (failure to recognize or identify objects), aphasia (language disturbance), and apraxia occur later; however, a mild amnestic aphasia may be an early finding.

In the early stages of Alzheimer's disease, a subjective memory deficit is difficult to distinguish from benign forgetfulness. Deficits in memory, language, concept formation, and visual spatial praxis evolve slowly. Later, patients with Alzheimer's disease become passive, coarse, and less spontaneous. Some become depressed. Depressed Alzheimer's patients often exhibit degeneration of the locus coeruleus or substantia nigra.

More than half of Alzheimer's patients with mild cognitive impairment present with at least one psychiatric symptom and one third present with two or more symptoms. After the initial stage of the disease, patients enter a stage of global cognitive impairment. Denial replaces anxiety, and cognitive deficits are noticeable to family and friends. In the final stages, patients become aimless, abulic (unable to make decisions), aphasic, and restless. At this stage, abnormal neurologic reflexes, such as the snout, palmomental, and grasp reflexes, are common.

B. Psychological Testing: The clinical assessment and staging of Alzheimer's disease have always been difficult. The MMSE is often used but sometimes seriously underestimates cognitive impairment. The Standardized MMSE has better reliability than the MMSE. The Blessed Dementia Scale uses collateral sources and correlates well with postmortem pathology. The interrater reliability of the Blessed Dementia Scale is low.

The Extended Scale for Dementia is a rating scale designed to distinguish the intellectual function of dementia patients from normal seniors. The Neurobehavioral Cognitive Status Examination (NCSE) is a tool that assesses a patient's cognitive abilities in a short amount of time. This instrument uses independent tests to estimate functioning within five major cognitive ability areas: language, constructions, memory, calculations, and reasoning. The Mattis Dementia Rating Scale (DRS) is useful in staging dementia. Both the NCSE and the DRS are sensitive, but they are more time consuming than the MMSE.

Comprehensive scales combine clinical judgment, objective data, and specific rating criteria. The Reisberg Brief Cognitive Rating Scale and the Global Deterioration Scale are brief comprehensive scales. The Clinical Dementia Rating Scale (CDR) is a more extensive instrument that includes subject interview, collateral interview, brief neuropsychological assessment, and interview impression. Patients with a CDR score of 0.5 are likely to have "very mild" Alzheimer's disease. The CDR has a complicated scoring algorithm and is best reserved for research.

The Alzheimer's Disease Assessment: Cognitive (ADAS COG) and the Behavioral Pathology in Alzheimer's Disease (Behave-AD) instruments are used in clinical drug trials to determine pharmacologic efficacy in cognitive areas or behavioral areas, respectively.

The Consortium to Establish a Registry for Alzheimer's Disease Criteria (CERAD) examination includes general physical and neurologic examinations as well as laboratory tests. Specified neuropsychological tests and a depression scale are also administered.

C. Laboratory Findings & Imaging: Although CT scans reveal atrophy in Alzheimer's patients as a group, atrophy alone does not reliably predict Alzheimer's disease in individual patients. Atrophy can be quantified using appropriate ratios and progresses on serial evaluation, but this information adds little to the patient's clinical care.

MRI region-of-interest techniques reveal reduced brain volume and higher CSF volume in patients with Alzheimer's disease. Alzheimer's disease may be associated with enlarged CSF spaces or atypical signal intensity in the medial temporal lobes. Patients with dementia may show a periventricular "halo" with a smooth margin that correlates with dementia severity. The halo is much more extensive than the periventricular hyperintensity encountered in normal aging. Lesion-brain ratios best express this pathology. These findings infer that advancing Alzheimer's disease is associated with increased brain water. Finally, volumetric studies may show hippocampal sclerosis in the brains of Alzheimer's patients. Hippocampal atrophy may be relatively specific to Alzheimer's disease and may eventually be useful for early detection and differential diagnosis.

^{31}P–nuclear magnetic resonance (NMR) spectroscopy profiles may be helpful in the evaluation of Alzheimer's disease. ^{31}P NMR profiles of Alzheimer's disease patients show elevated ratios of phosphomonoesterase to phosphodiesters in the temporoparietal region.

In the early stage of dementia, functional brain imaging (ie, PET and SPECT scans) is more sensitive than structural brain imaging (ie, MRI and CT scan). PET scans reveal changes in temporoparietal metabolism that differentiate patients with Alzheimer's disease from the normal elderly. PET scans reveal the following abnormalities in Alzheimer's disease: (1) reductions in whole-brain metabolism (paralleling dementia severity), (2) hypometabolism in the association cortex exceeding that in the primary sensorimotor cortex, and (3) metabolic asymmetry in suitable cortical areas accompanying neuropsychological deficits. In Alzheimer's disease metabolic deficits start in the temporoparietal cortex. Frontal metabolism decreases as dementia progresses. Alzheimer's disease spares the primary motor cortex, sensory cortex, and striatum.

SPECT scans can reveal information about regional brain function at a much lower cost and degree of complexity than PET scans, but the spatial resolution is not as good. In more advanced Alzheimer's disease cases, SPECT scans reveal decreased perfusion in the bilateral temporoparietal regions.

EEG abnormalities are not common early in Alzheimer's disease, but they develop as the disease progresses. Diffuse slow wave abnormalities occur first in the left temporal regions and become more frequent and longer as the disease progresses. EEG abnormalities that occur early in dementia suggest a coexisting delirium. Because dementia often presents first in association with delirium, infectious, toxic, or metabolic pathology should be considered.

Evoked potentials are an EEG technology that average many signals following a specific stimulus. In Alzheimer's disease, the auditory P300 amplitude in the posterior parietal regions is suppressed on evoked potential maps. Other studies have not demonstrated clinically useful abnormalities of the P300 component in dementia. Compared to control subjects, Alzheimer's disease patients show longer P100 latencies of pattern-reversal visual evoked potentials. The flash P100 distinguishes them only marginally. The long-latency auditory evoked potential helps differentiate between cortical and subcortical dementias. Patients with subcortical dementias exhibit prolonged latencies.

Differential Diagnosis

Clinicians have traditionally used a battery of laboratory tests to differentiate Alzheimer's disease from a variety of medical conditions that cause memory impairment. These tests include complete blood count, comprehensive metabolic panel, thyroid function tests, vitamin B_{12}, and rapid plasmin reagin. In many cases, a careful history and bedside mental status examination positively establish Alzheimer's disease and distinguish it from other forms of dementia. A detailed drug history is necessary because drugs, especially those with anticholinergic properties, can cause Alzheimer-like symptomatology. A normal neurologic examination is entirely consistent with Alzheimer's disease. Neurologic abnormalities are much more common in other dementing illnesses. The relationship between Alzheimer's disease and depression is complex and is discussed later in this chapter.

Memory loss is common in nondemented seniors. Many of these patients become terrified that they have Alzheimer's disease and seek medical help.

Physicians have difficulty distinguishing normal age-associated memory loss, benign forgetfulness, and early Alzheimer's disease. **Benign senile forgetfulness** is a condition that occurs when effects of aging on memory are greater than expected. Elderly patients with benign forgetfulness forget unimportant details. This contrasts with Alzheimer's patients, who forget events randomly. Seniors who experience benign senile forgetfulness have trouble remembering recent information; typically, Alzheimer's patients have difficulty with recent and remote memory. Benign senile forgetfulness usually qualifies as a mild cognitive impairment in accordance with DSM-IV. The most important aspect of the treatment of benign senile forgetfulness is reassurance, but cognitive retraining can sometimes be helpful. Some of these patients later develop more serious disorders, however.

Although Alzheimer's disease can be diagnosed accurately in clinical settings, inaccuracy of diagnosis continues to plague clinical care. Alzheimer's disease is overdiagnosed. Patients with frontal lobe dementia, Parkinson's disease, diffuse Lewy body disease, or even metabolic conditions mistakenly receive the diagnosis of Alzheimer's disease. Unfortunately, even patients taking multiple medications and those who have delirium may receive the diagnosis of Alzheimer's disease.

Treatment

The aim of pharmacotherapy in Alzheimer's disease is as follows: (1) to prevent the disease in asymptomatic individuals, (2) to alter the natural course of the disease in those already diagnosed, and (3) to enhance patients' cognition and memory. Treatment to enhance memory in Alzheimer's patients has focused on improving cholinergic activity. Cholinergic enhancement can occur through the administration of acetylcholine precursors, choline esterase inhibitors, and combinations of AChE with precursors, muscarinic agonists, nicotinic agonists, or drugs facilitating AChE release.

Early attempts to treat dementia with ergoloid mesylates were of limited benefit. Nevertheless, ergoloid mesylates were more effective than placebo. The dose-response relation suggests that the effective dosage may be higher than currently approved. Unfortunately, the original clinical trial designs were flawed, leaving persistent doubts about their benefit.

Attempts to enhance acetylcholine transmission with precursors such as lecithin and choline failed to show benefits in Alzheimer's disease. Cholinomimetic substances such as arecoline were more successful but have had limited use because of adverse side effects, short half-life, and narrow dose range. Physostigmine, an acetylcholinesterase inhibitor, has limited benefit because of its short half-life and significant side effects.

The first drug approved for use for in Alzheimer's disease is tetrahydroaminoacridine (Tacrine). Tacrine is a centrally acting, noncompetitive inhibitor of acetylcholinesterase that may cause cognitive improvement in patients with mild to moderate Alzheimer's disease. Tacrine acts on peripheral and central acetylcholinesterase. As a result, it also frequently causes adverse side effects, particularly gastrointestinal hyperactivity. Elevation of liver transaminase is another significant side effect. Of the patients who take Tacrine, 25% will experience elevations (up to three times the normal) in alanine amino transferase levels. The Tacrine dosage should be increased gradually from 40 mg/day to 160 mg/day, at 6-week intervals. At these dosages, about 70% of patients experience significant adverse reactions.

Second-generation cholinesterase inhibitors such as donepezil are more specific for CNS acetylcholinesterase than for peripheral acetylcholinesterase. These drugs do not have the limitations associated with Tacrine. Donepezil has the additional advantage of daily dosing. It does not cause significant hepatotoxicity. Rivastigmine is a cholinesterase inhibitor that has a relative specificity for a type of acetylcholinesterase that is present at high concentrations in the brains of patients with Alzheimer's disease. Metrifonate, another cholinesterase inhibitor, produces irreversible inhibition of acetylcholinesterase. The latter two drugs have a greater effect than donepezil but have not been approved by the FDA. They also produce a greater number of side effects. Muscarinic M_1 receptors are relatively intact despite the degeneration of presynaptic cholinergic innervation. Several muscarinic agonists now in clinical trials show promise. Finally, stimulation of nicotinic receptors appears to have a protective effect.

Therapeutic strategies intended to slow progression of Alzheimer's disease have not been very successful. A link between estrogen and Alzheimer's disease has been suggested because the incidence of Alzheimer's disease is reduced in postmenopausal women taking estrogen. Animal studies show that the cholinergic neurons of the basal forebrain contain estrogen; however, the exact mechanism for this reduced incidence has not been established. Nonsteroidal anti-inflammatory drugs also seem to slow the development of the disease. The use of these drugs has been limited by their gastrointestinal side effects. The new Cox II inhibitors may allow practical use of nonsteroidal anti-inflammatory agents for the prevention of Alzheimer's disease. Antioxidants such as vitamin E and selegiline have a beneficial effect. Nicotine has protective properties, but the toxic effect of the drug on other body systems currently precludes its use as treatment. Attempts to treat Alzheimer's disease with nerve growth factor have been limited by the inability of the substance to cross the blood-brain barrier.

Treatments that use an approach based on etiology are not available; however, a transgenic mouse has been developed. Amyloid accumulates in areas of the mouse brain in a manner that is similar to that occurring in the human brain in Alzheimer's disease. This and other animal models may lead to the development of therapies that prevent the disease in individuals who are at risk (eg, drugs that target amyloid production and plaque formation).

Prognosis & Course of Illness

An early-onset form of Alzheimer's disease occurs in some people in their 40s, 50s, or 60s. A prolonged, indolent, subtle deterioration in mental function characterizes the clinical course of illness. From the time of clinical diagnosis the course is variable, but survival is possible up to 20 years from clinical recognition. Early-onset cases tend to progress more rapidly. Ultimately, functional performance declines. The patient's ability to drive becomes impaired, and he or she becomes unable to manage personal finances or to produce a complete meal. Later, impairment of language and inability to recognize familiar people lead to agitation, restlessness, and wandering. Hallucinations and other disruptive behaviors may make management difficult. In the final stages of the disease, the patient is generally mute and completely devoid of comprehension. Death most often results from a comorbid illness such as pneumonia.

American College of Medical Genetics/American Society of Human Genetics Working Group on ApoE and Alzheimer Disease Consensus Statement: Statement on use of apolipoprotein testing for Alzheimer disease. J Am Med Assoc 1995;20:1627.

Chartier-Harlin MC et al: Early onset Alzheimer's disease by mutation at codon 17 of the beta-amyloid precursor protein gene. Nature 1991;353:844.

Cummings JL, Kaufer D: Neuropsychiatric aspects of Alzheimer's disease: the cholinergic hypothesis revisited. Neurology 1996;47:876.

Farlow MR, Evans RM: Pharmacologic treatment of cognition and Alzheimer's dementia. Neurology 1998;51 (Suppl 1):S36.

Schneider LS, Olin JT: Overview of clinical trials of hydergine in dementia. Arch Neurol 1994;51:787.

Roses AD: Apolipoprotein E affects the rate of Alzheimer disease expression: β-amyloid burden is a secondary consequence dependent on APO E genotype and duration of disease. J Neuropathol Exp Neurol 1994;53:429.

Small GW, Leiter F: Neuroimaging for diagnosis of dementia. J Clin Psychiatry 1998;59(Suppl 11):4.

Small GW et al: Diagnosis and treatment of Alzheimer disease and related disorders. Consensus statement of the American Association for Geriatric Psychiatry, the Alzheimer's Association, and the American Geriatrics Society. J Am Med Assoc 1997;278:1363.

Yankner BA et al: Neurotoxicity of a fragment of the amyloid precursor associated with Alzheimer's disease. Science 1989;245:417.

2. DEMENTIA DUE TO PICK'S DISEASE & OTHER FRONTAL LOBE DEMENTIAS

Essentials of Diagnosis

Frontal lobe dementias represent a cluster of related disorders associated with degeneration of the frontal lobe. Personality changes usually precede or overshadow the patient's cognitive problems. Many patients become apathetic and stop caring about hygiene or social involvement. Others become disinhibited or impulsive. Sexual inappropriateness is common. Executive functions such as planning and judgment may also be abnormal in some patients. Alternatively, patients may tend to exhibit anger, irritability, and even mania. In rare cases, the Klüver-Bucy syndrome may develop with hyperorality, hypersexuality, and a compulsion to attend to any visual stimulus. These patients also have impaired visual object recognition. Many frontal lobe dementia patients present with progressive aphasia.

The variety of presentations is the result of the segmental nature of the pathology. Some areas of the frontal lobe may be devastated, whereas adjacent areas may be entirely normal. Therefore, any behavioral syndrome compatible with damage to a specific frontal region is possible.

General Considerations

There is a fundamental lack of understanding of frontal lobe dementias. They represent about 10% of degenerative dementias. About 40% of patients with these disorders have a family history of dementia, which suggests dominantly inherited illness. Other risk factors include electroconvulsive therapy (ECT) and alcoholism. Pick's disease is the most recognized frontal lobe dementia. It is often familial.

Clinical Findings

A. Signs & Symptoms: Frontal lobe dementias are pathologically heterogeneous conditions. In some patients, neuropathologic evaluation shows no specific histopathologic changes. In other patients, frontal lobe dementia occurs simultaneously with lower motor neuron disease as in amyotrophic lateral sclerosis. Frontotemporal dementia associated with parkinsonism is a specific syndrome linked to chromosome 17. Lobar spongiform degeneration accounts for specific symptoms in yet another group of patients. The relationship between the variants of frontal lobe dementia is unclear.

Pick's disease is a form of frontal lobe dementia; however, not all patients with frontal lobe dementia have Pick's cells and bodies (irregularly shaped silver-staining, intracytoplasmic inclusion bodies that displace the nucleus toward the periphery). Despite the absence of Pick's cells and bodies, most patients with frontal lobe dementias exhibit many features in common with Pick's disease. As a result these dementias are often referred to as frontotemporal dementia. A consensus group recently defined three specific types of frontal lobe dementia: (1) frontotemporal dementia, (2) progressive nonfluent aphasia, and (3) semantic aphasia and associative agnosia.

Core features of frontal lobe dementias include insidious onset and gradual progression. There is early decline in social interpersonal conduct. Emotional blunting and apathy also occurs early without insight. There's a marked decline in personal hygiene and significant distractibility and motor impersistence (failure to maintain a motor activity). In the types associated with aphasia, language is affected more significantly than personality.

Personality change, lack of insight, and poor judgment dominate the early stages of frontal lobe dementias. Frontal lobe dementias cause patients to be apathetic when medial frontal damage occurs and disinhibited when basal-frontal dysfunction predominates. Social withdrawal and behavioral disinhibition may precede the onset of dementia by several years. Sometimes memory is impaired, but attention, language, and visuospatial skills are spared.

In patients whose frontal lobe dementia primarily affects frontal language, loss of spontaneity of speech is often the first noticeable symptom. Selective language defects may occur in the absence of significant cognitive decline. In these patients, the clinical picture resembles a progressive aphasia.

Most patients with frontal lobe dementias lack drive and motivation. Others are tactless or insensitive in the early stages of the illness. Some patients develop symptoms of Klüver-Bucy syndrome with hypersexuality and hyperorality, going on later to exhibit perseverative speech, apathy, or stereotyped behavior. The memory disorder of frontal lobe dementias is more prominent concerning recently acquired material. Remote memory remains intact until later in the disease. Behavioral symptoms are usually more prominent in frontal lobe dementias, whereas parietal lobe symptoms such as receptive aphasia and agnosia are less common.

B. Psychological Testing: On psychological testing, patients exhibit features consistent with frontal lobe dysfunction. Useful tests include the Wisconsin Card Sorting Test, the Stroop Test, the FAS test (in which the subject is asked to list words beginning with the letters F, A, and S and the response is timed), the Trail Making Test, and other tests designed to ferret out frontal lobe dysfunction. Some measures of aphasia should also be included in the neuropsychological test battery.

C. Laboratory Findings & Imaging: In classic cases of Pick's disease, the patient's brain exhibits marked atrophy of the frontal and temporal lobes, resulting in a knife-like appearance of the gyri. MRI may show a dramatic frontal pole or temporal pole atrophy that clearly differentiates Pick's and other frontal lobe dementias from the pattern of temporoparietal atrophy seen in Alzheimer's patients. In frontal lobe dementias, the EEG may remain normal despite severe pathology.

PET scans demonstrate that the metabolic profile of Pick's disease is distinct from that of Alzheimer's dementia and vascular dementias (discussed later in this chapter). Pick's disease is associated with bilateral frontal hypometabolism without temporoparietal defects. These findings are not always observed in early Pick's disease. In some patients the findings may be unilateral. In the later stages, functional imaging diagnosis can be more difficult because both Alzheimer's disease and vascular dementias show increasing frontality (ie, frontal lobe deficits). SPECT scans reveal findings similar to PET scans in Pick's disease. SPECT scans may demonstrate decreased frontotemporal perfusion.

At a microscopic level, cell loss is particularly marked in the outer layers of the cortex. Degenerating neurons may have Pick's bodies. The structural changes of Alzheimer's disease, including amyloid plaques and tangles, are entirely lacking. Frontal lobe dementias are not associated with Lewy bodies; however, areas of spongiform degeneration, similar to those found in Creutzfeldt-Jakob disease, may be observed. The pathology is patchy: Some frontal lobe areas remain normal. From a histopathologic point of view, frontal lobe dementia (Pick's disease) is characterized by gliosis, microvacuolation, neuronal atrophy loss, and 40–50% loss of synapses in three superficial cortical laminae of the frontal convexity and anterior temporal cortex. The deeper laminae are little changed.

Differential Diagnosis

Other conditions can present with frontal lobe behaviors and dementia, for example, vascular dementias, normal pressure hydrocephalus, Huntington's disease, and mass lesions. Butterfly gliomas are particularly likely to present with pure frontal lobe behaviors and dementia. Frontal lobe dementias can also be confused with personality disorder, mania, and depression. This is particularly true early in the course of the illness when the cognitive involvement is minimal.

Treatment

Treatment of frontal lobe dementias is limited to psychosocial interventions, such as protecting the patient from his or her indiscretions, and symptomatic psychiatric treatment. At times an associated depression occurs. Treatment of this depression with SSRIs may be helpful. Psychostimulants, such as methylphenidate, may help motivate apathetic patients. Carbamazepine may be helpful for Klüver-Bucy syndrome by reducing the frequency of behaviors. Olanzapine may be helpful when extreme disinhibition occurs. In patients with memory disorder, donepezil may be helpful.

Prognosis & Course of Illness

Frontal lobe dementias have primarily a presenile onset. Progression is quite variable but, generally speaking, slow. Memory functions may be retained until later in the illness. Patients with frontal lobe dementias can later develop motor neuron disease, although the clinical features of motor neuron disease may accompany or occasionally precede the onset of dementia.

Neary D et al: Frontotemporal lobar degeneration: a consensus on clinical diagnostic criteria. Neurology 1998;51: 1546.

3. DIFFUSE LEWY BODY DISEASE

Essentials of Diagnosis

Patients with Lewy body disease demonstrate fluctuating cognitive impairment that affects memory and higher cortical functions. There is both episodic confusion and intervals of lucidity. These patients may present with unexplained delirium. Associated features include visual or auditory hallucinations, mild extrapyramidal signs, or repeated and unexplained falls. Autonomic findings are common, and diffuse Lewy body disease may present as part of Shy-Dragger syndrome. The illness progresses at a variable rate to an end stage of severe dementia. Vascular dementias and other physical illness must be excluded.

General Considerations

The prevalence of diffuse Lewy body disease may have been underestimated in the past because of the difficulty of making the neuropathologic diagnosis. Lewy bodies may occur in the cortex or in subcortical regions. They may also be intermixed with plaques and tangles. When Lewy bodies occur together with the pathology of Alzheimer's disease, the term Lewy body variant of Alzheimer's disease is used. This condition is also referred to as the common form of Lewy body disease. The pure form of Lewy body disease lacks Alzheimer's pathologic features. This form is sometimes referred to as diffuse Lewy body disease. Diffuse Lewy body disease is also a common and important cause of the dementia associated with Parkinson's disease.

A. Epidemiology: The disease represents approximately 15% of dementias seen at autopsy. The age at onset is somewhat earlier than Alzheimer's and shows a greater degree of variability. There is substantial overlap with Alzheimer's disease, and many patients exhibit mixed pathology. The mean age at onset is 68 and at death is 75 years. Men are affected more often than women.

B. Genetics: The ApoE E4 allele is overly represented in patients with Lewy body disease. When it occurs there is a greater likelihood of neurofibrillary tangles. The mutant allele of *CYP2D6B* is a risk factor for both Parkinson's disease and Lewy body disease. This gene encodes an enzyme that is involved in detoxifying environmental toxins. The mutation eliminates the active form of the enzyme. This mutation may fail to inactivate a neurotoxin that has yet to be identified.

Clinical Findings

A. Signs & Symptoms: In the early stages of diffuse Lewy body disease, memory loss, inattention, and difficulty in sustaining a train of thought are characteristic. Psychiatric signs are prominent in many patients with diffuse Lewy body disease and may be the first indication of the disorder. Psychiatric symptoms include personality change, depression, hallucinations, or delusions. Weight loss is common. Extrapyramidal signs are less severe in diffuse Lewy body disease than in Parkinson's disease. Bradykinesia is more common than the tremor. Sometimes extrapyramidal signs are limited to the patient's gait. The anatomic location of the Lewy bodies explains some characteristics of the disorder. Diffuse Lewy body disease affects both cholinergic and dopaminergic systems.

B. Psychological Testing: Patients with diffuse Lewy body disease present with both cortical and subcortical neuropsychological findings. The subcortical features distinguish the condition from Alzheimer's disease. Although not a pure subcortical dementia, diffuse Lewy body disease has prominent subcortical features.

The primary symptoms of subcortical dementias include forgetfulness, slowed thinking, and apathy. In addition, the patient's ability to manage information efficiently is reduced. Executive functions are also diminished. Patients with subcortical dementias are unable to profit from feedback because of poor concentration and inability to maintain set. They have difficulty sequencing and conceptualizing ideas. Another symptom is perseveration. Memory problems and visual spatial disturbances are also common but are not as severe as in Alzheimer's disease. Subcortical dementias differ from Alzheimer's disease in that the former are not associated with aphasia, recognition deficits, and denial of illness.

C. Laboratory Findings & Imaging: The hallmark of diffuse Lewy body disease is extensive Lewy body formation in the neocortex. Lewy bodies are eosinophilic inclusions in the cytoplasm of neurons. They have dense cores surrounded by peripheral halos. The severity of dementia is related to the density of cortical Lewy bodies. Lewy bodies are usually found in the pigmented neurons of the substantia nigra in Parkinson's disease. Cortical Lewy bodies are much easier to overlook. Staining with anti-ubiquitin antibodies simplifies identification and increases the recognition of diffuse Lewy body disease. In contrast, Alz-50 immunoreactivity is small or nonexistent.

The EEG can be helpful in distinguishing between diffuse Lewy body disease and Alzheimer's disease. Diffuse slowing and frontal intermittent delta activity are common in Lewy body disease. Significant slowing and frontal intermittent rhythmic delta are not present in early Alzheimer's disease; however, slowing of the background EEG does occur in vascular dementias. Vascular dementias, particularly those caused by stroke, are likely to demonstrate focal EEG changes consistent with the underlying structural damage. Focal EEG findings are not consistent with either diffuse Lewy body disease or Alzheimer's disease. Even though the EEG may provide useful information, EEG alone cannot reliably differentiate vascular dementias from Alzheimer's disease or diffuse Lewy body disease.

Differential Diagnosis

A noninvasive diagnostic test does not exist for Lewy body disease. The most distinctive feature of the disease is the delirium-like episodes with psychotic features that occur and then remit spontaneously. Diffuse Lewy body disease shares some features with progressive supranuclear palsy, frontotemporal dementia, Parkinson's disease, Alzheimer's disease, and normal pressure hydrocephalus. The dementia caused by the later stages of small vessel disease may also bear a striking resemblance to Lewy body dementia. Late-life psychosis, delirium, syncope, and drug toxicity must also be considered.

Treatment

Because diffuse Lewy body disease affects neocortical dopamine systems, typical neuroleptic treatment of the psychiatric symptoms is usually not successful and can produce significant extrapyramidal side effects. Severe and often fatal neuroleptic sensitivity may occur in some elderly patients with dementia of the Lewy body type. Neuroleptic sensitivity may be manifested as neuroleptic malignant syndrome. Although the typical neuroleptics are not well tolerated, atypical neuroleptics such as olanzapine may produce significant antipsychotic effect without serious side effects.

The response to L-dopa is less dramatic than in other Parkinson's syndromes. Higher doses of L-dopa will often produce psychosis. In contrast, depression is treatable and responds readily to antidepressant agents, often with a corresponding improvement in cognition. Antidepressants that cause orthostasis should be avoided. Some patients may need fludrocortisone to support blood pressure. Donepezil will generally improve memory dysfunction and some behavioral problems, but often it worsens parkinsonian signs. Neuroprotective agents such as vitamin E or selegiline may be tried, but there is no proof of their benefit.

Prognosis & Course of Illness

Diffuse Lewy body disease has quite a variable course but generally progresses more rapidly than Alzheimer's disease. The average time from diagnosis to death is approximately 6 years. The disease often presents as a psychiatric condition because of the strange and complex hallucinations and delusions. The psychiatric symptoms occur much earlier in the course of diffuse Lewy body disease than in Alzheimer's disease. Cardinal features of fully developed Lewy body dementia include delirium, hallucinatory-delusional states, disturbed behavior, akinesia, rigidity, and orthostatic hypotension. Aphasia is notably absent. Although the cognitive impairment is progressive, there is marked daily variability. As the disease progresses, parkinsonian signs become more severe. Involuntary movements, myoclonus, quadriparesis in flexion, and dysphagia (difficulty swallowing) occur in the final stages.

Karla S, Bergeron C, Lang AE: Lewy body disease and dementia. Arch Intern Med 1996;156:487.

McKeith I et al: Neuroleptic sensitivity in patients with senile dementia of Lewy body type [see comments]. Br Med J 1992;305:673.

McKeith I et al: Consensus Guidelines for the Clinical and Pathological Diagnoses of Dementia with Lewy Bodies (Dlb): report of the Consortium on Dlb International Workshop. Neurology 1996;47:1113.

Schmidt ML et al: Epitope map of neurofilament protein domains in cortical and peripheral nervous system Lewy bodies. Am J Pathol 1991;139:53.

4. SUBCORTICAL DEMENTIAS

Essentials of Diagnosis

Patients with subcortical dementias have a diagnosed disorder of deeper brain structures in the presence of a relatively unaffected cerebral cortex. These patients have problems with arousal, attention, mood, motivation, language, and memory. Subcortical dementias may occur in Parkinson's disease, Huntington's disease, progressive supranuclear palsy, cortical basal ganglia degeneration, Hallervorden-Spatz disease, idiopathic basal ganglia calcification, and the spinocerebellar degenerations. Subcortical dementias have also been identified in inflammatory, infectious, vascular, and demyelinating illness.

General Considerations

The concept of subcortical dementias unifies conceptually those conditions affecting the relationship of deeper structures to the cortex. In subcortical dementias, cerebral cortical functioning is relatively intact, but the basal ganglia are dysfunctional or disconnected. Subcortical dementias are not entirely homogeneous entities, and specific features will depend on the pathologic causes. Thus the features of the cognitive disorder observed in Parkinson's disease is not exactly the same as that seen in Huntington's disease or in progressive supranuclear palsy.

A. Major Etiologic Theories: Subcortical dementias involve primarily the thalamus, basal ganglia, and related brainstem nuclei with relative sparing of the cerebral cortex. Patients with basal ganglia disease or with disease affecting basal ganglia frontal circuits develop subcortical dementias.

Parkinson's disease is always associated with neuronal loss in the substantia nigra, leading to destruction of dopaminergic connections to the basal ganglia. As a result, subcortico-cortical pathways function defectively. Striatal dopamine depletion disrupts the normal pattern of basal ganglia function in Parkinson's disease and, consequently, interrupts normal transmission of information through frontostriatal circuitry. Dopaminergic transmission, along the nigrostriatal pathway, may be implicated in sustaining various cognitive and motor processes.

In addition, neuronal loss occurs throughout the CNS. Patients with dementia due to Parkinson's disease have significant cell loss in many other CNS structures, particularly in the basal nucleus of Meynert. The depletion of acetylcholine in the cortex is less severe than in Alzheimer's disease. There is significant damage to the locus coeruleus, secondary loss of cortical norepinephrine, and cell loss in the raphe nucleus leading to serotonin depletion. This may explain the anxiety and depression so commonly associated with Parkinson's disease.

B. Epidemiology: Estimates of the prevalence of dementia in Parkinson's patients depends on the population studied and criteria used. Estimates ranging from 30% to 50% have frequently been reported, but if neuropsychological testing criteria are used, prevalence may reach 90%. The overall prevalence rate of Parkinson's disease with dementia is estimated to be about 40 per 100,000.

The prevalence of Huntington's disease is about six per 100,000. Dementia is a ubiquitous feature of Huntington's disease, but the severity of impairment varies greatly among patients.

There are other degenerative diseases of the basal ganglia frontal circuits that lead to subcortical dementia. Progressive supranuclear palsy, the disease in which subcortical dementia was first described, is less common than Parkinson's disease. Striatonigral degeneration and corticobasal degeneration can also cause subcortical dementia. These entities are more widely recognized with improved diagnostic techniques.

C. Genetics: Huntington's disease has an autosomal dominant mode of inheritance. An excess number of CAG trinucleotide repeats in the 5'-translated region of chromosome 4 causes Huntington's disease. A DNA test can detect the gene before symptoms appear. Virtually 100% of patients with more than 40 repeats of the gene will manifest the disease at some point in their lives; however, the age at which the disease manifests itself is quite variable. Huntington's disease exhibits an earlier onset in successive generations of a pedigree especially when transmitted through the father. There is greater variability of repeat length with paternal transmission, and the gene tends to have ever-increasing CAG repeats. The change in repeat length with paternal transmission is correlated significantly with decreasing age at onset between the father and offspring.

The genetics of progressive supranuclear palsy has recently been clarified. Studies suggest that progressive supranuclear palsy is an autosomal recessive condition that maps to a polymorphism in the tau gene. It has been reported that a genetic variant of tau, known as the A0 allele, was represented excessively in patients with progressive supranuclear palsy in comparison to control subjects. A highly significant overrepresentation of the A0/A0 genotype and a decrease in the frequency of the A0/A3 genotype were found in patients with progressive supranuclear palsy. The presence of the tau A0/A0 genotype is a risk factor for developing the disorder, whereas A3 may be protective.

Hallervorden-Spatz syndrome is a rare, autosomal recessive neurodegenerative disorder in which iron accumulates in the basal ganglia. Extrapyramidal signs are dominant and include dystonia. Mental deterioration occurs as the disease progresses. MRI reveals marked overall low signal from the globus pallidus.

The genetics of Parkinson's disease are extremely complex and reflect the fact that the disorder has multiple etiologies. Overwhelming evidence indicates a role for genetic factors in susceptibility to Parkinson's disease. In addition, it has long been believed that Parkinson's represents an interaction between genetic and environmental factors. A large twin study also suggests that genetic influences are less important in patients with disease beginning after the age of 50 years. In contrast, genetic influences are larger in earlier-onset disease.

Other more purely genetic forms of Parkinson's disease have been identified. The *g209a* mutation in the *alpha-synuclein* gene has been associated with autosomal dominant Parkinson's disease in a family from Contursi, Italy, and in three apparently unrelated Greek families. The g209a mutation is not detected in familial cases of Parkinson's disease in non-Greek or non-Italian populations. Another locus for autosomal dominantly inherited Parkinson's disease has been mapped to chromosome 2p13. Different mutations in the microtubule-associated tau protein gene have been identified in several families with hereditary frontotemporal dementia and parkinsonism (*ftdp-17*) linked to chromosome 17q21–22. Another gene, *Gstp1-1,* expressed in the blood-brain barrier, may influence response to neurotoxins and explain the susceptibility of some people to the parkinsonism-inducing effects of pesticides. The dopamine receptor gene has also been implicated in Parkinson's disease. Autosomal recessive juvenile parkinsonism and early-onset parkinsonism with diurnal fluctuation are other forms of Parkinson's disease with relatively clear genetic causes. Like Parkinson's disease, corticobasal degeneration is a pathologically and clinically heterogeneous disorder with substantial overlap with other neurodegenerative disorders.

General Clinical Findings

In contrast to cortical dementias such as Alzheimer's disease, subcortical dementias are relatively circumscribed syndromes. The principal features of subcortical dementias include slowed mentation, impairment of executive function, recall abnormalities, and visuospatial disturbances. Recall is better than in Alzheimer's disease, and overall memory impairment is not as severe. At each functional stage, patients with subcortical dementias are less intellectually impaired than are patients with Alzheimer's disease. Subcortical dementias do not involve aphasia, agnosia, or apraxia.

Subcortical dementias may constitute a group of partially treatable forms of dementia. Subcortical dementias create a cognitive picture similar to that of major affective disorder. Moreover, if the patient becomes depressed, his or her cognitive abilities are reduced even further. Psychiatric consultation may be obtained to treat depression and apathy. Depression aggravates the memory and language impairments associated with subcortical dementias. Antidepressants may improve cognition in subcortical syndromes. Specific subtypes of cognitive impairment are related directly to the neuropathology of each disease. In progressive supranuclear palsy, behavioral and cognitive changes resemble those associated with lesions of the frontal lobes.

Symptoms of subcortical dementias may respond to psychotropic medication. Mood disorders are extremely common in subcortical dementias and may respond to antidepressants. Sometimes the cognitive deficits improve along with the mood disorder. The response of psychotic symptoms to neuroleptics is more variable. The choice of neuroleptic must be thought out more carefully. Antipsychotics may be required to control psychotic symptoms and agitation; however, many of these patients have associated movement disorders and antipsychotics may affect motor symptoms in either a positive or a negative manner depending on the specific movement disorder.

The dementias associated with Parkinson's disease and Huntington's disease are discussed in detail in the sections that follow.

Dementia Due to Parkinson's Disease

A. Signs & Symptoms: Cognitive changes, particularly mild impairment in memory, executive functions, attention, and information processing, occur early in Parkinson's disease. The time required to make decisions is prolonged. These effects are more noticeable if the primary symptoms are bradykinesia and rigidity. Patients who complain primarily of tremors have fewer cognitive abnormalities. Cognition is worse if the primary motor symptoms are on the left side of the body rather than on the right.

Some Parkinson's patients have only a subcortical dementia. Others are more seriously mentally impaired, and these patients appear to have either cortical Lewy bodies or plaques and tangles, suggesting Alzheimer's disease. These patients also differ from others with the disorder in that they present a more marked severity of the extrapyramidal syndrome with predominant bradykinesia and an earlier deteriorating response to L-dopa treatment. The presence of dysphasia or other cortical deficits early in the course of the illness suggests the presence of coexisting Alzheimer's disease. These patients are also more likely to develop a significant depression early in the course of the illness. In the presence of depression, Parkinson's patients are more likely to develop a cognitive disorder that persists even when the depression is treated.

B. Psychological Testing: Very early in the disease course, Parkinson's patients demonstrate mild impairment on tests sensitive to information processing speed, maintaining set, and visuospatial discrimination. Neuropsychological tests suggest that an underlying perceptual motor deficit exists in Parkinson's disease. Personality changes occur early whereas recall abnormalities and apathy tend to occur later. These subtle cognitive difficulties might underlie the mental inflexibility and rigidity associated with Parkinson's disease and could be attributed to destruction of the ascending dopaminergic and mesocorticolimbic pathway.

Parkinson's patients whose disease develops relatively late in life are prone to develop comorbid dementing illness such as Alzheimer's disease, diffuse Lewy body disease, or vascular dementia. Neuropsychological testing can help determine whether these patients are developing a mixed syndrome, sometimes referred to as Parkinson's plus.

C. Laboratory Findings & Imaging: PET scans using [^{18}F]fluorodeoxyglucose will often show hypofrontality in nondemented Parkinson's patients or in those with mild subcortical dementia. The presence of bilateral temporoparietal deficits in addition to hypofrontality suggests the coexistence of either Lewy body disease or Alzheimer's disease.

PET scans can be used to examine glucose metabolism through the use of [^{18}F]fluorodeoxyglucose and to examine dopamine metabolic patterns through the use of [^{18}F]fluorodopa. [^{11}C]raclopride can be used to examine dopamine D_2 receptor binding. These techniques hold promise for future diagnostic clarification.

In Parkinson's patients, SPECT scans demonstrate decreased frontal lobe blood flow that is more significant on the left side than on the right. Basal ganglia decrements are also visible. These changes appear to be particularly accentuated in the early stages of Parkinson's disease with subcortical dementia.

SPECT binding studies demonstrate decreased basal ganglia binding in demented Parkinson's patients compared to nondemented Parkinson's patients. Bilateral temporoparietal deficits probably indicate concomitant Alzheimer's disease.

NMR spectroscopy indicates an increase in cerebral lactate in patients with Parkinson's disease, especially in those with dementia. Finally, evoked potential studies indicate some difference between Parkinson's patients with and without dementia. Reaction time is prolonged in both groups of patients. The event-related P300 evoked potential is normal in nondemented Parkinson's patients but is prolonged in demented Parkinson's patients. Visual evoked potentials show an increased latency of P100 in demented Parkinson's patients compared to nondemented Parkinson's patients.

Dementia Due to Huntington's Disease

A. Signs & Symptoms: Huntington's disease often has a delayed onset, with a mean age at onset of about 40 years. Progressive cognitive decline is a cardinal feature of Huntington's disease; however, mild deficits in cognitive function are an early finding. Severe mental deterioration is apparent later in the disease. The onset is proportional to the number of CAG repeats in the Huntington's disease allele, although the degree of cognitive deficit is not proportional to the number of CAG repeats but rather to chronicity of the illness.

Huntington's disease usually presents with choreiform movements, but it can present as incipient dementia or depression. As the disease progresses, all patients become demented. The cognitive changes are quite varied, even in the late stages of the illness.

The dementia develops slowly and is consistent with damage to pathways linking the frontal areas to the striatum. Prominent complaints are apathy, slow information processing, and problems in maintaining attention. Difficulty with attention and concentration is more pronounced than in Parkinson's disease. Compared to patients with Alzheimer's disease, those with Huntington's disease have less memory impairment. Cortical symptoms such as aphasia, agnosia, and apraxia are less common in Huntington's than in Alzheimer's disease.

Most patients with Huntington's disease develop prominent psychiatric symptoms. Depression is the most common symptom, but up to 10% of patients have symptoms resembling bipolar disorder. Irritability, personality change, and other behavioral problems are also common. Frontal lobe impairment results in poor judgment that may lead to embarrassing or even illegal activities. A paranoid psychosis is common in Huntington's patients.

B. Psychological Testing: Huntington's patients initially show difficulty with attention tasks. Other early deficits include psychomotor speed and the ability to shift set. Go/no-go tasks are impaired early as are other tasks that require internal cues. Huntington's patients are unable to maintain divided attention and to perform tasks in which multimodal sensory information is provided. When compared to Alzheimer's patients, Huntington's patients demonstrate greater impairment on the initiation/perseveration subscale of the DRS. Alzheimer's patients demonstrate greater impairment on the memory subscale than do Huntington's patients. Constructional praxis becomes apparent at moderate and severe levels of dementia in Huntington's patients but appears relatively early in Alzheimer's patients.

C. Laboratory Findings & Imaging: At autopsy, there is a marked decrease in small cholinergic neurons in the striatum, with low levels of choline acetyl transferase. The disease also damages the small cells containing GABA. Consequently the basal ganglia have decreased concentrations of GABA. Acetylcholine-containing neurons in the basal nucleus of Meynert are preserved. The dopaminergic system is also spared. In Huntington's disease, brain imaging reveals atrophy in the caudate nucleus, reflecting this loss of neurons.

CT scans and MRI show atrophy of the basal ganglia years before the development of symptoms. The putamen is less affected than the caudate. PET scans show striatal hypometabolism in the brains of Huntington's patients early in the course of the disease. Asymptomatic carriers can be identified with 86% sensitivity and 100% specificity. Glucose metabolism decreases at a rate of about 2% per year. Raclopride binding is decreased by about 6% per year and correlates with the number of CAG repeats.

Differential Diagnosis

A. Parkinson's Disease: Parkinson's disease with subcortical dementia must be distinguished first from Parkinson's disease with coexisting Alzheimer's or diffuse Lewy body disease. Functional imaging may help. Other conditions to consider include vascular dementias and other parkinsonian syndromes such as progressive supranuclear palsy.

B. Huntington's Disease: Huntington's disease must be differentiated from other choreiform disorders. The existence of a specific genetic test has aided greatly in diagnosis. The most compelling question of differential diagnosis is whether to perform this test on asymptomatic individuals who have not yet developed the disease.

Treatment

A. Parkinson's Disease: Many medications affect cognition in Parkinson's disease patients. As a rule, anticholinergic medication impairs cognition, whereas dopaminergic medication may mildly enhance it. The dosage of dopaminergic medication is important, because at higher dosages patients may become confused or hallucinate. Standard neuroleptics

may cause significant rigidity in patients with Parkinson's disease or diffuse Lewy body dementia. Atypical neuroleptics are usually preferred in these patients because standard neuroleptics cause extrapyramidal side effects, tardive dyskinesia, and neuroleptic malignant syndrome. Clozapine or quetiapine may be preferred neuroleptics for patients with subcortical dementias because these atypical agents may improve psychotic symptoms without adverse motor effects.

ECT has been used in the management of psychiatric complications in Parkinson's disease. Not only do affective symptoms respond, but motor symptoms improve. Unfortunately patients with dementia due to Parkinson's disease may develop post-ECT delirium. Nonetheless, ECT remains a viable treatment for intractable depression associated with Parkinson's disease. The dosage of antidepressant or number of ECT treatments should be considered together with antiparkinsonian therapies. Demented parkinsonian patients often experience side effects after taking antiparkinsonian medication. As a result, the clinician should be inclined to treat the motor symptoms conservatively in order to minimize cognitive side effects.

B. Huntington's Disease: Patients with Huntington's disease may experience an improvement in chorea from neuroleptics but may concurrently experience cognitive decline. Affective disorder is extremely common in Huntington's patients. Mood-stabilizing agents, particularly lithium, can be helpful. Ten percent of patients become psychotic. Clozapine can be used effectively in psychotic Huntington's patients. Other patients show prominent obsessive-compulsive features. Chlorimipramine may be effective for associated obsessive-compulsive disorder. An interesting finding is that psychiatric illness is increased significantly in patients who are at risk for the disease but in whom later genetic testing reveals the absence of the Huntington's disease gene. This finding emphasizes the need for considerable counseling and social support in this disease.

Prognosis & Course of Illness

A. Parkinson's Disease: Patients with Parkinson's disease who become demented are older, have a longer duration of disease, and a later age at onset than those who do not become demented. Age is the biggest risk factor. The development of dementia is strongly related to the age at which the patient developed motor manifestations. In some patients, cortical Lewy bodies cause the dementia. Although most patients with Parkinson's disease do not have Alzheimer's disease, some Parkinson's patients have dementia that is due to the coexistence of Alzheimer's disease. The dual diagnosis of Parkinson's and Alzheimer's disease is associated with a particularly poor prognosis.

The cognitive deficits evident in early Parkinson's disease do not progress to dementia in all patients. When dementia does develop, the symptoms are quite heterogeneous. Patients with Parkinson's dementia have a great deal of difficulty with tasks that involve visual and spatial orientation. Intellectual ability begins a global decline in Parkinson's disease with dementia, but memory is more severely impaired than are language and other cortical functions. Episodic memory (ie, memory for items relating to date and time) is especially distorted. Although the patient can drive an automobile, decline in spatial memory may make following directions difficult and slowed reaction time makes driving dangerous.

The association between depression and Parkinson's disease has been recognized for more than 150 years. Depression affects up to 50% of Parkinson's patients and is more pronounced during the early stages of the illness. Affective disorder aggravates the poor concentration and impaired information processing associated with Parkinson's disease. The treatment of depression tends to improve some of these cognitive deficiencies.

B. Huntington's Disease: The prognosis of Huntington's disease is universally fatal. The later the onset of Huntington's disease the greater the probability that cognitive decline will be minimal; however, 60% of Huntington's patients develop features typical of subcortical dementia. Initially chorea predominates, but later the patient becomes rigid. Striatal damage progresses at a rate that is determined by the length of the CAG repeat. If the patient is affected by psychiatric illness, particularly affective disorder, there is a high prevalence of suicide. The relationship between the severity of chorea and dementia is robust, particularly regarding memory loss. The degree of cognitive disability is ultimately related to the chronicity of the illness but not to the length of the CAG repeat.

Cummings JL: Depression and Parkinson's disease: a review. Am J Psychiatry 1992;149:443.

Foroud T et al: Cognitive scores in carriers of Huntington's disease gene compared to noncarriers. Ann Neurol 1995;37:657.

Pillon B et al: Severity and specificity of cognitive impairment in Alzheimer's, Huntington's, and Parkinson's diseases and progressive supranuclear palsy. Neurology 1991;41:634.

VASCULAR DEMENTIA

DSM-IV Diagnostic Criteria

A. The development of multiple cognitive deficits manifested by both
   (1) memory impairment (impaired ability to learn new information or to recall previously learned information)
   (2) one (or more) of the following cognitive disturbances:
       (a) aphasia (language disturbance)
       (b) apraxia (impaired ability to carry out motor activities despite intact motor function)
       (c) agnosia (failure to recognize or identify objects despite intact sensory function)
       (d) disturbance in executive functioning (ie, planning, organizing, sequencing, abstracting)
B. The cognitive deficits in Criteria A1 and A2 each cause significant impairment in social or occupational functioning and represent a significant decline from a previous level of functioning.
C. Focal neurological signs and symptoms or laboratory evidence indicative of cerebrovascular disease that are judged to be etiologically related to the disturbance.
D. The deficits do not occur exclusively during the course of a delirium.

Adapted, with permission, from *Diagnostic and Statistical Manual of Mental Disorders,* 4th ed. Copyright 1994 American Psychiatric Association.

Essentials of Diagnosis

Diagnostic subclassifications and the concept of vascular dementia are very much in flux. The Hachinski Scale is used primarily to exclude vascular dementia when studying Alzheimer's disease. The criteria from the National Institute of Neurological Disorders and Stroke and from the European Association Internationale pour la Recherche et l'Enseignement en Neurosciences are more specific in regard to etiology and are more flexible.

General Considerations

Because such a large number of possible etiologic mechanisms exist, the clinical features related to vascular dementia differ from one patient to another. Vascular dementias have many causes: small vessel disease, multi-infarct dementia, strategic strokes, cerebral hypoperfusion, vasculitis, subarachnoid hemorrhage, genetic causes, and cerebral amyloid angiopathy. Recent neuroimaging studies have revealed that vascular dementias may be more common than previously supposed.

Factors leading to cerebrovascular disease that produces a vascular dementia include (1) volume of lesion (eg, one large lesion or several small lesions), (2) number of cerebral injuries, (3) location of cerebral injury (eg, cortical lesions produce a different form of dementia than do subcortical lesions; strokes in strategic locations may produce dementia), (4) white-matter ischemia due to small vessel disease, and (5) co-occurrence of vascular disease and Alzheimer's disease or another dementing process.

Vascular dementias may be more amenable to prevention and treatment than is Alzheimer's disease. Generally, the risk factors for vascular dementias are the same as those for strokes: hypertension, diabetes mellitus, advanced age, male sex, smoking, and cardiac disease.

1. DEMENTIA DUE TO SMALL VESSEL DISEASE

Small vessel disease can cause a subcortical dementia syndrome. Personality and mood changes are frequent. Psychomotor retardation and poor judgment accompany memory deficits. Binswanger's disease is an extreme form of this condition and is characterized by pseudobulbar signs, abulia, and significant mood and behavior change. Binswanger's disease is associated with multiple small areas of hemispheric softening and demyelination. It occurs mainly in hypertensive males. In most cases, there is not only atherosclerosis of the extracranial arteries but also fibrous and muscular thickening of the small vessels.

Clinical Findings

Small vessel disease can cause cortical and subcortical lesions. Imaging studies can identify these lesions, often referred to as leukoariosis, or ischemic deep white-matter disease. Imaging studies identify excessive CNS water caused by damage to the capillaries and postcapillary venules: Collagen is deposited in the media and adventitia and may eventually block the lumen of the arteriole, ultimately affecting the regulation of blood flow in the brain parenchyma. The result is a characteristic pathologic change in the nervous system: rarefaction of the white matter. Anxiety, depression, and overall severity of neuropsychiatric symptoms are associated with white-matter ischemia.

The effects of small vessel disease are synergistic with lacunar infarcts. PET research has shown that reduction in cortical metabolism is related to the severity of subcortical pathology. Pathology in the subcortical nuclei greatly influences the metabolism of the frontal cortex.

2. MULTI-INFARCT DEMENTIA

Lacunar infarcts are small punctate lesions usually found in deep structures. Multiple lacunar strokes or a few larger strokes can lead to multi-infarct dementia. Hypertension is the greatest risk factor. Previous strokes or myocardial infarction often precede dementia. Previous strokes and cortical atrophy predict dementia.

Clinical Findings

Multi-infarct dementia advances in stepwise fashion. The clinical signs and symptoms of the disease are associated with changes in MRI, CT scan, and EEG. The Hachinski Scale is a rating scale based on clinical course and illness features that is intended to assess the probability of multi-infarct dementia. Mean Hachinski ischemic scores of 10 will predict infarcts in 93% of patients. Small, localized strokes in brain areas that are functionally important cause well-recognized conditions such as Weber's or Wallenberg's syndromes; however, these lesions may not cause dementia. In patients with multi-infarct dementia, the deep middle cerebral artery territory supplied by the lenticulostriate branches is most likely to be affected. Bilateral infarcts are very common.

A subcortical dementia can sometimes occur in vascular dementia. Paramedial mesencephalic and diencephalic infarcts cause cognitive and affective disorder closely resembling that associated with subcortical degenerative disorders. In these cases, CT scans or MRI sometimes delineate clinical anatomic relationships that account for specific constituents of the syndrome. The mechanism of dementia resulting from small deep infarctions is not understood. The current theory is that multiple lesions have a cumulative effect on mental function.

3. DEMENTIA DUE TO STRATEGIC STROKES

Strategic single infarcts in particular areas of the brain can cause dementia. Patients who have strokes in the left supramarginal or angular gyrus may develop profound difficulties with comprehension. Strategic strokes in the frontal lobes or in the nondominant parietal lobe can lead to significant reduction in cognitive abilities. One or more strategically placed strokes can therefore lead to dementia. For the most part, these strokes are in the territory of the middle cerebral artery; however, strokes in the anterior or posterior cerebral territories can also cause dementia.

Stroke patients are prone to affective disorder that can affect recovery. With left anterior infarcts, the severity of poststroke depression is linked to frontal pole proximity. Systemic vascular disease, drug therapy, and psychological reactions to disability contribute to poststroke depression. Subcortical atrophy may predispose to the development of poststroke depression. Patients with ventricular enlargement may be more likely than those without atrophy to develop major depression following a left frontal or left basal ganglia lesion. Whereas left-hemisphere injury leads to depression, right-hemisphere lesions and preexisting subcortical atrophy predispose to mania.

Clinical Findings

Each brain hemisphere has a different biochemical response to injury. PET scan findings suggest the biochemical response of the two hemispheres to stroke may be different. Right-hemisphere stroke increases serotonin-receptor binding. This does not occur following comparable left-hemisphere stroke. The lower the serotonin binding within the left hemisphere, the more severe the depression. This finding suggests that the right, not the left, hemisphere produces biochemical "compensation" for damage by increasing serotonin binding in the noninjured regions. After a stroke, depression may be a result of the failure to upregulate serotonin receptors. Nondepressed patients experience less cognitive impairment than do depressed patients. Structural neurologic damage may produce either classic affective disorder or disorders of affective expression and personality that bear little resemblance to classic affective disorder. Stroke patients with depression often respond to antidepressant treatment.

A. Right-Hemisphere Lesions: The expression and understanding of affect are right-hemisphere functions. Evaluation of mood disorders in patients with right-hemisphere damage requires consideration of alterations of affective communication. Depression may be underdiagnosed in patients with right temporoparietal lesions. These patients are often unable to understand nuances of affect. Common cognitive complications of right parietal dysfunction include denial of illness, hemi-inattention (lack of attention to one side of the body), constructional apraxia, and spatial discrimination. Patients with right posterior lesions may not verbally acknowledge depressed feelings. They may appear emotionally flat, or indifferent. A late-onset depression may occur in these patients.

Right frontal lobe damage causes expressive aprosodia (impairment in the normal variations of speech), an inability to express nuances of affect. Affective explosiveness, a temporal lobe function, is preserved. Depressed patients with expressive aprosodia do not appear depressed during a psychiatric interview.

B. Left-Hemisphere Lesions: With left-hemisphere lesions, language impairment complicates the diagnosis of affective disorder. Patients with Broca's aphasia exhibit nonfluent speech, impaired writing, defective naming, and (usually) hemiparesis (one-sided paralysis). Verbal acknowledgment of a depressed mood may be difficult to elicit. In spite of diagnostic difficulties, the incidence of depression in patients with unilateral left frontal lobe damage is striking. The putative mechanism is interruption of catecholamine axons to, and arborization in, the cerebral cortex.

C. Differentiating Frontal Lobe Disorder From Depression: Several characteristics differentiate frontal lobe disorder from depression. Frontal patients are apathetic and not deeply depressed. Frontal personality changes are more dramatic than are those in depression. Frontal lobe systems are responsible for affect modulation. When these systems disconnect from brainstem centers, pseudobulbar affect develops. Patients with pseudobulbar affect express emotions that are minimally connected to either a significant internal feeling state or a cognitive belief. The phrase "emotionally incontinent" is sometimes applied to these patients because of their inability to inhibit emotional expression. Frontal patients often have impaired insight and judgment. They are perseverative concerning some social responses, yet they may be unable to initiate others. As a result, they can appear bizarre in social settings.

Comprehension deficits in patients with posterior aphasia make accurate diagnosis of affective disorder difficult. Clinically, posterior aphasia can resemble either dementia or affective disorder. Speech is fluent and associated neurologic deficits often subtle; however, neologisms and paraphasic errors punctuate the speech of patients with Wernicke's aphasia. In addition, Wernicke's patients exhibit impaired reading, writing, naming, repetition, and comprehension. Patients with left posterior lesions display exaggerated affect because the main remaining vehicle of communication is affective expression. As a result, they often exhibit manic behavior.

Left parietal illness dysfunction can mimic Alzheimer's disease because it produces ideomotor apraxia, right-left disorientation, finger agnosia, amnestic aphasia, dyslexia (inability to read, spell, and write words), dysgraphia (difficulty in writing), and acalculia (inability to do simple arithmetic calculations). Right parietal dysfunction causes left spatial neglect and "dressing apraxia." These patients do not usually have as great a memory impairment as do Alzheimer's disease patients. Some visuospatial disruption attends normal aging. Neuropsychological evaluation distinguishes normal elders from those with parietal disorder or dementia.

Clinical deterioration may occur in brain-disordered patients without a new lesion. Erratic recovery and poor cooperation during rehabilitation suggest affective disorder. Pathologic laughing or crying, depressive propositional language, and perhaps abnormal dexamethasone suppression test suggest depression. Bilateral hemispheric dysfunction may cause excessive crying. Conversely, depression in some brain-injured people may cause pathologic affect.

4. DEMENTIA DUE TO CEREBRAL HYPOPERFUSION OF WATERSHED

Hypotension, decreased volume of body fluids, cardiac arrhythmias, and other causes of hypoperfusion can cause ischemia in the watershed areas between the major sources of cerebral arterial supply. Significant watershed strokes can lead to serious disconnection syndromes. Lesions circling Broca's area cause a transcortical motor aphasia. Transcortical motor aphasia displays elements of Broca's aphasia with intact repetition. Patients with transcortical motor aphasia have decreased speech production (abulia). Mild forms of the disorder can be identified by poor performance on the FAS test and on other frontal lobe tests.

Watershed lesions surrounding Wernicke's area cause transcortical sensory aphasia. This syndrome is similar to Wernicke's aphasia, but repetition remains intact. The most severe form of watershed infarct causes isolation of the speech area. In this condition the entire language apparatus is disconnected from other brain structures. Echolalia is the only form of speech of which the patient is capable.

Disconnection syndromes and the posterior circulation can cause visual agnosia, prosopagnosia (inability to recognize familiar faces), alexia without agraphia, and severe memory disorder. The cumulative effect of these disconnections can lead to dementia.

5. DEMENTIA DUE TO CEREBRAL VASCULITIS

Autoimmune vasculitis can cause dementia. Systemic vasculitis that affects the CNS occurs most often in conjunction with collagen vascular disease (eg, lupus erythematosus). A variety of antiphospholipid antibodies can also be associated with stroke syndromes. CNS vasculitis can occur in isolation (eg, granulomatous angiitis). Infectious diseases such as neurosyphilis and Lyme disease can cause CNS vasculitis, which can be extremely difficult to diagnose but should be considered in the presence of any rapidly progressing dementia.

6. DEMENTIA DUE TO SUBARACHNOID HEMORRHAGE

Subarachnoid hemorrhage causes intense vasospasm, which can lead to significant ischemia. This ischemia can cause a dementing syndrome that persists after the subarachnoid hemorrhage has resolved.

7. DEMENTIA DUE TO CEREBRAL AUTOSOMAL DOMINANT ARTERIOPATHY WITH SUBCORTICAL INFARCTS & LEUKOENCEPHALOPATHY (CADASIL)

CADASIL is an inherited arterial disease of the brain recently mapped to chromosome 19p13.1. Features of the disorder include recurrent subcortical ischemic events, progressive or stepwise subcortical dementia, pseudobulbar palsy, migraine with aura, and severe depressive episodes. Attacks of migraine with aura occur earlier in life than ischemic events. The diagnosis should be considered in patients with recurrent small subcortical infarcts leading to dementia who also have transient ischemic attacks, migraine with aura, and severe depression. Demented patients exhibit frontal, temporal, and basal ganglia deficits on SPECT scans despite the relative absence of focal neurologic findings.

8. DEMENTIA DUE TO CEREBRAL AMYLOID ANGIOPATHY

Cerebral amyloid angiopathy is the term given to a condition in which amyloid is deposited on the walls of small arteries and arterioles, weakening the blood vessels and leading to an increased incidence of intracerebral hemorrhage. Amyloid angiopathy may cause deep white-matter ischemic lesion. The hemorrhages are lobar, may be recurrent, and often occur in patients without hypertension. Cerebral amyloid angiopathy often occurs within the context of Alzheimer's disease and is a cause of mixed vascular-Alzheimer's dementia.

Clinical Findings in Vascular Dementias

A. Signs & Symptoms: See discussions of individual dementias.

B. Psychological Testing: The neuropsychological deficits in vascular dementias tend to be variable and depend on both the underlying pathology and the location of the lesion. Although memory is almost always affected, executive, subcortical, and frontal lobe functions may exhibit significant deterioration. Patients with vascular dementias generally have better language function and better memory than do those with Alzheimer's disease.

Neuropsychological findings in vascular dementias depend heavily on the volume and location of the infarct. Usually multiple forms of vascular pathology contribute concurrently to the overall findings of vascular cognitive impairment.

C. Laboratory Findings & Imaging: A variety of clinical laboratory findings may be indicated in the investigation of vascular dementias. A complete blood count, sedimentation rate, blood glucose, and ECG are obtained routinely. Often a carotid Doppler, transesophageal echocardiography, and Holter monitor (recording ambulatory ECG) add to the investigation. In some cases, coagulation screen, lipid profile, lupus anticoagulant, anticardiolipin antibodies, and autoantibody screens may be necessary. Cerebral angiography may be necessary to diagnose cerebral vasculitis but is not routinely obtained. If an infection or inflammation is suspected, then a spinal tap may be helpful.

MRI is the most helpful radiologic tool in the diagnosis of vascular dementias, but CT scans may be helpful in some cases. Patchy diffuse white-matter lucency on CT scan or hyperintensity on MRI suggests leukoariosis. Normal scans may show lesions that are punctate or partially confluent. The aging brain becomes susceptible to an assortment of changes in the periventricular and subcortical white matter. These changes are radiolucent on CT scans and hyperintense on T2-weighted MRI. White-matter changes are common in patients with chronic hypertension. Examination of affected tissues reveals dilated perivascular (Virchow-Robin) spaces, mild demyelination, gliosis, and diffuse neuropil vacuolation. The associated clinical abnormalities are usually not serious, but defects of attention, mental processing speed, and psychomotor control may be evident, although usually only through neuropsychological testing. As a result, significant overlap occurs between the scans of normal patients and those who have clinically significant vascular disease. These changes also appear in early Alzheimer's disease, making the interpretation of early disease more difficult. Leukoariosis is associated with increased age, hypertension, limb weakness, and extensor-plantar responses. Some patients have extensive deep white-matter brain lesions without detriment to cognitive, behavioral, or neurologic functioning.

Pathology becomes evident when periventricular capping and plaque-like hyperintensities become confluent. For example, the diagnosis of Binswanger's disease can be made readily based on T2-weighted MRI. Lesions that distinguish patients with vascular dementias include lacunar infarction, irregular periventricular hyperintensities extending into the deep white matter, and large confluent areas of deep white-matter hyperintensity. These abnormalities are associated with extensive arteriosclerosis, diffuse white-matter rarefication, and even necrosis. In contrast, the hyperintensities associated with Alzheimer's disease are punctate or smooth and halo-like.

A relationship exists between the extent of MRI abnormality and dementia, but because the pathology of dementia is usually multifactorial, the relationship between MRI findings and dementia is relatively loose. MRI abnormality is also related to the patient's history of hypertension; however, the associated clinical signs are variable, and one third of patients have no neurologic deficit. In CADASIL, MRI reveals prominent signal abnormalities in the subcortical white matter and basal ganglia. Cognitive impairment is linked to signal abnormalities and hypoperfusion in the basal ganglia.

^{31}P NMR spectroscopy profiles may be helpful in the evaluation of vascular dementias. Patients with vascular dementias exhibit elevations of the phosphocreatine/inorganic orthophosphate ratio in temporoparietal and frontal regions.

PET scans may be helpful in diagnosing vascular dementias. They may demonstrate focal areas of hypometabolism that correspond roughly to areas of impairment discovered on neuropsychological testing. Hypometabolism, even without atrophy, is visible on anatomic images. Areas of hypometabolism seen on PET scans conform to cortical high-signal intensity on MRI. In addition, cerebral metabolism is reduced globally because isolated lesions have extensive and distant metabolic effects. The pattern of hypometabolism observed in vascular dementias is distinct from that observed in Alzheimer's disease. Vascular dementias are associated with multiple defects in the cortex, deep nuclei, subcortical white matter, and cerebellum. Dementia increases as global and frontal hypometabolism evolve. Consequently, PET scans detect more widespread brain involvement than does structural imaging. SPECT scans of patients with vascular dementias show varying degrees of irregular uptake in the cerebral cortex, similar to that seen in PET scans. In SPECT studies of individuals affected with CADASIL, cerebral blood flow reduction matched with MRI signal abnormalities.

EEG often shows focal slowing corresponding to areas of cerebral ischemia or infarction. These areas of slowing may be demonstrated visually on EEG brain maps. Computer-analyzed EEGs use mathematical formulas to break the EEG into power distributions across frequencies. This technique reveals decreased alpha power and increased theta power and delta power that parallel the degree of dementia. The ratio of high-frequency to low-frequency electrical activity in the left temporal region is decreased. Compared to Alzheimer's disease, vascular dementias are associated with lower EEG frequency and reduced synchronization. Somatosensory evoked potentials show prolonged central conduction time and a reduction of the primary cortical response amplitude in multi-infarct dementia but not in Alzheimer's disease.

Treatment

Prevention is important in vascular dementias. Control of hypertension is probably the single most important preventive measure; however, caution must be taken not to lower the blood pressure too much and thus cause hypoperfusion. Control of diabetes and abstinence from cigarettes are also important. Treatment of atrial fibrillation can prevent embolic strokes. Although anticoagulants are highly effective for preventing cardioembolic strokes, their effectiveness in noncardioembolic strokes is uncertain. Diagnosis and surgical treatment of carotid disease is also important.

Daily aspirin stabilizes cerebral perfusion and cognition in vascular dementias. Ticlopidine is the most effective antiplatelet agent and may ultimately be useful in treating a variety of vascular dementias. The side effects of ticlopidine currently restrict its use. Pentoxifylline has been tested but has demonstrated limited efficacy. In cases of either systemic or cerebral vasculitis, high-dose corticosteroids may prevent further cognitive loss.

Prognosis & Course of Illness

Vascular dementias shorten life expectancy. Three-year mortality is almost three times greater in the very elderly than in age-matched controls. About one third of patients die from dementia itself; the others die from cerebral vascular disease, cardiac disease, or other, unrelated conditions.

Chabriat H et al: Clinical spectrum of CADASIL: a study of 7 families. Cerebral autosomal dominant arteriopathy with subcortical infarcts and leukoencephalopathy [see comments]. Lancet 1995;346:934.

Robinson RG, Starkstein SE: Mood disorders following stroke: new findings and future directions. J Geriatr Psychiatry 1989;22:1.

Roman GC et al: Vascular dementia: diagnostic criteria for research studies. Report of the NINDS-AIREN International Workshop. Neurology 1993;43:250.

Verhey FRJ et al: Comparison of seven sets of criteria used for the diagnosis of vascular dementia. Neuroepidemiology 1996;15:166.

Zhang WW et al: Structural and vasoactive factors influencing intracerebral arterioles in cases of vascular dementia and other cerebrovascular disease: a review. Immunohistochemical studies on expression of collagens, basal lamina components and endothelin-1. Dementia 1994;5:153.

DEMENTIA DUE TO CEREBRAL INFECTION & INFLAMMATION

Essentials of Diagnosis

Infectious processes can cause a sustained, progressive loss of intellectual function. The diagnosis of dementia due to cerebral infection or inflammation is made when the infectious process can be established as a causal agent of the dementia.

General Considerations

Neurosyphilis is the classic dementia due to an infectious process. More recently, the AIDS dementia complex has become the most common form of infectious dementia. Other viral causes of dementia include herpes simplex, progressive multifocal leukoencephalopathy, and subacute sclerosing panencephalitis. Any severe encephalitis can cause a subsequent dementia. Creutzfeldt-Jakob disease is an uncommon cause of rapidly developing dementia caused by a prion, a novel infectious entity that may be present for many years and then suddenly produces a spongiform encephalopathy.

1. DEMENTIA DUE TO HIV DISEASE, OPPORTUNISTIC INFECTION, OR MULTIFOCAL LEUKOENCEPHALOPATHY

Dementia due to HIV disease is often referred to as the AIDS dementia complex, which eventually affects about 15% of AIDS patients.

Clinical Findings

A. Signs & Symptoms: Early in HIV infection, patients are likely to experience an acute encephalitis or aseptic meningitis. In HIV-infected patients, impaired memory and reduced psychomotor speed are more common than is global intellectual deterioration. HIV-induced neuropsychological impairment does not correlate with subjective complaints, neurologic signs, reduced T4 lymphocytes, CSF abnormalities, EEG slowing, atrophy on brain CT scan, or nonspecific hyperintensities on brain MRI. Dementia, cancer of the CNS, and opportunistic infection present later in HIV infection.

AIDS dementia complex is characterized by a clinical triad of progressive cognitive decline, motor dysfunction, and behavioral abnormality. Early symptoms include memory difficulty and psychomotor slowing.

Behavioral symptoms include apathy and social withdrawal. It can be difficult to distinguish the AIDS dementia complex from depression. Eventually, cognitive and motor impairment progresses, leading in the final stages to global dementia and paraplegia. Although the AIDS dementia complex may present at any stage of HIV infection, it usually appears relatively late in the course of the disease. The mean survival time in patients with AIDS dementia complex was 7 months before the introduction of protease inhibitors.

B. Psychological Testing: Patients with the AIDS dementia complex have a neuropsychological profile consisting of decreased motor speed, decreased memory, and failure on frontal lobe tasks. The HIV Dementia Scale tests specific abilities including timed motor tasks, frontal lobe function, and memory. The test is easy to administer and may be used to follow the patient's progress and his or her response to treatment. Physical findings in the HIV dementia complex include hyperreflexia and hypertonia.

C. Laboratory Findings & Imaging: The AIDS dementia complex has a variable relationship to HIV infection. HIV probably enters the CNS through macrophages that cross the blood-brain barrier. These macrophages infect microglia. In the AIDS dementia complex, the HIV virus can be detected in macrophage- and glial-activated cells in the white matter and deep gray matter. Activated macrophages and microglia probably cause dementia through the secretion of neurotoxins that cause neuronal depopulation and a loss of dendritic arborization. The most common neuropathologic finding is a diffuse destruction of white matter and subcortical gray matter.

Sixty percent of patients show a slightly elevated spinal fluid protein. There may also be an elevated IgG fraction and oligoclonal bands. CSF lymphocytosis may occur; the CD4/CD8 ratio mirrors that of the peripheral blood. HIV can usually be isolated directly from the CSF.

Brain imaging is essential in the evaluation of patients with the AIDS dementia complex because infection with the human immunodeficiency virus-type 1 (HIV-1) predisposes the individual to a number of opportunistic CNS infections and tumors. In order to diagnose the AIDS dementia complex, the clinician must exclude these opportunistic infections, including progressive multifocal leukoencephalopathy, toxoplasmosis, tuberculosis, and cryptococcosis. On MRI and CT scans, the brains of patients with the AIDS dementia complex demonstrate atrophy. MRI shows scattered white-matter abnormalities.

Differential Diagnosis

Diagnostic uncertainty may exist in severe cases. Progressive multifocal leukoencephalopathy produces focal white-matter abnormalities due to multiple foci of demyelination. Radionucleotide brain imaging techniques help to distinguish opportunistic infections from intracerebral lymphoma.

Treatment

The most effective therapy is to reduce the number of viruses with antiretroviral agents such as 3′-azido-3′deoxythymidine (AZT). AZT can improve the mental function of HIV-infected patients. If AZT therapy is not initially effective, the dosage can be increased to the patient's ability to tolerate side effects or another antiviral agent can be added. Protease inhibitors would be expected to have a similar effect. Psychostimulants have been reported to provide symptomatic relief in some patients.

Prognosis & Course of Illness

In the early stages of the illness, the AIDS patient experiences forgetfulness, lapses in concentration, and social withdrawal. Cognitive and motor slowing are prominent. The memory problem is mild compared to that observed in Alzheimer's disease. Patients retain a relatively good sense of self-awareness and rarely experience the denial of illness that often occurs in other dementias. As the disease progresses patients become unable to perform activities of daily living. Motor function appears to be affected simultaneously. Patients become unable to walk or require a walker and personal assistance. In the final stages of the disease, patients are nearly vegetative.

2. DEMENTIA DUE TO OTHER VIRUSES

Herpes simplex encephalitis damages the temporal lobes. The disease can present initially with confusion or psychiatric symptomatology. Later the patient develops a severe headache and confusion. MRI and CSF examination are helpful for early diagnosis. A specific EEG pattern is associated with the disorder. Early recognition is essential so that antiviral therapy can be initiated. If the disease progresses, the patient may be left with rather severe deficits. Klüver-Bucy syndrome, an amnestic syndrome, or global dementia are common residuals of herpetic encephalitis.

Progressive multifocal leukoencephalopathy generally occurs in older immunocompromised patients. It may also occur in the later stages of AIDS. This disorder proceeds extremely rapidly, and death usually occurs within months. Subacute sclerosing panencephalitis is a rare disease of late childhood caused by measles virus. It has become even more rare since measles vaccine was introduced. Sporadic encephalitis is another uncommon cause of dementia.

3. DEMENTIA DUE TO NEUROSYPHILIS

Neurosyphilis, caused by the virus *Treponema pallidum,* is an infrequent cause of dementia. Neurosyphilis presents as a vascular occlusive disease. The meninges may appear thickened and inflamed. Neuroimaging may show infarction, arteritis, cortical lesions, or meningeal enhancement. The basal areas of the brain are preferentially affected leading to frontal and temporal lobe dysfunction.

Clinical Findings

A. Signs & Symptoms: Neurosyphilis frequently causes psychiatric symptoms such as labile affect, depression, or mania. Patients are usually moderately demented but experience a preponderance of personality disturbances. Although the Argyll Robertson pupil (ie, the pupil accommodates but does not react to light) is observed occasionally, many patients are demented without exhibiting this sign. Tabes dorsalis is an associated finding in some patients.

B. Laboratory Findings: A variety of screening tests are used to establish the possibility of syphilitic infection. Once the possibility of infection is established, a spinal tap is indicated. The diagnosis of neurosyphilis is made by performing the Venereal Disease Research Laboratory (VDRL) test on the patient's CSF.

Treatment

The principal mode of treatment for neurosyphilis is intravenous penicillin. The decision to retreat a patient who has already had a course of penicillin is difficult to make and is usually based on the patient's clinical response, CSF cell count, and protein concentration. Even after successful treatment of the infection, the patient may continue to have significant difficulties. VDRL titer may be an indicator of continued *T. pallidum* activity in patients without obvious clinical deterioration.

Prognosis & Course of Illness

Neurosyphilis can occur decades after the original infection. It is not uncommon for an elderly woman to present with this disorder, having been infected many years earlier by her spouse. Early symptoms include fatigue, personality change, and forgetfulness. Neurosyphilis is a great imitator and can produce almost any psychiatric or cognitive disorder. Late in the disease the patient becomes confused and disoriented. Myoclonus, seizures, and dysarthria are common.

4. DEMENTIA DUE TO LYME DISEASE

Lyme disease is a multisystemic illness that can affect the CNS, causing neurologic and psychiatric symptoms. It is caused by the spirochete *Borrelia burgdorferi,* which enters the host after a bite by a deer tick.

Clinical Findings

Lyme disease may involve either the peripheral or the central nervous system. Dissemination to the CNS can occur within the first few weeks after skin infection. Like syphilis, Lyme disease may have a latency period of months to years before symptoms of late infection emerge. A broad range of psychiatric reactions have been associated with Lyme disease including dementia, psychosis, and depression.

5. DEMENTIA DUE TO CREUTZFELDT-JAKOB DISEASE

An unusual infectious agent, known as a prion, leads to Creutzfeldt-Jakob disease, a condition associated with a rapidly progressive dementia. There are three forms of Creutzfeldt-Jakob disease: infectious, sporadic, and inherited. Until recently, the infectious variety was usually iatrogenic; however, the addition of sheep brain to cow feed in Britain has led to an outbreak of the disease among beefeaters in Britain (so-called mad-cow disease).

Clinical Findings

A. Signs & Symptoms: The majority of patients who present with dementia exhibit myoclonus and pyramidal signs. Although most cases are sporadic, 10–15% are familial. Gerstmann-Straussler syndrome is a rare familial dementia caused by a prion and related to Creutzfeldt-Jakob syndrome. It resembles olivopontocerebellar degeneration. Spongiform encephalopathy accompanies both Gerstmann-Straussler syndrome and Creutzfeldt-Jakob disease. Mutation in the prion protein (PrP) gene occurs in Gerstmann-Straussler syndrome. Fatal familial insomnia is another rare inherited dementia caused by the prion. Patients with this disorder experience a complete lack of sleep in the year or two prior to death. PrP gene analysis is potentially useful for diagnosis and genetic counseling.

B. Laboratory Findings: Creutzfeldt-Jakob disease is the only dementia that can be distinguished by characteristic electrical patterns. EEG shows triphasic bursts, sometimes correlating with myoclonic jerks. PrP genetic analysis can be helpful in some cases of prion disease.

Prognosis & Course of Illness

Prion disease is uniformly fatal. The time between diagnosis and death is generally less than 2 years. There are no treatments. Because the disease has been transmitted through careless production and processing of meat, primary prevention is possible.

Navia BA, Cho ES, Petito RW: The AIDS dementia complex: II. Neuropathology. Ann Neurol 1986;19:517.
Price RW: Management of AIDS dementia complex and HIV-1 brain infection. Clinical-virological correlations. Ann Neurol 1995;38:563.
Prusiner SB: Genetic and infectious prion diseases. Arch Neurol 1993;50:1129.

DEMENTIA DUE TO OTHER GENERAL MEDICAL CONDITIONS

Metabolic causes of dementia include dialysis dementia, repeated episodes of diabetic hypoglycemia, prolonged hepatic encephalopathy, hypothyroidism, and hypoxia. Many diseases can cause dementia in older people, for example, pernicious anemia, thyroid disorder, systemic infection, collagen disease, brain hypoxia, and toxic exposure.

Vitamin B_{12} deficiency causes subacute combined degeneration. Subacute combined degeneration causes demyelination in the posterior columns and loss of pyramidal cells in the motor strip. Often a peripheral neuropathy is present. Slow information processing, confusion, memory changes, delirium, hallucinations, delusions, depression, and psychosis have been observed in patients with vitamin B_{12} deficiency. Anemia is not necessary for the syndrome to develop. Sometimes a familial pattern occurs. Anti-parietal-cell antibodies are often present. Current state-of-the-art testing uses serum cobalamin levels as a screening test and serum or urine homocysteine and methylmalonic acid determinations as confirmatory tests. Homocysteine abnormalities are associated with neurologic deficits and psychiatric symptomatology. A Schilling test follows the patient's vitamin B_{12} level to help determine etiology.

Depression and dementia respond rapidly to the administration of vitamin B_{12} when the condition is diagnosed in its early stages. Vitamin B_{12} deficiency is treatable with monthly injections, daily oral supplements, or an intranasal gel. If the condition is not diagnosed in the early stages, neurologic, psychiatric, and cognitive impairment may persist and be irreversible. The prevalence of low cobalamin levels is significantly increased in Alzheimer's disease. Alzheimer's disease may be associated with alterations in brain transmethylation mechanisms. Unfortunately, vitamin B_{12} supplementation rarely leads to much improvement in primary dementia. Contrary to widely accepted beliefs, subnormal serum vitamin B_{12} levels are a rare cause of reversible dementia.

Older people frequently have mildly decreased thyroid function. This does not cause an irreversible dementia. In some people, hypothyroidism exacerbates a depression. Thyroid deficiency can also hasten a severe melancholic depression that causes a patient to appear demented. Consequently, thyroid function tests (including thyroid stimulating hormone level) should be obtained. On exceedingly rare occasions, hyperthyroidism or hypothyroidism cause a delirium that can be mistaken for dementia. Patients with vascular dementias often have hypothyroidism. The reason for this association is unclear, but thyroid replacement can improve the performance of patients who have this condition.

Patients who are undergoing dialysis may experience impaired mental functioning that can be secondary to a parathyroid hormone abnormality and its effect on calcium metabolism. Patients who have been on dialysis for extended periods may experience a general decline in intellectual function that is usually mild. True dialysis dementia has become rare since aluminum was eliminated from the dialysate.

Many toxins can cause dementia. Organic solvents inhaled in the workplace cause cognitive deficits. Organic solvents can occasionally cause dementia when used as intoxicants. Carbon monoxide is another common toxin that affects mental function. Heavy metals are yet another cause of toxic brain damage. Appropriate history, physical examination, and toxicology evaluation are necessary for the diagnosis of dementia due to toxins.

Dementia can be caused by the direct or indirect effect of cancer. Patients with cancer develop dementia as a result of intracranial tumors, cerebral metastases, carcinomatous meningitis, progressive multifocal leukoencephalitis, opportunistic infections, and paraneoplastic effects. Tumors can lead to noncommunicating hydrocephalus by obstructing the outflow of CSF. Some patients develop progressive dementia as a complication of whole-brain radiotherapy.

1. DEMENTIA DUE TO NORMAL PRESSURE HYDROCEPHALUS

Essentials of Diagnosis

Normal pressure hydrocephalus causes a relatively distinct syndrome consisting of gait apraxia, urinary incontinence, and dementia. Normal pressure hydrocephalus may be idiopathic, but it may follow a subarachnoid hemorrhage, meningitis, or other entity that can cause altered spinal fluid dynamics.

General Considerations

A. Major Etiologic Theories: Normal pressure hydrocephalus occurs when the arachnoid villi are not able to reabsorb CSF as rapidly as the choroid plexus produces it. Sometimes, normal pressure hydrocephalus follows subarachnoid hemorrhage, meningitis, or head trauma. In these cases, it is assumed that the arachnoid villi have become obstructed with blood or other proteinaceous material, forcing the CSF to be reabsorbed through the ventricles.

B. Epidemiology: Normal pressure hydrocephalus is the most common type of hydrocephalus diagnosed in people over age 60 years.

Clinical Findings

The clinical diagnosis of hydrocephalus as a cause of dementia is confusing because many conditions can cause similar symptoms. Nonetheless, a timely diagnosis is important because dementia caused by normal pressure hydrocephalus can sometimes be reversed if the diagnosis is made early enough.

A. Signs & Symptoms: The patient presents the classic triad of dementia, incontinence, and gait disturbance. The dementia develops at a rapid pace. The patient's gait becomes magnetic in quality, and he or she is likely to experience frequent falls.

B. Psychological Testing: Patients with normal pressure hydrocephalus are impaired on tests designed to detect frontal lobe involvement. The presence of aphasia on psychological testing suggests a poor prognosis. Successful shunt treatment improves the patient's distractibility and motor speed but not intelligence or memory.

C. Laboratory Findings & Imaging: The clinical picture associated with vascular dementias can closely resemble that associated with normal pressure hydrocephalus. Unfortunately, MRI findings in patients with normal pressure hydrocephalus overlap those seen in patients who have small vessel disease. Both conditions are associated with increased ventricular size and significant periventricular hyperintensity, as shown on T2-weighted MRI. Normal pressure hydrocephalus differs from small vessel disease in that in the former the MRI can show a large cerebral aqueduct when the pulsation of CSF creates a flow void.

When radioisotope-labeled albumin (RISA) is injected into the lumbar sac (the RISA cisternogram test), it usually diffuses readily over the cerebral convexities. Patients with normal pressure hydrocephalus have abnormal CSF dynamics: Radioactivity appears in the ventricles but is absent over the convexities. Although this test may sometimes be useful, it is not often used today.

Cerebral fluid drainage procedures are sometimes used to help predict whether surgery will be successful. If the patient's gait improves after removal of a large amount of CSF, then the patient is judged to be a better candidate for surgery. Lack of improvement militates against surgery.

Differential Diagnosis

Normal pressure hydrocephalus can be difficult to distinguish from vascular dementias and Alzheimer's disease. Although imaging tests help, there is some overlap between the findings of normal pressure hydrocephalus and other forms of dementia. Tests of spinal fluid dynamics help clarify the matter, but ultimately, improvement after shunt placement clarifies the issue. Unfortunately, shunt placement often does not result in any significant improvement.

Treatment

Dementia from normal pressure hydrocephalus may respond to shunting, the treatment of choice; however, shunting is associated with significant morbidity. Thus the procedure should probably be carried out only in cases in which the indications are clear and in which the dementia has not progressed significantly. Although shunting carries a substantial risk of morbidity, it is often done empirically in clinical practice and the diagnosis is made only when the patient improves.

Prognosis & Course of Illness

Patients whose normal pressure hydrocephalus has a defined etiology, such as previous head trauma or subarachnoid hemorrhage, do better than do patients with idiopathic hydrocephalus. Variables associated with a positive outcome from CSF shunting include CSF pressure, regional cerebral blood flow, duration of dementia, and gait abnormality preceding dementia.

2. DEMENTIA DUE TO TRAUMATIC BRAIN INJURY

Essentials of Diagnosis

Dementia due to traumatic brain injury refers to a wide range of alterations in thinking, mood, and behavior that are due to the specific neurologic damage associated with the brain trauma. Severity of the injury is an important dimension that helps determine outcome. Specific vulnerabilities such as age, preexisting neurologic or psychiatric disease, and social support determine the ultimate prognosis.

General Considerations

A. Major Etiologic Theories: Head trauma severe enough to cause brief loss of consciousness or posttraumatic amnesia can also produce long-lasting cognitive and behavioral changes.

The principle mechanisms causing the symptoms that follow head injury have been well established. Forces of deceleration and acceleration act within the cranial compartment to produce significant changes within the brain. The swirling movement of brain tissue causes diffuse injury to axons. Because the hippocampus is found near the sphenoid ridge, it is especially susceptible to damage when the brain is set in sudden motion. Memory mechanisms fail, and both anterograde and retrograde amnesia follow. The length of posttraumatic amnesia is closely related to the overall severity of diffuse brain damage. Closed head trauma causes diffuse brain damage, but brain contusion and laceration may also produce focal brain damage, with large and small infarcts throughout the brain. These lesions may be pronounced in the area of the brain opposite the side of impact. Subarachnoid hemorrhage and subdural hematoma may produce additional damage, and cerebral edema further complicates the picture.

Beyond structural changes, biochemical alterations may also occur. For example, free acetylcholine may appear in large quantities in the CSF, or anoxic damage may produce an increase in CSF lactate.

B. Epidemiology: The annual rate of traumatic brain injury among the general population is about 200 per 100,000 people in the United States. Traumatic brain injuries are most common among young adult males and most often are the result of automobile accidents. Older adults also represent a significant risk group. Falls are the most common cause of injury in children and older adults. Most head injuries are considered to be mild. Older adults are more likely than younger adults to have a severe injury.

Clinical Findings

A. Signs & Symptoms: Fatigue, headache, and dizziness may occur shortly after a mild head trauma. Later a postconcussive disorder may develop. The cognitive deficit involves impaired information processing and resembles other subcortical processes. The most significant features of postconcussive disorder are slowing of information processing, impaired attention, and poor memory.

Head injuries that are more severe may be rated according to the Glasgow coma scale. This is a measure of consciousness that analyzes eye opening response, verbal response, and motor response. Head trauma is categorized on this scale as mild, moderate, or severe. The Glasgow coma scale gives a rough judgment regarding prognosis.

Recovery from moderate and severe head trauma is an extremely long process. Recovery is most rapid during the first year or two, and it can continue for many years. In the initial stages of recovery, assessment of progress is accomplished through the Rancho Los Amigos scale. In the later stages of recovery, measurement of recovery is based on clinical indicators such as return to work.

Recovery from head trauma is also affected by secondary brain injury. Intracranial hematomas, brain edema, and vasospasm affect prognosis by causing occlusion of intracranial vessels, thus producing secondary strokes. Infection, seizures, or metabolic imbalance may affect the postinjury course. Traumatic brain injury produces physical disability ranging from sensory and motor deficits to posttraumatic epilepsy. In addition, there is usually some deterioration in cognitive ability. Emotional or behavioral deviation usually produces the most significant disability. Some individuals show personality disturbance characterized by anxiety, depression, or irritability. Others may demonstrate classic frontotemporal syndrome with memory impairment, apathy, lack of motivation, and indifference to the environment. Physicians must consider these emotional difficulties when providing treatment and rehabilitation to these patients.

B. Psychological Testing: Neuropsychological test data are used to develop treatment strategies tailored for an individual's strengths and deficits. Neuropsychological testing can sometimes reveal subtle changes in information processing in patients who otherwise appear normal. A commonly used test is the paced auditory serial addition task. During this exercise, subjects listen to digits presented at a standard rate and add each digit to the one immediately preceding. Head trauma patients are both slower and less accurate than are normal subjects.

Patients with mild to moderate postconcussive disorder may become irritable or even aggressive, and exhibit blunt affect, apathy, or lack of spontaneity. The effects of mild to moderate head trauma can be subtle, and both patients and practitioners may make light of the cognitive impairment associated with mild head trauma despite sometimes devastating consequences.

In more severe forms of head trauma, neuropsychological testing can be used to measure the extent of secondary injury. To some extent this helps establish the prognosis. Neuropsychological testing can then be used to measure progress. Because cognitive rehabilitation is an important part of recovery, neuropsychological testing can help the behavioral psychologist focus on the particular areas that need work.

C. Laboratory Findings & Imaging: The EEG is sensitive to brain changes following trauma. Local suppression of the alpha rhythm may extend bilaterally. In more severe injury, EEG discharges become progressively slower and delta activity may predominate. The EEG is not a reliable guide to prognosis, and other clinical features must be considered. An EEG that becomes normal early in the course of the illness usually predicts good recovery following head trauma.

Treatment

Recovery from head trauma is a dynamic process rather than a static one. As a result, treatment evolves during the course of recovery. In mild head trauma, treatment consists in determining the neuropsychological deficit and giving appropriate counsel. In addition, symptomatic treatment of headaches, dizziness, and mood alteration is useful. Intervention with the patient's employer may help foster understanding and help encourage work conditions that are more conducive to success.

In moderate or severe head trauma, the goals of treatment change as the patient recovers. The early stages of treatment may be oriented to merely suppressing violent outbursts and improving sleep. Later on therapy becomes more tailored to improving memory, impulsiveness, irritability, and affective disorder. Both pharmacotherapy and psychotherapy are useful in this regard. Carbamazepine is generally useful for impulsiveness and may be combined with an atypical neuroleptic. Sleep disturbance may respond to trazodone. The affective disorders respond to SSRIs and other antidepressants. In general, dosing should be started low. Increases of psychopharmacologic agents should be made gradually. Head trauma patients tend to have greater sensitivity to medication side effects.

Complications

Depression and anxiety are common in outpatients with traumatic brain injuries. These symptoms add to the morbidity of closed head trauma because depressed or anxious patients perceive themselves as more severely disabled. Death by suicide is a risk after head injury.

Alcohol and substance abuse also alter the outcome of traumatic brain injury. Alcohol intoxication is present in up to one half of patients hospitalized for brain injury. Two thirds of rehabilitation patients have a history of substance abuse preceding their injuries. Untreated substance abuse adversely affects cognitive status in rehabilitation patients.

Repeated head trauma in boxers produces dementia pugilistica. In its fully developed form, the disorder consists of cerebellar, pyramidal, and extrapyramidal features, along with intellectual deterioration. The syndrome may progress even after the boxer has retired from the sport.

Prognosis & Course of Illness

Periods of unconsciousness may last several hours yet still be compatible with complete recovery. The longer the patient is unconscious, the poorer the outcome. As the patient recovers from severe head trauma, a period of confusion may follow lasting from hours to months. Some patients pass through a period of extremely disturbed behavior that poses severe management problems. The patient may be abusive, aggressive, or uncooperative. The patient may appear delirious during this time with vivid audiovisual hallucinations. When head trauma is associated with prolonged unconsciousness, recovery is usually followed by some degree of dementia. Recovery from mild to moderate head trauma is more variable and difficult to predict.

Graff-Radford NR, Godersky JC, Jones MP: Variables predicting surgical outcome in symptomatic hydrocephalus in the elderly. Neurology 1989;39:1601.
Levin HS et al: Serial MRI and neurobehavioral findings after mild to moderate closed head injury. J Neurol Neurosurg Psychiatry 1992;55:255.

DEMENTIA & DEPRESSION

Depressed seniors often deny mood disorder and focus on memory problems, complaining of memory loss disproportionate to their actual decrement in memory functioning. Because depressed seniors commonly exhibit impaired attention, perception, problem solving, or memory, psychometric testing may not distinguish depression from Alzheimer's disease. This lack of diagnostic clarity has led to the term **pseudodementia.** This term creates unrealistic expectations for a psychiatric cure for dementia. Cognitive disorder seen during late-life affective disorder is real and not simulated. **Depressive dementia** is a more accurate term.

The cognitive decline encountered in depressed older people is more precipitous than in demented patients. Patient history often reveals previous depression. The combined effects of age and depression produce a pattern of deficits distinct from that found in younger depressed patients and less severe than that in Alzheimer's patients. The actual memory impairment is modest in depressed patients, but the level of subjective complaint is high. In contrast, organically impaired patients have more memory loss and less frequent subjective complaints. The cognitive dysfunction encountered in depressed patients is probably secondary to decreased arousal with associated deficits in motivation and attention. Depressed patients do well on simple tasks but poorly on tasks requiring increased exertion. Following drug treatment, their performance improves. Patients' cognitive complaints correlate with depressive symptoms rather than with MMSE scores.

Patients with depressive dementia often exhibit early morning awakening, anxiety, weight loss, psychomotor retardation, and decreased libido. Patients with dementia present with disorientation, and their daily activities are more seriously impaired. Despite these differences, there is no definitive diagnostic tool. Cognitive decline in depressed older people commonly has a multifactorial etiology. In fact, depression may be the presenting symptom of a degenerative disorder.

The dexamethasone suppression test is not useful in discriminating between depression and dementia or between subtypes of dementia. Sleep studies distinguish depression from dementia with about 85% accuracy. Depressed seniors experience shorter rapid eye movement (REM) latency, higher REM sleep percentage, less non-REM sleep disturbance, and early morning awakening. Patients with Alzheimer's disease experience less REM sleep. Computerized techniques, including amplitude frequency measures and spectral analyses, permit new approaches to the examination of delta sleep. Many depressed patients show lower delta wave intensity during the first non-REM period than during the second period.

Several studies have shown an association between depressive dementia and degenerative dementia. The longer the follow-up, the more likely that depressive dementia will evolve into degenerative dementia. Elderly depressed patients also display a remarkable increase in prevalence of cortical infarcts and leukoencephalopathy. Depressed patients tend also to have basal ganglia lesions, sulcal atrophy, large cerebral ventricles, and subcortical white-matter lesions. Nevertheless, Alzheimer's disease patients have more prominent cortical atrophy compared to those with major depression.

PET scans distinguish dementia from late-life depression more clearly than does structural imaging (ie, CT scan and MRI). The temporoparietal pattern observed in patients with primary degenerative dementia is not observed in those with affective disorder. In severely depressed patients, PET scans show left-right prefrontal asymmetry in resting-state cerebral metabolic rates. Successful drug therapy reduces the asym-

metry. In depression, the decrease in glucose metabolism is more pronounced in prefrontal areas, and these changes persist despite clinical improvement, suggesting that the abnormality is not state dependent.

Both mania and depression can present as pseudodelirium. Vegetative signs are not helpful in distinguishing depression from delirium. Laboratory investigations are required. Mania may present with symptoms of dementia, but delirium is more common. About one quarter of manic patients over age 65 years have no history of affective illness. Cognitive changes often persist even after the patient has "switched" into depression. Treatment with lithium, carbamazepine, or valproate resolves both mania and cognitive impairment. Antidepressant medication for affective disorder is usually effective; however, side effects are troublesome in older patients. Previous treatment response should help guide therapy. Tricyclic plasma levels must be monitored in order to avoid overmedication. Unfortunately, one third of the seniors hospitalized for mania experience a permanent decline in their MMSE scores. This suggests that late-life mania is related to structural changes in the brain.

Because TCAs are likely to cause adverse drug reactions in seniors, alternatives should be considered such as SSRIs, monoamine oxidase inhibitors, alprazolam, and bupropion. For mild depression, SSRIs are first-line agents. When TCAs are required, nortriptyline and desipramine are the preferred agents. Lithium or triiodothyronine may be useful adjutants in patients whose depression is resistant to TCA treatment. Reduced kidney function makes lithium more difficult to manage. Psychostimulants such as methylphenidate and dextroamphetamine present yet another treatment option. These drugs appear to be of particular benefit when used in the short term for the treatment of depression that complicates medical illness.

Lithium is effective in treating bipolar disorder, but its side effect of impairing renal function limits its use. In elderly patients, lithium has a very narrow therapeutic index. Lithium toxicity can occur quickly, damaging already-compromised kidneys. Valproate may be preferred if the patient has a new-onset illness and has not previously been exposed to treatment. If lithium is used, very close monitoring is required. When other therapies have failed, ECT may reverse pseudodementia or pseudodelirium dramatically. ECT is safe and effective, even in patients older than 80 years or in those with poststroke depression. Common complications of ECT in the elderly include severe confusion, falls, and cardiorespiratory problems.

DELUSIONS & BEHAVIORAL DISTURBANCE

As dementia worsens, behavioral problems emerge. Problem behavior often stems from the inability of staff to understand patients' needs. It is important to identify the cause of the dementia before rushing into pharmacologic treatment. Patients can exhibit problems because they are hungry, thirsty, bored, constipated, tired, sexually aroused, or in pain. Patients with dementia need to feel loved. They benefit from opportunities to develop self-esteem. An initial psychosocial approach to these problematic patients should assess whether these needs are being met.

A multidisciplinary team setting is the most appropriate format for setting treatment goals that are then communicated to the family. It is essential to involve the family in order to educate them and to initiate social interventions. Patients and family members need to believe that a meaningful life is possible despite dementia. This is particularly true if family members are taught to validate the patient's emotional experience. Very little can be gained by approaches aimed at reorientation or enforcing confrontation with reality. Support groups help family members learn not only to cope with the negative outcomes but also to understand their loved one in the context of the illness.

The Omnibus Reconciliation Act of 1990 introduced specific restrictions on the use of psychotropic medication in the care of nursing home residents. Nonetheless, pharmacotherapy is often essential for treatment of the behavioral disorders that accompany dementia. Psychiatrists are frequently asked to treat agitation in demented patients. Antipsychotics, antidepressants, and sedative-hypnotics are used widely for this purpose; however, data from double-blind clinical trials are limited. Neuroleptics are modestly effective, but no particular neuroleptic stands out. A clearly positive clinical response is the exception rather than the rule in elderly patients who have dementia. Only 18% of agitated demented patients benefit from treatment with a neuroleptic. As a result, many other drugs have been used to treat agitation in demented patients. Neuroleptics must be used continuously in small doses for best effect. High-potency drugs such as haloperidol have the advantage of fewer anticholinergic side effects. In the clinical setting, neuroleptics should be reduced periodically or discontinued in order to determine ongoing need. Patients may show improved effect without any deterioration of behavior when neuroleptics are discontinued. Attempts to wean the patient off the drug gradually are important because tardive dyskinesia is a significant risk in the elderly.

Atypical agents such as olanzapine and quetiapine have been introduced. These newer drugs demonstrate many of the benefits of the older agents without as many side effects. Notably, tardive dyskinesia risk is substantially reduced and fewer extrapyramidal reactions occur. As a result, concomitant anticholinergic medication is not required.

Short-acting benzodiazepines control agitation and may be used on occasion in the short term to treat agitation or as a hypnotic in severely demented patients. They can be used in conjunction with antipsychotics.

Benzodiazepines are effective for only a minority of patients and then side effects frequently make patients worse. Even when used only at night, these drugs have an adverse effect on cognition and are a common cause of incoordination and falls in older hospitalized patients. Their use should be reserved for the management of short-term crisis situations in which a rapid response is necessary.

Trazodone has been used to control aggression in demented patients on the theory that aggression is related to serotonergic depletion. Patients generally receive a mild benefit in dosages of 150–300 mg/day. Because some elderly patients experience gait disturbances immediately after the nighttime dose, fall precautions must be taken. Buspirone reduces agitation in dementia in dosages of 20–40 mg/day. Some patients respond preferentially to valproic acid. These patients often have manic symptoms associated with agitation, including pressured speech, flight of ideas, and sleeplessness.

There are almost no placebo-controlled studies of the drugs used to treat agitation in older people, but the use of psychopharmacology is common in patients who have failed conventional treatment. Carbamazepine or valproate may be best for patients with manic symptoms, buspirone for patients with anxiety, and antidepressants for patients who appear depressed. Because these medications often are given to dementia patients for prolonged periods, studies are needed to define their long-term clinical efficacy.

Some behaviors such as wandering, purposeless repetitive activity, stealing, and screaming are not amenable to pharmacologic intervention. These behaviors must be dealt with by environmental design such as the wander-guard system (a wristband alarm system) or appropriate sound-proofing. Clinicians can reduce the occurrence of sundowning by promoting daytime activity, preventing daytime napping, and enforcing a regular sleep schedule. The medical treatment of sundowning can be frustrating; however, sedatives are sometimes helpful.

Burke WJ: Neuroleptic drug use in the nursing home: the impact of OBRA. Am Fam Physician 1991;43:2125.

Flint AJ, van Reekum R: The pharmacologic treatment of Alzheimer's disease: a guide for the general psychiatrist [see comments]. Can J Psychiatry 1998;43:689.

AMNESTIC DISORDERS

MEMORY FUNCTION

The study of memory is a great challenge because the systems that underlie memory function are complex and not well understood. Patients are diagnosed with an amnestic disorder when they are unable to learn new information or recall previously learned facts or events. To diagnose an amnestic disorder, dementia or delirium must be excluded. An amnestic disorder may be due to a general medical condition or induced by a particular toxin. An amnestic disorder due to a general medical disorder must be the direct consequence of that disorder. The physician must report the responsible medical condition as part of the Axis I diagnosis. Amnestic disorders are difficult to categorize and may be difficult to distinguish from mild generalized cognitive impairment.

A. Short-Term Versus Long-Term Memory: There is much controversy about the nature and measurement of memory. **Short-term memory** consists of registration and immediate memory. **Registration** holds information very briefly for about 1 or 2 seconds. **Immediate or working memory** is retained for 30 seconds to a few minutes. Immediate memory retains information in reverberating neural circuits involving the frontal lobes. If it is not converted to long-term storage, data is lost. Memories are stored in long-term memory through a process called **consolidation.** The long-term memory store is organized in the brain according to meaning. Long-term memory is a biochemical process that depends on protein synthesis and the development of dendritic connections.

Patients who have difficulty with short-term memory generally have **anterograde amnesia** and are unable to learn new material. Patients who have difficulty recalling information stored before the onset of an illness or injury have **retrograde amnesia** due to impairment in long-term memory. The retention of material in long-term storage depends on that part of the cerebral cortex related to the specific sensory modality involved. Thus if both the occipital and occipital-parietal cortices are involved in an injury, visual memories may be impaired significantly.

B. Implicit Versus Explicit Memory: Cognitive neuroscience has provided strong support for the idea that multiple memory systems exist. One system divides memory into explicit and implicit types. **Explicit memory** is synonymous with declarative memory. Declarative memory reflects a conscious recollection of the past. Recall and recognition are defined as explicit memory functions. **Declarative memory** is concerned with the accumulation of facts. It is used, for example, to remember the facts in this chapter. Declarative memory contains facts not only about verbal material but about all sensory modalities. Declarative memory is ultimately about relationships. An example of declarative memory would be the recollection that a certain bird has blue feathers and is 4 inches tall. Declarative memory combines information about the bird with its attributes. Declarative memories are consciously known and are therefore explicit. Explicit memory disorders are well recognized clinically. Lesions in the medial temporal lobes, midline diencephalon, or basal forebrain can impair

declarative memory because relationships between sensory modalities are processed through the hippocampal diencephalic system.

Declarative memory can be divided into episodic memory and semantic memory. **Episodic memory** contains information about events specific to an individual's personal experience. **Semantic memory** refers to memory concerning objects, people, and events of the world. Patients with deficits in semantic memory lose the language ability because the meaning of words, people, and events becomes impoverished. Semantic memories can be modality specific (visual, auditory, sensory) or category specific (living things versus nonliving things).

Patients with semantic deficits may retain factual autobiographical information. The retention of this information implies that episodic memory is intact. Patients with the classic amnestic syndromes often have impairment of episodic memory. In contrast, patients with Alzheimer's disease have significant deficiencies in semantic memory.

Nondeclarative memory is sometimes called implicit memory. **Implicit memory** implies that a person may be able to know something without being able to actively remember it. Implicit memory is not usually tested clinically. It requires neuropsychological testing. Implicit memory does not involve the conscious recollection of recent experiences for the execution of tasks. Procedural learning (eg, how to drive a car) is an example of implicit memory. Apraxia exemplifies a deficit in implicit memory. Amnestic patients can learn certain skills or acquire problem-solving abilities, even though the amnestic patient has no memory of having learned the behavior.

Procedural learning is a form of implicit memory. This form of learning is involved in complicated psychomotor procedures such as driving a car or shooting a basketball. The basal ganglia, cerebellum, and frontal lobes have been linked to procedural learning. Procedural learning does not involve the hippocampal diencephalic system. Procedural learning is most affected in subcortical dementias such as Huntington's and Parkinson's diseases.

Additional examples of implicit learning include classical conditioning (stimulus-response) and operant conditioning (reinforcing behaviors). Even people who do not have amnestic disorders learn by classical conditioning but may not be able to recollect the experience. People who have severe declarative memory disorders are quite capable of learning through stimulus-response and reinforcement paradigms. The cerebellum is heavily involved in this type of memory.

Yet another form of memory is **probabilistic learning,** in which we learn from past experiences to predict the future. This form of memory is also relatively independent of medial temporal lobe functions.

All memories are influenced heavily by emotions. Memory for emotionally arousing events is modulated by an endogenous memory-modulating system consisting of stress hormones and the amygdala. This system is an adaptive method of creating memory strength that is proportional to memory importance. In addition, some memory is state specific so that these memories can be recalled only during emotional states similar to the ones present when they were created.

It is important for the practitioner to realize that memory is highly complex and difficult to quantify at the bedside. It is equally important to recognize that in patients with amnestic syndromes, neuropsychological testing reveals normal perception, language, motor functions, and preserved intellectual skills.

C. Theories of Memory: Recently neural network theories of memory have been proposed. These theories rely on mathematical and logical descriptions of the network architectures of computer programs. In these models, dissociable systems mediate learning through different modalities and work together to form memories. Distinct neural networks mediate different memory modalities. Neural networks are based on the idea that streams of information are combined by forming, strengthening, or pruning connections between neurons to form new representations that can later be retrieved. This process is mediated by neurons that possess connections of modifiable strength. Evidence for this process comes from the fact that damage to specific areas of the association cortex affects individual sensory memory modalities. Currently research in functional brain imaging is being combined with these theories to provide a new source of information about how memory systems function.

CLINICAL SYNDROMES

Clinical bedside diagnosis of amnestic disorders is generally limited to processes that damage the medial temporal lobe. The severity of memory impairment depends heavily on the location and extent of damage in these brain structures. The thalamus, basal ganglia, cerebellum, frontal lobe, and other cortical structures have a role.

The autonomic structures affected in amnestic disorders include the medial temporal lobes, mammillary bodies, fornix, medial dorsal thalamus, and frontal lobes. Damage to these pathways by neurologic insults or toxins causes clinical memory problems. Injuries and toxic exposures can produce either reversible or irreversible amnestic conditions.

SUBSTANCE-INDUCED PERSISTING AMNESTIC DISORDER

DSM-IV Diagnostic Criteria

A. The development of memory impairment as manifested by impairment in the ability to learn new

information or the inability to recall previously learned information.

B. The memory disturbance causes significant impairment in social or occupational functioning and represents a significant decline from a previous level of functioning.

C. The memory disturbance does not occur exclusively during the course of a delirium or a dementia and persists beyond the usual duration of substance intoxication or withdrawal.

D. There is evidence from the history, physical examination, or laboratory findings that the memory disturbance is etiologically related to persisting effects of substance use (eg, a drug of abuse, a medication).

Reprinted, with permission, from *Diagnostic and Statistical Manual of Mental Disorders,* 4th ed. Copyright 1994 American Psychiatric Association.

1. KORSAKOFF'S SYNDROME

Korsakoff's syndrome is a severe anterograde learning defect associated with confabulations. Korsakoff's patients have difficulty encoding and consolidating explicit memory. Storage is mildly impaired, but retrieval and new learning are severely impaired. When Korsakoff's patients learn new material, they will forget it at a normal rate, but learning the new material is extremely difficult and in severe cases new learning is impossible. Retrograde memory is also impaired in Korsakoff's syndrome, but the impairment of retrograde memory is not as severe as that of anterograde memory. Korsakoff's patients have retrograde amnesia back to the onset of illness, as severe as their anterograde loss. The most remote memories prior to the onset of illness are spared. As a result, Korsakoff's patients retain more distant memories dramatically more proficiently than they learn new material.

Korsakoff's patients have little impairment in implicit memory, and their ability to perform motor procedures remains intact. They may retain the capacity to complete complex motor tasks. Typically general intelligence, perceptual skills, and language remain relatively normal. The cardinal symptom of Korsakoff's syndrome is confabulation. Although remote memory for events before the neurologic insult is often surprisingly intact, Korsakoff's patients are unable to organize memories in a temporal context. Because they distort the relationships between facts, Korsakoff's patients have remote memory deficits.

Korsakoff's syndrome commonly follows an episode of Wernicke's encephalopathy. This neurologic condition is manifested by confusion, ataxia, and nystagmus; thiamin deficiency is its direct cause. If thiamin is given during the acute stage of Wernicke's encephalopathy, Korsakoff's syndrome can be prevented. The administration of glucose-containing fluid must be avoided, for it will hasten Korsakoff's syndrome unless the patient has been adequately dosed with thiamin and recovery has begun. Alcohol abuse causes the conditions that lead to Korsakoff's syndrome, but malnutrition alone can cause the disorder. The lesions caused by thiamin deficiency occur in the hippocampus, the mammillary bodies, and the anterior and dorsal nucleus of the thalamus, and disrupt a critical circuit between the hippocampus and the frontal lobes.

2. AMNESIA FROM DRUGS & TOXINS

Patients prescribed sedatives, hypnotics, and anxiolytics can develop substance-induced amnestic disorders. Amnestic syndromes usually follow intense continuous use of these drugs, but recovery usually occurs when the patient stops using the offending agent. Toxins can also cause amnestic disorders. Neurotransmitters involved in memory include acetylcholine, catecholamines, GABA, and glutamic acid. Disruption of these transmitter systems by drugs or toxins also disrupts specific memory functions. Drugs having this effect include benzodiazepines, anticonvulsants, and antiarrhythmics. Amnesia is a characteristic of all the benzodiazepines, with the effect depending on the route of administration, dose, and pharmacokinetics of the particular drug. The amnestic effects of benzodiazepines are sometimes used for therapeutic purposes during surgical procedures. Toxins that affect memory include organophosphates, carbon monoxide, and organic solvents. Chronic exposure to these and other neurotoxins may also affect memory. The patient's ability to recover memory functions depends on the substance, the length of exposure, and other comorbidities.

AMNESTIC DISORDER DUE TO A GENERAL MEDICAL CONDITION

DSM-IV Diagnostic Criteria

A. The development of memory impairment as manifested by impairment in the ability to learn new information or the inability to recall previously learned information.

B. The memory disturbance causes significant impairment in social or occupational functioning and represents a significant decline from a previous level of functioning.

C. The memory disturbance does not occur exclusively during the course of a delirium or a dementia.

D. There is evidence from the history, physical examination, or laboratory findings that the disturbance is the direct physiological consequence of a general medical condition (including physical trauma).

Specify if:

Transient: if memory impairment lasts for 1 month or less. When the diagnosis is made within the first month without waiting for recovery, the term "provisional" may be added.
Chronic: if memory impairment lasts for more than 1 month.

Reprinted, with permission, from *Diagnostic and Statistical Manual of Mental Disorders,* 4th ed. Copyright 1994 American Psychiatric Association.

1. TEMPORAL LOBE MEMORY SYNDROMES

The medial temporal lobe system consists of the hippocampus and adjacent, anatomically related entorhinal, perirhinal, and parahippocampal cortices. These structures have widespread and reciprocal connections with the neocortex. Medial temporal structures are essential for consolidating long-term memory for facts and events; however, the function of this system is temporary. As time passes, memory stored in the neocortex becomes independent of the medial temporal lobe. Lesions that involve the medial temporal lobes are the most important clinical cause of the amnestic syndrome. Disease of the posterior cerebral artery or bilateral medial temporal lobectomy for epilepsy can produce bilateral temporal lobe lesions. Patients with bilateral temporal lobe damage can develop Korsakoff's syndrome with profound deficits in learning and retention. Lesions of the fornix and bilateral paramedial thalamic lesions also disrupt temporal lobe memory circuits, causing patterns of amnesia that resemble Korsakoff's syndrome.

Unilateral damage to the medial temporal lobe produces distinct temporal lobe memory syndromes. These memory deficits are commonly observed in patients with hippocampal sclerosis. Deficits may be specific for verbal material if the lesion is in the left temporal lobe or for nonverbal material if the right temporal lobe is involved. Patients with these deficits often have complex partial seizures as well as memory problems. When the seizure disorder is highly active, the memory deficit may be more profound.

Other temporal lobe memory syndromes exist. Damage to the lateral temporal lobe causes retrograde amnesia. Temporal lobe lesions that disconnect the hippocampus from the association cortex can produce memory disorders specific for a sensory modality such as vision or touch. Temporal lobe damage can result from prolonged seizures, anoxia, trauma, ischemia, or basilar meningitis. Whatever the cause, medial temporal damage produces anterograde amnesia.

2. FRONTAL LOBE MEMORY SYNDROMES

The frontal thalamic and striatum system mediates the executive component of working memory, which plays an important role in some forms of sensorimotor skill learning. In patients with frontal lobe damage, memory for procedural steps may be impaired. This is sometimes called "forgetting to remember." Patients with frontal memory problems have difficulty maintaining set. They interpret the world concretely. Not only do they have a tendency to become distracted, they also perseverate. Working memory may be particularly impaired in patients with frontal lobe damage. Patients with left frontal lobe damage have difficulty with rote verbal learning. Patients with right frontal lobe damage may have difficulty keeping memories preserved in a visuospatial sketch pad for rehearsal and learning of spatial relationships.

3. TRANSIENT GLOBAL AMNESIA

Transient global amnesia is a benign neurologic syndrome characterized by global memory loss. Consciousness and self-awareness are preserved. Associated behavioral changes include repetitive questioning. The syndrome generally resolves within 24 hours. Mild brainstem symptoms are often present during the attack, but major neurologic abnormalities never occur. After the attack the only remaining symptom is a permanent amnestic gap for the duration of the episode. The syndrome may be recurrent.

Transient global amnesia was originally thought to have cerebrovascular etiology; however, the disorder is not associated with the conventional risk factors for cerebrovascular disease. Migraine is much more common in transient global amnesia patients. A significant minority of transient global amnesia patients will develop epilepsy.

4. POST-ECT MEMORY DISORDERS

Memory loss is a well-known side effect of ECT. Anterograde memory loss for events during the series of treatments is to be expected. Mild retrograde amnesia also occurs. Memory complaints are more common in individuals who receive bilateral ECT. Bilateral ECT produces greater anterograde memory loss than does right unilateral ECT. Bilateral ECT also produces more extensive retrograde amnesia. Nondominant unilateral ECT has been shown in a small number of poorly designed studies to improve memory in some depressed patients; however, it is often less efficacious than bilateral ECT.

The long-term memory problems associated with ECT are more troubling to patients than are the short-term ones. ECT creates a persistent storage deficit that results in accelerated forgetting. Capacity for new learning recovers substantially by several months after ECT, but accelerated forgetting can be documented for up to 6 months post-ECT.

5. AMNESTIC DISORDERS DUE TO HEAD TRAUMA

Memory problems are frequent after head trauma. The pattern of memory deficits depends on the nature of the injury. Patients who are severely injured have damage to multiple cortical structures. How much brain is destroyed has a profound impact on the recovery of memory function. The variability of the damage is so great that no single pattern of amnestic disorder occurs after head trauma. Mild head trauma produces memory deficits that are prominent in the initial months after the injury but then recover. More severe damage may cause deficits that prevent the patient from returning to school or to work. Because damage to structures involved in the maintenance of attention interferes with the patient's ability to learn new material, frontal lobe damage can contribute to the memory deficits observed in closed head trauma. Other neurologic damage, emotional difficulties, and psychiatric disorder may contribute significantly to the memory disorder observed in head trauma patients. Finally, head trauma patients are frequently involved in legal action; therefore, some individuals intentionally exaggerate deficits to derive secondary gain.

Because closed head injury often affects the medial temporal lobe, both anterograde and retrograde memory deficits may occur. Anterograde deficits depend on the amount of damage to temporal lobe structures. If the temporal structures recover, anterograde deficits improve. Persisting disorders are the result of destruction of medial temporal lobe structures from infarction or surgery. Because head injury patients have difficulty focusing attention, their recall is often distorted. This applies to both new learning and to remote memory.

Retrograde deficits after closed head injury last for variable amounts of time, with a characteristic pattern of greatest deficits immediately after injury and improvement during the 2 years that follow. "Shrinking retrograde amnesia" has been described, in which memories more distant from the injury are recovered first. More recent events are recovered later. A focal retrograde amnesia, in which patients are unable to remember specific events, has also been described. This focal retrograde amnesia has involved autobiographical information in some patients. The severity of retrograde memory deficit serves as a marker for injury severity. Posttraumatic amnesia is related both to deficits in information processing speed and to cognitive outcome. Length of loss of consciousness and length of retrograde amnesia are correlated with severity of anterograde amnesia.

Haslam C et al: Post-coma disturbance and post-traumatic amnesia as nonlinear predictors of cognitive outcome following severe closed head injury: findings from the Westmead Head Injury Project. Brain Inj 1994;8:519.

Hodges JR, Warlow CP: The aetiology of transient global amnesia. A case-control study of 114 cases with prospective follow-up. Brain 1990;113:639.

Kopelman MD: The Korsakoff syndrome. Br J Psychiatry 1995;166:154.

Milner B: Some cognitive effects of frontal-lobe lesions in man. Phil Trans R Soc Lond (Biol) 1982;298:211.

Polster MR: Drug-induced amnesia: implications for cognitive neuropsychological investigations of memory. Psychol Bull 1993;114:477.

Ross ED: Sensory-specific and fractional disorders of recent memory in man. II. Unilateral loss of tactile recent memory. Arch Neurol 1980;37:267.

Squire LR: ECT and memory loss. Am J Psychiatry 1977;134:997.

CONCLUSION

The psychiatrist must use the medical model skillfully to participate fully in the care of patients who have delirium, dementia, or other cognitive disorders. The dual diagnosis of neurologic and affective disorders is more the rule than the exception. In many patients, affective disorder and optimal cognitive functioning are mutually dependent. The diagnostic skills obtained through the practice of general psychiatry have tremendous value. Treatment of affective disorders and other psychiatric conditions contribute significantly to the patient's ultimate cognitive outcome.

In the care of patients who have delirium and dementia, the boundary between neurology and psychiatry is blurred. Specific neurologic disorders not only have psychiatric implications but even cause specific psychiatric disorders. Although diagnosis does not determine a cure, it does suggest an appropriate clinical treatment plan. The cost-effective treatment of neuropsychiatric disorders has the potential to remove patients from inappropriately expensive placements. Nonetheless, psychological treatments require a basic understanding of the biological limitations placed on patients. To understand properly these limitations, the psychiatrist must have a thorough understanding of the effects of normal aging. Unfortunately, the major limitation placed on geriatric patients is often dementia. Eventually research will uncover prevention techniques based on diet, exercise, antioxidants, or other yet undiscovered compounds. Until then, the medical model remains the most useful method for the treatment of these mental disorders.

Substance-Related Disorders[1]

18

Peter R. Martin, MD, & John R. Hubbard, MD, PhD

DSM-IV Diagnostic Criteria

Substance Dependence

A maladaptive pattern of substance use, leading to clinically significant impairment or distress, as manifested by three (or more) of the following, occurring at any time in the same 12-month period:

(1) tolerance
(2) withdrawal
(3) the substance is often taken in larger amounts or over a longer period than was intended
(4) there is a persistent desire or unsuccessful efforts to cut down or control substance use
(5) a great deal of time is spent in activities necessary to obtain the substance, use the substance, or recover from its effects
(6) important social, occupational, or recreational activities are given up or reduced because of substance use
(7) the substance use is continued despite knowledge of having a persistent or recurrent physical or psychological problem that is likely to have been caused or exacerbated by the substance

Substance Abuse

A. A maladaptive pattern of substance use leading to clinically significant impairment or distress, as manifested by one (or more) of the following, occurring within a 12-month period:
   (1) recurrent substance use resulting in failure to fulfill major role obligations at work, school, or home
   (2) recurrent substance use in situations in which it is physically hazardous
   (3) recurrent substance-related legal problems
   (4) continued substance use despite having persistent or recurrent social or interpersonal problems caused or exacerbated by the effects of the substance

B. The symptoms have never met the criteria for substance dependence for this class of substance.

Substance Intoxication

A. The development of a reversible substance-specific syndrome due to recent ingestion of (or exposure to) a substance.
B. Clinically significant maladaptive behavioral or psychological changes that are due to the effect of the substance on the central nervous system.
C. The symptoms are not due to a general medical condition and are not better accounted for by another mental disorder.

Substance Withdrawal

A. The development of a substance-specific syndrome due to the cessation of (or reduction in) substance use that has been heavy and prolonged.
B. The substance-specific syndrome causes clinically significant distress or impairment in social, occupational, or other important areas of functioning.
C. The symptoms are not due to a general medical condition and are not better accounted for by another mental disorder.

Adapted, with permission, from *Diagnostic and Statistical Manual of Mental Disorders,* 4th ed. Copyright 1994 American Psychiatric Association.

Classification of Substance-Related Disorders

The substance-related disorders are classified into two categories: (1) substance use disorders and (2) substance-induced disorders (Table 18–1). The substance use disorders are (somewhat arbitrarily) dichotomized into substance abuse and substance dependence based on the number of relevant symptoms that the patient exhibits. The *Diagnostic and Statistical Manual of Mental Disorders,* 4th edition (DSM-IV) specifies substance use disorders that result from the self-administration of several different drugs of abuse (Table 18–2).

The specific criteria for diagnosis of substance use disorders draw heavily on the concept of the **depen-**

[1] This work was supported in part by the National Institute on Alcohol Abuse and Alcoholism (RO1 AA08492, RO1 AA10433, and TO1 AA07515).

Table 18–1. Substance-related disorders as classified in DSM-IV.

Substance use disorders
Substance dependence
Substance abuse
Substance-induced disorders
Substance-induced intoxication
Substance withdrawal
Substance-induced delirium
Substance-induced persisting dementia
Substance-induced persisting amnestic disorder
Substance-induced psychotic disorder
Substance-induced mood disorder
Substance-induced anxiety disorder
Substance-induced sexual dysfunction
Substance-induced sleep disorder

dence syndrome. This important advance in our thinking about these disorders frames the interactions among the pharmacologic actions of the drug, individual psychopathology, and the effects of the environment in a clinically meaningful construct that is generalizable to all drugs of abuse. This concept is derived from the clinical observation that patients may have maladaptive behavior as a result of drug use without the presence of neurophysiologic adaptive changes such as tolerance or withdrawal (also referred to as **neuroadaptation**). Neuroadaptation is not necessarily dysfunctional if there is no concomitant inappropriate desire to continue the use of the drug (**drug seeking**). For example, driving while drunk may have devastating consequences, particularly in the sporadi-cally drinking young driver who has not acquired tolerance to ethanol. In another example, the postsurgical patient who has been receiving morphine for pain relief clearly exhibits neuroadaptation but is not likely to develop the dependence syndrome.

Fundamental to the concept of the dependence syndrome is the priority of drug-seeking over other behaviors in the maintenance of dysfunctional drug use. Lesser weight is attributed to the presence of tolerance or withdrawal. In general, three (or more) individual symptoms from among the following three symptom clusters need to be part of the clinical presentation for the diagnosis of substance dependence: (1) loss of control (ie, the substance is taken in larger amounts or over a longer period than intended, or there are unsuccessful efforts to reduce use); (2) salience to the behavioral repertoire (ie, a great deal of time is spent in substance-related activities at the expense of important social, occupational, or recreational activities that are reduced or given up, or there is continued substance use despite knowledge of having a persistent or recurrent physical or psychological problem likely to have been caused or exacerbated by the substance); and (3) neuroadaptation (ie, the presence of tolerance or withdrawal).

Diagnosis of a substance use disorder by the presence of a given number of symptoms provides at best an incomplete picture of various clinically important features of the illness, such as severity, course, and prognosis, as well as indicated treatment for this heterogeneous patient population. The issue of illness

Table 18–2. Classes of substances of abuse in DSM-IV.

Class	Common Examples
Alcohol	Beer, wine, sherry, whiskey, vodka, gin
Amphetamine and amphetamine-like substances	Amphetamine, dextroamphetamine, methamphetamine, methylphenidate, diet pills, khat
Caffeine	Coffee, tea, soft drinks, analgesics, cold remedies, stimulants, diet pills
Cannabis	Marijuana, hashish, delta-9-tetrahydrocannabinol (THC)
Cocaine	Coca leaves or paste, cocaine hydrochloride, cocaine alkaloid (crack)
Hallucinogens	Lysergic acid diethylamide (LSD), psilocybin, dimethyltryptamine, mescaline
Inhalants	Aliphatic, aromatic, and halogenated hydrocarbons (eg, gasoline, glue, paint, paint thinners, other volatile compounds)
Nicotine	Cigarettes and other types of tobacco products
Opioids	Heroin, morphine, methadone, codeine, hydromorphone, oxycodone, meperidine, fentanyl, pentazocine, buprenorphine
Phencyclidine and phencyclidine-like substances	Phencyclidine, ketamine
Sedatives, hypnotics, and anxiolytics	Benzodiazepines (eg, diazepam, oxazepam, chlordiazepoxide, alprazolam, midazolam, clonazepam), barbiturates (eg, secobarbital, amobarbital, pentobarbital, phenobarbital), nonbarbiturate hypnosedatives (eg, ethchlorvynol, glutethimide, chloral hydrate, methaqualone)
Other	Anabolic steroids, nitrite inhalants, nitrous oxide, and various over-the-counter and prescription drugs that do not readily fall into the other categories

severity is addressed in DSM-IV primarily by a distinction between substance abuse and dependence. The importance of diagnostic criteria for drug abuse is evident: they identify the substantial minority of individuals who have a history of substance use but do not progress to dependence despite continuing substance abuse and developing certain associated problems. However, the distinction between drug abuse and dependence may not be practical, or possible, if substance use disorders are considered in terms of continuities rather than categorically. As a result, substance abuse is a residual category, applied only to individuals who do not meet criteria for substance dependence (for the given class of substance) but still experience clinically significant impairment or distress in life functioning as a result of substance use. In order to augment diagnostic sensitivity and also maintain the primacy of drug-seeking behavior, a person can be diagnosed as substance dependent without ever having exhibited tolerance or withdrawal. In DSM-IV, dependence is formally subtyped according to whether or not there is physiologic dependence (ie, the presence of tolerance or withdrawal). Finally, to better characterize individual patients, certain descriptive terms, or **course specifiers,** have been added to distinguish among different clinical courses of the dependence syndrome. For example, a dependent patient may be in remission (which may be early or sustained, full or partial), on agonist therapy (eg, methadone), or in a controlled environment (eg, locked hospital ward).

It may be exceedingly difficult to establish whether psychopathology in a given individual who has a substance use disorder is a consequence of drug use or is due to an additional psychiatric diagnosis. Table 18–3 indicates the broad overlap between substance-induced disorders and other psychiatric syndromes con-

sidered in this book. For example, diverse psychiatric signs and symptoms, including those of delirium (see Chapter 17), psychotic disorders (see Chapters 19 and 20), mood disorders (see Chapter 21), anxiety disorders (see Chapter 22), sexual dysfunction (see Chapter 28), and sleep disorders (see Chapter 30), can have their onset during intoxication or withdrawal. Dementia, amnestic disorder, and flashbacks (recurrences of the intoxicating effects of the drug that may occur years after use) associated with hallucinogen use may persist long after the acute effects of intoxication and withdrawal have abated. Accordingly, it is helpful to determine, preferably by longitudinal observation or by history, the timing of the onset of psychopathology with respect to the initiation of drug use, and whether it is still present when drug use has ceased, recognizing that the duration of abstinence can be a determining variable.

Pharmacotherapy of a complicating psychiatric disorder is currently considered appropriate only if it is independent (ie, a primary disorder), but not if it is a consequence (ie, a secondary disorder), of a substance use disorder. The distinction between whether a complicating psychiatric disorder is primary or secondary to substance dependence is not easily made, particularly if both disorders started early in life or are historically closely intertwined. Nevertheless, the use of medications with dependence liability (eg, benzodiazepines, methylphenidate, barbiturates, anticholinergics) for the treatment of a coexisting psychiatric disorder, or the failure to address the primary disorder (ie, substance dependence), may be severely detrimental to the patient.

Integration via a multiaxial diagnostic classification system of the physical, psychological, and social domains of each patient's clinical presentation is an im-

Table 18–3. Substance-induced psychiatric syndromes associated with psychoactive substances.[1]

Psychiatric Syndrome	Psychoactive Substance[2]
Delirium	Depressants (I/W), stimulants (I), opioids (I), cannabinoids (I), hallucinogens (I), arylcyclohexylamines (I), inhalants (I)
Dementia	Depressants (P), inhalants (P)
Amnestic disorder	Depressants (P)
Psychotic disorders	Depressants (I/W), stimulants (I), opioids (I), cannabinoids (I), hallucinogens (I/P), arylcyclohexylamines (I), inhalants (I)
Mood disorders	Depressants (I/W), stimulants (I/W), opioids (I), hallucinogens (I), arylcyclohexylamines (I), inhalants (I)
Anxiety disorders	Depressants (I/W), stimulants (I/W), caffeine (I), cannabinoids (I), hallucinogens (I), arylcyclohexylamines (I), inhalants (I)
Sexual dysfunction	Depressants (I), stimulants (I), opioids (I)
Sleep disorders	Depressants (I/W), stimulants (I/W), opioids (I/W), caffeine (I)

[1] Adapted, with permission, from American Psychiatric Association: *Diagnostic and Statistical Manual of Mental Disorders,* 4th ed. American Psychiatric Association, 1994.
[2] Letters in parentheses denote that the disorder has its onset during intoxication (I), withdrawal (W), intoxication or withdrawal (I/W), or the disturbance persists (P) long after the acute effects of intoxication or withdrawal. Depressants include alcohol, sedatives, hypnotics, and anxiolytics; stimulants include cocaine and amphetamine and amphetamine-like substances.

portant feature of DSM-IV. However, this classification approach is not always adequate to describe fully how the dependence syndrome may be modified by diverse factors such as complex drug use patterns (ie, more than one drug via different routes of administration), disabilities resulting from drug use (eg, mood disorders, brain dysfunction, medical complications), or various personality disorders and the sociocultural context of drug use. Physicians cannot ignore these more difficult issues as they communicate with each other and with other health care professionals or as they serve as legal consultants, perform disability assessments, and help develop health care policy.

A. Use of Psychoactive Substances: Throughout history, members of almost every society have used indigenous psychoactive substances (eg, opium, stimulants, cannabis, tobacco) for widely accepted medical, religious, or recreational purposes. In more recent times, a wide range of substances (eg, central nervous system [CNS] depressants and stimulants, hallucinogens, and dissociative anesthetics), synthesized de novo or structurally modified from naturally occurring psychoactive compounds, have also become available for self-administration.

Descriptors of the magnitude and context of psychoactive drug use (eg, excessive use, abuse, misuse, addiction) represent difficult value judgments. Even if such terms are defined explicitly, they are not likely to be readily generalizable from one society (or group within the society) to another. To demonstrate the arbitrary nature of these terms one needs only to examine the changes in perceptions of drug use in the United States since the 1960s.

B. Maladaptive Patterns of Drug Use: Maladaptive patterns of use involve the self-administration of psychoactive agents to alter one's subjective state and experience of the environment, under inappropriate circumstances or in greater amounts than generally considered acceptable within the social constraints of one's culture. Medical diagnosis of substance-related disorders requires meaningful diagnostic criteria that are generalizable across cultures and drugs of abuse. Definition of maladaptive patterns of use in terms of their consequences, presumably less influenced by value judgments, has provided the conceptual basis for DSM-IV diagnostic criteria. Accordingly, considerable weight is placed on behavioral factors rather than on purely medical complications of use or physiologic effects. This conceptual advance, theoretically consistent with the biopsychosocial model of health care, is readily amenable to prevention and has important implications for treatment. The diagnostic focus has shifted from the drug per se to the interactions of drug, individual, and societal factors. Such a perspective is quite different from the traditional medical model of considering drug use as merely a bad "habit" until organ damage is diagnosable, or the social model in which use sufficient to cause physical complications is not considered an illness.

General Considerations

A. Major Etiologic Theories: The etiology of substance use disorders has been conceptualized in terms of an integration of biological, psychological, and social theories.

1. Individual vulnerabilities—The major goal of any etiologic theory is to explain why, in the face of widespread availability of drugs and alcohol, certain individuals develop a substance use disorder, and others do not. This is a gargantuan task because these are complex and multifaceted disorders. Substance abuse and dependence are heterogeneous disorders that represent the final common pathway for a variety of behavioral difficulties in diverse sociocultural contexts. Also, circumstances that lead to these complex and multifaceted disorders differ among individuals. Equally difficult to understand is why in some patients substance use disorders continue inexorably to death in spite of treatment, whereas in other patients drug use can be decreased or stopped (either spontaneously or with treatment). Therefore, substance use disorders are perhaps most usefully conceptualized in terms of multiple simultaneous variables interacting over time.

The fact that not all individuals who self-administer psychoactive agents, during given developmental stages or life circumstances, progress to repeated problematic use, has led to the search for factors that determine individual vulnerability. Biological factors that may contribute to the development of substance use disorders include interindividual differences in (1) susceptibility to acute psychopharmacologic effects of a given drug; (2) metabolism of the drug; (3) cellular adaptation within the CNS to chronic exposure to the drug; (4) predisposing personality characteristics (eg, sensation seeking or antisocial traits); and (5) susceptibility to medical and neuropsychiatric complications of chronic drug self-administration. Psychological factors—such as the presence of comorbid psychopathology (eg, depression, anxiety, attention-deficit/hyperactivity disorder, psychosis); medical illnesses (eg, chronic pain, essential tremor); or past or present severe stress (eg, resulting from crime, battle exposure, sexual trauma, or economic difficulties)—have received considerable attention as potential causes for "self-medication." The possibility exists that susceptibility to psychological stressors and substance use disorders may have similar etiologies. For example, some of the etiologic factors that predispose an individual to depression following major losses (eg, dysregulation of noradrenergic neurotransmission or the hypothalamic-pituitary-adrenal axis) may also contribute to the development of substance use disorders. Finally, social factors also contribute to the initiation of drug use and progression of substance use disorders. Such social factors include peer group attitudes toward, and shared expectations of the benefits of, drug use (such as enhanced pleasurable activities with drug use); the availability of competing reinforcers in the form of educational, recreational, and occupational alternatives to substance use; and the availability of drugs during particular developmental stages.

The fact that individuals often use more than one drug simultaneously, or give a history of having used different drugs sequentially during their lifetime, has led to an emphasis on the similarities rather than the differences among abused substances with respect to the ontogeny of drug use behaviors. Further, the stepwise development of different substance use disorders over time suggests common mechanisms of susceptibility and generalizable diagnostic criteria and treatment strategies.

a. Drug-seeking behavior. Conceptualization of substance use disorders in terms of the biopsychosocial model, rather than as simply the physiologic consequences of chronic drug use, has led to recognition of the central role of conditioning and learning in drug dependence. This behavioral perspective provides a framework for understanding the entire spectrum of psychoactive substance use, from its initiation to its progression to compulsive drug use,

as well as the acquisition of tolerance and physical dependence. Psychopharmacologic processes that initiate, maintain, and regulate drug-seeking behavior include (1) the positive reinforcing and discriminative effects of drugs; (2) the environmental stimuli associated with drug effects (which facilitate drug seeking), and (3) the aversive effects of drugs (which extinguish drug seeking). These processes are modulated by social, environmental, and genetic factors such as the individual's personal history, the presence of psychopathology (eg, anxiety, depression, thought disorders), and the individual's previous exposure to (expectancy of) psychoactive drugs (Figure 18–1). The neural mechanisms and behavioral factors that influence psychoactive drug use are amenable to detailed analysis using drug self-administration models in laboratory animals, in which the neuropharmacology and neuroanatomy of the brain systems that mediate reward can be explored.

b. Drug intoxication. Individual factors that affect the quality and magnitude of intoxication also influence drug reinforcement, and ultimately, the development of substance use disorders. Among these are

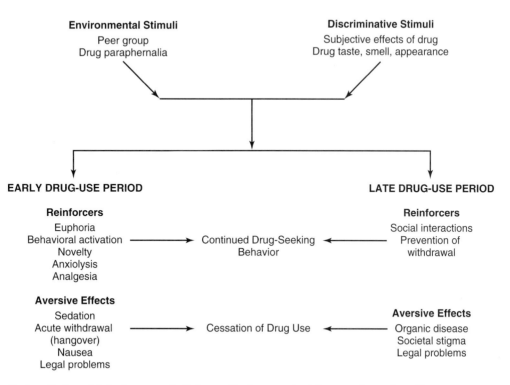

Factors that modulate drug use at all stages: Socioeconomic status; genetic predisposition to drug abuse; success or failure in career/family; social and cultural milieu; psychologic stress; health; financial and legal problems.

Figure 18–1. Factors contributing to drug-seeking behavior. Adapted, with permission, from Martin PR, Lovinger DM, Breese GR: Alcohol and other abused substances. Pages 417–452 in Munson P, Mueller RA, Breese GR (editors): *Principles of Pharmacology: Basic Concepts and Clinical Applications.* Chapman & Hall, 1995.

variables such as initial tolerance, previous experience with the drug, social context of administration, and presence of disorders that affect the CNS or other organs that determine the brain concentration of the drug. Direct adverse consequences of acute intoxication are predictable based on the pharmacologic actions of the drug. For example, CNS depressants have a spectrum of dose-related effects from initial disinhibition at low doses to stupor and coma at higher doses. Similarly, CNS stimulants enhance arousal, attention, and performance at low doses but can lead to psychomotor agitation, psychotic disorganization, and convulsions at higher doses. Often the most serious consequences of these agents are indirect effects, namely impaired performance or judgment, which can cause automobile or work-related accidents, drug-related violence, or unprotected sexual activity. Finally, the route of drug administration can greatly influence intoxication. For example, both intravenous administration and smoking result in rapid entry of the drug into the brain with intense but relatively short-lived euphoria; for highly reinforcing drugs (eg, cocaine, opioids) this can result in compulsive, binge-like use. Nasal insufflation, subcutaneous administration (so-called "skin popping"), and oral ingestion result in relatively slower access to the drug's site of action in the brain, with greater variability in drug bioavailability and lesser reinforcement.

c. Neural mechanisms. Investigation of the neural pathways that mediate the powerful (positive) reinforcing effects of drugs of abuse have implicated dopamine, opioid, and gamma-amino butyric acid (GABA) systems within a midbrain-forebrain-extrapyramidal reward circuit with its focus in the nucleus accumbens. The connections of the ventral midbrain and forebrain, commonly called the medial forebrain bundle, are a major conduit for hypothalamic afferents and efferents and also support (more than any other brain region) the repeated self-administration of current through electrodes (an intracranial self-stimulation model of addiction). This system modulates, or filters, signals from the limbic system that mediate basic biological drives and motivational variables, convert emotion into motivated action and movement via the extrapyramidal system, and may also be the neuronal substrate for the rewarding effects of drugs of abuse. It has been hypothesized that the mesocorticolimbic dopamine system may be critical in motor arousal associated with anticipation of reward, and that all addictive drugs have a psychostimulant (dopaminergic) action as a common underlying mechanism that contributes to reinforcement.

d. Behavioral mechanisms. Behavioral effects of drugs that mediate their positive reinforcing effects are desired changes in mood (euphoria), alleviation of negative affective states (eg, anxiety, depression), functional enhancement (eg, improved psychomotor or cognitive performance), and alleviation of withdrawal. It is difficult to understand why certain psy-

choactive drugs with profound aversive effects can nonetheless maintain drug-seeking behavior and have dependence liability. Aversive effects of drugs counteract the tendency toward self-administration and may limit drug use if they result in dose-dependent toxicity. For example, initial exposure to nicotine in the form of cigarettes often results in distressing symptoms, such as coughing, nausea, and lightheadedness, which may terminate smoking. Similarly, severe gastritis in the chronic alcoholic patient may result in attempts to cut down drinking or limit continued alcohol ingestion. It is now recognized that the stimulus properties of most drugs of abuse, a major determinant of drug-seeking behavior, are complex and multifaceted. Specifically, their pharmacologic profiles include both positive reinforcing and aversive components, and their effects are modified readily by associated environmental stimuli and interindividual differences among drug users.

If a drug is repeatedly administered under given circumstances (situation, time, place), environmental stimuli can become associated with effects of the drug by means of classical (Pavlovian) conditioning processes. Subsequently, the circumstances under which the drug was administered (without actual presentation of the drug) comprise certain environmental (conditioned) stimuli that can modify drug-seeking behavior, subjective state, or psychophysiologic responses (conditioned reinforcement). For example, patients who have been abstinent from intravenous heroin for many years can experience a desire to use heroin when they return to the location where they previously used or when they view a film that portrays others who are injecting drugs intravenously. Using positron emission tomography (PET), researchers have shown that in dependent patients, dopaminergic activation accompanies the presentation of relevant cues from the environment or the anticipation of drug (without its administration). The importance of conditioned stimuli in the response to drugs is also demonstrated readily in laboratory animals by the greater tolerance present when a drug is tested in an environment in which it was administered previously than in a distinctly different environment.

2. Neuroadaptation—Neuroadaptation refers to the neuronal changes and consequent clinical signs and symptoms that result from repeated drug administration independent of drug-seeking behavior or use-related organ damage. It encompasses the biological substrata of tolerance and physical (as opposed to psychological) dependence.

a. Tolerance. After repeated exposure to many psychopharmacologic agents, individuals require a larger dose to produce intoxication of the magnitude that was experienced when the drug was first administered. Conversely, a smaller degree of intoxication results from doses of the drug that were used initially. This phenomenon, called tolerance, is a pharmacologic characteristic shared by many of the substances of abuse considered in DSM-IV (particularly the CNS depressants and the opioids). Tolerance allows and may promote progressively greater doses to be self-administered. (After repeated exposure to CNS stimulants, reverse tolerance, or a greater pharmacologic effect, may be observed.) Tolerance is an adaptive physiologic response of the intact organism that opposes the pharmacologic effects of the drug. The mechanistic underpinnings reside in molecular changes at the cellular level and in the interactions of the organ systems of the body. For example, separable components of tolerance include (1) increased capacity for clearance of a drug by metabolizing enzymes in the liver (pharmacokinetic or metabolic tolerance), (2) reduced response from the same drug concentration (functional or pharmacodynamic tolerance), and (3) accommodation to drug effects through learning (behavioral or learned tolerance). Tolerance to one CNS depressant usually results in some cross-tolerance to other (sometimes chemically unrelated) CNS depressants. Acquisition of tolerance accelerates the development of dose-related complications of drug use.

Acquired tolerance should be distinguished from sensitivity to a given drug on first administration and from acute tolerance that develops over the course of a single exposure to the drug. Differences in the population in initial or acute tolerance to a given drug are innate characteristics of the CNS that may influence individual vulnerability to development of psychoactive substance use disorders.

b. Dependence. Traditionally, dependence has referred to both the neuronal changes that develop after repeated exposure to a given agent and the clinical syndrome characterized by compulsive drug use and serious biopsychosocial consequences that accompanies these neuronal changes. At present, dependence can be defined only indirectly in terms of (1) the presence of tolerance or the emergence of a withdrawal syndrome (immediate and protracted) upon drug discontinuation (physical dependence) and (2) the craving experienced or drug-seeking behavior manifested as a result of conditioned stimuli (psychological dependence). The dependence syndrome represents the elements of psychological dependence, including drug-seeking and psychosocial consequences of drug use. Physical dependence usually develops in concert with tolerance, and controversy remains over whether physical dependence and tolerance are simply different manifestations of the same neuronal changes. The reacquisition of both tolerance and physical dependence are accelerated following repeated cycles of drug administration and withdrawal, suggesting certain similarities between these phenomena and learning and memory. Furthermore, reinforcing and aversive affects of drugs may differ considerably at different stages in the course of a substance use disorder (see Figure 18–1).

c. Withdrawal. Upon discontinuation of chronic administration of many psychoactive agents (or administration of a specific antagonist), a withdrawal (abstinence) syndrome emerges as drug concentrations (or receptor occupancy) at the pharmacologic sites of action decline. This syndrome is characterized by a spectrum of signs and symptoms that are generally opposite to those of intoxication and whose severity is related to the cumulative dose (dosage and duration of administration). For example, withdrawal from CNS depressants results in CNS hyperexcitability, whereas withdrawal from psychostimulants causes CNS depression. For most drugs of abuse, the withdrawal syndrome also involves homeostatic responses to the reversal of neuroadaptive changes that have occurred as a result of long-term drug administration with significant activation of the autonomic nervous system.

d. Cellular & molecular mechanisms of neuroadaptation. Advances in neuroscience, such as the development of specific receptor antagonists, electrophysiologic and brain imaging techniques, and molecular methods to measure subtle cellular alterations, have enhanced our fundamental understanding of neuroadaptation. Neuroadaptation can be conceptualized not only in terms of the intact organism (of particular relevance to understanding the clinical signs and symptoms of withdrawal) but also at the level of neuronal signal transduction, which can be studied in vitro. Changes in synaptic membrane composition, receptor function, and postreceptor intracellular events have all been proposed as the basis of neuroadaptation to psychoactive drugs of abuse. For example, acute alcohol exposure fluidizes cell membranes, but chronic alcohol exposure results in alterations in the lipid composition that render synaptic membranes more rigid. The inhibition by cocaine of dopamine reuptake leads to increased intrasynaptic dopamine, subsequent depletion of presynaptic dopamine due to reduced synthesis of the neurotransmitter, and eventual upregulation, or enhanced sensitivity, of postsynaptic dopamine receptors. Finally, in rats, chronic morphine administration increases G proteins, cyclic adenosine monophosphate–dependent protein kinase, and the phosphorylation of a number of proteins. Several of these adaptive mechanisms likely occur during the development of tolerance or physical dependence, but it is not clear whether one final common pathway exists. Such a common pathway of responses to all psychoactive substances of abuse might be akin to the molecular-level alterations that occur during learning and memory. Keys to molecular changes during neuroadaptation have clear implications for the pharmacotherapy of dependence and withdrawal.

B. Epidemiology: Surveys conducted by various government agencies at fixed intervals since the 1960s have monitored changes in population attitudes, prevalences of different types of drug use, health consequences and estimated costs to society, and treatment outcome. Cross-sectional epidemiologic studies are valuable to the clinician, because knowledge concerning the prevalence of drug-related problems can suggest the likelihood with which these problems may be encountered in the patient population they serve. For example, a physician may be assisted in the management of an overdose or other drug-related emergency by knowing "what's on the street" at that point in time. Longitudinal population studies of cohorts of drug users are particularly informative with respect to understanding antecedents of substance use disorders, dose-response relationships for consequences of use, and determinants of effective treatment outcome.

1. Prevalence of drug use—Patterns of drug use change over time, and contemporaneous prevalence rates can vary according to the epidemiologic survey quoted. Epidemiologic surveys in the United States documented epidemics of marijuana abuse in the 1960s, heroin in the 1970s, and cocaine in the 1980s, with a background of an upward trend in the usage of all drugs and alcohol during the 1970s, followed by a downward trend in the 1980s. Recent reports suggest that the reductions in drug use in the 1980s reversed in the 1990s. Although more Americans use alcohol than any other drug (Table 18–4), younger individuals tend to combine alcohol with multiple other drugs, whereas older cohorts (age 35 years and older) predominantly use alcohol alone. National data have consistently shown that substance use, abuse, and dependence are most prevalent among the young (age 18–34 years) and that the highest rates are observed for young men.

2. Prevalence of substance use disorders— According to the most extensive community survey in which a reliable interview schedule was administered to representative samples of the entire U.S. population, the lifetime prevalence rate of a substance use disorder (except for use of nicotine or caffeine) was 16.7 per 100 persons 18 years and older, higher than for any other mental illness. Alcohol abuse or dependence was identified in 13.5% of the population during their lifetime, and drug abuse or dependence was identified in 6.1% of the population (Table 18–5). In the one sample in this study in which cigarette smok-

Table 18–5. Lifetime prevalence of substance use disorders (per 100 persons aged 18 years or older).[1]

Substance Use Disorders[2]	Lifetime Prevalence
Any substance use disorder	16.7
Any alcohol disorder	13.5
Any drug disorder	6.1
Marijuana dependence or abuse	4.3
Cocaine dependence or abuse	0.2
Opioid dependence or abuse	0.7
Barbiturate dependence or abuse	1.2
Amphetamine dependence or abuse	1.7
Hallucinogen dependence or abuse	0.3

[1] Adapted, with permission, from Regier DA, Kramer ME, Rae DS: Comorbidity of mental disorders with alcohol and other drug abuse: results from the Epidemiologic Catchment Area study. J Am Med Assoc 1990;264:2511.
[2] Diagnoses in the study were based on DSM-III and were obtained using the Diagnostic Interview Schedule, which lay interviewers administered between 1980 and 1984 to a representative sampling of the entire U.S. population.

ing was surveyed, the reported lifetime prevalence was 36.0%. Lifetime prevalence rates for abuse of or dependence on other psychoactive substances were 4.3% for marijuana, 1.7% for amphetamines, 1.2% for barbiturates, 0.7% for opioids, 0.3% for hallucinogens, and 0.2% for cocaine.

3. Risk of comorbid psychiatric diagnoses— The odds of having a mental disorder were 2.7 times greater if one also had substance abuse or dependence (excluding nicotine or caffeine) in comparison with no drug use disorder. Drug use disorders occurred at higher rates in individuals who had alcohol abuse or dependence (21.5%) than in those who did not (3.7%). Alcohol use disorders were more prevalent among those who met criteria for drug abuse or dependence (47.3%) than among those who did not (11.3%). Specific psychiatric diagnoses, such as major depressive disorder, bipolar affective disorder, schizophrenia, anxiety disorders, and antisocial personality disorder, have been associated with substance use disorders, leading to theories of common pathogenesis. This association suggests that the clinician should have a high index of suspicion for diagnosing substance use disorders when dealing with certain clinical populations and should be circumspect about prescribing psychoactive medications to patients who have dependence liability.

C. Genetics: The clinical features and course of alcohol dependence have been studied more extensively than have those of other substance use disorders. Hence, alcohol dependence is a heuristically useful paradigm for understanding the genetic factors that can contribute to the development of most substance use disorders. As discussed earlier in this chap-

Table 18–4. Prevalence rates of psychoactive substance use in the general population (persons aged 18 years or older).[1]

Drug	Percentage Using in Past Year	
	Male (%)	Female (%)
Alcohol	73	64
Cigarettes	35	30
Marijuana	12	8
Psychostimulants	6	3
Tranquilizers	2	2
Any illicit drug	15	11

[1] Adapted, with permission, from Kandel DB: Epidemiology of drug use and abuse. Pages 1–30 in Michels R et al (editors): *Psychiatry.* Vol 3. JB Lippincott, 1992.

ter, individual vulnerabilities to substance use disorders span biological, psychological, and social domains. These domains are tightly interrelated and can influence one another, such that it may be difficult to unravel the role(s) of single variables. Furthermore, substance abuse or dependence in family members disrupts family life in countless ways, thereby affecting developmental processes in children within the family. It is not surprising, therefore, that higher than normal rates of alcohol or drug dependence, as well as of other forms of psychopathology, exist among children of these families. In addition to these environmental factors, genetic factors also play a role in the familial predisposition to substance use disorders.

1. Inheritance of alcohol dependence—Findings from twin and adoption studies demonstrate the relative contributions of genetic and environmental factors in predisposition to alcohol dependence. For example, the concordance rate for alcohol dependence is substantially higher in monozygotic (0.70) than dizygotic (0.33) twins, whereas concordance rates are no different for less severe forms of the disorder or for alcohol abuse (0.8 for both monozygotic and dizygotic twins). Adoption studies show that adopted-away men with alcoholic biological parents have an increased likelihood of developing alcoholism regardless of whether they are raised in an alcoholic environment. In general, the severity of parental alcoholism tends to influence the prevalence of alcoholism in adopted-away sons; patients with the most severe alcoholism have the highest rates of alcohol dependence in their offspring. These studies suggest that the relative contributions of environmental and genetic factors in development of alcoholism may vary with the severity or type of alcohol dependence.

2. Heterogeneity of alcohol dependence— As discussed earlier in this chapter, large differences exist among groups of alcohol-dependent patients. The challenge in genetic studies of alcoholism has been to identify more homogenous subgroups of alcohol-dependent patients. Such clearly circumscribed subgroupings of patients (and their families) could then be studied in depth to identify predictors of etiology, longitudinal course, and response to different treatment modalities. One heuristically useful classification is based predominantly on the age at onset of alcohol dependence, namely, onset after age 25 (Type 1) and onset before age 25 (Type 2). Reliably different clusters of alcohol-related problems and personality traits tend to occur with these two types of alcohol dependence. In general, patients with Type 2 alcoholism are characterized by greater thrill-seeking, impulsiveness, and aggressiveness than are patients with Type 1 alcoholism, who have a greater tendency to become anxious and depressed as a result of their drinking. Type 2 alcoholism tends to be more recalcitrant to treatment than is Type 1 alcoholism.

Both genetic predisposition and an alcoholic rearing environment were required for adopted-away sons of fathers with Type 1 alcoholism to express Type 1 alcoholism. In contrast, adopted-away sons of fathers with Type 2 alcoholism were significantly more likely to manifest this type of alcohol dependence than were offspring of fathers without Type 2 alcoholism, whether or not they were raised in an alcoholic family. This observation indicates that the genetic loading for alcohol dependence is influenced profoundly by the environment for late-onset alcohol dependence, whereas environmental background is relatively less important for early-onset alcohol dependence.

3. Women & addiction—There are distinct differences between the genders in the inheritance, clinical presentation, and longitudinal course of alcohol dependence. It is particularly important to understand alcohol use disorders in women because of the adverse effects of drinking on the developing fetus, and the disruptive effects of alcohol use or dependence on the mother-child relationship. Both of these consequences of alcohol consumption in women can perpetuate the transmission of alcohol use disorders from one generation to the next via nongenetic means.

Women still have lower rates of alcohol dependence compared to men, although these rates are rising at a disquieting pace. Lower rates of alcohol dependence result in part from the lower amounts of alcohol consumed by women in general for a number of psychosocial and biological reasons. Even though women start drinking later than men do, they tend to develop, at about the same age as men, more serious physical complications. These observations suggest greater intrinsic toxicity of ethanol to the liver, brain, and possibly other organ systems in women compared to men. Established gender-related differences in predisposition to comorbid psychopathology (eg, depression and somatic anxiety) may complicate and exacerbate alcohol dependence. Daughters of fathers with Type 1 alcoholism are at increased risk for alcoholism but not for other psychopathology; daughters of fathers with Type 2 alcoholism are at higher risk only for somatization disorder.

4. Genetic factors in development of alcoholism—Although genetic studies suggest that genetic factors are important contributors to the development of alcoholism, the mechanisms involved remain to be elucidated. This is an exciting area of research, but the clinical application of the proposed hypotheses is not clear. For example, it has been suggested that children of alcoholic fathers are less sensitive to the intoxicating effects of ethanol than are children of nonalcoholic fathers. Presumably, these children would have to drink more than would children of nonalcoholic fathers in order to become intoxicated and, thus, may be more likely to become alcohol dependent. The abilities of researchers to match subjects in terms of lifetime exposure to, and experience with, alcohol are important limitations of these studies. Such limitations can be overcome only by carefully conducted longitudinal investigations beginning in childhood. Early notions that differences in innate tolerance to ethanol or susceptibility to alcohol dependence were based on differences in ethanol metabolism have not been firmly established. More recently, researchers have focused on interindividual differences in brain biogenic amine metabolism as predisposing to development of alcohol dependence. Specifically, considerable preclinical and human data implicate low brain serotonergic activity in stimulating alcohol consumption and in producing the aggressive and impulsive behavior often associated with Type 2 alcoholism. In addition, the impaired ability to allocate significance to targeted stimuli, as manifested by a reduced amplitude of the late positive component of event-related electroencephalographic (EEG) potential, has been identified in children of fathers with Type 2 alcoholism, and thus, is considered a predisposing factor to development of alcohol dependence.

5. Inheritance of substance use disorders other than alcohol dependence—It is unknown whether the genetic mechanisms that predispose individuals to alcohol dependence also influence the development of other substance use disorders. Common causality is suggested (though difficult to prove) because many, particularly younger individuals tend to combine (often indiscriminately) alcohol and other drugs of abuse.

The twin and adoption studies described earlier in this chapter provide guidelines for how to study this question in patients with drug abuse or dependence. For example, in one adoption study of genetic and environmental factors in drug abuse, drug abuse in adult adoptees was associated in equivalent proportions with (1) antisocial personality in the adoptees, related to a biological background of antisocial personality; (2) no antisocial personality in the adoptees but with a biological background of alcoholism; and (3) neither antisocial personality nor alcoholism in either the adoptee or the biological background but psychosocial factors such as divorce and psychiatric illness in the adopting family environment. Such studies show that interactions of genetic and environmental factors are as important in the development of other substance use disorders as they are for alcohol dependence. A shared underlying mechanism seems most likely to involve abnormalities of brain functioning or the presence of, or vulnerability to, depression, anxiety, or related psychopathology.

Cloninger CR: Neurogenetic adaptive mechanisms in alcoholism. Science 1987;236:410.

Crabbe JC, Belknap JK, Buck KJ: Genetic animal models of alcohol and drug abuse. Science 1994;264:1715.

O'Brien CP et al: A learning model of addiction. Pages 157–177 in O'Brien CP, Jaffe JH (editors): *Addictive States.* Raven, 1992.

Robinson TE, Berridge KC: The neural basis of drug craving: an incentive-sensitization theory of addiction. Brain Res Rev 1993;18:247.

Patterns of Use

1. Alcohol & other CNS depressants—The CNS depressants include brewed or distilled alcoholic beverages and various pharmaceutical agents prescribed for treatment of insomnia, anxiety, depression, and less frequently for control of seizure disorders or as muscle relaxants (see Table 18–2). Although new CNS depressants (eg, alprazolam, buspirone, zolpidem) may initially be marketed with claims of pharmacologic novelty, no CNS depressant has been developed to date that is totally free of abuse liability and the potential for a significant withdrawal syndrome upon drug discontinuation, problems they share with alcoholic beverages.

Alcoholic beverages are readily available at affordable cost with minimal legal restrictions. Accordingly, there is widespread use of alcohol in diverse recreational and work-related circumstances, and traumatic injuries sustained while under the influence of elevated blood alcohol concentrations are among the most common public health problems today. Youngsters with little experience with drinking are particularly vulnerable as they first begin to participate in high-risk activities such as sports, sexuality, and driving. Also, heavy drinkers, who often have blood alcohol concentrations that impair judgment and motor skills or who use other drugs in combination with alcohol, are particularly at risk for alcohol-related violence, traumatic injury, and death.

The benzodiazepines are currently (as barbiturates were previously) among the most widely prescribed medications and the most commonly misused or abused type of prescription drug. With continued use, individuals develop tolerance and need larger doses to achieve symptomatic relief. If the physician does not educate the patient and provide careful prescription monitoring, the patient may eventually receive large doses of these medications with attendant side effects such as mood disorders, cognitive dysfunction, social difficulties, impaired work performance, and traumatic injury due to falls or vehicular accidents. In order to maintain symptomatic relief in the face of tighter controls by the prescribing physician, the patient may combine alcohol or other prescribed medications or illicit drugs (eg, marijuana, opioids) with the prescribed dose of CNS depressant, seek other physicians to provide additional prescriptions (so-called doctor shopping), or engage in illegal activities such as forging prescriptions. The combination of alcohol with other CNS depressants greatly increases the risk associated with its use and is the most common clinical cause of severe drug overdoses. Cessation of drug use leads to undesirable, and potentially harmful, withdrawal symptoms (such as seizures). Thus drug-seeking behavior and repeated drug use is often continued in order to prevent these effects. Fulminant withdrawal occasionally results in patients who discontinue CNS depressant use because of illness or other unforeseen circumstances such as hospitalization for a motor vehicle accident.

2. Psychostimulants: cocaine & amphetamines—The alkaloid cocaine is derived from *Erythroxylon coca,* a plant indigenous to South America, where since time immemorial its leaves have been chewed for their stimulating effects. Because the only contemporary medical use for cocaine is as a local anesthetic, the drug is almost always purchased illegally by users. Amphetamine and amphetamine-like stimulants may be obtained by prescription for the treatment of obesity, attention-deficit/hyperactivity disorder, and narcolepsy; therefore, diversion of prescribed stimulants into the illegal market is relatively common (see Table 18–2). The current epidemic of cocaine use started in the late 1970s, preceded by a period in which cocaine was thought not to be particularly dangerous. Cocaine's significant dependence liability came to be recognized later, resulting in a recent diminution in use of the drug.

Abuse of amphetamine-like compounds has continued unabated because of their widespread availability and relatively low cost. Recently, illegally manufactured methamphetamine derivatives (so-called designer drugs), including a crystallized, smokable form called "ice," have become available on the illegal market.

Cocaine and other stimulants are almost always used with other psychoactive substances, most commonly alcohol but also other CNS depressants or opioids. Alcohol is considered a gateway drug for cocaine and other stimulant use. It can accentuate the "high" obtained from stimulants, alleviate some of the adverse effects (eg, "wired" feelings), and is a readily available (ie, legal) substitute. Heroin (sometimes called "speedball") is another drug that is commonly combined with cocaine and is reported to increase cocaine euphoria.

Methods of use include inhalation via the nostrils (snorting), subcutaneous or intravenous injection, and smoking (free basing). Inhalation is the most common and least dangerous method, but it does not provide the ecstatic sensation associated with smoking or injection. These latter routes of administration give the drug rapid access to the brain, thereby increasing its reinforcing effect and its toxicity.

3. Opioids—Opioid use and addiction has occurred for centuries, and many opioid compounds are abused throughout the world (see Table 18–2). Opioid abuse may start with initially appropriate use for medical analgesia. Some drugs such as codeine and pentazocine can be found in nonprescription medications such as cough syrup and may be abused when more potent illicit drugs are not readily available. Illicit heroin use has surpassed that of morphine in most Western countries. About 1.3% of the U.S. population used heroin in 1991. According to one study, urban dwellers are the most frequent abusers of opioids, and about half of these live in New York City. Medical

professionals with easy access to opioids are also at increased risk. In Asia, frequent opium use is still popular.

Unrefined opium is often smoked using a water pipe. Intravenous use of heroin (mainlining) and morphine is popular because of the short-lived (less than a minute), sudden "rush" produced. Subcutaneous injection is sometimes used, especially if veins have become unusable because of frequent injections. Refined opioids can also be inhaled, a method often preferred by new users. Although the euphoric state of opioid intake is short, the sedative and analgesic effects can continue for hours. Street drugs are frequently "cut" (mixed or combined) with other substances, such as caffeine, powdered milk, quinine, and strychnine, to dilute the concentration of the active ingredient. These other substances can lead to altered clinical effects and medical difficulties beyond those associated with the opioid.

4. Cannabinoids—Marijuana is the common name for the plant *Cannabis sativa.* Other names for the plant or its products include hemp, hashish, chasra, bhang, ganja, and daga. The highest concentrations of the psychoactive cannabinoids are found in the flowering tops of both male and female plants. Most commonly the plant is cut, dried, chopped, and then incorporated into cigarettes. The primary psychoactive constituent of marijuana is delta-9-tetrahydrocannabinol, although many other active cannabinoids are known. The hemp plant synthesizes at least 400 of these chemicals.

As of 1991, marijuana was the most commonly used illicit substance. About 33% of adults in the United States have used marijuana, and approximately 5% use it on a regular basis. In North America, teenagers and young adults often use marijuana (whether in school or otherwise). Marijuana is often the first illicit drug, other than alcohol, that youngsters try. Marijuana use has been declining among young adults, and for the first time in history, use rates in females appear to be higher than in males. The likelihood of having used cocaine increases with the extent of marijuana use in all age groups. The epidemiology of marijuana use, therefore, can be viewed as a predictor of cocaine-related problems in a given population.

5. Nicotine & tobacco—Tobacco is a substance commonly used in many countries and across age groups, from early teens to the elderly. Almost 75% of the U.S. population have used cigarettes at some point during their lifetime. Comparatively high use is found in males, although use in females is increasing. Cigarette smoking is the most common method of use, although cigar smoking, pipe smoking, and smokeless tobacco (snuff) use each have had varying levels of popularity at different times and among different groups. Primarily because of educational programs, use of tobacco products has declined over the past 20 years in North America, although about 36% of the population continues to use tobacco products and use increased recently in some subpopulations, such as teenage girls.

According to studies that alter nicotine and tar content of cigarettes, user satisfaction appears to be related to nicotine content, suggesting that this agent is responsible for the reinforcing effects. Heated debate, litigation, changes in laws, and greater enforcement of existing laws regulating the cigarette industry have occurred recently.

6. Hallucinogens & volatile inhalants—Hallucinogens are subdivided into two major categories: the indoalkylamines (such as D-lysergic acid diethylamide [LSD], dimethyltryptamine [DMT], psilocin, psilocybin, and diethyltryptamine [DET]) and the phenylethylamines (such as trimethoxyphenylethylamine [mescaline], 3,4-methylenedioxy methamphetamine [MDMA; called "ecstasy" on the streets], 2,5-dimethoxytryptamine [DOM, STP], and 3,4-methylenedioxy amphetamine [MDA]). Other hallucinogens include peyote (mescaline, from Mexican cactus), *Myristica fragrans* (nutmeg), and morning-glory seeds (similar to LSD). Arylcyclohexylamines include phencyclidine (PCP; called "angel dust," "crystal," "weed," and "hog" on the streets) and ketamine. Ketamine is most commonly used as an anesthetic in veterinary medicine; PCP has no current medical uses.

Volatile inhalants include aromatic, aliphatic, and halogenated hydrocarbon compounds such as gasoline, solvents (eg, acetone), paints, glues, refrigerants (eg, Freon), and paint thinners (eg, turpentine). Nitrous oxide (an anesthetic) and amyl nitrite (a vasodilator; called "poppers" on the streets) are also often included.

Native Americans used psychedelic drugs such as mushrooms (psilocybin and psilocin) and peyote before the Spanish exploration of Mexico. Hoffman reported the hallucinogenic effects of LSD in 1943. Scopolamine (and other belladonna alkaloids), mescaline (a plant product), and amphetamine designer drugs have similar effects. Use of hallucinogens in the United States was most popular in the 1960s and early 1970s, with a dramatic decline shortly afterward. The use of these drugs has continued, however, at a fairly constant level since the late 1970s. An increase of use, particularly of the designer drugs, has been noted among teens and young adults. Some Native Americans and other groups continue to use certain of the plant hallucinogens in their mystic ceremonies. PCP is used most commonly in urban areas.

Users of volatile inhalants are most often in their preteen and teenage years. Professionals, such as dentists, who have easy access to substances such as nitrous oxide are also at increased risk of use. Use of volatile inhalants was perhaps greatest in the late 1970s and early 1980s.

Clinical Findings

A. Signs & Symptoms:
1. Alcohol & other CNS depressants—
a. Intoxication. Alcohol and other CNS depressant intoxication proceeds in stages that depend on dosage and time following administration. Apparent CNS stimulation, which occurs early in alcohol or CNS depressant intoxication or at low dosages, results from depression of inhibitory control mechanisms. The most sensitive parts of the brain are the polysynaptic structures of the reticular activating system and the cortex, depression of which causes euphoria and dulling of performance that depends on training and previous experience. Excitation resulting from intoxication is characterized by increased activity, verbal communication, and often aggression (Table 18–6). Euphoric feelings or calming effects are typically the expressed reason for drug self-administration. Higher blood concentrations of alcohol or other CNS depressants cause mild impairment of motor skills and slowing of reaction time, followed by sedation, decreased motor coordination, impaired judgment, diminished memory and other cognitive deficits, and eventually diminished psychomotor activity and sleep. At still higher concentrations, alcohol and most CNS depressants can induce stupor, and ultimately coma and death, by progressive depression of midbrain functions and interference with spinal reflexes, temperature regulation, and the medullary cen-

Table 18–6. Signs and symptoms of CNS depressant intoxication and withdrawal.

Intoxication	Withdrawal
Disinhibition (eg, inappropriate sexual or aggressive behavior, impaired judgment, mood lability)	Anxiety or psychomotor agitation
Somnolence, stupor, or coma	Tremor
Impaired attention or memory	Craving
Slurred speech	Autonomic hyperactivity (eg, tachycardia, hypertension, sweating, hyperthermia, arrhythmia)
Incoordination	Insomnia
Unsteady gait	Sensory distortions or hallucinations (eg, transient visual, tactile, or auditory)
Nystagmus	Nausea or vomiting
	Seizures
	Delirium

ters controlling cardiorespiratory functions. Death due to benzodiazepine overdose is very unlikely unless combined with alcohol or other CNS depressants.

The dose-response curve of ethanol has been studied in greater depth than has any other CNS depressant. Sensitivity to alcohol intoxication varies widely within the population as a whole. For example, at blood ethanol concentrations of 50, 100–150, and 200 mg/100 mL, it is estimated that approximately 10%, 64%, and almost all of the general population, respectively, would appear overtly intoxicated. In contrast, at a blood ethanol concentration of 300 mg/100 mL, some alcoholic individuals may appear only mildly intoxicated even though their psychomotor performance and judgment are impaired significantly. According to the Council of Scientific Affairs of the American Medical Association, blood alcohol concentrations of 60, 100, and 150 mg/100 mL increase an individual's relative probability of causing an automobile accident 2-, 6-, and 25-fold, respectively. Legal limits of blood ethanol concentration for automobile drivers are 100 mg/100 mL (the term in common use is 0.10) for most states in the United States, 80 mg/100 mL for most countries in Western Europe, and between 0 and 50 mg/100 mL for Scandinavian and Eastern European countries.

b. Drug-seeking behavior. The classic sedative-hypnotic actions of ethanol, barbiturates, and benzodiazepines correlate well with their shared ability to modulate GABA-induced chloride anion fluxes in vitro. These drugs can also act as anxiolytics; however, benzodiazepines are unique among CNS depressants because of their ability to reduce anxiety while causing minimal sedation. It is believed that the reinforcing actions and abuse potential of CNS depressants reside primarily in their anxiolytic and tension-reducing properties mediated by activation of $GABA_A$ receptors. Furthermore, in animal models, established GABA efferents from the nucleus accumbens to the substantia innominata-ventral pallidum can influence expression of cocaine- or opioid-induced behavioral stimulation. This may explain why alcohol and other CNS depressants are often used by addicted individuals along with cocaine or opioids.

c. Neuroadaptation. Adaptive neuronal changes resulting from the continued presence of alcohol or other CNS depressants involve a decrease in inhibitory functions of the nervous system. Although the molecular basis of such neuronal adaptation has not been elucidated fully, the clinical consequences are well characterized and include the development of tolerance and dependence, which usually proceed in parallel. Although pharmacokinetic differences among CNS depressants may alter the duration of time the agent is present at its site of pharmacologic action, and subtle molecular differences may influence the precise interactions of the different agents with their binding site(s) and the complement of neuronal receptors occupied, the neuroadaptive changes that eventually re-

sult from chronic ingestion of alcohol, benzodiazepines, barbiturates, or nonbarbiturate hypnosedatives are for practical purposes much the same.

The development of tolerance to, and dependence on, CNS depressants can occur after only a few days of repeated ingestion and, as with all drugs, is determined by dosage and frequency of use. For example, a drug dosage that initially caused sedation and anxiolysis may in time be insufficient to induce sleep or reduce anxiety; thus, higher dosages are needed to attain these therapeutic goals. Tolerance may not develop at the same rate to all actions of a CNS depressant. For example, whereas sedation usually diminishes after the first few days of treatment with most benzodiazepines, anxiolytic effects may persist for months without the need to increase the dosage. Euphoric effects may not be as predictable, which can cause rapid increases in dosage if the drug is being self-administered for this purpose. In general, for alcohol and other CNS depressants there is no marked elevation of the lethal dosage with repeated use, and respiratory depression may be superimposed on chronic consumption with a severe, acute overdose.

d. Withdrawal. Cessation of alcohol or CNS depressant intake after prolonged use is associated with a syndrome of neuronal hyperexcitability with increased noradrenergic and adrenocortical activity. This syndrome is initially characterized by anxiety, apprehension, restlessness, irritability, and insomnia with clinically apparent tremor and hyperreflexia (see Table 18–6). Moderately severe cases progress to signs of autonomic hyperactivity with tachycardia, hypertension, diaphoresis, hyperthermia, and muscle fasciculations. Often patients experience anorexia, nausea, or vomiting with subsequent dehydration and electrolyte disturbances. Paroxysmal EEG discharges may precede generalized tonic-clonic seizure activity. Patients with the most severe cases may develop delirium (agitation, disorientation, fluctuating level of consciousness, visual and auditory hallucinations, and intense autonomic arousal).

Among the CNS depressants, the most severe and potentially dangerous withdrawal syndrome results from barbiturates and nonbarbiturate hypnosedatives; alcohol withdrawal is of intermediate severity; and withdrawal from benzodiazepines poses the least risk. The onset, severity, and duration of the withdrawal syndrome in a given class of CNS depressants are determined by the rate of elimination of the drug and metabolites from the body. In the alcohol withdrawal syndrome, generalized tonic-clonic seizures typically occur 12–48 hours after the last drink, and delirium tremens begins at 48–72 hours. The signs of acute alcohol withdrawal typically abate by 3–5 days after the last drink, but subtle brain abnormalities may persist for an undetermined period. Among the barbiturates, nonbarbiturate hypnosedatives, and benzodiazepines, withdrawal usually begins within 12 hours and is most severe for rapidly eliminated compounds (eg, amobarbital, methyprylon, triazolam). For slowly metabolized compounds (eg, phenobarbital, diazepam, clonazepam), the syndrome may be delayed for several days after drug discontinuation. More protracted effects of withdrawal from CNS depressants have not been well studied, but residual problems related to cognitive impairment, anxiety and depressive symptoms, and insomnia may result.

2. Psychostimulants: cocaine & amphetamines—

a. Intoxication. The main clinically relevant pharmacologic action of cocaine and amphetamine-related stimulants is the blockade of reuptake of the catecholamine neurotransmitters norepinephrine and dopamine. The consequences of noradrenergic reuptake blockade include tachycardia, hypertension, vasoconstriction, mydriasis, diaphoresis, and tremor. The effects of dopamine reuptake blockade include self-stimulation, anorexia, stereotyped movements, hyperactivity, and sexual excitement. As a result, many of the signs and symptoms of cocaine and amphetamine intoxication are similar (Table 18–7). CNS stimulation and a subjective "high" are accompanied by an increased sense of energy, psychomotor agitation, and autonomic arousal.

The psychoactive effects of most amphetamine-like substances last longer than those of cocaine. Furthermore, because cocaine has local anesthetic actions, the risk of it causing severe medical complications such as cardiac arrhythmia and seizures is greater than for amphetamine-like stimulants. Amphetamine-related compounds therefore remain popular in the stimulant-abusing population.

b. Drug-seeking behavior. The most striking pharmacologic characteristic of cocaine is its tremendous reinforcing effect. Women who are cocaine dependent have higher rates of primary major depression than do cocaine-dependent men, consistent with drug use as a form of self-medication. Men with cocaine dependence have higher rates of comorbid antisocial personality disorder than do cocaine-dependent women. Studies in animal models have shown that animals will self-administer cocaine preferentially over food, leading to emaciation and death (in contrast to other highly reinforcing agents such as opioids). Dopamine seems to be the primary neurotransmitter involved in the positive reinforcement of cocaine.

c. Neuroadaptation. Although not well-understood, neuroadaptation appears to occur in response to chronic psychostimulant use. Users develop acute tolerance to the subjective effects of cocaine, which can play a major role in dose escalation and subsequent toxicity. Sensitization appears to play a role in cocaine-induced panic attacks, paranoia, and lethality.

d. Withdrawal. In humans, discontinuation of cocaine leads to dysphoria (a so-called crash). Hypersomnolence and anergia are also common (see Table 18–7). In rats, termination of repeated cocaine administration produces interoceptive stimuli that are similar to the discriminative stimulus effects of pentetrazole, a drug that is anxiogenic in humans. As a result, the typical cycle of use consists of binges, each followed by a crash (lasting 9 hours to 4 days), followed by withdrawal (lasting 1–10 weeks), during which craving and relapse is common.

3. Opioids—

a. Intoxication. The characteristic pharmacologic action of opioids is analgesia. Centrally, opioids are activating at low dosages and sedating at higher dosages. Other major features of intoxication are feelings of euphoria or dysphoria, feelings of warmth, facial flushing, itchy face, dry mouth, and pupil constriction (Table 18–8). Intravenous use can cause lower abdominal sensations described as an orgasm-like "rush." This is followed by a feeling of sedation (called the "nod") and dreaming. Severe intoxication may cause respiratory suppression, areflexia, hypotension, tachycardia, apnea, cyanosis, and death.

b. Drug-seeking behavior. Addiction to opioids (particularly heroin) can be severe and often leads individuals to dysfunctional behaviors to sup-

Table 18–7. Signs and symptoms of psychostimulant intoxication and withdrawal.

Intoxication	Withdrawal
Stimulation (euphoria, hypervigilance, anxiety, tension, anger, impaired judgment)	Depression (dysphoria)
Psychomotor agitation (stereotyped behaviors, dyskinesias, dystonias)	Psychomotor retardation
Energy (decreased need for sleep)	Fatigue (increased need for sleep)
Anorexia (nausea or vomiting, weight loss)	Increased appetite
Autonomic arousal (tachycardia, hypertension, pupillary dilation, perspiration or chills)	Craving
Chest pain, cardiac arrhythmias, respiratory depression	
Confusion	
Seizures	

port their habit. Animals tend to prolong and repeat opioid self-administration.

Self-administered opioid compounds affect the endogenous opioid systems of the body. Endogenous opioid peptides are distributed throughout the brain and form three major functional systems defined by their precursor molecules: β-endorphin from pro-opiomelanocortin, enkephalins from proenkephalin, and dynorphin from prodynorphin. The endogenous opioids modulate nociceptive responses to painful stimuli, stressors, reward, and homeostatic adaptive functions such as hunger, thirst, and temperature regulation. Rats will self-administer opioid peptides into the ventral tegmental area (VTA) and nucleus accumbens, suggesting that these regions may, at least in part, be responsible for the reinforcing properties of opioids (and cocaine). Other regions supporting rewarding effects for opioids are the hippocampus and hypothalamus. Endogenous opioid tone contributes to maintenance of normal mood and a nondopaminergic system of opioid reward.

Three main types of opioid receptors may be distinguished pharmacologically: μ, δ, and κ. These G protein–coupled proteins inhibit adenyl cyclases in various tissues and cause their pharmacologic actions by reducing cyclic adenosine monophosphate levels. The μ-opioid receptor subtype appears to be important for the reinforcing actions of opioids, whereas δ-opioid receptors may play a role in the opioid motor stimulation that is dopamine (D$_1$ receptor) dependent. Like other substances of abuse, opioids can increase dopamine release in the nucleus accumbens as measured by in vivo microdialysis in awake, freely moving animals, but the reinforcing effect of opioids in the nucleus accumbens can be independent of dopamine release. Therefore, the reinforcing actions of opioids may involve both a dopamine-dependent (VTA) and a dopamine-independent (nucleus accumbens) mechanism.

c. Neuroadaptation. Neuroadaptation occurs in response to regular opioid use. For example, when chronically abused by humans, heroin rapidly loses its aversive properties while increasing its reinforcing ones. The tolerance that develops when opioids are administered repeatedly appears to be receptor selective. It has been theorized that μ-receptors couple less well to G proteins in rat locus coeruleus neurons that have been chronically treated with morphine. Tolerance occurs both to specific opioid effects such as analgesia and motor inhibition and to the generally depressant properties of opioids, whereas the psychomotor effects are potentiated. Behavioral sensitization to opioids can be modeled by intra-VTA, but not intra-accumbens, morphine (or psychostimulants) and is related to an increased activation of VTA dopaminergic neurons.

d. Withdrawal. Withdrawal of opioids is characterized by hyperalgesia, photophobia, goose flesh, diarrhea, tachycardia, increased blood pressure, gastrointestinal cramps, joint and muscle aches, and anxiety and depressed mood (see Table 18–8). Spontaneous withdrawal results in intense craving because of the reduction of dopamine release in the nucleus accumbens, but the degree of physical dependence does not predict the severity of craving. The motivational (affective) properties of withdrawal are independent of the intensity and pattern of the physical symptoms. Because opioids can counteract both the withdrawal dysphoria and the reduction of dopaminergic transmission, these changes may contribute to maintenance of opioid addiction.

4. Cannabinoids—

a. Intoxication. The subjective effects of marijuana intoxication vary from individual to individual determined in part by highly variable pharmacokinetic variables, dosage, route of administration, setting, experience and expectation, and individual vul-

Table 18–8. Signs and symptoms of opioid intoxication and withdrawal.

Intoxication	Withdrawal
Activation or "rush" (early or with low dosages) and sedation/apathy or "nod" (late or with high dosages)	Depressed mood and anxiety Dysphoria
Euphoria or dysphoria	Craving
Feelings of warmth, facial flushing, or itching	Piloerection ("goose flesh") Lacrimation or rhinorrhea
Impaired judgment, attention, or memory	
Analgesia	Hyperalgia, joint and muscle aches
Constipation	Diarrhea and gastrointestinal cramping, nausea, or vomiting
Pupillary constriction	Pupillary dilation and photophobia
Drowsiness	Insomnia
Respiratory depression, areflexia, hypotension, tachycardia	Autonomic hyperactivity (eg, tachypnea, hyperreflexia, tachycardia, hypertension, sweating, hyperthermia)
Apnea, cyanosis, coma	Yawning

Table 18–9. Signs and symptoms of cannabis intoxication.

Euphoria, drowsiness, or sedation
Sensation of slowed time
Auditory or visual distortions, dissociation
Impaired judgment, motor coordination, attention, or memory
Slowed reaction time
Conjunctival injection
Tachycardia
Increased appetite
Anxiety, acute panic reactions, paranoia, illusions, or agitation

nerability to certain psychotoxic effects. Typically, intoxication is characterized by an initial period of "high" that has been described as a sense of well-being and happiness (Table 18–9). This euphoria is followed frequently by a period of drowsiness or sedation. Perception of time is altered and hearing and vision are distorted. The subjective effects of intoxication often include dissociation reactions. Impaired functioning occurs in a variety of cognitive and performance tasks, including memory, reaction time, concept formation, learning, perception, motor coordination, attention, and signal detection. At dosages equivalent to one or two joints (marijuana cigarettes), processes involved in the operation of motor vehicles or airplanes are impaired. The impairment persists for 4–8 hours, long after the user perceives the subjective effects of the drug. The impairment produced by alcohol is additive to that produced by marijuana. Tolerant individuals may exhibit somewhat lesser performance decrements.

Physically, dilation of conjunctival blood vessels and tachycardia may be noted. Blood pressure remains relatively unchanged unless high dosages are used, in which case orthostatic hypotension ensues. Increased appetite is often attributed to marijuana but has not been observed consistently in controlled studies. At higher dosages, acute panic reactions, paranoia, hallucinations, illusions, thought disorganization, and agitation have been observed. With extremely high dosages, an acute toxic psychosis is accompanied by depersonalization and loss of insight.

b. Drug-seeking behavior. In chronic cannabinoid users, dependence and degree of drug-seeking behaviors is controversial. In some patients, drug-seeking behavior appears to be manifested primarily as drug craving. The psychological or physiologic mechanisms underpinning this craving are not certain. Laboratory animals do not self-administer the drug.

c. Neuroadaptation. Neuroadaptation in response to cannabinoid use has been more difficult to document than in some of the other drugs of abuse. Tolerance to cannabinoids appears to develop in animals and in humans, although it does not seem to be as profound as with some other drugs and occurs mostly with heavy use.

d. Withdrawal. Cannabinoid withdrawal does not produce well-characterized withdrawal symptoms, and DSM-IV does not include cannabis withdrawal. Some patients have reported insomnia, irritability, dysphoria, anorexia, hand tremor, mild fever, or slight nausea with discontinuation of use. This occurs primarily in patients who smoke very potent preparations.

5. Nicotine & tobacco—

a. Intoxication. Nicotine intoxication is not a DSM-IV diagnosis. However, nicotine intake has multiple effects. For example, many users report improved mood, skeletal muscle relaxation, and diminished anxiety and appetite. In addition, cognitive effects including enhanced attention, problem solving, learning, and memory have been reported.

b. Drug-seeking behavior. Users of tobacco products frequently exhibit substance-seeking behaviors. Smokers often describe strong cravings for tobacco, especially in specific situations such as after eating or while experiencing stress. The degree of craving appears to differ among individuals, and the ability to discontinue tobacco products also varies greatly.

c. Neuroadaptation. Nicotine is thought to be the primary substance in tobacco that causes neuroadaptation. Tolerance to nicotine has been shown in both laboratory animals and humans. Dependence is indicated by the difficulty of discontinuing use of nicotine products despite a desire to quit.

The primary pharmacologic actions of nicotine appear to occur via nicotine binding to acetylcholine receptors in the brain and autonomic ganglia. Several subtypes of nicotinic cholinergic receptors are found in the CNS. Activation of these receptors appears to cause the reinforcing effects and diminished appetite associated with nicotine. Some of the reinforcing actions of nicotine may be due to effects of nicotine on dopamine pathways projecting from the VTA to the limbic system and the cerebral cortex. Stimulation of peripheral nicotine receptors causes many of the autonomic effects associated with nicotine use. Short-term use of tobacco appears to increase cerebral blood flow, whereas long-term use has the opposite effect. Aspects of neuroadaptation to nicotine may also be secondary to release of hormones such as β-endorphin, adrenocorticotropic hormone (ACTH), cortisol, epinephrine, norepinephrine, and vasopressin.

d. Withdrawal. Withdrawal symptoms often occur with abrupt discontinuation of nicotine intake. Symptoms include craving, anxiety, depression, irritability, headaches, poor concentration, sleep disturbances, enhanced blood pressure, and increased heart rate. In some cases, craving may last for years under appropriate circumstances.

6. Hallucinogens & volatile inhalants—

a. Intoxication. Intoxication with hallucinogens causes effects that vary greatly and may last 8–12 hours, with flashbacks possible after termination of use (Table 18–10). The cardinal features of hallucinogen intoxication include visual hallucinations and disturbance of thoughts and perception in multiple sensory modalities. These features can lead to devas-

Table 18–10. Signs and symptoms
of hallucinogen intoxication.

Marked anxiety or depression
Perceptual changes (eg, intense perceptions, depersonalization, derealization, illusions, hallucinations, synesthesias)
Thought disorders (eg, ideas of reference, paranoia, impaired reality testing)
Impaired judgment
Autonomic arousal (eg, pupillary dilation, tachycardia, sweating, palpitations, blurring of vision, tremors, incoordination)

---

tating consequences if they occur in dangerous situations (eg, when driving or when standing in potential fall areas such as on a balcony). Other features include sensory changes (eg, colors, shapes), synesthesia (the misperception of a sensory stimulus of one modality with that of a different one), delusions, paranoia, derealization, depersonalization, cognitive impairment, coordination problems, behavioral changes, euphoria (or dysphoria), nausea, tremors, time distortion, dizziness, weakness, and giddiness. A "bad trip" may occur with striking dysphoria. Visual hallucinations with perception of various light patterns or incorrect movement perception or object recognition have been reported. Augmented sensory perception (particularly tactile), which can be pleasurable (thus the term "ecstasy" for MDMA), often occurs with methamphetamine use. Other symptoms such as ataxia, dizziness, nausea, perspiration, and bruxism can occur with use. Many complications are related to hallucinogen use (eg, panic reactions, seizures, exacerbation of psychiatric illnesses). Suicidal or homicidal tendencies may be enhanced.

Anticholinergic drugs of abuse include antihistamines and the belladonna alkaloids such as scopolamine and atropine. Anticholinergic drugs are characterized by "dream-like" states, feelings of euphoria, heightened social interaction, and sedation. At high dosages, disorientation or paranoia may occur. These substances are sometimes used with mild opioids (called "Juice and Beans" or "T's and Blues" on the streets) to enhance the euphoric effect.

Arylcyclohexylamines, such as PCP, act as dissociative anesthetics. Behavioral alterations include paranoia, mood shifts, agitation, catalepsy, and violence. PCP may be smoked, snorted, or injected and causes reddening of the skin, pupillary changes, dissociation, delusions, amnesia, dry skin, dizziness, poor coordination, excitement, and nystagmus. Increased blood pressure and tachycardia may also occur.

Intoxication by volatile inhalants generally lasts only several minutes. Confusion, sedation, and possible euphoria often may result from use. Physical effects include analgesia, respiratory depression, hypotension, and ataxia. Nitrous oxide is associated with production of euphoric sensations and laughter and thus is called "laughing gas."

b. Drug-seeking behavior. Psychedelic substances produce little or no dependence, and regular use is not common. Animals generally do not self-administer these drugs (except for MDMA-like compounds), and frequent users generally do not report craving. Tolerance to LSD occurs after only days of use; however, the intoxicating effects return after a few days without use. Other indolamines are cross-tolerant with LSD, but the phenylethylamine hallucinogens are not. Tolerance to anticholinergic drugs can also occur but usually requires prolonged use.

c. Neuroadaptation. Little is known about the mechanism(s) of neuroadaptation to the actions of hallucinogens. Phenylalkylamines and indolamines are serotonin receptor agonists, which probably relates to their clinical effects. Phosphatidylinositol hydrolysis is stimulated after receptor binding and leads to enhanced excitability of certain neurons in the limbic system, cerebral cortex, and brainstem.

The phenylisopropylamines inhibit reuptake of catecholamine and indolamine neurotransmitters and may be transported into serotonin neurons. It is hypothesized that the serotonergic actions of these drugs may account for their hallucinogenic effects (as with other hallucinogens), while the effect on catecholamines causes arousal.

Anticholinergic drugs such as scopolamine and atropine act as antagonists of muscarinic receptors. These receptors are found in the cerebral cortex, and several subtypes have been reported. Stimulation may excite or inhibit neuronal activity including effects on serotonin receptors.

Arylcyclohexylamines, such as PCP, act as antagonists to the N-methyl-D-aspartate class of glutamate receptors, which are themselves ion channels. PCP also binds to σ-type opioid receptors and inhibits catecholamine reuptake.

d. Withdrawal. Withdrawal symptoms are not common with these drugs; however, the anticholinergic substances may cause tachycardia, sweating, depression, anxiety, or psychomotor agitation after use has been discontinued.

B. Psychological Testing: Alcohol and other substances of abuse can cause both transient and enduring damage to the brain. Neuropsychological testing is important in the overall assessment of some patients with substance-related disorders. Most of these tests are readily available, noninvasive, and of reasonable cost. They require the full participation of the patient; therefore, they may not be as objective as blood chemistries or radiologic procedures. Neuropsychological tests are preferably conducted at least 3 weeks after the most recent substance use so that lasting brain dysfunction can be characterized. Although these tests are useful, many factors may influence them, including medications, comorbid medical conditions, comorbid psychiatric disorders, and patient compliance with testing.

Intelligence tests such as the Wechsler Adult Intelligence Scale (WAIS) are useful in determining the patient's global behavioral and adaptive potential. The WAIS is predictive of the patient's likely success in activities such as work and school. Other intelligence tests may be more appropriate for specific patient populations. Different aspects of cognition may be evaluated by specific tests. For example, the Wechsler Memory Scale is useful for patients who have possible substance-induced memory impairment.

Neuropsychological batteries such as the Halstead-Reitan Neuropsychological Test Battery and the Luria-Nebraska Neuropsychological Battery can provide comprehensive information about many aspects of brain functioning. In alcoholic patients, the Halstead-Reitan Battery frequently reveals impairment on many of the individual tests such as the Tactual Performance Test, Categories (visual-spatial abstracting), Trails B (perceptual motor speed), and Tactual Performance Test-Location (incidental memory for spatial relationships).

Some assessment tools have been developed for evaluation of substance abuse itself (as opposed to possible causes or consequences thereof). One of the major difficulties in using such measures is in distinguishing use from abuse. The four-question CAGE assessment is used to screen patients for alcoholism. CAGE stands for an acronym reflecting (1) the need to **c**ut down, (2) being **a**nnoyed at other people when they comment on his or her drinking, (3) feelings of **g**uilt over use, and (4) the need for an **e**ye opener. Generally, two out of four yes answers are considered a positive screen. Sensitivity and specificity are high for most populations. The more involved Michigan Alcoholism Screening Test (MAST) is often used in assessment of alcohol intake and consequences of consumption. It has 25 differentially weighted items in a true-false format. Sensitivity, specificity, and validity testing have all been favorable. Shorter 10- and 13-item forms are also available with reasonably good validity. A similar test of good reliability to evaluate the consumption and consequences of drug abuse is the Drug Abuse Screening Test. It has 28 items (unlike the MAST, not differentially weighted) in a true-false format. Other useful instruments include the Alcohol Dependence Scale. This scale has 25 multiple-choice items and is concerned primarily with the loss of ability to control drinking.

Because comorbid psychiatric illnesses are common in substance abusers, many other psychological tests may be of value in certain patients. For example, the Minnesota Multiphasic Personality Inventory, a commonly used assessment tool with over 500 items (with results formatted into 10 clinical scales and 3 validity scales) tends to give typical profiles for substance-dependent patients.

C. Laboratory Findings & Imaging: A number of laboratory findings are of use in the evaluation and care of substance abuse patients. Urine drug screens and blood alcohol levels provide objective information as to what drugs are in the patient's system and at what current concentration. The relative degree of intoxication or withdrawal at specific drug levels may also provide clues as to the patient's level of tolerance and dependence. A complete evaluation should consider whether specific drugs are detectable in urine as well as the length of time that they are detectable. This will vary according to many factors, including the dosage or duration of use and the metabolic and renal clearance rates of the individual. Some average upper limits on urine detection times are given in Table 18–11.

Many other blood chemistries are useful, particularly in the evaluation of alcoholic patients. The toxic effects of alcohol on the liver are evaluated with liver function tests, such as SGOT (serum glutamic oxaloacetic transaminase) and SGPT (serum glutamic pyruvic transaminase). GGT (γ-glutamyl transpeptidase) is perhaps the most sensitive monitor of alcohol consumption. Alcohol-induced hepatitis classically presents with a SGOT:SGPT ratio of about 2:1. Viral hepatitis screens can help differentiate causes of abnormalities in hepatic function. Serum amylase is valuable in the detection of pancreatitis. A complete blood cell count can monitor bone marrow functioning; mild, macrocytic anemia is often observed in alcohol-abusing patients. Low potassium and bicarbonate are consistent with drug-related diarrhea. Chloride deficiencies are associated with chronic vomiting. Although total body stores of magnesium may be difficult to assess, alcohol-induced magnesium wasting in the urine may lead to detectable extracellular deficiencies. Protein, albumin, potassium, and phosphorus are helpful indicators of nutritional status.

Intellectual impairment is perhaps the earliest complication of chronic alcoholism. Computed tomography or magnetic resonance imaging studies of patients with 2–36 weeks of abstinence have shown that a large proportion of alcoholic patients have detectable cerebral and cerebellar atrophy and ventricular dilation.

Table 18–11. The upper limit of urine detection.

Drug	Limit
Alcohol	12 hours
Amphetamine	2 days
Cannabis	4 weeks
Cocaine	8 hours (4 days for metabolites)
Opioids	3 days
Phencyclidine (PCP)	8 days
Benzodiazepines	3 days
Barbiturates	1 day (short-acting); 3 weeks (long-acting)
Codeine	2 days

Benowitz NL: Pharmacology of nicotine: addiction and therapeutics. Annu Rev Pharmacol Toxicol 1996;36:597.

Martin PR, Lovinger DM, Breese GR: Alcohol and other abused substances. Pages 417–452 in Munson P, Mueller RA, Breese GR (editors): *Principles of Pharmacology: Basic Concepts and Clinical Applications.* Chapman & Hall, 1995.

Differential Diagnosis

Patients are unlikely to present to physicians complaining of difficulties with their use of psychoactive substances. Rather they present for treatment of the complications of substance use. Such patients are unlikely to offer information that they use psychoactive agents, much less admit to problematic drug use. They may deny that they have a drug problem when questioned. The nonspecificity and wide variety of symptoms that accompany these psychoactive substances, as well as the unreliability of patient reports, make the diagnosis of these disorders difficult. The physician must approach, with a high index of suspicion, patients who exhibit signs and symptoms consistent with a substance use disorder. Only if the physician is open to making the diagnosis will it be made appropriately.

Because of the multiple clinical manifestations of substance use disorders, the physician must consider these disorders in the differential diagnosis of myriad medical and psychiatric illnesses. For example, a withdrawal-induced delirium must be differentiated from the almost endless number of other causes of delirium, ranging from CNS infections and metabolic disturbances, to medication toxicity. Similarly, numerous medical problems must be reasonably eliminated before a physician can assume that all the signs and symptoms exhibited by a drug-abusing patient are the result of a substance of abuse (even if one or more is known to have been used). For example, an intoxicated individual may have fallen and be suffering from a closed head injury or may be in diabetic ketoacidosis.

Numerous similar presentations can be cited. For example, patients with hyperthyroidism or bipolar affective disorder may have similar initial clinical features as a person on stimulants, and vice versa. Patients with psychosis (eg, schizophrenia, bipolar affective disorder, or major depressive disorder with psychotic features) may exhibit signs and symptoms similar to those of a person on hallucinogens, or vice versa.

A common problem is the differential diagnosis of the anxious or depressed alcoholic patient. The physician may need to determine whether the patient has a primary mood or anxiety disorder with subsequent substance abuse or a substance-induced mood disorder. In such circumstances, the only way the physician can differentiate the cause(s) of the patient's depressed mood or anxiety may be by taking a careful history or by observing the patient's response to treatment.

In the differential diagnosis of substance abuse, the physician must be aware that the patient may be in denial, in which case the reported history may be intentionally or unintentionally inaccurate or incomplete. This may result in unexpected medical or psychiatric problems or concomitant drug abuse.

Book H et al: The ASAM and Green Spring Alcohol and Drug Detoxification and Rehabilitation Criteria for Utilization Review. Am J Addict 1995;4:187.

Litten RZ, Allen J, Fertig J: Pharmacotherapies for alcohol problems: a review of research with focus on developments since 1991. Alcohol Clin Exp Res 1996;20:859.

Mendelson JH, Mello NK: Management of cocaine abuse and dependence. N Engl J Med 1996;334:965.

Treatment

The treatment of substance use disorders is perhaps more influenced by the widely held societal attributions of responsibility for causation of the problem and for its solution than by any meaningful understanding of etiology. In simplified terms, such attributions can lead to a broad range of responses, the most extreme forms of which include viewing the addicted individual as either a patient or a criminal, and hence, as moral or immoral, innocent or guilty, victim or perpetrator.

A corollary of this viewpoint is that the rehabilitation of individuals who have substance use disorders is perceived as belonging either in the realm of medicine or within the criminal justice system. However, the social control mechanisms used for prevention of or deterrence from substance use disorders are not so easily dichotomized. There are distinct inconsistencies and tensions between the medical (ie, prevention) and legal (ie, deterrence) systems as evidenced by the lack of a straightforward relationship between the pharmacologic properties and health risks of a drug, and whether it is considered legal or illicit within criminal law. For example, drugs such as alcohol and nicotine (as smoked in tobacco)—which cause the greatest expenses for our health care system—are currently freely available, and heated debate has existed concerning how, or whether, other drugs that present societal problems should be legally controlled. In general, the more alternatives there are to the law—derived from the individual, family, or community—for controlling dysfunctional drug use, the less legal regulation is required. Attitudinal changes in society have contributed to the reemergence over time of so-called epidemics of drug use, currently brought to the forefront with respect to cocaine but observed in the past century for most other psychoactive drugs. For example, there are historical examples of failed attempts at prohibition of caffeine and nicotine, and the focuses of intensive legal suppression during the 20th century have been, in turn, alcohol, heroin, cannabis, and cocaine.

Treatment of substance abuse requires a multistage process. Generally patients must go through detoxification, rehabilitation, and then relapse prevention (aftercare). Emphasis is now on the similarities—such as common neurochemical mechanisms of drug-seeking behavior and underlying psychopathology—rather than the differences (as had been the case in the past) among substances of abuse. Thus patients who abuse different drugs can receive treatment in the same programs, and abstinence from all substances of abuse is promoted. In addition, treatment of comorbid psychiatric and medical problems should be started simultaneously with treatment of the substance use disorder, as one problem frequently affects the other. Pharmacologic treatment of concomitant psychiatric disorders requires careful diagnosis and avoidance of potentially addicting psychoactive substances, for example, treatment of panic attacks with alprazolam.

The biopsychosocial model is a useful guide to the treatment of substance use disorders. As a result, both pharmacologic and nonpharmacologic approaches are important in the treatment of substance abuse.

A. Nonpharmacologic Treatments: Whereas detoxification (treatment of withdrawal) varies among individual drugs of abuse because of differing pharmacologic profiles, long-term management is more similar than different for the numerous substances of abuse (Table 18–12).

The degree of outside social support and the reliability and stability of the patient's social circumstances are the major determinants of whether inpatient or outpatient treatment is indicated. After initial detoxification (usually inpatient, but increasingly outpatient if appropriate), a rehabilitation program should be initiated. Substance abuse education (of the patient and family) is very helpful and can be achieved in formal or informal settings. Refinement of coping skills and relaxation training (eg, biofeedback) are also of great value to many patients who have a comorbid anxiety problem. Both inpatient and outpatient treatment should include appropriately selected psychotherapies (eg, social/milieu, insight-oriented, behavioral, individual, cognitive, and group,

Table 18–12. Nonpharmacologic modalities of substance abuse treatment.

Education
12-Step support program facilitation (eg, Alcoholics Anonymous, Narcotics Anonymous, Cocaine Anonymous)
Enhancement of coping strategies
Relaxation training
Family therapy
Lifestyle change (avoiding drug use trigger situations)
Psychotherapy (usually cognitive, relational, or supportive, in a group or individual setting)
Vocational and physical rehabilitation
Recreational therapy
Sexual education
Health and nutritional counseling
Spiritual growth
Aftercare

in various combinations) and should encourage patients to participate in self-support groups.

Health maintenance issues should be addressed with an emphasis on smoking cessation, hygiene, exercise, diet, sex education (eg, HIV and other sexually transmitted diseases), among other areas. Use of non-addicting medications for conditions such as chronic pain should be encouraged, and physicians should attempt to coordinate their care for each patient. In addition, examination of spirituality should be encouraged as appropriate for the needs of the patient.

Aftercare is as important as the initial treatment program (if not more so). Participation in organized aftercare groups following formal treatment keeps patients engaged with the treatment professionals and peer groups with whom care was initiated and allows patients to monitor their relative progress. Individuals with disorganized family situations or no outside supports may benefit from structured living situations such as halfway houses. Lifestyle changes often are needed that require the patient to remove himself or herself from people and situations that promote drug use or stimulate craving. Vocational rehabilitation may be valuable to help the patient develop ways to fill previously unproductive and drug-using time. Twelve-step programs, such as Alcoholics Anonymous and Narcotics Anonymous, and other support groups are helpful to many individuals in preventing relapse and redirecting patients' lives to help others with substance abuse problems.

Psychiatric treatment of comorbid conditions, such as depression, anxiety disorders, bipolar affective disorder, and chronic pain disorders, may be vitally important in preventing relapse if the patient is using addictive drugs in an attempt at misguided self-medication. Appropriate pharmacologic and nonpharmacologic therapies should be initiated, but potentially addicting medications should be avoided. Education about the commonly used medications that are mood altering and may lead to relapse may help the patient deal with the incidental aches and pains of life.

B. Pharmacologic Approaches: The following sections describe some of the well-accepted pharmacologic approaches to treatment of withdrawal from various drugs of abuse (Table 18–13). Development of pharmacologic strategies for longer-term treatment of substance use disorders is an exciting new field of research, but its clinical utility remains limited and will not be discussed here.

1. Alcohol & other CNS depressants— Cross-tolerance and cross-dependence among alcohol and other CNS depressants indicates shared cellular and molecular mechanisms of action and provides the rationale for pharmacologic treatment of CNS depressant withdrawal. The general approach is to administer a CNS depressant that has a longer elimination half-life than the drug from which the patient is being withdrawn once obvious clinical signs of withdrawal are apparent. A long-acting benzodiazepine, such as

Table 18–13. Pharmacologic treatment of withdrawal syndromes from substances of abuse.

Substance	Agent and Dosage	Other Treatments
Alcohol	Diazepam, 10–20 mg/1–2 hours (typical dosage required, 60 mg)	Thiamin, 100 mg intramuscularly or 100 mg by mouth, and multivitamin tablets for 3 days
Other CNS depressants	Phenobarbital, 120 mg/hour (typical dosage, 900–1500 mg)	
Stimulants	Not usually needed	Anxiolytics or neuroleptics acutely for agitation
Opioids	5–10 day taper of clonidine (0.1–0.3 mg every 4–6 hours) or the abused opioid Alternatively, methadone taper dosed at 10–20 mg every 12 hours initially, over a 5–10 day period to reduce withdrawal symptoms (1 mg of methadone is equivalent to 1 mg of heroin, 3 mg of morphine, or 20 mg of meperidine)	Ibuprofen for muscle cramps, loperamide for loose stools, and promethazine for nausea or vomiting Typical maintenance doses: methadone, 40–120 mg/day; LAAM, 30–80 mg 3 times/week
Nicotine and tobacco	Nicotine patch or gum	Clonidine or antidepressants
Cannabinoids	Not usually needed	Anxiolytics acutely only in cases of severe agitation or anxiety
Hallucinogens	Not usually needed	Neuroleptics or anxiolytics in cases of acute severe toxic psychosis

diazepam (or chlordiazepoxide), is the treatment of choice for alcohol withdrawal, and the slowly eliminated barbiturate phenobarbital is optimal for the other CNS depressants (see Table 18–13). Hourly doses are administered until the withdrawal symptoms are suppressed (for treatment of alcohol withdrawal) or until the patient manifests signs of mild intoxication (for other CNS depressant withdrawal). Physicians sometimes use a tapering dose of the abused benzodiazepine for detoxification, although the phenobarbital loading dose strategy appears to be the better treatment option. For example, alprazolam tapers are generally very slow (about 10% per week) because of the risk of significant withdrawal reactions and are often associated with relapse.

All drugs currently used for the treatment of CNS depressant withdrawal have dependence liability. When prescribing these medications, careful patient education is needed concerning the risks and benefits, particularly with regard to the potential for dependence. Problems may occur if the patient is not monitored carefully, or if the patient takes the medication(s) in excess of that prescribed. The treating physician may not be aware that the patient is obtaining prescriptions of the same (or similar) drug(s) from other doctors in a pattern of abuse and possible dependence. A major challenge for pharmacologists is to develop agents that can ease CNS depressant withdrawal but have little liability for abuse and dependence.

Patients in alcohol detoxification should be prescribed thiamin and multiple vitamins to prevent some of the neurologic, hematopoietic, and cognitive effects of chronic drinking. The FDA has approved administration of naltrexone as a pharmacologic ap-

proach to help prevent alcohol craving and relapse. Aversion therapy with disulfiram has also been used; however, the method's long-term effectiveness has not been established, and patients must be carefully educated and monitored because of the potential for serious reactions if disulfiram is taken with alcohol (see "Adverse Outcomes of Treatment" section).

2. Psychostimulants: cocaine & amphetamines—The treatment of stimulant intoxication is usually supportive care. Anxiolytics or neuroleptics may be needed for agitation. Psychostimulants can be highly addicting, and chronic users must address causes of relapse and strategies for relapse prevention. Pharmacologic agents such as carbamazepine, phenytoin, and tricyclic antidepressants may help prevent relapse, but controlled studies are inconclusive. Although cocaine is clearly a highly efficacious positive reinforcer, in animal models environmental manipulations such as inflicting punishment, increasing the amount of effort required to obtain the drug, or offering alternative reinforcers are effective in decreasing its self-administration. Such behavioral observations have guided clinical treatment approaches. Only if the patient can maintain abstinence beyond the withdrawal period can extinction and ultimate abstinence follow. Therefore, treatment should address the conditions that lead to relapse, that is, reducing the effects of conditioned cues that trigger craving (such as persons with whom, or situations in which, the individual has used cocaine and the availability of cocaine in one's neighborhood).

If an overdose of these medications occurs, further treatment may be needed. In the case of amphetamines, the patient's urine can be acidified with ammonium chloride to increase excretion of the substance. An α-adrenergic antagonist can be used to decrease elevated blood pressure, and antipsychotics, such as chlorpromazine, may be needed to diminish CNS overstimulation.

Cocaine overdoses can be more complicated because of the greater potential for cardiac arrhythmia, respiratory failure, and seizures. Chlorpromazine may be useful in reducing CNS and cardiovascular problems (as it has some α-adrenergic-inhibiting action). Artificial respiration or cardiac life support may be needed.

3. Opioids—Opioid withdrawal and dependence may be treated in several ways. Often a slow taper of methadone (a long-acting opioid that has addiction potential and that currently requires special licensure for use) is given at approved facilities. In other circumstances, a 5–10 day taper of the abused opioid or clonidine is used to reduce withdrawal symptoms. Clonidine has the advantage of not being an opioid and not having addicting properties, but it may not provide as smooth a withdrawal. Baseline blood pressure and regular monitoring of blood pressure is advised. Other agents, such as ibuprofen for muscle cramps, loperamide for loose stools, and promethazine for nausea can be helpful adjunctive medications.

Methadone maintenance programs (for 1–2 years or longer) are used in some locations to help reduce the patient's risk of reentering the drug and crime cultures. Some patients on methadone maintenance use other drugs, such as alcohol and cocaine, and may sell the methadone they receive on the streets to support their drug use. A longer-acting opioid called L-alpha-acetylmethadol (LAMM) has also been used for maintenance treatment. Other pharmacologic means of relapse prevention are being investigated and currently include buprenorphine and naltrexone. In the treatment of chronic pain, nonaddicting medications (eg, carbamazepine and certain antidepressants) and other modalities (eg, physical therapy, nerve blocks) should be used in appropriate patients to minimize the likelihood of relapse to opioid use.

4. Cannabinoids—The treatment of cannabinoid intoxication usually requires only a safe, calm environment. Anxiolytic medications are used only acutely in cases of severe agitation or anxiety. Educational programs are important, particularly among younger populations.

5. Nicotine & tobacco—Nonpharmacologic approaches are frequently used to help tobacco users quit smoking. Issues such as weight gain and mood lability may need to be addressed, and strategies may need to be developed to help users get through the day without the need for tobacco use. Clonidine can help reduce withdrawal symptoms. Nicotine-containing products such as dermal patches and gum can be used to help titrate smokers off the nicotine. Antidepressants and limited anxiolytic drug therapy have also been helpful in some patients.

6. Hallucinogens & volatile inhalants—Detoxification from low dosages of hallucinogens can often be achieved with a safe, structured environment and emotional support. Anxiolytics and possibly neuroleptics (such as haloperidol, but not phenothiazines because of possible side effects) may be needed. If respiratory suppression occurs, emergency oxygen may be required. The primary treatment for arylcyclohexylamine overdose is removal from sensory stimulation, and possibly treatment with benzodiazepines or neuroleptics.

Comorbidity

Psychoactive substance abuse can contribute to or result from various forms of psychopathology. Physicians are most likely to encounter patients with substance use disorders when they present for treatment of a complicating or associated physical or emotional illness. Medical and psychiatric complications of drug use are attributable to either direct pharmacologic actions of the substance (eg, overdose, organ toxicity, metabolic consequences) or indirect effects of drug self-administration on lifestyle. Indirect effects include use of other than the primary drug of abuse (including tobacco), inappropriate use of prescribed medications such as analgesics or anxiolytics, malnutrition, trauma, infection, neglect, or lack of compliance with the medical regimen for coexistent illnesses. Treatment of severe medical complications clearly takes precedence if the illness is life threatening or incapacitating. However, unless the underlying substance use disorder and emotional concomitants are recognized and addressed, initial treatment efforts may be for naught.

Regier DA, Kramer ME, Rae DS: Comorbidity of mental disorders with alcohol and other drug abuse: results from the Epidemiologic Catchment Area study. J Am Med Assoc 1990;264:2511.

Complications

1. Alcohol—The medical complications of chronic alcoholism derive from the pharmacologic effects of ethanol, the changes in intermediary metabolism resulting from its biotransformation to acetaldehyde in the liver, and the toxic effects of this metabolite in various body tissues (Table 18–14).

Ethanol metabolism leads to conversion of pyruvate to lactate and to the formation of acetoacetate, acetone, and β-hydroxybutyrate. These chemicals can interfere with renal tubular secretion of uric acid, causing modest increases in blood urate and thus exacerbating gout.

Heavy drinking after a period of not eating can cause severe, sometimes fatal, hypoglycemia. This is the result of the combination of low hepatic glycogen stores and inhibition by ethanol of gluconeogenesis. Fatty liver can be caused by single episodes of ethanol bingeing. Chronic fatty liver, probably in combination

Table 18–14. Medical complications of alcoholism.

Metabolic and malnutrition
  Gout
  Hyperlipidemia and fatty liver
  Hypoglycemia
  Weight loss or obesity
  Immune compromise (opportunistic infections)
  Impaired protein synthesis
  Mineral and electrolyte imbalances
  Vitamin deficiencies
  Decreased blood clotting
Gastrointestinal
  Esophagitis
  Gastritis or ulcer
  Pancreatitis
  Liver disease (alcoholic hepatitis, cirrhosis)
  Malabsorption
  Altered drug and carcinogen metabolism
  Increased cancer incidence
Endocrine
  Pancreatic insufficiency (glucose intolerance)
  Increased ACTH, glucocorticoid, or catecholamine release
  Inhibited testosterone synthesis (male hypogonadism)
  Inhibition of ADH, oxytocin release
Neurologic
  Dementia
  Amnesia
  Cerebellar degeneration
  Fetal alcohol effects
  Neuropathy
Cardiovascular
  Hypertension
  Stroke
  Arrhythmias
  Coronary heart disease

with nutritional deficiencies, progresses to alcoholic hepatitis and finally cirrhosis. Ethanol can induce an isozyme of cytochrome P-450 that converts some chemicals to hepatotoxic metabolites. Alcoholic cirrhosis is the second most common cause of death among individuals aged 24–44 years in large urban areas and the third most common cause of death among individuals aged 45–64 years.

The diuresis associated with drinking alcoholic beverages is caused primarily by inhibition of ADH release from the posterior pituitary. Alcohol also increases the release of ACTH, glucocorticoids, and catecholamines. The synthesis of testosterone is inhibited, and its hepatic metabolism is increased. Men with chronic alcoholism often have signs of hypogonadism and feminization (eg, gynecomastia).

Ethanol stimulates the secretion of gastric and pancreatic juices. This effect on gastric juices and the direct irritant action of concentrated solutions of ethanol help to explain why one of every three heavy drinkers has chronic gastritis. High dosages of ethanol may cause vomiting to occur independent of any local irritation. Alcohol abuse is associated with acute and chronic pancreatitis and esophagitis. An increased incidence of carcinoma of the pharynx, larynx, and esophagus has been found among heavy users of alcoholic beverages. Nutritional problems are common

among alcoholic patients and are manifested by weight loss or obesity, impaired protein synthesis, altered amino acid metabolism, immune incompetence, mineral and electrolyte imbalance, and vitamin deficiencies.

2. Psychostimulants: cocaine & amphetamines—Physical consequences of cocaine abuse include sleep problems, chronic fatigue, severe headaches, nasal sores and bleeding, chronic cough and sore throat, nausea, and vomiting (Table 18–15).

Cocaine abuse can lead to seizures, cerebrovascular accident, cerebrovasculitis, hyperpyrexia and rhabdomyolysis, and dystonias. Possible mechanisms for neuropsychiatric complications include cerebrovascular vasoconstriction, neurotransmitter depletion, and reduced limbic seizure threshold resulting from repeated subconvulsant stimulation.

Cocaine abuse is particularly dangerous because of the devastating cardiovascular effects that can occur in healthy and young individuals. These effects include angina pectoris, myocardial infarction, syncope, aortic dissection, pulmonary edema, and sudden arrhythmic death.

3. Opioids—Opioid abuse can lead to many serious medical complications in addition to dependence (Table 18–16). For example, injuries may result from sedation, especially if an individual drives or uses dangerous machinery while taking an opioid medication. The analgesic effect may block natural mechanisms that alert the user of physical injury. Decreased respiratory drive, vomiting, and death (from respiratory suppression) may occur with overdose. Shared needle use in intravenous users enhances the risk of HIV infection, hepatitis, brain abscess, thrombophlebitis, pulmonary emboli, pulmonary infection,

Table 18–15. Medical complications of psychostimulant abuse.

General health
  Chronic fatigue
  Sleep problems
  Nasal congestion, ulceration, or bleeding
  Chronic cough or sore throat
  Nausea or vomiting
  Sexual disinterest
  Intravenously or sexually transmitted hepatitis or HIV
  Traumatic injuries and overdose
Neurologic
  Seizure
  Cerebrovascular accident
  Hyperpyrexia and rhabdomyolysis
  Headaches
  Dystonias
  Cerebrovasculitis
Cardiovascular
  Arrhythmia
  Angina pectoris
  Myocardial infarction
  Syncope
  Pulmonary edema
  Aortic dissection

Table 18–16. Medical complications of opioid abuse.

General health
 Chronic fatigue
 Sleep problems
 Nausea or vomiting
 Sexual disinterest
 Traumatic injuries
Pulmonary
 Pulmonary edema
 Overdose
 Respiratory depression
 Death
Infectious diseases
 Intravenously or sexually transmitted hepatitis or HIV
 Thrombophlebitis
 Pulmonary emboli or abscess

acute endocarditis, septic arthritis, and other infectious diseases. Substances added to opioid street preparations (eg, strychnine) can lead to peripheral neuropathy, myelopathy, and amblyopia. It has been estimated that over 25% of street opioid addicts are dead within 10–20 years of abuse.

4. Cannabinoids—A controversial amotivational syndrome has been described in the literature, wherein chronic marijuana users have been noted to exhibit apathy; dullness; impairment of judgment, concentration, and memory; and loss of interest in personal appearance and pursuit of conventional goals. Well-controlled clinical studies have not provided strong evidence that an amotivational syndrome is a direct consequence of marijuana use; however, such symptoms would be of particular concern to school-aged children. There is evidence of alterations in heart rate, blood pressure, reproductive system function, immune system function, and pulmonary function. Cannabinoid-induced testosterone suppression is an issue of concern particularly in adolescents.

5. Nicotine & tobacco—The complications of tobacco use are considerable. Much has been written and debated about the adverse effects of tobacco use. It is generally accepted that users have significantly increased risk of many serious illnesses including pulmonary disease (eg, emphysema, lung cancer); cardiovascular disease (eg, coronary artery disease); peripheral vascular disease, particularly with chronic use; dental disease (eg, oral cancer, especially with smokeless tobacco), nicotine stomatitis, and stained teeth; and diminished birth weight in babies of mothers who smoke. Many of these complications can be lethal. Some researchers have estimated that as many as 25% of deaths in the United States are associated with tobacco use. High concentrations of nicotine, such as is found in some insecticides, can cause diarrhea, nausea, vomiting, irritability, headache, convulsions, tachypnea, coma, or death.

6. Hallucinogens & volatile inhalants—Acute effects of hallucinogens include sympathomimetic actions such as high blood pressure and seizures, particularly with use of phenylisopropylamine compounds. Autonomic blockade by anticholinergic substances can cause amnesia, hallucinations, dry mouth, constipation, bronchodilation, tachycardia, urinary retention, diminished penile erection, photophobia, increased intraocular pressure, and blurred vision (from dilated pupils). Long-term complications include flashbacks, which seem to be stimulated by stress and fatigue.

PCP use may lead to paranoid hallucinations, violent behaviors, and self-abuse. Medical effects include hypersalivation, catalepsy, perspiration, rigidity, myoclonus, stereotyped movements, hyperreflexia, cardiac arrhythmia, hypertension, and convulsions.

Intoxication with volatile inhalants can be associated with dizziness and syncope. Cardiac arrhythmia, pulmonary edema, liver damage, asphyxiation, and renal dysfunction may occur. Neurotoxic effects can lead to dementia.

Brewer RD et al: The risk of dying in alcohol-related automobile crashes among habitual drunk drivers. N Engl J Med 1994;331:513.

Brust JCM: *Neurological Aspects of Substance Abuse.* Butterworth-Heinemann, 1993.

Lieber CS: Medical disorders of alcoholism. N Engl J Med 1995;333:1058.

Marzuk PM: Fatal injuries after cocaine use as a leading cause of death among young adults in New York City. N Engl J Med 1995;332:1753.

Adverse Outcomes of Treatment

A. Unrecognized or Untreated Medical Complications: Patients with alcohol and drug dependence often are inappropriately triaged to treatment facilities that lack the medical expertise needed to manage significant medical complications. This may be because intoxicated patients cannot provide adequate histories or because of negative attitudes among treating professionals. All substance-dependent patients deserve a meticulous history, physical examination, and appropriate laboratory examinations to rule out common medical complications. Medical and surgical consultation and joint management are often necessary for more complex cases. In addition, it is important to recognize addictive disorders in patients who have medical disorders that typically can complicate alcohol or drug abuse or in those patients who are recalcitrant to usually effective treatments. These points are discussed in greater detail in the "Differential Diagnosis" section.

B. Unrecognized or Untreated Other Psychiatric Disorders: It can be devastating if a treatable psychiatric disorder is overlooked in a substance-abusing patient. Many jurisdictions artificially separate the psychiatric care of patients with addictions from those with other psychiatric disorders. Some 12-step support groups proscribe the use of all psychopharmacologic agents, even if they have no known abuse liability and are potentially beneficial.

This is in large part the result of a mistrust of psychiatrists, who until recently avoided care of patients with substance use disorders. All psychiatrists should develop the expertise needed for the diagnosis and appropriate treatment or referral of substance-dependent patients and should develop collaborative relationships with community resources such as 12-step programs.

C. Drug Interactions: Disulfiram inhibits aldehyde dehydrogenase (involved in alcohol metabolism), and its effects in the drinker are largely if not entirely due to accumulation of acetaldehyde. Taken alone, disulfiram causes little or no effects. With alcohol, it causes intense flushing of the face and neck, tachycardia, hypotension, nausea, and vomiting. It has caused death. In treating alcoholism, physicians must use disulfiram with caution and combined with psychosocial treatment modalities.

Disulfiram inhibits other drug-metabolizing enzymes and increases the elimination half-life of several drugs, including phenytoin, warfarin, thiopental, and caffeine. Calcium carbimide, which is available in Canada and other countries but not in the United States, also inhibits aldehyde dehydrogenase and is said by some to be less toxic than disulfiram.

Although alcohol can alter absorption of some drugs (eg, it increases the absorption of diazepam), the demonstrated basis for most pharmacokinetic ethanol-drug interactions involves the alcohol dehydrogenase pathway and liver microsomes. Microsomal drug metabolism (cytochrome P-450) is inhibited in the presence of high concentrations of ethanol. Therefore, when ethanol and prescribed drugs are taken together, the drug's effect may be augmented (in the case of phenytoin and warfarin) or the alcohol effect may be prolonged (in the case of chloral hydrate, chlorpromazine, or cimetidine). Microsomal induction after long-term alcohol consumption contributes to accelerated ethanol metabolism at high blood ethanol concentrations. Increased drug metabolism and activation of xenobiotics (eg, carcinogens) because of microsomal induction results in lower than therapeutic blood levels (in the case of barbiturates, phenytoin, isoniazid, meprobamate, methadone, and warfarin) or increased production of toxic metabolites (in the case of acetaminophen). Common mechanisms for pharmacodynamic ethanol-drug interactions include increased drug effects when an individual is intoxicated with ethanol, because of additive CNS depression (in the case of antihistamines, other CNS depressants, opioids, antipsychotics, and antidepressants); or diminished drug effects when the individual has not been drinking, because of the presence of cross-tolerance to other CNS depressants.

Metabolism of methadone can be altered by the coadministration of medications that induce cytochrome P-450 (eg, rifampin, phenytoin, barbiturates, carbamazepine), thereby complicating dosing during methadone maintenance.

Prognosis & Course of Illness

The prognosis and course of illness in substance abuse disorders depends on numerous factors involving a complex interaction of biological, psychological, and environmental elements. The specific substance(s) used, the duration and dosage of substance use, psychiatric and medical comorbidity, coping skills, developmental history, socioeconomic status, social support, genetic predispositions, treatment choices, and other aspects are all important. The prognosis for individuals who abuse drugs other than alcohol is complicated by a lifestyle in conflict with the legal system. In addition, intravenous use of those drugs (as well as sex-for-drugs transactions) increases the risk and spread of life-threatening illnesses such as AIDS and hepatitis.

The outcome of treatment of substance-related problems is enhanced by emphasis on relapse prevention using nonpharmacologic approaches involving psychotherapy and self-help groups (such as Alcoholics Anonymous). Appropriate adjunctive pharmacologic treatments have been shown to be effective in combination with psychosocial treatments to prevent relapse.

Treatment of comorbid psychiatric illnesses may be important in improving prognosis. The majority of alcoholic patients also have another psychiatric illness, including affective and anxiety disorders and personality disorders, which can worsen the prognosis if not addressed. Psychiatric comorbidity is also high in other substance use disorders. Complete psychiatric evaluation and treatment is therefore essential in patients with substance and related disorders.

1. Alcohol & other CNS depressants—Naltrexone is the only medication approved by the FDA to directly help prevent alcohol relapse. Naltrexone seems to lower alcohol craving and reduce the reinforcing effects of alcohol. It should be used in conjunction with psychosocial forms of therapy. Naltrexone reduces relapse by approximately half that of control subjects over a 2- to 3-month period (down to a rate of about 20–25%). (Patients who are unable to remain totally abstinent may obtain more relative benefit from this medication.) The type of psychotherapy used with naltrexone appears to influence treatment outcome. Thus lower rates of relapse have been reported in patients using supportive therapy compared to coping skills therapy. For those patients who are unable to maintain total abstinence, the rate of relapse is reduced when naltrexone is combined with coping skills therapy. About 60% of patients on combined naltrexone and supportive therapy remain abstinent over a 2- to 3-month period, in comparison with about 20% of patients on supportive therapy alone. These results underscore the significant improvements of prognosis that can be obtained with optimal treatment of alcoholism.

Other medications are currently being investigated for alcohol relapse prevention. For example, acamprosate (calcium bisacetylhomotaurinate), a chemical analog of L-glutamic acid, has binding affinity for $GABA_A$ and $GABA_B$ receptor sites. Initial findings suggest that acamprosate increases the mean duration of abstinence over a 200-day period. Without acamprosate treatment, about 20% of alcoholic patients can maintain extended abstinence; with adequate treatment, 65% of typical alcoholic patients maintain abstinence for at least 1 year.

2. Psychostimulants: cocaine & amphetamines—Users of stimulants such as cocaine and amphetamines often have patterns of either nearly daily use (in low or high dosages) or intermittent use (eg, weekend binges). Binge use of high dosages of psychostimulants often leads to dependence. Daily users often increase rapidly the dosage taken. Intravenous use or smoking of cocaine can lead to dependence in a matter of only weeks to months, whereas dependence may take a longer period to develop in individuals who nasally insufflate the drug. Preliminary studies indicate that cognitive-behavioral therapy may be more effective than interpersonal psychotherapy in prevention of relapse in cocaine-dependent patients (with abstinence rates over a 3-week period of 60% and 33%, respectively). Behavioral treatment (including contracting, counseling, community reinforcement, and so on) increases abstinence to about 40% in a 3- to 4-month period compared to 5% participating in drug counseling only. In addition, some preliminary trials suggest that patients with cocaine dependence may benefit from antidepressants such as desipramine and from anticonvulsants such as carbamazepine.

3. Opioids—Opioid dependence is often characterized by short periods of abstinence followed by relapse. Even after years of forced abstinence by incarceration, many subjects relapse after being released from jail. Relapse often occurs after patients fail to inform their physician about their addictions and opioids are prescribed for medical ailments. Psychosocial therapies for opioid dependence are often helpful. Agonist substitution with methadone is well established to benefit the most severely addicted patient population when provided in methadone maintenance programs. When specific modalities have been compared in patients on methadone maintenance (for opioid dependence) similar benefits have been found between standard outpatient counseling or psychotherapy compared to therapeutic communities. Subjects who remain in this combined treatment have lower relapse rates than do those who drop out. Psychodynamic therapy and cognitive therapy have been of greater benefit than standard drug counseling alone. Interestingly, limited monthly interactions with a psychotherapist appear to be as effective as more intensive and frequent interpersonal psychotherapy when combined with methadone maintenance.

4. Cannabinoids—Cannabis dependence occurs slowly in those who develop patterns of increasing dosage and frequency of use. The pleasurable effects of cannabis often diminish with regular heavy use. In patients with marijuana dependence, manual-guided individual treatment and group therapy appear to have similar beneficial effects. Marijuana use dropped about 50% in response to these treatment modalities.

5. Nicotine & tobacco—Tobacco smokers usually start in their early teen years, often in social settings. These children are at increased risk if their parents or close friends smoke. Since the 1970s, smoking has decreased in the U.S. population but to a much lesser degree in females than males. The greatest prevalence rate of smoking is in the psychiatric population, especially among patients with schizophrenia or depression. Smoking is very reinforcing, and although some people can stop smoking "cold turkey," overall failure rates of treatment are high (over 70% at 1 year).

6. Hallucinogens & volatile inhalants—Onset of hallucinogen use is highly dependent on availability, social and cultural setting, and perceived expectations. Use is often experimental and intermittent, but chronic or heavy use can lead to long-term consequences such as flashbacks, mood lability, personality disturbances, and dementia.

Kandel DB: Epidemiology of drug use and abuse. Pages 1–30 in Michels R et al (editors): *Psychiatry.* Vol 3. JB Lippincott, 1992.

Vaillant GE: A long-term follow-up of male alcohol abuse. Arch Gen Psychiatry 1996;53:243.

CONCLUSION

The substance-related disorders exact an immense toll on the mental and physical well-being of many individuals in our society. Consequently, they jeopardize the integrity of the family and other social institutions. Because of the prevalence of substance-related disorders, and because they can masquerade as diverse medical and other psychiatric disorders, their recognition and initial treatment are relevant to all physicians, in particular, to psychiatrists. Substance-related disorders are heterogeneous in terms of the interactions between the manifest psychopathology of the individual patient and the psychopharmacologic actions of a given drug, within the relevant sociocultural context. This perspective is useful in seeking an etiologic understanding of these disorders, conducting a clinical assessment, planning for the initial treatment of the direct consequences of drug use, and developing and implementing a comprehensive treatment strategy for patients.

Future directions in substance abuse treatment research are likely to focus on understanding issues of comorbid psychiatric conditions, developing new psychopharmacologic treatment options, and combining the use of pharmacotherapy and psychotherapy in the management of these disorders. Agents that can help reduce drug craving and relapse are of particular interest. Overall, considerably more research is needed on the optimal combination of treatment modalities to prevent relapse in substance-dependent patients and improve prognosis.

19

Schizophrenia

Herbert Y. Meltzer, MD, & S. Hossein Fatemi, MD, PhD

DSM-IV Diagnostic Criteria

A. *Characteristic symptoms:* Two (or more) of the following, each present for a significant portion of time during a 1-month period (or less if successfully treated):
   (1) delusions
   (2) hallucinations
   (3) disorganized speech (eg, frequent derailment or incoherence)
   (4) grossly disorganized or catatonic behavior
   (5) negative symptoms, ie, affective flattening, alogia, or avolition

Note: Only one Criterion A symptom is required if delusions are bizarre or hallucinations consist of a voice keeping up a running commentary on the person's behavior or thoughts, or two or more voices conversing with each other.

B. *Social/occupational dysfunction:* For a significant portion of the time since the onset of the disturbance, one or more major areas of functioning such as work, interpersonal relations, or self-care are markedly below the level achieved prior to the onset (or when the onset is in childhood or adolescence, failure to achieve expected level of interpersonal, academic, or occupational achievement).

C. *Duration:* Continuous signs of the disturbance persist for at least 6 months. This 6-month period must include at least 1 month of symptoms (or less if successfully treated) that meet Criterion A (ie, active-phase symptoms) and may include periods of prodromal or residual symptoms. During these prodromal or residual periods, the signs of the disturbance may be manifested by only negative symptoms or two or more symptoms listed in Criterion A present in an attenuated form (eg, odd beliefs, unusual perceptual experiences).

D. *Schizoaffective and mood disorder exclusion:* Schizoaffective disorder and mood disorder with psychotic features have been ruled out because either (1) no major depressive, manic, or mixed episodes have occurred concurrently with the active-phase symptoms; or (2) if mood episodes have occurred during active-phase symptoms, their total duration has been brief relative to the duration of the active and residual periods.

E. *Substance/general medical condition exclusion:* The disturbance is not due to the direct physiological effects of a substance (eg, a drug of abuse, a medication) or a general medical condition.

F. *Relationship to a pervasive developmental disorder:* If there is a history of autistic disorder or another pervasive developmental disorder, the additional diagnosis of schizophrenia is made only if prominent delusions or hallucinations are also present for at least a month (or less if successfully treated).

Adapted, with permission, from *Diagnostic and Statistical Manual of Mental Disorders,* 4th ed. Copyright 1994 American Psychiatric Association.

Schizophrenia is one of the major forms of psychotic disorder. Psychosis, in its narrow definition, is restricted to delusions (false, fixed beliefs) or hallucinations in the absence of insight into their pathologic nature. The concept of schizophrenia as a diagnostic entity is still evolving, even though the criteria in use today have been fairly stable for nearly a decade. The current concept of schizophrenia has its origins in the pioneering clinical observations of Emil Kraepelin and Eugen Bleuler. Kraepelin's great contribution was to distinguish manic-depressive illness (now called bipolar disorder) as a remitting, noncognitively impairing, relatively late-onset psychosis (usually occurring in the fourth decade of life or later) with a usually good vocational and social outcome, from an early-onset psychosis (usually occurring in the second or third decade), which could affect cognition permanently and usually led to poor outcome. This latter psychosis was labeled **dementia praecox,** the direct precursor of schizophrenia. Bleuler's major contribution was to suggest schizophrenia as a more appropriate name than dementia praecox because of his observation that the outcome of this illness was neither universally poor nor associated with severe dementia and to suggest that splitting of thought and affect was the central feature of the illness. Bleuler specifically identified four components that described the essence of the syndrome: autism, ambivalence, flat affect, and disturbance of volition. Kurt Schneider contributed the concept of **first-rank symptoms** (eg, thought diffusion, thought insertion, voices arguing and commenting), which he believed were pathognomonic of schizophrenia. It is now known that the first-rank symptoms are not specific for schizophrenia.

Amador XF et al: Psychopathologic domains and insight in schizophrenia. Psychiatr Clin N Am 1998;21:27.

General Considerations

The current definition of schizophrenia in use in the United States is the product of extensive empirical testing to refine the diagnostic category in order to obtain specificity, reliability, and validity. The *Diagnostic and Statistical Manual of Mental Disorders,* 4th edition (DSM-IV) requires at least two of five types of positive and negative symptoms. The four positive symptoms—delusions, hallucinations, disorganized speech, and grossly disorganized or catatonic behavior—are considered to be psychotic in that these beliefs, precepts, and behaviors are inconsistent with the experiences of normal humans. They are considered to be positive symptoms because they represent the product of an abnormal disease process. The fifth group of symptoms consists of withdrawal, anhedonia (decreased capacity for pleasure), anergia (diminished energy), and affective flattening—considered negative symptoms because they represent a deficit of normal function and are not psychotic per se. Neither positive nor negative symptoms are unique to schizophrenia; they are also found in bipolar disorder, in some drug-induced states, and in various psychoses due to general medical conditions.

Impairment in psychosocial function is an essential feature of schizophrenia, in the absence of effective treatment or spontaneous remission. None of these symptoms is present in all schizophrenic patients, but some patients exhibit all of these symptoms at one time or another. Clinical features can vary greatly over time within the same patient. One or more of the positive symptoms must be present in the absence of effective treatment for at least 1 month prior to establishing the diagnosis of schizophrenia. Continuous signs of disturbance must be present over a 6-month period. Schizophrenia is a diagnosis of exclusion in that the criteria for major depression or mania must not be fulfilled during the same period when psychotic symptoms are present. Schizoaffective disorder and mood disorder with psychotic features should be ruled out by assessing whether criteria for major depressive, manic, or mixed episodes have occurred simultaneously with the psychotic symptoms or were brief relative to the prodrome (the period before active psychosis) and active psychotic periods.

A. The Three Syndromes: Large factor analytic studies have identified three independent syndromes or types of psychopathology in schizophrenia. These are positive, negative, and disorganization symptoms.

Positive symptoms include delusions, hallucinations, and formal thought disorder. Delusions in schizophrenia are most often paranoid and suspicious, or bizarre in nature, but some patients experience grandiose, depressive, manic, somatic, or tactile delusions. Hallucinations are usually auditory in nature and are experienced as coming from within the brain or from external sources. Distinct voices or amorphous sounds may be experienced at intervals of greatly variable frequency. Disorganization was historically referred to as hebephrenia. It consists of incoherence, loose associations, inappropriate affect, and poverty of thought content. The thought disorder in schizophrenia consists of a disorder of content (ie, delusions and disorders of the form of thought). This disorder consists of loose associations and poverty of speech content. Thus the thought disorder in schizophrenia may be part of the positive or disorganization syndromes.

Negative symptoms are often present throughout the illness. They are most evident as affective flattening, loss of spontaneity, lack of initiative or willed action, anergia, and anhedonia. They may be difficult to distinguish from depression and extrapyramidal side effects (EPS) due to neuroleptic treatment.

Most patients will manifest mixtures of all three forms of psychopathology at some time during the illness, but only one or two of the forms may be present at a given time.

B. Subtyping in Schizophrenia: Schizophrenia has also been subdivided on the basis of psychopathology, course, and response to treatment (Table 19–1). Historically, subtyping by form of psychopathology was the most important. **Paranoid schizophrenia** is characterized by prominent persecutory or grandiose delusions. It is the most common form of the illness. The next most frequent form is **undifferentiated schizophrenia,** in which delusions and hallucinations of any type are prominent and are accompanied by incoherence and grossly disorganized behavior. **Disorganized schizophrenia** is characterized by the absence of systematized delusions and the presence of incoherence and inappropriate affect. **Residual schizophrenia** is a form of the illness in which positive symptoms are minimal and negative symptoms predominate. A rare form of the illness is **catatonic schizophrenia,** in which motor disturbance is the dominant feature, consisting of either agitated hyperactivity or a decrease in gross motor activity

Table 19–1. Subtyping of schizophrenia.

Basis for Subtyping	Types	Characteristics
Psychopathology	Paranoid	+ Delusions or auditory hallucinations − Disorganized speech or behavior − Flat or inappropriate affect − Catatonic behavior
	Disorganized	+ Disorganized speech or behavior + Flat or inappropriate affect − Catatonic behavior
	Catatonic (minimum of two symptoms)	+ Motoric immobility (ie, catalepsy or stupor) + Excessive motor activity + Extreme negativism or mutism + Posturing, or stereotypy, mannerisms, grimacing + Echolalia or echopraxia
	Undifferentiated	+ Criterion A symptoms − Paranoid, disorganized or catatonic symptoms
	Residual	− Delusions, hallucinations, disorganized speech or behavior, catatonia + Negative symptoms or + Attenuated forms of 2 or more Criterion A symptoms (ie, odd beliefs, unusual perceptual experience)
Duration	Acute Chronic	Recent appearance or exacerbation of positive symptoms Persistent disability for 2 years or longer
Genetics	Familial	+ Concordance rate of 46% in monozygotic twins + Concordance rate of 14% in dizygotic twins + Family history of psychosis
	Nonfamilial	− Family history of psychosis + Evidence for neurodevelopmental symptoms
Prognosis	Good/poor	See Table 19–4.
Symptomatology	Positive Negative Disorganized	+ Delusions, hallucinations + Flat affect, alogia, anhedonia, avolition + Disorganized speech or behavior, inappropriate affect

with stupor, rigidity, or bizarre postures (so-called waxy flexibility). It is seen much less frequently now than in previous years.

Coleman N, Gillberg C (editors): *The Schizophrenias: A Biological Approach to the Schizophrenia Spectrum Disorders.* Springer-Verlag, 1996.
Hirsch SR, Weinberger DR (editors): *Schizophrenia.* Blackwell Scientific, 1995.
Keshaven MS, Murray RM (editors): *Neurodevelopment and Adult Psychopathology.* Cambridge University Press, 1997.

A. Major Etiologic Theories: Kraepelin, Bleuler, and Freud believed that schizophrenia was caused by a biological abnormality, even though all attempts to identify that abnormality in their era were unsuccessful. These attempts involved neuropathologic studies, including those of Alois Alzheimer, which led to the admonition that "schizophrenia is the graveyard of neuropathology." In the middle of the 20th century, the view that schizophrenia was the result of specific disturbances in child-rearing received considerable attention. In particular, communication deviance between parents and the child who was diagnosed with schizophrenia was considered by some clinicians to be a sufficient cause of schizophrenia. Although communication deviance in families with a schizophrenic child was demonstrated in a number of studies, evidence that this feature was specific for schizophrenia or caused the disorder was unconvincing. Nevertheless, this line of research led to a continual interest in how family (and other caregiver) interactions can contribute to or diminish the stress and coping skills of patients with schizophrenia and, thus, modulate the course of the illness. Factors influencing the course of illness include the timing of the first episode of psychosis, the patient's compliance with and response to treatment, the patient's social skills and interpersonal function, and the frequency of relapse. These studies were the precursors for subsequent research on the effect of **expressed emotion** (ie, in which family members express hostility and are overly controlling), which leads to an increase in relapse rates.

The effect of these familial behaviors is muted if patients are receiving neuroleptic drugs. The view that schizophrenia is a brain disease prevailed after evidence for a genetic basis for schizophrenia was found. Investigators conducted studies of adoptees with a biological parent who had schizophrenia, adoptees with no familial schizophrenia who were adopted into a family with a schizophrenic parent, or twins who were monozygotic (MZ) or dizygotic (DZ) and concordant or discordant for schizophrenia. These studies established unequivocally that there was a genetic basis for schizophrenia and that being raised by a parent with schizophrenia had little effect on an individual's likelihood of becoming schizophrenic or on the outcome of the disorder. Recently, the possibility that genetic factors may influence family interactions and the individual's ability to cope with the environment has again focused interest on the environment as a cause of expression of the genetic predisposition to develop schizophrenia.

1. Dopamine hypothesis—The most widely accepted original hypothesis of the etiology of schizophrenia and of the action of antipsychotic drugs has implicated the neurotransmitter dopamine (DA). Dopaminergic neurons arise from two midbrain nuclei: (1) The nigrostriatal tract originates in the substantia nigra, terminates in the striatum, and is involved in modulation of motoric behavior, cognition, and sensory gating; and (2) the mesolimbic and mesocortical tracts originate in the ventral tegmental area and terminate in limbic and cortical structures, respectively, affecting cognitive, motivational, and reward systems. The dopamine 1 (D_1) receptor family, which includes D_1 and D_5 receptors, is present in high concentration in the cortex and striatum. The dopamine 2 (D_2) receptor family consists of D_2, D_3, and D_4 receptors and is concentrated in the limbic and striatal regions. Presynaptic DA receptors (ie, D_2 and D_3) can consist of either somatodendritic autoreceptors localized to cell bodies in the substantia nigra and ventral tegmental area or terminal autoreceptors limited to axons of these DA cells. The somatodendritic and terminal autoreceptors affect firing of DA cells and synthesis and release of DA, respectively. Decreased DA activity in the prefrontal cortex may mediate the negative symptoms and cognitive dysfunction associated with schizophrenia.

The DA hypothesis of schizophrenia, as originally postulated, proposed that schizophrenia was due to an excess of DA activity in limbic brain areas, especially the nucleus accumbens, as well as the stria terminalis, lateral septum, and olfactory tubercle. This hypothesis was based on evidence that chronic administration of the stimulant D-amphetamine produced a psychosis that resembled paranoid schizophrenia. D-Amphetamine increased the release of DA and norepinephrine (NE) and inhibited their reuptake. Isomers of D-amphetamine with different effects on the availability of NE and DA in rodents were used to show that increased locomotor activity, which correlates best with psychosis in humans, was due to an increased release of DA rather than NE.

The second line of evidence relating DA to schizophrenia was that drugs that proved to be antipsychotics decreased DA activity by receptor blockade (reserpine)

and depletion (neuroleptics). The most compelling evidence that linked DA to the positive symptoms of schizophrenia was the finding that chlorpromazine was an effective antipsychotic drug and that it blocked DA receptors in vivo, which inhibited the effect of D-amphetamine on locomotor activity. The discovery that a number of different chemical classes of DA-receptor antagonists were effective as antipsychotic drugs and that there was a high correlation between the drug's average daily dosage and its affinity for the D_2 receptor family led to the view that increased stimulation of these receptors caused schizophrenia.

The concept of increased DA activity as the core deficit in schizophrenia was developed at the time when delusions and hallucinations were central to the diagnosis of schizophrenia and negative symptoms, affective symptoms, and cognitive dysfunction were relegated to a secondary role. These latter aspects of schizophrenia have never been associated with excessive DA activity. As mentioned earlier in this chapter, researchers have proposed that decreased DA activity may lead to cognitive impairment and possibly depression. There is little evidence that blockade of D_2 or D_4 receptors induces depression or cognitive impairment. Recent studies in primates have implicated the D_1 receptor family in the control of working memory, a cognitive function that is impaired in schizophrenia.

Postmortem studies of patients with schizophrenia have not found consistent abnormalities in the density of any of the five DA receptors or changes in their affinities for DA, with the possible exception of the D_3 receptor, which may have an abnormal form. Several research groups have also reported a link between D_3 polymorphisms and schizophrenia. There is no reliable evidence, from either postmortem studies or positron emission tomography (PET) studies, for an increase in the density of D_2 receptors in schizophrenia. Recent PET studies of the release of DA in the striatum of patients with schizophrenia have suggested that the extracellular concentration of DA in this region is increased compared to normal subjects. Plasma and cerebrospinal fluid (CSF) levels of homovanillic acid, the major metabolite of DA, are not elevated in patients who have schizophrenia. Some researchers have suggested that DA receptor sensitization occurs in schizophrenia, but only indirect evidence supports this hypothesis.

Jaskiw GE, Weinberger DR: Dopamine and schizophrenia: a cortically correct perspective. Semin Neurosci 1992; 4:179.

2. Serotonin hypothesis—Serotonin (5-HT) neurons originate in the midbrain dorsal and median raphe nuclei, which project to the cortex, striatum, hippocampus, and other limbic regions. There are at least 15 types of 5-HT receptors; of these, the most relevant to schizophrenia are the 5-HT_1, 5-HT_{1D}, 5-HT_2, 5-HT_3, 5-HT_6, and 5-HT_7 receptors. Somatodendritic autoreceptors (of the 5-HT_{1A} type) are present on the cell bodies of 5-HT raphe neurons and inhibit firing of serotonergic neurons. Terminal autoreceptors ($5-HT_{1D}$ in humans) regulate the synthesis and release of 5-HT. $5-HT_3$ receptors stimulate DA release. Postsynaptic $5-HT_{2A}$ receptors are localized on pyramidal neurons in mesocortical areas. The complex interaction between 5-HT and DA varies by brain region and by types of 5-HT and DA receptors.

An early theory of the etiology of schizophrenia was that it was due to an excess of brain serotonergic activity. This theory was based on the belief that the psychotomimetic properties of lysergic acid diethylamide (LSD), an indole compound, were due to its 5-HT agonist properties. This led to a search for endogenous indole hallucinogens in the brain, blood, and urine of schizophrenic patients. The enzymes that synthesize and catabolize indoles, of which 5-HT is the most important, were also studied in detail; however, none of the putative abnormalities was confirmed by subsequent careful study.

The notion that the effects of LSD and other indole hallucinogens, such as psilocybin and N,N-dimethyltryptamine, provide an adequate model of schizophrenia was also rejected because the primary effect of these drugs is to cause visual hallucinations. The potency of these agents as hallucinogens is highly correlated with their $5-HT_{2A}$-receptor antagonist affinity. The thought disorder, auditory hallucinations, and bizarre behavior usually present in schizophrenia are generally absent in normal individuals who are given these agents. However, ingestion of these agents can cause an exacerbation of positive symptoms in schizophrenic patients. Neuroleptic drugs are not particularly useful in decreasing the effects of the indole hallucinogens. Newer antipsychotic drugs such as clozapine, olanzapine, risperidone, quetiapine, and sertindole are potent antagonists of the $5-HT_{2A}$ receptor. Some of the advantages of these drugs may result from their greater potency as $5-HT_{2A}$-receptor antagonists, relative to D_2-receptor blockade. The most likely advantages of these drugs, related to their higher affinity to $5-HT_{2A}$ versus DA receptors, are their low D_2-induced EPS profile and their ability to improve negative symptoms. Increased stimulation of $5-HT_{2A}$ receptors may be important in the etiology of negative symptoms and EPS. Although this concept of the role of 5-HT in schizophrenia is no longer considered viable, alternative theories of the role of 5-HT are of interest and are discussed in subsequent sections.

Meltzer HY, Fatemi SH: The role of serotonin in schizophrenia and the mechanisms of action of antipsychotic drugs. Pages 77–107 in Kane JM, Möller HJ, Awouters F (editors): *Serotonin in Antipsychotic Treatment: Mechanisms and Clinical Practice.* Marcel Dekker, 1996.

3. Glutamate hypothesis—Clinical and experimental evidence has supported a complex role for glutamate in the etiology of schizophrenia. Evidence indicates that decreased glutamatergic activity is the result of decreased levels of glutamate receptors of the N-methyl-D-aspartate (NMDA) subtype. Decreased levels of glutamate in the CSF of patients with schizophrenia have also been reported. Consistent with the role of glutamate in schizophrenia, three noncompetitive antagonists of NMDA receptors (phencyclidine [PCP], ketamine, and MK-801), and three competitive antagonists (CPP, CPP-ene, and CGS 19755), can produce a range of positive and negative symptoms and cognitive dysfunction in normal control subjects and in schizophrenic patients. Neuroleptics can block some of the clinical effects of PCP. The ability of the $5-HT_{2A}$- and D_2-receptor antagonists, such as clozapine and olanzapine, to block the clinical effects of these NMDA-receptor antagonists is unknown. However, the preclinical effects of PCP, such as disruption of sensory gatings, can be blocked by selective $5-HT_{2A}$-receptor antagonists, such as MDL100907, and by clozapine. Glycine, which can enhance the ability of glutamate to stimulate the glutamate receptor, has been reported to decrease negative but not positive symptoms in patients with schizophrenia when administered in conjunction with typical neuroleptic drugs. It has also been suggested that increased levels of glutamate can have neurotoxic effects on various neurons; however, there is no conclusive evidence for neurodegenerative changes in schizophrenia. A recent report shows that mice expressing 5% of normal NMDARI levels exhibit schizophrenia-like behavioral abnormalities when they reach adulthood supporting a hypoglutamatergic hypothesis of schizophrenia.

Mohn AR et al: Mice with reduced NMDA receptor expression display behaviors related to schizophrenia. CELL 1999;98:427.
Olney JW, Farber NB: Glutamate receptor dysfunction and schizophrenia. Arch Gen Psychiatry 1995;52:998.

4. Neurodevelopmental hypothesis—According to the neurodevelopmental hypothesis, the etiology of schizophrenia may involve pathologic processes that begin before the brain approaches its adult anatomical state in adolescence. These neurodevelopmental abnormalities, developing in utero for some and thereafter for others, have been suggested to lead to the activation of pathologic neural circuits during adolescence or young adulthood (sometimes owing to severe stress), which leads to the emergence of positive or negative symptoms, or both. Earlier neuropathologic work indicated that some cases of schizophrenia result from embryologic maldevelopment. E. Slater also referred to maldevelopmental similarities between temporal lobe epilepsy and schizophrenia and stressed their possible neuropathologic basis. The emergence of evidence for cortical maldevelopment in schizophrenia and the development of several plausible animal models of schizophrenia, which are based on neonatal lesions that produce behavioral abnormalities or altered sensitivity to dopaminergic drugs only in adolescent or adult animals, have strengthened the link between maldevelopment and schizophrenia. The concept of schizophrenia as a neurodevelopmental disorder is also consistent with other epidemiologic and clinical lines of evidence, discussed in the following sections.

a. Obstetric and perinatal complications. An association between obstetric complications and later development of schizophrenia has been found. Some studies have found that obstetric complications were more common in early-onset, male, and chronic schizophrenic patients than in control subjects. Such an association has not been found in late-onset, female, and acute schizophrenic patients. The complications observed include periventricular hemorrhages, hypoxia, and ischemic injuries, which presumably cause subsequent abnormal connections in the brains of schizophrenic subjects. It is not clear whether obstetric abnormalities cause schizophrenia or whether preschizophrenic fetal abnormalities predispose to obstetric complications. The frequency of such complications is at most twice the rate found in control populations and may be thought of as one of many risk factors.

b. Structural abnormalities based on in vivo brain imaging. A consistent finding in schizophrenia is cerebral ventricular enlargement. A large number of computed tomography (CT) and magnetic resonance imaging (MRI) studies indicate lateral and third ventricular enlargement and widening of cortical fissures and sulci. Because these abnormalities are present at the onset of the illness and progress very slowly if at all, they are unrelated to the duration of illness or treatment received. In sets of MZ twins in which only one twin has schizophrenia, the affected twins have larger ventricles than do the unaffected twins. The loss of gray matter is correlated with poor premorbid social and educational adjustment during early childhood and with obstetric complications.

c. Postmortem studies. Postmortem studies of the brains of schizophrenic patients have revealed several possible abnormalities including decreased volume of limbic and temporal structures, such as the amygdala, hippocampus, parahippocampal gyrus, entorhinal cortex, and internal palladium. Volumes of various hippocampal fields are also reduced. There is brain tissue loss of approximately 5% in schizophrenic patients compared to age- and sex-matched control subjects. Hemispheric asymmetries, consistent with second-trimester developmental anomalies, have been identified in the lengths of the sylvian fissures and in the widths of the occipital lobes. Finally, agenesis of the corpus callosum has been noted in the brains of schizophrenic patients. None of these abnormalities can be considered pathognomonic for schizophrenia, and they are not present in all patients.

Several postmortem histopathologic findings also have been identified in the brains of schizophrenic subjects. There are reductions in the granule cell layer of the dentate gyrus and in the hippocampus (more in the left CA4 region), mediodorsal thalamus, nucleus accumbens, cingulate cortex, prefrontal area, motor cortex, and superficial layers of the entorhinal cortex. Some investigators have identified a disarray of pyramidal hippocampal cells in some schizophrenic patients. Heterotopic displacement of single pre-alpha cells in upper parahippocampal gyrus without evidence of brain injury or glial reaction (gliosis) suggests disruption of neuronal migration during the second trimester. An increased distance between the pial surface of the entorhinal cortex and the center of pre-alpha cell clusters suggests disruption of pre-alpha cell migration. Finally, disruption, displacement, and paucity of neurons in superficial layers of the entorhinal cortex suggests excessive synaptic pruning, which may lead to decreased connectivity between neurons.

Several recent cytoarchitectural studies give credence to the idea of early abnormal laminar organization and orientation of neurons: (1) decreased entorhinal cellularity in superficial layers I and II, incomplete clustering of neurons in layer II, and the presence of clusters in deeper layers where they are normally not found; (2) findings similar to those in the entorhinal cortices in prefrontal and cingulate cortices; and (3) reduced NADPH-diaphorase (nitric oxide synthase)–positive cells (remnants of the embryonic subplate zone) in cortical layers I and II, and increased density in deep layers (subcortical white layer or the putative vestigial subplate zone) in dorsolateral prefrontal, hippocampal, and lateral temporal cortices. Such defects in the inside-out organization of neurons may be due to defects in the neuronal migration process.

d. Synaptic marker anomalies. Biological markers consistent with potential neurodevelopmental lesions in schizophrenia include changes in the normal expression of proteins that are involved in early migration of neurons, cell proliferation, axonal outgrowth, and synaptogenesis (Table 19–2). Of considerable value is the recent finding of reductions of 40–50% in Reelin mRNA and protein in the brains of schizophrenic patients. Reelin is an important secretory protein that is responsible for normal lamination of the brain during early growth. Prenatal human influenza viral infection, a potential risk factor for schizophrenia, can also result in decreased expression of Reelin, supporting the epidemiologic evidence linking fetal brain insult and later increase in incidence of schizophrenia.

e. Adverse environmental events in utero. Epidemiologic data consistently show that schizophrenic patients have an increased likelihood of having been born in the late winter and spring months. An explanation for this seasonal effect has been linked to epidemics of influenza or viral infections that occur more frequently during winter months. A number of epidemiologic studies have attributed the increased rate of schizophrenic births to maternal influenza or other viral infections during the second trimester. Maternal influenza during the second trimester may

Table 19–2. Neurodevelopmental markers and schizophrenia.

Neurodevelopmental Event	Molecule	Findings in Schizophrenia
Cell migration	PSA-NCAM	↓ in dentate hilar area
	Reelin	↓ in mRNA and protein of neocortex, hippocampus, and cerebellum
Synaptogenesis and axonal growth	SNAP-25	↓ in hippocampus and frontal cortex
	GAP-43	↑ in prefrontal and inferior temporal cortex; ↓ dentate gyrus
	Synaptophysin	↓ in prefrontal cortex and hippocampus
	Synapsin	↓ in hippocampus
Survival of connections	BDNF	↓ in hippocampus
Neuronal cytoskeletal proteins	MAP-2	↓ in subiculum and entorhinal cortex
	MAP-5	↓ in subiculum

impair fetal growth and predispose to obstetric complications and lower birth weight in about 2% of individuals destined to develop schizophrenia. Recent epidemiologic evidence based on 2669 cases of schizophrenia in a population cohort of 1.75 million persons showed significant relative risks of developing schizophrenia with increased urbanization and season of birth. The highest association was for births in the months of February and March, presumably due to increased risk of viral infection during pregnancy.

Other complicating factors such as maternal malnutrition and Rh incompatibility during gestation have been associated with an individual's increased vulnerability to schizophrenia.

Fatemi SH et al: Defective corticogenesis and reduction in Reelin immunoreactivity in cortex and hippocampus of prenatally infected neonatal mice. Mol Psychiatry 1999;4:145.
Mortensen PB et al: Effects of family history and place and season of birth on the risk of schizophrenia. N Engl J Med 1999;340:603.

f. The absence of gliosis. Gliosis is the scar tissue in the brain that signifies cellular loss, degeneration, or inflammation in the developed brain. Absence of gliosis in the postmortem brain specimens of schizophrenic patients implies that neuron loss occurred during the early gestational period, prior to development of glial cells, or by programmed cell death (apoptosis) after birth, in which case gliosis would not be present.

g. Congenital anomalies. Incidental anomalies indicative of neurodevelopmental deviations have been found in schizophrenic patients. These anomalies may include corpus callosum agenesis, aqueduct stenosis, cerebral hamartomas, and cavum septum pellucidum. Other minor physical anomalies such as low-set ears, epicanthal eye folds, and wide spaces between the first and second toes, which are found in a small proportion of patients with schizophrenia, are suggestive of first trimester anomalies. Schizophrenic patients may have abnormal dermatoglyphics (a second trimester event) or decreased birth weight.

h. Developmental neurologic and biopsychosocial dysfunction. Several reports indicate the presence of premorbid neurologic soft signs in children who later develop schizophrenia. Fish et al used the term **pandysmaturation syndrome** to refer to a series of disorders of skeletal growth, arousal, tonus, motility, proprioception, and vestibular and vasovegetative functions seen in preschizophrenic children. Slight posturing of hands and transient choreoathetoid movements have been observed during the first 2 years of life in affected siblings who later developed schizophrenia. Additionally, poor performance on tests of attention and neuromotor performance, affective and social impairment, and excessive anxiety have been reported to occur more frequently in high-risk children with a schizophrenic parent. All of these findings are consistent with abnormalities of brain development.

Brown AS: The neurodevelopmental hypothesis of schizophrenia. Psychiatr Ann 1999;29:123.
Impagnatiello F et al: A decrease of Reelin expression as a putative vulnerability factor in schizophrenia. Proc Natl Acad Sci U S A 1998;95:15718.
Weickert CS et al: A candidate molecule approach to defining developmental pathology in schizophrenia. Schizophr Bull 1998;24:303.

B. Epidemiology: Schizophrenia affects 1% of the adult population. The incidence is comparable in all societies. Individuals in lower socioeconomic classes have higher rates of schizophrenia because of the markedly impaired work function of patients with this illness. Lower income is to be expected in the families of schizophrenics because 10% of the parents of schizophrenic patients have schizophrenia themselves, and other parents may have subclinical forms of the illness, including cognitive impairments and Axis II pathology, which may impair their ability to earn income.

Schizophrenia is slightly more common in males than in females. The impairment in male patients is, on average, greater than in female patients because male patients tend to have a poorer response to neuroleptic treatment. Male patients whose schizophrenia is not treatment resistant have a younger age at onset and are more likely to have comorbid substance abuse.

The age at onset of schizophrenia is gender related in some types of schizophrenia. Female patients, especially those with the paranoid subtype of schizophrenia, have an age at onset that is, on average, 5 years later than in male patients. The mean age for female patients is 25 years with a range of 15–30 years being the most common. For male patients, the mean age is 20 years with a range of 10–24 years. Patients with poor outcome, as indicated by poor response to currently available therapies, have an earlier age at onset than do those who are more responsive to treatment. The average age at onset of neuroleptic-resistant schizophrenia in female patients may be 4–5 years less than in female patients with neuroleptic-responsive schizophrenia, but male and female patients with neuroleptic-resistant schizophrenia have similar ages at onset: 20–21 years, on average, according to one study.

C. Genetics: Recent evidence indicates that schizophrenia is a familial disorder with a complex mode of inheritance and variable phenotypic expressivity. Twin studies of schizophrenia found concordance rates of 46% for MZ twins and 14% for DZ twins. The lifetime expectancy of manifesting schizophrenia in the relatives of schizophrenic patients varies as a function of the closeness of the relationship. Among first-degree relatives, lifetime expectancies are as follows: 5.6% for a parent, 10.1% for a sibling, 16.7% for a sibling with one schizophrenic parent, and 46.3% for children with two schizophrenic parents. In second-degree and third-degree relatives, the expectancies are 3.3% and 2.4%, respectively. Furthermore, adoption studies show a lifetime prevalence of 9.4% in the adopted-away offspring of schizophrenic parents and a lifetime prevalence of 1.2% in control adoptees.

The exact mode of transmission in schizophrenia is unknown; family studies have ruled out single dominant gene defects. A multifactorial threshold model (ie, additive effects of numerous genes at different loci) or a mixed model (ie, interaction between a single major gene with a number of other genes) are the most likely modes. Ongoing subpair studies seem likely to identify the genetic basis for this disorder within the next few years.

Linkage and association studies have produced conflicting results that point to chromosomes 6, 11, 21, and X as potential sites in the genetic transmission of schizophrenia. Candidate genes such as the D_2 and D_4 genes have been ruled out. Some of the candidate association sites have included the porphobilinogen deaminase gene (for porphyria), the long arm of chromosome 11, and the association between the HLA9 marker and paranoid schizophrenia. More interesting, linkage studies of the gene for the D_3 receptor, which has restricted expression in the limbic regions and has been localized to the long arm of chromosome 3, have often been positive.

Recent findings and association studies point to several susceptibility loci on chromosomes 6, 8, and 22. A mutation involving the function of ubiquitin fusion-degradation 1 like (Udf1L), an important molecule normally expressed in neural-crest-derived embryonic tissues, leads to development of an autosomal dominant syndrome (velo-cardio-facial syndrome) that is associated with an increased risk of developing schizophrenia. Patients with this syndrome also exhibit congenital abnormalities involving heart, thymus, and craniofacial development. More recently haploinsufficiency of UFD1L gene product has been identified in a cohort of schizophrenic patients giving credence to potential involvement of this protein in schizophrenia.

Asherson P, Mant R, McGiffin P: Genetics and schizophrenia. Pages 253–274 in Hirsch SR, Weinberger DR (editors): *Schizophrenia.* Blackwell Scientific, 1995.
Dunham I et al: The DNA sequence of human chromosome 22. Nature 1999;402:489.
Gothelf D et al: Clinical characteristics of schizophrenia associated with velo-cardio-facial syndrome. Schizophr Res 1999;35:105.
Moldin SO et al: At issue: genes, experience, and chance in schizophrenia—positioning for the 21st century. Schizophr Bull 1997;23:547.
Pasini A et al: Association between schizophrenia and the UFD1L promtes polymorphism-277 A/G. Society for Neuroscience 1999;25:571 (Abs. 232.1).
Yamagishi H et al: A molecular pathway revealing a genetic basis for human cardiac and craniofacial defects. Science 1999;283:1158.

Clinical Findings

A. Signs & Symptoms: In contrast to other medical conditions, no one sign or symptom is diagnostic of schizophrenia. Thus it is important to obtain as much information as possible about the patient's medical and psychiatric history, mental status examination, family and social history as well as other pertinent information from family and friends.

Some families of schizophrenic patients report progressive behavioral disturbances in childhood and adolescence in males and early adulthood in females. These disturbances include social withdrawal and academic and personal problems. An individual who develops schizophrenia may have been labeled as introverted, shy, and asocial, with few or no friends, as a child. Such individuals may first complain of somatic symptoms. Later, he or she may become involved in highly unusual hobbies, such as the occult. The individual may exhibit bizarre thinking, unusual speech, or abnormal affect mixed with hallucinatory experiences. A transient psychotic episode may lead to a referral of the patient to a physician or a psychiatrist. However, many patients with schizophrenia show no abnormalities until the beginning of the prodromal period. This period may last from months to years, during which time a change occurs in some aspect of the patient's behavior or cognitive function. Parents and patients report personality changes, withdrawal, decreased academic performance, less interest in sex and other previously enjoyable activities, obsessive-compulsive and ritualistic behavior, less care for hygiene, moodiness and flat affect, magical thinking, and increased aggressiveness. Because these symptoms are often part of normal adolescence, it is difficult, even for professionals, to identify an impending psychosis.

Upon examination, schizophrenic patients may appear disheveled, and they may show evidence of poor self-care and grooming. They often relate poorly to the examiner, appearing uninvolved and suspicious. These behaviors are described in more detail later in this section. Some patients may exhibit bizarre postures, stereotyped behaviors, grimacing, athetosis, mutism, or catatonia (either agitation or stupor). It may be difficult for some patients to tolerate more than a brief interview. The schizophrenic patient's affect is often incongruent with his or her state of mind and may be best described as inappropriate. For example, patients may exhibit a happy affect while talking about a sad event. The patient's affect may be devoid of emotional tone or, when present, may be described as blunted or flat. Flat affect may be secondary to EPS. It is essential for clinicians to recognize serious depression in schizophrenic patients because of the risk of suicide.

Patients' thoughts may be loose, illogical, or bizarre in form and content. Their speech may reflect circumstantiality, tangentiality, slang associations, neologisms, perseveration, and poverty of content. Patients may repeat others' words (echolalia), become mute, show thought blocking (ie, a sudden stop in the middle of a conversation), and be unable to understand abstract concepts.

Schizophrenic patients experience visual or auditory hallucinations. Hallucinations based on every type of sensory modality (eg, auditory, visual, gustatory, olfactory, tactile, and cenesthesic [altered body states]) have been reported. Auditory hallucinations occur more frequently than other hallucinations. They may be well-tolerated by some patients, whereas in other patients the frequency and intensity of hallucinations may be very debilitating and even lead to suicide.

Schizophrenic patients may exhibit delusions that reflect ideas of persecution, grandiosity, outside control, or reference. Patients may experience the belief that their thoughts are being broadcast or controlled. They may claim that outside forces are able to insert thoughts into or withdraw thoughts from their brains.

Patients may exhibit stereotyped behavior whereupon they repeat various functions or gestures. They may imitate others' movements (echopraxia), refuse to cooperate (negativism), remain motionless for a long time (catatonic stupor), and maintain their limbs or trunks in unusual positions (waxy flexibility, or catalepsy) for various lengths of time. Schizophrenic

patients may cause self-induced water intoxication or avoid eating because of certain delusional beliefs. They may stoically refuse to admit any pain or may complain of unusual emotions (eg, rotting of intestines or burning of their brains).

A preponderance of evidence shows a link between neurologic soft signs and the neurodevelopmental origin of schizophrenia. Mild neurologic deficits have been noted, including abnormal body movements, gait, mannerisms, or reflexes; increased or decreased muscle tone; abnormal rapid eye movements (saccades); frequent blinking; dysdiadochokinesia; astereognosis; and poor right-left discrimination.

Cognitive dysfunction is a cardinal feature of schizophrenia. On average, the intelligence quotient (IQ) of schizophrenic patients, when first diagnosed with the disorder, is 10 points lower than comparison groups, including unaffected siblings or cotwins. Children at risk for schizophrenia have lower IQs than do control subjects and show abnormalities in attention and concentration. Patients in their first episode of schizophrenia exhibit impairments in attention, working memory, visual-spatial memory, semantic memory, recall memory, and executive functions.

The diverse nature of the cognitive disturbance in schizophrenia suggests that the disturbance is based on diffuse rather than localized brain disease. With treatment, that impairment might improve slightly, but there is little evidence that antipsychotic drugs, with the exception of clozapine, have a significant effect on the cognitive disturbance in schizophrenia. Cognitive impairment is often independent of positive and negative symptoms and even of the disorganization syndrome. Over the course of the illness, a small percentage of schizophrenic patients experience a great worsening in cognition and reach the levels of impairment of patients with a variety of senile psychoses, including Alzheimer's disease. The majority of schizophrenic patients do not exhibit marked change in cognitive dysfunction. Specific types of cognitive disturbance play a major role in limiting social and occupational performance in schizophrenic patients. For this reason, therapies that target the cognitive disturbance in schizophrenia are likely to be of immense value.

B. Neuropsychological Testing: The presence of significant cognitive abnormalities in schizophrenic patients warrants the use of neuropsychological testing to establish evidence of brain disorder early during the diagnosis of the disease. Formal neuropsychological assessment using objective tests, such as the Halstead-Reitan Battery, the Luria-Nebraska Battery, the Wechsler Adult Intelligence Scale, the Wechsler Intelligence Scale for Children, and the Wisconsin Card Sorting Test (WCST), can identify the presence of various abnormalities involving the frontotemporal areas of the brain. The usefulness of projective and personality tests in the diagnosis of schizophrenia may be limited because these tests indicate the presence of bizarre ideations or abnormal personality traits and are more prone to biased subjective interpretations.

C. Laboratory Findings & Imaging:

1. Cerebral ventricular enlargement—Early descriptions of ventricular enlargement in the brains of some schizophrenic subjects demonstrated by pneumoencephalography has now been replicated by a large number of CT and MRI studies. Moreover, the ventricular enlargement has been associated with reductions in cerebral brain tissue. Despite the large body of supportive imaging studies, other studies have reported on the nonspecificity of brain ventricular enlargement. Meta-analyses of studies of ventricular enlargement and cortical sulcal prominence in groups of patients with mood disorders and schizophrenia compared to control subjects found that ventricular enlargement and increased sulcal prominence is not limited to patients with schizophrenia but can also be observed in patients with mood disorders. Further, patients with mood disorders have less ventricular enlargement when compared to schizophrenic patients, but the magnitude of the difference is small.

2. Other brain abnormalities—A number of other brain abnormalities have been identified based on in vivo imaging. These abnormalities include smaller cerebral and cranial sizes; smaller medial temporal structures, specifically hippocampi; enlargement of lenticular nucleus; cerebellar vermal dysplasia; and association of brain changes with a family history of schizophrenia. One study reported that the size of the thalamus was smaller in schizophrenic patients when compared to normal control subjects. This study also confirmed that schizophrenic patients had more CSF and less brain tissue.

3. Functional brain abnormalities—Recent improvements in accurate measurement of regional cranial blood flow and brain glucose metabolism, using PET and single photon emission computed tomography (SPECT), have added to the identification of various brain abnormalities not previously known in schizophrenia. Generally, simple sensory or motor tasks are associated with various regional cerebral blood flow changes. Comparison of normal and schizophrenic brain blood flow studies either at rest or following specific neuropsychological testing can help to pinpoint any major differences. PET studies of schizophrenic patients on medications enabled the correlation of certain cerebral blood flow patterns with three stable symptom complexes in schizophrenic patients: (1) **Psychomotor poverty** (ie, negative symptoms) correlates with decreased blood flow in left parietal cortex and prefrontal areas, whereas increased flow is associated with caudate nuclei; (2) **reality distortion** (ie, positive symptoms) is associated with increased flow in the medial temporal cortex and decreased flow in the posterior cingulate and left lateral lobe; and (3) **disorganization syndrome** correlates with increased flow in the right anterior cingulate and decreased flow

in the right anterior prefrontal cortex. These results support other studies that found that positive symptoms such as hallucinations and delusions correlate with increased flow in the left temporal lobe, whereas negative symptoms are associated with bilateral frontal hypoperfusion. The functional significance of these changes in blood flow for the activity of specific types of neurons remains to be determined. In another study, researchers used PET to localize the sources of auditory hallucinations to several subcortical nuclei including thalamus, striatum, limbic (hippocampal), and paralimbic (parahippocampal and cingulate gyri orbitofrontal cortices) areas. Schizophrenic patients who hallucinated exhibited significantly different patterns of main blood flow in some of these areas, even when they were not hallucinating, compared to those who did not hallucinate. If confirmed, such data may indicate biologically unique subtypes of schizophrenia. A recent report using functional MRI to analyze brain regions that activate during auditory hallucinations shows that although in normal volunteer subjects inner speech is not associated with activity in primary auditory cortex, in hallucinating schizophrenic patients, inner speech activates primary auditory cortex and is falsely attributed by the patient to the voice of an external source.

Another way to localize sites of brain function is to activate specific cortical areas with cognitive tests. For example, investigators used the WCST to identify impaired frontal function in schizophrenic patients. In the schizophrenic population in this study, flexibility in problem solving, as measured by the WCST, was abnormal and was correlated with a lesser degree of activation of dorsolateral prefrontal cortex when compared to normal control subjects. Decreased prefrontal activation was correlated with reduced hippocampal volume and reduced dopaminergic activity, which could be reversed by the DA agonist apomorphine.

Other researchers used PET to study the role of DA as a regulatory agent on cortical function in schizophrenic patients. During a verbal fluency test and under basal conditions, schizophrenic patients showed a relative failure of flow increase in anterior cingulate cortex. Following administration of apomorphine (a mixed D_1, D_2, D_3 agonist), a larger than normal activation of anterior cingulate cortex was observed, consistent with the enhanced sensitivity of schizophrenia to DA.

Andreasen NC et al: Thalamic abnormalities in schizophrenia visualized through magnetic resonance image averaging. Science 1994;266:294.

Dolan RJ et al: Dopaminergic modulation of impaired cognitive activation in the anterior cingulate cortex in schizophrenia. Nature 1995;378:180.

Elkis H et al: Meta-analyses of studies of ventricular enlargement and cortical sulcal prominence in mood disorders. Comparisons with controls or patients with schizophrenia. Arch Gen Psychiatry 1995;52:735.

Frith C: How hallucinations make themselves heard. Neuron 1999;4:4.

Liddle PF: Brain imaging. Pages 425–439 in Hirsch SR, Weinberger DR (editors): *Schizophrenia.* Blackwell Scientific, 1995.

Liddle PF et al: Patterns of cerebral blood flow in schizophrenia. Br J Psychiatry 1992;160:179.

Silbersweig DA et al: A functional neuroanatomy of hallucinations in schizophrenia. Nature 1995;378:176.

Weinberger DR: Schizophrenia as a neurodevelopmental disorder. Pages 293–323 in Hirsch SR, Weinberger DR (editors): *Schizophrenia.* Blackwell Scientific, 1995.

Differential Diagnosis

Psychotic symptoms may be present in a number of disorders other than schizophrenia. Before giving a patient the diagnosis of schizophrenia, the clinician must exclude all other possibilities through a careful history, physical examination, mental status examination, and laboratory testing.

A. Mood Disorders: Manic or severely depressed patients may exhibit psychotic symptoms during the peak of their disease states (see Chapter 21). These symptoms may include hallucinations or delusions that can be either mood congruent or mood incongruent. Accurate historical and clinical data should help to differentiate schizophrenia from mania-related psychotic features in the presence of other symptoms such as increased energy levels, grandiosity, hypersexuality, irritability, pressured speech, and distractibility. By the same token, psychosis may accompany the depressed phase of bipolar disorder or unipolar depression. These disorders should be differentiated from schizophrenia by the presence of other criteria for mood disorder. When psychotic symptoms, which may be indistinguishable from those of schizophrenia, occur exclusively during periods of mood disturbance, the diagnosis should be mood disorder with psychotic features or schizoaffective disorder.

B. Psychotic Disorders Due to a General Medical or Neurologic Condition & Substance-Induced Psychotic Disorders: Many conditions can cause schizophrenia-like symptoms. Clinicians must carefully evaluate the chronology of symptoms in relation to the inciting cause and note whether symptoms improve or worsen in relation to such cause. Substances that can produce psychotic symptoms include amphetamines (eg, substituted amphetamines such as 3,4-methylenedioxy methamphetamine, or "ecstasy"), hallucinogens, belladonna alkaloids, alcohol, barbiturates (in withdrawal), cocaine, ketamine, and PCP.

Patients with a number of medical or neurologic conditions may exhibit psychosis before developing other symptoms. Examples include temporal lobe epilepsy, neoplasms, frontal or limbic trauma, cerebrovascular accidents, AIDS, acute intermittent porphyria, vitamin B_{12} deficiency, carbon monoxide poisoning, Creutzfeldt-Jakob disease, Fabry's disease, Fahr's disease, Hallervorden-Spatz disease, heavy metal poisoning, herpes encephalitis, homocystinuria, Huntington's disease, metachromatic leukodystrophy, neurosyphilis, normal pressure hydrocephalus, pellagra, systemic lupus erythematosus, Wernicke-Korsakoff syndrome, and Wilson's disease. The clinical course, patient history, and pertinent laboratory testing may help the clinician to identify the causative illness and rule out schizophrenia.

C. Other Psychotic Disorders: There is controversy over how to classify patients with delusions or hallucinations of a schizophrenic type with concomitant mood symptoms (either depressive or manic in nature) in the absence of a primary mood disorder. Such patients are diagnosed as having schizoaffective disorder, manic or depressed type (see Chapter 20). The essential features of schizoaffective disorder are an uninterrupted period of illness during which time criteria for a major depressive, mixed, or manic episode occur together with at least two of the five major symptoms of schizophrenia. In addition, delusions or hallucinations must be present for at least 2 weeks in the absence of prominent mood symptoms. Furthermore, the mood symptoms must be present for a substantial portion of the total duration of the illness. According to DSM-IV, this disorder does not constitute a subtype of schizophrenia but is a separate form of psychotic illness. There is likely considerable overlap in etiology and pathophysiology between schizoaffective disorder and schizophrenia on the one hand and between psychotic mood disorders and schizophrenia on the other.

Other types of psychotic illness distinguished from schizophrenia are brief reactive psychosis (schizophrenic-type symptoms for at least 1 day but less than 4 weeks that follow a major stressor), schizophreniform disorder (prodromal, active, and residual symptoms for at least 1 month but less than 6 months), and psychotic disorders not otherwise specified (for psychotic disorders that do not meet the criteria for any specific psychotic disorder or about which there is inadequate information to make a specific diagnosis). Schizophreniform illness is more often associated with a good outcome than is schizophrenia. The diagnosis should be made on a provisional basis unless all symptoms resolve within the 6-month period. If symptoms persist, the diagnosis should be changed to schizophrenia. Schizophreniform disorder may be specified as with good prognostic features if at least two of the following features are present: onset of prominent psychotic symptoms within 4 weeks of the first distinct deviation from usual functioning, confusion or perplexity at the peak of the positive symptoms, good premorbid social and vocational functioning, and absence of blunted or flat affect. In the absence of at least two of the above, schizophreniform disorder is specified as without good prognostic features. Delusional disorder refers to nonbizarre delusions in the absence of hallucinations, disorganized speech, and behavior or prominent negative symptoms or a mood disorder.

D. Personality Disorders: Schizotypal, schizoid, paranoid, and borderline personality disorders share some features with schizophrenia (eg, paranoid ideation, magical thinking, social avoidance, vague speech). In personality disorders these symptoms are mild, can be present throughout the patient's life, and have no exact date of onset (see Chapter 33).

Treatment

A. Pharmacologic Treatments:

1. Initiation of treatment—In general, neuroleptics are best commenced at a low dosage (ie, 10 mg/day haloperidol equivalent). The dosage should not be increased for 4–6 weeks unless psychotic or aggressive symptoms or sleeplessness are severe. Raising dosages rapidly increases the risk of EPS and secondary negative symptoms without conveying added antipsychotic benefit. Routine use of short-acting parenteral medication for newly hospitalized patients is to be avoided. Long-acting medication should not be given initially except to those patients with a history of noncompliance with other forms of treatment. The use of higher dosages (greater than 40 mg haloperidol equivalents) for the acute treatment of schizophrenia is no more effective than the use of neuroleptics at a more moderate dosage (5–10 haloperidol equivalents).

Some patients may respond to antipsychotics within the first week of treatment or even on the first day. Most patients may not respond for 2–6 weeks. Accordingly, it is inadvisable to discontinue a drug prematurely and substitute a different class of neuroleptic agent before the optimal 4–6 weeks of therapy has passed, unless significant side effects or EPS develop that are not amenable to treatment.

The use of several neuroleptics at the same time should be avoided. In particular, there is no justification for the concomitant use of two classes of typical neuroleptic drugs (eg, a parenteral and an oral antipsychotic drug) unless the patient's treatment is being converted from intramuscular to oral administration. In some instances, particularly when a neuroleptic is not adequately controlling anxiety and agitation, the adjunctive use of benzodiazepines may be helpful.

2. Typical antipsychotic drugs—The discovery of chlorpromazine in 1950 revolutionized the treatment of schizophrenia. Chlorpromazine and similar antipsychotic agents decrease positive symptoms of schizophrenia, but they have a limited effect on negative symptoms (eg, apathy, anhedonia, asociality, avolition, loss of affect, alogia, or poverty of thought) or on cognition or mood disturbance. A comparison of the outcome of schizophrenia before and after the introduction of neuroleptics found that the proportion of patient benefits in the good treatment responsiveness group, as defined by minimal symptoms and adequate social functioning, increased only about 15%. This finding does not detract from the significance of an-

tipsychotic treatment, which dramatically reduces positive symptoms in 60–70% of patients and enables many patients to live in the community, albeit unprepared for the outside world.

The effectiveness of neuroleptic drugs in ameliorating the positive symptoms of schizophrenia has been demonstrated in numerous double-blind, controlled studies. The first generation of these drugs were called neuroleptics because they produce neurologic side effects such as catalepsy in rodents and EPS in humans. These effects are secondary to their ability to decrease dopaminergic activity due to blockade of the D_2 receptor family. With prolonged administration (7–21 days) inactivation of mesolimbic and mesocortical DA neurons (which originate in the ventral tegmentum) and substantia nigra DA neurons (which project to the striatum) may contribute to the antipsychotic effects and EPS, respectively. With the exception of the substituted benzamides, such as sulpiride and amisulpride, which are highly selective D_2-receptor antagonists, these drugs also have variable affinities for binding to other neurotransmitter receptors (see "Dopamine Hypothesis" section earlier in this chapter). Because of the similarity in their fundamental mechanisms of action, these agents show little difference in efficacy in clinical practice.

As mentioned earlier in this section, up to 70% of patients with schizophrenia (and other psychotic disorders) will experience clinically significant amelioration of positive symptoms and disorganization when treated with these agents for 4–6 weeks at appropriate dosages (Table 19–3). The choice of which typical neuroleptic drug to use is based on a variety of considerations, including the availability of long-acting preparations. The low-potency drugs (ie, those in which the upper end of the dosage range is 300 mg/day or greater—eg, chlorpromazine, thioridazine, mesoridazine) are more sedative and more hypotensive than are the high-potency drugs such as haloperidol and fluphenazine. The latter agents produce more EPS than do the low-potency agents (see Table 19–3). Both low and high-potency agents decrease agitation and combative behavior.

If the patient's history of drug response does not indicate an unusual sensitivity to EPS, high-potency agents such as haloperidol and fluphenazine are often the treatments of choice. If EPS develop, anticholinergic agents such as benztropine, biperiden, or trihexyphenidyl may be used or the patient may be switched from to a medium-potency drug (eg, trifluoperazine) or to a low-potency drug (eg, thioridazine). One of the atypical antipsychotics (eg, clozapine, olanzapine, risperidone, sertindole, ziprasidone) may be the treatment of choice if patients are particularly sensitive to EPS (see next section). Untreated EPS may be the cause of negative symptoms and noncompliance. Some evidence indicates that prolonged delays in starting antipsychotic treatment may predict a poorer outcome, presumably because some aspects of

Table 19–3. Commonly used antipsychotic drugs.

Class and Drug Name	Dosage Range (mg)	Approximate Oral Dose Equivalents (mg)	Parenteral Dosage (mg)	Galenic Forms[1]
Conventional Drugs				
Butyrophenone				
Haloperidol (Haldol)	5–30	2	5–10	O,L,I
Haloperidol decanoate (Haldol-D)	NA	NA	25–100 every 1–4 weeks	NA
Dibenzoxazepine				
Loxapine succinate (Loxitane)	40–100	15	25	O,L,I
Diphenylbutylpiperidine				
Pimozide (Orap)	2–6	1	NA	O
Dihydroindolone				
Molindone hydrochloride (Moban)	50–225	10	NA	O,L
Phenothiazines				
Chlorpromazine (Thorazine)	200–800	100	25–50	O,L,I,S
Thioridazine (Mellaril)	150–800	100	NA	O,L
Mesoridazine (Serentil)	75–300	50	25	O,L,I
Perphenazine (Trilafon)	8–32	10	5–10	O,L,I
Trifluoperazine (Stelazine)	5–20	5	1–2	O,L,I
Fluphenazine hydrochloride (Prolixin)	2–60	2	1.25–2.5	O,L,I
Fluphenazine decanoate (Prolixin-D)	NA	NA	12.5–50 every 1–4 weeks	NA
Fluphenazine enanthate (Prolixin-E)	NA	NA	12.5–50 every 1–4 weeks	NA
Thioxanthenes				
Thiothixene hydrochloride (Navane)	5–30	5	2–4	O,L,I
Atypical Drugs				
Benzisothiazolyl piperazine[2]				
Ziprasidone (Zeldox)	40–160	40	10	O,L,I
Benzisoxazole				
Risperidone (Risperdal)	4–8	1	NA	O,L
Dibenzothiazepine				
Quetiapine fumarate (Seroquel)	150–600	100	NA	O
Dibenzodiazepine				
Clozapine (Clozaril)	100–900	50	NA	O
Imidazolidinone[2]				
Sertindole (Serlect)	12–24	4	NA	O
Thienobenzodiazepine				
Olanzapine (Zyprexa)	10–20	4	NA	O

[1] O, oral; L, liquid; I, injection; S = suppository.
[2] Under FDA investigation.

the process of psychosis may be biologically toxic to brain structure.

The affinities that antipsychotic agents have for D_2, 5-HT_{2A}, and muscarinic receptors are key determinants of their liability to cause EPS. D_2-receptor affinities predict levels of susceptibility to EPS. Elevated serum prolactin and sedative and hypotensive side effects reflect histaminergic (H_1) and adrenergic (α_2)–receptor antagonist properties. Other side effects of typical neuroleptics such as gynecomastia, impotence, and amenorrhea are also due to DA-receptor blockade. Weight gain is due to 5-HT_{2C}- and H_1-receptor blockade. Hematologic effects, jaundice, cardiac effects, photosensitivity, and retinitis result from toxic effects in specific target tissues. Plasma levels of antipsychotics and their metabolites vary greatly between patients. The only agents with probable therapeutic windows are haloperidol and clozapine. For haloperidol, a steady-state plasma range of 12–17 ng/liter has been associated with optimal antipsychotic action. Evidence suggests that lower dosages of typical antipsychotics (eg, haloperidol, risperidone) can bring relief to patients rapidly, more efficiently, and without any bothersome side effects. For instance, daily dosages of 5–10 mg of haloperidol may be adequate for many, if not most, patients with acute psychosis. Higher dosages should not be tried until at least 4 weeks of treatment have elapsed. In contrast, risperidone dosages of 1–4 mg/day avoids the unnecessary increase in EPS with higher dosages.

In chronically noncompliant patients who are unwilling to take oral medication, biweekly or monthly injections of fluphenazine decanoate or haloperidol decanoate (given at clinics or by visiting nurses) often decrease relapse rates significantly.

3. Atypical antipsychotics—

a. Clozapine is the only antipsychotic drug shown in controlled clinical trials to effectively reduce positive and negative symptoms in patients who fail to respond to typical neuroleptic drugs. It also produces almost no EPS, including akathisia. It has been used in several hundred thousand patients in Western countries for more than 20 years with no definite cases of tardive dyskinesia being reported. The onset of a significant response to clozapine may be delayed for up to 6 months. Primary negative symptoms tend to improve more slowly than do other types of symptoms. The response to clozapine is usually only partial, but for patients whose symptoms have been severely nonresponsive to all other therapies, the change may be dramatic.

The remarkable advantages of clozapine (described later in this section) must be considered in light of its ability to cause granulocytopenia, or agranulocytosis, in 1% of patients. As a result, clozapine has been approved in the United States only for patients with schizophrenia who have failed to respond adequately to typical neuroleptic drugs or who are intolerant of typical neuroleptic drugs because of EPS or tardive

dyskinesia. Just what is an adequate response to an antipsychotic agent should be left to the judgment of the patient, his or her family, and mental health workers. Poor work function and residual negative symptoms may be considered a poor response, even if only mild positive symptoms are present.

Agranulocytosis during clozapine treatment generally occurs within 4–18 weeks after initiation of treatment, but it can occur rarely at later times. In the United States, the patient's white blood cell count must be monitored every 2 weeks on an indefinite basis, even though the risk is very small after 12 months. When the white blood cell count falls below 3000 cells per mm^3, clozapine should be stopped and not restarted. If agranulocytosis has developed, granulocyte colony stimulating factor or some other growth factors can be used to hasten the recovery process. Recovery generally takes 7–14 days. Hospitalization to prevent or treat sepsis is essential. To date, the death rate from clozapine due to agranulocytosis has been about 1 per 10,000 patients. Clozapine can also cause leukocytosis and eosinophilia in the early stages. The development of these disorders does not predict later development of agranulocytosis. Other side effects of clozapine include sedation, weight gain, major motor seizures, obsessive-compulsive symptoms or treatment-emergent obsessive-compulsive disorder, hypersalivation, tachycardia, hypotension, hypertension, stuttering, neuroleptic malignant syndrome, urinary incontinence, constipation, and hyperglycemia. These side effects can generally be managed by reducing the dosage. Seizures often must be treated with an anticonvulsant such as valproic acid.

The dosage of clozapine ranges from 100 to 900 mg/day for most patients. It must be titrated slowly because of tachycardia and hypotensive side effects, with a starting dosage of 25 mg/day. The average dosage is 400–500 mg/day. It is usually given twice daily. Plasma levels of 350–400 ng/ml are more likely to be associated with clinical response than are lower levels.

Clozapine has been shown to reduce depression and suicidality. The latter effect leads to a major decrease in the overall mortality rate associated with treatment, despite the slight increase due to agranulocytosis. Four studies have reported that clozapine can improve some aspects of cognitive function, especially verbal fluency, attention, and recall memory. This effect appears to be unrelated to the drug's lack of effect on motor function. Several cost-effectiveness studies have indicated that the cost of clozapine ($3000–5000/year plus monitoring costs) is offset by the decreased need for hospitalization. Clozapine has also been shown to improve work function and quality of life, which may justify its premium price. Clozapine is effective in reducing water intoxication and violence in patients with schizophrenia. There are no data regarding the effectiveness of clozapine in treating schizotypal or schizoid personality disorders.

Clozapine has a very complex pharmacologic profile. It has a high affinity for serotonergic (5-$HT_{2A,2C,6,7}$), adrenergic ($\alpha_{1,2}$), muscarinic, and histaminergic receptors. Its strong affinity for 5-HT_{2A} and weak affinity for D_{2A} receptors likely contribute to its low EPS profile. Other atypical antipsychotic agents (described in the next sections) with the same relative affinities for 5-HT_{2A} and D_2 receptors have low EPS profiles at clinically effective dosages.

b. Risperidone has been found in multicenter trials with schizophrenic inpatients to be more effective than haloperidol in decreasing total psychopathology and positive and negative symptoms at dosages of 4–8 mg/day. There is no evidence yet that risperidone is effective in a significant proportion of patients who fail to respond adequately to typical neuroleptic drugs. Recent evidence indicates that risperidone can improve some types of cognitive function. The potential for risperidone to cause tardive dyskinesia has not been established, but a few cases have been reported. In this regard, chronic administration of low dosages of risperidone may have some advantage over typical neuroleptic drugs.

The recommended dosage of risperidone is 4–8 mg/day, but some patients will respond to 2 mg/day and some will require up to 10–16 mg/day. At dosages of 2–4 mg/day, EPS are generally mild, one of the major advantages of risperidone in clinical practice. Risperidone in vivo produces higher occupancy of D_2 receptors than does clozapine. This observation contributes to risperidone's higher propensity to cause EPS. Risperidone is usually given twice daily because of its shorter half-life.

Some cost-effectiveness data indicate that in clinical practice risperidone has the advantages previously reported in clinical trials and that these advantages lead to an overall reduction in health care costs. This is important because a year's supply of risperidone in the United States may cost $2000–4000, depending on the dosage. The higher cost in comparison to a generic neuroleptic is offset by decreased hospitalization; however, cost minimization should not be the only basis for evaluation of a therapy. Cost-utility (ie, the analysis of costs in relation to benefits) is the optimal basis for evaluation of all antipsychotic drugs. There is no evidence to indicate that the lower EPS potential of risperidone will lead to greater compliance, but this seems like a realistic possibility, and it, too, will reduce costs. Risperidone is a reasonable choice for patients who respond to typical neuroleptics with a reduction in positive symptoms but who experience troublesome EPS and secondary negative symptoms. There is also some evidence that risperidone is effective in suppressing the symptoms of established tardive dyskinesia. Side effects of risperidone other than EPS include akathisia, weight gain, sexual dysfunction, decreased libido, and galactorrhea. Unlike clozapine, risperidone increases serum prolactin levels. There is no evidence

that risperidone has any increased risk of causing agranulocytosis.

c. Olanzapine is one of the newest atypical antipsychotic agents to be marketed worldwide and to receive FDA approval in the United States. This novel agent exhibits nanomolar affinity at dopaminergic (D_{1-4}), serotonergic (5-$HT_{2,3,6}$), muscarinic (M_{1-5}), adrenergic (α_1), and histaminergic (H_1) receptor sites. Olanzapine may enhance glutamatergic activity indirectly as indicated by its ability to reverse PCP- or MK-801-induced behaviors.

Behavioral pharmacologic experiments demonstrated that olanzapine has several characteristics of an atypical antipsychotic, such as low propensity for EPS, structural similarity to clozapine, effectiveness in the treatment of negative symptoms, minimal effect on prolactin levels, and broad efficacy. Double-blind clinical studies indicated that olanzapine is more effective than placebo in improving positive and negative symptoms and is as effective as haloperidol in reducing positive symptoms. It is more effective than haloperidol in improving negative symptoms. The recommended starting dosage is 10 mg/day, once daily. Many patients will require 10–25 mg/day, but the dosage should be raised slowly. As with clozapine, response may be delayed for several months.

Olanzapine produces fewer EPS than does haloperidol. It may reduce the risk of tardive dyskinesia. The major side effects for olanzapine are weight gain and sedation. Other side effects include dizziness and transient asymptomatic liver transaminase elevations. Olanzapine produces only transient increases in serum prolactin levels.

d. Quetiapine, sertindole, & ziprasidone—three novel antipsychotic drugs (the latter two under evaluation by the FDA)—are able to produce fewer EPS at clinically effective dosages, in comparison to typical neuroleptics. Like clozapine, risperidone, and olanzapine, these three agents are more potent as 5-HT_{2A}-receptor antagonists than as D_2 antagonists. However, they differ in other pharmacologic features. For example, ziprasidone is a potent 5-HT_{1A} agonist and 5-HT_{1D} antagonist. It also inhibits 5-HT and NE reuptake. These effects may contribute to the drug's low EPS profile and to its antidepressant action. One large-scale dose-response study found sertindole to have greater efficacy than haloperidol in reducing negative symptoms. This has not yet been demonstrated with ziprasidone or quetiapine. Because these drugs require titration, they will be somewhat less convenient for patients to use than olanzapine. Nevertheless, only head-to-head clinical trials can determine which, if any, are more effective and better tolerated in the clinic. This determination will likely require trials of one or more of these agents to determine which agent produces optimal response for a given patient.

Quetiapine is a dibenzothiazepine with high affinity for serotonergic (5-HT_{2A}), adrenergic (α_1), and histaminergic (H_1) receptors. It also has moderate affinity for D_2 and low affinity for muscarinic (M_1) receptors. Quetiapine was recently shown to be superior to placebo and equal to chlorpromazine in hospitalized patients. At 150–180 mg/day, the drug improves negative and positive symptoms. The most common side effects of quetiapine include drowsiness, dry mouth, weight gain, agitation, constipation, mild elevations of alanine aminotransferase and aspartate aminotransferase levels, and orthostatic hypotension. Because of its short half-life (6–9 hours), quetiapine should be administered 2–3 times daily.

Sertindole is an imidazolidonone compound that shows high affinity for serotonergic (5-HT_{2A}), dopaminergic (D_2), and adrenergic (α_1) receptors. Additionally, it exhibits lower affinity for adrenergic (α_2) receptors and minimal affinity for histaminergic (H_1) receptors. For decreasing positive symptoms, sertindole in daily dosages of 12–24 mg/day is superior to placebo and similar to 4–16 mg/day of haloperidol. Sertindole, at dosages of 20–24 mg/day, has a greater effect on negative symptoms than does haloperidol. This action may be due in part to the low EPS profile of sertindole. Side effects of sertindole include headaches, tachycardia, mild prolongation of Q-T interval (15–25 msec), decreased ejaculatory volume, weight gain, nasal congestion, nausea, and insomnia. Sertindole has a half-life of 1–4 days, which makes this agent suitable for once-daily dosing.

Ziprasidone has a 10-fold higher affinity for the 5-HT_{2A} receptor compared to its D_2 receptor. Ziprasidone also has a relatively high affinity for the 5-HT_{2C}, 5-HT_{1D}, 5-HT_{1A}, and D_3 receptors. It has a weak affinity for the muscarinic and histaminergic (H_1) receptors. This pharmacologic profile leads to a low EPS profile at clinically effective dosages. Because of a relatively short half-life (approximately 6 hours), the drug should be given twice daily. In double-blind trials, it appears to be as effective as haloperidol and produces fewer EPS. Early trials show that ziprasidone is effective in treating positive and negative symptoms in patients experiencing acute exacerbations of schizophrenic symptoms. The major side effect is sedation. Its relatively high affinity for the 5-HT_{1A} and D_3 receptors could make it more effective than other 5-HT_{2A}- and D_2-receptor antagonists in specific patients. There are no data as to its ability to suppress tardive dyskinesia or to have a lesser tendency to cause tardive dyskinesia than typical neuroleptics.

B. Electroconvulsive Treatment: Electroconvulsive treatment (ECT) is used infrequently today because of the ease of administration of antipsychotics and the need for maintenance treatment, which is difficult to provide on an outpatient basis. A short course of ECT (eg, 6–12 treatments) may be useful as an adjunctive treatment to antipsychotic drugs of all classes, including clozapine, for patients with limited response to treatment and particularly when very rapid control of agitated behavior is necessary. Excited catatonia and severe agitation will often respond to antipsychotics, benzodiazepines, reduced environmental stimulation, seclusion, and physical restraint. If these methods fail, ECT should be administered. There is inadequate data to recommend maintenance ECT for schizophrenia.

C. Psychosocial Treatments: Although antipsychotic drugs are the mainstay of treatment of schizophrenia, important nonpharmacologic treatments are also available. These treatments are aimed at improving compliance with drug therapy, supporting the patients, fostering independent living skills, improving psychosocial and work functioning, and reducing caretaker burden. Providing education and support to family members is a crucial component of a comprehensive treatment approach.

In most mental health systems, a program of case management has been developed to provide low-cost support to patients living in the community, many of whom were formerly chronically institutionalized. Case managers may help patients find housing; manage financial resources; get access to psychiatric clinics, rehabilitation services, and crisis intervention; and comply with medication regimens. Such assistance may enable patients to live in settings with no or minimal mental health worker–provided supervision. As mentioned earlier in this chapter, expressed emotion predicts relapse of schizophrenia. Relapse rates may be twice as high among families in which expressed emotion is high, in comparison to families in which expressed emotion is low. Family treatment that reduces expressed emotion reduces the likelihood of relapse, especially if the patient's response to antipsychotic medication is less than optimal.

Fatemi SH, Roth BL, Meltzer HY: Atypical antipsychotic drugs: clinical and preclinical studies. Pages 77–115 in Csernansky JG (editor): *Handbook of Experimental Pharmacology.* Vol 120. Springer-Verlag, 1996.

Krueger RB, Sackeim HA: Electroconvulsive therapy and schizophrenia. Pages 503–545 in Hirsch SR, Weinberger DR (editors): *Schizophrenia.* Blackwell Scientific, 1995.

Liberman RP, Spaulding WD, Corrigan PW: Cognitive-behavioral therapies in psychiatric rehabilitation. Pages 605–625 in Hirsch SR, Weinberger DR (editors): *Schizophrenia.* Blackwell Scientific, 1995.

Meltzer HY, Fatemi SH: Suicide in schizophrenia: the effect of clozapine. Clin Neuropharmacol 1996;18(Suppl 3):S18.

Meltzer HY, Fatemi SH: Treatment of schizophrenia. Pages 747–787 in Schatzberg AF, Nemeroff CB (editors): *The American Psychiatric Press Textbook of Psychopharmacology.* American Psychiatric Press, 1998.

Muerer KT, Bellack AS: Psychotherapy for schizophrenia. Pages 626–648 in Hirsch SR, Weinberger DR (editors): *Schizophrenia.* Blackwell Scientific, 1995.

Complications, Comorbidity, & Adverse Outcomes of Treatment

The generally poor outcome of schizophrenia from the perspective of social and work function and persistence of major types of psychopathology has been well documented. Although psychosis remits in some patients in their 60s or 70s, the more common outcome is a persistence of psychosis and negative symptoms and a marginal existence, due in no small measure to persistent cognitive deficits. A small proportion of patients progress to a dementia that may be as severe as that in senile dementia, Alzheimer's type, but that is not associated with the neuropathologic changes of that disorder or any other gross or microscopic findings.

Patients with schizophrenia often experience comorbid substance abuse and addiction to tobacco. Alcohol, marijuana, and cocaine are the most frequently abused agents, but schizophrenic patients may also abuse amphetamines and PCP if they have access to them. Psychostimulants such as cocaine and amphetamines and dissociative agents such as PCP usually exacerbate positive and disorganization symptoms. Cocaine and amphetamines can induce euphoria and alleviate depression transiently in patients with schizophrenia, as they can in the general population. Alcohol abuse does not specifically induce an exacerbation of psychosis, but it leads to depression, nutritional disturbances, failure to take antipsychotic medication, and in severe cases, liver damage, which may interfere with the metabolism of antipsychotic drugs. The outcome in schizophrenic patients who have comorbid substance abuse is generally poorer than for schizophrenic patients who do not abuse alcohol or drugs. This poor outcome results largely from noncompliance with antipsychotic medication and poor nutrition, as in the case of those who abuse alcohol. Treatment should include substance abuse counseling and the use of adjunctive measures such as Alcoholics Anonymous.

Schizophrenic patients smoke more heavily than does the general population. There may be a physiologic reason for this observation: Nicotine increases the release of dopamine in the nucleus accumbens and other limbic areas. Antipsychotic drugs are for the most part ineffective in diminishing the craving for tobacco; however, some preliminary studies have reported that clozapine may do so.

Significant morbidity and mortality is associated with schizophrenia. Patients with schizophrenia are at increased risk for cardiovascular events such as arrhythmias and myocardial infarction. The latter may be the result of poor nutrition and lack of exercise as well as increased stress. Institutionalized patients are at increased risk for infectious diseases. Typical neuroleptics and clozapine increase the risk of major motor seizures and weight gain.

Suicide is the major factor limiting the life of patients with schizophrenia. Suicide occurs in 9–13% of patients with this illness, which is only slightly less than the suicide rate associated with major depression. There were nearly 8000 reported deaths due to suicide in schizophrenic patients in the United States in 1994, which represents an estimated rate of about 0.33% per year. This rate is less than other reported annual rates, which range from 0.4% to 1.1%. On a lifetime basis, the suicide attempt rate is 25–50%.

Several risk factors have been identified for suicide. The foremost risk factor is a previous suicide attempt. Most patients who complete suicide have generally failed on previous attempts. Suicide is more common in male patients than in female patients and occurs more commonly during the first decade of the illness but can occur at any time during the patient's life span. Patients often exhibit depression and hopelessness prior to a suicide attempt. Schizophrenic patients who abuse substances are at increased risk. Patients who have made suicide attempts should receive more intensive treatment. The addition of an antidepressant medication may be indicated. Evidence indicates that clozapine may reduce the rate of attempted and completed suicide, but further study is indicated.

Meltzer HY, Okayli G: The reduction of suicidality during clozapine treatment in neuroleptic-resistant schizophrenia: impact on risk-benefit assessment. Am J Psychiatry 1995;152:183.

Prognosis & Course of Illness

The modern concept of the prognosis of schizophrenia is based on multiple outcome measures. Four types of outcome measures have been identified: psychopathology, work function, social function, and rehospitalization. These measures could vary independently in schizophrenia, and although they are central to evaluating outcome in schizophrenia, other measures such as cognitive function, general health, and suicide are also important.

Outcome in schizophrenia can be predicted partially by age at onset and by the nature of the prodrome and first episode (Table 19–4). Early age at onset (eg, 14–18 years) is often associated with a worse outcome than is later age at onset. An insidious rather than an abrupt onset is also associated with a poor outcome. If the initial clinical presentation is characterized mainly by negative symptoms, outcome is likely to be poor, both in the short and long term. Conversely, florid psychosis and an abrupt onset are both likely to be associated with a good prognosis because antipsychotic drugs are much more effective against positive symptoms and disorganization than they are against negative symptoms and cognitive disturbance.

Despite some variability in methods of diagnosing schizophrenia and outcome criteria, the course of schizophrenia over 10 and 30 years is as follows: (1) Over a 10-year period, 25% of patients recover completely, 25% improve greatly and become relatively independent, 25% improve but require extensive help, 15% remain hospitalized and do not improve, and finally, 10% die mostly by suicide. (2) Over a 30-year period, 25% of patients recover fully, 35% improve significantly and reach relative independence,

Table 19–4. Predictors of course and outcome in schizophrenia.

Factor	Good Outcome	Poor Outcome
Age at onset	About 20–25	Below 20
Sex	Possibly females	Possibly males
Socioeconomic status	Middle, high	Low
Occupational record	Stable	Irregular
Other adverse social factors	Absent	Present
Family history of mental illness	Affective	Schizophrenia
Precipitating factors	Present	Absent
Onset	Acute, late	Insidious
Rate of progression	Rapid	Slow
Length of episode prior to assessment	Months or less	Years
Initial clinical symptoms	Catatonia, paranoia, depression, schizoaffective diagnosis, atypical symptoms, confusion	Negative symptoms (eg, flat affect, poverty of thought, apathy, asociality); obsessive-compulsive symptoms
CT/MRI studies	Normal morphology	Dilated ventricles, brain atrophy
Early treatment with medications	Present	Absent
Response to medications initially	Present	Absent

15% improve but require extensive support, 10% remain hospitalized and unimproved, and finally, 15% die mostly as a result of suicide.

Generally, the overall prognosis of schizophrenia is more favorable now than before neuroleptics were introduced, mostly because of improvements in pharmacologic therapies and, to some degree, changes in psychosocial treatment strategies. The increased mortality in patients with schizophrenia is the result of suicide, accidents, and diseases (eg, infections, type II diabetes, heart disease, and in females, breast cancer).

Carpenter WT et al: The prediction of outcome in schizophrenia, IV: eleven-year follow-up of the Washington IPSS cohort. J Nerv Ment Dis 1991;179:517.

Torrey EF: Pages 125–139 in *Surviving Schizophrenia: A Manual for Families, Consumers, and Providers,* 3rd ed. Harper Collins, 1995.

Torrey EF et al: *Schizophrenia and Manic Depression Disorders: The Biological Roots of Mental Illness As Revealed By a Landmark Study of Identical Twins.* Basic Books, 1994.

Other Psychotic Disorders

Richard C. Shelton, MD

SCHIZOPHRENIFORM DISORDER

DSM-IV Diagnostic Criteria

A. Criteria A, D, and E of schizophrenia must be met.

B. An episode of the disorder (including prodromal, active, and residual phases) lasts at least 1 month but less than 6 months. When the diagnosis must be made without waiting for recovery, it should be qualified as "provisional."

Specify if:

> *Without good prognostic features*
> *With good prognostic features:* as evidenced by two (or more) of the following:

> (1) onset of prominent psychotic symptoms within 4 weeks of the first noticeable change in usual behavior or functioning
> (2) confusion or perplexity at the height of the psychotic episode
> (3) good premorbid social and occupational functioning
> (4) absence of blunted or flat affect

Reprinted, with permission, from *Diagnostic and Statistical Manual of Mental Disorders,* 4th ed. Copyright 1994 American Psychiatric Association.

General Considerations

A. Major Etiologic Theories: Schizophreniform disorder is a heterogeneous category; therefore, in all likelihood it has several distinct etiologies. Because most patients with this disorder will proceed on to meet diagnostic criteria for schizophrenia, the etiologies will be the same as for that condition, discussed in detail in Chapter 19. Some patients with this disorder appear to recover significantly and thus represent a manifestation that is distinct from typical schizophrenia.

B. Epidemiology: Diagnostically, schizophreniform disorder is "sandwiched" in time between brief psychotic disorder (discussed later in this chapter), which lasts 1 month or less, and schizophrenia (see Chapter 19), which by definition continues beyond 6 months. Although many patients eventually will be shown to have schizophrenia, a small but significant proportion of patients with persisting psychotic disorders will show complete recovery of their illness. The extent of recovery is likely to be small, although the exact proportion is unknown. Those who do show recovery typically exhibit characteristics known to predict better outcome in other diagnostic categories (eg, acute onset, brief prodrome, lack of psychosocial deterioration, and prominent mood symptoms).

C. Genetics: Because schizophreniform disorder is likely to be an etiologically heterogeneous disorder, genetic relationships are unclear. Those persons who proceed on to manifest typical schizophrenia show genetic predispositions that are similar to this condition. Those who recover completely may have increased family histories of both psychotic and affective disorders, especially bipolar disorder.

Clinical Findings

A. Signs & Symptoms: Patients with schizophreniform disorder exhibit symptoms consistent with Criterion A of schizophrenia (ie, typically hallucinations; delusions; negative symptoms; disorganization of thought, speech, and behavior) that last between 1 and 6 months. Patients with these symptoms may proceed on to a typical pattern of schizophrenia and should be diagnosed as such if the symptoms are present for more than 6 months. However, others may proceed to complete or near-complete resolution of their symptoms. These patients generally have good premorbid function, acute onset (often after a stressor), and complete resolution without residual deficits in psychosocial function. In addition, mood symptoms tend to be more prominent and a family history of mood disorder is common in these patients.

B. Psychological Testing: Psychological testing will reveal a pattern of symptoms more typical of schizophrenia (see Chapter 19). These findings will include the common symptoms of thought disorganization, hallucinations, and delusions. However, overt cognitive impairment (including memory problems) is uncommon, and prominent mood symptoms may occur. Persons with schizophreniform disorder may demonstrate frontal cortical regional deficits such as impaired performance on the Wisconsin Card Sorting Test.

C. Laboratory Findings & Imaging: Deficits in frontal cortical, especially left frontal, activation have been reported in schizophreniform disorder, much like that shown in schizophrenia. These results should not be surprising because many patients eventually will develop schizophrenia. As also occurs in schizophrenia, brain imaging studies may show enlargement of the cerebral ventricular system.

Treatment

The treatment of schizophreniform disorder is similar to that of schizophrenia (see Chapter 19). Hospitalization is usually required in the acute stages of overt psychotic symptoms. Antipsychotic drugs represent the mainstay of symptomatic management, and resolution of psychosis often is fairly rapid. Sedative agents, especially benzodiazepines, may be needed to manage acute agitation. Psychosocial support and rehabilitation is critical with these patients to help reduce the deterioration in function more typical of schizophrenia. Therefore, rapid treatment of symptoms and social reintegration of the patient is important.

After the resolution of the acute symptoms, psychological, social, and occupational or educational treatment becomes the main focus of treatment. An acute schizophreniform psychotic episode represents a catastrophic event in the life of the patient, and psychotherapy is needed to help the patient understand the event and gain a sense of control over future episodes. A variety of issues should be discussed with the patient and his or her family or significant other: (1) the fundamental biological nature of the disorder; (2) the role of medication in controlling current and future symptoms, particularly the possible effect of symptom management on the evolution of the disorder; (3) the early-warning signs that indicate a return of psychosis; (4) the impact of the disturbance on the person's life and that of the family; (5) the need for gradual reintegration into work or school; and (6) the importance of future psychosocial management, including intensive case management or occupational or educational rehabilitation.

Prognosis & Course of Illness

As noted earlier in this chapter, schizophreniform disorder often follows a course typical of schizophrenia. If symptoms are present for more than 6 months, psychological and social deterioration typically associated with schizophrenia may occur. Antipsychotics such as haloperidol reduce the symptoms of the illness but will not prevent deterioration if the symptoms are present for more than 6 months. The potential beneficial effects of newer, atypical antipsychotics (eg, clozapine, risperidone, olanzapine, quetiapine) in preventing psychosocial deterioration or cognitive impairment is unknown.

Most individuals with schizophreniform disorder are simply in the early stages of the development of more typical schizophrenia. The 6-month cutoff for the diagnosis of schizophreniform disorder acknowledges that although patients with typical schizophrenic symptoms sometimes show complete resolution, this seldom occurs when the symptoms have been present for 6 months or more. Almost all patients will then proceed to a course more consistent with schizophrenia, with persistent deterioration and impairment in psychosocial functioning. Exceptions to this rule are very rare.

Strakowski SM: Diagnostic validity of schizophreniform disorder. Am J Psychiatry 1994;151:815.

SCHIZOAFFECTIVE DISORDER

DSM-IV Diagnostic Criteria

A. An uninterrupted period of illness during which, at some time, there is either a major depressive disorder, a manic episode, or a mixed episode concurrent with symptoms that meet Criterion A for schizophrenia.

Note: The major depressive episode must include Criterion A1: depressed mood.

B. During the same period of illness, there have been delusions or hallucinations for at least 2 weeks in the absence of prominent mood symptoms.
C. Symptoms that meet criteria for a mood episode are present for a substantial portion of the total duration of the active and residual periods of the illness.
D. The disturbance is not due to the direct physiological effects of a substance (eg, a drug of abuse, a medication) or a general medical condition.

Specify type:

Bipolar type: if the disturbance includes a manic or a mixed episode (or a manic or a mixed episode and major depressive episodes)
Depressive type: if the disturbance only includes major depressive episodes

Reprinted, with permission, from *Diagnostic and Statistical Manual of Mental Disorders,* 4th ed. Copyright 1994 American Psychiatric Association.

General Considerations

Schizoaffective disorder is characterized by prominent mood symptoms (mania or depression) occurring during the course of a chronic psychotic disorder. The phenomenology of schizoaffective disorder can be thought of as standing in the middle ground between mood disorder, especially psychotic mood disorder, and the chronic psychotic disorders such as schizophrenia. The debate continues over whether schizoaffective disorder "belongs" to the spectrum of either schizophrenic or affective disorders or represents a distinct category. Schizoaffective disorder likely represents a heterogeneous disorder with multiple distinct etiologies.

Recent research indicates that there appear to be distinct etiologies and outcomes depending on whether the course of schizoaffective disorder is typified by episodes of bipolar-type cycling or simple depressive episodes in the absence of mania. In the bipolar variant, there is an increased proportion of family history of bipolar disorder (but not schizophrenia) and a better overall outcome. Although a family history of affective disorder is observed in the depressive variant, a history of psychotic disorder seems to be more common and outcome is poorer than in the bipolar form. Both variants usually have a better prognosis than does schizophrenia without prominent mood symptoms.

Clinical Findings

A. Signs & Symptoms: Patients with schizoaffective disorder exhibit symptoms consistent with DSM-IV diagnostic Criterion A for schizophrenia. However, during the course of illness, there are superimposed episodes of full depressive or manic symptoms. These patients would be diagnosed as having schizoaffective disorder, depressed or manic types, respectively. However, psychotic symptoms consistent with schizophrenia must be present for at least 2 weeks independently of the mania or depression syndromes.

Schizoaffective disorder, bipolar type, usually involves cycling of mania, depression, or mixed states in a way that is consistent with bipolar disorder. Similarly, patients with schizoaffective disorder, depressive type, may have repeated episodes of major depression, as in major depressive disorder. However, unlike depressive or bipolar disorders, there are consistent symptoms of schizophrenia in the absence of overt mood disorder. In schizoaffective disorder, depressive type, depressive episodes in which the patient meets full diagnostic criteria for major depression must be distinguished from the mood and negative symptoms associated with schizophrenia. For example, DSM-IV criteria require the presence of persisting depressed mood for this diagnosis. Similarly, care should be taken to avoid misdiagnosing as mania agitation, hostility, insomnia, and other symptoms of an acute exacerbation of schizophrenia.

B. Psychological Testing: The results of psychological tests depend on the state of illness of a given patient. That is, although the typical results of schizophrenia usually are present (see Chapter 19), characteristics of mood disorders also may be present. For example, psychological testing results will be consistent with depression or mania during corresponding episodes of illness. However, schizoaffective disorder, bipolar type, may be associated with less psychosocial and cognitive impairments than are schizophrenia or schizoaffective disorder, depressive type.

Differential Diagnosis

Persons with schizophrenia are not immune to the occurrence of mood symptoms. When these features meet the diagnostic criteria for a mood disorder concurrently with features of schizophrenia, the diagnosis of schizoaffective disorder may be made. However, great care must be exercised in the evaluation in order to provide appropriate management of the disorder. For example, depressive symptoms not meeting full diagnostic criteria for a major depressive episode are common in schizophrenia and do not warrant a diagnosis of schizoaffective disorder per se. In fact, treatment of schizophrenia, especially management with atypical antipsychotics, may reduce these symptoms in many patients without reliance on antidepressants. Alternatively, the negative symptoms of schizophrenia (eg, apathy, withdrawal, avolition, blunted affect) may be confused with the symptoms of depression. Again, these symptoms generally are treated more effectively with atypical antipsychotics. Finally, the agitation, insomnia, and grandiose delusions of an acutely psychotic patient with schizophrenia sometimes can be confused with mania. However, a careful examination of the course of illness, prodromal symptoms, and acute presentation can be helpful in making the diagnosis. For example, the acutely agitated patient who presents for treatment after a period of progressive withdrawal, isolation, and bizarre behavior is unlikely to have mania. A good diagnostic rule of thumb is to evaluate the patient for the presence of current or past mood disorder by excluding the symptoms of schizophrenia, prior to confirming the diagnosis of schizoaffective disorder.

Psychotic mood disorders also may present with a confusing picture. DSM-IV diagnostic criteria are written to aid the clinician in making this distinction. The presence of mood symptoms concurrent with psychosis, even symptoms that otherwise appear to be more typically schizophrenic (ie, bizarre behavior or disorganized speech) are not adequate to make the diagnosis of schizoaffective disorder. This condition is understood as representing a mood disorder superimposed on a course of schizophrenia. Therefore, the criteria require the symptoms of schizophrenia to be present for at least 2 weeks in the absence of prominent mood symptoms meeting diagnostic criteria for major depression, mania, or mixed state. A course consistent with dysthymia concurrent with schizophrenia does not constitute a diagnosis of schizophrenia.

Treatment

Once a definite diagnosis of schizoaffective disorder is made, treatment must take into consideration the necessity of managing both mood symptoms and psychotic symptoms (Table 20–1). Antipsychotics are required for the management of the psychotic features (see Chapter 19). However, the focus of care is generally on the treatment of depression or mania. Antidepressant drugs should be used as required in a manner similar to that discussed in Chapter 21 for the treatment of major depression. Alternatively, mood-stabilizing agents such as lithium, carbamazepine, valproate, or divalproex usually are required for the treatment of mood cycling. Finally, psychosocial management often is needed in much the same fashion as with schizophrenia or schizophreniform disorder to aid in social reintegration.

Prognosis & Course of Illness

Generally, persons with schizoaffective disorder have a course of illness that is intermediate between the mood disorders (with a relatively better prognosis) and schizophrenia (with marked residual psychosocial deterioration). However, distinctions also can be made for patients within the schizoaffective spectrum. Patients with schizoaffective disorder, bipolar type (ie, those with a history of manic or mixed bipolar episode), have a course of illness that is more similar to bipolar disorder. These patients often have better functioning between acute episodes of illness than either persons with schizophrenia or schizoaffective disorder, depressive type. Patients with schizoaffective disorder, depressive type, tend to exhibit more typical schizophrenic symptoms and course, although when the disorder is managed properly, the prognosis may be better than typical schizophrenia without comorbid depression. Regardless of the category, certain factors are associated with a worse outcome. These features include insidious onset prior to the first psychotic episode; earlier onset of illness; poor or deteriorating premorbid functioning; the absence of a clear precipitating stressor; prominent negative symptoms in the prodromal, acute, or residual phases of illness; and a family history of schizophrenia. These characteristics often are associated with a poorer outcome in persons with schizophrenia without prominent mood symptoms.

Keck PE Jr., McElroy SL, Strakowski SM: New developments in the pharmacologic treatment of schizoaffective disorder. J Clin Psychiatry 1996;57(Suppl 9):41.

Lapensee MA: A review of schizoaffective disorder: I. Current concepts. Can J Psychiatry 1992;37:335.

DELUSIONAL DISORDER

DSM-IV Diagnostic Criteria

A. Nonbizarre delusions (ie, involving situations that occur in real life, such as being followed, poisoned, infected, loved at a distance, or deceived by spouse or lover, or having a disease) of at least 1 month's duration.

B. Criterion A for schizophrenia has never been met.

Note: Tactile and olfactory hallucinations may be present in delusional disorder if they are related to the delusional theme.

C. Apart from the impact of the delusion(s) or its ramifications, functioning is not markedly impaired and behavior is not obviously odd or bizarre.

D. If mood episodes have occurred concurrently with delusions, their total duration has been brief relative to the duration of the delusional periods.

E. The disturbance is not due to the direct physiological effects of a substance (eg, a drug of abuse, a medication) or a general medical condition.

Specify type (the following types are assigned based on the predominant delusional theme):

Erotomanic type: delusions that another person, usually of higher status, is in love with the individual

Grandiose type: delusions of inflated worth, power, knowledge, identity, or special relationship to a deity or famous person

Jealous type: delusions that the individual's sexual partner is unfaithful

Persecutory type: delusions that the person (or someone to whom the person is close) is being malevolently treated in some way

Somatic type: delusions that the person has some physical defect or general medical condition

Mixed type: delusions characteristic of more than one of the above types but no one theme predominates

Table 20–1. Principles of management of schizoaffective disorder.

Acute and chronic antipsychotic drug therapies usually are required for psychotic symptoms.

Atypical antipsychotics may be more effective in managing psychotic and mood symptoms.

Mood stabilizers often are helpful for patients with a history of mania.

Antidepressants will sometimes be required for both depressive and bipolar types; however, exposure to antidepressant medications should be minimized for patients with a history of mania.

Psychological, social, educational, and occupational support and rehabilitation usually are needed as with schizophrenia.

General Considerations

A. Major Etiologic Theories: Etiologic theories about the development of delusional disorder abound, but systematic study is sparse. Early concepts of etiology focused on the denial and projection of unacceptable impulses. Hence, as examples, homosexual attraction would be reformulated unconsciously to homosexual delusions or a belief in a love relationship with a famous person. Other theories focus on projection of unacceptable sexual and aggressive drives, leading to paranoid fears of others. These and other psychodynamic theories have certain heuristic appeal, but little systematic study has been done to support these conjectures.

B. Epidemiology: A very small proportion of the population (roughly 0.03%) experience persistent, relatively fixed delusions in the absence of the characteristic features of other psychotic disorders.

C. Genetics: Little is known about the genetics of delusional disorder. Family studies have suggested a decided lack of increased family history of psychotic or mood disorder.

Clinical Findings

A. Signs & Symptoms: Delusional disorder is characterized by nonbizarre delusions. Most often the delusional content is plausible. For example, people with this condition may have fixed delusions that they are in an unrequited love relationship with a famous person or that they are being watched by the CIA, but not that their movements are being controlled by beings from another planet. Persons with this condition may appear otherwise quite normal. They often hold jobs and may be married. The oddness and eccentricity of their beliefs and behavior may manifest itself only around the topic of the delusion.

The diagnosis of delusional disorder depends on the presence of nonbizarre delusions in the absence of meeting Criterion A for schizophrenia (see Chapter 19). Specifically, there should not be significant hallucinatory experiences, marked thought disorder, prominent negative symptoms, or psychosocial deterioration. Except for the behaviors associated with the delusions (eg, delusional accusations of unfaithfulness in the spouse), the actions of the individual are not otherwise impaired. Although people with delusional disorder may have comorbid major depression or bipolar disorder, the delusions should be present at times when a mood disorder is not present and not just concurrently with an episode of depression or mania.

Specific types of delusional disorder have distinguishing features. The most familiar is the so-called persecutory type, in which patients experience fixed paranoid delusions that other persons are intending harm in some way. These patients may believe that they are being watched or followed, or that malevolent parties are engaging in other persecutory or threatening behavior. The affected person will act in a way that is consistent with the content of the persecutory delusion but will otherwise be normal.

Another common variant is the jealous type. These patients exhibit delusional beliefs that their significant other is being unfaithful. As with the persecutory type, the plausible nature of the belief system makes it difficult at times to distinguish delusional beliefs from normal fears or real experiences. Patients with delusional disorder, jealous type, either have beliefs that cross the threshold of credibility or refuse to accept reasonable reassurances. For example, a 90-year-old man who believes that his 88-year-old wife is having sex regularly with teenage or young adult men may be suffering from delusional disorder.

In delusional disorder, erotomanic type (sometimes referred to as de Clerambault syndrome), the delusion is that another person, usually someone who is famous or of higher social status, is in love with the affected individual. These beliefs may be highly elaborate, although plausibility is maintained. For example, a young woman with delusional disorder, erotomanic type, may travel around the country to attend the concerts of a famous performer. She may believe that the performer gives her secret signals during his concert that indicate his love. However, she also may believe that there is some external reason that he cannot express his love more directly, for example, because he is married, or has an ill mother, or some other reason. Persons with this condition seldom make direct contact with their paramour, although they may, occasionally, engage in more aggressive stalking behavior. Whenever the disorder occurs, it typically becomes the central focus of the person's life.

In the grandiose type of the disorder, the person experiences fixed, false beliefs of power (eg, being the owner of a major corporation), money, identity (eg, being the Prince of England), a special relationship with God (eg, being Jesus Christ) or famous people, or some other distinguishing characteristic. These patients may be quietly psychotic but may come to treatment as a result of a contact with a government agency or other organization. For example, a person who believes that he is the President of the United States may be picked up wandering the grounds of the White House.

The somatic type of delusional disorder involves a fixed belief of some physical abnormality or characteristic. Distinguishing this disorder from simple hypochondriasis may be difficult and generally depends of the content of the belief and the degree to which the belief is held in spite of evidence to the contrary. People with somatoform disorders such as hypochondriasis or body dysmorphic disorder may have a fixed belief regarding a specific, serious, but plausible physical illness, such as cancer or AIDS. In hypochondriasis, these beliefs often relate to specific symptoms, such as pain, stiffness, or swelling. Patients with delusional disorder, somatic type, may have beliefs about other, more unusual conditions. These delusions may involve beliefs about contamination with toxic substances, infestations of insects or other vermin, foul body odors, malfunctions of specific body parts such as the liver or intestines, or other unusual content.

Finally, the mixed type of delusional disorder involves more than one of the types described above, without one taking prominence, and the unspecified type involves delusions that do not fall into one of the other categories.

B. Psychological Testing: Psychological testing will reveal the presence of the delusional psychotic material in these patients but, most often, little else. The cognitive impairments or social deterioration seen in schizophrenia are absent; if such impairments are present, the diagnosis of schizophrenia should be considered. Similarly, prominent mood symptoms might suggest a diagnosis of a psychotic mood disorder.

C. Laboratory Findings & Imaging: There is very little brain imaging data on delusional disorder. Limited data indicate that persons with delusional disorder show reduced cortical gray matter and increased ventricular and sulcal size similar to that seen in schizophrenia. However, there has been little systemic study of this condition.

Differential Diagnosis

The differential diagnosis of delusional disorder encompasses broad categories of disorders. For example, delusional thinking may occur in patients with other psychotic disorders such as schizophrenia, schizoaffective disorder, mood disorders (bipolar disorder, manic or depressed type or major depression) with psychotic features, psychotic disorders due to a general medical condition, or substance-induced psychotic disorder. In delusional disorder, however, important features of those conditions will be absent. For example, the prominent hallucinations, negative symptoms, thought disorder, or social deterioration consistent with schizophrenia will be absent. Similarly, mood symptoms, if present, are not prominent. The delusional thinking should not be accounted for by the presence of a medical condition or substance, including substances of abuse. For example, a young patient with a history of stimulant abuse who exhibits paranoid ideation after a recent cocaine binge would not necessarily have delusional disorder.

A delusional diagnosis also may be easily confused with the obsessions of obsessive-compulsive disorder (OCD; see Chapter 24); however, in OCD the patient almost always has at least some insight into the exaggerated nature of the thoughts. Further, obsessions associated with OCD most often involve an inappropriate or exaggerated appraisal of a real threat. This could include a fear of contamination, loss of control

of impulses, loss of important documents, and similar threats. When delusional disorder involves a fear of a specific threat, the fears are more typically paranoid or persecutory in nature.

Somatization disorders are easily confused with delusional disorder, somatic type (see Chapter 25). As noted earlier, delusional disorder, somatic type, generally differs in both degree and type of belief. That is, in delusional disorder the beliefs are held tenaciously, and often will involve implausible content.

Paranoid personality disorder also may be confused with delusional disorder (see Chapter 33). Two significant characteristics distinguish these disorders. In paranoid personality disorder, the hostility and paranoid thinking most often are generalized and affect multiple areas of the person's life. For example, the patient may be jealous of the spouse but also will exhibit hypersensitive thinking at work and in other areas. By contrast, the psychotic thoughts of delusional disorder usually are focused in a single area with remarkable preservation of other areas of thinking and functioning. Another feature distinguishing the disorders is the tenacity of the delusional belief. Persons with delusional disorder most often will maintain a stable but false belief system for long periods. Alternatively, the threatening beliefs of the person with paranoid personality disorder do not reach delusional proportions and often wax and wane in intensity.

Treatment

The treatment of delusional disorder relies heavily on the use of antipsychotic drugs; however, little systematic study has examined the effectiveness of this approach. Pharmacotherapy should be undertaken with caution: Patients with delusional disorder are convinced of the delusional beliefs and will usually resist medication management. Drug treatment should only be undertaken in the context of an ongoing therapeutic relationship in which there has been an effort to establish rapport, collaboration, and shared goals. For example, it is of little use to try to convince patients who have persecutory delusions that medicine will help them by changing how they think about the feared situation. Patients may be willing to take a drug that will calm the anxiety that has resulted from the persecution. Certain medicines such as pimozide may be preferentially helpful. Individual supportive psychotherapy as well as family therapy may also be required.

Complications, Comorbidity, & Adverse Outcomes of Treatment

The main complication of delusional disorder has to do with whether the affected person acts on the delusion in some way. Most people with this disorder lead quiet, uneventful lives otherwise. However, a sudden, unexpected event may intervene, such as the stalking of a famous person. These events may lead to incarceration or involuntary hospitalization, which may surprise friends and coworkers. These actions are consistent with the content of the delusion. Unfortunately, treatment, at least in the short term, often is ineffective, leading to a repetition of the behaviors related to the false beliefs.

Prognosis & Course of Illness

Occasionally, patients with delusional disorder will go on to develop schizophrenia. This is an exception, though; most patients maintain the delusional diagnosis. About half of patients recover fully and about one-third improve significantly. Only about 20% maintain the delusion indefinitely.

Hart JJ: Paranoid states: classification and management. Br J Hosp Med 1990;44:34.

Manschreck TC: Delusional disorder: the recognition and management of paranoia. J Clin Psychiatry 1996; 57(Suppl 3):32, 49.

BRIEF PSYCHOTIC DISORDER

DSM-IV Diagnostic Criteria

A. Presence of one or more of the following symptoms:
   (1) delusions
   (2) hallucinations
   (3) disorganized speech (eg, frequent derailment or incoherence)
   (4) grossly disorganized or catatonic behavior

   Note: Do not include a symptom if it is a culturally sanctioned response pattern.

B. Duration of an episode of the disturbance is at least 1 day but less than 1 month, with eventual full return to premorbid level of functioning.

C. The disturbance is not better accounted for by a mood disorder with psychotic features, schizoaffective disorder, or schizophrenia and is not due to the direct physiological effects of a substance (eg, a drug of abuse, a medication) or a general medical condition.

Specify if:

With marked stressor(s) (brief reactive psychosis): if symptoms occur shortly after and apparently in response to events that, singly or together, would be markedly stressful to almost anyone in similar circumstances in the person's culture

Without marked stressor(s): if psychotic symptoms do not occur shortly after, or are not apparently in response to events that, singly or together, would be markedly stressful to almost anyone in similar circumstances in the person's culture.

With postpartum onset: if onset within 4 weeks postpartum

Reprinted, with permission, from *Diagnostic and Statistical Manual of Mental Disorders,* 4th ed. Copyright 1994 American Psychiatric Association.

General Considerations

The emergence of transient psychotic symptoms, particularly after a severe psychological or social stressor such as a move or loss of a loved one, is not rare. Brief psychotic symptoms in the absence of a clear stressor is less common but also may occur. This disorder is generally associated with very acute onset and florid symptoms that decline relatively rapidly even in the absence of the use of antipsychotic drugs. A diagnosis of brief psychotic disorder should be considered if a psychotic patient has a history of good premorbid functioning and an acute onset that resolves rapidly and completely in response to antipsychotic therapy.

A. Major Etiologic Theories: A variety of stressors may occur prior to the onset of brief psychotic disorder. If the onset occurs within 4 weeks of giving birth, the specifier *with postpartum onset* is used. Many other stressors may predispose to the occurrence of this condition. For example, the disorder may occur after the death of a loved one, after a move to a new country (culture shock), during a natural disaster, or during combat or other military activity. A variety of factors are associated with the occurrence of brief psychotic disorder. They can be associated either with an increased likelihood of experiencing a stressor (eg, lower socioeconomic status, refugee or immigrant status, presence in a war zone) or limitations in coping skills (eg, persons with personality disorders, children or adolescents). However, the problem may also occur in people experiencing mild or no stressor and without predisposing characteristics.

B. Epidemiology: Reliable estimates of the frequency of this disorder are not available; however, an increased frequency is observed in populations that have experienced significant life stresses (eg, immigrants, refugees, military recruits, and persons who have experienced a disaster such as an earthquake or hurricane). Predisposing variables include comorbidity of personality disorder, substance use disorder, or dementia, or low socioeconomic status. Socioeconomic status may be associated with brief psychotic disorder in part because persons of lower social class may be at increased risk for major life stresses.

C. Genetics: Family history relationships are unclear; however, there may be an increased risk of psychotic disorder (including brief psychotic episodes) or affective disorder in relatives of persons with this condition.

Clinical Findings

Psychotic symptoms occurring for 1 month or less with complete resolution constitute brief psychotic disorder. This condition occurs most often after a significant external stressor, although DSM-IV allows the diagnosis without an obvious stress. The presentation is usually particularly florid. Patients can exhibit confusion, marked agitation or catatonia, emotional lability, and psychotic symptoms such as hallucinations or delusions. The symptoms may be so severe as to mimic the appearance of delirium.

Differential Diagnosis

The diagnosis of brief psychotic disorder is often difficult to make, and corroborative information from a family member or friend may be required to distinguish this problem from another psychotic disorder or cognitive disorder such as delirium.

A variety of disorders should be considered in the differential, including schizophrenia spectrum disorders (ie, schizophreniform disorder, schizophrenia, or schizoaffective disorder), psychotic affective disorder, delusional disorder, personality disorder, substance use disorder (including withdrawal), delirium, psychotic disorder due to medical condition, or substance-induced psychotic disorder. Schizophrenia and related disorders (including delusional disorder) are distinguished by the duration of psychotic symptoms and impairments. Persons with brief psychotic disorder show complete resolution of their psychotic symptoms and impairments within the 30 days allotted for the diagnosis. The symptoms of persons with delusional disorder are more confined to the delusional content and are not as pervasive as that usually seen in brief psychotic disorder.

A diagnosis of psychotic affective disorder should be considered in the presence of prominent mood symptoms such as mania or depression. This distinction may be difficult to make, especially in highly agitated or otherwise distressed patients. The mood, psychotic, and behavioral symptoms of affective psychosis rarely resolve completely within 30 days of initiation of treatment; therefore, if patients show complete return of baseline function within this time frame, a diagnosis of brief psychotic disorder should be considered, especially in the absence of a history of mood disorder.

Patients with personality disorder may present transient episodes of psychosis, sometimes referred to as "quasi-psychotic states" or "micropsychotic episodes." This is particularly true of borderline personality disorder but may be seen in other disorders, including histrionic, schizotypal, or obsessive-compulsive personality. These events almost always follow a significant stressor, especially an interpersonal stressful event. These occurrences may be very brief (ie, less than 1 day) and would be included in the category of psychotic disorder not otherwise classified. However, if they occur for more than 1 day but less than 1 month, the patient should be given a diagnosis of brief psychotic disorder along with the personality disorder diagnosis. Finally, if the psychotic symptoms seem related to substance use or withdrawal or to a medical condition, the alternatives of substance use disorder (including substance-induced psychotic disorder) or psychotic disorder due to medical condition should be given diagnostic primacy.

Treatment

Treatment proceeds as with any other form of psychosis (Table 20–2). Hospitalization is usually required, and a reduction in sensory stimulation is helpful. Antipsychotics and sedatives help to ameliorate the symptoms, especially by inducing sleep. Response to antipsychotic drug treatment is often rapid and complete. If complete resolution of psychotic symptoms occurs, the total duration of antipsychotic drug therapy should be brief in order to minimize adverse events such as tardive dyskinesia.

Subsequent psychotherapeutic management should be aimed at three goals. The first goal of treatment is to help the person understand the nature of the problem, especially as it relates to the reaction to a specific stressor (if any). An acute onset of a major psychotic episode is a highly disruptive and disturbing event. Any person so affected needs to make sense of the experience. The second goal is rapid reintegration into the environment. Third, longer-term goals include the development of coping skills to help prevent subsequent episodes of illness. Because the problem may recur, it is important to help the patient and family recognize early prodromal signs (eg, sleeplessness) of an impending episode.

Table 20–2. Principles of management of brief psychotic disorder.

Hospitalization usually is indicated.
Undertake a thorough psychiatric and medical evaluation and laboratory testing to rule out other major psychiatric, medical, or substance use disorders.
Attempt to identify and eliminate or modify significant stressors.
Antipsychotic and sedative drugs (such as benzodiazepines) often are indicated in acute management; however, long-term treatment with these medicines should be avoided when the diagnosis of brief psychotic disorder is clear and the patient experiences complete resolution of symptoms.
Long-term treatment should focus on several major elements:
  Improving coping skills
  Eliminating or stabilizing ongoing psychological or social stressors
  Establishing a network of social support
  Managing comorbid conditions, including personality disorders
  Reintegrating the patient into the social, educational, or occupational milieu
  Helping the patient and social network to understand the condition and to recognize early prodromal symptoms of impending psychosis, especially sleeplessness
  Facilitating sleep, nutrition, and hygiene

Complications, Comorbidity, & Adverse Outcomes

The principal complications of brief psychotic disorder have to do with the disruptions of social function, including employment, that may occur. As a result, rapid but stepwise reintegration is indicated in most patients. Careful attention should be paid to predisposing variables, including ongoing stressors (eg, relationship stress, especially abuse) and comorbid disorders (eg, comorbid personality or substance use disorders or medical conditions). Longer-term adverse outcomes may be more related to the outcome of these predisposing variables (especially personality disorder) than to the brief psychotic disorder per se. Some patients will never experience another psychotic event, whereas others will experience recurrences.

Prognosis & Course of Illness

By definition, the short-term outcome of this disorder is good. Symptoms should resolve completely; however, recurrence of psychotic events often occurs, especially in the face of ongoing stressors or comorbid conditions such as personality disorder. When recurrence is frequent, long-term management with an antipsychotic (usually an atypical antipsychotic agent) may be indicated.

Jorgensen P: Long-term course of acute reactive paranoid psychosis: a follow-up study. Acta Psychiatr Scand 1988;71:332.

SHARED PSYCHOTIC DISORDER

DSM-IV Diagnostic Criteria

A. A delusion develops in the context of a close relationship with another person(s), who has an already-established delusion.
B. The delusion is similar in content to that of the person who already has the established delusion.
C. The disturbance is not better accounted for by another psychotic disorder (eg, schizophrenia) or a mood disorder with psychotic features and is not due to the direct physiological effects of a substance (eg, a drug of abuse, a medication) or a general medical condition.

Reprinted, with permission, from *Diagnostic and Statistical Manual of Mental Disorders,* 4th ed. Copyright 1994 American Psychiatric Association.

General Considerations

Shared psychotic disorder, commonly referred to as *folie à deux,* occurs when a delusion develops in a person who has a close relationship with another person who already has a fixed delusion in the context of another psychotic illness such as schizophrenia or delusional disorder. Most often the person experiencing shared psychotic disorder is in a dependent or submissive position. This would include, as examples, the position of a dependent wife or child of a psychotic person. Further, specific factors such as social isolation or family history of schizophrenia, physical disability, or mental retardation in the submissive person may enhance the likelihood of the occurrence. Most cases involve members of a family, although it may occur in other situations (eg, religious cults).

A. Major Etiologic Theories: The etiology of shared psychotic disorder is generally thought to be psychological. The dominant, psychotic person simply imposes the delusional belief on the submissive party.

B. Epidemiology: The exact frequency of shared psychotic disorder is not known. It may occur with greater frequency in certain groups or situations, especially with social isolation of the involved parties.

Prognosis & Treatment

In the most common situation, simple separation results in resolution of the delusional belief in the submissive member *(folie imposée).* Less commonly, the delusion fails to remit in either of the parties at separation *(folie simultanée).* In the most rare form, the dominant person induces a delusion in a second person, but that person goes on to develop his or her own additional delusional ideation *(folie communiquée).* In the latter two conditions, antipsychotic drug therapy may be required to help reduce the psychosis of the submissive person. Table 20–3 summarizes the treatment options.

Mentjox R, et al: Induced psychotic disorder: clinical aspects, theoretical considerations, and some guidelines for treatment. Compr Psychiatry 1993;34:120.
Silveira JM, Seeman MV: Shared psychotic disorder: a critical review of the literature. Can J Psychiatry 1995; 40:389.

Table 20–3. Principles of management of shared psychotic disorder.

Separate the involved persons. Make an effort to maintain separation if possible.
Hospitalization or alternative community residence (such as respite care) may be needed.
Avoid the use of medications if possible.
Provide ongoing psychological and social support after acute treatment.
Ongoing psychological treatment should focus on the development of coping skills and social independence.
Social monitoring and intervention (including family therapy) are indicated if the patient is going to return to the same environment.

PSYCHOTIC DISORDER DUE TO A GENERAL MEDICAL CONDITION & SUBSTANCE-INDUCED PSYCHOTIC DISORDER

DSM-IV Diagnostic Criteria

Psychotic Disorder Due to a General Medical Condition

A. Prominent hallucinations or delusions.
B. There is evidence from the history, physical examination, or laboratory findings that the disturbance is the direct physiological consequence of a general medical condition.
C. The disturbance is not better accounted for by another mental disorder.
D. The disturbance does not occur exclusively during the course of a delirium.

Substance-Induced Psychotic Disorder

A. Prominent hallucinations or delusions.

Note: Do not include hallucinations if the person has insight that they are substance induced.

B. There is evidence from the history, physical examination, or laboratory findings of either (1) or (2):
    (1) the symptoms in Criterion A developed during, or within a month of, substance intoxication or withdrawal
    (2) medication use is etiologically related to the disturbance
C. The disturbance is not better accounted for by a psychotic disorder that is not substance induced. Evidence that the symptoms are better accounted for by a psychotic disorder that is not substance induced might include the following: the symptoms precede the onset of the use (or medication use); the symptoms persist for a substantial period of time (eg, about a month) after the cessation of acute withdrawal or severe intoxication, or are substantially in excess of what would be expected given the duration of use; or there is other evidence that suggests the existence of an independent non-substance-induced psychotic disorder (eg, a history of recurrent non-substance-related episodes).
D. The disturbance does not occur exclusively during the course of delirium.

Reprinted, with permission, from *Diagnostic and Statistical Manual of Mental Disorders,* 4th ed. Copyright 1994 American Psychiatric Association.

General Considerations

Many medical illnesses and drugs can induce psychotic symptoms (Tables 20–4 and 20–5). Other med-

Table 20–4. Medical conditions associated with psychotic symptoms.

Brain neoplasm
Cerebrovascular accident
Creutzfeldt-Jakob disease
Deficiency states (vitamin B_{12}, folate, thiamin, niacin)
Dementias (eg, Alzheimer's disease, Pick's disease)
Fabry's disease
Fahr's disease
Hallervorden-Spatz disease
Heavy metal poisoning
Herpes encephalitis
HIV/AIDS
Huntington's disease
Metachromatic leukodystrophy
Neurosyphilis
Porphyria
Seizure disorder (complex partial seizures)
Systemic lupus erythematosus
Wilson's disease

ical conditions, toxins, and drugs should be considered with any patient presenting with psychosis or with an exacerbation of a preexisting psychotic disorder. Psychotic conditions related to medical conditions are very common, especially in the hospital setting. Clinicians should be prepared to treat these conditions vigorously.

Clinical Findings

Hallucinations and delusions are common; however, the hallucinations of illness-related psychosis tend to be fairly specific to the underlying illness. For example, olfactory (smell) and gustatory (taste) hallucinations are associated with basal lesions of the brain or seizure disorders involving the temporal lobe or hippocampus. Alcohol or other sedative withdrawal may result in tactile (touch) hallucinations. Visual hallucinations may be reported in psychotic states induced by dopamine agonists, sympathomimetics, anticholinergics, or hallucinogenic drugs.

Treatment

The management of these disorders requires identification and aggressive management of the underlying illness or drug that has induced the psychosis (Table 20–6). In addition, antipsychotics such as haloperidol

Table 20–5. Drugs associated with the induction of psychosis.

Anticholinergics (atropine)
Antidepressants
Dopamine agonists (L-dopa, bromocriptine, pramipexole)
Hallucinogens (D-lysergic acid diethylamide, phencyclidine, cannabis, mescaline)
Histamine-2 antagonists (cimetidine)
Inhalants (toluene)
Psychostimulants (cocaine, amphetamine, sympathomimetics)
Sedative-hypnotic, alcohol, or anxiolytic withdrawal

Table 20–6. Management of psychotic disorder due to medical condition and substance-induced psychotic disorder.

Evaluate all psychotic patients for medical or substance-induced causes, even those with chronic psychotic conditions.
Identify and vigorously treat the underlying medical or substance use disorder (including withdrawal).
Minimize exposure to all drugs.
Judiciously use antipsychotics or sedatives (including benzodiazepines).
Drug management may include low-dose typical (eg, haloperidol 0.5–2 mg/day) or atypical (eg, risperidone 0.5–2 mg/day, olanzapine 2.5–5 mg/day) antipsychotics or low-dose, short-acting benzodiazepines (eg, alprazolam, lorazepam 0.25–1 mg/day).
Lower the dose or discontinue psychotropic medications as soon as possible.
Longer-term management should focus on the vigorous treatment of the underlying condition. In addition, special attention should be paid to sleep hygiene.

at low doses may be required to treat the psychotic symptoms acutely. Generally, elimination of the offending illness or drug will resolve the psychotic state. Drug treatment should be conservative and targeted to the offending symptoms, such as psychosis, insomnia, or agitation.

Prognosis & Course of Illness

The long-term prognosis of these conditions relates to the course of the underlying illness. Psychosis in the face of medical conditions does not portend a favorable outcome in many patients. In addition, psychosis may recur if the fundamental medical disorder recurs.

Fricchione GL, Carbone L, Bennett WI: Psychotic disorder caused by a general medical condition, with delusions. Secondary "organic" delusional syndromes. Psychiatr Clin N Am 1995;18:363.

PSYCHOTIC DISORDER NOT OTHERWISE SPECIFIED (NOS)

Certain psychotic states cannot be classified into one of the foregoing categories of psychoses and are referred to as psychotic disorder NOS.

Kendler KS, Walsh D: Schizophreniform disorder, delusional disorder and psychotic disorder not otherwise specified: clinical features, outcome and familial psychopathology. Acta Psychiatr Scand 1995;91:370.

DSM-IV Diagnostic Criteria

This category includes psychotic symptomatology (ie, delusions, hallucinations, disorganized speech, grossly disorganized or catatonic behavior) about which there is inadequate information to make a spe-

cific diagnosis or about which there is contradictory information, or disorders with psychotic symptoms that do not meet the criteria for any specific psychotic disorder.

Examples include:

1. Postpartum psychosis that does not meet criteria for mood disorder with psychotic features, brief psychotic disorder, psychotic disorder due to a general disorder
2. Psychotic symptoms that have lasted for less than 1 month but that have not yet remitted, so that the criteria for brief psychotic disorder are not met
3. Persistent auditory hallucinations in the absence of any other features
4. Persistent nonbizarre delusions with periods of overlapping mood episodes that have been present for a substantial portion of the delusional disturbance
5. Situations in which the clinician has concluded that a psychotic disorder is present, but is unable to determine whether it is primary, due to a general medical condition, or substance induced

Reprinted, with permission, from *Diagnostic and Statistical Manual of Mental Disorders,* 4th ed. Copyright 1994 American Psychiatric Association.

OTHER SPECIFIED OR CULTURE-BOUND PSYCHOTIC DISORDERS

Several psychotic disorders have specific presentations or are contained within certain demographic groups. These disorders are widely recognized but are not accorded formal diagnostic status in DSM-IV.

A. Capgras Syndrome (delusion of doubles): This disorder represents a fixed belief that familiar persons have been replaced by identical imposters who behave identically to the original person.

B. Lycanthropy: This is a delusion that the person is a werewolf or other animal.

C. Frégoli's Phenomenon: In this delusion, a persecutor (who usually is following the person) changes faces or makeup to avoid detection.

D. Cotard's Syndrome (*délire de négation*): A false perception of having lost everything, including money, status, strength, health, but also internal organs. This may be seen in schizophrenia or psychotic depression and responds to treatment of the underlying condition.

E. Autoscopic Psychosis: The main symptom is a visual hallucination of a transparent phantom of one's own body.

F. Koro: This disorder in males is characterized by a sudden belief that the penis is shrinking and may disappear into the abdomen. An associated feature may be the belief that when this occurs the person will die. A similar condition may be seen in women with fears of the loss of the genitals or breasts. Although this problem is seen more commonly in Asia, presentations in Western countries occur occasionally.

G. Amok: The amok syndrome consists of an abrupt onset of unprovoked and uncontrolled rage in which the affected person may run about savagely attacking and even killing people and animals in his or her way. It is seen most often in Malayan natives but has been reported in other cultures. In some circumstances, this problem is observed in individuals with preexisting psychotic disorders.

H. Piblokto (Arctic hysteria): This disorder occurs among the Eskimos and is characterized by a sudden onset of screaming, crying, and tearing off of clothes. The affected person may then run or roll about in the snow. It usually resolves rapidly, and the person will usually have no memory of the event.

I. Windigo (witigo): Specific North American Indian tribes, including the Cree and Ojibwa, manifest this rare psychotic state. People affected may believe that they are possessed by a demon or monster that murders and eats human flesh. Trivial symptoms including hunger or nausea may induce intense agitation because of a fear of transformation into the demon.

Bernstein RL, Gaw AC: Koro: proposed classification for DSM-IV. Am J Psychiatry 1990;147:1670.

Berrios GE, Luque R: Cotard's syndrome: analysis of 100 cases. Acta Psychiatr Scand 1995;91:185.

Koehler K, Ebel H, Vartzopoulos D: Lycanthropy and demonomania: some psychopathological issues. Psychol Med 1990;20:629.

Kon Y: Amok. Br J Psychiatry 1994;165:685.

Mojtabai R: Fregoli syndrome. Aust N Z J Psychiatry 1994;28:458.

21

Mood Disorders

Peter T. Loosen, MD, PhD, John L. Beyer, MD, Sam R. Sells, MD,
Harry E. Gwirtsman, MD, Richard C. Shelton, MD, R. Pryor Baird, MD, PhD, & James L. Nash, MD

I. MAJOR DEPRESSIVE DISORDER

John L. Beyer, MD, James Nash, MD, Richard Shelton, MD, & Peter T. Loosen, MD

DSM-IV Diagnostic Criteria

Major Depressive Episode

A. Five (or more) of the following symptoms have been present during the same 2-week period and represent a change from previous functioning; at least one of the symptoms is either (1) depressed mood or (2) loss of interest or pleasure.

Note: Do not include symptoms that are clearly due to a general medical condition, or mood-incongruent delusions and hallucinations.

  (1) depressed mood
  (2) loss of interest or pleasure (anhedonia)
  (3) significant weight loss when not dieting or weight gain, or decrease or increase in appetite
  (4) insomnia or hypersomnia
  (5) psychomotor agitation or retardation
  (6) fatigue or loss of energy
  (7) feelings of worthlessness or inappropriate/excessive guilt
  (8) diminished ability to think or concentrate, or indecisiveness
  (9) recurrent thoughts of death or suicide

B. The symptoms do not meet criteria for a mixed episode.

C. The symptoms cause significant distress or impairment in social, occupational, or other important areas of functioning.

D. The symptoms are not due to the direct physiological effects of a substance (eg, drug of abuse) or a general medical condition (eg, hypothyroidism).

E. The symptoms are not better accounted for by bereavement (ie, depressive/grief symptoms lasting less than 2 months).

Adapted, with permission, from *Diagnostic and Statistical Manual of Mental Disorders*, 4th ed. Copyright 1994 American Psychiatric Association.

General Considerations

A. Major Etiologic Theories: Despite intensive attempts to establish its etiologic or pathophysiologic basis, the precise cause of major depressive disorder is not known. There is consensus that multiple etiologic factors—genetic, biochemical, psychodynamic, and socioenvironmental—may interact in complex ways and that the modern-day understanding of depressive disorder requires a sophisticated understanding of the interrelationships among these factors.

  1. Life events—Recent evidence confirms that crucial life events, particularly the death or loss of a loved one, can precede the onset of depression. However, such losses precede only a small (though substantial) number of cases of depression. Fewer than 20% of individuals experiencing losses become clinically depressed. These observations argue strongly for a predisposing factor, possibly genetic, psychosocial, or characterological in nature.

  2. Biological theories—
  a. Neurotransmitters. Associations between mood and monoamines (ie, norepinephrine, serotonin, and dopamine) were first indicated serendipitously by the mood-altering effects of isoniazid (used initially for the treatment of tuberculosis) and later by reports that isoniazid affects monoamine concentrations in the brains of laboratory animals. We now know that all clinically effective antidepressants increase neurotransmitter concentrations at postsynaptic receptor sites by inhibiting their reuptake (into the presynaptic neuron) from the synaptic cleft. This action has led to the hypothesis that depression is caused by a neurotransmitter deficiency and that antidepressants exert their clinical effect by treating this imbalance.

  In the late 1970s, emphasis shifted from acute presynaptic to delayed postsynaptic receptor–mediated events after it was shown that most chronic antidepressant treatments (including pharmacotherapy and electroconvulsive therapy [ECT]) cause subsensitivity of the norepinephrine receptor–coupled adenylate cyclase system in brain. This desensitization of norepinephrine receptor systems was linked to a decrease in the density of β-adrenoceptors. More important, it paralleled the delayed onset of action common to all antidepressants. It was also shown that glucocorticoid hormones can alter norepinephrine receptor sensitivity in brain. Glucocorticoid hormones represent, in concert with catecholamines and indolamines, the third physiologically important group of regulators of the β-adrenoceptor-coupled adenylate cyclase system in brain: the serotonin–norepinephrine–glucocorticoid link hypothesis of affective disorders. The link hypothesis evolving from the original deficiency hypotheses now emphasizes the integration of multiple intracellular signals that regulate neuronal response (ie, changes in G protein, cyclic adenosine monophosphate, or protein kinase and the induction of gene transcription). It is possible that the serotonin-linked and glucocorticoid-responsive β-adrenoreceptor system may amplify or adapt in a more general way stimulus transcription coupling and regulation of specific gene expression. However, it has also become clear that other neurotransmitters (eg, acetylcholine, gamma amino butyric acid, melatonin, glycine, histamine), hormones (eg, thyroid and adrenal hormones), and neuropeptides (eg, endorphins, enkephalins, vasopressin, cholecystokinin, substance P) may play significant roles in the modulation of mood.

b. Neuroendocrine factors. Emotional trauma often precedes the onset of depression. Emotional trauma can also precede the onset of endocrine disorders such as hyperthyroidism and Cushing's disease, both of which are commonly associated with psychological disturbance, most commonly in mood and cognition. When endocrine changes are associated with psychological disturbance it is often unclear whether such changes are precipitants, perpetuating influences, or secondary effects.

The two endocrine systems most extensively studied in psychiatry are the hypothalamic-pituitary-adrenal (HPA) axis and the hypothalamic-pituitary-thyroid (HPT) axis. About half of patients with major depression exhibit cortisol hypersecretion that returns to normal once the depression is cured. Human studies have also demonstrated a profound effect of thyroid hormones on brain development, maturation, and connectivity. The effects of thyroid hormones on mature brain function, as they pertain to mood, are less marked. The most common effects are as follows: (1) Depression and cognitive decline are the most frequently observed psychiatric symptoms in patients who have adult hypothyroidism. (2) A small dose of thyroid hormone, preferably triiodothyronine (T_3), will accelerate the therapeutic effect of various antidepressants in women and will convert antidepressant nonresponders into responders in both sexes. (3) Most longitudinal studies have revealed dynamic reductions in serum thyroxine (T_4) concentrations in depressed patients during a wide range of somatic treatments, including various antidepressants, lithium, sleep deprivation, and ECT. (4) Administration of thyrotropin-releasing hormone (TRH) may induce an increased sense of well-being and relaxation in normal subjects and in patients with neurologic and psychiatric disease, especially depression. (5) Although overt thyroid disease is rare in major depression, subtle forms of thyroid dysfunction are common—for example, absence or flattening of the diurnal thyroid-stimulating hormone (TSH) curve, often caused by a reduction in the nocturnal TSH surge; a blunted TSH response after administration of TRH (discussed in greater detail later in this section); and subclinical hypothyroidism or positive antithyroid antibodies.

Ahmed N, Loosen PT: Thyroid hormones in major depressive and bipolar disorders. In: Casper R (editor): *Women's Health and Emotion.* Cambridge University Press, 1997.

Goodwin FK, Jamison KR: *Manic Depressive Illness.* Oxford University Press, 1990.

Loosen PT: Hormones of the hypothalamic-pituitary-thyroid axis: a psychoneuroendocrine perspective. Pharmacopsychiatry 1986;19:401.

Musselman DL et al: Biology of mood disorders. In: Schatzberg AF, Nemeroff CB (editors): *Textbook of Psychopharmacology,* 2nd ed. American Psychiatric Press, 1998.

Nemeroff CB, Loosen PT (editors): *Handbook of Clinical Psychoneuroendocrinology.* Guilford Press, 1987.

Pearson Murphy BE: Steroids and depression. J Steroid Biochem Mol Biol 1991;38:537.

Pryor JC, Sulser F: Evolution of the monoamine hypothesis of depression. In Horton RW, Katona CLE (editors): *Biological Aspects of Affective Disorders.* Academic Press, 1991.

3. Psychosocial theories—
a. Psychoanalytic and psychodynamic models. In the early 20th century psychoanalytic interpretations of mental illness were prominent (see Chapter 4). They did not distinguish consistently between depression as a transitory (or characterologically persistent) affect and depression (melancholia) as a psychopathologic syndrome. Karl Abraham (1911) wrote the first important psychoanalytic paper on depression, demonstrating that depression is unconsciously motivated and the result of repressed sexual and aggressive drives. Abraham's later writings were influenced heavily by the concurrent writings of Sigmund Freud. Depression and, to a less successful extent, mania were understood as precipitated by loss and manifested by regressions to anal and oral phases of libidinal development. These regressions in adult life resulted from an unfortunate combination of predisposition (constitutional overaccentuation of oral eroticism) and critical childhood disappointments. Armed with Freud's concepts on the role of introjection in normal mourning and in melancholia, Abraham wrote of the "severe

conflict of ambivalent feelings from which [the patient] can only escape by turning against himself the hostility he originally felt towards his object."

The precepts that depression is the result of a loss and that it symptomatically represents "anger turned against the self" are part of the enduring legacy of classic psychoanalytic thinking. Freud believed that the real, threatened, or imagined loss of a narcissistic object choice (meaning that the individual's love of the object was equivalent to love of the self) would trigger a withdrawal of libido away from the object and back into the self through introjection of the ambivalently cathected object. The patient then would attack himself (depressive symptoms) as though for misdeeds that were the doing of the lost object. In other words, the depressed patient experiences a loss as a narcissistic wound; suicide becomes an unconscious attempt to destroy the now hated object that dwells in the patient's ego by means of introjection. Like Abraham, Freud also emphasized the importance of somatic factors in predisposing the individual to depression and in the clinical picture itself. Diurnal variation of mood, for example, was beyond psychological explanation. Later psychoanalytic writers (eg, M. Klein, D. W. Winicott, E. Bibring) sought to expand on Freud's thinking, incorporating further developments in ego psychology, object relations theory, and self psychology.

b. Behavioral models. In the mid-1900s, three models based on behavioral theory emerged (see Chapter 2). Peter Lewinsohn showed that depression can be caused by inadequate or insufficient positive reinforcement. In everyday life, this can occur in two main ways: (1) if an environment lacks positive reinforcement (eg, through individual or mass unemployment) or (2) if the person is not able to take advantage of reinforcement (eg, through isolation induced by poor social skills). Inadequate positive reinforcement may lead to a self-perpetuating cycle consisting of dysphoria, a reduction in behaviors that would normally obtain the reinforcement, lowered self-esteem and increased hopelessness, and increased isolation.

Martin Seligman developed the theory of learned helplessness as he was searching for an animal model of depression. Laboratory animals given random shocks from which they cannot escape develop apathy to any stimulus. Generalizing this observation to humans, Seligman's theory suggests that depression can result from situations in which a person has lost (actual or imagined) control over negative life events.

The cognitive-behavioral model of depression developed by Aaron Beck suggests that depression develops when the patient cognitively misinterprets life events. The conceptual core of this model consists of the cognitive triad of depression: (1) a negative self-view (ie, "things are bad because I am bad"), (2) a negative interpretation of experience (ie, "everything has always been bad"), and (3) a negative view of the future (ie, "everything will always be bad"). It is a

basic tenet of this theory that a depressed person interprets the world through depressive schemata that distort experiences in a negative direction. Typical cognitive distortions include arbitrary inference (in which the person assumes a negative event was caused by himself or herself), selective abstraction (in which the person focuses on the negative element in an otherwise positive set of information), magnification and minimization (in which the person overemphasizes negatives and underemphasizes positives), and inexact labeling (in which the person gives a distorted label to an event and then reacts to the label rather than to the event).

Freud S: Mourning and melancholia (1917). Pages 237–260 in Strachey J (editor and translator): *Standard Edition of the Complete Psychological Works of Sigmund Freud.* Vol 14. Hogarth, 1957.

Roose S: Depression. Pages 301–318 in Nersessian E, Kopff R (editors): *Textbook of Psychoanalysis.* American Psychiatric Press, 1996.

B. Epidemiology: Early reviews of epidemiologic studies acknowledge and reflect the problem of case definition (eg, the use of imprecise definitions of diagnostic terms and/or the lack of standardized methods of collecting data) (see Chapter 5). Because depression grades into normalcy, and because people with depression who are not bipolar constitute a heterogeneous group, it has been proposed that the depression spectrum be divided into three categories: (1) depressive symptoms (ie, patients with depressive symptoms that are not sufficiently severe to warrant clinical diagnosis or intervention), (2) bipolar disorder (defined by one or more episodes of mania), and (3) non–bipolar disorder.

The separation into bipolar and non–bipolar disorder has proved clinically and diagnostically useful. It is supported by family studies, twin studies, and biological studies. It is supported further by differential clinical responses to treatment and differential disease onsets and outcomes. To these factors we can add the epidemiologic risk factors detailed in Table 21–1.

Symptoms and disorders of the depression spectrum are rather common. Lifetime prevalence rates for depressive symptoms are 13–20% and for major depressive disorder 3.7–6.7%. Major depressive disorder is about two to three times as common in adolescent and adult females as in adolescent and adult males. In prepubertal children, boys and girls are affected equally. Rates in women and men are highest in the 25- to 44-year-old age group.

Boyd JH, Weissman MM: Epidemiology. Pages 109–125 in Paykel ES (editor): *Handbook of Affective Disorders.* Guilford Press, 1982.

Weissman MN, Livingston Bruce M, Leaf PJ, Florio LP, Holzer C: Affective Disorders. Pages 53-80 in Robins LN, Regier DA (editors): *Psychiatric Disorders in America.* Free Press, 1991.

Table 21–1. Risk factors for major depressive disorder.

Family history	High risk in families with history of depression (7%) or alcoholism (8%)
Social class	No relationship
Race	Less common in blacks
Life events	Recent negative life events may precede episode
Personality	Insecure, worried, introverted, stress sensitive, obsessive, unassertive, dependent
Childhood experience	Early loss, disruptive, hostile, negative environment
Postpartum	Depressive episodes common
Menopause	No relationship
Lack of intimate relationships	Common risk factor

C. Genetics: Mood disorders are familial, but the exact mode of transmission is not well understood (see Chapter 6).

Clinical Findings

A. Signs & Symptoms:

1. Major depressive episode—The cardinal feature of a major depressive episode is a depressed mood or the loss of interest or pleasure (see items *a* and *b* below) that predominates for at least 2 weeks and causes significant distress or impairment in the individual's social, occupational, or other important areas of functioning. During this time, the individual must also exhibit at least four additional symptoms (ie, other than depressed mood or anhedonia), drawn from the following common features of depression:

a. Depressed mood. Depressed mood is the most characteristic symptom, occurring in over 90% of patients. The patient usually describes himself or herself as feeling sad, low, empty, hopeless, gloomy, or down in the dumps. The quality of mood is likely to be portrayed as different from a normal sense of sadness or grief. The physician often observes changes in the patient's posture, speech, facies (eg, a melancholic expression known as facies melancholica), dress, and grooming consistent with the patient's self-report. Many depressed patients state that they are unable to cry, whereas others report frequent weeping spells that occur without significant precipitants.

A small percentage of patients do not report a depressed mood, usually referred to as **masked depression.** These patients are usually brought to their physician by family members or coworkers who have noticed the patients' social withdrawal or decreased activity. Similarly, some children and adolescents do not exhibit a sad demeanor, presenting instead as irritable or cranky.

b. Anhedonia. An inability to enjoy usual activities is almost universal among depressed patients. The patient or his or her family may report markedly diminished interest in all, or almost all, activities previously enjoyed such as sex, hobbies, and daily routines.

c. Change in appetite. About 70% of patients observe a reduction in appetite with accompanying weight loss; only a minority of patients experience an increase in appetite, often associated with cravings for particular foods such as sweets.

d. Change in sleep. About 80% of depressed patients complain of some type of sleep disturbance, the most common being insomnia. Insomnia is usually classified as initial (ie, problems in falling asleep), middle (ie, problems of staying asleep with frequent awakenings throughout the night), or late (ie, early morning awakening). The most common and unpleasant form of sleep disturbance in major depressive disorder is late insomnia, with awakenings in the early morning (usually around 4 A.M. to 5 A.M.) and significant worsening of depressive symptoms in the first part of the day. In contrast, initial insomnia is especially common in those with significant comorbid anxiety. Some patients complain of hypersomnia rather than insomnia; hypersomnia is common in atypical depression and seasonal affective disorder and is often associated with hyperphagia.

e. Change in body activity. About one half of depressed patients develop a slowing, or retardation, of their normal level of activity. They may exhibit a slowness in thinking, speaking, or body movement or a decrease in volume or content of speech, with long pauses before answering. In about 75% of depressed women and 50% of depressed men, anxiety is expressed in the form of psychomotor agitation, with pacing, an inability to sit still, and hand-wringing.

f. Loss of energy. Almost all depressed patients report a significant loss of energy (anergia), unusual fatigue or tiredness, and a general lack of efficiency even in small or elementary tasks.

g. Feelings of worthlessness and excessive or inappropriate guilt. A depressed individual may experience a marked (and often unrealistic) decrease in self-esteem. In European cultures, well over half of depressed patients exhibit some guilt, ranging from a vague feeling that their current condition is the result of something they have done, to frank delusions and hallucinations of poverty or of having committed an unpardonable sin. In other cultures, shame or humiliation is experienced.

h. Indecisiveness or decreased concentration. About one half of depressed patients complain of or exhibit a slowing of thought. They may feel that they are not able to think as well as before, that they cannot concentrate, or that they are easily distracted. Frequently they will doubt their ability to make good judgments and find themselves unable to make even small decisions. On formal psychological testing, the patient's accuracy is usually retained, but speed and performance are slow. In severe forms, called **pseudodementia,** particularly among the elderly, memory deficits may be mistaken for early signs of dementia. In contrast to dementia, pseudodementia usually reverses after treatment of the underlying depression.

i. Suicidal ideation. Many depressed individuals experience recurrent thoughts of death, ranging from transient feelings that others would be better off without them, to the actual planning and implementing of suicide. Up to 15% of patients with severe major depressive disorder are likely to die by suicide. The risk of suicide is present throughout a depressive episode but is probably highest immediately after initiation of treatment and during the 6–9 month period following symptomatic recovery. Table 21–2 lists common predictors of suicide risk.

2. Melancholia subtype—The symptoms of melancholia are similar to those of a major depressive episode, but at least five of nine symptoms are present: (1) loss of interest or pleasure, (2) lack of reactivity to usually pleasurable stimuli, (3) depression regularly worse in the morning, (4) early morning awakening, (5) psychomotor agitation or retardation, (6) significant anorexia or weight loss, (7) no personality disturbance before first episode, (8) one or more previous episodes followed by complete remission, and (9) previous good response to specific and adequate somatic antidepressant therapy (eg, ECT, tricyclic antidepressants [TCAs], monoamine oxidase inhibitors [MAOIs], lithium).

3. Seasonal affective disorder—Occasionally patients experience depressive episodes at characteristic times of the year. Most commonly the episodes of seasonal affective disorder (SAD) begin in fall or winter and remit in spring, but occasionally they can also be observed in summer. SAD with prevalence during the winter months (winter depression) appears to vary with latitude, age, and sex. SAD is more common in colder climates and among younger people, particularly in females. SAD is characterized clinically by hypersomnia, anergia, and a craving for sweets. SAD responds particularly well to light therapy and serotonergic agents (ie, selective serotonin reuptake inhibitors [SSRIs]).

B. Laboratory Findings & Imaging: No laboratory findings are diagnostic of a major depressive episode; however, several laboratory findings are abnormal in some patients with major depression, compared to the general population. It appears that most laboratory abnormalities are state dependent (ie, they occur while patients are depressed), but some findings may precede the onset of an episode or persist after its remission.

1. Hypothalamic-pituitary-adrenal axis—

a. Dexamethasone suppression test. Although the dexamethasone suppression test (DST) has little use as a clinical marker for depression, it is worth mentioning some of the more pertinent DST findings: (1) The overall sensitivity (ie, positive DST outcome) was 44% among all patients with major depression given 1 mg dexamethasone; sensitivity was significantly higher (65%) in elderly depressed patients but dropped to 31% in a smaller group of patients who received 2 mg of dexamethasone. (2) Within the depression spectrum, the rates of DST nonsuppression increased strikingly from grief reactions (10%) and dysthymic disorders (23%), to major depressive disorders (44%), major depressive disorders with melancholia (50%), psychotic affective disorders (69%), and depression with serious suicidality (78%). (3) In some depressed patients, the DST allowed researchers to predict or monitor long-term treatment outcome. (4) DST-positive patients appeared to respond more favorably to biological interventions such as antidepressants or ECT. (5) Among depressed patients, abnormal DST results correlated mostly with initial insomnia, weight loss, loss of sexual interest, ruminative thinking, and psychomotor retardation or agitation. (6) HPA axis dysregulation contributed to cognitive dysfunction, although it is not known whether hypercortisolemia and cognitive impairment in depression are related indirectly or causally.

A hyperactive HPA axis has been observed in stroke patients with major depression; in pain patients with major depression; and in patients with anorexia nervosa, bulimia nervosa, alcoholism, obsessive-compulsive disorder, or anxiety disorders. It has not been observed in schizophrenic patients.

b. Corticotropin-releasing hormone test. A blunted adrenocorticotropic hormone response after corticotropin-releasing hormone administration is another HPA axis abnormality commonly observed in major depression.

Table 21–2. Common predictors of suicide risk.

Older than 45 years, male, white (ie, risk is greater in males, especially white males, where it appears to increase with age)
Prior suicide attempt
Detailed plan for suicide
Chronic self-destructive pattern
Recent severe loss
Inability to accept help
Lack of available support from society
Poor health or fear of poor health
Psychotic symptoms
Comorbid alcoholism or drug abuse

2. Hypothalamic-pituitary-thyroid axis—

a. Serum thyroxine concentrations. Most depressed patients appear to be euthyroid; however, longitudinal studies consistently found significant serum T_4 reductions during a wide range of somatic treatments, including various antidepressants, lithium, sleep deprivation, or ECT. Evidence indicates that the T_4 reduction was greater in treatment responders than in nonresponders. It is not known whether the initial T_4 increase in depression is part of the pathophysiology of the illness, or whether it is a compensatory mechanism by which the organism delivers thyroid hormone to the brain.

b. Subclinical hypothyroidism. Subtle thyroid dysfunctions are common in depression. Between 1% and 4% of patients show evidence of overt hypothyroidism, and between 4% and 40% show evidence of subclinical hypothyroidism. Comorbid subclinical hypothyroidism can be associated with cognitive dysfunction or with a diminished response to standard psychiatric treatments. Some depressed patients with subclinical hypothyroidism may respond behaviorally to thyroid hormone substitution.

c. Thyrotropin-releasing hormone test. The TRH test (ie, measurement of serum TSH following TRH administration) has been used widely in psychiatry. More than 3000 patients have been studied, the majority of whom had major depressive disorder. Approximately 30% of patients had a blunted TSH response during depression, and a smaller number showed TSH blunting during remission; however, definitions of TSH blunting have varied among studies, different assays have been used, and a standard amount of TRH has not always been injected.

There appears to be no association between the TRH-induced TSH response and (1) the patient's body surface or age, (2) serum thyroid hormone or cortisol concentrations, (3) severity of depression, or (4) previous intake of antidepressant drugs (excluding long-term lithium administration). Further, the TRH test does not aid in the distinction between primary and secondary depression or between unipolar and bipolar subgroups. Preliminary evidence suggests that TSH blunting may be associated with a more prolonged course of depression and with a history of violent suicidal behavior.

Within psychiatric disorders, TSH blunting can also occur in some patients who have borderline personality disorder, anorexia nervosa, panic disorder, primary degenerative dementia, chronic pain, premenstrual syndrome, or alcoholism, both during acute withdrawal and after prolonged abstinence. The absence of TSH blunting in both schizophrenic patients and phobic patients during exposure therapy suggests that the abnormality is not a mere correlate of mental distress.

3. Sleep electroencephalogram—Most depressed patients have insomnia. Sleep problems commonly reported include interruptions throughout the night, early morning awakenings, and less frequently, difficulty falling asleep. Sleep electroencephalogram (EEG) recordings reveal the following: (1) a shortened rapid eye movement (REM) latency (ie, a shorter than normal interval between sleep onset and first REM period), more common in elderly depressed patients and often associated with unipolar depression; (2) a shift of slow-wave sleep (ie, sleep stages 3 and 4), normally occurring during the first non-REM period, into the second non-REM period; and (3) an increased REM density (ie, more frequent REM episodes) during the first few hours of sleep.

Because most of these sleep EEG abnormalities can be found in other illnesses, and some accompany normal aging, there is no agreement as to whether these abnormalities constitute diagnostic markers of depression or whether they reflect abnormal functioning in sleep-related processes but lack diagnostic specificity (see Chapter 30). There is evidence that EEG sleep variables are normal in depressed patients 6 months after an acute episode.

4. Brain imaging—Brain imaging studies are less uniform in depression than they are in schizophrenia. Moreover, most studies do not take into account the unipolar-bipolar distinction, and only a few longitudinal studies include patients who are well and not taking medications.

Depression tends to be associated with lesions in the left frontotemporal or right parieto-occipital regions. This concept is consistent with neuroanatomical and behavioral findings in stroke patients. Patients with dominant anterior or nondominant posterior strokes are especially vulnerable to secondary depressions, whereas patients with nondominant anterior or dominant posterior strokes are especially vulnerable to mania or hypomania. It has been suggested that findings implicating left-hemispheric dysfunction in depression and right-hemispheric dysfunction in mania merely reflect characteristics of the frontotemporal regions, and that the left (ie, dominant) prefrontal cortex may play a key role in the neurobiology of depression. The data are also consistent with the literature on laterality, which proposes that the two hemispheres serve different functions in terms of information processing and cognition. Laterality studies in depression have shown that relative functional deficits can be found in the nondominant hemisphere. Neuroimaging findings do not allow one to infer causal relationships between neuroanatomical lesion or deficit and observed behavior.

Ahmed N, Loosen PT: Thyroid hormones in major depressive and bipolar disorders. In: Casper R (editor): *Women's Health and Emotion.* Cambridge University Press, 1997.

Goodwin FK, Jamison KR: *Manic Depressive Illness.* Oxford University Press, 1990.

Loosen PT: Hormones of the hypothalamic-pituitary-thyroid axis: a psychoneuroendocrine perspective. Pharmacopsychiatry 1986;19:401.

Musselman DL et al: Biology of mood disorders. In: Schatzberg AF, Nemeroff CB (editors): *Textbook of Psychopharmacology,* 2nd ed. American Psychiatric Press, 1998.

Nemeroff CB, Loosen PT (editors): *Handbook of Clinical Psychoneuroendocrinology.* Guilford Press, 1987.

Pearson Murphy BE: Steroids and depression. J Steroid Biochem Mol Biol 1991;38:537.

Pryor JC, Sulser F: Evolution of the monoamine hypothesis of depression. In: Horton RW, Katona CLE (editors): *Biological Aspects of Affective Disorders.* Academic Press, 1991.

Differential Diagnosis

A diagnosis of depression is made if the individual is significantly impaired by the depressive symptoms outlined in the preceding section, and if three exclusion criteria are met: (1) the illness is not due to the effects of a substance (eg, drug of abuse or medication) or a general medical condition, (2) the illness is not part of a mixed episode (see section on Bipolar Disorders later in this chapter), and (3) the symptoms are not better accounted for by bereavement.

A. Medical Conditions: Most patients with depression will initially present not to a psychiatrist but to their general medical practitioner and often with a somatic complaint (ie, "I can't sleep," or "I have no energy") rather than a psychiatric complaint (ie, "I'm depressed"). This is especially true for elderly patients. It is also true that many medications and medical disorders commonly produce symptoms of depression (Table 21–3). Most of these sources of depression can be detected by a thorough review of a patient's history, a complete physical and neurologic examination, and standard laboratory tests. If an etiologic relationship exists between one of these causes and a mood disturbance, the diagnosis will be mood disorder due to a general medical condition (see section on Mood Disorder Due to a General Medical Condition later in this chapter).

B. Other Psychiatric Disorders: Depression can be a feature of almost all other psychiatric disorders; however, the diagnosis should not be made if the episode is part of a bipolar disorder or schizoaffective disorder.

Table 21–3. Organic causes of depression.

Medications
Analgesics (eg, indomethacin, opiates)
Antibiotics (eg, ampicillin)
Antihypertensive agents (eg, propranolol, reserpine, α-methyldopa, clonidine)
Antineoplastic agents (eg, cycloserine, vincristine, vinblastine)
Cimetidine
L-Dopa
Insecticides
Mercury, lead
Oral contraceptives
Sedative-hypnotics (eg, barbiturates, benzodiazepines, chloral hydrate, phenothiazines)

Substances of abuse
Alcohol
Cocaine
Opiates

Neurologic disease
Chronic subdural hematoma
Dementias
Huntington's disease
Migraine headaches
Multiple sclerosis
Normal pressure hydrocephalus
Parkinson's disease
Strokes
Temporal lobe epilepsy
Wilson's disease

Infectious disease
Brucellosis
Encephalitis
HIV
Infectious hepatitis
Influenza
Mononucleosis
Subacute bacterial endocarditis
Syphilis
Tuberculosis
Viral pneumonia

Neoplasms
Bronchogenic carcinoma
CNS tumors
Disseminated carcinomatosis
Lymphoma
Pancreatic cancer

Metabolic and endocrine disorders
Addison's disease
Anemia
Apathetic hyperthyroidism
Cushing's disease
Diabetes
Hepatic disease
Hypokalemia
Hyponatremia
Hypoparathyroidism
Hypopituitarism (Sheehan's disease)
Hypothyroidism
Pellagra
Pernicious anemia
Porphyria
Thiamine, vitamin B_{12}, and folate deficiencies
Uremia

Collagen-vascular conditions
Giant cell arteritis
Rheumatoid arthritis
Systemic lupus erythematosus

Cardiovascular conditions
Chronic heart failure
Hypoxia
Mitral valve prolapse

Miscellaneous
Chronic pyelonephritis
Pancreatitis
Peptic ulcer disease
Postpartum depression

C. Uncomplicated Bereavement: Bereavement generally refers to the grief symptoms experienced after the loss of a loved one. Bereavement is not considered a mental disorder even though it may have symptoms characteristic of a major depressive episode (eg, sadness, insomnia, loss of appetite, weight loss, feelings of guilt or hopelessness). Data indicate that almost 25% of bereaved individuals meet criteria for major depression at 2 months and again at 7 months and that many of these people continue to do so at 13 months. Patients with more prolonged symptoms tend to be younger and tend to have a history of major depression. Antidepressant treatment is justified in bereavement when the behavioral symptoms are prolonged or if they are associated with continued functional impairment.

Treatment

An important aspect of the treatment of depression is for the physician to discuss with patients and their families the illness, its symptoms and course, and particularly its recurrent nature. Patients should recognize that the illness may recur; they—and their close family members—should be cognizant of the premonitory signs and symptoms of an impending episode (ie, insomnia, especially early morning awakening, loss of energy, loss of appetite and libido, and diurnal changes in well-being); and they should be told to return to their physician as soon as they have noticed any combination of the premonitory signs for, say, longer than 1 week. This, of course, is best achieved if patients are followed up closely in and out of episodes, if the communication between the physician and the patient or patient's family is open and continuous, and if all parties are thoroughly aware that the nature of the illness necessitates both close, continuous observation of its course and early, decisive intervention to prevent relapse. It is also important to recognize that clinical features often have significant treatment implications. A summary of these features and their suggested solutions is provided in Table 21–4.

A. Pharmacologic Treatments:

1. Clinical pharmacology—

a. Principles of use. The following general principles provide a useful framework for the clinical use of antidepressants in major depressive disorder: (1) diagnose properly; (2) avoid treatment of symptoms (eg, agitation, insomnia, memory disturbances) if possible, because most symptoms fit into specific diagnostic entities; and (3) be aware of the cycling course of the disease, because it necessitates different treatment approaches: acute treatment for florid symptoms; continuation therapy to prevent early relapse; and maintenance therapy to make relapse (ie, recurrence) less likely or, if it occurs, less severe.

b. Indications. Antidepressant drugs are used successfully to treat a variety of psychiatric and other conditions (Table 21–5). In mood disorders, they are used most widely in the treatment of major depressive disorder, but they also have some (albeit reduced) therapeutic activity in treating dysthymic disorder and bipolar disorder (see sections on Dysthymic Disorders and Bipolar Disorders later in this chapter).

The effectiveness of antidepressants in young patients remains controversial, because controlled clinical trials failed to show consistent beneficial effects in children and adolescents. Even though mitigating factors such as different study designs, medication compliance, and the impact of exogenous factors (eg, family discord) on symptom manifestation limit the interpretation of these studies, antidepressant drugs are used widely in depressed children and adolescents.

In contrast, antidepressants are very useful in elderly depressed patients, in whom daily dosage requirements are normally reduced because of pharmacokinetic changes associated with aging (ie, reductions in both hepatic clearance and protein binding).

Antidepressants are usually initiated at a low dosage and increased over a 7- to 10-day period to achieve the initial target dosage. The dosage may have to be increased further in some patients in order to achieve the best results. With suicidal patients, the physician must take extra care early in the treatment because behavioral activation can precede observable mood effects, providing patients with sufficient energy to act on suicidal impulses.

Once a therapeutic effect is achieved, the antidepressant medication should be continued through the period of high vulnerability for relapse (ie, at least 6 months for continuation therapy). Because more than 60% of depressed patients will eventually relapse, especially if unprotected by medication, and because future episodes are more severe, it has been proposed that some depressed patients be placed on long-term or indefinite treatment. Such maintenance therapy for extended periods of time (even years) should be considered if (1) the patient is older than 40 years and had two or more prior episodes of illness, (2) the first episode occurred at age 50 years or older, (3) the patient has a history of three or more depressive episodes, or (4) the patient has been depressed or dysthymic for 2 or more years before treatment.

Slow tapering of the antidepressant medication can be considered after at least 5 years of treatment if the patient is completely asymptomatic and is not experiencing or anticipating significant stressors. Some patients prefer lifetime treatment rather than risking a return of depression.

2. Adverse effects—Table 21–6 lists common adverse effects associated with antidepressant drugs, their possible mechanisms, and their management. Table 21–7 indicates the relative potency of antidepressants at producing these effects.

a. Monoamine oxidase inhibitors. Common side effects of MAOIs include those associated with

Table 21–4. Clinical features influencing treatment and their solutions.[1,2]

Features	Treatment Considerations
Severity	Even mild depression, if unresponsive to nonsomatic treatment, should be considered for antidepressants.
Recurrent depression	Consider for maintenance therapy.
Prior mania or hypomania	Somatic treatments may provoke (hypo)manic episodes in approximately 5–20% of patients (most have a history of bipolar disorder). Such treatments may also precipitate rapid-cycling bipolar disorder. The treatments of choice are lithium alone or in combination with an MAOI or bupropion.
Depression with psychotic features	Carries a higher risk of suicide and recurrent depression. Combine a neuroleptic with an antidepressant or use amoxapine.
Depression with catatonic features	If intravenous injections of lorazepam or amobarbital are not immediately helpful, consider ECT.
Depression with atypical features	Features include anxiety, reverse polarity (eg, hypersomnia, hyperphagia, marked mood reactivity), and a sense of severe fatigue. TCAs are useful in only 35–50% of patients; in contrast, MAOIs yield response rates of 55–75%.
Depression with alcohol and/or substance abuse	A patient who has major depression with comorbid addiction is more likely to require hospitalization, more likely to attempt suicide, and less likely to comply with treatment than is a patient without such comorbidity. Advisable to detoxify the patient before initiating antidepressant treatment.
Depression with panic and/or anxiety disorder	Panic disorder complicates major depression in 15–30% of cases. Good response to non-MAOI antidepressants, especially imipramine.
Pseudodementia	Lacks the signs of cortical dysfunction seen in true dementia (eg, aphasia, apraxia, agnosia); treat early and aggressively.
Postpsychotic depression	Depressive symptoms complicate the course of schizophrenia in 25% of cases. Add antidepressant to neuroleptic regimen.
Depression during or after pregnancy	Carefully assess the benefit-risk ratio, especially if treatment is prescribed during the first trimester. If possible, avoid pharmacologic treatment in nursing mothers. Be aware of the possible teratogenic effects of benzodiazepines (ie, cleft lip and palate) and lithium (ie, cardiac malformations). Consider ECT as alternative treatment.
Depression superimposed on dysthymia	Antidepressant treatment may resolve both major depression and underlying dysthymia. SSRIs and MAOIs may be the most helpful.
Depression superimposed on personality disorder	Frequently associated with atypical features; more likely to respond to MAOIs or SSRIs. Patients usually show less satisfactory treatment response in regard to both social functioning and residual depressive symptoms.

[1] Modified and reproduced, with permission, from American Psychiatric Association: Practice guidelines for major depressive disorder in adults. Am J Psychiatry 1993;150(Suppl):4.
[2] ECT, electroconvulsive therapy; MAOIs, monoamine oxidase inhibitors; SSRIs, selective serotonin reuptake inhibitors; TCAs, tricyclic antidepressants.

Table 21–5. Common clinical uses of antidepressants.

Major Indications	Secondary Indications
Major depressive disorder Dysthymia Bipolar disorder, depressed type Panic disorder (with or without agoraphobia)	Obsessive-compulsive disorder[1] Generalized anxiety disorder Social phobia Bulimia nervosa Attention-deficit/hyperactivity disorder[2] Diabetic polyneuropathy[1] Chronic pain syndromes[1] Sleep disorders Enuresis[3]

[1] Mainly serotonergic antidepressants.
[2] Especially tricyclic antidepressants such as imipramine and desipramine.
[3] Specific for the use of imipramine in children.

α_1-adrenergic or muscarinic/cholinergic antagonism (see Table 21–6). They are generally manageable by slowing the dose titration or by adjusting the maximum dosage. Less common reactions include ataxia, color blindness, hepatotoxicity, or induction of mania in bipolar patients. Withdrawal reactions—including anxiety, restlessness, insomnia, nausea, agitation, myoclonus, and in extreme cases, the induction of mania—may occur after abrupt discontinuation.

The most serious side effect associated with MAOI use is the development of an acute hypertensive crisis. The metabolism of certain dietary amino acids, especially tyramine, is blocked by MAOIs. The resulting increase in neurotransmitter availability can lead to an acute hypertensive crisis, with patients complaining about pounding headaches and presenting with flush-

Table 21–6. Mechanisms and management of common side effects of antidepressants.[1,2]

Mechanism	Side Effects	Management	Drug Examples
Muscarinic/cholinergic blockade	Dry mouth, blurred vision, constipation, urinary retention, mild sinus tachycardia, memory problems.	*Dry mouth:* candy, sugarless gum. *Constipation:* hydration, bulk laxatives. *Urinary retention:* bethanechol, 30–200 mg/day. Use bupropion, sertraline, or trazodone.	TCAs, MAOIs
α_1-adrenergic antagonism	Orthostatic hypotension, dizziness, reflex tachycardia, flushing, diaphoresis, potentiation of the antihypertensive effect of prazosin.	*Orthostatic hypotension:* increase dosage slowly, use safer agents such as nortriptyline, desipramine, bupropion, or SSRIs. Exert especial caution in elderly patients who are susceptible to falls and fractures.	TCAs, MAOIs, trazodone, nefazodone
Histaminic (H_1) antagonism	Somnolence, weight gain, hypotension, and potentiation of CNS depressants.	*Weight gain:* bupropion, fluoxetine, sertraline, and trazodone are alternatives; bupropion and fluoxetine may reduce weight.	TCAs
NE reuptake blockade	Tremor, tachycardia, insomnia, anxiety, erectile and orgasmic dysfunction, blockade of the antihypertensive effect of guanethidine and guanadrel.		TCAs, most heterocyclics
5-HT reuptake blockade	Nausea, diarrhea, anorexia, anxiety, headache, insomnia, sexual dysfunction (loss of erectile or ejaculatory function in men, loss of libido and anorgasmia in women).	*Sexual dysfunction:* neostigmine, 7.5–15.0 mg taken 30 minutes before intercourse, will enhance libido and reverse delayed ejaculation. Cyproheptadine, 4 mg/day orally, may reverse anorgasmia.	SSRIs, clomipramine, venlafaxine, MAOIs
DA reuptake blockade	Psychomotor activation, insomnia, anxiety, aggravation of psychosis, potentiation of antiparkinsonian agents.	NA	TCAs (weak), bupropion
DA$_2$- receptor blockade	Parkinsonian (ie, extrapyramidal) effects, elevation of prolactin with gynecomastia and galactorrhea.	NA	Amoxapine, TCAs (weak)
5-HT$_2$-receptor antagonism	Hypotension, somnolence.	NA	Trazodone, nefazodone, amitriptyline
Effects like those of class I antiarrhythmic agents	Neurologic side effects: seizures, mild myoclonus, toxic confusional state.	*Seizures:* fluoxetine, sertraline, trazodone, and MAOIs carry a lower risk to induce seizures. *Myoclonus:* clonazepam, 0.25 mg three times daily. *Toxic confusional state:* seen at higher dose and blood levels, responds to lowering the dose.	TCAs
	Cardiovascular effects: TCAs may induce symptomatic conduction defects and orthostatic hypotension among patients with preexisting but asymptomatic conduction defects. TCAs may also provoke arrhythmia in patients with subclinical sinus node dysfunction.	Monitor those patients carefully who already take another class I antiarrhythmic agent. Evaluate patients for preexisting but asymptomatic conduction defects such as interventricular conduction delay and bundle branch block. Be aware that patients with prolonged Q-T intervals, whether preexisting or drug-induced, are predisposed to the development of ventricular tachycardia. Obtain ECG in all patients older than 40 years before initiating treatment.	TCAs, trazodone
	Insomnia and anxiety.	Minimize anxiety by starting at a low dose. Manage insomnia by adding trazodone, 100 mg at bedtime (be aware that trazodone can induce priapism in some patients).	Fluoxetine (anxiety and insomnia); desipramine and bupropion (anxiety)

[1] Modified and reproduced, with permission, from American Psychiatric Association: Practice guidelines for major depressive disorder in adults. Am J Psychiatry 1993;150(Suppl):4.
[2] 5-HT, serotonin; CNS, central nervous system; DA, dopamine; ECG, electrocardiogram; MAOIs, monoamine oxidase inhibitors; NA, not applicable; NE, norepinephrine; SSRIs, selective serotonin reuptake inhibitors; TCAs, tricyclic antidepressants.

ing and blood vessel distention. The reaction must be considered a medical emergency to be treated with slow intravenous administration of the α-adrenergic antagonist phentolamine, 5 mg (which may be repeated hourly as needed).

MAOIs may also produce acute toxicity by interfering with the metabolic removal of other drugs, including general anesthetics, barbiturates and other sedatives, antihistamines, alcohol, narcotics, anticholinergic agents, TCAs, sympathomimetic amines (eg, pseudoephedrine and phenylpropanolamine used commonly in decongestants), and the narcotic meperidine.

Coadministration of MAOIs with either SSRIs or L-tryptophan can provoke a central serotonin syndrome, characterized by acute mental status changes (eg, confusion, hypomania), restlessness, myoclonus, diaphoresis, tremor, diarrhea, hyperreflexia, and occasionally, seizures, coma, and death. The syndrome is usually mild in nature and resolves within 24 hours

after drug discontinuation. MAOIs should therefore not be started within 2 weeks of discontinuation of most SSRIs (5 weeks in the case of fluoxetine, because of its long half-life time [see next section]).

Coadministration of TCAs and MAOIs (used occasionally for the management of treatment-refractory depression) can produce serious side effects, including delirium and hypertension. It is therefore advisable to wait at least 2 weeks after discontinuing TCAs before initiating treatment with MAOIs. Table 21–8 lists foods and drugs that can produce serious adverse effects. Patients should be given a copy of this list before beginning treatment with MAOIs.

b. Tricyclic antidepressants & related antidepressants. Tricyclic-induced side effects are the result of their binding to both specific (eg, norepinephrine or serotonin) and nonspecific (eg, histamine, muscarinic) sites. Table 21–6 summarizes these actions and their consequences.

The tertiary amine TCAs—amitriptyline, imip-

Table 21–7. Clinical characteristics of antidepressants.[1,2]

Drug	Dose Range (mg)	Central Action[3]	Side Effects[4]				
			ACh	A$_1$	H$_1$	S$_2$	Quin
Tricyclics							
Amitriptyline	100–300	NE (5-HT)	VH	VH	H	M	+
Clomipramine[5]	100–250	5-HT (NE)	VH	M	M	M	+
Desipramine	100–300	NE	M	L	L	L	+
Doxepin	100–300	NE (5-HT)	H	VH	VH	M	+
Imipramine	100–300	NE (5-HT)	H	M	M	L	+
Nortriptyline	50–200	NE (5-HT)	M	M	M	M	+
Protriptyline	20–60	NE	VH	L	M	L	+
Trimipramine	75–300	NE (5-HT)	H	VH	VH	M	+
Heterocyclics							
Amoxapine	100–400	NE	L	M	M	VH	+
Bupropion	300–450	DA(?)	VL	VL	VL	VL	–
Maprotiline	100–225	NE	L	M	H	L	+
Nefazodone	100–500	5-HT$_2$ antagonism (NE, 5-HT)	H	VL	H	VL	–
Trazodone	150–400	5-HT$_2$ antagonism (NE, 5-HT)	L	H	L	H	+
Venlafaxine	75–375	5-HT	VL	VL	VL	VL	–
SSRIs							
Fluoxetine[5]	20–80	5-HT	L	VL	VL	VL	–
Fluvoxamine[5]	100–300	5-HT	VL	VL	M	VL	–
Paroxetine	20–80	5-HT	L	VL	VL	VL	–
Sertraline	50–200	5-HT	VL	VL	VL	VL	–
MAOIs							
Phenelzine	30–90	MAO inhibition	L	M	H	(?)	–
Tranylcypromine	10–40	MAO inhibition	L	M	H	(?)	–

[1] Modified and reproduced, with permission, from American Psychiatric Association: Practice guidelines for major depressive disorder in adults. Am J Psychiatry 1993;150(Suppl):4; and from Hardman JG, Limbird LE: *The Pharmacological Basis of Therapeutics.* McGraw-Hill, 1996.
[2] NE, norepinephrine; 5-HT, 5-hydroxytryptamine (serotonin); DA, dopamine; MAOIs, monoamine oxidase inhibitors; ACh, acetylcholine; A$_1$, alpha, adrenergic; H$_1$, histamine-1; S$_2$, 5-HT$_2$; Quin, quinidine-like effect; HTN, hypertensive; VH, very high; H, high; M, medium; L, low; VL, very low.
[3] Reuptake inhibition, except as otherwise indicated. Less significant clinical effects are shown in parentheses.
[4] Side effects are listed on a mg/kg basis (K$_d$); always multiply by the total dose to get the true clinical side effect profile.
[5] Established benefit in obsessive-compulsive disorder.

Table 21–8. Dietary and drug restrictions associated with monoamine oxidase inhibitor antidepressants.[1]

	Foods	Drugs
Very dangerous (must be avoided under all circumstances)	All cheese (cottage cheese, cream cheese, and yogurt are safe) Sauerkraut	Amphetamines Asthma inhalants (*pure* steroid inhalants are safe) Cyclopentamine Decongestants, cold, and sinus medications Ephedrine Meperidine Metaraminol Methylphenidate Phenylephrine Phenylpropanolamine Pseudoephedrine Serotonin-active antidepressants (eg, clomipramine, fluoxetine, sertraline, paroxetine, fluvoxamine)
Moderately dangerous (should be avoided)	All fermented or aged foods (eg, aged corned beef, salami, fermented sausage, pepperoni, summer sausage, pickled herring) Fermented alcoholic beverages (eg, red wine, sherry, vermouth, cognac, beer, and ale) (clear alcoholic drinks are permitted in true moderation) Broad bean pods (eg, English broad beans, Chinese pea pods) Liver (chicken, beef, or pork) or liverwurst Meat or yeast extracts Spoiled fruit (eg, spoiled bananas, pineapples, avocados, figs, raisins)	Antihistamines Dopamine L-Dopa Local anesthetics with epinephrine (safe without epinephrine—eg, carbocaine) Narcotics (codeine is safe) Tricyclic antidepressants (eg, imipramine, amitriptyline, nortriptyline, desipramine, doxepin)
Minimal danger (rarely associated with hypertensive episodes and can be eaten in small amounts)	Anchovies Beets Caviar Chocolate Coffee Colas Curry powder Figs Junket Licorice Mushrooms Rhubarb Snails Soy sauce Worcestershire sauce	

[1] Diabetics taking insulin may have increased hypoglycemia, requiring adjustment in dose of insulin (otherwise safe); patients taking hypotensive agents for high blood pressure may have more hypotension, also requiring adjustment (but also otherwise safe).

ramine, and doxepin—tend to be more potent at unspecific binding sites and therefore produce more severe side effects than the secondary amine TCAs nortriptyline and desipramine (see Tables 21–6 and 21–7).

TCAs and trazodone can affect the heart in the same way as the class 1 antiarrhythmics quinidine or procainamide, inducing atrioventricular (A-V) conduction delays. Special care should be taken with patients who have a first-degree A-V block (a relative contraindication) or a second-degree A-V block (an absolute contraindication) (see Table 21–6). As type 1 antiarrhythmics, these antidepressants may pose greater long-term risk than previously thought. The primary antiarrhythmics can increase the risk of sudden death from a presumed arrhythmic source. This may explain the long-standing observation of increased risk of sudden death in patients treated chronically with TCAs.

Maprotiline is associated with an increased risk for seizures at higher dosages and plasma levels and has never gained wide use in the United States. Venlafaxine, a mixed norepinephrine and serotonin reuptake inhibitor, can produce mild hypertensive reactions, especially at dosages greater than 300 mg/day. Risk factors for hypertension, such as age, race, or preexisting renal or hypertensive disorder, are usually not associated with this effect.

c. Selective serotonin reuptake inhibitors.
SSRIs potently and selectively block the uptake of serotonin, thereby producing characteristic side effects such as nausea, diarrhea, anorexia, anxiety, headache, insomnia, and orgasmic dysfunction (see Table 21–6). Sexual dysfunction is troublesome and can be persistent. It can be managed by reducing the dosage or by switching to bupropion or nefazodone. Cyproheptadine, yohimbine, or methylphenidate are also occasionally useful in reversing these effects.

3. Pharmacokinetics—
a. Absorption. All antidepressant drugs are highly lipophilic and are absorbed readily from the gastrointestinal tract. Plasma peaks typically occur within 30–60 minutes and remain unbound for 30 minutes.

b. Distribution. Most (80–90%) antidepressants are highly protein bound, although individual differences in binding can produce a fourfold variation in the amount of free drug. Tissue distribution and demethylation, the first step in metabolism of tertiary heterocyclics, occur rapidly. All antidepressants can be displaced by other drugs with similar protein-binding characteristics. Similarly, antidepressants will displace other compounds that are highly protein bound (eg, the anticoagulant warfarin); this can increase the free fraction of these drugs and, therefore, both its therapeutic and its adverse effects.

c. Metabolism. Antidepressants are metabolized mainly in the liver. Metabolism includes demethylation, hydroxylation, and glucuronide conjugation. Individual differences in a patient's microsomal enzyme activity produce steady-state plasma concentrations (bound and unbound) that may vary as much as 40-fold. During the first pass through the liver, about 80% of the drug is degraded (the so-called **first-pass effect**). The first demethylation of imipramine and amitriptyline produces (the clinically highly active) desipramine and nortriptyline, respectively; these and other drugs have active metabolites that significantly prolong their biological half-lives. Glucuronide conjugation occurs after hydroxylation and makes the derivative water soluble; approximately 65% of the drug

Table 21–9. Half-life times of common antidepressants.

Drug	Half-life Time (hours)
Trazodone	5
Imipramine	16
Amitriptyline	16
Paroxetine	20
Desipramine	22
Nortriptyline	24
Amoxapine	30
Citalopram	33
Maprotiline	47
Fluoxetine	24–72
Clomipramine	54–77
Protriptyline	126

is eventually eliminated in the urine. Plasma clearance is slow.

Impairment of hepatic or renal function will reduce plasma clearance of antidepressants and thus potentiate their effects. Antipsychotics, by competing for metabolism, can have a similar effect. Conversely carbamazepine and barbiturates, by inducing metabolism, can reduce their therapeutic efficacy.

d. Half-life times. After a single oral dose, distribution is most important in regard to clinical efficacy; after chronic dosing, half-life time (HLT) becomes more important. The HLTs of the most commonly used antidepressants are given in Table 21–9.

4. Predicting treatment response & managing treatment failure—Several factors are useful in predicting a patient's clinical response (positive and negative) to an antidepressant (Table 21–10).

Between 60% and 70% of persons with major depressive disorder respond well to an adequate antidepressant drug trial, but the remainder do not. The reasons for treatment failure include inadequate dose

Table 21–10. Predictors of antidepressant response.

Positive Predictors	Negative Predictors
Vegetative symptoms (anorexia, weight loss, middle and late insomnia) Diurnal mood variation Psychomotor agitation or retardation Autonomous and pervasive symptoms Acute onset Family history of depression Dose of imipramine (or equivalent dose of another heterocyclic) above 125–150 mg/day Blood levels of desipramine (or imipramine and desipramine) above 200 ng/mL, and nortriptyline between 50 and 150 ng/mL	Coexistence of other significant psychiatric disturbances (particularly with hysterical or externalizing features) Chronic symptoms Psychotic features Hypochondriacal concerns or predominant somatic features Previous drug trial failure(s) History of sensitivity to adverse reactions

and/or serum level, inadequate duration of treatment (minimum 6 weeks), prominent side effects, noncompliance, and incorrect diagnosis.

Because single doses of antidepressants can produce widely varying drug serum levels, the patient's plasma levels should be measured in order to ensure optimal dosing. Associations between plasma levels and clinical response are known for several antidepressants (Table 21–11). The monitoring of the plasma level of nortriptyline is particularly important because there appears to be a therapeutic window in which the drug is most effective. Plasma levels can also be assessed for other antidepressants, including fluoxetine, but the relationship between plasma levels and clinical response is less well understood for these agents. Indications for monitoring drug levels of antidepressants are (1) failure to respond to a presumably adequate trial in terms of dose and duration; (2) concurrent physical illness, especially cardiovascular disease; (3) use of higher than usual doses (ie, greater than 300 mg/day of imipramine); (4) treatment in the very young or old (or in any patient with decreased protein binding); (5) the presence of side effects uncertainly related to drug treatment; and (6) drug overdose.

When a true treatment failure has occurred, the physician needs to consider an alternative approach. This may involve trying another treatment approach (eg, ECT or combining TCAs with an MAOI) or using one of several augmentation strategies (Table 21–12). A large body of evidence supports these strategies, and particularly in tertiary care centers (to which most nonresponders normally are referred) they are widely and safely used.

Lithium carbonate, thyroid hormone (preferably T_3), or sleep deprivation are most effective in augmenting the therapeutic effects of TCAs. Among these strategies, sleep deprivation is the least invasive and most easily conducted technique. Its antidepressant effects, observed in about 65% of patients after only one night of wakefulness, are immediate; it is entirely free of side effects; and patients can repeat it easily and safely even after they have been discharged from the hospital. Lithium can be titrated to standard serum levels and T_3 started at 25 µg/day; both augmentation strategies should be maintained for a minimum of 3 weeks in the absence of therapeutic response. About half of patients who have not responded to standard antidepressants will experience

Table 21–11. Therapeutic plasma levels of antidepressants.

Drug	Plasma Concentration (ng/mL)
Amitriptyline (plus nortriptyline)	150–250
Nortriptyline	50–150[1]
Imipramine (plus desipramine)	150–250
Desipramine	50–150
Doxepin (plus desmethyldoxepin)	>100

[1] Therapeutic window.

Table 21–12. Alternative therapies for treatment-resistant depression.[1,2]

Augmentation of TCAs or MAOIs with
  Sleep deprivation [I]
  Lithium [I]
  Thyroid hormone [II]
  L-Tryptophan [III]
  Psychostimulants (amphetamine, methylphenidate—in combination with TCAs only) [III]
  Carbamazepine [II]
TCA/MAOI combination (use with extreme care) [II]
ECT (reserved primarily for severe intractable depression or when the patient is acutely suicidal) [I]
Phototherapy or light therapy [II]
Psychostimulants alone (reserved largely for treatment in elderly depressed patients) [III]
Psychotherapy (cognitive-behavioral and interpersonal psychotherapy) alone or in combination with TCAs [II]

[1] Modified and reproduced, with permission, from American Psychiatric Association: Practice guidelines for major depressive disorder in adults. Am J Psychiatry 1993;150(Suppl):4.
[2] [I] indicates recommended with substantial clinical confidence; [II] indicates recommended with moderate clinical confidence; [III] indicates options that may be recommended on the basis of individual circumstances. MAOI, monoamine oxidase inhibitor; TCA, tricyclic antidepressant.

sudden clinical improvement. It is not known whether lithium or T_3 should be continued after a clinical response has occurred, or whether they are as effective in augmenting SSRIs as they are in augmenting TCAs. T_3, lithium, and sleep deprivation may be most important in triggering or facilitating the acute response to an antidepressant, because there is little evidence that their continued administration is useful in maintaining remission or preventing relapse.

Alternative methods for treating refractory depression include the use of a combination of a noradrenergic antidepressant such as desipramine with a serotonergic one such as fluoxetine. Care must be taken to measure the plasma level of the TCA because SSRIs compete for their metabolic removal, thereby raising the plasma level of the TCA. Psychostimulants such as amphetamine or methylphenidate may be useful in some patients but in a more limited way.

If these techniques are ineffective, two other options remain. The first is to use a TCA and an MAOI together, but this strategy bears some risk of acute and potentially serious side effects. Imipramine and phenelzine are commonly employed. Each drug is started at a low level, and the dosages are increased slowly in an alternating fashion until a therapeutic level is achieved. Patients must be cautioned regarding potential negative consequences, including hypertensive reactions. If none of the aforementioned strategies is helpful, ECT remains as a final, but highly effective and safe alternative.

American Psychiatric Association: Practice guidelines for major depressive disorder in adults. Am J Psychiatry 1993;150(Suppl):4.

Baldessarini RJ: Drugs and the treatment of psychiatric disorders, depression and mania. Pages 431–459 in Hardman JG, Limbird LE (editors): *The Pharmacological Basis of Therapeutics.* McGraw-Hill, 1996.

Charney DS, Berman RM, Miller HL: Treatment of depression. In: Schatzberg AF, Nemeroff CB (editors): *Textbook of Psychopharmacology,* 2nd ed. American Psychiatric Press, 1998.

Glassman AH, Roose SP, Bigger JT Jr.: The safety of tricyclic antidepressants in cardiac patients: risk-benefit reconsidered. J Am Med Assoc 1993;269:2673.

Goodwin FK, Jamison KR: *Manic Depressive Illness.* Oxford University Press, 1990.

Schatzberg AF, Nemeroff CB (editors): *Textbook of Psychopharmacology,* 2nd ed. American Psychiatric Press, 1998.

B. Electroconvulsive Therapy: Between 80% and 90% of all ECT treatments in the United States are performed for the treatment of major depressive disorder. Although ECT appears to be most effective in the most severely depressed patients, attempts to use clinical symptoms, patient history, demographics, or other factors as predictors of clinical response have been largely unsuccessful.

ECT has shown efficacy in all types of major depressive disorder. Recent evidence suggests that it is less useful in patients whose depressive episodes occur in the context of a concurrent mental or medical disease (ie, secondary depression) or in the treatment of depression that has been refractory to medications during the present episode.

1. When to use electroconvulsive therapy— The decision to refer a patient for treatment with ECT is made only after careful considerations of its risks and benefits. ECT is used as primary treatment when (1) an urgent need (either psychiatrically or medically) for a rapid response exists, (2) there is less risk with ECT than with other treatment alternatives, (3) there is a patient history of better response to ECT, or (4) there is a strong patient preference for its use. A majority of patients referred for ECT do not meet these criteria. ECT is used as a secondary treatment when (1) the patient has responded poorly to or is intolerant of alternative treatments or (2) the patient has deteriorated to the point at which a rapid response is needed urgently.

2. Contraindications—There are no absolute contraindications to the use of ECT, but some conditions are relative contraindications (Table 21–13). If treatment with ECT becomes necessary on a life-saving basis, these risks can generally be minimized

Table 21–13. Relative contraindications to electroconvulsive therapy.

Conditions with increased intracranial pressure
Intracerebral hemorrhage
Pheochromocytoma
Recent myocardial infarction
Space-occupying intracerebral lesions (except for small, slow growing tumors without edema or other mass effect)
Unstable vascular aneurysms or malformations

to some extent using appropriate pharmacologic interventions. With appropriate preparation, ECT can be used effectively and safely in both pregnant and elderly patients.

3. Adverse outcomes of treatment—

a. Mortality. The overall mortality rate of ECT is extremely low; it approximates that of brief general anesthesia. Estimates range between 1 in 10,000 (0.01%) and 1 in 1,000 (0.1%) patients.

b. Cognitive changes. There is no relationship between ECT and brain damage; however, temporary cognitive changes do occur and are often the most notable and most distressing side effects. Three types of cognitive change may be observed:

Postictal confusion. Because ECT induces seizure activity, all patients experience some transient confusion, lasting from a few minutes to a few hours, after they awaken from the ECT treatment. Most patients usually will not remember the immediate postictal period and will not experience the cognitive changes following a seizure as a significant disturbance. Reassurance, support, and avoidance of cognitive demands during the acute postictal period are typically all that is necessary for treatment. Postictal sedation with a short-acting benzodiazepine such as midazolam may be necessary if the patient becomes agitated.

Interictal confusion. Occasionally postictal confusion may not disappear fully, and when severe, it may develop into an interictal confusional state or delirium. This phenomenon, which is uncommon, may be cumulative over the ECT course but disappears rapidly over a period of days after the conclusion of treatments.

Memory impairment. Amnesia often occurs with ECT and varies considerably in both severity and persistence. Memory disturbances consist of both retrograde amnesia (ie, difficulty in recalling information learned prior to the ECT course) and anterograde amnesia (ie, difficulty in retaining newly learned information). When present, anterograde and retrograde amnesia disappear rapidly over a period of days to weeks after completion of the ECT course.

A small group of patients report that their memory never returned to normal after ECT. The etiology for this phenomenon is unclear, and objective memory testing generally does not substantiate the subjective complaint.

c. Cardiovascular complications. During the seizure and acute postictal period, the sympathetic and parasympathetic autonomic systems are stimulated sequentially. Activation of the sympathetic system increases heart rate, blood pressure, and myocardial oxygen consumption, placing an increased demand on the cardiovascular system. Activation of the parasympathetic system causes a transient reduction in cardiac rate. These changes in heart rate and cardiac output challenge the cardiovascular system, occasionally giving rise to transient arrhythmias and, in susceptible individuals, transient ischemic changes.

Most cardiovascular changes are minor, and the risk of complications can be diminished greatly by the use of oxygen and appropriate medications in susceptible patients.

d. Other adverse effects. General somatic complaints (ie, headaches, nausea, muscle soreness) are common after ECT. Analgesics may be given prophylactically prior to ECT to patients who routinely have post-ECT headaches. The dosage of muscle relaxant should be increased if muscle soreness and headaches are due to inadequate relaxation.

About 7% of depressed bipolar patients switch into a manic or mixed state after ECT. This state can be managed by either continuing ECT or stopping ECT and administering an antimanic agent.

4. Course of treatment—
a. Number of treatments. A typical ECT course involves 6–12 treatments, but the number required may be as low as 3 or as high as 20. Alterations in the ECT course should be considered for nonresponders or for patients whose clinical progress is minimal after approximately six treatments. Alterations may include changing from unilateral to bilateral electrode placement, increasing stimulus intensity, or potentiating the seizure pharmacologically. If there is still no response after three or four additional treatments, or if the patient's response has reached a plateau below a full level of remission, the ECT course should be terminated.

b. Multiple monitored electroconvulsive therapy. Multiple monitored electroconvulsive therapy (MMECT) was developed in an attempt to decrease the average length of the treatment course by inducing multiple seizures (usually 2–10) during a single treatment. MMECT appears to be associated with a more rapid clinical response, but the total number of seizures required is greater. There is also evidence that MMECT is associated with a higher frequency of prolonged seizure activity, exaggerated cardiovascular responses, and increased cognitive side effects.

c. Frequency of treatments. In the United States, most ECT treatments are given three times a week (eg, Monday, Wednesday, and Friday). An increase in the frequency is associated with a more rapid response but also increased cognitive side effects.

d. Continuation treatment. Most psychiatrists agree that after the remission of a depressive or manic episode, ECT treatment should be continued for at least 6–12 months. After the conclusion of a course of ECT, there are three options for continued treatment: (1) administration of appropriate psychotropic medications (eg, antidepressants); (2) continuation of ECT; or (3) psychotherapy, combined with pharmacotherapy or ECT.

e. Maintenance treatment. Because of the severity and chronicity of some patients' illnesses, many practitioners now prophylactically continue pharmacotherapy or ECT for longer time periods, par-

ticularly when attempts to discontinue treatment have resulted in a recurrence of the illness. Maintenance ECT treatments are given monthly, although some individuals require more frequent administration. There is no lifetime maximum number of treatments that a patient may have. Cumulative amnestic effects are not usually seen.

American Psychiatric Association: The Practice of ECT: Recommendations for Treatment, Training, and Privileging. American Psychiatric Press, 1990.
Weiner RD, Coffey CE: Electroconvulsive therapy in the medical and neurologic patient. Pages 207–224 in Stoudemire A, Fogel BS (editors): *Psychiatric Care of the Medical Patient.* Oxford University Press, 1993.

C. Nonpharmacologic Treatments: The establishment and maintenance of a supportive therapeutic relationship, wherein the therapist gains the patient's confidence and is available in times of crisis, is crucial in the treatment of depression. Beyond pure psychotherapeutic management the therapeutic relationship contains other important factors. These include observing emerging destructive impulses toward self or others; providing ongoing education, knowledge, and feedback about the patient's illness, its prognosis, and treatment; discouraging the patient from making major life changes while he or she is depressed; setting realistic, attainable, and tangible goals; and enlisting the support of others in the patient's social network.

Depression is often treated with psychotherapy, either alone or in combination with antidepressants. This is particularly true for unipolar depression. The psychosocial interventions that have fared well in controlled trials relative to antidepressants include interpersonal psychotherapy, cognitive-behavioral therapy, and some of the marital and family interventions. Traditional dynamic psychotherapy has not proved effective but may not have been evaluated adequately.

1. Interpersonal psychotherapy—Interpersonal psychotherapy seeks to recognize and explore depressive precipitants that involve interpersonal losses, role disputes and transitions, social isolation, or deficits in social skills. It focuses on current interpersonal problems and deemphasizes childhood antecedents or extensive attention to transference in the therapeutic relationship. Interpersonal psychotherapy can be effective in reducing depressive symptoms in the acute phase of nonmelancholic major depression of lesser severity. It seems to produce a greater change in social functioning than antidepressants; this change may not appear until after several months of treatment (or until several months after treatment is over).

2. Cognitive-behavioral therapy—Cognitive-behavioral therapy is based on the premise that helping patients recognize and correct erroneous beliefs can relieve their affective distress. It also can be effective in reducing depressive symptoms in the acute phase of nonmelancholic major depression of lesser severity but appears not to be significantly different from pill placebo coupled with clinical management. Cognitive-behavioral therapy may have an enduring effect that protects the patient against subsequent relapse following treatment termination, but no firm conclusions have been reached at this time. In the treatment of more severe depression in outpatients neither interpersonal therapy nor cognitive-behavioral therapy are as effective as antidepressant drugs.

3. Marital therapy & family therapy—Marital and family problems are common in the course of mood disorders. They may be a consequence of depression but may also increase the patient's vulnerability to depression and in some instances retard recovery. Research suggests that marital therapy and family therapy may reduce depressive symptoms and the risk of relapse in patients with marital or family problems.

4. Selection of specific therapies—Patient preference plays a large role in the selection of a particular form of psychotherapy. In choosing the most appropriate form, the psychiatrist should consider that an interpersonal approach may be more useful for patients who are in the midst of conflicts with significant others and for those having difficulty adjusting to an altered career or social role or other life transition. A cognitive approach can be helpful for patients who seek and are able to tolerate explicit, structured guidance from another party. A psychodynamic or psychotherapeutic approach may best help those who have a chronic sense of emptiness; harsh self-expectations and self-underestimation; a history of childhood abuses, losses, or separations; chronic interpersonal conflicts; or coexisting Axis II disorders or traits. Factors contributing to the success of a psychodynamic or psychoanalytic modality include mild to moderate illness; a stable environment; and the patient's motivation, capacity for insight, psychological mindedness, and capacity to form a relationship.

Hollon SD, Shelton RC, Loosen PT: Cognitive therapy and pharmacotherapy for depression. J Consult Clin Psychol 1991;59:88.

Jarrett RB, Rush AJ: Short-term psychotherapy of depressive disorders: current status and future directions. Psychiatry 1994;57:115.

Weissman MM, Markowitz JC: Interpersonal psychotherapy: current status. Arch Gen Psychiatry 1994;51:599.

Complications, Comorbidity, & Adverse Outcomes of Treatment

Major depressive disorder is associated with a high level of morbidity and mortality. Up to 15% of patients with severe major depressive disorder commit suicide (among patients with recurrent depression, death by suicide occurs at the rate of about 1% per year). Among patients with major depressive disorder who are older than 55 years, the death rate is increased fourfold. Compared to nondepressive subjects, patients with major depressive disorder admit-

ted to a nursing home are more likely to die within the first 5 years. Among patients in general medical settings, physically ill patients with depression have increased pain and physical illness and decreased social and role functioning. In fact, deterioration of functioning associated with depression or depressive symptoms can be equal to or worse than that associated with severe medical conditions. The combination of advanced coronary artery disease and depressive symptoms was associated with roughly twice the reduction in social functioning as with either condition alone, suggesting that the effects of depressive symptoms and chronic medical conditions on functioning can be additive.

Major depressive disorder exacts a large toll on patients, family members, and society, because of its high level of morbidity and mortality. It may account for more bed days than any other physical disorder except cardiovascular disease, and it may be more costly to the economy than chronic respiratory illness, diabetes, arthritis, or hypertension. It has been estimated that depression and other mood disorders account for $43.7 billion in direct costs (ie, treatment) and indirect costs (ie, lost productivity through illness, absenteeism, or suicide). Before modern treatments, depressed patients typically spent one fourth of their adult lives in the hospital and fully one half of their lives disabled.

Goodwin FK, Jamison KR: *Manic Depressive Illness.* Oxford University Press, 1990.

Course & Prognosis of Illness

Major depressive disorder may be preceded by dysthymic disorder (10% in community samples, and 15–25% in clinical samples). Table 21–14 summarizes the course and prognosis of both non–bipolar disorders and bipolar disorders.

Major depressive disorder may begin at any age, with an average age at onset in the middle to late 20s. Symptoms typically develop over days to weeks, and prodromal symptoms (eg, generalized anxiety, panic attacks, phobias, subthreshold depressive symptoms) are common. Although some patients have only a single episode, with full return to premorbid functioning, approximately 50% of patients with such episodes will eventually have another episode, at which time they will meet criteria for recurrent depression.

The course of recurrent depression is variable. Some patients have a few isolated episodes separated by stable intervals (years) of normal functioning. Others have clusters of episodes, and still others have increasingly frequent episodes with shortening of the interepisode interval and generally increased disease severity. About 50% of patients with one depressive episode will have three or more episodes, and about 90% of patients who have had three episodes can be expected to have a fourth. Thus the number of past episodes can serve as a predictor of the future (ie, as

Table 21–14. Course and prognosis of mood disorders.[1]

	Non–Bipolar Disorders	Bipolar Disorders
Age at onset	38–45 years	28–33 years
Duration of episode	Before 1960: 24% develop episodes lasting more than 1 year; after 1960: 18% develop episodes lasting more than 1 year	Before 1960: 7–13 months; after 1960: 2–4 months
Recovery	5–10% do not recover from index episode	5–10% do not recover from index episode
Long-term outcome	More benign in one third of patients, length of cycle shortens with more frequent episodes	More chronic course, more episodes, length of cycle shortens with more frequent episodes
Mortality and suicide	Up to 15% commit suicide	Completed suicide occurs in 10–15% of patients with bipolar I disorder

[1] Non–bipolar disorders refers to the clinical category under which major depressive disorders are classified.

the number of recurrences increases, the episodes lengthen in duration and increase in both frequency and intensity). The average number of lifetime episodes is around five. About 5–10% of patients with an initial diagnosis of major depressive disorder subsequently develop a manic episode.

Depressive episodes may remit completely, partially, or not at all. The patient's functioning usually returns to the premorbid level between episodes, but 20–35% of patients show persistent residual symptoms and social or occupational impairment. Data from the pre-psychopharmacology era (ie, before 1960) suggest that, if untreated, a depressive episode may last about 12 months. Relapse is common. Almost 25% of patients relapse within the first 6 months of remission, especially if they have discontinued their antidepressant medications; 30–50% relapse in the first 2 years; and 50–75% relapse within the first 5 years. The risk of relapse during early remission can be reduced significantly by maintaining patients on antidepressants for at least 6 months—a regimen now generally viewed as important in managing the cycling nature of the illness.

A major depressive episode often follows acute psychosocial stressors, such as death, loss of a loved one, divorce, or acute medical illness. There is evidence that psychosocial stressors are more important in triggering or facilitating the first two depressive episodes and that their influence becomes less important in subsequent episodes.

Major depressive disorder is not a benign disease, but careful management, including early, aggressive therapeutic intervention can largely improve its otherwise poor prognosis. Although the literature on long-term outcome has produced variable results because of study design (ie, short duration of observation, focus on hospitalized episodes, exclusion of episodes preceding the index episode, and retrospective rather than prospective analysis) and different case definitions, the IOWA 500 study, involving 35 years of retrospective follow-up of patients initially presenting with a manic episode, found that outcome was good in 64% of pa-

tients, fair in 14%, and poor in 22%. Compared to well-matched patients with minor surgery or schizophrenia, the depressed patients' outcome was intermediate (ie, better than that of schizophrenic patients but worse than that of surgery patients).

Positive prognostic indicators include an absence of psychotic symptoms, a short hospitalization or duration of depression, and good family functioning. Poor prognostic indicators include a comorbid psychiatric disorder, substance abuse, early age at onset, long duration of the index episode, and inpatient hospitalization. A patient who has major depression with comorbid addiction is more likely to require hospitalization, more likely to attempt suicide, and less likely to comply with treatment than is a patient with depression of similar severity not complicated by comorbid addiction.

Clinicians have noted substantially increased mortality rates in major depressive disorder and bipolar disorder for more than 60 years. They recognized suicide as the most significant factor contributing to mortality, although other factors (eg, malnutrition, comorbid medical illness) are likely to contribute. Early studies reported up to six times the mortality rates expected for a normal population of the same age, but later studies found a less striking yet still significant increase in mortality, averaging about two times the expected rates.

II. DYSTHYMIC DISORDER

Harry E. Gwirtsman, MD, & Peter T. Loosen, MD

DSM-IV Diagnostic Criteria

A. Depressed mood for most of the day, for more days than not, as indicated either by subjective account or observation made by others, for at least 2 years.

Note: In children and adolescents, mood can be irritable and duration must be at least 1 year.

B. Presence, while depressed, of two (or more) of the following:
   (1) poor appetite or overeating
   (2) insomnia or hypersomnia
   (3) low energy or fatigue
   (4) low self-esteem
   (5) poor concentration or difficulty making decisions
   (6) feelings of hopelessness
C. During the 2-year period (1 year for children or adolescents) of the disturbance, the person has never been without the symptoms in Criteria A and B for more than 2 months at a time.
D. No major depressive episode has been present during the first 2 years of the disturbance (1 year for children and adolescents); ie, the disturbance is not better accounted for by chronic major depressive disorder, or major depressive disorder, in partial remission.

Note: There may have been a previous major depressive episode provided there was a full remission (no significant signs or symptoms for 2 months) before development of the dysthymic disorder. In addition, after the initial 2 years (1 year in children and adolescents) of dysthymic disorder, there may be superimposed episodes of major depressive disorder, in which case both diagnoses may be given when the criteria are met for a major depressive episode.

E. There has never been a manic episode, a mixed episode, or a hypomanic episode, and criteria have never been met for cyclothymic disorder.
F. The disturbance does not occur exclusively during the course of a chronic psychotic disorder, such as schizophrenia or delusional disorder.
G. The symptoms are not due to the direct effects of a substance (eg, drugs of abuse, a medication) or a general medical condition (eg, hypothyroidism).
H. The symptoms cause clinically significant distress or impairment in social, occupational, or other important areas of functioning.

Reprinted, with permission, from *Diagnostic and Statistical Manual of Mental Disorders,* 4th ed. Copyright 1994 American Psychiatric Association.

General Considerations

The term **dysthymia** is derived from the Greek word *thymos,* and its literal meaning is "disordered mood." The classic dysthymic patient has been described by Akiskal as "ill-humored . . . (having the) . . . disposition to low-grade dysphoria . . . habitually brooding, overcontentious, incapable of fun, and preoccupied with personal inadequacy" (1995, p. 1073). The term **dysthymic disorder** was first used in the *Diagnostic and Statistical Manual of Mental Disorders,* 3rd edition (DSM-III), which attempted to create a diagnostic concept under which a heterogeneous group of disorders previously referred to as depressive

neurosis could be subsumed. The creation of this diagnostic entity as separate from major depressive disorder has been an impetus for increased research activity.

Despite our improved understanding of this condition, dysthymic disorder, as Max Hamilton stated just before his death in 1989, "lies on the border between the normal and pathological." Because patients with dysthymic disorder experience symptoms that are of a lower intensity than those associated with major depression, the term **subsyndromal mood disorder** has been applied. In a rural primary care population, 3.8–6.0% of patients were classified as having low-grade or intermittent depressions according to research diagnostic criteria (which were used mainly for research purposes and preceded the development of the DSM-III), and almost twice as many patients (11.2%) had a psychiatric disorder with significant depressive symptomatology that did not fit into a specific depressive disorder category. (The diagnosis of intermittent depression using research diagnostic criteria can be seen as the precursor of the diagnosis of dysthymic disorder in DSM-III.) The data suggest that dysthymic disorder is the tip of a very large iceberg of subsyndromal mood states.

A. Major Etiologic Theories:

1. Life events—Personality features may be involved in the pathogenesis of dysthymic disorder. Psychoanalytic theorists have stressed the concept of inordinate interpersonal dependency, in which the patient's self-esteem is excessively reliant on approval, reassurance, attention, and love from others. Thus when such interpersonal concern from others wanes or terminates, depression ensues.

Cognitive theorists ascribe the symptoms of depression to disordered basic cognitive schema, or dysfunctional thoughts, that are developed early in life. The learned helplessness model holds that after repeated, inescapable shock, experimental animals will not initiate avoidance from aversive stimuli, even when avenues of escape are readily available. Even when faced with major traumatic events and losses, most people do not progress from grief to pathologic depression, suggesting that adverse life events and an underlying vulnerability interact to produce symptoms of chronic depression. It is also true that mood disorders create adverse conditions, such as separation, divorce, and suicide. When such conditions occur in parents, an already predisposed child is exposed to environmentally determined object losses that might precipitate more severe illness or earlier onset of depressive episodes.

2. Biological theories—Family studies demonstrate that patients with dysthymic disorder and patients with major depression exhibit similar rates of mood disorders in first-degree relatives. Patients with dysthymic disorder also exhibit shortened REM latency during sleep onset, as do patients with major depression. Thus there may be a biological or familial relationship between these two disorders.

Personality inventories of patients with dysthymic disorder often reveal a disturbed personality structure; dependent, avoidant, borderline, and narcissistic personality disorders are the most common. Little is known about the exact biological determinants of dysthymic disorder. Many dysthymic individuals respond well to antidepressants, although the percentage of those who respond and the magnitude of their response are generally less than that observed in patients with major depression.

B. Epidemiology: Table 21–15 summarizes the relevant risk factors. The lifetime prevalence of dysthymic disorder in the general population (3.2%) is exceeded only by that for major depression (4.9%). Even more dramatic are the 1-month point prevalence rate estimates from the Epidemiologic Catchment Area (ECA) survey, which at 3.3% rank dysthymic disorder second only to phobia and more common than alcoholism and all other mental disorders assessed. The protracted course of dysthymic disorder makes it the most commonly encountered form of mood disorder. It affects women more often than men, with a ratio of nearly 2 to 1. Dysthymic disorder usually sets in before the age of 45 years. Although dysthymic disorder appears to be the least common among African Americans (2.5%), the ECA survey noted the largest number of depressive and dysthymic symptoms in that population. This finding may imply either denial of illness by some respondents or a higher rate of subsyndromal mood disorder (currently diagnosed as depressive disorder not otherwise specified or the proposed depressive personality disorder).

C. Genetics: Family studies support a genetic link between dysthymic disorder and major depression. Twin studies have not corroborated a strong relationship between dysthymic disorder and other personality disorders, with the exception of the depressive personality disorder. Depressive personality disorder is a construct noted in the DSM-IV, in which individuals demonstrate a pervasive pattern of depressive cognitions and behaviors beginning in early adulthood but do not develop dysthymic disorder or major depressive episodes. Depressive personality disorder may be a condition that subsumes the persistent trait-like qualities of the depressive disorders. Preliminary evidence from family studies indicates that this disorder is related to the major mood disorders such as dysthymic disorder.

Thus far, research has not identified any specific gene or set of genes associated with dysthymic disorder.

Akiskal HS: Mood disorders: Introduction and overview. In: Kaplan HI, Sadock BJ (editors): *Comprehensive Textbook of Psychiatry.* Vol 1, 6th ed. Williams & Wilkins, 1995.

Barrett JE et al: The prevalence of psychiatric disorders in a primary care practice. Arch Gen Psychiatry 1988; 45:1100.

Hamilton M: Foreword. In: Burton SW, Akiskal HS (editors): *Dysthymic Disorder.* Royal College of Psychiatrists, 1990.

Kessler RC: Dysthymia in the community and its comorbidity with psychiatric and substance use disorders. NIMH Sponsored Workshop: Subsyndromal Mood Disorders: Dysthymia and Cyclothymia. Bethesda, MD, April 26, 1993.

Regier DA et al: One-month prevalence of mental disorders in the United States. Arch Gen Psychiatry 1988;45:977.

Weissman MN, Livingston Bruce M, Leaf PJ, Florio LP, Holzer C: Affective Disorders. Pages 53-80 in Robins LN, Regier DA (editors): *Psychiatric Disorders in America.* Free Press, 1991.

Clinical Findings

A. Signs & Symptoms: Although there has been some controversy concerning the symptoms that best define dysthymic disorder, recent studies suggest that the symptoms most commonly encountered in dysthymic disorder may be those found in the alternative DSM-IV research criterion B for dysthymic disorder (Table 21–16).

In children, dysthymic disorder often results in impaired social interaction and school performance. Children and adolescents with dysthymic disorder are usually irritable, pessimistic, cranky, and depressed and have low self-esteem and poor social skills.

B. Psychological Testing: Patients with dysthymic disorder have increased scores for neuroticism and introversion on the Maudsley Personality Inventory; these abnormalities persist even after recovery.

C. Laboratory Findings & Imaging: About 25–50% of adults with dysthymic disorder have EEG abnormalities similar to those found in major depressive disorder (eg, reduced REM latency, increased

Table 21–15. Risk factors for dysthymic disorder.

Familial pattern	Dysthymic disorder is more common among first-degree relatives of people with major depression than among the general population.
Social class	No relationship.
Race	Possibly low occurrence in African Americans (2.5% versus 3.3% in whites).

Table 21–16. Symptoms most commonly encountered in dysthymic disorder.[1]

Low self-esteem or self-confidence, or feelings of inadequacy
Feelings of pessimism, despair, or hopelessness
Generalized loss of interest or pleasure
Social withdrawal
Chronic fatigue or tiredness
Feelings of guilt, brooding about past
Subjective feelings of irritability or excessive anger
Decreased activity, effectiveness, or productivity
Difficulty in thinking, reflected by poor concentration, poor memory, or indecisiveness

[1] Modified and reproduced, with permission, from *Diagnostic and Statistical Manual of Mental Disorders,* 4th ed. Copyright 1994 American Psychiatric Association.

REM density, reduced slow-wave sleep, impaired sleep continuity). Dysthymic patients with these abnormalities have a positive family history for major depressive disorder more often than do patients without these abnormalities; they also appear to respond better to antidepressant medications. It is not clear whether EEG abnormalities can also be observed in patients with pure dysthymic disorder (ie, in those with no history of major depressive episodes). An abnormal DST is not common in dysthymic disorder, unless criteria are also met for a major depressive episode.

Differential Diagnosis

Major depressive disorder usually consists of one or more discrete episodes of depression that can be distinguished, by both onset and duration, from the person's usual functioning. During these episodes vegetative symptoms such as insomnia, loss of appetite, loss of libido, weight loss, and psychomotor symptoms are common. In contrast, dysthymic disorder is characterized by chronic, less severe depressive symptoms that can persist for 2 or more years; vegetative symptoms are less common in dysthymic disorder than in major depressive disorder.

Depressive symptoms may be associated with chronic psychotic disorders and are not considered to indicate dysthymic disorder if they occur only during the course of the psychotic disorder (including residual phases). If mood disturbance is judged to be the direct physiologic consequence of a specific, usually chronic, general medical condition (eg, multiple sclerosis), then the diagnosis is mood disorder due to a general medical condition. Similarly, substance-induced mood disorder is diagnosed when the depressive symptoms are thought to result from the ingestion of a drug of abuse or a medication or from exposure to a toxin.

Treatment

A. Pharmacologic Treatments: Substantial evidence from controlled treatment trials indicates that antidepressants are useful in the treatment of dysthymic disorder, with or without comorbid major depression (Table 21–17). TCAs, MAOIs, and SSRIs all appear to be effective treatments. Rates of response have varied, and there is currently no information assessing the rates of response to a second antidepressant if the first trial was unsuccessful. Controlled maintenance treatment studies are under way. Most dys-

thymic patients, if they respond to an antidepressant, require continued treatment for at least 6–12 months.

Because dysthymic patients with mild symptoms are not likely to tolerate side effects, the clinician should initiate treatment with an SSRI, because it produces less anticholinergic and sedating side effects and less weight gain. This is particularly important in women receiving long-term treatment. SSRIs can produce a number of mild and time-limited side effects, including gastrointestinal symptoms, insomnia, nervousness, sweating, tremor, dizziness, occasional somnolence, and sexual dysfunction. In patients who do not respond to SSRIs, imipramine and desipramine are effective. Among nonselective MAOIs, phenelzine is particularly beneficial for those with atypical reversed vegetative symptoms (eg, hypersomnia, hyperphagia).

Many of the controlled medication trials reported only partial responses in some subjects with dysthymic disorder. Such patients might benefit from augmentation with a second antidepressant, lithium, thyroid hormone, or combined treatment with psychotherapy. However, there have been no controlled studies of pharmacologic augmentation strategies, nor of combined pharmacotherapy and psychotherapy approaches.

B. Nonpharmacologic Treatments: Although antidepressants are effective in treating dysthymic disorder, a substantial proportion of patients either fail to respond or are unable to tolerate the side effects. Psychotherapy should be used to address impairments in social and occupational functioning, chronic pessimism and hopelessness, and lack of assertiveness (see Table 21–17). Interpersonal psychotherapy and cognitive-behavioral therapy are useful in treating major depression. Recent modifications of these approaches for dysthymic disorder have been investigated in small naturalistic studies, with successful results. Both therapies are typically time-limited (ie, lasting less than 6 months).

Interpersonal psychotherapy emphasizes the interaction between the individual and his or her psychosocial environment. Interpersonal psychotherapy has the dual therapeutic goals of reducing depressive symptoms and developing more effective strategies for dealing with social and interpersonal relations. As applied to dysthymic disorder, interpersonal psychotherapy has a major focus on the therapeutic rela-

Table 21–17. Treatment of dysthymic disorder.

Treatment Approach	Primary Method	Secondary Methods
Behavioral	Interpersonal psychotherapy, cognitive-behavioral therapy	None
Pharmacologic	SSRIs (eg, fluoxetine, paroxetine, sertraline, venlafaxine)[1]	TCAs (eg, desipramine, nortriptyline), MAOIs (eg, phenelzine)[1]

[1] See Table 21–6 for the normal dosage range.
[2] MAOIs, monoamine oxidase inhibitors; SSRIs, selective serotonin reuptake inhibitors; TCAs, tricyclic antidepressants.

tionship, which is used as a model for other interpersonal interactions. The therapist encourages the patient to engage in occupational and social activities and helps the patient to identify personal needs, to assert those needs, and to set limits.

Cognitive-behavioral therapy is based on the assertion that depression is associated with negative thought patterns, cognitive errors, and faulty information processing that can be altered by specific psychotherapeutic strategies. These strategies help the patient to identify and test negative cognitions and to replace them with alternative, more flexible schemata, which are subsequently rehearsed and studied. As applied to dysthymic disorder, chronic beliefs of helplessness and lack of control are challenged and modified by the experience of mastery in producing desired outcomes, especially in the area of interactions with others.

Charney DS, Berman RM, Miller HL: Treatment of depression. In: Schatzberg AF, Nemeroff CB (editors): *Textbook of Psychopharmacology,* 2nd ed. American Psychiatric Press, 1998.

Harrison WA, Stewart JW: Pharmacotherapy of dysthymia. Psychiatr Ann 1993;23:638.

Hirschfeld RMA, Shea MT: Mood disorders: psychosocial treatments. Pages 1178–1187 in Kaplan HI, Sadock BJ (editors): *Comprehensive Textbook of Psychiatry,* 6th ed. Williams & Wilkins, 1995.

Complications, Comorbidity, & Adverse Outcomes of Treatment

Pure dysthymic disorder without prior major depressive disorder is a risk factor for developing major depressive disorder. Ten percent of patients with pure dysthymic disorder will develop major depressive disorder over the ensuing year. In clinical settings, individuals with dysthymic disorder frequently have superimposed major depressive disorder, which is often the reason for seeking treatment.

The condition that cooccurs most frequently with dysthymic disorder is major depressive disorder. The ECA studies estimated that 3.5% of the population had major depression only, 1.8% had dysthymic disorder only, and 1.4% of the population had both disorders, or double depression, at some point in their lives. Moreover, major depressive disorder occurred in 42% of patients with dysthymic disorder, and dysthymic disorders occurred in 28% of patients with major depressive disorder.

The National Comorbidity Survey (NCS) has confirmed that patients with dysthymic disorder have high rates of coexisting psychopathology. In that sample, only 8% of dysthymic patients were unaffected by another Axis I disorder. Besides major depression, the NCS revealed high rates of social phobia, posttraumatic stress disorder, and generalized anxiety disorder. Eating disorders, especially bulimia nervosa, are also associated with nonendogenous depression of only moderate severity. Furthermore, subjective observations and objective investigations have found that depressive symptoms in bulimia are highly reactive, unstable, short lived, and temporally related to bingeing and purging episodes.

Chronic mood symptoms can contribute to interpersonal problems or be associated with distorted self-perception. Thus the assessment of features of a personality disorder is difficult in such individuals. Nevertheless, concomitant personality disorders—especially cluster C personality diagnosis (ie, avoidant, obsessive-compulsive, and dependent)—can complicate dysthymic disorder. The disorder can also be associated with the cluster B personality diagnoses (ie, borderline, histrionic, and narcissistic).

Other chronic Axis I disorders (eg, substance dependence) or chronic psychosocial stressors can be associated with dysthymic disorder in adults. In children, dysthymic disorder can be comorbid with attention-deficit/hyperactivity disorder (ADHD), conduct disorder, anxiety disorders, learning disorders, and mental retardation.

Kessler RC: Dysthymia in the community and its comorbidity with psychiatric and substance use disorders. NIMH Sponsored Workshop: Subsyndromal Mood Disorders: Dysthymia and Cyclothymia. Bethesda, MD, April 26, 1993.

Weissman MN, Livingston Bruce M, Leaf PJ, Florio LP, Holzer C: Affective Disorders. Pages 53-80 in Robins LN, Regier DA (editors): *Psychiatric Disorders in America.* Free Press, 1991.

Prognosis & Course of Illness

Dysthymic disorder often has an early and insidious onset (ie, in childhood, adolescence, or early adult life) and a chronic course. Disease onset is usually before age 45, but a sizable subgroup of patients develop the disorder in late life (45% after age 45, and 19% after age 65). If dysthymic disorder precedes the onset of major depressive disorder, there is less probability that there will be spontaneous full recovery between major depressive episodes and a greater likelihood of having more frequent subsequent major depressive episodes.

The outcome literature of dysthymic disorder is not encouraging: Of dysthymic inpatients, only about 40% recovered after 2 years of follow-up, and only about 30% after 5 years of follow-up. Thus one can conclude that the available treatments for dysthymic disorder, as currently delivered, are only modestly effective and that relapse is quite common.

III. BIPOLAR DISORDERS

Sam R. Sells, MD, & Peter T. Loosen, MD

DSM-IV Diagnostic Criteria

Hypomanic Episode

A. A distinct period of abnormally and persistently elevated, expansive, or irritable mood lasting at least

1 week (or any duration if hospitalization is necessary).

B. During the period of mood disturbance, three (or more) of the following symptoms have persisted (four if the mood is only irritable) and have been present to a significant degree:

(1) inflated self-esteem or grandiosity

(2) decreased need for sleep (eg, feels rested after only 3 hours of sleep)

(3) more talkative than usual or pressure to keep talking

(4) flight of ideas or subjective experience that thoughts are racing

(5) distractibility (ie, attention too easily drawn to unimportant or irrelevant external stimuli)

(6) increase in goal-directed activity (either socially, at work or school, or sexually) or psychomotor agitation

(7) excessive involvement in pleasurable activities that have a high potential for painful consequences (eg, engaging in unrestrained buying sprees, sexual indiscretions, or foolish business investments)

C. The symptoms do not meet the criteria for a mixed episode.

D. The mood disturbance is sufficiently severe to cause marked impairment in occupational functioning or in usual social activities or relationships with others, or to necessitate hospitalization to prevent harm to self or others, or there are psychotic features.

E. The symptoms are not due to the direct physiological effects of a substance (eg, a drug of abuse, a medication, or other treatment) or a general medical condition (eg, hyperthyroidism).

Note: Manic-like episodes that are clearly caused by somatic antidepressant treatment (eg, medication, electroconvulsive treatment, light therapy) should not count toward a diagnosis of bipolar I disorder.

Reprinted, with permission, from *Diagnostic and Statistical Manual of Mental Disorders,* 4th ed. Copyright 1994 American Psychiatric Association.

General Considerations

Bipolar disorders can be conceptualized into three distinct entities: **bipolar I disorder,** consisting of episodes of mania cycling with depressive episodes; **bipolar II disorder,** consisting of episodes of hypomania cycling with depressive episodes; and **cyclothymic disorder,** consisting of hypomania and less severe episodes of depression (see section on Cyclothymic Disorder later in this chapter). Very few patients have only manic episodes.

A. Major Etiologic Theories: Despite intensive attempts to establish its etiologic or pathophysiologic basis, the precise cause of bipolar disorder is not known. As in major depressive disorder, there is consensus that multiple etiologic factors—genetic, bio-chemical, psychodynamic, and socioenvironmental—may interact in complex ways.

1. Life events—Although psychosocial stressors can occasionally precede the onset of bipolar disorder, there is no clear association between life events and the onset of manic or hypomanic episodes.

2. Biological theories—

a. Neurotransmitters. Neurotransmitter theories initially conceptualized that depression and mania are on the opposite ends of the same continuum. For example, the norepinephrine hypothesis of affective illness centered around the availability of norepinephrine at synaptic sites, with less norepinephrine being available in depression, and more in mania. This theory, and later modifications of it, especially as they pertain to the separation of unipolar and bipolar disorders, are discussed earlier in this chapter.

b. Neuroendocrine factors. Abnormalities in the HPA axis and, more so, in the HPT axis are common in bipolar disorder; they are discussed later in this section.

3. Psychosocial theories—Psychosocial theories pertaining to the etiology of bipolar disorders are the same as those described for major depressive disorder (see section on Major Depressive Disorder earlier in this chapter).

a. Kindling. Environmental conditions contribute more to the timing of a bipolar episode than to the patient's underlying vulnerability. In other words, more stressful life events appear to precede early episodes than later ones, and there is a pattern of increased frequency over time. It is possible that early precipitating events merely activate preexisting vulnerability, thereby making an individual more vulnerable for future episodes.

This clinical observation is supported conceptually by the **kindling model.** In laboratory animals, repeated kindling of the amygdala will lead to the development of a spontaneous seizure disorder, in which seizures occur without external stimulation. Applied to bipolar disorder, this model provides a better understanding of several phenomena inherent in the illness, including the above-mentioned effects of repeated episodes on disease severity and outcome (eg, rapid-cycling bipolar disorder usually develops late in the course of the illness) and the acute and prophylactic treatment effects of ECT and anticonvulsants such as carbamazepine and valproic acid. Because these therapies inhibit kindling in laboratory animals, their therapeutic effect in bipolar disorder may involve interruption of kindling.

The kindling model also has enormous treatment implications. Because it suggests that preventing or treating early episodes will favorably affect outcome, it stresses the need for early identification and intervention techniques. This pertains particularly to younger patients, because the risk of kindling is highest during adolescence.

B. Epidemiology: Table 21–18 summarizes the relevant risk factors. Among the key risk factors for

Table 21–18. Risk factors for bipolar disorder.[1]

Social class	Found more frequently in the upper socioeconomic class.
Race	No relationship.
Life events	No relationship.
Personality	No relationship.
Childhood experience	No relationship.
Marital status	Data not uniform.
Family history	Bipolar patients have both bipolar and unipolar first-degree relatives in roughly equal proportions.

[1] Modified and reproduced, with permission, from Paykel ES: *Handbook of Affective Disorders.* Guilford Press, 1982; and from Robins LN, Regier DA: *Psychiatric Disorders in America. The Epidemiologic Catchment Area Study.* Free Press, 1991.

bipolar disorder are being female, having a family history of bipolar disorder, and coming from an upper socioeconomic class. Data also suggest that people under age 50 years are at higher risk of a first attack of bipolar disorder, whereas someone who already has the disorder faces an increasing risk of a recurrent manic or depressive episode as he or she grows older.

Epidemiologic Catchment Area (ECA) studies support a lifetime prevalence of bipolar disorder ranging from 0.6% to 1.1% (between 0.8% and 1.1% in men, and between 0.5% and 1.3% in women). Estimates from community samples range from 0.4% to 1.6%. The disorder affects over 3 million persons in the United States. Bipolar disorder accounts for one quarter of all mood disorders. It is likely that prevalence rates of bipolar disorders are underestimated, because of problems in identifying manic and, more so, hypomanic episodes.

Bipolar disorders are about equally distributed among males and females, but there are more females with more serious bipolar disorder, especially rapid-cycling bipolar disorder. Higher rates of hypothyroidism, greater use of antidepressant medication, and changes in reproductive status and gonadal steroids may account for the greater prevalence of rapid-cycling bipolar disorder among women.

Approximately 10–15% of adolescents with recurrent major depression will go on to develop bipolar I disorder. Mixed episodes appear to be more likely in adolescents and young adults than in older adults. An age at onset for a first manic episode after age 40 years should alert the clinician to the possibility that the symptoms may be due to a general medical condition or substance use. Bipolar disorder is often misdiagnosed in adolescents (eg, as ADHD). Patients with early-onset bipolar disorder are more likely to display psychotic symptoms and to have a poorer prognosis in terms of lifetime outcome.

Mood disorders often have seasonal patterns. Acute episodes of depression are common in spring and fall, whereas mania appears to cluster in the summer months. Corresponding data on suicides also show a peak in the spring and a (smaller) peak in the late fall.

C. Genetics: Twin and family studies provide strong evidence for a genetic component in bipolar disorder, but the precise mechanisms of inheritance are not known. In monozygotic twins, the concordance rate is higher for bipolar disorder (80%) than for unipolar disorder (54%). In dizygotic twins, concordance rates are 24% for bipolar disorder and 19% for unipolar disorder. Adoption studies have shown that the biological children of affected parents have an increased risk for developing a mood disorder, even when reared by unaffected parents, although the data are not uniform. Finally, first-degree biological relatives of bipolar I patients have elevated rates of bipolar I disorder (4–20%), bipolar II disorder (1–5%), and major depressive disorder (4–24%).

Ahmed N, Loosen PT: Thyroid hormones in major depressive and bipolar disorders. In: Casper R (editor): *Women's Health and Emotion.* Cambridge University Press, 1997.

Arana GW, Baldessarini RJ, Ornsteen M: The dexamethasone suppression test for diagnosis and prognosis in psychiatry. Commentary and review. Arch Gen Psychiatry 1985;42:1193.

Boyd JH, Weissman MM: Epidemiology. Pages 109–125 in Paykel ES (editor): *Handbook of Affective Disorders.* Guilford Press, 1982.

Goodwin FK, Jamison KR: *Manic Depressive Illness.* Oxford University Press, 1990.

Musselman DL et al: Biology of mood disorders. In: Schatzberg AF, Nemeroff CB (editors): *Textbook of Psychopharmacology,* 2nd ed. American Psychiatric Press, 1998.

Weissman MN, Livingston Bruce M, Leaf PJ, Florio LP, Holzer C: Affective Disorders. Pages 53-80 in Robins LN, Regier DA (editors): *Psychiatric Disorders in America.* Free Press, 1991.

Clinical Findings

A. Signs & Symptoms: Bipolar disorders can be subdivided into two diagnostic entities: bipolar I disorder (recurrent major depressive episodes with manic episodes) and bipolar II disorder (recurrent major depressive episodes with hypomanic episodes). The symptoms of both bipolar disorders involve changes in mood, cognition, and behavior (Table 21–19).

Table 21–19. Stages of mania.[1]

	Stage I	Stage II	Stage III
Mood	Labile affect; euphoria predominates; irritability if demands not satisfied	Increased dysphoria and depression; open hostility and anger	Very dysphoric; panic-stricken; hopeless
Cognition	Expansive, grandiose, overconfident; thoughts coherent but occasionally tangential; sexual and religious preoccupation; racing thoughts	Flight of ideas; disorganization of cognition; delusions	Incoherent, definite loosening of associations; bizarre and idiosyncratic delusions; hallucinations in one third of patients; disorientation to time and place; occasional ideas of reference
Behavior	Increased psychomotor activity; increased rate of speech; increased spending, smoking, telephone use	Increased psychomotor activity; pressured speech; occasional assaultive behavior	Frenzied, frequently bizarre psychomotor activity

[1] Adapted, with permission, from Goodwin FK, Jamison KR: *Manic Depressive Illness.* Oxford University Press, 1990.

1. Bipolar I disorder—Episodes typically begin suddenly, with a rapid escalation through the stages summarized in Table 21–19. In 50–60% of cases, a depressive episode immediately precedes or follows a manic episode. Pure (or monopolar) mania is very rare. The hallmark of a manic episode is abnormally and persistently elevated, expansive, or irritable mood. The elevated mood can be described as euphoric, cheerful, and with indiscriminate enthusiasm and optimism; therefore, others often perceive it as infectious. Although the patient's mood may be predominantly elevated, it may quickly become irritable, especially after demands are not satisfied.

a. Somatic features. Bipolar patients' sleep varies with their clinical state. When depressed, bipolar patients may sleep too much; when manic, they sleep little or not at all and typically report feeling fully rested nevertheless. As the manic episode intensifies, patients may go without sleep for nights, their insomnia further intensifying the manic syndrome. There is speculation as to whether the insomnia precedes, and perhaps triggers or fuels, the manic episode. It is difficult to control an acute manic episode clinically if one cannot control the associated insomnia. Conversely, some bipolar patients may experience a manic or hypomanic episode after a single night of sleep deprivation.

b. Behavioral features. Patients are initially social, outgoing, self-confident, and talkative and can be difficult to interrupt. Their speech is full of puns, jokes, and irrelevancies. Patients are often hypersexual, promiscuous, disinhibited, and seductive; they may present to an emergency room setting dressed in colorful, flamboyant, and inappropriate clothing. As the manic episode intensifies, their speech becomes loud, intrusive, rapid, and difficult to follow, and they can become irritable, assaultive, and threatening.

c. Cognitive features. Manic patients are easily distracted. Their thought processes are difficult to follow because of racing thoughts and flight of ideas.

They appear to have an unrestrained and accelerated flow of thoughts and ideas, which are often unrelated. Patients can be overly self-confident and become preoccupied with political, personal, religious, and sexual themes. They may exhibit an inappropriate increase in self-esteem and open grandiosity. Their judgment is impaired significantly, resulting in buying sprees, sexual indiscretions, and unwise business investments. Psychotic features such as paranoia, delusions, and hallucinations are often present, not unlike those seen in patients with schizophrenia.

d. Risk of suicide. Bipolar patients are at a substantial risk for suicide, with a mortality rate 2–3 times higher than the general population. Evidence indicates that lithium maintenance treatment can markedly attenuate the risk of suicide attempts and completions. When 16,800 bipolar patients were followed for a 2-year period, the annual risk of suicide or suicide attempts was 0.26 ± 0.4 with lithium and 1.68 ± 1.5 without lithium. Risk factors for suicide among bipolar patients include previous suicide attempts, comorbid substance abuse, mixed episode, current depressive episode, and a history of rapid-cycling bipolar disorder.

2. Bipolar II disorder—Characterized by recurrent episodes of major depression and hypomania, bipolar II disorder has been identified as a distinct disorder only in DSM-IV. Hypomanic symptoms are similar to manic symptoms but typically do not reach the same level of symptom severity or social impairment (ie, the patient's capacity to function vocationally is seldom compromised). Hypomania, though associated with, say, elated mood and increased self-assuredness, does not usually present with psychotic symptoms, racing thoughts, or marked psychomotor agitation. Hypomanic patients thus do not perceive themselves as being ill and are likely to minimize their symptoms and to resist treatment.

3. Rapid-cycling bipolar disorder—By definition, patients with rapid-cycling bipolar disorder experience four or more affective episodes per year. Approximately 10–15% of bipolar patients experience rapid cycling. Although similar to other bipolar patients nosologically and demographically, patients with rapid-cycling bipolar disorder tend to have a longer duration of illness, and the illness has a more refractory course. Women are represented disproportionately, making up 80–95% of rapid-cycling patients, compared to about 50% of non-rapid-cycling patients. A variety of factors may predispose bipolar illness to a rapid-cycling course, including treatment with TCAs, MAOIs, lithium, and antipsychotics. The development of clinical or subclinical hypothyroidism (spontaneously or during lithium treatment) in a manic patient predisposes to a more rapidly cycling course. The kindling hypothesis, invoked to conceptualize these changes pathophysiologically, receives further confirmation by the clinical usefulness of the anticonvulsants valproic acid and carbamazepine.

B. Laboratory Findings & Imaging: No laboratory findings are diagnostic of a bipolar disorder or of a manic or hypomanic episode; however, several laboratory findings have been noted to be abnormal in groups of individuals with bipolar disorder. Compared to the wealth of findings in major depressive disorder, research findings in bipolar disorder are in general scarce and inconclusive. For one thing, bipolar disorder is not as common as major depressive disorder. Beyond that, patients with acute manic states are not as likely to collaborate in research studies; they experience lack of insight, agitation, irritability, and racing thoughts, among other symptoms; and they are normally in need of rapid containment of symptoms.

1. Hypothalamic-pituitary-adrenal axis—The few available cross-sectional and longitudinal studies reveal increased plasma cortisol levels in some depressed bipolar patients. Abnormalities in the DST have also been noted. DST nonsuppression occurs more frequently in the mixed phase of the illness (78%) but also occurs in bipolar depression (38%) and mania (49%). Both hypercortisolemia and DST results normalize after the acute episode subsides, suggesting that these abnormalities are state and not trait dependent. Although these abnormalities are not specific for bipolar disorder or even major depression, their pathophysiology is suggestive of central (ie, hypothalamic) rather than peripheral dysregulation of cortisol.

2. Hypothalamic-pituitary-thyroid axis—HPT axis abnormalities are rather common in bipolar disorder, especially in rapid-cycling bipolar disorder, but the precise relationship of these abnormalities with the illness and its various clinical presentations is not known. Among these abnormalities are an attenuated nocturnal TSH peak, a blunted TSH response to TRH administration, and a high prevalence of various degrees of hypothyroidism.

There are intriguing associations among thyroid function, bipolar disorder, and gender. Hypothy-roidism is very common in patients with bipolar disorder; it is especially common in female patients who present with a rapid-cycling course. Treatment with hypermetabolic doses of T_4 has shown some promise in that it may reduce acute symptoms, number of relapses, and duration of hospitalizations.

Two main conclusions can be drawn from these observations. Clinically, comorbid hypothyroidism seems to negatively affect disease outcome by predisposing the individual patient to a rapid-cycling course. Substitution with T_4 has proven useful in some patients, but often high doses are necessary to induce clinical response. Conceptually these findings support the hypothesis that a relative central thyroid hormone deficit may predispose to the marked and frequent mood swings that characterize rapid-cycling bipolar disorder. We may ask whether the central thyroid hormone deficit serves only as a risk factor for the development of rapid cycling in a known bipolar patient, or whether it can predispose most affectively ill patients to any major behavioral change (ie, the switch from depression into recovery, from recovery into depression, or from depression into mania).

3. Sleep electroencephalogram—Sleep EEG recordings have revealed normal results in acutely ill bipolar patients, including normal REM latencies, but not all studies agree. These data, of course, are in stark contrast to those reported in major depressive disorder, in which shortened REM latencies are common. However, bipolar patients in full clinical remission can exhibit an increased density and percentage of REM and a sleep architecture more sensitive to arecoline (an acetylcholine agonist known to produce a shortened REM latency). The discrepancies between unipolar and bipolar patients are thought to be the result of different levels of clinical severity, variable proportions of bipolar I and bipolar II patients, and age differences.

4. Brain imaging—Patients with right (ie, nondominant) frontotemporal or left (ie, dominant) parieto-occipital lesions are especially vulnerable to mania or hypomania. These observations are consistent with the literature on laterality, which indicates right-sided dysfunction in mania. It is not known whether manic symptoms occurring after such lesions represent a new emergence of mania, or whether the lesions triggered a manic episode in vulnerable individuals.

Ahmed N, Loosen PT: Thyroid hormones in major depressive and bipolar disorders. In: Casper R (editor): *Women's Health and Emotion.* Cambridge University Press, 1997.

Arana GW, Baldessarini RJ, Ornsteen M: The dexamethasone suppression test for diagnosis and prognosis in psychiatry; commentary and review. Arch Gen Psychiatry 1985;42:1193.

Bauer MS, Whybrow PC: Thyroid hormones and the central nervous system in affective illness: interactions that may have clinical significance. Integr Psychiatry 1988;6:75.

Goodwin FK, Jamison KR: *Manic Depressive Illness.* Oxford University Press, 1990.

Musselman DL, et al: Biology of mood disorders. In: Schatzberg AF, Nemeroff CB (editors): *Textbook of Psychopharmacology,* 2nd ed. American Psychiatric Press, 1998.

Differential Diagnosis

A. Medical Disorders: Numerous medical disorders and medications can induce or mimic the clinical picture of bipolar disorder, exacerbate its course and severity, or complicate its treatment. It has been widely noted that psychopharmacologic interventions are less successful if the bipolar disorder is due to a primary medical condition; whenever possible, it is advisable to attempt to correct the underlying medical disorder before beginning psychopharmacologic treatment.

DSM-IV criteria specify that to make a diagnosis of bipolar disorder, the symptoms cannot be the direct result of a substance or a general medical condition. A late onset of the first manic episode (over age 50) should prompt the clinician to carefully exclude a possible medical cause. Table 21–20 lists the many organic causes of mania and hypomania.

B. Psychiatric Disorders: The Axis I and Axis II disorders associated with hypomanic or manic symptoms need to be included in the differential diagnosis of bipolar disorders (Table 21–21). First, the psychotic features associated with schizophrenia or schizoaffective disorder are often indistinguishable from those associated with acute mania. Second, major depressive episodes may be associated prominently with irritable mood and may thus be difficult to distinguish from a mixed bipolar episode. Third, in children and adolescents, ADHD and mania are both characterized by overactivity, impulsive behavior, poor judgment and academic performance, and psychological denial. Fourth, patients with certain personality disorders (eg, borderline or histrionic personality disorders) can exhibit impulsivity, affective instability, and paranoid ideations, as do manic patients.

Finally, substance abuse is exceedingly common in patients with bipolar disorder. As many as 41% of bipolar patients abuse or are dependent on drugs, 46% abuse or are dependent on alcohol, and as many as 61% abuse or are dependent on any substance. Careful etiologic evaluation, and a drug-free washout period after intoxication, are often necessary to distinguish whether the mood disturbance is the consequence of substance abuse or whether the substance abuse is the consequence of a mood disturbance. Such differentiation is important because psychiatric comorbidity complicates the acute manic

---

Table 21–20. Organic causes of mania and hypomania.[1]

Medications	**Neurologic disorders**
Anticonvulsants	Huntington's disease
Barbiturates	Multiple sclerosis
Benzodiazepines	Poststroke
Bromide	Right hemisphere damage
Bronchodilators	Right temporal lobe seizures
Calcium replacement	Seizure disorders
Cimetidine	
Cocaine	**Infectious diseases**
Corticosteroids and adrenocorticotropic hormone	Herpes simplex encephalitis
Decongestants	HIV infection
Disulfiram	Influenza
L-Dopa	Neurosyphilis
Hallucinogens	Q fever
Isoniazid	
Metoclopramide	**Neoplasms**
Phencyclidine	Diencephalic glioma
Procarbazine	Parasagittal meningioma
Procyclidine	Right intraventricular meningioma
Sympathomimetic amines	Right temporoparietal occipital metastases
Tricyclic antidepressants	Suprasellar craniopharyngioma
	Tumor of floor of the fourth ventricle
Metabolic disturbances	
Addison's disease	**Other conditions**
Dialysis	Delirium
Hemodialysis	Post-ECT
Hyperthyroidism	Postisolation syndrome
Iatrogenic Cushing's disease	Posttraumatic confusion
Postinfection states	Right temporal lobectomy
Postoperative states	Serotonin syndrome
Vitamin B_{12}	

[1] Modified and reproduced, with permission, from Goodwin FK, Jamison KR: *Manic Depressive Illness.* Oxford University Press, 1990.

Table 21–21. Axis I and Axis II disorders that may be associated with manic or hypomanic symptoms.

Axis I
Attention-deficit/hyperactivity disorder
Conduct disorder
Cyclothymic disorder
Delirium
Delusional disorders
Dementia
Factitious disorder
Malingering
Psychotic disorder not otherwise specified
Schizoaffective disorder
Schizophrenia
Substance-related disorders

Axis II
Borderline personality disorder
Histrionic personality disorder

state and negatively affects disease outcome. The mood disorders complicated by substance abuse are therefore treated in units especially designed to treat aspects of dual diagnosis.

Treatment

The clinical management of bipolar disorder involves treatment of the acute episodes and maintenance therapy. Acute bipolar episodes usually demand immediate symptom containment, which is achieved most easily using pharmacologic means (Table 21–22). Acute depressive episodes are treated best with SSRIs or bupropion, because these medications are less likely to trigger the switch into mania or hypomania frequently caused by TCAs. Acute manic episodes can be managed with lithium, valproic acid, or carbamazepine. If delusional symptoms and agitation are present, antipsychotics (eg, haloperidol) or benzodiazepines (eg, clonazepam) need to be added. Maintenance treatment of bipolar disorder, aimed at course stabilization and prevention of further episodes, includes lithium, valproic acid, or carbamazepine.

Most patients are likely to receive a combination of drugs (eg, lithium and valproic acid or carbamazepine) rather than monotherapy (see Table 21–22).

Other general treatment principles include mood charting, optimizing sleep, and eliminating mood destabilizers. Mood charting, though cumbersome and time consuming, allows careful delineation of the frequency and severity of episodes and of the drug's efficacy, including evidence of partial response patterns or loss of efficacy. Benzodiazepines (eg, clonazepam or lorazepam) are often useful in relieving the insomnia and agitation associated with acute illness. Clinicians agree that control of insomnia is paramount in treating acute bipolar illness, and there is speculation that continued insomnia may fuel the illness. Finally, agents with the propensity to destabilize mood (eg, TCAs, steroids, alcohol, stimulants) need to be identified and discontinued.

A. Lithium:
1. Indications—There are two main indications for lithium in patients with bipolar disorder: (1) for the management of the acute manic or hypomanic episode, and (2) for the prevention of further episodes of both mania and depression. Lithium is also useful in potentiating or augmenting the effects of antidepressants (mainly in refractory depression, as noted earlier in this chapter); in managing impulse-control disorders (especially episodic violence); in the long-term prophylactic treatment of cluster headaches; and in treating schizophrenia in a limited number of patients, particularly if they experience prominent affective symptoms (in which case a neuroleptic is also needed to treat the intrinsic schizophrenic symptoms).

a. Acute management of (hypo)mania. Lithium is useful in acute manic episodes. Approximately 80% of manic patients show at least a partial response to lithium monotherapy. Lithium also has some acute antidepressant effects, but these actions tend to be incomplete and require 3–4 weeks of treatment to achieve

Table 21–22. Treatment of bipolar disorder.[1]

Condition	Primary Method	Secondary Methods
Acute depressive episode	SSRI, bupropion	ECT, MAOIs, TCAs
Acute manic episode	Lithium (not useful in mixed episode); valproic acid or carbamazepine, with or without antipsychotic (eg, haloperidol) or benzodiazepines (eg, clonazepam)[2]	Verapamil, ECT
Maintenance treatment	Lithium, valproic acid, or carbamazepine; in difficult cases, lithium plus valproic acid or carbamazepine	Educational and structured psychosocial support

[1] ECT, electroconvulsive therapy; MAOIs, monoamine oxidase inhibitors; TCAs, tricyclic antidepressants.
[2] Lithium should be initiated at 300 mg twice daily and titrated with frequent blood-level monitoring to achieve levels between 0.8 and 1.2 nmol/L acutely (0.6 to 0.8 nmol/L during maintenance). Carbamazepine should be started at 200 mg twice daily with a gradual increase to plasma levels of 3–14 μg/mL. Valproic acid should be started in the 500–750-mg/day range and titrated in 250-mg increments to achieve plasma levels of 40–110 μg/mL, a range therapeutically effective yet well tolerated.

maximal effect. Often antidepressants are needed to effectively treat or prevent depressive episodes, but their use is always associated with the risk of precipitating (hypo)manic episodes or of destabilizing the illness course. Bupropion or SSRIs are least likely to produce these unwanted side effects. In acute manic states, lithium monotherapy can be beneficial in a matter of days, but usually there is a 5- to 10-day latency of response. Because of this delayed response lithium has not become the sole agent in everyday clinical practice. Most clinicians now use neuroleptics or benzodiazepines in addition to lithium in the acute phase of mania to control psychosis, hyperactivity, insomnia, and agitation. Neuroleptics appear to be superior to lithium only in the initial management of the acute state (ie, in the first few days of treatment).

Once the acute manic episode is resolved, lithium should be continued for at least 6–12 months—the time span during which the risk of relapse is highest. At this time, the clinician should carefully explain to the patient that he or she may have a chronic condition, that a manic or depressive episode is likely to recur in the future, that it is necessary to be cognizant of the early symptoms of a developing episode (eg, insomnia, elation or depression of mood, increased or decreased activity), and that treatment should be sought as soon as such symptoms occur. It is also important to point out, ideally to both the patient and family members, that patients are not likely to seek treatment in the early hypomanic states because the

associated self-assuredness, mood elation, and boundless energy are generally perceived as pleasant. When lithium is withdrawn abruptly, approximately 50% of patients relapse within 5 months.

b. Prevention of relapse. The efficacy of lithium in the long-term prophylactic treatment of bipolar disorder has been well documented; it appears to involve a reduction in both the number of episodes and their intensity. The preventive effects of lithium are most robust when there is evidence that the interval between episodes has shortened, that is, when the course of bipolar disorder has intensified in both severity of symptoms and frequency of episodes.

c. Management of breakthrough depression. A depressive episode sometimes "breaks through" lithium maintenance treatment. If this occurs, the following steps should be taken: (1) Increase lithium dose; (2) maximize thyroid function; (3) add an SSRI (the drug of choice), bupropion, or an MAOI; (4) consider treatment alternatives (eg, valproic acid, carbamazepine); and (5) consider sleep deprivation or ECT for severe depression. Because acute side effects and toxicity are common with lithium treatment, a thorough pretreatment and follow-up evaluation are necessary (Table 21–23).

In healthy patients, lithium carbonate can be initiated at 300 mg twice daily and titrated with frequent blood level monitoring. The blood level should be adjusted and maintained in a range of 0.6–1.2 mmol/L. This will require widely varying doses (600–1800

Table 21–23. Medical monitoring of healthy patients on maintenance lithium.[1]

Minimum recommendations	Frequency
Plasma lithium	4–8 weeks[2]
Thyroxine, free thyroxine, thyroid-stimulating hormone	6 months
Creatinine	12 months
Urinalysis	12 months
Optional recommendations	**Frequency**
24-Hour urine volume	6–12 months
Creatinine clearance	6–12 months
Urine osmolality	6–12 months
Complete blood count	6–12 months
Electrocardiogram (over age 50 years)	6–12 months

Special circumstances that can alter dose/blood-level relationships

Medical illness, especially with diarrhea, vomiting, or anorexia
Surgery
Crash dieting
Strenuous exercise
Very hot climate
Advanced age
Pregnancy and delivery

[1] Modified and reproduced, with permission, from Goodwin FK, Jamison KR: *Manic Depressive Illness*. Oxford University Press, 1990.
[2] This frequency can be reduced over time, especially with reliable patients.

mg/day). However, most patients are maintained effectively at 900–1200 mg/day.

Occasionally treatment calls for the use of medication in liquid form. Lithium citrate, a suspension form of the drug is available. Not only does this preparation allow for finer gradations of titration, but it reduces the likelihood of nausea and vomiting, which are associated with lithium treatment.

2. Adverse effects—Lithium is well tolerated by most patients. However, careful management of lithium plasma concentrations is required because of its narrow therapeutic window and because of the close association between plasma levels and toxicity (Table 21–24). Within the normal range of lithium plasma levels, one can commonly observe persistent but benign side effects, including increased thirst or urination, fine tremor, weight gain, and edema. Above the normal range of lithium plasma levels, serious side effects can occur rapidly; they include (with increasing plasma concentrations and symptom severity) nausea, vomiting, diarrhea, drowsiness and mental dullness, slurred speech, confusion, coarse tremor and twitching, muscle weakness, and above levels of 3.0 mmol/L, seizures, coma and death.

The major side effects of lithium affect the endocrine, renal, hematologic, cardiovascular, cutaneous gastrointestinal, ocular, and nervous systems (Table 21–25). Side effects are usually dosage dependent and transient in nature. Lithium has teratogenic effects, particularly when taken during the first trimester of pregnancy. The risk factors predisposing to lithium side effects and toxicity include renal disease or reduced renal clearance with age; organic brain disorder; dehydration after vomiting, diarrhea, increased perspiration, and strenuous exercise; low sodium intake or high sodium excretion; prolonged dieting, especially salt-restriction diets; and early pregnancy (see Table 21–23).

a. Management of lithium side effects. Because most side effects are dosage dependent, reduction of lithium intake will quickly ameliorate the acute symptoms, but this may increase the risk of relapse (see Table 21–25). Nausea, vomiting, and diarrhea can be reduced in some patients by switching from the carbonate to the citrate salt of lithium. Poly-

dipsia and polyuria can be managed by giving the entire daily dosage of lithium at bedtime. Tremor is often responsive to β-blockers such as atenolol or propranolol. These and other common side effects (ie, memory problems, weight gain, and tremor)—although not immediately harmful and dangerous—can be quite troublesome, may be intolerable to patients, and often negatively affect compliance. Goodwin and Jamison (1990), pooling percentages from 12 studies including 1094 patients, showed that subjective complaints were common. Among the most frequent were thirst (36%), polyuria (30%), memory problems (28%), tremor (27%), weight gain (19%), drowsiness (12%), and diarrhea (9%). Only 26% of patients had no complaints. Memory problems were most likely to cause noncompliance, followed by weight gain, tremor, polyuria, and drowsiness.

Thyroid dysfunction can be associated with lithium treatment. A small proportion of patients receiving chronic lithium treatment will develop thyroid enlargement with elevations in plasma TSH concentrations. Few patients, however, develop frank hypothyroidism. When this occurs, lithium may be discontinued, if possible, or thyroid hormone supplementation may be initiated.

The most common renal problems in patients taking lithium are polydipsia and polyuria, both of which are usually reversible. Occasionally patients develop diabetes insipidus or structural kidney damage (see Table 21–25), both of which require regular monitoring of kidney functioning (see Table 21–23). We now use lower plasma concentrations during maintenance therapy (ie, 0.6–0.8 nmol/L) than, say, two decades ago; this reduction in lithium dosing has resulted in a lower side-effect profile, especially of renal side effects.

Serious cardiac side effects are uncommon (see Table 21–25). T-wave flattening or inversion occur often and are not associated with negative treatment outcome. Some patients taking lithium over the long-term may experience sudden death of presumed cardiac origin. In particular, sinoatrial node dysfunction (sick sinus syndrome) can occur with increased frequency in these patients. Routine monitoring of the patient's electrocardiogram and pulse is necessary in order to minimize cardiac risk.

The use of lithium during pregnancy is controversial (see Table 21–25). Mild transient hypothyroidism and somnolence are common in newborns exposed in utero. The concentration of lithium in breast milk may also adversely affect nursing infants. The possibility of cardiovascular abnormalities in some infants exposed to lithium during the first trimester in utero necessitates both a careful initial risk-benefit analysis and close monitoring.

b. Contraindications to lithium. Relative or absolute contraindications to lithium are severe renal disease, acute myocardial infarction (in which complications may occur owing to arrhythmias, use of di-

Table 21–24. Associations between lithium plasma levels and toxicity.

Lithium Level (mmol/L)	Side Effects
1.0–1.5	Fine tremor, nausea
1.5–2.0	Cogwheeling tremor, nausea and vomiting, somnolence
2.0–2.5	Ataxia, confusion
2.5–3.0	Dysarthria, gross tremor
>3.0	Delirium, seizures, coma, death

Table 21–25. Common side effects of lithium.[1]

Affected System	Side Effect	Comments
Endocrine	Thyroid dysfunction	Lithium inhibits iodine uptake by the thyroid gland, iodination of tyrosine, release of T_4 and T_3, the peripheral degradation of thyroid hormones, and the stimulating effects of TSH. Approximately 5% of patients taking lithium develop signs of hypothyroidism; another 3% have elevated TSH levels or abnormal clinical signs and symptoms.
	Diabetes mellitus	Lithium may alter glucose tolerance, leading to mild diabetes status in some patients.
Renal	Polydipsia and polyuria	Lithium causes polydipsia and polyuria in about 60% of patients; it persists in 20% –25%. Usually these symptoms appear early in treatment and may reappear after several months. This adverse reaction is likely to be the result of an inhibition of the interaction between antidiuretic hormone and adenylate cyclase in the renal tubule and collecting duct system; it is usually reversible.
	Diabetes insipidus	Occasionally a nephrogenic diabetes insipidus–like syndrome develops in which the patient cannot concentrate urine. Excretion of urine is greater than 3 L/day, and patients must drink comparable amounts of water to avoid dehydration. This condition is almost always reversible.
	Structural kidney damage	This chronic tubulointerstitial nephropathy, perhaps the most worrisome adverse reaction occurring after long-term lithium administration, may be characterized by focal glomerular atrophy, interstitial fibrosis, and significant impairment of tubular functioning. Damage correlates roughly with the length of exposure to lithium. Persistent polyuria may be an early warning sign, but because many patients develop polyuria during maintenance treatment, the physician is often faced with a difficult problem.
	Other kidney effects	Lithium and sodium are managed similarly by the kidney. Perspiration, diarrhea, vomiting, thiazide diuretics, and salt-free diets may thus produce a significant increase in the lithium level, necessitating careful monitoring.
Hematologic	White blood cell count elevation	Because this effect involves a true proliferative response of the bone marrow, lithium can be useful in conditions associated with neutropenia (ie, radiotherapy or chemotherapy).
Cardiovascular	Significant effects on the heart (eg, T-wave flattening, U-waves)	Adverse reactions are rare. Several types of conduction problems have appeared, including first-degree atrioventricular block, irregular or slowed sinus node rhythms, and increased numbers of ventricular premature contractions.
Cutaneous	Pruritic, maculopapular rash	May appear during first month of treatment.
Gastrointestinal	Gastric irritation, anorexia, abdominal cramps, nausea, vomiting, diarrhea	Common.
CNS and neuromuscular	Mental dullness, decreased memory and concentration, headaches, fatigue and lethargy, muscle weakness, and tremor	Frequent at therapeutic dosages. A fine hand tremor of irregular rhythm and frequency occurs in about 50% of patients; worsened by caffeine, anxiety, and muscle tension; decreases over time. If it persists, propranolol, 20–160 mg/day, may help.
Ocular	Tearing, itching, burning, or blurring of vision	Rare. May occur during first week of treatment.
Other effects	Weight gain	Between 20% and 60% of patients are said to gain more than 20 pounds during treatment. Etiology unknown.
Pregnancy	Various congenital abnormalities, particularly of the heart and great vessels (Epstein's anomaly)	May occur in babies exposed to lithium in utero during the first trimester. The risk of major congenital malformations with first trimester lithium use is 4–12%; prenatal diagnosis by fetal echocardiogram and high-resolution ultrasound examination at 16–18 weeks' gestation is suggested. The alternatives to lithium—carbamazepine or sodium valproate—are associated with a marked increase in spina bifida. These agents should be avoided during pregnancy. If this is not possible, a thorough risk-benefit analysis is necessary before prescribing any of these drugs during pregnancy.

[1] T_3, triiodothyronine; T_4, thyroxine; TSH, thyroid-stimulating hormone; CNS, central nervous system.

uretics and digoxin, reduced fluid or salt intake, cardiac failure, and reduced renal function), myasthenia gravis (in which lithium interferes with the release of acetylcholine and the depolarization and repolarization of the motor endplate), first trimester of pregnancy, and breast-feeding mothers.

3. Management of lithium treatment failure. About 60% of bipolar patients respond to lithium treatment alone. If patients do not respond to lithium treatment, the clinician has several alternative options. The first is to change the medication schedule to one of two anticonvulsants, carbamazepine or sodium valproate. These can be administered with or without continuing lithium, and the majority of patients will respond to one or the other. Table 21–26 summarizes other, less common options.

The efficacy of the anticonvulsants carbamazepine or sodium valproate in bipolar disorder is well demonstrated. Preliminary evidence indicates that maintenance treatment with anticonvulsants may carry a higher risk of suicide than maintenance treatment with lithium, but no firm conclusions can be drawn yet. The following are predictors of a good response to anticonvulsants: rapid-cycling course of the illness, mixed episode, previous poor response to lithium, secondary mania, and recurrent substance abuse.

a. Carbamazepine. Of the two anticonvulsants, carbamazepine has been used clinically for a longer period of time. Doses are typically started at 200–400 mg/day and titrated to achieve a plasma concentration of 3–14 μg/mL. Common side effects include somnolence, dizziness, nausea and vomiting, and mild ataxia; these effects can be managed effectively with dosage reduction or slow dosage titration. Mild elevations of liver enzymes and mildly reduced white blood counts are also common. These problems typically improve or resolve with time. Finally, rash is common and usually requires discontinuation.

Two potentially serious adverse reactions associated with carbamazepine treatment require close and regular monitoring during treatment (Table 21–27).

Table 21–26. Alternative or adjunctive treatments for patients who respond poorly to lithium.

Assessment of present treatment
Evaluate possible cycle-inducing effect of adjunctive antidepressant or antimanic medication
Evaluate contribution of drug or alcohol abuse

Change of pharmacologic strategy
Anticonvulsants (eg, carbamazepine or valproate)
Monoamine oxidase inhibitor (eg, clorgiline)
Thyroxine (hypermetabolic doses)
L-Tryptophan
Calcium channel blockers (eg, verapamil and others)
Magnesium aspartate

Other approaches
Maintenance electroconvulsive therapy
Periodic sleep deprivation

Table 21–27. Pretreatment and posttreatment evaluation for carbamazepine.

Complete blood count, including platelets, white blood count, reticulocyte, and serum iron[1]
Liver function tests[2]
Electrolytes
Thyroid functions: triiodothyronine, thyroxine, and thyrotropin-stimulating hormone
Complete urinalysis and blood urea nitrogen
Rule out history of cardiac, hepatic, or renal damage
Rule out history of adverse hematologic response to other drugs

[1] Repeat at 2 and 4 weeks, and quarterly thereafter.
[2] Repeat at 1, 3, 6, and 12 months, and biannually thereafter.

Carbamazepine can acutely damage the liver, resulting in marked increases in liver enzymes and sometimes frank jaundice. Hepatic failure, however, is rare.

Blood dyscrasias, including granulocytopenia, agranulocytosis, or aplastic anemia, pose a second category of problems. Although rare (the incidence of agranulocytosis is approximately six per million population per year, whereas aplastic anemia occurs in two per million per year), the possibility of these adverse reactions necessitates that the patient have a complete blood count taken regularly (see Table 21–27). If the patient's absolute neutrophil count falls below 2000, the count should be monitored at least weekly until a rebound is observed. At below 1500, the carbamazepine dosage should be lowered quickly to about 50% of previous dosage and the count monitored weekly until it rebounds. If the count falls below 1000, carbamazepine should be discontinued and the patient monitored under hospital conditions until the count rebounds.

The teratogenic effects of carbamazepine are well known. Carbamazepine appears to induce neural tube defects such as spina bifida at high rates (about 1% of exposures); therefore, it should not be used in pregnant women. Human chorionic gonadotropin testing is indicated in women of childbearing potential who are to be started on this agent.

b. Valproic acid. Recent clinical trials have established the effectiveness of valproic acid in the acute management of mania, but long-term maintenance studies are lacking. The agent is available as regular sodium valproate or as a dimer molecule. The latter dissociates in the gastrointestinal tract to form free valproate, which is then absorbed. This delays absorption, prolonging the drug's effective half-life.

Sodium valproate is started in the 500–750 mg/day range and titrated in 250 mg increments to achieve an adequate plasma level. The therapeutic plasma-level range is 50–125 μg/mL. The higher end of the plasma-level range is indicated for patients whose illness is poorly controlled on lower levels.

Common side effects associated with sodium valproate include nausea and vomiting, diarrhea or constipation, mild elevations of liver enzymes, mild drowsiness or fatigue, and skin rash. More serious reactions are rare. Hepatic failure has been reported and has resulted in fatalities; it is especially prevalent in young children. Liver function studies are required at baseline and within the first month of treatment. They should be repeated at 3 and 6 months, then biannually thereafter. Mild elevations of liver enzymes are an indication for more frequent monitoring. Clotting abnormalities also have been reported. Finally, like carbamazepine, valproate may produce spina bifida in infants exposed in utero. Use in pregnancy must be avoided.

c. Other options. If both lithium and anticonvulsant therapy fail, other alternatives can be considered. The anticonvulsant lamotrigine may be effective, although formal clinical trials are needed to establish its effectiveness. In addition, verapamil can be effective in the acute and maintenance phases of treatment, but it has never gained broad acceptance. The combined use of lithium with either carbamazepine or sodium valproate (each is used in the usual therapeutic plasma-level range) has not been tested adequately in clinical trials but is common nonetheless. Finally, lithium or an anticonvulsant can be used in combination with a typical or atypical antipsychotic in order to manage the psychosis associated with the manic or depressive state or to control intractable cycling.

B. Psychotherapy: Little is known about the role of psychotherapy in the treatment of bipolar disorder. Efforts are currently under way to evaluate whether treatments such as interpersonal psychotherapy or cognitive therapy work as well in bipolar patients as they do in unipolar patients. Preliminary evidence indicates that family education may reduce the risk for relapse and that cognitive therapy may enhance compliance with medications. On the whole, some of the newer psychosocial interventions appear to represent a viable alternative or valuable adjunct to pharmacotherapy in mild to moderate unipolar disorder. Whether those advantages apply to more severely depressed unipolar patients or to patients with bipolar disorders remains to be determined.

C. Electroconvulsive Therapy: Approximately 80% of manic patients show substantial improvement after ECT, but the widespread (and successful) use of lithium and other antimanic agents, often in combination with antipsychotic medications, has limited ECT to patients who are intolerant of medications or whose illness is refractory to medications. ECT has proven especially useful for those manic patients who did not respond to medication and for those in mixed states who present with a high risk for suicide and are thus in need of acute symptom containment.

Baldessarini RJ: Drugs and the treatment of psychiatric disorders, depression and mania. Pages 431–459 in Hardman JG, Limbird LE (editors): *The Pharmacological Basis of Therapeutics.* McGraw-Hill, 1996.

Bowden C: Treatment of bipolar disorder. In: Schatzberg AF, Nemeroff CB (editors): *Textbook of Psychopharmacology,* 2nd ed. American Psychiatric Press, 1998.
Keck PE, McElroy SL: Antiepileptic drugs. In: Schatzberg AF, Nemeroff CB (editors): *Textbook of Psychopharmacology,* 2nd ed. American Psychiatric Press, 1998.
Lenox RH, Manji HK: Lithium. In: Schatzberg AF, Nemeroff CB (editors): *Textbook of Psychopharmacology,* 2nd ed. American Psychiatric Press, 1998.

Course of Illness & Prognosis

The natural course of bipolar disorders is variable. Patients usually experience their first manic episode in their early 20s, but bipolar disorders sometimes start in adolescence or after age 40 years. Manic episodes typically begin suddenly, with a rapid escalation of symptoms over a few days; often they are triggered by psychosocial stressors. In about 50% of patients a depressive episode immediately precedes a manic episode.

It appears that the availability of treatment for bipolar disorder has significantly affected the length of an average episode. Before 1960 (ie, before the introduction of psychopharmacologic medications such as lithium), episode length averaged 7–13 months; thereafter, it averaged 2–4 months. With the emergence of early intervention and successful treatment of the illness, the effects of kindling on outcome (described earlier in this section) may have been interrupted, resulting in fewer episodes over time and reduced cycle length. Early disease onset suggests poor prognosis; patients who experience their initial episode in their late teens are likely to have a less favorable outcome than patients who experience their initial episode in their early 30s. Patients with early-onset bipolar disorder should be quickly identified and targeted for aggressive treatment intervention.

Although medications are effective in treating acute episodes and in maintaining patients in remission, they are not completely effective in preventing future episodes. Studies have shown that patients maintained with lithium levels of 0.8–1.0 ng/mL are less likely to have a recurrence than are patients maintained on lower lithium levels (0.4–0.6 ng/mL). Combinations of lithium and anticonvulsants have shown promise in maintaining euthymia and increasing cycle intervals.

As discussed earlier in this section, somatic interventions can have a marked effect on the prognosis of bipolar disorder. Comorbidity with substance abuse, antisocial behavior, and personality disorders often complicates the clinical outcome. Substantial psychosocial morbidity can affect marriage, children, occupation, and other aspects of the patient's life. Divorce rates are two to three times higher in bipolar patients than in the general population, and occupational status is twice as likely to deteriorate. Completed suicide rates approximate 15% in bipolar patients, and suicide is more common among females and is usually associated with a depressive or mixed episode.

IV. CYCLOTHYMIC DISORDER

Harry E. Gwirtsman, MD, & Peter T. Loosen, MD

DSM-IV Diagnostic Criteria

A. For at least 2 years, the presence of numerous periods with hypomanic symptoms and numerous periods with depressive symptoms that do not meet criteria for a major depressive episode.

Note: In children and adolescents, the duration must be at least 1 year.

B. During the above 2-year period (1 year in children and adolescents), the person has not been without the symptoms in Criterion A for more than 2 months at a time.

C. No major depressive episode, manic episode, or mixed episode has been present during the first 2 years of the disturbance.

Note: After the initial 2 years (1 year in children and adolescents) of cyclothymic disorder, there may be superimposed manic or mixed episodes (in which case both bipolar I disorder and cyclothymic disorder may be diagnosed) or major depressive episodes (in which case both bipolar II disorder and cyclothymic disorder may be diagnosed).

D. The symptoms in Criterion A are not better accounted for by schizoaffective disorder, and are not superimposed on schizophrenia, schizophreniform disorder, delusional disorder, or psychotic disorder not otherwise specified.

E. The symptoms are not due to the direct physiological effects of a substance (eg, drugs of abuse, a medication) or a general medical condition (eg, hyperthyroidism).

F. The symptoms cause clinically significant distress or impairment in social, occupational, or other important areas of functioning.

Reprinted, with permission, from *Diagnostic and Statistical Manual of Mental Disorders,* 4th ed. Copyright 1994 American Psychiatric Association.

General Considerations

A. Major Etiologic Theories: Cyclothymic individuals alternate between the extremes of dysthymia (gloomy and depressed) and hyperthymia (cheerful and uninhibited). They can be moody, impulsive, erratic, and volatile but usually do not meet the full syndromal criteria for bipolar disorder. Repeated romantic or conjugal failures occurring in the context of interpersonal and social disturbances are common. Cyclothymia first received an operational definition in the *Diagnostic and Statistical Manual of Mental Disorders,* 3rd edition.

There is still considerable controversy concerning the association between cyclothymic disorder and both other mood disorders and cluster B personality disorders. However, current research favors the conceptualization of cyclothymic disorder as a bona fide mood disorder.

B. Epidemiology: Cyclothymic disorder often begins early in life. Lifetime prevalence rates for this disorder range between 0.4% and 1.0% in the general population, and between 3% and 5% in mood disorder clinics. In community samples, cyclothymic disorder is equally common in men and women, but women are more prevalent in clinical settings (in a ratio of approximately 3 to 2).

C. Genetics: Among first-degree relatives of cyclothymic patients, the diagnoses of major depressive disorder and bipolar I and II disorders are more common than in the general population (Table 21–28). There may also be an increased familial risk of substance-related disorders.

Akiskal HS: Depression in cyclothymic and related temperaments: clinical and pharmacologic considerations. J Clin Psychiatry Monogr 1992;10:37.

Weissman MN, Livingston Bruce M, Leaf PJ, Florio LP, Holzer C: Affective Disorders. Pages 53-80 in Robins LN, Regier DA (editors): *Psychiatric Disorders in America.* Free Press, 1991.

Clinical Findings

Cyclothymic disorder is characterized by periods of depression alternating with periods of hypomania, which are generally of less severity or shorter duration than those associated with bipolar I disorder. The changes in mood tend to be irregular and abrupt, sometimes occurring within hours of each other. Approximately 50% of patients with cyclothymic disorder are predominantly depressed; a minority have primarily hypomanic symptoms and are unlikely to consult a mental health practitioner. Almost all individuals with cyclothymic disorder have periods of mixed symptoms with marked irritability, leading to unprovoked disagreements with friends, family, and coworkers. Cyclothymic individuals may have a history of multiple geographical moves, involvement in religious cults, or inability to maintain a career pathway.

Hypomania can be triggered by interpersonal stressors or by losses. Although most individuals with cyclothymic disorder seek psychiatric help for depres-

Table 21–28. Risk factors for cyclothymic disorder.

Familial pattern	Approximately 30% of cyclothymic patients have first-degree relatives with bipolar I disorder (a rate similar to that for bipolar I patients). Cyclothymic disorder also occurs more frequently in relatives of bipolar I disorder patients than in relatives of other psychiatrically ill patients.
Social class	Not known.
Race	Not known.

sion, their problems are often related to the interpersonal and behavioral crises (eg, romantic failures) caused by their hypomanic episodes. The unpredictable nature of the mood changes causes a great deal of stress, and patients will often feel as if their moods are out of control. Patients will also present with disorganization and work productivity problems following hypomanic episodes.

Howland RH, Thase ME: A comprehensive review of cyclothymic disorder. J Nerv Ment Dis 1993;181:485.

Differential Diagnosis

When the mood disturbance is judged to be the direct physiologic consequence of a specific, usually chronic general medical condition (eg, hypothyroidism), then the diagnosis should be mood disorder due to a general medical condition (see below). If substances, such as stimulants, are judged to be etiologically related to the mood disturbance, then a substance-induced mood disorder should be diagnosed. The mood swings suggestive of substance-induced mood disorder usually dissipate following cessation of drug use.

Although cyclothymic disorder may resemble bipolar I or II disorders with rapid cycling, the mood states in cyclothymic disorder do not meet the criteria for a manic, major depressive, or mixed episode. Borderline personality disorder is frequently confused with cyclothymic disorder, because of its strong affective component with marked shifts in mood. If criteria are met for each disorder, both may be diagnosed. In children and adolescents, ADHD can be clinically difficult to differentiate from cyclothymic disorder, but a pharmacologic trial of stimulants might be diagnostic, as stimulants tend to improve the symptoms of ADHD but worsen the mood swings of cyclothymic disorder.

Treatment

There are no systematic data on the treatment of cyclothymic disorder. Lithium has been used to suppress the hypomanic cycles, but most patients seek treatment for their labile, irritable moods and their anxious, dysphoric depressions. Some of these patients may shift into acute manic states or may develop rapid cycling if their depressions are treated solely with TCAs. In this case, bupropion, MAOIs, and low-dose SSRIs, in conjunction with lithium or other mood stabilizers, may be appropriate. Other alternatives include sodium valproate or thyroid augmentation. The latter appears to be especially promising in female patients.

Although traditional insight-oriented psychotherapeutic approaches have been used to treat the so-called temperamental and Axis II comorbid features of cyclothymic disorder, experts now also advocate psychoeducational and interpersonal strategies as adjuncts to pharmacotherapy directed at the affective instability.

Akiskal HS: Dysthymic and cyclothymic depressions: therapeutic considerations. J Clin Psychiatry 1994;55(Suppl):46.

Howland RH, Thase ME: A comprehensive review of cyclothymic disorder. J Nerv Ment Dis 1993;181:485.

Complications, Comorbidity, & Adverse Outcomes of Treatment

There are several sources of comorbidity for cyclothymic disorder. For example, mood disorders, especially major depressive disorder and bipolar II disorder, may follow the onset of cyclothymic disorder. Other comorbid disorders include personality disorders, especially borderline personality disorder (in 10–20% of patients), impulse-control disorders such as intermittent explosive disorder, and substance-related disorders (in 5–10% of patients). Patients may use substances such as alcohol and sedatives to self-medicate the fluctuating moods, or they may ingest stimulants in order to achieve even further stimulation. Sleep disorders (such as problems initiating and maintaining sleep) are occasionally present.

Prognosis & Course of Illness

Cyclothymic disorder usually appears in adolescence or early adult life; its onset is insidious and its course chronic. The disorder is considered by some to reflect a temperamental predisposition to other mood disorders, and there is a 15–50% risk that a bipolar I or II disorder will develop subsequently.

V. MOOD DISORDER DUE TO A GENERAL MEDICAL CONDITION

Pryor Baird, MD, & Peter T. Loosen, MD

DSM-IV Diagnostic Criteria

A. A prominent and persistent disturbance in mood predominates in the clinical picture and is characterized by either (or both) of the following:
   (1) depressed mood or markedly diminished interest or pleasure in all, or almost all, activities
   (2) elevated, expansive, or irritable mood
B. There is evidence from the history, physical examination, or laboratory findings that the disturbance is the direct physiological consequence of a general medical condition.
C. The disturbance is not accounted for by another mental disorder (eg, adjustment disorder with depressed mood in response to the stress of having a general medical condition).
D. The disturbance does not occur exclusively during the course of a delirium.
E. The symptoms cause clinically significant distress or impairment in social, occupational, or other important areas of functioning.

Reprinted, with permission, from *Diagnostic and Statistical Manual of Mental Disorders,* 4th ed. Copyright 1994 American Psychiatric Association.

General Considerations

A. Associated Medical Conditions: A variety of general medical conditions may cause mood symptoms (see Tables 21–3 and 21–4). For example, the clinical signs and symptoms of pancreatic cancer, especially cancer of the pancreas head, are often preceded by depression. If a mood disorder due to a general medical condition is suspected, and if other more immediate causes have been eliminated, it is advisable to obtain a computed tomography scan of the pancreas in order to rule out this possibility.

Endocrine diseases commonly associated with depression are Cushing's disease, primary hypothyroidism (1–6% prevalence in middle-aged females), diabetes mellitus, and Addison's disease. Depression may be among the earliest symptoms of endogenous Cushing's disease, sometimes preceding its final diagnosis by years. It is noteworthy that patients with endogenous Cushing's disease usually present with depression (prevalence rates are as high as 65%), whereas patients with iatrogenic Cushing's disease (eg, resulting after high doses of glucocorticoids for allergic or autoimmune conditions) are more likely to present with mood elevation. If diabetes mellitus is associated with comorbid depression, it may be difficult to appropriately control the endocrine aspects of the disease. Converging evidence indicates that comorbid depression can be associated with a less predictable course and wider fluctuations of blood glucose levels, often necessitating a more intensive treatment approach.

B. Epidemiology: Approximately 25–40% of patients with certain neurologic conditions (eg, Parkinson's disease, multiple sclerosis, systemic lupus erythematosus) develop symptoms of severe depression at some point during their illness. For medical conditions that do not directly affect the brain, prevalence rates appear to be more variable, ranging from 40% (for primary hypothyroidism) to less than 8% (for chronic renal disease).

Clinical Findings

The diagnostic criteria for mood disorder due to a general medical condition are less vigorous than those for the primarily psychiatric mood disorders and require only the presence of depressed mood/diminished enjoyment or elevated, expansive, or irritable mood (manic symptoms). Regarding the medical illness, the required signs, symptoms, and laboratory findings are simply those that, in conjunction with the clinical history, yield the medical diagnosis. Furthermore, history, physical examination, or laboratory results must suggest that the mood disturbance is a physiologic consequence of the medical illness.

Differential Diagnosis

The differential diagnosis of a mood disorder due to a general medical condition must include delirium (a separate diagnosis of mood disorder due to a general medical condition is not given if the mood disturbance is part of a delirium), dementia of the Alzheimer's type, vascular dementia, substance-induced mood disorder, and the other major mood disorders.

Treatment

Treatment approaches are directed primarily at the medical condition. It is noteworthy that particularly in endocrine disorders behavioral remission often does not parallel medical remission, that is, patients may continue to be depressed even after they have been cured endocrinologically. It is possible that in some patients (ie, in those with a genetic vulnerability for developing depression) the mood disorder was simply triggered by the general medical condition, whereas in others it was more causally linked.

The psychopharmacologic treatment of comorbid mood disorders in medically ill patients requires a careful risk-benefit assessment. The considerations necessary for such assessment include the following: (1) side effects of psychotropic agents that may complicate existing medical illness (examples include the use of TCAs in patients with hypothyroidism, orthostatic hypotension, chronic heart disease including myocardial infarction and congestive heart failure, prostatic hypertrophy, or narrow-angle glaucoma); (2) potential interactions of psychotropic agents (eg, antidepressants) with drugs used to treat medical disorders; and (3) the effects of impaired renal, hepatic, or gastrointestinal functioning on psychotropic drug absorption and metabolism. Medically ill patients are often older and more sensitive to drugs, they require lower dosages, and they metabolize drugs slower than do younger individuals. Therefore, when treating mood disorders in elderly, medically ill patients, clinicians should use low dosages of antidepressants at the beginning of treatment and raise the dosages gradually depending on the patient's toleration of side effects and response to treatment. The following sections summarize the management of comorbid depression in specific medical conditions:

A. Asthma: MAOIs should be administered with caution to patients who have asthma because of interactions with sympathomimetic bronchodilators. Other antidepressants appear to be safe.

B. Cardiac Disease: Because of their quinidine-like effects, the TCAs have antiarrhythmic properties and prolong the Q-T interval. A prolonged Q-T interval (ie, >0.440 seconds) presents a relative contraindication for the use of TCAs. Among patients with preexisting but asymptomatic conduction defects, TCAs may induce symptomatic conduction defects and orthostatic hypotension. TCAs may also provoke arrhythmia in patients with subclinical sinus node dysfunction. SSRIs, trazodone, and bupropion present safer alternatives for treating depression in patients with cardiac disease. It is also advisable to monitor carefully those patients who already take another class I antiarrhythmic agent; to evaluate patients for preexisting but asymptomatic conduction defects such as interventricular conduction delay and bundle branch block; to be aware that patients with prolonged Q-T intervals, whether preexisting or drug induced, are predisposed to the development of ventricular tachycardia; and to obtain an EKG for all patients over age 40 years before initiating treatment.

C. Dementia: Patients with dementia are particularly sensitive to the toxic effects of anticholinergic agents on memory and attention. Antidepressants with low anticholinergic profiles are the drugs of choice (eg, SSRIs, bupropion, trazodone, desipramine, nortriptyline). Stimulants can be useful occasionally. ECT can be used if medications are either contraindicated or not tolerated, and if immediate resolution of depressive symptoms is medically indicated.

D. Hypertension: Antihypertensive medications and antidepressants may interact in various ways, either intensifying or weakening the effects of the antihypertensive therapy. The antihypertensive effect of prazosin is intensified by TCAs, because both block the α-receptors. In contrast, TCAs antagonize the therapeutic actions of guanethidine, clonidine, or α-methyldopa. Orthostatic hypotension can occur when antihypertensives, especially diuretics, are combined with TCAs, trazodone, or MAOIs. β-Blockers, especially propranolol, are known to cause depression in some individuals; the situation is remedied by changing to another antihypertensive medication.

E. Narrow-Angle Glaucoma: The anticholinergic side effects of TCAs can acutely exacerbate narrow-angle glaucoma in susceptible individuals (ie, in those with shallow anterior chambers). Patients who receive miotics for their glaucoma may take antidepressants, including those with strong anticholinergic effects, provided that their intraocular pressure is monitored. SSRIs, trazodone, and bupropion present safer alternatives. Trazodone, however, can produce priapism in some patients (about 1 in 7000 men treated); priapism may necessitate surgical intervention, which is often associated with impotence or erectile problems.

F. Obstructive Uropathy: Prostate enlargement and other forms of bladder outlet obstruction present relative contraindications to the use of antidepressants with strong anticholinergic effects. Benzodiazepines, trazodone, and MAOIs may also retard bladder emptying. The drugs of choice in this case are SSRIs, bupropion, and desipramine.

G. Orthostatic Hypotension: A common side effect of TCAs is orthostatic hypotension, particularly in elderly patients or in patients with preexisting hypotension, impaired left ventricular function, or bundle branch block. Good treatment alternatives are SSRIs and bupropion. They have little affinity for histaminic, muscarinic, and α-adrenergic receptors and are thus not likely to significantly affect pulse rate or blood pressure. Clinicians should advise elderly patients of the potential serious risk of acute orthostatic hypotension (eg, femur neck fractures) and discuss with them possible ways of avoiding such risk (eg, not changing positions too rapidly; sitting up in bed before standing up, particularly at night when patients awake because of the need to urinate).

H. Parkinson's Disease: Depression is common in patients with Parkinson's disease; 40–50% of patients are so afflicted. The management of depression in this condition often presents great difficulty, and there is no evidence that any particular antidepressant is more efficacious than others. Amoxapine and lithium should be avoided because both can exacerbate neurologic symptoms. MAOIs may adversely interact with L-dopa. The beneficial effects of anticholinergic agents are offset by their induction of memory impairment. ECT may be of transient benefit.

I. Seizure Disorders: The effects of antidepressants on the seizure threshold are not completely understood. Two antidepressants, maprotiline and bupropion, are associated with an increased risk for seizures, especially if administered in high dosages. In patients receiving treatment for seizure disorder, fluoxetine may dramatically increase the plasma levels of carbamazepine, whereas TCAs may lower the levels. The plasma levels of TCAs can be increased by valproic acid. ECT can be safely used in patients with seizure disorder.

Complications, Comorbidity, & Adverse Outcomes of Treatment

Comorbid depression is not a clinically benign condition. In diabetes mellitus, comorbid depression can significantly complicate the acute treatment of the illness or negatively affect its outcome. Among patients in a general medical setting, those with comorbid depression report increased pain, more severe physical illness, decreased social functioning, and increased mortality. The deterioration of functioning associated with depression or depressive symptoms may be equal to or worse than that associated with severe medical conditions. Evidence indicates that the combination of current advanced coronary artery disease and depressive symptoms can be associated with roughly twice the reduction in social functioning as with either condition alone, suggesting that the effects of depressive symptoms and chronic medical conditions on functioning can be additive. In chronic heart disease, the diagnosis of comorbid depression may be associated with an increased likelihood of medical complications, a more protracted course, and sudden death. It is important to identify such comorbidity early and to treat it aggressively.

Cassem NH, Stern TA, Rosenbaum JF (editors): *Massachusetts General Hospital Handbook of General Hospital Psychiatry.* Mosby, 1997.

Goodwin FK, Jamison KR: *Manic Depressive Illness.* Oxford University Press, 1990.

Harrison TR, Fauci AS, Braunwald E, Hauser SL (editors): *Harrison's Principles of Internal Medicine.* McGraw-Hill, 1997.

Stoudemire A, Fogel BS: *Principles of Medical Psychiatry.* Grune & Stratton, 1987.

Stoudemire A, Moran MG: Psychopharmacology in the medically ill patient. In: Schatzberg AF, Nemeroff CB (editors): *Textbook of Psychopharmacology,* 2nd ed. American Psychiatric Press, 1998.

22

Anxiety Disorders

Richard C. Shelton, MD

Anxiety disorders range in severity from common, mild phobias (eg, fear of insects, heights, or storms) to chronic, disabling conditions such as panic disorder or obsessive-compulsive disorder (OCD). Anxiety diagnoses are made according to the specific symptomatic manifestation of each disorder. Table 22–1 lists the anxiety disorder diagnoses included in the *Diagnostic and Statistical Manual of Mental Disorders,* 4th edition (DSM-IV). Posttraumatic stress disorder and acute stress disorder are covered in Chapter 23, and OCD is covered in Chapter 24.

Anxiety is characterized by heightened arousal (ie, physical symptoms such as tension, tachycardia, tachypnea, tremor) accompanied by apprehension, fear, obsessions, or the like. Anxiety disorders are different from normal fears, although the symptoms can be similar. Generally speaking, normal fears represent emotional reactions to real, external threats, and the emotional response is appropriately related to the actual danger. In contrast, the symptoms of anxiety disorders occur either without obvious external threat or when the response to the threat is excessive. When an extreme or inappropriate fear or worry is present and is coupled with some degree of life impairment, the diagnosis of anxiety disorder should be considered.

A. Major Etiologic Theories:

1. Psychodynamic theory—Traditional psychoanalytic theory describes anxiety disorders as being rooted in unconscious conflict. Freud originally used the term "angst" (literally, "fear") to describe the simple intrapsychic response to either internal or external

threat. He later derived the concept of the pleasure principle, which describes the tendency of the psychic apparatus to seek immediate discharge of impulses. In his earliest organized theory of anxiety, Freud postulated that conflicts or inhibitions result in the failure to dissipate libidinal (ie, sexual) drives. These restrictions on sexual expression could occur because of external threat and would subsequently result in a fear of the loss of control of the drive. The damming-up of the impulses, along with the fear of loss of control, would result in anxiety.

Freud soon began to see the limitations of this theory and later proposed that anxiety was central to the concept of neurosis. He acknowledged that anxiety was a natural, biologically derived response mechanism required for survival. He abandoned the concept of the transformation of sexual drive (energy) into anxiety and accepted the prevailing notion of the time: that anxiety was a result of threat. He recognized two sources of such threat. The first, termed **traumatic situations,** involved stimuli that were too severe for the person to manage effectively and could be considered the common or natural fear response. The second, called **danger situations,** resulted from the recognition or anticipation of upcoming trauma, whether internal (by loss of control of drives) or external. The response to these threats resulted in what was called **signal anxiety,** which was an attenuated and therefore more manageable anxiety response not directly related to trauma. Signal anxiety could be seen as anxiety that resulted from the avoidance of threat.

The structural hypothesis of mental function—which includes the id as the seat of drives, the superego as the location of inhibitions, and the ego as the apparatus for managing drives and inhibitions—evolved during this time period. Central to this hypothesis is the concept of **defense mechanisms.** Psychological defenses are thought to be primarily a function of the ego, which uses these defenses to manage id impulses and superego demands. **Repression** is formulated as the primary defense mechanism, in which unacceptable drive states are maintained

Table 22–1. DSM-IV anxiety disorders.

Panic disorder (with or without agoraphobia)
Specific phobia
Social phobia
Generalized anxiety disorder
Obsessive-compulsive disorder
Acute stress disorder
Posttraumatic stress disorder
Anxiety disorder due to medical condition
Substance-induced anxiety disorder

largely outside of awareness. Failure of repression could result in anxiety and the use of secondary mechanisms to maintain intrapsychic stability.

The concept of the primacy of the defense mechanism to both generate and manage the anxiety has remained central to psychoanalysis for much of its history. Further, psychoanalytic treatment has focused on the need to uncover childhood trauma, releasing unnecessary defensive inhibitions and developing psychological competence. A number of schools of thought have been elaborated from classical Freudian psychoanalysis, including ego psychology, object relations theory, and self psychology (see Chapter 4).

2. Learning theory—The basic principles of learning theory as they relate to human development are rooted in the work of developmental psychologists, especially Jean Piaget (see Chapter 1). Piaget's observations of children led to an understanding of the progress of development through a series of predictable stages, referred to as epigenesis. Developmental milestones represent an interaction between the maturing brain substrate and environmental influences. Hence children learn according to both the capacity of the brain to manage incoming stimuli and the nature of the stimuli themselves. Appropriate environmental responses facilitate a normal learning process, and aberrant reactions produce problems in development.

As stimuli are assimilated and processed, learning takes place. Learning theory proposes two forms of learning: classical conditioning and operant conditioning (see Chapter 3). The classical conditioning model depends on the pairing of a stimulus that evokes a response (the unconditioned stimulus) with a neutral environmental object or event (the conditioned stimulus). The repeated pairing of the two stimuli would lead to the ability of the conditioned stimulus to elicit the same response as the unconditioned stimulus (the conditioned response).

Whereas classical conditioning views the organism as a relatively passive participant in the learning process, operant conditioning views stimuli as a series of either positive or negative events that influence subsequent behavior. Positive reinforcement occurs when a particular behavior results in a reward. Alternatively, negative reinforcement results when a specific behavior leads to the successful avoidance of an aversive event (ie, punishment). Positive or negative reinforcements would then enhance the likelihood that the behavior would be repeated. Reinforcements of behaviors, whether they are achievements of rewards or avoidance of pain, underlie learning.

According to learning theory, an anxiety disorder develops when environmental cues become associated with anxiety-producing events during development. Within the construct of generalized anxiety disorder (GAD), for example, worry and fear become conditioned and are repeated in order to avoid intermittent

negative reinforcement. Hence the periodic successful avoidance of a negative outcome reinforces the behavior. For example, an individual's fear (and subsequent avoidance) of air travel would be enhanced by reading about occasional air disasters.

Traditional behavioral therapy of anxiety involves the uncoupling of the unconditioned response from the associated stimulus. Wolpe postulated that actions that inhibited anxiety (ie, relaxation) in the face of the conditioned stimulus would reduce symptoms. Behavioral treatment of anxiety uses **systematic desensitization** (progressive exposure to an anxiety-evoking stimulus). This type of treatment has been used successfully to treat anxiety disorders such as phobias and OCD, but it has had limited systematic study in other anxiety disorders.

3. Cognitive theory—In a subsequent elaboration of learning theory, a cognitive theory of the etiology of depressive and anxiety disorders has evolved (see Chapter 2). Although several theories have been advanced, Beck's concept of the cognitive triad has gained the broadest acceptance and application. In this view, abnormal emotional states, such as anxiety and depression, are a result of distorted beliefs about the self, the world, and the future. Anxiety disorders, therefore, involve incorrect beliefs that interpret events in an exaggeratedly dangerous or threatening manner. These fundamental belief systems, or schema, result in automatic thought responses to external or internal cues that trigger anxiety. As such, anxiety disorders consistently involve abnormalities of information processing that result in symptom formation.

Cognitive-behavioral therapy involves elements of classical behavioral approaches such as systematic desensitization; however, treatment is extended to the discovery and correction of distorted cognitive schema. The absence of exaggerated misinterpretations of cues leads to a reduction in symptom formation. Cognitive-behavioral psychotherapy has been used successfully to treat a variety of anxiety disorders, including panic disorder, phobias, and OCD.

4. Biological theories—From a biological standpoint, anxiety and fear have high adaptive value in all animals by increasing the animal's capacity for survival. The emotion of anxiety drives a number of highly adaptive behaviors, including escape from threat. The normal brain functions that underlie the anxiety response have been elucidated gradually over the past 50 years. The current understanding of the biological nature of anxiety has been prompted in part by an elucidation of the actions of drugs that reduce the symptoms of anxiety disorders. These observations can be divided into three broad areas: the gamma amino butyric acid (GABA) receptor–benzodiazepine receptor–chloride channel complex; the noradrenergic nucleus locus coeruleus and related brain stem nuclei; and the serotonin system, especially the raphe nuclei and their projections. Abnormalities in the functioning of these areas have been associated with various anxiety disorders.

Gray and colleagues have developed a general theory of a **neural behavioral-inhibition system** that mediates anxiety. The purpose of this system is to evaluate stimuli—consistent with punishment, nonreward, novelty, or fear—that simultaneously produce behavioral inhibition and increase arousal and attention. Antianxiety drugs inhibit responses in these areas. Using pharmacologic and lesioning studies, researchers have related anxiety to several interconnected anatomical areas. Sensory stimuli activate the hippocampus, especially the entorhinal cortex, which secondarily produces habituation by actions on the lateral and medial septal areas. Behavioral inhibition is achieved by projections to the cingulate gyrus. These areas are then influenced by noradrenergic activity of the locus coeruleus and are modulated both by serotonergic innervations from the raphe and by $GABA_A$ receptor activity. Antianxiety drugs work via mechanisms that influence these areas and receptors. These mechanisms include noradrenergic activation (eg, tricyclic antidepressants), serotonergic activity (eg, selective serotonin reuptake inhibitors or buspirone), or benzodiazepine interactions with GABA receptors.

B. Epidemiology: Anxiety disorders are among the most common of psychiatric disorders, affecting upward of 15% of the population at any time. Individual anxiety disorders occur frequently. Phobic disorders (ie, specific or social phobia) may affect as much as 8–10% of the population. GAD is found in about 5% of the population, and OCD and panic disorder are each seen in about 1–3% of the population. Although posttraumatic stress disorder probably is common, its specific frequency is unknown (see Chapter 23). The comorbidity of anxiety disorders with other psychiatric disorders is high. For example, about 40% of patients with primary anxiety disorders will have a lifetime history of a DSM-IV depressive disorder. Further, in patients who have other psychiatric disorders, significant anxiety symptoms often are associated with those disorders. Therefore, clinically significant anxiety symptoms will occur frequently in patients seen in clinical practice.

C. Genetics: The data from genetic studies of anxiety disorders are quite limited; however, existing research indicates that there is a strong genetic component to these disorders. For example, half or more of persons with panic disorder have a family history for the disorder. The genetic relationships sometimes are complex. The frequency of family history in OCD is low; however, family members of persons with this condition have a higher than expected rate of tic disorders, indicating a possible genetic linkage between OCD and complex tic disorders. This relationship also is supported by the observation of an increased frequency of tic disorders in persons with OCD and vice versa.

Identification of Pathologic Anxiety

Anxiety is a normal emotion, a common reaction to the stresses of everyday life. At what point does anxiety become pathologic? In order to make this distinction, one must define the key characteristics of the disorders and recognize that in pathologic anxiety normal psychological adaptive processes have been overwhelmed to the point that daily functioning has been impaired. Anxiety disorders begin at the point of impairment. For example, everyone worries occasionally. When this worry begins to preoccupy a person's thoughts to the point that psychosocial functioning is impeded, an anxiety disorder may be diagnosed.

Anxiety is commonly associated with other medical or psychiatric conditions. Other conditions that give rise to anxiety have their own diagnostic categories: anxiety disorder due to medical condition and substance-induced anxiety disorder. These differential diagnoses, along with other psychiatric disorders that can manifest significant anxiety, are listed in Table 22–2.

PANIC DISORDER WITH OR WITHOUT AGORAPHOBIA

DSM-IV Diagnostic Criteria

A. Both (1) and (2):
  (1) recurrent, unexpected panic attacks (see below)
  (2) at least one of the attacks has been followed by 1 month (or more) of one (or more) of the following:
    (a) persistent concern about having additional attacks
    (b) worry about the implications of the attack or its consequences (eg, losing control, having a heart attack, "going crazy")
    (c) A significant change in behavior related to the attacks
B. The presence or absence of agoraphobia (see below).
C. The panic attacks are not due to the direct physiological effects of a substance or a general medical condition.
D. The panic attacks are not better accounted for by another mental disorder, such as social phobia, specific phobia, obsessive-compulsive disorder, posttraumatic stress disorder, or separation anxiety disorder.

Criteria for Panic Attack (not a separate diagnostic category)

A discrete period of intense fear or discomfort, in which four (or more) of the following symptoms developed abruptly and reached a peak within 10 minutes:

Table 22–2. Differential diagnosis of anxiety disorders.

Medical Illnesses	Substance Use/Abuse	Psychiatric Disorders
Cardiac Angina Arrhythmias Congestive failure Infarction Mitral valve prolapse Paroxysmal atrial tachycardia	**Prescription or over-the-counter drug use** Antidepressants Fenfluramine/phentermine Psychostimulants (eg, methylphenidate, amphetamine) Steroids Sympathomimetics	Adjustment disorders Affective disorder Dissociative disorders Personality disorders Somatoform disorders Schizophrenia (and other psychotic disorders)
Endocrinologic Hyperthyroidism Cushing's disease Hyperparathyroidism Hypoglycemia Premenstrual syndrome	**Substance abuse** Alcohol/sedative withdrawal Caffeine Hallucinogen Stimulant abuse (eg, cocaine)	
Neoplastic Carcinoid Insulinoma Pheocromocytoma		
Neurologic Huntington's disease Meniere's disease Migraine Multiple sclerosis Seizure disorder Transient ischemic attack Vertigo Wilson's disease		
Pulmonary Asthma Embolism Obstruction Obstructive pulmonary disease		
Other Porphyria Uremia		

(1) palpitations, pounding heart, or accelerated heart rate
(2) sweating
(3) trembling or shaking
(4) sensations of shortness of breath or smothering
(5) feeling of choking
(6) chest pain or discomfort
(7) nausea or abdominal distress
(8) feeling dizzy, unsteady, lightheaded, or faint
(9) derealization or depersonalization
(10) fear of losing control or going crazy
(11) fear of dying
(12) paresthesias (numbness or tingling)
(13) chills or hot flashes

Criteria for Agoraphobia (not a separate diagnostic category)

A. Anxiety about being in places or situations from which escape might be difficult (or embarrassing) or in which help may not be available in the event of having an unexpected or situationally predisposed panic attack or panic-like symptoms. Agoraphobic fears typically involve characteristic clusters of situations that include being outside the home alone; being in a crowd or standing in a line; being on a bridge; and traveling on a bus, train, or automobile.

B. The situations are avoided or endured with marked distress or with anxiety about having a panic attack or panic-like symptoms, or require the presence of a companion.

C. The anxiety of phobic avoidance is not better accounted for by another mental disorder, such as social phobia, specific phobia, obsessive-compulsive disorder, posttraumatic stress disorder, or separation anxiety disorder.

Adapted, with permission, from *Diagnostic and Statistical Manual of Mental Disorders*, 4th ed. Copyright 1994 American Psychiatric Association.

General Considerations

A. Major Etiologic Theories: Although there have been many theories about the genesis of panic, two dominant (and not mutually exclusive) frameworks have been proposed. There is strong evidence to support a biological foundation. For example, some antidepressant and antianxiety drugs can block the attacks. Further, specific substances known as panicogens (eg, intravenous sodium lactate or inhalation of 5–35% carbon dioxide) can induce panic attacks in persons with panic disorder while sparing those without such a history. These agents collectively activate brain stem nuclei such as the locus coeruleus. Klein and colleagues have postulated that panic attacks are a result of a misperception of suffocation, referred to as a false suffocation response.

There also is support for a cognitive theory of the disorder. Persons with panic disorder often exhibit common cognitive characteristics, with a strong sensitivity to, and misinterpretation of, physical sensations. Cognitive theory suggests that mild physical symptoms are misinterpreted as dangerous. Cognitive-behavioral psychotherapy, with its emphasis on recognizing and correcting catastrophic thoughts, reduces both agoraphobic avoidance and the panic attacks themselves.

B. Epidemiology: Panic disorder occurs in 1–3% of the population and is about twice as common in women as men. Panic-related phenomena, such as isolated panic attacks or limited-symptom attacks, are much more common. Panic may develop at any time in the life span, although the median age at onset is in the mid-20s. Panic disorder in childhood may be underrecognized or misdiagnosed as a conduct disorder or school avoidance. Children with panic disorder often exhibit considerable avoidance behavior with associated educational disability. Panic disorder may flare up in childhood, become quiescent in the teenage years and early adult life, only to reemerge later.

Clinical Findings

Although the symptoms of panic disorder have been described for over a century, and effective treatment has been available for more than 30 years, the disorder has been recognized widely for only about the last 15 years. Panic disorder is characterized by recurring, spontaneous, unexpected anxiety attacks with rapid onset and short duration. Because of the physical symptoms of the attacks, patients are likely to fear that they are experiencing a heart attack, stroke, or the like. Occasionally patients will think that they are going "crazy" or "out of control." Patients with panic disorder typically fear further attacks, worry about the implications of the attacks (eg, that the attacks indicate a serious undiagnosed physical illness), and change their behavior as a result.

Panic attacks involve severe anxiety symptoms of rapid onset. These symptoms climb to maximum severity within 10 minutes but can peak within a few seconds. Typical symptoms include shortness of breath, tachypnea, tachycardia, tremor, dizziness, hot or cold sensations, chest discomfort, and feelings of depersonalization or derealization. A minimum of four symptoms is required to meet the diagnosis of panic attack. The symptoms usually last for less than 1 hour and most commonly diminish within 30 minutes.

People who experience a panic attack will usually seek help, often at a hospital emergency room. Although this condition is readily diagnosable by clinical signs and symptoms, most cases are not diagnosed initially. This is unfortunate because early detection and treatment can usually prevent disability.

Left untreated, the panic attacks will likely continue. Repeated visits to physicians (of various specialties) and emergency rooms are common. Patients often seek help from many professionals, counselors, therapists, and others. If the diagnosis is not made and treatment is not started, the disorder usually progresses. Patients begin to avoid settings in which panic attacks have happened in the past, particularly social settings such as theaters, malls, grocery stores, churches, and other places where escape might be difficult or embarrassing. Extensive phobic avoidance is referred to as **agoraphobia.**

Agoraphobia is intimately linked with the development of panic disorder. Panic disorder can occur without any significant agoraphobia. This is seen when the panic attacks are relatively mild or are truly spontaneous in nature. However, most people with panic disorder find that particular situations stimulate panic; therefore, they avoid these situations. Most patients find that the likelihood of having an attack is reduced in "safe places" (eg, at home) or with "safe people" (eg, a spouse or parent) who will help in the event of an attack. Phobic avoidance is promoted further by anticipatory anxiety, which occurs when patients envision going into a situation in which an attack might occur.

Agoraphobia rarely occurs without a history of frank panic attacks. When it does occur, it is most often accompanied by so-called **limited-symptom attacks** (panic-like attacks that do not meet the full four-symptom criteria for panic attack). Recurrent limited-symptom attacks often predate full panic attacks in many people with panic disorder.

Differential Diagnosis

Panic disorder and agoraphobia share features with other mental disorders. Persons with OCD, specific and social phobias, posttraumatic stress disorder, major depression, psychotic disorders, and some personality disorders (eg, avoidant, paranoid, dependent, schizoid) exhibit social avoidance. These disorders, however, do not share the features of spontaneous panic attacks. The absence of spontaneous panic attacks also distinguishes other disorders with somatic fears including obsessive-compulsive spectrum disorders (eg, somatic obsessions and body dysmorphic disorder), GAD, and somatization disorders. Although persons with specific and social phobias may have situationally bound panic attacks, recurring unexpected panic attacks do not occur.

Although the diagnosis is usually straightforward, many patients with panic disorder undergo extensive, unnecessary medical evaluation. Some differential diagnostic possibilities for panic attacks include paroxysmal atrial tachycardia, pulmonary embolus, seizure disorder, Meniere's disease, transient ischemic attack, carcinoid syndrome, Cushing's disease, hyperthyroidism, true hypoglycemia, and pheochromocytoma. Extensive medical evaluation for these disorders is indicated only when other features suggest physical disease.

Treatment

A. Pharmacologic Treatment: Panic in many relatively mildly ill patients requires no medication and can be managed with psychotherapy alone. When drug therapy is required, a short course of a low dosage of a benzodiazepine may facilitate behavioral treatment. Behavioral or cognitive-behavioral therapy is the treatment of choice. Medications in combination with psychotherapy should be reserved for more severely ill patients.

Medication should be considered if the panic disorder impairs functioning, for example, (1) if agoraphobia is present or developing, (2) if major depression (currently or by history) or a personality disorder is present, (3) if the patient reports significant suicidal ideation, or (4) if the patient voices a strong preference for medication management. The last option is intended to facilitate the development of the therapeutic alliance and to encourage the patient's involvement in therapy. Many patients with this condition fear behavioral therapy because of the need for exposure to the phobic stimuli.

Tricyclic antidepressants, especially imipramine, have the best-established research record. In fact, imipramine is the standard against which other agents are usually compared. The physician must warn patients about the potential for the development of transient anxiety, along with other side effects (Table 22–3). The dosage should start low and be titrated upward slowly. High plasma levels appear to worsen outcome.

Amitriptyline and clomipramine also have reasonable empirical support for their effectiveness; however, these drugs tend to produce significantly more side effects and are not used widely. Other drugs such as nortriptyline or doxepin have limited support. There is some evidence that other antidepressants, such as desipramine, maprotiline, trazodone, and bupropion, are less effective than imipramine.

The monoamine oxidase inhibitors, especially phenelzine, have relatively strong empirical support. Like imipramine, phenelzine reduces the frequency and intensity of panic attacks. It also appears to have a substantial antianxiety and antiphobic effect. Unfortunately, the effectiveness of phenelzine is limited by its side effects and safety problems. Besides the side effects listed in Table 22–3, hypertensive reactions can occur when the patient's diet has a high tyramine content. Further, toxicity can be produced when this drug is taken with other agents, such as meperidine or sympathomimetic amines. Although such toxic effects can generally be avoided, patients with panic disorder are especially fearful of them.

Research data support the effectiveness of SSRI antidepressants, including paroxetine, fluoxetine, and sertraline, in the treatment of panic disorder. These drugs have become more popular in recent years and

Table 22–3. Drugs used for the treatment of panic disorder.

Drug	Starting Dosage	Daily Dosing Range	Maximum Dosage	Common Side Effects
Imipramine (or other tricyclic antidepressants)	25 mg at bedtime	50–100 mg	150 mg	Dry mouth, blurred vision, constipation, urinary hesitancy, orthostasis, somnolence, anxiety, sexual dysfunction
Phenelzine	15 mg twice daily	30–90 mg	90 mg	Dry mouth, drowsiness, nausea, anxiety/nervousness, orthostatic hypotension, myoclonus, hypertensive reactions
Fluoxetine	10 mg	20–40 mg	60 mg	Nausea, diarrhea, anxiety/nervousness, sexual dysfunction
Paroxetine	10 mg	20–40 mg	60 mg	Nausea, diarrhea, anxiety/nervousness, sexual dysfunction, somnolence
Sertraline	25 mg	25–150 mg	200 mg	Nausea, diarrhea, anxiety/nervousness, sexual dysfunction
Alprazolam	0.25–0.5 mg three times daily	1.5–4.0 mg	6 mg/day	Somnolence, ataxia, memory problems, physical dependence, withdrawal reactions
Clonazepam	0.25–0.5 mg twice daily	1.5–4.0 mg	6 mg/day	Somnolence, ataxia, memory problems, physical dependence, withdrawal reactions

have supplanted other antidepressants and benzodiazepines in the treatment of panic disorder; however, in standard antidepressant dosages, these drugs may not be tolerated because of increased anxiety. Dosages should be started low and titrating upward slowly.

As mentioned earlier, low-dose benzodiazepine management can be used on an as-needed basis to reduce anticipatory anxiety and facilitate exposure activities. Virtually any benzodiazepine can be used successfully in this way. The high-potency benzodiazepines alprazolam and clonazepam have specific antipanic effects. Within the usual dosing range, most patients with panic experience a substantial reduction in panic attacks and also experience a reduction in anticipatory anxiety.

The likelihood of benzodiazepine abuse is low in carefully selected patients; however, nearly all patients eventually develop some degree of physical dependency. On withdrawal, classical withdrawal effects can occur, such as a rebound return of panic symptoms. Many patients find it very difficult to withdraw completely. As many as 60% of patients with panic disorder will stay on these medications indefinitely. Moderate- to high-dose benzodiazepine therapy should be reserved for patients who require pharmacotherapy and who have failed on antidepressant treatment, for those who are unable to tolerate antidepressants, or for those for whom antidepressant medications are otherwise inappropriate.

The medications discussed in this section generally reduce the intensity and frequency of panic symptoms as long as they are taken. After discontinuation, most patients relapse. Relapse often occurs during dosage tapering, even with benzodiazepines. As a result, behavioral or cognitive-behavioral therapy with exposure should be combined with pharmacotherapy.

B. Psychotherapy: A variety of therapies have been used to treat panic disorder. Only traditional behavioral treatments and cognitive-behavioral psychotherapy have significant empirical evidence to support their effectiveness. Considerable evidence supports the effectiveness of cognitive-behavioral therapy for treatment of panic disorder. This approach helps patients to recognize the relationships between specific thoughts (ie, cognitions) and the anxiety that they experience. These thoughts represent misinterpretations of external, or more commonly internal, cues as being threatening. For example, feeling mildly short of breath, slightly tremulous, or having a small increase in heart rate can be misinterpreted as an indication that a catastrophic physical event (eg, heart attack) is occurring. Successful treatment, then, would help the patient to discover the true relationship between specific internal or external cues and their anxiety, and to correctly interpret the cues as benign.

An elaboration of cognitive-behavioral therapy includes **interoceptive exposure** as part of the treatment. This method uses experimental manipulations of physical sensations to induce symptoms that are commonly misinterpreted. Exposure techniques may include spinning in place, hyperventilating voluntarily, or ingesting large amounts of caffeine in order to simulate the physical cues that stimulate anxiety. This technique helps the therapist to uncover the catastrophic cognitions and help the client to interpret them correctly.

The last component of cognitive-behavioral therapy of panic disorder involves more traditional relaxation and exposure activities, in which patients gradually and systematically expose themselves to situations that induce anxiety, thereby desensitizing themselves.

Prognosis & Comorbidity

Overall, the long-term prognosis for panic disorder is good, although a significant proportion of patients will develop disability associated with the condition. Major depression occurs in about 40% of patients. Although both depression and panic symptoms respond to antidepressant drugs, comorbid depression worsens the outcome of panic disorder and increases the rate of suicide. About 7% of patients with panic disorder commit suicide, and more than 20% of patients with panic disorder and comorbid psychiatric disorders will eventually commit suicide. Substance abuse, especially alcoholism, also occurs at an increased frequency in panic disorder relative to the general population.

Ballenger JC et al: Alprazolam in panic disorder and agoraphobia: results from a multicenter trial. I. Efficacy in short-term treatment. Arch Gen Psychiatry 1988;45:413.

Burrows GD, Judd FK, Norman TR: Long-term drug treatment of panic disorder. J Psychiatr Res 1993;27(Suppl 1):111.

Hirschfeld RM: Panic disorder: diagnosis, epidemiology, and clinical course. J Clin Psychiatry 1996;57(Suppl 10):3.

Katon W: Panic disorder: relationship to high medical utilization, unexplained physical symptoms, and medical costs. J Clin Psychiatry 1996;57(Suppl 10):11.

Mavissakalian MR, Perel JM: Imipramine treatment of panic disorder with agoraphobia: dose ranging and plasma level-response relationships. Am J Psychiatry 1995;152:673.

Pollack MH, Otto MW: Long-term course and outcome of panic disorder. J Clin Psychiatry 1997;58(Suppl 2):57.

Rosenbaum JF et al: Integrated treatment of panic disorder. Bull Menninger Clin 1995;59(2 Suppl A):A4.

PHOBIC DISORDERS: SPECIFIC PHOBIA & SOCIAL PHOBIA

DSM-IV Diagnostic Criteria

Specific Phobia

A. A marked and persistent fear that is excessive or unreasonable, cued by the presence or anticipation of a specific object or situation.

B. Exposure to the phobic stimulus almost invariably provokes an immediate anxiety response, which may take the form of a situationally bound or situationally predisposed panic attack.

Note: In children, the anxiety may be expressed by crying, tantrums, freezing, or clinging.

C. The person recognizes that the fear is excessive or unreasonable.

Note: In children, this feature may be absent.

D. The object or situation is avoided or else is endured with intense anxiety or distress.

E. The avoidance, anxious anticipation, or distress in the feared situation(s) interferes significantly with the person's normal routine, occupational (or academic) functioning, or social activities or relationships, or there is marked distress about having the phobia.

F. In individuals under age 18 years, the duration is at least 6 months.

G. The anxiety, panic attacks, or phobic avoidance associated with the specific object or situation are not better accounted for by another mental disorder, such as obsessive-compulsive disorder, posttraumatic stress disorder, separation anxiety disorder, social phobia, panic disorder with agoraphobia, or agoraphobia without history of panic disorder.

Specify type:

Animal type: if the fear is cued by animals or insects. This subtype generally has a childhood onset.

Natural environment type: if the fear is cued by objects in the natural environment, such as storms, heights, or water. This subtype generally has a childhood onset.

Blood-injection-injury type: if the fear is cued by seeing blood or an injury or by receiving an injection or other invasive medical procedure. This subtype is highly familial and is often characterized by a strong vasovagal response.

Situational type: if the fear is cued by a specific situation such as public transportation, tunnels, bridges, elevators, flying, driving, or enclosed places. This subtype has a bimodal age-at-onset distribution, with one peak in childhood and another peak in the mid-20s. This subtype appears to be similar to panic disorder with agoraphobia in its characteristic sex ratios, familial aggregation pattern, and age at onset.

Other type: if the fear is cued by other stimuli. These stimuli might include the fear or avoidance of situations that might lead to choking, vomiting, or contracting an illness; "space" phobia (ie, the individual is afraid of falling down if away from walls or other means of physical support); and children's fears of loud sounds or costumed characters.

Social Phobia

A. A marked and persistent fear of one or more social or performance situations in which the person is exposed to unfamiliar people or to possible scrutiny by others. The individual fears that he or she will act in a way (or show anxiety symptoms) that will be humiliating or embarrassing.

Note: In children, there must be evidence of the capacity for age-appropriate social relationships with familiar people and the anxiety must occur in peer settings, not just in interactions with adults.

B. Exposure to the feared social situation almost invariably provokes anxiety, which may take the form of a situationally bound or situationally predisposed panic attack.

Note: In children, the anxiety may be expressed by crying, tantrums, freezing, or shrinking from social situations with unfamiliar people.

C. The person recognizes that the fear is excessive or unreasonable.

Note: In children, this feature may be absent.

D. The social or performance situation is avoided or else is endured with intense anxiety or distress.

E. The avoidance, anxious anticipation, or distress in the feared social or performance situation(s) interferes significantly with the person's normal routine, occupational (or academic) functioning, or social activities or relationships, or there is marked distress about having the phobia.

F. In individuals under age 18 years, the duration is at least 6 months.

G. The fear or avoidance is not due to the direct physiological effects of a substance or a general medical condition and is not better accounted for by another mental disorder.

H. If a general medical condition or another mental disorder is present, the fear in Criterion A is unrelated to it, eg, the fear is not of stuttering, trembling in Parkinson's disease, or exhibiting abnormal eating behavior in anorexia nervosa or bulimia nervosa.

Specify if:

Generalized: if the fears include most social situations.

Note: Also consider the additional diagnosis of avoidant personality disorder.

Adapted, with permission, from *Diagnostic and Statistical Manual of Mental Disorders,* 4th ed. Copyright 1994 American Psychiatric Association.

General Considerations

Phobic disorders are among the most common of all psychiatric disorders. Specific phobia affects 5–10% of the general population, and social phobia affects about 3%. The onset is typically in childhood or early adult life, and the condition is usually chronic. Many people with specific phobia learn to "live around" the feared stimulus. Social phobia is often more disabling.

Phobic disorders may develop because of a pairing of anxiety with specific environmental events or experiences. For example, emotional trauma accompanying experiences such as riding in a car or speaking in public may produce a phobia. The majority of individuals with these problems, however, do not report that particular events have led to the disorder. Under these circumstances, the etiology is unknown.

Clinical Findings

A specific phobia is an intense, irrational fear or aversion to a particular object or situation, other than a social situation. Typical specific phobias are fears of animals (especially insects or spiders); the natural environment (eg, storms); blood, injection, or injury; or situations (eg, heights, closed places, elevators, airplane travel). Most people deal with this problem by simply avoiding the feared stimulus, although this is not always possible. For example, people who have a fear of insects or spiders may avoid basements, attics, or closets; however, the emotional reactions or avoidance behavior may cause more serious problems. People who have a fear of flying may be unable to perform certain kinds of work. People who have a blood-injection-injury phobia may experience vasodilation, bradycardia, orthostatic hypotension, or fainting on exposure.

Social phobia is characterized by an extreme anxiety response in situations in which the affected person may be observed by others. People with social phobia usually fear that they will act in an embarrassing or humiliating manner. As with a specific phobia, social situations are avoided or endured with severe anxiety. Common phobic situations include speaking in public, eating in public, using public restrooms, writing while others are observing, and performing publicly. Rarely, people with this condition suffer from generalized social phobia, in which most or all social situations are avoided.

Differential Diagnosis

DSM-IV diagnostic criteria allow the inclusion of a situationally confined panic attack in the category of phobic disorders. Therefore, panic disorder (with or without accompanying agoraphobia) must be distinguished from phobic disorders. In phobic disorders, anxiety or fear is restricted to a particular object or situation. Panic disorder, by definition, is characterized by severe, unexpected anxiety attacks during at least some phase of the disorder. Agoraphobia is distinguished by its association with panic disorder. This condition is differentiated by anxiety that occurs in situations in which help might not be available in case of a panic attack.

Avoidant personality disorder shares many features with and is often comorbid with social phobia. The generalized form of social phobia is especially difficult to distinguish from avoidant personality. Avoidant personality disorder is in many ways equivalent to patho-

logic shyness and is characterized in DSM-IV by "a pervasive pattern of social inhibition, feelings of inadequacy, and hypersensitivity to negative evaluation." Like social phobia, avoidant personality disorder is usually associated with a fear of being shamed or ridiculed; however, in social phobia the fear is generally confined to performance situations, with a relative sparing of other social interactions. For example, a person with social phobia may find it quite impossible to speak or write in public, whereas he or she could conduct a casual conversation with ease. This would not be true of someone with avoidant personality disorder.

People with psychotic or paranoid disorders may experience abnormal fears and avoid others. Patients with somatoform disorders (eg, hypochondriasis) may exhibit anxiety and avoidance that can be confused with phobic disorders. However, unlike patients with somatoform disorder, those with specific or social phobias retain insight into the irrationality of their condition. OCD or major depression can sometimes be confused with phobic disorders.

Treatment

A. Pharmacologic Treatment: Although treatments for phobic disorders typically are psychotherapeutic, some drug treatments have been used (Table 22–4). Benzodiazepines are commonly used to reduce the anxiety associated with specific and social phobias. β-Blockers such as propranolol have been used with success to reduce the autonomic hyperarousal and tremor associated with performance situations. β-Blockers can also be helpful in blood-injection-injury phobia. These medications all have attendant side effects and are often unnecessary because behavioral treatments are so effective. Controlled clinical trials have shown antidepressants, such as imipramine, to be beneficial in treating social phobia, especially the generalized type of social phobia.

B. Psychotherapy: Behavioral or cognitive-behavioral psychotherapies are the treatments of choice. A typical treatment regimen involves relaxation training, usually coupled with visualization of the phobic stimulus, followed by progressive desensitization through repeated controlled exposure to the phobic cue. This regimen is generally followed by extinction of the anxiety response. A cognitive-behavioral approach adds the dimension of managing the catastrophic thoughts associated with exposure to the situation.

Complications, Comorbidity, & Adverse Outcomes of Treatment

Specific and social phobias are common and usually fairly benign conditions. Many people experience specific fears but learn to live around them. That is, most people with phobias simply avoid situations in which they may be exposed to a phobic stimulus. Phobias occasionally have a disabling effect. For example, a business executive with a fear of public speaking or flying may find that the phobia restricts his or

Table 22–4. Pharmacologic treatment of social phobia.

Drug	Starting Dosage	Daily Dosing Range	Maximum Dosage	Common Side Effects
Imipramine	50 mg at bedtime	100–250 mg	250 mg	Dry mouth, blurred vision, constipation, urinary hesitancy, orthostasis, somnolence, anxiety, sexual dysfunction
Phenelzine	15 mg twice daily	30–90 mg	90 mg	Dry mouth, drowsiness, nausea, anxiety/nervousness, orthostatic hypotension, myoclonus, hypertensive reactions
Paroxetine	20 mg	20–40 mg	60 mg	Nausea, diarrhea, anxiety/nervousness, sexual dysfunction, somnolence
Fluoxetine	20 mg	20–60 mg	80 mg	Nausea, diarrhea, anxiety/nervousness, sexual dysfunction
Sertraline	50 mg	50–150 mg	200 mg	Nausea, diarrhea, anxiety/nervousness, sexual dysfunction
Benzodiazepines (various)	—	—	—	Somnolence, ataxia, memory problems, nausea, physical dependence, withdrawal reactions
Propranolol	10 mg as needed	10–40 mg as needed	240 mg/day	Drowsiness, headache, orthostatic hypotension, bradycardia, exacerbation of asthma or obstructive pulmonary disease

her ability to benefit from career advancement. Although behavioral treatments may be anxiety provoking, they often produce significant results. Some individuals use substances of abuse, especially alcohol, to endure their anxiety; therefore, a careful alcohol and drug history is important in the evaluation of patients with phobic disorders.

Prognosis & Course of Illness

Relatively little is known about the long-term course of phobic disorders; however, untreated, phobias often are chronic conditions.

Curtis GC et al: Specific fears and phobias. Epidemiology and classification. Br J Psychiatry 1998;173:212.
Liebowitz MR: Pharmacotherapy of social phobia. J Clin Psychiatry 1993;54(Suppl):31.
Marks I: Blood-injury phobia: a review. Am J Psychiatry 1988;145:1207.
Rapaport MH, Paniccia G, Judd LL: A review of social phobia. Psychopharmacol Bull 1995;31:125.

GENERALIZED ANXIETY DISORDER

DSM-IV Diagnostic Criteria

A. Excessive anxiety and worry (apprehensive expectation), occurring more days than not for at least 6 months about a number of events or activities (such as work or school performance).

B. The person finds it difficult to control the worry.

C. The anxiety and worry are associated with three (or more) of the following six symptoms (with at least some symptoms present for more days than not for the past 6 months).

Note: Only one item is required in children.

(1) restlessness or feeling keyed up—on edge
(2) easily fatigued
(3) difficulty concentrating or mind going blank
(4) irritability
(5) muscle tension
(6) sleep disturbance

D. The focus of the anxiety and worry is not confined to features of an Axis I disorder, eg, the anxiety or worry is not about having a panic attack (as in panic disorder), being contaminated (as in obsessive-compulsive disorder), being away from home or close relatives (as in separation anxiety disorder), gaining weight (as in anorexia nervosa), having multiple physical complaints (as in somatization disorder), or having a serious illness (as in hypochondriasis), and the anxiety and worry do not occur exclusively during posttraumatic stress disorder.

E. The anxiety, worry, or physical symptoms cause clinically significant distress or impairment in social, occupational, or other important areas of functioning.

F. The disturbance is not due to the direct physiological effects of a substance (eg, a drug of abuse, a medication) or medical condition (eg, hypothyroidism) and does not occur exclusively during a mood disorder, a psychotic disorder, or a pervasive developmental disorder.

Reprinted, with permission, from *Diagnostic and Statistical Manual of Mental Disorders,* 4th ed. Copyright 1994 American Psychiatric Association.

General Considerations

GAD typically begins in early adult life, is seen slightly more commonly in women, and is usually chronic. Although this disorder is fairly common, it is seen more frequently in general medical practice than in psychiatry practice. Patients with GAD typically experience persistent worry of variable severity across time that often leads them to their primary care clinician for help. Continuity of care across time is critical to the recognition and treatment of this disorder. Further, patients with GAD have a high rate of comorbidity with major depression. GAD comes closest to the classic concept of the anxiety neurosis. Peter Tyrer and colleagues have discussed the broader concept of the so-called **general neurotic syndrome,** in which there is persisting anxiety and worry that is associated with inhibited or dependent personality characteristics. This syndrome can occur in the absence of major life events. Within this theoretical construct, there can be a change in the primary diagnosis over time. That is, the patient may experience bouts of depression or other psychiatric disorders superimposed on a chronic pattern of anxiety, fear, or worry.

Tyrer P, Seivewright N, Ferguson B, et al: The general neurotic syndrome: a coaxial diagnosis of anxiety, depression, and personality disorder. Acta Psychiatr Scand 1992;85:201.

Clinical Findings

GAD is a syndrome of persistent worry coupled with symptoms of hyperarousal. Most patients with GAD do not recognize themselves as having a psychiatric disorder, even though the symptoms can be quite disabling. These patients are much more likely to present in a general medical setting than in a psychiatrist's office. For this reason, primary care clinicians must be particularly sensitive to patients' emotional needs.

Differential Diagnosis

Persistent hyperarousal coupled with obsessive thoughts are common to other psychiatric disorders (eg, major depression). In some ways, GAD could be considered to be major depression without persistently depressed mood or anhedonia (see Chapter 21). In fact, GAD often responds well to treatment with tricyclic antidepressants, as discussed later in this chapter. If the patient worries chronically, depression should always be considered in the differential diagnosis. Other psychiatric disorders with obsessive thinking (eg, OCD; panic disorder; somatoform disorders; psychotic disorders, especially paranoid subtypes; eating disorders, particularly anorexia nervosa; and many personality disorders) are associated with persistent fear, apprehension, or worry that can be confused with GAD. The focus of the worry should not be related primarily to one of these conditions. For example, if a patient fears the occurrence of a panic attack, the obvious cause of the problem is panic disorder, even if other associated worries (eg, personal health or the well-being of a significant other) are present. Similarly, if the central concern is physical health, without panic attacks, then somatoform disorder is likely to be the primary diagnosis.

Treatment

The management of GAD should consider the long-standing nature of the problem. Treatment should deal with the underlying causes of the condition, such as persistently distorted cognitions. Unfortunately, several factors work against treatment. GAD tends to be underrecognized. Even when it is identified, the problem is often not taken as seriously as the degree of disability associated with the condition would suggest. If treatment is provided, it is likely to be brief. Finally, insurance coverage tends to discriminate against the treatment of this problem. Together, these factors conspire to ensure that most patients with this problem do not get appropriate treatment.

A. Pharmacologic Treatment: Patients with GAD are likely to receive benzodiazepines, even though psychotherapies and other medications are clearly beneficial. Although benzodiazepines are helpful, GAD is a chronic condition and benzodiazepines are not curative. If benzodiazepines alone are used, long-term management is required to prevent symptoms from returning. Benzodiazepines generally should not be used alone to treat GAD, but they can be helpful adjuncts to treatment, particularly when the symptoms are severe. Short-term, low-to-moderate dosages of benzodiazepines can facilitate psychotherapy. Benzodiazepines can also be used to reduce symptoms and to return the patient to normal functioning. After a few weeks, the benzodiazepine should be reduced and eventually discontinued.

Most clinicians worry about the potential for benzodiazepine abuse. Epidemiologic studies, however, demonstrate that legitimate clinical use far outweighs any abuse. True abuse is relatively uncommon. Benzodiazepine abuse is seen most often in three situations: (1) when they are used by persons to counteract the adverse effects of psychostimulants such as cocaine, (2) when they are used to augment the euphoric effects of other sedative drugs such as alcohol, or (3) when they are used for self-medication in alcohol or other sedative withdrawal.

Benzodiazepines should not be given to patients who have a personal history or strong first-degree family history of drug or alcohol abuse. Even though the primary abuse of benzodiazepines is uncommon, some patients develop psychological and physiologic dependence. Physiologic dependence becomes an increasing problem when these drugs have been given continuously for 3 months or more, although mild withdrawal reactions can occur after shorter treatment periods. Clinicians who are considering treating GAD with benzodiazepines should first weigh the alternatives (described later in this section). In general, brief, interrupted courses of benzodiazepine treatment should be given as psychotherapeutic management is being initiated; prescription refills should be monitored carefully; and the drug should then be tapered if continuous use exceeds 1 month. Problems can generally be avoided under these circumstances.

Benzodiazepines can produce other adverse effects, such as daytime sedation, ataxia (which can cause dangerous falls in the elderly), accident proneness (eg, motor vehicle accidents), headaches, memory problems (ranging from short-term memory problems to brief periods of profound memory loss), and occasionally, paradoxical excitement or anxiety. These problems are especially prominent in the elderly, in whom drug metabolites can accumulate and produce high plasma levels.

The anxiolytic buspirone, a serotonin 1_A receptor partial agonist, is an alternative to benzodiazepines (Table 22–5). Buspirone has several advantages. It produces no motor, memory, or concentration impairments. It has no abuse potential, and it does not cause dependency or withdrawal, even after long periods of exposure. It does not produce drug interactions. It appears to be an almost ideal anxiolytic; however, it has some disadvantages. In contrast to the benzodiazepines, which are often experienced by patients as having an immediate effect, buspirone requires at least 3 weeks to mitigate anxiety. Patients with severe anxiety, especially those who previously received benzodiazepines, may have a reduced level of response. Further, buspirone stimulates the locus coeruleus, which may be associated with a paradoxical increase in anxiety in some patients. Despite these disadvantages, buspirone should be considered a practical alternative to benzodiazepines. Although not adequately tested empirically, this drug is often used for long-term treatment.

The tricyclic antidepressant imipramine and the heterocyclic antidepressant venlafaxine have demonstrated significant benefit in the treatment of GAD. Like buspirone, the therapeutic effect is delayed, but severely anxious patients appear to improve.

Other tricyclic antidepressants or selective serotonin reuptake inhibitors (SSRIs) may be helpful but have not been tested adequately. β-Blockers and clonidine have been reported to be helpful in treating GAD. Although these drugs can reduce anxiety, side effects of hypotension and depression are prominent. Antipsychotic drugs, such as chlorpromazine or haloperidol, reduce anxiety, but the risk of tardive dyskinesia outweighs the potential benefit.

B. Psychotherapy: Two psychotherapeutic approaches are helpful in treating GAD. Behavioral therapy can teach patients progressive deep muscle relaxation while they imagine anxiety-inducing stimuli. If the patient avoids situations that generate significant anxiety, progressive desensitization can be helpful.

An alternative is cognitive-behavioral therapy. This treatment adds a cognitive component to basic behavioral therapy on the assumption that the anxiety associated with GAD is a result of persistent distortions about the self, other people, and the future. Misinterpretations, especially catastrophic misperceptions of threat or danger, contribute significantly to anxiety. Cognitive-behavioral therapy helps patients to recognize the relationships between specific situations and pathogenic distortions of thinking. Further, the treatment helps to elucidate the faulty fundamental belief systems that underlie the distorted thinking. Patients learn to recognize and counter the distortions with alternative thoughts that eventually become automatic.

Other interventions may be needed, such as marital, family, or occupational therapy. Other primary therapies (eg, psychodynamic, client-centered, or interpersonal therapy) have little or no empirical support.

Complications & Comorbidity

GAD is a highly comorbid condition. The most common comorbid diagnosis is major depression. As noted earlier in this chapter, diagnostic primacy may

Table 22–5. Pharmacologic treatment of generalized anxiety disorder.

Drug	Starting Dosage	Daily Dosing Range	Maximum Dosage	Common Side Effects
Buspirone	5 mg three times daily	15–40 mg	60 mg	Anxiety/nervousness, headache, nausea
Imipramine	25 mg at bedtime	25–150 mg	200 mg	Dry mouth, blurred vision, constipation, urinary hesitancy, orthostasis, somnolence, anxiety
Venlafaxine	37.5 mg in the morning	37.5–225 mg	300 mg	Anxiety/nervousness, nausea, diarrhea, sexual dysfunction, withdrawal reactions
Benzodiazepines (various)	—	—	—	Somnolence, ataxia, memory problems, nausea, physical dependence, withdrawal reactions

shift frequently across the patient's lifetime in a more chronic neurotic pattern between the more typical depressive and anxious symptoms. GAD may be comorbid with other conditions, including personality disorders (eg, obsessive-compulsive, schizoid, histrionic, avoidant) or other anxiety disorders (eg, OCD, panic disorder). The diagnosis of GAD should be given only if the diagnosis is clearly independent of other Axis I or Axis II disorders. For example, the diagnosis would not be given to a patient who has a history of persistent anxiety or worry occurring only in the context of major depression. Similarly, the diagnosis is excluded if the worries or fears are clearly related to the pattern of OCD, social phobia, or panic disorder. However, the diagnosis can be given if the symptoms of GAD predate the onset of these other conditions or are otherwise definitely temporally independent. Because the frequency of comorbidity is high, the existence of comorbid disorders should be examined whenever the diagnosis of GAD is considered.

Prognosis & Course of Illness

DSM-IV diagnostic criteria require the characteristic features of GAD to be present for at least 6 months before the diagnosis can be made. However, most patients are chronically ill, often for decades. Untreated, GAD typically follows a chronic pattern, with waxing and waning severity. Comorbid conditions may contribute to chronicity. Pharmacologic treatments will relieve symptoms, but the syndrome usually reemerges after treatment has been discontinued. Psychotherapeutic management (with or without symptomatic treatment with medications) often is helpful in reducing the chronicity associated with GAD.

Barlow DH, Wincze J: DSM-IV and beyond: what is generalized anxiety disorder? Acta Psychiatr Scand 1998; 393(Suppl):23.

Rickels K et al: Antidepressants for the treatment of generalized anxiety disorder. Arch Gen Psychiatry 1993; 50:884.

GENERAL REFERENCES

Chambless DL, Gillis: Cognitive therapy of anxiety disorders. J Consult Clin Psychol 1993;61:248.

Sellers EM et al: Alprazolam and benzodiazepine dependence. J Clin Psychiatry 1993;54(Suppl):64.

Posttraumatic Stress Disorder & Acute Stress Disorder

23

Gregory M. Gillette, MD, & Elliot M. Fielstein, PhD

POSTTRAUMATIC STRESS DISORDER

DSM-IV Diagnostic Criteria

A. The person has been exposed to a traumatic event in which both of the following were present:
   (1) the person experienced, witnessed, or was confronted with an event or events that involved actual or threatened death or serious injury, or a threat to the physical integrity of self or others
   (2) the person's response involved fear, helplessness, or horror
B. The traumatic event is persistently reexperienced in one (or more) of the following ways:
   (1) recurrent and intrusive distressing recollections of the event, including images, thoughts, or perceptions
   (2) recurrent distressing dreams of the event
   (3) acting or feeling as if the traumatic event were recurring (includes a sense of reliving the experience, illusions, hallucinations, and dissociative flashback episodes, including those that occur on awakening or when intoxicated)
   (4) intense psychological distress at exposure to internal or external cues that symbolize or resemble an aspect of the traumatic event
   (5) physiological reactivity on exposure to internal or external cues that symbolize or resemble an aspect of the traumatic event
C. Persistent avoidance of stimuli associated with the trauma and numbing of general responsiveness (not present before the trauma), as indicated by three (or more) of the following:
   (1) efforts to avoid thoughts, feelings, or conversations associated with the trauma
   (2) efforts to avoid activities, places, or people that arouse recollections of the trauma
   (3) inability to recall an important aspect of the trauma

(4) markedly diminished interest or participation in significant activities
(5) feeling of detachment or estrangement from others
(6) restricted range of affect (eg, unable to have loving feelings)
(7) sense of a foreshortened future (eg, does not expect to have a career, marriage, children, or a normal life span)
D. Persistent symptoms of increased arousal (not present before the trauma), as indicated by two (or more) of the following:
   (1) difficulty falling or staying asleep
   (2) irritability or outbursts of anger
   (3) difficulty concentrating
   (4) hypervigilance
   (5) exaggerated startle response
E. Duration of the disturbance (symptoms in Criteria B, C, and D) is more than 1 month.
F. The disturbance causes clinically significant distress or impairment in social, occupational, or other important areas of functioning.

Reprinted, with permission, from *Diagnostic and Statistical Manual of Mental Disorders,* 4th ed. Copyright 1994 American Psychiatric Association.

General Considerations

A. Major Etiologic Theories: By definition a patient cannot have posttraumatic stress disorder without having already experienced a traumatic event or events; therefore, such events must somehow be involved in the etiology of posttraumatic stress disorder. Much of the initial impetus for codifying the disorder in the *Diagnostic and Statistical Manual of Mental Disorders,* 3rd edition (DSM-III) came from mental health professionals with a strong sense of advocacy on behalf of Vietnam combat veterans whose mental afflictions seemed inadequately captured by the diagnostic nosologies extant before 1980. Consequently, at the time criteria for the disorder were being codified in 1980, there was a strong theoretical bias toward portraying posttraumatic stress disorder as the inevitable consequence of overwhelming traumatic events themselves. Allied to this assumption was the concept that symptoms of the disorder occurring months, years, or even decades after the initial traumatic events represented the persistence or recurrence in nontraumatic situations of reactions to overwhelming traumatic events that were normal reactions at the time of these events.

Because fewer than half of persons exposed to comparable traumatic events, whether military or civilian, develop posttraumatic stress disorder, early theoretical assumptions regarding the exclusive role of the traumatic events themselves have come under scrutiny. The role of pretraumatic biological or psychological vulnerability, either constitutional or developmental, has become an important focus, as has the possibility that even immediate responses to traumatic events may have been abnormal or poorly adaptive at the time of the events. Such questions are currently being investigated in twin-based studies.

Concerning neurobiological theories of posttraumatic stress disorder, the neurotransmitter system of predominant interest has been the noradrenergic cerebral cortical projection from the brain stem locus coeruleus, studied extensively by investigators at Yale University. Recent findings suggest excessive noradrenergic tone in the locus coeruleus, possibly accounting for both hyperarousal and reexperiencing symptoms. Other neurotransmitters (eg, dopamine, N-methyl-D-aspartate, acetylcholine) and neuropeptides (eg, opioids, corticotropin-releasing hormone, thyrotropin-releasing hormone) have also been implicated as having a possible role in the mechanistic etiology of posttraumatic stress disorder. Post and colleagues have proposed a model attempting to integrate the variety of biochemical findings in posttraumatic stress disorder, based on analogy or homology with the preclinical amygdala-kindled-seizures model of recurrent affective disorders. This model will no doubt prompt reconsideration of the complexity of the biological underpinnings of posttraumatic stress disorder.

B. Epidemiology: As yet, there are no epidemiologic data based on DSM-IV diagnostic criteria for posttraumatic stress disorder. According to the National Comorbidity Survey, based on DSM-III-R diagnostic criteria, American men aged 15–54 years had a lifetime prevalence of exposure to qualifying traumatic events of 60.7%, with a lifetime prevalence of having developed posttraumatic stress disorder of 5.0%. Women in the same age range exhibited a 51.2% lifetime prevalence of trauma exposure and 10.4% lifetime prevalence of posttraumatic stress disorder, suggesting that women are more than twice as likely as men to develop posttraumatic stress disorder after exposure to a traumatic event. This skewed gender ratio must be interpreted with caution, however,

given differences in the type of traumas to which men and women report exposure. Among men, the traumas most commonly associated with posttraumatic stress disorder are combat exposure and witnessing overt violence, whereas among women the most commonly associated traumas are rape and sexual molestation.

C. Genetics: Several twin-based studies indicate an important role for genetic vulnerability in the development of combat-related posttraumatic stress disorder. Another study currently under way is investigating the role of genetic factors in determining biological variables or markers putatively associated with combat-related posttraumatic stress disorder (ie, exaggerated startle response, mid-latency and long-latency auditory evoked brain potentials, and hypocortisolemia). Twin-based studies have not been performed in a comparable manner to elucidate the genetic influence on posttraumatic stress disorder related to civilian traumas.

Charney DS et al: Neural circuits and mechanisms of post-traumatic stress disorder. In: Friedman MJ, Charney DS, Deutch AY (editors): *Neurobiological and Clinical Consequences of Stress: From Normal Adaptation to Post-Traumatic Stress Disorder.* Lippincott-Raven, 1995.

McFarlane AC: The aetiology of post-traumatic morbidity: predisposing, precipitating and perpetuating factors. Br J Psychiatry 1989;154:221.

Post RM, Weiss SRB, Smith MA: Sensitization and kindling: implications for the evolving neural substrates of post-traumatic stress disorder. In: Friedman MJ, Charney DS, Deutch AY (editors): *Neurobiological and Clinical Consequences of Stress: From Normal Adaptation to Post-Traumatic Stress Disorder.* Lippincott-Raven, 1995.

Yehuda R, McFarlane AC: Conflict between current knowledge about posttraumatic stress disorder and its original conceptual basis. Am J Psychiatry 1995;152:1705.

Clinical Findings

A. Signs & Symptoms: Most prominent and pathognomonic among the variety of symptoms listed in the DSM-IV diagnostic criteria for posttraumatic stress disorder are those representing the reexperiencing of traumatic event(s) in the form of dreams, flashbacks, and intrusive memories of these events. What makes all of these perceptions pathologic is that they are recurrent, intrusive, and distressful. Additional reexperiencing symptoms include intense emotional distress or physiologic reactivity subsequent to exposure to trauma reminders. Despite some possibly important symptom profile differences among posttraumatic stress disorder patients with differing traumatic events, the primacy of reexperiencing symptoms in the development of the disorder has been confirmed in patient populations as diverse as World War II holocaust survivors, Israeli combatants from the 1982 Lebanon war, volunteer firefighters in the devastating bushfires in Australia in 1983, and American women survivors of rape and assault. Findings in two diverse traumatized populations (Persian Gulf War veterans and female victims of rape and nonsexual assault) suggest that symptoms of hyperarousal may be most universal and most severe in the first months after trauma exposure but may not necessarily discriminate those who will progress to diagnosable posttraumatic stress disorder from those who will not.

Some DSM-IV hyperarousal symptoms of posttraumatic stress disorder may be difficult to distinguish from symptoms in the reexperiencing and avoidance clusters. For example, difficulty falling or staying asleep may overlap with recurrent distressing dreams insofar as anticipating trauma-related dreams may result in a patient's reluctance to fall asleep, or such dreams may in and of themselves result in awakenings from sleep. Outbursts of anger may mimic or be indistinguishable from reenactment flashbacks of the victim's behavior in traumatic situations of combat or sexual assault. Difficulty concentrating may overlap in presentation with inability to recall an important aspect of the trauma or markedly diminished interest or participation in significant activities. Hypervigilance and exaggerated startle response may overlap with physiologic reactivity to reminders.

B. Psychological Testing:

1. Self-report questionnaires—A variety of self-report questionnaires have been developed for assistance in both making the diagnosis of posttraumatic stress disorder and measuring the severity of its symptoms. Some of these instruments have been adapted from general psychopathology scales, whereas others have been constructed specifically for assessing posttraumatic stress disorder. Advantages of self-report measures lie in their brevity and efficiency, requiring minimum clinician time. Limitations of such measures include vulnerability to feigned or exaggerated symptoms, and dependency on intact cognition. The next several sections describe selected self-report measures for posttraumatic stress disorder.

a. Minnesota Multiphasic Personality Inventory-Posttraumatic Stress Disorder (MMPI-PTSD) subscale. The MMPI-PTSD subscale, developed by Keane and colleagues, has demonstrated improved diagnostic accuracy compared with clinical scale profiles derived from the entire MMPI, but it remains vulnerable to the weakness of the latter: It often identifies as having posttraumatic disorder individuals who do not have it (ie, false positives) but who exhibit elevations on this subscale because of high levels of general distress.

b. Rorschach inkblot test. The Rorschach inkblot test is one of the original psychological tests used to assess psychopathology. In recent years, standardization has been applied to administration and scoring of the test, increasing its reliability. The Rorschach is a projective technique, designed to assess unconscious processes, revealed through their projection as meaningful percepts upon ambiguous stimuli such as inkblots. Investigators have studied Rorschach responses in diverse posttraumatic stress disorder populations, revealing relatively consistent patterns of impaired reality perception, affect dysregulation, low stress tolerance with impulsivity, and emotional distancing, corresponding with certain DSM-IV posttraumatic stress disorder diagnostic criteria on symptom checklists and interview questions, where obvious symptom descriptions are readily subject to volitional exaggeration or even fabrication.

c. Mississippi Scale for Combat-Related Posttraumatic Stress Disorder. Keane and colleagues developed this scale specifically to measure DSM-III posttraumatic stress disorder symptoms in male combat veterans. Alternate forms are available for use with civilians and women. Several analyses of its diagnostic utility have been encouraging for detection of posttraumatic stress disorder in both treatment-seeking patients and community samples. Its primary weakness lies in the fact that an informed respondent can easily determine which items are posttraumatic stress disorder symptoms, rendering it vulnerable to deliberate exaggeration or fabrication of symptoms.

d. Impact of Events Scale (IES). Horowitz and colleagues developed the IES to measure the psychological impact of traumatic events before DSM-III criteria were introduced. It was derived from an empirically validated model of stress response syndromes, and it focuses on intrusion and avoidance symptoms. The IES has been standardized with a predominantly female and civilian traumatized population. Diagnostic studies indicate the IES is highly sensitive but only moderately specific.

2. Measures of traumatic stressors—To date, less attention has been devoted to development of objective measures to characterize traumatic stressor events than to development of instruments to measure symptom severity. Most measures of traumatic stressors currently available have been developed for male Vietnam combat veterans. The most widely used of these, the Combat Exposure Scale, is a seven-item instrument that rates the degree of exposure to combat-related life-threatening events. A more extensive measure of Vietnam combat trauma has been developed for use in large-scale community-based studies of posttraumatic stress disorder. It includes 100 items measuring a variety of dimensions of combat-related traumatic stress. A war zone scale appropriate for female Vietnam veterans, the Women's Wartime Stressor Scale, covers potentially traumatizing events in professional, environmental, and psychosocial domains.

A comprehensive structured diagnostic interview for psychiatric disorders ideally should be able to aid in the diagnosis of both posttraumatic stress disorder and other Axis I and Axis II disorders at the level of symptom presence or absence, if not severity, and it should be able to aid in the determination of whether symptoms are present following trauma that are not subsumed under the posttraumatic stress disorder diagnostic criteria. A common limitation of currently available structured or semistructured clinical diagnostic interviews is their failure to provide measures of symptom severity. Rating scales are still more useful for this purpose.

a. Structured Clinical Interview for DSM-IV (SCID), Posttraumatic Stress Disorder Module (SCID-PTSD). The SCID is a semistructured interview system for comprehensive diagnosis of all major DSM-IV Axis I and Axis II disorders, including posttraumatic stress disorder. The posttraumatic stress disorder module consists of an initial open-ended narrative by the patient to identify traumatic exposure, which then serves as the basis for assessment of signs and symptoms. Diagnostic criteria are presented with probe questions formatted to determine severity of each symptom. A trained clinician must administer the SCID. The SCID-PTSD has been used in a large-scale community-based study of Vietnam veterans and has demonstrated satisfactory interrater reliability and close correspondence with the Mississippi Scale for posttraumatic stress disorder and the MMPI-PTSD subscale. The time required for this interview (up to 1–3 hours in complicated cases with psychiatric comorbidity) makes it inefficient for routine clinical practice.

b. Clinician Administered Posttraumatic Stress Disorder Scale (CAPS). This structured interview is a comprehensive, DSM-IV-based diagnostic instrument. A unique feature of the CAPS is its provision of both intensity and frequency ratings for severity of each symptom. The CAPS assesses related features of the disorder such as anxiety, depression, and suicidality and provides supplemental measures of social and occupational impairments. Current and lifetime versions of the scale are available.

c. Posttraumatic Stress Disorder Interview (PTSD-I). The PTSD-I was developed to reflect DSM-III-R criteria and to provide both dichotomous and continuous measures of posttraumatic stress disorder symptom severity. This interview differs from semistructured interviews described earlier in this section in that the patient, not the interviewer, rates symptom severity. This feature makes it possible for the interview to be administered by a nonprofessional. Validation studies with Vietnam veterans reveal high correlations with posttraumatic stress disorder–related psychometric instruments and good sensitivity and specificity for diagnosis of posttraumatic stress disorder.

3. Assessment of cognitive disturbance—A relatively recent focus for research in psychological assessment of posttraumatic stress disorder has been investigation of apparent cognitive disturbances in patients who have posttraumatic stress disorder. Neurobiological research suggests that exposure to chronic stress is associated with disturbances in neurochemical systems that may damage brain structures involved in cognitive processes such as attention, memory, and learning. Psychological treatment

for posttraumatic stress disorder, including most currently applied psychotherapy techniques, requires not only the basic cognitive capacities of attention and memory but also a substantial degree of reasoning and problem-solving ability. Neuropsychological tests of attention, memory, learning, and problem solving have been applied to the study of posttraumatic stress disorder. These tests have been shown to be sensitive to brain damage by virtue of validity studies on patients with structural brain lesions, although their validity as measures of brain function in psychiatric conditions has not been investigated thoroughly. In the clinical context, the primary benefit of these tests lies in their ability to measure current level of cognitive functioning to determine capability to manage educational, vocational, and psychotherapeutic environments.

C. Laboratory Findings & Imaging: Although numerous studies have enriched our preliminary understanding of the neurobiology underlying posttraumatic stress disorder, no laboratory or imaging findings have yet been sufficiently replicated and validated to render them clinically applicable to posttraumatic stress disorder. Study approaches in humans have included baseline serum catecholamines, cortisol, growth hormone, thyroid hormones; urinary catecholamines and cortisol; stimulated serum catecholamines, cortisol, adrenocorticotropic hormone, thyroid hormones, and thyroid-stimulating hormone; yohimbine and lactate challenges for provocation of panic attacks or flashbacks; polysomnography; electrophysiologic measures (startle, skin conductance, mid- and long-latency auditory evoked potentials); and neuroimaging, both functional (trauma-related script-driven magnetic resonance imaging [MRI]) and structural (hippocampal volume MRI and FLAIR MRI).

Orr SP: An overview of psychophysiological studies in posttraumatic stress disorder. Posttraumatic Stress Disorder Research Quarterly 1994;5:1.

Differential Diagnosis

The differential diagnosis for posttraumatic stress disorder may be divided into those disorders with a stressor of an extreme or overwhelming nature and those disorders with more normative stressor severity. Among the first category must be included acute stress disorder (described later in this chapter), some cases of adjustment disorder, many cases of borderline personality disorder, and most if not all cases of dissociative identity disorder. Cases of acute stress disorder may be distinguished from those of posttraumatic stress disorder primarily by their symptomatic onset and remission within 4 weeks of the traumatic stressor. Cases of adjustment disorder, borderline personality disorder, and dissociative identity disorder resulting from exposure to an extreme or overwhelming traumatic stressor may be distinguished from those of posttraumatic stress disorder primarily by their failure to meet diagnostic criteria for the latter, most notably by the absence of intrusive traumatic reexperiencing symptoms as predominant clinical manifestations. Many cases of adjustment disorder and bereavement are distinguished from posttraumatic stress disorder by the less extreme nature of the stressor, which may represent relatively normative conflicts and losses of everyday life.

Treatment

A. Pharmacologic Treatment: No medications have been developed primarily for the purpose of treating posttraumatic stress disorder. All medication trials to date for posttraumatic stress disorder, whether methodologically rigorous (double-blind, placebo-controlled) or not (open-label or anecdotal), have involved medications originally developed and marketed for treatment of other disorders, including anxiety or mood disorders, seizure disorders, and hypertension. This situation becomes even more complicated when high rates of comorbidity of mood disorders and other anxiety disorders with posttraumatic stress disorder are considered. To date, no medication trial utilizing antipsychotic agents has been conducted with posttraumatic stress disorder patients.

Table 23–1 summarizes results of published double-blind, placebo-controlled studies in posttraumatic stress disorder. These studies have utilized one benzodiazepine anxiolytic (alprazolam), one selective serotonin reuptake inhibitor antidepressant (fluoxetine), two monoamine oxidase inhibitor antidepressants (phenelzine and brofaromine), and three tricyclic antidepressants (amitriptyline, imipramine, and desipramine). Results are generally disappointing, with improvements in reexperiencing symptoms with phenelzine, imipramine, and amitriptyline, in descend-

Table 23–1. Controlled drug trials for treatment of posttraumatic stress disorder.[1]

Investigator	Subjects	Agent(s)/Dosage	Treatment Length/ Design	Results
Shestatzky et al 1988	13 patients, DSM-III PTSD, varied trauma	Phenelzine, 45–75 mg	Greater than 4 weeks/crossover	No difference in response between phenelzine and placebo.
Frank et al 1988	46 male veterans, DSM-III-R PTSD	Imipramine, 50–300 mg; phenelzine, 15–75 mg	Mean 6.4 weeks	IES intrusion subscale scores decreased substantially with phenelzine, also decreased with imipramine; no decrease in avoidance subscale with any group; no difference in measures with placebo group.
Reist et al 1989	21 male veterans, DSM-III PTSD, most with other concurrent diagnoses	Desipramine, 100–200 mg	4 weeks/crossover	Significant improvement on IES intrusion subscale and depressive symptoms only for group with concurrent major depression ($n = 7$); no change overall in anxiety or PTSD symptoms.
Davidson et al 1990, 1993	62 male veterans, DSM-III	Amitriptyline, 50–300 mg	8 weeks	Amitriptyline superior to placebo on Hamilton anxiety scale; marginally significant improvement on IES avoidance and intrusion subscales.
Braun et al 1990	16 Israeli patients, DSM-III PTSD, varied trauma	Alprazolam, 2.5–6 mg	5 weeks	Alprazolam superior to placebo on Hamilton anxiety scale; no difference on IES or Hamilton depression scale.
Van der Kolk 1994	31 veterans, 33 civilian trauma victims	Fluoxetine, 20–40 mg	5 weeks double-blind, 5 weeks open	Significant reduction in symptoms, including intrusive symptoms and numbing. One half no longer met criteria for PTSD.
Baker et al 1995	118 patients, DSM-III-R PTSD, varied trauma	Brofaromine, 150 mg	12 weeks double-blind, randomized, placebo-controlled parallel groups	Both brofaromine and placebo groups showed significant CAPS score reductions, with no significant differences between groups.

[1] PTSD, posttraumatic stress disorder; IES, Impact of Events Scale; CAPS, Clinician Administered Posttraumatic Stress Disorder Scale.

ing order of apparent efficacy. Phenelzine is a problematic medication for many patients with posttraumatic stress disorder because of the necessary dietary restrictions and the high rate of comorbid alcohol abuse and dependence in this patient population. Desipramine improved reexperiencing symptoms only in posttraumatic stress disorder patients with comorbid major depression. Fluoxetine improved numbing and arousal symptoms mainly in patients who experienced civilian traumas and acute posttraumatic stress disorder, but not in patients with combat-related chronic posttraumatic stress disorder. Brofaromine and alprazolam were no more effective than placebo for treatment of core posttraumatic stress disorder symptoms.

Uncontrolled, open-label trials have suggested potential efficacy for sertraline, fluvoxamine, paroxetine, and moclobemide. Small uncontrolled trials and case reports have suggested possible efficacy for a variety of other medications, including lithium, carbamazepine, valproic acid, clonidine propranolol, clonazepam, doxepin, clomipramine, nortriptyline, buspirone, trazodone, nefazodone, venlafaxine, cyproheptadine, clozapine, risperidone, olanzapine, and naltrexone. This list should be viewed with caution, given the methodologic limitations of the reports involved, and the absence of Food and Drug Administration (FDA) indication for any medication specifically for the treatment of posttraumatic stress disorder. Given the relative paucity of scientifically valid and replicated data on pharmacologic treatment of posttraumatic stress disorder, a prudent approach must consider and weigh heavily considerations of medical and psychiatric comorbidities and their own validated pharmacologic treatments.

B. Psychological Treatment: Psychological treatment approaches to posttraumatic stress disorder may be categorized by the psychological theory on which each is based. The theories are often presented as distinctive, but careful review reveals commonalities, and many treatments overlap in content and technique.

1. Psychodynamic approaches—Psychodynamic approaches to posttraumatic stress disorder have been adapted from psychodynamic treatments of anxiety and affective disorder. Horowitz has posited three phases in the stress response: (1) initial phase, characterized by a painful realization of the event and intense ventilation of anger, sadness, and grief; (2) denial phase, characterized as a defense against intrusion of memories of the traumatic event, in which the victim exhibits impaired memory for the event, inattention to reminders of the event, and the use of fantasy to counteract perception of the reality of the event; and (3) intrusive phase, characterized by hypervigilance, exaggerated startle, sleeping and dreaming disturbances, intrusive and repetitive trauma-related thoughts, and confusion. Posttraumatic stress disorder develops if these phases are not worked through sufficiently. Horowitz advocated a brief psychodynamic psychotherapy model in which the treatment is geared

to the adaptation phase of the patient and is targeted to the denial and intrusion phases specifically. Effectiveness of treatment depends largely on the reinterpretation of the traumatic event, altering destructive attribution and developing more realistic interpretations. Despite the popularity of the psychodynamic treatment approach, there have been few outcome studies documenting objectively its effectiveness.

2. Cognitive-behavioral approaches—Cognitive-behavioral treatments of posttraumatic stress disorder have also been adapted from techniques for treating other anxiety disorders. Learning theory models incorporate classical and operant conditioning to explain the development and persistence of posttraumatic stress disorder symptoms. Cognitive theory was advanced to supplement learning theory in order to help explain why perceived threat was a more powerful trigger of posttraumatic stress disorder symptoms than was actual threat. Personal meanings attributed to trauma events are the focus of cognitive-behavioral treatments. Additional interventions, such as coping skills training or assertiveness training, have been used to manage refractory symptoms or to provide more adaptive reactions to fear and anxiety.

At the core of cognitive-behavioral treatment of posttraumatic stress disorder lies an array of treatments that utilize repetitive exposure to trauma-relevant fear stimuli to reduce anxiety. The degree of exposure may be graduated or intensive and may or may not be accompanied by efforts to maintain a fear-antagonistic state. Systematic desensitization involves graduated exposure accompanied by maintenance of a fear-antagonistic state (ie, relaxation). By contrast, flooding (see next section) involves intensive exposure not accompanied by maintenance of a fear-antagonistic state. The form of exposure may be in vivo (eg, return to the original location of the traumatic event) or in imagination (eg, self-generated memory of the traumatic event assisted by verbal cues to produce affective associations). Through a process of extinction resulting from multiple repeated exposures to fear-producing stimuli associated with the trauma, anxiety may habituate and previous triggers to anxiety may lose potency.

3. Flooding techniques—Controlled clinical trials utilizing flooding techniques in chronic combat-related posttraumatic stress disorder have produced positive results immediately posttreatment, which were maintained at subsequent follow-up. Other controlled studies, utilizing a clinical variant of therapeutic exposure, systematic desensitization, or guided exposure techniques, have shown similar symptom reductions. Unfortunately these studies have often combined exposure techniques with other treatment procedures, making it unclear what independent effects exposure itself produced. This confounding of treatments has been addressed in several well-controlled studies with more acute civilian sexual assault victims, suggesting that therapeutic exposure alone may improve intrusive and hyperarousal symptoms immediately posttreatment and at subsequent follow-up. However, avoidant symptoms seem more refractory to these treatments. A more serious reservation concerning exposure treatment lies in the observation that a subset of veterans show increased symptom severity after receiving treatment with flooding techniques.

4. Training in coping skills—Another behavioral approach applied to posttraumatic stress disorder involves training in coping skills for improved self-control of symptoms and improved adaptive responses to anxiety. One example, Stress Inoculation Training (SIT) involves an educational phase and a coping skills phase. The educational phase provides a rationale for the treatment and begins the process of establishing confidence in the treatment and rapport with the therapist. The coping skills phase incorporates training in relaxation techniques, thought-stopping techniques to counteract negative rumination, and guided self-dialogue narration to enhance self-esteem and self-control. Skills are developed through practice within sessions and through homework assignments to be completed outside of sessions. In addition to the specific packaging of skills training in SIT, a range of other specific interventions are available to be provided individually or in clinically meaningful combinations such as anger management training, assertiveness training, cognitive therapy to counteract cognitive distortions, and problem-solving training.

The clinical outcome of SIT has been studied by several groups. In each study, outcomes of SIT were compared against those resulting from established alternative treatment and no treatment controls. SIT, along with the other treatments, has been found to be effective in reducing posttraumatic stress disorder re-experiencing, intrusion, and avoidance symptoms in a study of rape victims. Foa and colleagues have conducted several carefully controlled clinical trials comparing SIT with prolonged exposure, both in vivo and imaginal, in the treatment of rape-related posttraumatic stress disorder. They report that at the end of treatment, only the SIT group showed declines in symptom severity compared to the no-treatment group, but at follow-up, subjects in the prolonged exposure group showed superior symptom reduction compared with those of the SIT group. These provocative findings may indicate limited effectiveness of the anxiety management skills and more long-term benefits for exposure, but replication is necessary to draw any firm conclusions.

5. Eye movement desensitization reprocessing (EMDR)—Shapiro recently introduced EMDR treatment as an innovative approach to the treatment of posttraumatic stress disorder. The EMDR technique involves imaginal exposure to the traumatic event with eyes open, during which there is simultaneous verbalization of trauma-related cognitions and emotions, accompanied by continuous visual saccadic eye movements. According to Shapiro, this treatment is atheoretical, although it has been suggested that the eye movements in EMDR may be analogous to REM sleep–related eye movements hypothesized to serve a stress reducing function during sleep. An alternative hypothesis has been offered in which the saccadic eye movements produce a fear-antagonistic state and therefore play a counterconditioning role similar to the coupling of relaxation within systematic desensitization. Results of controlled investigations have been mixed. Further study of this relatively new technique is needed to determine its effectiveness with posttraumatic stress disorder populations.

In response to the high prevalence of posttraumatic stress disorder among Vietnam veterans, the Veterans Administration developed a comprehensive set of treatment programs. Specialized inpatient units were established around the country as intensive treatment programs for veterans with combat-related posttraumatic stress disorder. The treatment approaches vary by site, but the interdisciplinary emphasis of these programs assures multicomponent treatment strategies. In the first carefully controlled outcome study, the cohort of patients studied exhibited an increase in symptoms from admission to follow-up. Although interpersonal and family relations improved, and overall morale increased at discharge, these gains were lost at subsequent follow-up. This study highlights the treatment refractoriness of chronic posttraumatic stress disorder, despite extensive and intensive multimodal treatment efforts, and suggests the need for identifying characteristics of individual patients that could be used to match the patients with specific treatments most likely to benefit them.

Foa E, Olasov Rothbaum B, Molnar C: Cognitive-behavioral therapy of post-traumatic stress disorder. In: Friedman MJ, Charney DS, Deutch AY (editors): *Neurobiological and Clinical Consequences of Stress: From Normal Adaptation to Post-Traumatic Stress Disorder.* Lippincott-Raven, 1995.

Friedman MJ. Drug treatment for PTSD. Ann NY Acad Sci 1997;821:359.

Marshall RD et al: A pharmacotherapy algorithm in the treatment of posttraumatic stress disorder. Psychiatr Ann 1996;26:217.

Comorbidity

Several studies have suggested that patients with posttraumatic stress disorder also experience a disproportionate degree of medical illness. For example, firefighters with posttraumatic stress disorder after their involvement in the 1983 bushfire disaster in Australia reported significantly more neurologic, musculoskeletal, cardiovascular, and respiratory problems than those without posttraumatic stress disorder. Consistent with these findings are those suggesting that Vietnam combat veterans exhibit an unexpectedly high prevalence of soft neurologic signs and symptoms. Finally, two DSM-IV diagnostic criteria for posttraumatic stress disorder refer directly to disturbances of sleep: recurrent distressing dreams of the [traumatic] event and difficulty falling or staying asleep. Neither of these criteria captures the full range of parasomniac phenomena commonly occurring in patients with posttraumatic stress disorder, but such parasomnias constitute comorbid medical conditions when diagnosed concurrently with posttraumatic stress disorder.

Studies of both genders, in numerous clinical and community population samples and utilizing diverse diagnostic methods, have universally found a high prevalence of comorbidity of additional psychiatric disorders with posttraumatic stress disorder, ranging from 62% to 99%. The most commonly reported comorbid psychiatric disorders include mood disorders, especially major depression; anxiety disorders, especially phobias; substance use disorders, especially alcohol abuse and dependence; and conduct disorder or cluster B personality disorder, especially antisocial and borderline personality disorders. Kessler and colleagues, using data from the National Comorbidity Survey, have attempted to address the issue of whether posttraumatic stress disorder is primary or secondary relative to comorbid psychiatric diagnoses, using temporal precedence as indicating the primary diagnosis. They suggest that posttraumatic stress disorder is usually primary with respect to mood and substance use disorders in both genders and with respect to conduct disorder among women. Conduct disorder is usually primary with respect to posttraumatic stress disorder among men, and comorbid anxiety disorders are usually primary among both genders.

Adverse Outcomes of Treatment

Evidence that inpatient rehabilitation programs for combat-related posttraumatic stress disorder show disappointing results has already been cited earlier in this chapter, as has evidence that flooding psychotherapies may exacerbate symptoms in some patients, in contrast to their apparent efficacy in female, civilian, sexually traumatized posttraumatic stress disorder patients. A more critical issue involves the question whether Vietnam combat veterans with posttraumatic stress disorder exhibit a sustained high prevalence of suicide reaching epidemic proportions. An epidemiologic study failed to find evidence to support this belief and cited proportionate mortality rates for suicide ranging from 0.93 to 1.24 for in-country Vietnam veterans compared to other Vietnam-era veterans and ranging from 0.99 to 1.46 for in-country Vietnam veterans compared to nonveterans and U.S. males in general. A more recent study of attempted suicide among Vietnam veterans concluded that "the etiology of attempted suicide among Vietnam veterans remains largely unexplained. A partial explanation is that the predominant and direct causes spring from general psychiatric disorders rather than from traumatic exposure, posttraumatic stress disorder, or substance abuse. Traumatic exposure contributes directly to the development of posttraumatic stress disorder and general psychiatric disorders but only indirectly to making a suicide attempt" (Fontanta & Rosenheck, p. 102).

Fontana A, Rosenheck R: Attempted suicide among Vietnam veterans: a model of etiology in a community sample. Am J Psychiatry 1995;152:102.

Pollock DA et al: Estimating the number of suicides among Vietnam veterans. Am J Psychiatry 1990;147:772.

Prognosis & Course of Illness

Prognosis for full recovery from posttraumatic stress disorder remains incompletely understood. Most studies addressing prognosis have been conducted retrospectively and, therefore, are subject to distortion in reporting by subjects. However, some prospective studies are currently under way, and findings to date are consistent with those of retrospective studies. One study found that Persian Gulf War veterans meeting diagnostic criteria at 3 months posttrauma still meet criteria at 2 years posttrauma. Another study found that in the two decades since returning from war, approximately one third of Vietnam combat veterans have experienced posttraumatic stress disorder at some point in time, and approximately one half of those who have ever met full diagnostic criteria still do so two decades posttrauma. Both sets of findings in two different populations of combat veterans are consistent with those of the National Comorbidity Survey, which found that recovery rates from posttraumatic stress disorder were highest in the first 12 months after onset of symptoms and had leveled off permanently by 6 years after symptom onset. The average duration of symptoms for those with posttraumatic stress disorder who had ever obtained treatment was 36 months, compared to 64 months for those never treated. However, irrespective of treatment status, more than one third of persons who had ever experienced posttraumatic stress disorder had never fully remitted 6 years after onset of symptoms, with an apparently permanent leveling off of the recovery rate curve for both treated and untreated subjects. Regardless of issues mentioned throughout this chapter concerning genetic or developmental pretraumatic predisposition to posttraumatic stress disorder, both retrospective and prospective evidence currently available suggest that once posttraumatic stress disorder has developed, there is a 33–50% probability that it will become a chronic psychiatric disorder, perhaps irrespective of treatment status. Much work remains to be done to place posttraumatic stress disorder among those psychiatric disorders with a good prognosis.

Johnson D et al: Outcome of intensive inpatient treatment for combat-related posttraumatic stress disorder. Am J Psychiatry 1996;153:771.

Kessler RC et al: Posttraumatic stress disorder in the National Comorbidity Survey. Arch Gen Psychiatry 1995; 52:1048.

ACUTE STRESS DISORDER

DSM-IV Diagnostic Criteria

A. The person has been exposed to a traumatic event in which both of the following were present:
 (1) the person experienced, witnessed, or was confronted with an event or events that involved actual or threatened death or serious injury, or a threat to the physical integrity of self or others
 (2) the person's response involved fear, helplessness, or horror

B. Either while experiencing or after experiencing the distressing event, the individual has three (or more) of the following dissociative symptoms:
 (1) a subjective sense of numbing, detachment, or absence of emotional responsiveness
 (2) a reduction in awareness of his or her surroundings (eg, "being in a daze")
 (3) derealization
 (4) depersonalization
 (5) dissociative amnesia (ie, inability to recall an important aspect of the trauma

C. The traumatic event is persistently reexperienced in at least one of the following ways: recurrent images, thoughts, dreams, illusions, flashback episodes, or a sense of reliving the experience; or distress on exposure to reminders of the traumatic event.

D. Marked avoidance of stimuli that arouse recollections of the trauma.

E. Marked symptoms of anxiety or increased arousal (eg, difficulty sleeping, irritability, poor concentration, hypervigilance, exaggerated startle response, motor restlessness).

F. The disturbance causes clinically significant distress or impairment in social, occupational, or other important areas of functioning.

G. The disturbance lasts for a minimum of 2 days and a maximum of 4 weeks and occurs within 4 weeks of the traumatic event.

H. The disturbance is not due to the direct physiological effects of a substance or a general medical condition, is not better accounted for by brief psychotic disorder, and is not merely an exacerbation of a preexisting Axis I or Axis II disorder.

Adapted, with permission, from *Diagnostic and Statistical Manual of Mental Disorders,* 4th ed. Copyright 1994 American Psychiatric Association.

General Considerations

 Although conceptualized as a potential antecedent to posttraumatic stress disorder in individual patients, acute stress disorder was codified as a discrete disorder later than posttraumatic stress disorder. Consequently vastly less research has been conducted concerning acute stress disorder, and much less definitive is known about its clinical phenomena, differential diagnosis, treatment, and prognosis in comparison to posttraumatic stress disorder. Although the clinical phenomena of acute stress disorder superficially resemble those of posttraumatic stress disorder, even these differ significantly, and the two disorders have been studied for the most part in different patient populations. Most research on posttraumatic stress disorder has been conducted on male combat veterans years after trauma exposure, a population difficult or impossible to study reliably retrospectively for acute stress disorder. Conversely the populations most studied for acute stress disorder include predominantly motor vehicle accident survivors and, to a lesser extent, violent crime witnesses or victims, and survivors of natural disasters.

Clinical Findings

 The impetus for defining acute stress disorder stemmed largely from the failure of posttraumatic stress disorder criteria to capture individuals with a similar syndrome in the virtually immediate aftermath of the type of traumas that were acknowledged to potentially result in posttraumatic stress disorder. Investigators discovered that the experience of dissociative phenomena either during or immediately after the traumatic situation seemed to identify those individuals who would eventually develop posttraumatic stress disorder. This discovery led to dissociative signs and symptoms playing a large role in the diagnostic criteria for acute stress disorder. This prominent role of dissociative phenomena represents the greatest difference between criteria for acute stress disorder and posttraumatic stress disorder, other than the time course variables of onset of pathology.

Differential Diagnosis

 Other recognized conditions that may follow an acute stressor and must be considered in the differential diagnosis of patients presenting symptomatically in this situation would include brief psychotic disorder (differentiated by presence of psychotic features), major depressive episode (typically an additional diagnosis that develops in the context of an already recognizable acute stress disorder), dissociative fugue (which involves travel and amnesia), adjustment disorder (for pathologic stress responses that do not meet full criteria for acute stress disorder), and posttraumatic stress disorder (less acute onset or persistence longer than 1 month).

Treatment & Prognosis

 Little is known about treatment of acute stress disorder, but one small study suggested that cognitive-behavioral therapy was superior to supportive counseling. Anxiolytic medications targeted at hyperarousal symptoms such as insomnia and irritability may be indicated in individual cases.

Acute stress disorder has a limited duration by definition, so it has no prognosis beyond 1 month. However, a growing number of studies have indicated that meeting criteria for acute stress disorder in the month following a traumatic event strongly predicts later development of posttraumatic stress disorder or at least some of its features. This should not be surprising, because peritraumatic dissociative phenomena, which are not diagnostic criteria for posttraumatic stress disorder per se, but which were known to predict later development of posttraumatic stress disorder, were the very symptoms emphasized in constructing the criteria for acute stress disorder.

Bremner JD: Acute and chronic responses to psychological trauma: where do we go from here? Am J Psychiatry 1999;156:349.

Obsessive-Compulsive Disorder 24

William A. Hewlett, PhD, MD

DSM-IV Diagnostic Criteria

A. Either obsessions or compulsions:

Obsessions as defined by (1), (2), (3), and (4):

(1) recurrent and persistent thoughts, impulses, or images that are experienced, at some time during the disturbance, as intrusive and inappropriate and that cause marked anxiety or distress

(2) the thoughts, impulses, or images are not simply excessive worries about real-life problems

(3) the person attempts to ignore or suppress such thoughts, impulses, or images or neutralize them with some other thought or action

(4) the person recognizes that the thoughts, impulses, or images are a product of his or her own mind (not imposed from without as in thought insertion)

Compulsions as defined by (1) and (2):

(1) repetitive behaviors (eg, hand washing, ordering, checking) or mental acts (eg, praying, counting, repeating works silently) that the person feels driven to perform in response to an obsession, or according to rules that must be applied rigidly

(2) the behavior or mental acts are aimed at preventing or reducing distress or preventing some dreaded event or situation; however, these behaviors or mental acts either are not connected in a realistic way with what they are designed to neutralize or prevent or are clearly excessive

B. At some point during the course of the disorder, the person has recognized that the obsessions or compulsions are excessive or unreasonable.

Note: This does not apply to children.

C. The obsessions or compulsions cause marked distress, are time consuming (takes more than 1 hour/day) or significantly interfere with the person's normal routine, occupation (or academic functioning), or usual social activities or relationships.

D. If another Axis I disorder is present, the content of the obsessions or compulsions is not restricted to it.

E. The disturbance is not due to the direct physiological effects of a substance (eg, a drug of abuse, a medication) or a general medical condition.

Specify if:

With poor insight: if, for most of the time during the current episode, the person does not recognize that the obsessions and compulsions are excessive or unreasonable.

Reprinted, with permission, from *Diagnostic and Statistical Manual of Mental Disorders,* 4th ed. Copyright. 1994 American Psychiatric Association.

General Considerations

Obsessions are unwanted aversive cognitive experiences usually associated with feelings of dread, loathing, or a disturbing sense that something is not right. The individual recognizes (at some point in time) that these concerns are inappropriate in relation to reality and will generally attempt to ignore or suppress them. Compulsions are overt behaviors or covert mental acts performed to reduce the intensity of the aversive obsessions. They may occur as behaviors that are governed by rigid, but often irrelevant, internal specifications. They are inappropriate in nature or intensity in relation to the external circumstances that provoked them.

A. Major Etiologic Theories: Theories of etiology have invoked psychoanalytic (ie, relating to early childhood experiences), cognitive, posttraumatic, epileptic, traumatic (ie, brain injury), genetic, and postinfectious processes. The psychoanalytic view has fallen into disfavor in recent years. Likewise, it is no longer thought that symptoms of obsessive-compulsive disorder (OCD) are a consequence of psychic trauma. In cases where psychic trauma is associated with the onset of symptoms, the experience is thought to potentiate a propensity for developing OCD symptoms in susceptible individuals and does not create the pathology itself.

OCD can result from pathologic processes affecting cerebral functioning. For example, severe head trauma and epilepsy have been associated with the obsessive-compulsive symptoms. Disorders affecting the functioning of the basal ganglia have also been associated with OCD, and a postinfectious autoimmune-related form of OCD has been described in children. OCD symptoms in these children frequently occur after an infection with type A β-hemolytic *Streptococcus* bacteria, with or without classical symptoms of rheumatic fever. In the acute phase of this illness, antibodies directed at streptococcal M-protein react with specific brain proteins located primarily in the basal ganglia and may induce Sydenham's chorea (also called St. Vitus' dance). Obsessions, compulsions, or vocal and motor tics indistinguishable from those seen in Tourette's syndrome can be prominent when the chorea is present, although the child may not speak of them if not directly questioned. Sydenham's chorea is associated with swelling of the head of the caudate nucleus on magnetic resonance imaging (MRI).

Poststreptococcal antineuronal antibodies have also been detected in cases of abrupt-onset OCD that do not exhibit the symptoms of Sydenham's chorea nor any other manifestation of rheumatic fever. OCD symptoms appear in conjunction with increasing antibody titers and remit as titers fall. Autoimmune-related OCD has been described only in children. Adults with OCD, however, may have reduced volume in the caudate region of the basal ganglia. It is conceivable that neuropathologic processes, such as repeated autoimmune inflammation, could irreversibly damage central nervous system (CNS) tissue and result in a chronic form of OCD in adults. It is also possible that certain cases of familial OCD or Tourette's syndrome could be related to heritable proteins involved in the autoimmune process.

B. Epidemiology:

1. Population frequencies—OCD has lifetime prevalence rates of 2–3% in the United States, although rates may be slightly lower in certain mainland ethnic subgroups, including African Americans and possibly Hispanics. The U.S. prevalence rates are consistent with estimates of lifetime prevalence (approximately 2%) in Europe, Africa, Canada, and the Middle East, although estimates in certain Asian countries (ie, India and Taiwan) are somewhat lower (0.5–0.9%). Lower prevalence rates in selected U.S. and other national populations could be related to cultural conditions that result in an underreporting of symptoms in these groups or could be related to biological factors such as increased resistance to basal gangliar disease. Although OCD is thought to be a lifetime illness, lifetime prevalence rates in young adults are over twice those seen in the elderly. It is unclear whether this observation represents a reporting bias, a waning of symptoms with advancing age, a shorter life expectancy in patients with OCD, or a changing environmental factor relating to the etiology of the illness.

The usual onset of OCD is in childhood or early adulthood. Two thirds of cases have their onset prior to age 25, and only 15% occur after the age of 35. Approximately one third of OCD cases have their onset in childhood or early adolescence. There is a 2:1 preponderance of males in this population. In the adult population, OCD is slightly more predominant in women. The frequency of OCD in psychiatric practice may be significantly lower than in the general population. Indeed, the incidence of OCD was previously thought to be as low as 0.05% based on psychiatric samples. This low estimation of frequency may be related to the intense shame and secrecy associated with this illness and the subsequent reluctance of these patients to divulge their symptomatology.

The frequency of specific obsessions and compulsions is fairly constant across populations. Contamination fears are present in approximately 50% of all patients with OCD. Unwarranted fears that something is wrong (called pathologic doubt) also have high prevalence (40%). Other obsessions, including needs for symmetry, fears of harm to self or others, and unwanted sexual concerns, occur at lower frequencies (25–30%). Checking and decontamination rituals are the predominant rituals in OCD (50–60%). Other rituals, such as arranging, counting, repeating, and repetitive superstitious acts, occur less frequently (30–35%). Most patients with OCD (60%) have multiple obsessions or compulsions.

2. Population subtypes—The only subtype recognized in the *Diagnostic and Statistical Manual of Mental Disorders,* 4th edition (DSM-IV) is OCD with poor insight. Adults given this diagnosis were previously aware that they were symptomatic but became convinced of the validity of their fears and the necessity of their compulsions as their illness progressed. Children with this diagnosis have not yet developed insight regarding their symptoms.

It has not proved helpful to classify OCD according to symptom dyad (eg, contamination-washing) as a means of predicting the course of the illness, therapeutic outcome, or other relevant measures. Indeed, most individuals have multiple obsessions and compulsions, and symptom clusters can be exchanged over time (eg, a compulsive hand-washer will lose fear of contamination and develop fears of harming others). It has been more useful to classify subtypes of patients according to their underlying experiences. Patients with OCD can be divided into two subgroups based on experiences of (1) pathologic doubt (eg, dread and uncertainty) or (2) incompletion, or "not-just-right," perceptions. Individuals within these two subgroups appear to share common symptom clusters, comorbidities, and treatment prognoses.

OCD can also be classified on the basis of the presence or absence of tics. Patients with tics may respond to a different treatment regimen than do those who do not have tics. Because of the relationship between Tourette's syndrome and OCD, these patients may also have other symptoms found in the families of Tourette's syndrome patients, such as urges to carry out maladaptive acts and problems with impulse control.

Finally, a subset of OCD patients with schizotypal personality disorder has been characterized. These patients are often mistakenly diagnosed as having schizophrenia; however, they lack true category A symptoms. They are more likely to have poor insight and poor social functioning. OCD in this group of patients may require a different treatment regimen and is often refractory to treatment.

C. Genetics: OCD occurs with greater frequency in family members of OCD patients (10%), as compared to the general population. When combined with subclinical obsessions and compulsions, symptom prevalence rates approach 20% in first-degree relatives. Interestingly, familial rates of OCD are significantly higher in patients with childhood OCD than in family members of adult OCD patients. This may be related to a heritable tic-related form of OCD with onset in childhood. Although there have been no systematic twin studies of sufficient size to draw conclusions, 65–85% of monozygotic twin pairs with one twin having OCD are concordant for OCD symptoms, whereas only 15–45% of dizygotic twin pairs are so concordant.

OCD has been linked to the proposed autosomal dominant Tourette's syndrome *(Ts)* gene. This gene is associated with chronic motor tics, vocal tics, and OCD. Under this genetic model, males carrying the proposed gene have a 90–95% probability of developing at least one of these behaviors. Females carrying the *Ts* gene have a lower expression rate (approximately 60%), but a higher proportion will develop OCD. The *Ts* gene locus has not been identified. Some familial forms of OCD with partial penetrance do not appear to be related to the *Ts* gene. The genetic determinant of this form has not been identified.

Geller DA et al: Obsessive-compulsive disorder in children and adolescents: a review. Harv Rev Psychiatry 1998; 5:260.

Jenike MA et al: *Obsessive Compulsive Disorders: Theory and Management,* 2nd ed. Mosby Year-Book, 1990.

Karno M et al: The epidemiology of obsessive-compulsive disorder in five US communities. Arch Gen Psychiatry 1988;45:1094.

Pauls DL: The genetics of obsessive compulsive disorder and Gilles de la Tourette's syndrome. Psychiatr Clin N Am 1992;15:759.

Rasmussen SA, Eisen JL: The epidemiology and differential diagnosis of obsessive compulsive disorder. J Clin Psychiatry 1994;55(10 Suppl):5.

Swedo SE et al: Childhood-onset obsessive compulsive disorder. Psychiatr Clin N Am 1992;15:767.

Swedo SE et al: Pediatric autoimmune neuropsychiatric disorders associated with streptococcal infections: clinical description of the first 50 cases. Am J Psychiatry 1998;155:264. [Published erratum appears in Am J Psychiatry 1998;155:578.]

Clinical Findings

A. Signs & Symptoms: The clinical hallmarks of obsessions are aversive experiences of dread and uncertainty, or the disturbing sense that something is not right or is incomplete. Obsessive thoughts are the particular ideas associated with obsessive experiences. They are often bizarre or inadequate as explanations for these experiences. Obsessions can take the form of aversive mental images, dread and disgust related to perceived defilement, feelings that something very bad has either happened or is about to happen, or an urgent sense that something that needs to be done has not yet been completed. A sense of immediacy and urgency is almost always associated with the aversive experiences. Obsessions can be present without compulsions, most frequently when the individual recognizes that no action can alleviate the aversive experience. Under such circumstances the individual may only seek reassurance that his or her fears are unfounded or unrealistic.

Compulsions take the form of willed responses directed at reducing the aversive circumstances associated with the obsessive thoughts. They are generally carried out in concordance with the ideation surrounding the obsessions. They can take the form of overt behaviors or silent mental acts such as checking, praying, counting, or some other mental ritual. Mental compulsions differ from obsessive experiences in that they are willed mental acts performed for a purpose, rather than sensory or ideational experiences. Compulsions are usually carried out in a repetitive or stereotyped fashion, although they can be situation specific, dependent on the content of the obsessive thought. Compulsions can also be carried out in the absence of specific obsessive thoughts. In such cases they are usually responses to an urgent sense that something is not right or is incomplete.

Most adults with OCD recognize that their fears and behaviors are unrealistic or excessive. Insight in OCD can vary, however, from states of full awareness that the symptoms are absurd, with a few lingering doubts, through equivocal acknowledgment, to a delusional state in which the individual is convinced of the validity of his or her fear and the necessity of the consequent behavior. Some adults lose insight only during exacerbations of their illness. Others, often with schizotypal personalities, may have true insight only early in the illness, or transiently when their illness is quiescent. The term "overvalued idea" was used in the past to denote an obsessive thought firmly held to be valid. This term is no longer accepted as a construct, because it cannot be practically differentiated from delusional ideation. Patients who have lost insight regarding their symptoms are considered to have a diagnostic subclass of OCD.

Avoidance may be a prominent secondary symptom in OCD. The OCD patient will avoid circumstances that trigger particularly aversive obsessions or lead to time-consuming compulsions. Avoidance, itself, is not a compulsion; but when the illness is severe it can be a prominent clinical feature. In the course of treatment, as avoidance is reduced, a temporary, paradoxical increase in compulsions can occur because of increased exposure to circumstances that trigger them.

B. Associated Experiences: OCD stands out among psychiatric disorders in the degree to which the patient's thoughts and concerns diverge from their awareness of reality. Most OCD patients recognize the absurd nature of their behavior and are acutely aware of demeaning perceptions that others might have if they knew the degree to which they were affected by their illness. They have a strong fear that they will be considered crazy. Ashamed and embarrassed, they are reluctant to disclose their symptoms to anyone who might not understand their illness. As a result, individuals with OCD tend to be highly secretive.

Early in the illness, they will try to hide their symptoms from those who know them. They may delay seeking treatment until their symptoms are noticed by those around them. Many patients will not reveal their illness to their primary physicians. Therapists sometimes will care for a patient for several years before discovering that the patient has OCD. This is particularly true for patients who experience horrific sexual, blasphemous, or violent thoughts and images. These individuals fear that the therapist will believe that they want these scenarios to occur and that they might act inappropriately in concordance with their obsessive thoughts. In short, they fear that the physician will confirm their own fears and self-condemnation. They may leave a therapeutic relationship if they sense that the therapist does not understand the illness.

The combination of secrecy, avoidance of contact with others, and the time-consuming nature of the compulsions may lead to social isolation and secondary depression. Most patients with OCD also experience a heightened sense of internal tension and distress. When their OCD is worse they will describe feelings of desperation and despair, as they are unable to relieve their feelings of dread and uncertainty. It is these feelings that may lead the patient to seek initial treatment.

Patients who have OCD may also have an unreasonable fear of losing control. These feelings can be exacerbated by a perceived inability to control their compulsive behavior. The individual with OCD fears that he or she will lose control of natural inhibitions and act in a socially or personally maladaptive manner. These issues with control differ significantly from those of individuals with obsessive-compulsive personality disorder (OCPD), in that the latter individuals want control for the positive sense of mastery that it engenders. Patients with OCD often shun true control and responsibility because of their unrealistic fears that they might misuse or abuse it.

C. Pathologic Relationships: The individual with OCD frequently has a parent or life partner who is involved in the illness. There are two pathologic forms of such involvement. The first involves facilitation. By pleading, nagging, demanding, or threatening, the patient will induce others to accommodate to his or her fears and concerns. The facilitator may perform rituals for the patient or permit the patient to control the environment or common time. Facilitation allows the illness to flourish without normal constraints.

The second pathologic interaction is the antagonistic-defensive dyad. Such relationships are adversarial. The antagonistic partner acts in a caustic, demeaning manner and does not understand or accept the nature of the illness. The OCD symptoms are viewed as willful antagonism. The patient reacts in a hostile, defensive manner that aggravates the partner. The hostility, instability, loss of self-esteem, and stress in these interactions exacerbate the symptoms of OCD and lead to further antagonism.

In both forms of pathologic relationship, the patient may use his or her symptoms to control the other person. This can be an unconscious or pseudo-conscious process. Facilitating interactions can lead to circumstances in which the patient uses his or her illness to obtain material and emotional benefits. In antagonistic-defensive interactions, symptoms may serve to irritate and frustrate the hostile partner—one of the few mechanisms available to the patient to "get back at" that partner. In both pathologic interactive modes, the secondary gains associated with the symptoms can further ingrain the disorder.

D. Psychological Testing & Instruments for Diagnosis and Measurement: There is no good diagnostic instrument for OCD. The Structured Interview for DSM-IV Diagnosis has only rudimentary questions regarding OCD symptoms, and good clinical judgment is required if the proper diagnosis is to be made. Psychological testing has little value in the diagnosis of OCD or in predicting treatment outcome or course of the illness.

Valid, reliable, and sensitive scales for the measurement of OCD symptom severity have been available only since the late 1980s. The best is the Yale-Brown Obsessive Compulsive Scale (YBOCS). This semistructured interview consists of three parts: a symptom checklist, a symptom hierarchy list, and the Yale-Brown Obsessive Compulsive Scale. The rating scale evaluates severity of obsessions and compulsions on an ordinal scale from 0 to 4 (on the basis of time spent, interference, distress, resistance, and degree of control). The maximum score for this scale is 40. Patients with scores above 31 are considered to have extreme symptoms. Scores of 24–31 indicate severe symptoms, and scores of 16–23 indicate moderate symptoms. Patients with scores below 16 are considered to have mild to subclinical symptoms that often do not require treatment. The average YBOCS score for individuals with untreated OCD who are entering an OCD clinic is typically 23–25. The YBOCS also rates certain ancillary symptoms for informational purposes and provides for global assessments of severity and improvement.

Other scales that rate severity of symptoms include the Comprehensive Psychopathological Rating Scale and the obsessive-compulsive subsection of the Hopkins Symptoms Check List-90 (SCL-90). Neither of these is sensitive to changes in symptom intensity. Both scales include measures that are highly influenced by other factors such as mood. The Clinical Global Scale and the National Institute of Mental Health global rating scale belong to another class of scales that involve clinical judgments of either global or OCD-specific illness severity or changes in severity. They are based on categories such as mild, moderate, much improved, and so on. An older group of scales (eg, Leyton Obsessional Inventory or the Maudsley Obsessive and Compulsive Inventory) consist of lists of obsessions and compulsions, without true measures of severity.

E. Laboratory Findings & Imaging: Using magnetic resonance imaging (MRI) or computerized tomography (CT), certain studies have found decreased gray matter volume either unilaterally or bilaterally in the head of the caudate nucleus. Positron emission tomography (PET) studies have found increased resting metabolic activity in the orbitomedial prefrontal cortex, especially in the right hemisphere. Increased metabolic activity has also been found in the basal ganglia, particularly in the anterior caudate nucleus. Effective treatment of OCD by either pharmacologic or behavioral means can be associated with regionally specific decreases in resting metabolic activity. This has led to the suggestion that neural circuits between the orbitomedial prefrontal cortex and the basal ganglia are hyperactive in OCD, and that treatments that modulate this activity may be effective in OCD. Imaging procedures are primarily of research interest, however, and have little diagnostic value at this time.

Other studies have found biochemical, neuroendocrine, and physiologic alterations associated with the neurotransmitter serotonin. Again, no clinically useful tests have resulted from this work. Finally, abnormal neurologic soft signs, eye-tracking, and electroencephalogram (EEG) measurements have been associated with OCD. These observations have little clinical value, although the severity of soft signs may correlate with the severity of OCD.

Goodman WK et al: The Yale-Brown Obsessive Compulsive Scale. I. Development, use, and reliability. Arch Gen Psychiatry 1989;46:1006.

Pato MT, Eisen JL, Pato CN: Rating scales for obsessive compulsive disorder. Pages 77–92 in Hollander E et al (editors): *Current Insights in Obsessive Compulsive Disorder.* John Wiley & Sons, 1994.

Schwartz JM et al: Systematic changes in cerebral glucose metabolic rate after successful behavior modification treatment of obsessive-compulsive disorder. Arch Gen Psychiatry 1996;53:109.

Stein DJ et al: The neuropsychiatry of OCD. In: Hollander EH, Stein D (editors): *Obsessive Compulsive Disorders.* Marcel Dekker, 1996.

Differential Diagnosis of Obsessions & Compulsions

The differential diagnosis of OCD is one of the most complex in psychiatry because of confusion over the meanings of the terms "obsessions" and "compulsions," a confusion made worse by the fact that OCPD is associated with a cognitive style and behavior unrelated to OCD. It is important to recognize cognitive and behavioral phenomena that are often confused with true obsessions and compulsions. Table 24–1 summarizes these phenomena, and they are described in more detail in the next several sections.

A. Cognitive Differentiations: Numerous intrusive or persistent mental experiences have no relation to OCD. The experiences listed in this section are often confused with obsessions but can be distinguished on the basis of careful examination.

1. Anxious ruminations & excessive worries—Anxious ruminations and excessive worries are persistent intrusive concerns about adverse circumstances in the future. They are characterized by

Table 24–1. Differential symptomatology.

Cognitive Differentiations	Behavioral Differentiations
Anxious ruminations and excessive worries	Impulsions
Pathologic guilt	Meticulousness or perfectionism
Depressive ruminations	Pathologic atonement
Aggressive ruminations	Repetitive displacement behavior
Fantasies	Perseverative behavior
Paranoid fears	Stereotypic behavior
Flashbacks	Self-injurious behavior
Pathologic attraction	Pathologic overinvolvement
Rigid thinking	Pathologic persistence
Pathologic indecision	Hoarding
Realistic fears or concerns	Complex tics

preparative cognitive processing designed to deal with those circumstances. They differ from obsessions in that they are realistic in their nature, although they may be excessive. Worries can be fleeting or semi-conscious mental experiences associated with feelings of anxiety, whereas anxious ruminations are drawn out in time as the mind reviews potential adverse scenarios. They are not associated with rituals. In contrast to anxious ruminations, obsessions are immediate, aversive sensory experiences, often accompanied by incongruous dreadful mental images and specific unrealistic fears that those circumstances might occur or might have already occurred. While an individual may take preparatory actions in association with anxious ruminations, the experience lacks the dreadful immediacy of obsessive fears and the sense of urgency that drives the compulsive behaviors. Obsessions and worries can coexist when an obsession triggers not only an immediate sense of dread but also cognitive mental processing related to future untoward consequences of the dreaded event. Excessive worries and anxious ruminations also occur in generalized anxiety disorder and in OCPD. They are generally responsive to benzodiazepines. Obsessions, as a rule, are not.

2. Pathologic guilt—Pathologic guilt involves a heightened experience of responsibility for misfortune or harm. The perceived responsibility is usually excessive for the circumstance and can be delusional in nature. It is almost always associated with depressed mood. It differs from an obsession in that the individual truly believes that he or she bears responsibility for an adverse circumstance and experiences excessive remorse. Patients with OCD may have fears that they are responsible for horrific circumstances but usually recognize that their fears are unrealistic. Their experience is one of dread or horror at the notion that they might have done something harmful, often accompanied by significant anxiety relating to future ramifications of such events. Except in cases of delusional OCD, patients with OCD rarely experience remorse or regret in association with their obsessions, because they recognize at some level the absurdity of their concern. Many patients with OCD do become depressed and may have both obsessive concerns and pathologic guilt. Pathologic guilt can occur in patients with low self-esteem and almost always occurs in patients with significant depression.

3. Depressive ruminations—Depressive ruminations involve the persistent cognitive reprocessing of past memories and experiences, associated with sadness, a sense of loss, or regret. These ruminations are active, continuous mental processes, drawn out in time. The individual ponders past events and often experiences significant guilt or remorse, without dread or uncertainty. If a sense of incompletion is present, it is associated with regret that things were not done satisfactorily in the past. There is no sense of urgency that the situation must be remedied.

4. Aggressive ruminations—Aggressive ruminations are anger-related mental processes involving either past or future ego injuries. Individuals perceive rightly or wrongly that they either were or will be offended in some way, and they replay the events surrounding these circumstances over and over in their minds. Aggressive ruminations may be associated with vengeful fantasies and paranoid ideation. Ruminations may involve envisioning past events as the individual would have preferred them to have occurred. In ruminating about the future, the individual may envision an anticipated scenario in which he or she will be slighted or wronged and may envision various responses to such indignities. In some cases the individual may have difficulty escaping from the ruminative process, leading to interference in the individual's ability to function effectively. Aggressive ruminations differ from aggressive obsessions in that the former are ego-syntonic processes, associated with anger, in which the individual is cognitively involved as an active participant. By contrast, aggressive obsessions involve horrific sensory images or unrealistic fears of acting on destructive impulses, unaccompanied by feelings of anger. The individual tries to avoid these horrific images or fears by putting the thoughts out of mind or by taking steps to make sure that they do not occur. Aggressive ruminations typically occur in individuals with personality disorders (eg, paranoid, obsessive-compulsive, or narcissistic personality disorders) and in individuals with passive-aggressive personality traits. They may also occur in certain patients with psychotic disorders.

5. Fantasies—Fantasies are mental stories that the individual entertains, extending over a period of time. Fantasies almost always have an attractive component; however, the individual usually realizes that imagined events are unlikely to occur. In pathologic cases, the individual feels locked into the fantasies, envisioning complicated sequences of events, and is unable to withdraw from the mental experience. This may result in mental absences, delays, or impaired performance. Erotic, angry, persecutory, or paranoid fantasies should not be confused with sexual, violent, or aggressive obsessions. Erotic fantasies are associated with a sense of pleasure or captivation and are not experienced as horrific and aversive. Paranoid and anger-related fantasies involve escalating vengeful interactions with an imagined adversary and are not accompanied by doubt, dread, or uncertainty that the acts have occurred in reality. Unlike obsessions, fantasies do not drive the individual to carry out compulsions in the real world. Excessive fantasies can occur in patients with cluster A personality disorders or with OCPD.

6. Paranoid fears—Paranoid fears are concerns that somebody else harbors malevolent intent toward the affected individual. They may be associated with anger and may lead to avoidant, preparatory, or violent preemptive measures, designed to protect the individual from human attack. Preventive measures are taken in order to prepare for or protect against attack, not to alleviate the circumstances causing the fear. Patients with OCD sometimes have fears of being harmed by others, as in fears of being poisoned; however, these patients fear that they may be random victims and not specific targets of someone harboring malevolence against them in particular. Violent acts do not occur as a primary consequence of the obsessions of uncomplicated OCD.

7. Flashbacks—Flashbacks are intense, intrusive experiences associated with memories of past traumatic events. The individual usually reexperiences these events in association with a related trigger. Flashbacks often occupy the individual's entire awareness, as though the individual were reliving these events in the here and now. They differ from obsessions in that they spring from memories of past experiences and not from inexplicable horrific images unrelated to previous experience. During the flashback, the individual behaves appropriately within the context of the flashback. The individual may not be aware that the behavior is inappropriate in the present time. In some circumstances traumatic events can lead to time-consuming rituals that are excessive or unrealistic in relation to the degree of psychological trauma. Such rituals should be considered compulsions.

8. Pathologic attraction—Pathologic attraction occurs as cognitive and visceral experiences draw an individual toward a maladaptive behavior. It can be associated with feelings of desire, longing, yearning, or a need for the release of tension. It is usually accompanied by an urge to satisfy or gratify that desire. Pathologic attraction differs from an obsession in that the latter is by nature an intensely aversive experience and triggers behavior based on escape rather than gratification. Pathologic attraction is often associated with impulsions (see "Behavioral Differentiations" section later in this chapter) and is generally present in patients with impulse-control disorders.

9. Rigid thinking—Rigid thinking occurs when an individual is unable to switch sets and adopt a new perspective. It is usually ego syntonic and may be delusional in nature. People with rigid thinking may be argumentative, repeat themselves, or return to the same point again and again. They are generally unable to adopt the perspective of another individual and cannot be dissuaded from their point of view. Rigid thinking differs from obsessional concerns in that in the former there is no uncertainty or dread and little or no awareness of defect. Rigid thinking can occur in OCPD, in individuals with reduced intelligence, in geriatric populations, and in patients with organic and psychotic illness.

10. Pathologic indecision—Pathologic indecision occurs when an individual is unable to make choices with potential outcomes of unknown or mixed valence. In some cases individuals become paralyzed because they cannot make any decisions. Although there can be a sense of dreadful uncertainty associated with not knowing the outcome, in OCD the sense of dread tends to motivate decisions (including the decision not to act). Pathologic indecision can be seen in the setting of depression and is common in some forms of OCPD in which the individual wants to optimize an outcome without sufficient information. Such a condition can lead to significant procrastination and delayed commitments.

11. Realistic fears or concerns—Individuals with realistic fears or concerns may simulate a picture of OCD. Individuals with a history of violence or pathologic absent-mindedness or inattention may have realistic concerns that these problems will recur and may take special steps appropriate for their own circumstances (eg, removing dangerous weapons, checking the stove to be sure it is off) to reduce such recurrences. The clinician must establish that such fears or concerns have no realistic basis, or are clearly excessive, before diagnosing such concerns as obsessions.

B. Behavioral Differentiations:

1. Impulsions—Impulsions are maladaptive behaviors that an individual is attracted to or feels impelled to perform. They are associated with an urge for gratification, satisfaction, or release of tension. The individual may derive a sense of pleasure from the completion of the act. Impulsions can take the form of violent or destructive behaviors that release the tension associated with poorly controlled anger. Impulsions differ from compulsions in that in the former the individual is drawn to the act and derives inherent (not secondary) pleasure, satisfaction, gratification, or release of tension from its completion. By contrast, compulsions are performed to escape aversive circumstances or to prevent something terrible from happening. Compulsions in uncomplicated OCD never involve the willful performance of violent or harmful acts. Impulsions cross diagnostic lines in that maladaptive acts such as drug abuse, binge eating, serial homicide, sexual paraphilias, and impulse-control disorders all fall into this category on the basis of their underlying motivation. Some behaviors can have both gratifying and compulsive components, such as hot showers extended for both pleasure and a sense of incompletion. The clinician must separate impulsions from OCD symptoms.

2. Meticulousness or perfectionism—Meticulousness, or perfectionism, is motivated by a positive sense of accomplishment in completing activities in the proper or optimal manner. The individual achieves a sense of satisfaction and believes that the act is beneficial or rewarding in some way. The individual often believes that others should behave in a similar manner, whether or not the behavior of these others affects the perfectionist. Perfectionism differs from obsessions with symmetry, exactness, or order in that the former is reinforced by favorable consequences. The ordering, arranging, and "just-right" compulsions of OCD are carried out because of a sense that something is, or will be, very wrong if they are not done. These patients with OCD are intensely disturbed by a sense of misalignment, and experience an aversive sense of incompletion while the behavior is in progress. They generally recognize the absurd and uniquely personal nature of the behavior and do not believe that others need to carry out the same behavior, unless it directly affects their own circumstances. Perfectionism is often associated with OCPD.

3. Pathologic atonement—Pathologic atonement is motivated by guilt or fear of punishment. Individuals may regret past actions and seek to reduce their discomfort in the performance of penitent behavior. Pathologic atonement can take the form of religious rituals, self-punitive tasks, or in severe cases, self-injurious acts, such as flagellation or self-mutilation. This behavior differs from a compulsion of OCD in that the behavior is not motivated by doubt or incompletion but is willfully carried out to reduce the experience of guilt or to avoid an anticipated punishment of greater significance.

Under certain circumstances, an individual may have pathologic uncertainty as to whether the atonement was sufficiently or properly completed and will carry out the behavior repeatedly or excessively for that reason. In such cases the behavior is not driven so much by guilt as it is by the unreasonable sense that the action has not been carried out properly or completely. In such cases a diagnosis of OCD may be considered. Pathologic atonement can be observed in patients with severe depression, hyperreligiosity, severe personality disorders, or psychosis.

4. Repetitive displacement behavior—Repetitive displacement behavior is performed to escape or numb an aversive experience associated with an affective state such as depression or extreme anxiety. The process of carrying out and focusing attention on the act reduces the individual's awareness of the primary aversive condition. Repetitive displacement behavior can mimic OCD, as in cases where depressed or anxious individuals engage in repetitive cleaning or straightening to reduce their affective experience. Although repetitive and seemingly purposeless, the function of the behavior is to numb the psychic distress associated with the primary condition. In contrast to the compulsions of OCD, consequences of the behavior are relatively unimportant. Repetitive displacement behavior can be observed in avoidant, anxious, or depressed individuals and in patients with OCPD.

5. Perseverative behavior—Perseverative behavior involves the repetition of thoughts, speech, or brief behavioral sequences. Perseverative behavior can be carried out without conscious thought or may occur because it reduces an awareness of anxiety or other aversive experiences. It may occur in response to an urge without any affective component. It differs from repeating compulsions in that it is carried out without purpose. Perseverative behavior is not performed as a corrective or preventive measure nor is it driven by a sense of incompletion.

6. Stereotypic behavior—Stereotypic behavior is a form of perseverative motor behavior that is rhythmic in nature. Typically simpler than other perseverative behavior, it may be associated with primary reward or with a reduction of awareness of anxiety or another aversive experience. Stereotypic behavior is frequently seen in the mentally retarded, in patients with organic illnesses, and in very disturbed individuals, often with schizophrenia. It also may occur in normal children.

7. Self-injurious behavior—Self-injurious behavior can occur in several psychological settings. It frequently occurs as an escape behavior to reduce the intensity of a highly aversive affective experience. It can also occur as a pathologic manipulative process. Finally, as mentioned earlier, it may be carried out as a self-punitive process in pathologic atonement. When carried out as an escape behavior, the individual will describe a release of tension associated with the act, particularly upon visualization of the self-injurious process. The pain or shock of the injury appears to reduce or block out the awareness of the aversive affective experience that triggers the behavior. By contrast, compulsions of uncomplicated OCD never involve direct self-harm. Self-injurious behavior is observed in patients with borderline personality disorder, severe depression, or some organic or psychotic syndromes.

8. Pathologic overinvolvement—Pathologic overinvolvement occurs when an individual is preoccupied with a single process or set of processes to the exclusion of others. Overinvolvement is generally ego syntonic as the individual carries out the process upon which attention is focused. Each step of the process leads to the desire to carry out the next step. The individual experiences gratification from the process as it is occurring or upon completion, and the behavior is carried out because the individual values the achievement. The original purpose of the behavior may be lost. Overinvolvement becomes pathologic when the individual neglects or is unable to attend to more important tasks or social responsibilities. Pathologic overinvolvement differs from OCD in that the individual is attracted to the engagement and is not motivated by aversive experience. It can be prominent in patients with stimulant intoxication and hypomania and can occur in patients with OCPD.

9. Pathologic persistence—Pathologic persistence is observed when an individual continues to pursue an endeavor or interaction despite repeated failure or rebuff. It can be associated with rigidity of thought or related to an individual's inability to accept unwanted circumstances. It is often associated with an overvaluing of a personal agenda, relative to the agendas of others. It can result in mutually irritating interactions with those around the individual. Pathologic persistence is goal directed, and although there may be a concomitant sense of incompleteness or unfinished business, the behavior is motivated by some other purpose, such as a desire to win, have one's own way, or accomplish one's goals. Pathologic persistence differs from OCD in that the former behavior is ego syntonic. The individual seeks a favorable resolution of his or her pursuits and is not trying to escape an experience of dread or uncertainty. Pathologic persistence occurs in patients with OCPD, narcissistic personality disorder, borderline personality disorder, hypomania, and in some cases of stimulant intoxication.

10. Hoarding—Hoarding is observed in numerous syndromes other than OCD. These include anorexia nervosa, Tourette's syndrome, autism, Prader-Willi syndrome, OCPD, stimulant abuse, schizotypal personality disorder, and schizophrenia. In Prader-Willi syndrome, anorexia nervosa, and some cases of autism, hoarding occurs in secrecy. These patients have hidden stashes of items that they have collected, often by stealing or other surreptitious means. Collected items may have little tangible importance to the individual, as in food collected by the anorexic individual that will never be eaten. Collecting in OCPD is performed because of a sense that items may have positive value at some point in the future. The accumulation of possessions itself is important. The possessions are an extension of the individual, and the individual feels a sense of loss or waste if called upon to discard them. In OCD, by contrast, collecting is motivated by one of two different processes. It may be associated with an unreasonable urge to obtain an item, without any underlying reason (eg, picking up bird feathers or empty bottles on the street). Such collecting can be indistinguishable from that seen in Tourette's syndrome, autism, schizophrenia, and schizotypal personality disorder. The diagnosis is made on the basis of other associated pathology. Alternatively, hoarding or collecting in OCD may be associated with an unreasonable concern that the item, although unimportant now, might be needed in the future. The patient with OCD has a sense that there may be a time when not having the item will result in a distressing circumstance that should be protected against.

11. Complex tics—Complex tics occur in the setting of a tic disorder and are usually motivated by unwanted urges without rational motivation. Although some complex tics are confined to localized muscle groups, others can mimic the compulsions of OCD. Most often these latter tics involve "just-right" perceptions, accompanied by urges to order, align, or arrange. In addition, patients with Tourette's syndrome can have obsessions associated with their tics, such that they fear something terrible will happen if they do not give in to the urge to tic. These tics can be indistinguishable from the compulsive behavior of OCD. In such cases it is best to classify the behavior

as both a tic and a compulsion (an OCD-tic). Because treatment decisions can be affected by the presence of tics, the clinician should always observe the patient for such processes and should ask the patient about distinctive habits or mannerisms they might make or might have had previously, particularly in childhood.

Baer L, Jenike MA: Personality disorders in obsessive compulsive disorder. Psychiatr Clin N Am 1992;15:803.
Pigott TA et al: Obsessive compulsive disorder: comorbid conditions. J Clin Psychiatry 1994;55(10 Suppl):15.
Swedo SE et al: Pediatric autoimmune neuropsychiatric disorders associated with streptococcal infections: clinical description of the first 50 cases. Am J Psychiatry 1998;155:264. [Published erratum appears in Am J Psychiatry 1998;155:578.]

Differential Psychiatric Diagnoses

A number of psychiatric disorders have been confused with OCD on the basis of some common phenomenologic components. The differential psychiatric diagnosis for OCD is summarized in Table 24–2.

A. Obsessive-Compulsive Personality Disorder (OCPD): OCPD is an Axis II disorder that has a name that sounds similar to OCD but is associated with meticulousness, persistence, rigidity, and personal isolation. As noted earlier in this chapter, only a small minority of OCD patients have concurrent OCPD. This confusion may relate historically to Sigmund Freud's characterization of obsessions and compulsions in his work with the "Rat Man." Unfortunately, the Rat Man had both OCD and OCPD, leading Freud to entangle the two entities in his interpretations. The key difference between elements of OCPD and OCD is the ego-syntonic nature of the experiences and behavior in OCPD. There is no dread but rather a desire that others conform to the individual's standards or desires.

B. Specific Phobias: Specific phobias involve excessive fears of specific situations or circumstances. They often involve fears of situations that others might experience as mildly aversive or anxiety provoking (eg, contact with snakes or spiders), but the phobic individual has an excessive reaction to those circumstances. Avoidance is prominent and effective in allaying anxiety. In OCD, fears can be situation specific; however, there is usually a sense of doubt or uncertainty associated with the dread (eg, uncertainty

Table 24–2. Differential psychiatric diagnosis for obsessive-compulsive disorder.

Anorexia nervosa
Body dysmorphic disorder
Hypochondriasis
Obsessive-compulsive personality disorder
Pathologic skin-picking
Specific phobias
Trichotillomania

whether germs are present), as the individual cannot be certain he or she has successfully avoided the aversive circumstance. No rituals are involved in simple phobias.

C. Hypochondriasis: Hypochondriasis is an unreasonable, persistent concern that something is wrong with the body. It can lead to repeated requests for medical care or reassurance. Hypochondriasis can mimic the obsessions of OCD; however, hypochondriacal concerns are limited to the body, and there are no other obsessions and compulsions. The individual is usually not delusional and may recognize that the behavior is excessive. Patients with hypochondriasis usually lack the sense of immediacy that exists in OCD. The individual experiences worries about longterm health rather than short-term immediate dread. Hypochondriasis can be associated with abnormal somatic perceptions, which are unusual in OCD.

D. Body Dysmorphic Disorder: Body dysmorphic disorder (BDD) involves the unreasonable sense that something about the body is malformed, inadequate, or offensive to others. The individual may spend excessive time looking at, or seeking medical or surgical treatment for, the affected area. BDD differs from OCD in the degree of insight, as the individual with BDD truly believes that the body area is abnormal. There is no sense of incompletion or dread that something terrible will happen. The driven behaviors associated with BDD involve corrective measures to hide or alter an imagined defect and are not carried out with a sense that something has not been completed. The distinction between BDD and OCD can be difficult when the individual experiences "justright" perceptions related to the body or when the individual has a fear of having an offensive body odor. In such cases the diagnosis of OCD may be warranted.

E. Trichotillomania: Trichotillomania is characterized by urges to pull hairs from the body. The hair is most frequently pulled out singly, and the act of pulling is associated with an experience of pleasure or a release of tension. Binges of hair pulling result in large bald patches. Trichotillomania differs from OCD in that the former involves no obsessions, and the behavior is rewarding.

F. Pathologic Skin-Picking: Pathologic skinpicking can occur as an unconscious habit or as a response to an exaggerated concern about the texture of the skin. The individual may be drawn to the behavior by an attractive process that is hard to overcome. Skin-pickers are typically aware that what they are doing is destructive; however, they are unable to overcome the desire to carry out the behavior. Such picking is similar to trichotillomania in this regard. It differs from OCD in that in pathologic skin-picking there is no sense of dread, uncertainty, or incompletion, and the behavior is not carried out to prevent something bad from happening. It also differs from OCD in that pathologic skin-picking has a self-

destructive or mutilative component that is rarely seen in uncomplicated OCD.

G. Anorexia Nervosa: Anorexia nervosa involves an excessive concern with body image, accompanied by a refusal to eat, with purposeful behavior directed at maintaining a low body weight. In anorexia nervosa, there is a delusional perception that the body is overweight. Unlike in OCD, the anorexic individual has no insight regarding this concern. Feelings of dread, uncertainty, or incompletion are absent or are not prominent. Driven behaviors are performed with the intention of maintaining or exacerbating a desired condition. Although hoarding may be observed, no true compulsions are associated with the primary illness. Individuals with OCD can experience significant weight loss in conjunction with fears associated with food contamination. These individuals, however, do not typically have concerns about their body image and often acknowledge the absurdity of their condition.

Complications & Secondary Diagnoses

As mentioned earlier in this chapter, OCD has been associated with diseases of the basal ganglia. A significant number of children who developed Economo's disease after an influenza epidemic early in the 20th century experienced OCD symptoms, and there was a significant increase in the prevalence of chronic OCD in survivors of the epidemic. OCD has also been described in Huntington's disease, parkinsonism, and carbon monoxide poisoning associated with destruction of the globus pallidus. There is a higher incidence of rheumatic fever in family members of patients with OCD. Adults with a history of Sydenham's chorea have a higher incidence of OCD than does the population at large.

There is a high prevalence of vocal and motor tics in OCD (20%) and in the families of patients with OCD (20%). The full-fledged Tourette's syndrome is present in only 5–7% of adult patients with OCD. Over 60% of children with OCD will experience at least transient tics, and as many as 15% will develop the full Tourette's syndrome. For children with an early onset of symptoms, OCD may be the first manifestation of Tourette's syndrome. OCD symptoms occur in 40–70% of individuals with Tourette's syndrome and in 12% of family members of Tourette's syndrome patients who do not themselves have Tourette's syndrome.

OCD patients often have comorbid Axis I disorders. Depression is the most common secondary diagnosis in OCD. Approximately 50% of individuals with OCD will develop a major depressive episode in their lifetime. The depression occurs because OCD symptoms prevent the individual from carrying out activities important for self-esteem, and because attempts to resist the symptoms, or adequately meet the demands of the illness, inevitably fail. OCD can engender continual conflict with significant others and is often associated with social isolation. Effective treatment of the OCD in these cases often leads to resolution of the depressive episode.

Patients with OCD also have a high prevalence of panic disorder, secondary agoraphobia, social phobia, and alcohol and other substance abuse. Agoraphobia can result from a patient's attempts to avoid circumstances that trigger obsessions. In some cases the patient may be trapped at home because he or she is unable to tolerate the obsessions and compulsions that are triggered by contact with the outside world.

Anxiety can complicate OCD, as the individual worries about both the consequences of having OCD and the consequences of being unable to complete compulsions. Patients with OCD may describe panic-like attacks that are not true panic attacks. Rather, they are attacks of severe anxiety related to violation of an obsessive concern. For example, when an individual who has contamination fears discovers that he or she has been severely contaminated, the individual may experience an overwhelming sense of dread, anxiety, and despair, related to the impossible task of decontaminating everything that he or she has defiled. This patient might mislabel these experiences as panic attacks. The clinician must be aware of this process to avoid unnecessarily complicating the patient's diagnostic picture.

There is also a high prevalence of personality disorders in patients with OCD (50–70%). Avoidant, dependent, borderline, histrionic, and schizotypal personality disorders occur most frequently. OCPD occurs in only a small minority of patients, with estimates as low as 6% of OCD cases. This observation argues against an older view that OCD was an extreme variant of OCPD. Interestingly, although personality disorder symptoms are thought to be lifelong fixed traits, effective treatment of OCD will eliminate personality disorder symptoms in a majority of OCD patients, suggesting that the dysfunctional Axis II symptoms may in part be secondary to stress and tension associated with the Axis I disorder.

The diagnosis of avoidant personality disorder may be secondary to the individual's primary pathology, combined with an ambiguity in the DSM-IV diagnostic criteria for the personality disorder. An unreasonable concern of being the target of disapproval of others is a DSM-IV criterion for avoidant personality disorder. Individuals with OCD who fear they may be responsible for something bad happening may also fear that they will be the subject of consequent disapproval or ridicule. These patients have unreasonable concerns that they might in fact be at fault. Individuals with the true personality disorder (ie, those who do not have OCD) are unreasonably hypersensitive to the criticism itself. As individuals with OCD improve they often no longer meet criteria for this diagnosis.

Likewise, the dependent personality disorder can occur in patients with OCD who feel that they need assistance from others in carrying out their compulsions or who need reassurance that their obsessive concerns are not valid. Such assistance relieves them of the responsibility for carrying out acts that might have dreadful consequences. These individuals are dependent on their significant other, and they experience significant discomfort when that person is not available for these purposes. These patients will meet criteria for this personality disorder as a result of the nature of their OCD. As their OCD improves, many will no longer meet criteria for this diagnosis.

Treatment

Treatment ranges from simple stress reduction to neurosurgery (Tables 24–3 and 24–4). Mild forms of OCD (ie, with YBOCS scores of less than 16) that occur in association with temporary stress may respond to stress reduction and supportive measures. Most OCD seen by psychiatrists, however, requires more definitive treatment.

A. Behavioral Therapy: Behavioral therapy for OCD involves exposure and response prevention. According to learning theorists, patients with OCD have learned an inappropriate active avoidance response to anxiety associated with circumstances that trigger their OCD symptoms. The clinician must encourage the patient to experience the aversive condition (exposure) without performing the compulsion (response prevention). Chronic exposure alone will reduce the anxiety associated with the exposure, but the compulsions will remain if not specifically restricted. Response prevention is critical. Typically the individual is asked to order his or her fears as a hierarchy. A decision is then made as to which obsessive-compulsive dyad will be addressed. The patient is exposed by increasing degrees to the feared stimulus and is prohibited from carrying out the compulsive behavior. Anxiety with initial exposure is usually intense and enduring; however, with repeated exposure, the intensity and duration decrease. When it is not possible to expose the patient in the office, the therapist may accompany the patient to a location, such as the home or the street, where the feared stimuli are more prevalent. In an outpatient session the patient is typically instructed to repeatedly expose himself or herself to a specified set of circumstances on a proscribed number of occasions as "homework" between sessions. The patient should be encouraged to assess or question the validity of his or her obsessive thoughts as an adjunct to treatment. Such a cognitive approach may increase compliance, and when no compulsions are present, or when exposure is impractical, it may be the primary adjunct to treatment. In other cases, exposure to the actual fear (eg, killing one's child) is not practicable, and the patient must engage in imaginal exposure. Typically the therapist and patient will work on one symptom complex until the symptom has been reduced to an agreeable level or until a joint decision is made to address another symptom.

Table 24–3. Pharmacologic treatments for obsessive-compulsive disorder.

First line—PSRIs	Dosage (mg/day)
SSRIs	
Fluvoxamine	100–300
Fluoxetine	20–80
Sertraline	75–225
Paroxetine	20–60
Citalopram	20–60
Clomipramine	150–250
Adjuncts	
SSRI/clomipramine	Various
Neuroleptics (tics, family history of tics, schizotypal personality disorder)[1]	
Risperidone	1–3
Olanzapine	2.5–7.5
Pimozide	0.5–4
Haloperidol	0.5–4
Clonazepam (seizures, panic, anxiety, insomnia)[1]	1–6
For nonresponders	
MAOIs (panic, phobias, refractory depression)[1]	
Phenylzine	60–90
Tranylcypromine	20–60
Venlafaxine (refractory depression)[1]	150–300
Mirtazepine (refractory depression, anxiety)[1]	15–30
Trazodone (high-dose; for refractory depression)[1]	400–600
Clonazepam (high-dose; for seizures, panic, anxiety)[1]	4–10
Carbamazepine (abnormal EEG)[1]	Blood-level dependent

[1] Special circumstances that might favor this treatment option.

Table 24–4. Other treatments for obsessive-compulsive disorder.

Interactive treatments
  Behavioral therapy (exposure and response prevention)[1]
  Family therapy (eg, contracts, positive reinforcement, defacilitation)

Neurosurgical treatments (extreme, refractory cases only)[1]
  Anterior cingulotomy
  Limbic leukotomy
  Anterior capsulotomy
  Subcaudate tractotomy

Experimental treatments
  Intravenous clomipramine
  Plasmapheresis (autoimmune-related OCD)[1]
  Immunoglobulin (autoimmune-related OCD)[1]
  Chronic penicillin (streptococcal autoimmune-related OCD)[1]

[1] Special circumstances that might favor this treatment option.

Many physicians have neither the time nor the experience to carry out behavioral therapy themselves and should refer the patient to a specialist in this area. Symptoms most amenable to behavior therapy involve contamination concerns and fears that evoke behavior that can be elicited in the office. Behavioral therapy is most difficult to carry out with individuals who have only obsessions or whose compulsions involve only mental activities such as counting or mental checking. Individuals with poor insight, and those who cannot tolerate exposure, tend to have more difficulty with this treatment method.

Behavioral therapy is effective in roughly 70% of individuals who agree to undergo the process. However, approximately 30% of individuals with OCD will decline this form of treatment. Behavioral therapy may be better tolerated if the patient has appropriate pharmacologic treatment. In some circumstances symptoms can disappear completely; however, they often return over a 6-month period, and an additional short course of behavioral therapy may be needed to effectively treat the symptoms.

B. Pharmacologic Treatment:

1. Preferential serotonergic reuptake inhibitors—

Preferential serotonergic reuptake inhibitors (PSRIs), the medications most effective in treating OCD, preferentially inhibit the uptake of the neurotransmitter serotonin into nerve cells (see Table 24–3). These medications include clomipramine, together with the selective serotonergic reuptake inhibitors (SSRIs) fluoxetine, sertraline, paroxetine, citalopram, and fluvoxamine. Medications with noradrenergic reuptake inhibition have no benefit and may counteract or diminish the efficacy of serotonergic reuptake inhibition. Among the PSRIs, clomipramine alone is a tricyclic antidepressant and has significant anticholinergic, antihistaminic, and anti-α-adrenergic side effects. Clomipramine is also metabolized to desmethyl clomipramine, a metabolite that will inhibit the uptake of noradrenaline. Meta-analyses of efficacy suggest that clomipramine may be more effective than other PSRIs in treating OCD; however, there is no direct evidence that any one of the PSRIs is more effective than any other. Except in the case of fluvoxamine, each of the multicenter trials for PSRIs showed nonsignificant trends for higher doses to be more effective in treating OCD, suggesting that the optimal doses for these medications may be at the higher end of the permissible prescription range.

Unlike in depression, PSRIs do not exert their main effects until after 4–6 weeks of treatment and must be administered for up to 12 weeks to determine the benefit that can be achieved. Withdrawal from medication is frequently associated with relapse within 2–3 weeks, so that patients should be advised that they may need to stay on their medication to maintain benefits. Tolerance to the beneficial effects of the PSRIs rarely occurs.

The medications used to treat OCD rarely eliminate the OCD symptoms. Symptoms typically are reduced by 35% in aggregate and by 50–70% in most responders. Such figures underestimate the benefits for patients taking the medications. Although symptom levels may fall by less than half of their baseline levels, such patients can experience a significant improvement in the quality of their lives and can function more effectively in society. Approximately 50–60% of those initially undertaking a trial of a PSRI will achieve a clinically significant response. The medications allow the patients to tolerate the obsessions, and the urges to carry out the compulsions, without acting on them. The combination of behavioral therapy with medication appears to be optimal for most OCD patients, as up to 25% of patients who fail one modality will respond to joint treatment.

If a patient has no response to medication after 8 weeks, or has an inadequate response after 12 weeks, the clinician should consider trying a different PSRI. Approximately 20% of patients who do not respond to one PSRI will respond to another. If the patient has not responded to a second PSRI, a third PSRI trial should be attempted. One of the three PSRI trials should involve clomipramine.

2. Adjunctive medications—

If a patient does not achieve an adequate response with proper trials of PSRIs, a second medication should be added. The combination of an SSRI and clomipramine should be considered in this context. The combination of clomipramine and fluvoxamine may significantly augment serotonin uptake inhibition because fluvoxamine can inhibit the conversion of clomipramine to its noradrenergic desmethyl metabolite. Alternatively, low-dose, high-potency neuroleptics (eg, risperidone, olanzapine, pimozide, haloperidol) may be used to augment PSRI treatment, particularly if the patient has comorbid tics, a family history of tics, or features of a schizotypal personality disorder. OCD symptoms in the latter group of patients can be refractory to conventional treatments but may have a significant response to augmentation with a neuroleptic. For patients whose OCD has a significant anxiety component, patients with a history of seizures, and patients with additional symptoms consistent with partial complex seizures, the addition of clonazepam (0.5–6 mg) should be considered. Clonazepam can also be considered as an adjunct to high-dose clomipramine treatment (greater than 250 mg daily) as a means of reducing the potential for seizures. Both low-dose neuroleptics and clonazepam should be added after the patient has been taking the optimal PSRI for at least 6–8 weeks and is on the maximal dose tolerated. These adjuncts may have beneficial effects within 1 week; however, an adequate adjunctive trial should be 4–6 weeks. Other medications that have been used as adjunctive treatments include tryptophan, pindolol plus tryptophan, mirtazapine, gabapentin, and fenfluramine. Lithium, buspirone, and pindolol appear to have little benefit as augmenting agents in the treatment of OCD.

3. Alternative pharmacologic monotherapies—

Alternative medication trials must be considered for those patients who fail to respond to adequate trials of PSRIs and adjuncts in conjunction with appropriate behavioral therapy. A trial of a monoamine oxidase inhibitor (MAOI) should be considered for patients with panic or phobic symptoms. Patients with a seizure history, an abnormal EEG, or suspected partial complex seizures might be considered for a trial of clonazepam or carbamazepine as a monotherapy. High-dose clonazepam as a monotherapy has a success rate of 20–30% in the treatment of OCD. Low-dose clonazepam does not appear to be effective as a monotherapy. Clonazepam treatment can bring on or exacerbate a depressive episode. If this occurs, the trial should be discontinued because it will not alleviate OCD symptoms. Clonazepam treatment may also interfere with the efficiency of a behavioral therapy. Certain medications affecting serotonergic neurotransmission may also have efficacy as monotherapies in isolated cases. These medications include mirtazapine, venlafaxine, high-dose trazodone, and buspirone. Clonidine has no benefit for adults with OCD; however, it has been used effectively to reduce OCD symptoms in children who have combined Tourette's syndrome and OCD. Lithium, methylphenidate, neuroleptics, other heterocyclic antidepressants, and other benzodiazepines including alprazolam, have little benefit as monotherapies in OCD.

C. Family Therapy: Family members can unwittingly interfere with the success of traditional treatments. As mentioned earlier in this chapter, families can facilitate the OCD symptoms or antagonize the patient. In such cases, family therapy can be helpful. At the very least, education regarding the patient's condition and the appropriate responses to that condition should be attempted. In general, family members should not assist the patient in the OCD rituals, nor should they significantly alter or compromise the quality of their lives to accommodate the symptoms of the illness. The family should be supportive of reductions in symptoms but not critical of exacerbations. Family members should avoid disparaging remarks related to the OCD. More extensive family therapy involves mutually acceptable contracts between the patient and affected family members regarding behaviors targeted for suppression. OCD behaviors outside the contract that do not compromise the lives of family members should be dealt with only in a positive and constructive manner. Family members should be aware that behavior therapy is a stepwise process and that behavior that is currently not a part of the contract can be addressed in the future. In addition to interventions directed at the OCD, internal family conflicts may need to be addressed in therapy because these can exacerbate the OCD symptoms and impair the quality of life of all concerned.

D. Neurosurgery: Neurosurgery is the treatment of last resort. Neurosurgical procedures include bilateral cingulotomy, limbic leukotomy, anterior capsulotomy, and subcaudate tractotomy. Estimates of clinically significant improvement are 25–90%, although controlled studies have not been undertaken. There is some disagreement regarding the optimal site of the lesion. In intractable cases, however, neurosurgery is a treatment that may offer relief from disabling symptoms and from extreme psychic pain. Improvement after surgery is not immediate but may occur over a period of up to 1 year. Adverse effects include seizures, disinhibition syndromes, and the attendant risks of general anesthesia.

Patients should not be referred for surgery unless they have had full trials of at least three PSRIs at appropriate dosages, including one trial of clomipramine, as well as trials of both a neuroleptic and clonazepam as adjunctive medications. A trial of an MAOI should have been attempted. The patient should have had a course of behavioral therapy with a qualified therapist, preferably occurring while the patient was receiving optimal pharmacologic treatment. Additionally, the OCD or its complications should have life-threatening consequences for the patient or cause extreme dysfunction or severe psychic pain. Patients should be referred to centers that have stringent presurgical entrance criteria and extensive experience with this treatment modality.

E. Experimental Treatments:

1. Intravenous clomipramine—It is ironic that intravenous clomipramine treatment is considered an experimental treatment when most of the early work in Europe demonstrating the efficacy of clomipramine was completed using this parenteral preparation. Intravenous clomipramine treatment is currently receiving attention in the United States and may have significant promise in the treatment of OCD that does not respond to PSRIs. Specific clinical recommendations for this treatment modality are not yet available.

2. Immunosuppressant & antistreptococcal treatment—Recurrent, episodic, postinfectious OCD in children has been treated with immunosuppressive measures including steroids, plasmapheresis, and immunoglobulin treatment. In addition, children with repeated poststreptococcal episodes have been placed experimentally on prophylactic penicillin treatment. Although initial trials of immunosuppressants seem positive, specific clinical recommendations regarding these treatments are not available. As a rule, these treatments are not effective in treating OCD in adults.

Allen AJ et al: Case study: a new infection-triggered, autoimmune subtype of pediatric OCD and Tourette's syndrome. J Am Acad Child Adolesc Psychiatry 1995; 34:307.

Baer L: *Getting Control: Overcoming Your Obsessions and Compulsions.* Penguin, New York, 1991.

Foa EB: *Stop Obsessing: How to Overcome Your Obsessions and Compulsions.* Bantam Books, New York, 1991.

Hewlett WA: Novel pharmacologic treatments of obsessive compulsive disorder. In: Hollander EH, Stein D (editors): *Obsessive Compulsive Disorders.* Marcel Dekker, 1996.

Koran LM et al: Rapid benefit of intravenous pulse loading of clomipramine in obsessive-compulsive disorder. Am J Psychiatry 1997;154:396.

March JS et al: The Expert Consensus Guideline Series: treatment of obsessive compulsive disorder. J Clin Psychiatry 1997;(suppl 4):3.

Marks I: Behavior therapy for obsessive-compulsive disorder: a decade of progress. Can J Psychiatry 1997;42: 1021.

McDougle CJ: Update on pharmacologic management of OCD: agents and augmentation. J Clin Psychiatry 1997;12:11.

Mindus P et al: Neurosurgical treatment for refractory obsessive-compulsive disorder: implications for understanding frontal lobe function. J Neuropsychiatry Clin Neurosci 1994;6:467.

Ravizza L et al: Predictors of drug treatment response in obsessive-compulsive disorder. J Clin Psychiatry 1995;56: 368.

Prognosis & Course of Illness

There is no cure for OCD. The best that can be expected is a temporary remission of certain symptom complexes with appropriate behavioral therapy, and partial remission of symptoms with pharmacotherapy or neurosurgery. Even such partial remission is a welcome relief for patients plagued by this illness and often allows them to function with some effort at a full capacity. Overall, 75–85% of patients seeking treatment will achieve a significant clinical response with optimal combined treatments. Individuals with schizotypal features or neurologic soft signs have a poorer response prognosis, and the former group may not respond to either pharmacotherapy or behavioral interventions. Individuals who will not or cannot tolerate medications and behavioral measures likewise have a poor prognosis. Most biological research on OCD has been carried out only in the past decade, and new treatments such as immunosuppressive therapy, prophylactic penicillin, and intravenous clomipramine show promise for the future. The clinician should be optimistic that although at present there is no cure, the future may provide far more effective treatments.

25

Somatoform Disorders

Charles V. Ford, MD

Patients who somatize psychosocial distress commonly present in medical clinical settings. Approximately 25% of patients in primary care demonstrate some degree of somatization, and at least 10% of medical or surgical patients have no evidence of a disease process. Somatizing patients use a disproportionately large amount of medical services and frustrate their physicians, who often do not recognize the true nature of these patients' underlying problems. Somatizers rarely seek help from psychiatrists at their own initiative, and they may resent any implication that their physical distress is related to psychological problems. Despite the psychogenic etiology of their illnesses, these patients continue to seek medical care in nonpsychiatric settings where their somatization is often unrecognized.

Somatization is not an either-or proposition. Rather, many patients have some evidence of biological disease but overrespond to their symptoms or believe themselves to be more disabled than objective evidence would indicate. Medical or surgical patients who have concurrent anxiety or depressive disorders use medical services at a rate two to three times greater than that of persons with the same diseases who do not have a comorbid psychiatric disorder.

Despite the illusion that somatoform disorders are specific entities, as is implied by the use of specific diagnostic criteria from *Diagnostic and Statistical Manual of Mental Disorders,* 4th edition (DSM-IV), the symptoms most of these patients experience fail to meet the diagnostic criteria of the formal somatoform disorders. Further, over time, patients' symptoms tend to be fluid, and patients may be best described as having one disorder at one time and another disorder at some other time. Somatization is caused or facilitated by numerous interrelated factors (Table 25–1), and for an individual patient a particular symptom may have multiple etiologies. In other words, these disorders are heterogeneous both in clinical presentation and in etiology.

Somatoform disorders are generally multidetermined, and because they represent final common symptomatic pathways of many etiologic factors, each patient must be evaluated carefully so that an individualized treatment plan can be developed.

Ford CV: Dimensions of somatization and hypochondriasis. Neurol Clin N Am 1995;13:241.

Ford CV (section editor): Somatoform and factitious disorders. Pages 1711–1836 in Gabbard GO (editor): *Treatments of Psychiatric Disorders.* Vol 2, 2nd ed. American Psychiatric Press, 1995.

Noyes R, Holt CS, Kathol RG: Somatization: diagnosis and management. Arch Fam Med 1995;4:790.

CONVERSION DISORDER

DSM-IV Diagnostic Criteria

A. One or more symptoms or deficits affecting voluntary motor or sensory function that suggest a neurological or other general medical condition.

B. Psychological factors are judged to be associated with the symptom or deficit because the initiation or exacerbation of the symptom or deficit is preceded by conflicts or other stressors.

C. The symptom or deficit is not intentionally produced or feigned (as in factitious disorder or malingering).

D. The symptoms or deficit cannot, after appropriate investigation, be fully explained by a general medical condition, or by the direct effects of a substance, or as a culturally sanctioned behavior or experience.

E. The symptom or deficit causes clinically significant distress or impairment in social, occupational, or other important areas of functioning or warrants medical evaluation.

F. The symptom or deficit is not limited to pain or sexual dysfunction, does not occur exclusively during the course of somatization disorder, and is not better accounted for by another mental disorder.

Specify type of symptom or deficit:

With motor symptom or deficit (eg, impaired coordination or balance, paralysis, or localized weakness, difficulty swallowing or "lump in throat," aphonia, and urinary retention).

Table 25–1. Causes of somatization.

Illness allows a socially isolated person access to an auxiliary social support system.
The sick role can be used as a rationalization for failures in occupational, social, or sexual roles.
Illness can be a means of obtaining nurturance.
Illness can be used as a source of power to manipulate other people or social situations.
Somatic symptoms may be used as a communication or as a cry for help.
The somatic symptoms of certain psychological disorders (eg, major depression and panic disorder) may be incorrectly attributed to physical disease.
Because physical illness is less stigmatizing than psychiatric illness, many patients prefer to attribute psychological symptoms to physical causes.
Some individuals may be hypersensitive to somatic symptoms and amplify them. Such hypersensitivity is often related to concurrent emotions such as depression and anxiety.
Somatic symptoms can represent behavior learned in childhood, in that some parenting styles may emphasize attention to illness.
The sick role can provide incentives such as disability payments, the avoidance of social responsibilities, and solutions to intrapsychic conflicts.
Trauma, particularly childhood physical or sexual abuse, appears to predispose individuals to the use of somatic symptoms as a communication of psychosocial distress.
Physicians can inadvertently reinforce the concept of physical disease by symptomatic treatment or through so-called fashionable diagnoses, such as multiple chemical sensitivities or reactive hypoglycemia.

With sensory symptom or deficit (eg, loss of touch or pain sensation, double vision, blindness, deafness, and hallucinations).

With seizures or convulsions: includes seizures or convulsions with voluntary motor or sensory components.

With mixed presentation: if symptoms of more than one category are evident.

Reprinted, with permission, from *Diagnostic and Statistical Manual of Mental Disorders,* 4th ed. Copyright 1994 American Psychiatric Association.

General Considerations

Some phenomena that have traditionally been associated with conversion, such as symbolism, *la belle indifférence* (an inappropriate lack of concern for the disability), and histrionic personality, do not reliably differentiate conversion from physical disease.

A. Major Etiologic Theories: Some authors have viewed conversion as more of a symptom than a diagnosis, with the implication that another underlying psychiatric disorder is usually present. It is likely that conversion is heterogeneous and that for some patients there is more than one cause. Among proposed etiologies are suggestions that the symptoms resolve an intrapsychic conflict expressed symbolically through a somatic symptom. For example, a person with a conflict over anger may experience paralysis of a right arm. Interpersonal issues have also been implicated. That is, the symptom may manipulate the behavior of other persons and elicit attention, sympathy, and nurturance.

Conversion often follows a traumatic event and may be a psychological mechanism evoked to cope with acute stress. Conversion symptoms are frequently found in patients receiving treatment on neurologic services and in patients with cerebral dysfunction. It seems likely that underlying neurologic dysfunction fa-

cilitates the emergence of conversion symptoms, perhaps as a result of impairment in the patient's ability to articulate distress. Conversion may also be viewed as a learned behavior. For example, a person who has genuine epileptic convulsions may learn that seizures have a profound effect on others and may develop pseudoseizures. In this case the individual may have both genuine epileptic seizures and pseudoseizures, and distinguishing between the two may be difficult.

Current theories about the etiology of conversion emphasize the role of communication. People who have difficulty in verbally articulating psychosocial distress, for any reason, may use conversion symptoms as a way of communicating their distress.

B. Epidemiology: The reported incidence of conversion symptoms varies widely depending on the populations studied. The lifetime incidence of conversion disorder in women is approximately 33%; however, most of these symptoms remit spontaneously, and the incidence in tertiary-care settings is considerably lower. The incidence in men is unknown. Patients with conversion symptoms comprise 1–3% of patients seen by neurologists. Conversion is diagnosed in 5–10% of hospitalized medical or surgical patients who are referred for psychiatric consultation. Conversion symptoms occur in all age ranges from early childhood to advanced age. The disorder occurs with an approximately equal frequency in prepubertal boys and girls, but it is diagnosed much more frequently in adult women than in men.

Conversion symptoms appear to occur more frequently in people of lower intelligence, in those with less education or less social sophistication, and in those with any condition or situation in which verbal communication may be impeded.

C. Genetics: According to one nonreplicated Scandinavian study, relatives of patients with conversion disorder were at much higher risk for conversion symptoms. Polygenic transmission was proposed.

Clinical Findings

A. Signs & Symptoms: A conversion symptom, by definition, mimics dysfunction in the voluntary motor or sensory system. Common symptoms include pseudoseizures, vocal cord dysfunction (eg, aphonia), blindness, tunnel vision, deafness, and a variety of anesthesias and paralyses. On careful clinical examination and with the aid of laboratory investigations, these symptoms prove to be nonphysiologic. A clinical example is the presence of normal deep tendon reflexes in a person with a "paralyzed" arm.

Contrary to popular belief, patients with conversion disorder may be depressed or anxious about the symptom. *La belle indifference* should not be used as a differentiating sign because individuals with genuine physical disease may be stoic and appear less emotionally disturbed than they are.

B. Psychological Testing: Psychological tests often demonstrate comorbid psychiatric illness associated with tendencies to deny or repress psychological distress. A characteristic finding on the Minnesota Multiphasic Personality Inventory (MMPI) is the presence of the "conversion V," in which the hypochondriasis and hysteria scales are elevated above the depression scale, forming a "V" in the profile. However, such a finding is not pathognomonic for conversion.

C. Laboratory Findings & Imaging: Most conversion symptoms are, by definition, pseudoneurologic. Laboratory examinations, such as nerve conduction speed, electromyograms, and visual and auditory evoked potentials, demonstrate that the sensory and nervous system is intact despite the clinical symptoms. Simultaneous electromyographic and video recording of a patient with pseudoseizures can be diagnostic when the patient has epileptic-like movements while the simultaneous electroencephalogram (EEG) tracing demonstrates normal electrical activity in the brain. There have been no reported neuroimaging studies specific to conversion disorder.

Differential Diagnosis & Comorbidity

The differential diagnosis of conversion disorder always involves the possibility of physical disease. Even when conversion is obvious, the patient may have underlying neurologic or other disease that he or she has unconsciously amplified or elaborated. Table 25–2 lists conditions that often cause errors in diagnosis.

Table 25–2. Differential diagnosis for conversion disorder.

Frontal lobe tumor
Guillain-Barré syndrome
Multiple sclerosis
Pituitary tumor
Spinal cord tumor
Stroke (amnesia)
Torsion dystonia
Torticollis

Malingering must also be considered. The primary difference between malingering and conversion is that the degree of conscious motivation is higher in malingering. Systematic studies of conversion disorder suggest that it is often accompanied by other psychiatric disorders. Depression is common; and schizophrenia has also been reported, though rarely. Patients with conversion disorder may be responding to overwhelming environmental stressors that they cannot articulate, such as concurrent sexual or physical abuse or the feeling of being overwhelmed with responsibilities. Dissociative syndromes are also often associated with conversion, particularly pseudoseizures, which are regarded by some clinicians to be dissociative episodes. Some clinicians have proposed that dissociative disorders and conversion disorders involve the same mechanisms: dissociation reflects mental symptoms and conversion represents somatic symptoms. Conversion is grouped with the dissociative disorders in *International Classification of Disease,* 10th edition (ICD-10).

Treatment

The treatment of conversion disorder is often multimodal and varies according to the acuteness of the symptom. If the symptom is acute, symptom relief often occurs spontaneously or with suggestive techniques. If the symptom is chronic, it is often being reinforced by factors in the patient's environment; therefore, behavioral modification techniques are necessary.

A. Treatment of Comorbid Disorders: When identified, comorbid disorders must be treated concurrently. Conversion symptoms may respond, for example, to treatment for an underlying depression.

B. Hypnosis & Amobarbital (Amytal) Interviews: An acute conversion symptom may remit with suggestions through hypnosis or by the use of an Amytal (or lorazepam) interview that creates an altered state of consciousness. Such techniques may be useful in determining underlying psychological stressors, but caution must be exercised so that patients do not incorporate the interviewer's suggestions as a part of their own history.

C. Behavioral Therapy: Patients with chronic conversion symptoms generally require behavioral modification for symptom relief. Such behavioral therapy can be offered in the form of physical or speech therapy. This approach provides a face-saving mechanism by which patients can gradually discard their symptoms. Patients receive positive reinforcement for symptomatic improvement and are ignored, to avoid reinforcement, at times of symptom expression.

D. Environmental Manipulation: When the conversion symptom represents "a cry for help" because of environmental pressures, it may be necessary to manipulate these stressors in order to produce symptomatic relief. For example, the pseudoseizures of a teenage girl might be a cry for help because she is involved in an incestuous relationship with her stepfather. Obviously, symptom relief will require attention to the sexual abuse.

Complications & Adverse Outcomes of Treatment

Remission, with treatment of a conversion symptom, does not rule out the possibility that the patient has an underlying physical disease to which he or she was reacting with exaggeration or elaboration. Thus each patient must receive a careful medical evaluation. Conversely, a failure to consider conversion disorder and to continue to provide treatment as though the patient has a physical disease reinforces the symptom and can lead to permanent invalidism.

Prognosis & Course of Illness

Most conversion symptoms remit quickly, often spontaneously. They are often transient reactions to acute psychosocial stressors. When symptoms are more prolonged, they are generally accompanied by environmental reinforcers and are more resistant to treatment. A good prognosis is associated with symptoms precipitated by stressful events and preceded by good premorbid psychological health and with the absence of comorbid neurologic or psychiatric disorders. In a minority of patients, symptoms recur or substitution occurs.

Over a period of several years, an underlying neurologic disease will emerge in about 25% of patients with conversion disorder. This does not mean that the original symptom was neurologic in nature; rather, the patient may have been responding with a psychological symptom to an unrecognized, underlying neurologic dysfunction.

Griffith JL, Polles A, Griffith ME: Pseudo seizures, families and unspeakable dilemmas. Psychosomatics 1998;39:144.

SOMATIZATION DISORDER & UNDIFFERENTIATED SOMATIZATION DISORDER

DSM-IV Diagnostic Criteria

Somatization Disorder

A. A history of many physical complaints beginning before age 30 years that occur over a period of several years and result in treatment being sought or significant impairment in social, occupational, or other important areas of functioning.
B. Each of the following criteria must have been met, with individual symptoms occurring at any time during the course of the disturbance:
   (1) *four pain symptoms:* a history of pain related to at least four different sites or functions (eg,

head, abdomen, back, joints, extremities, chest, rectum, during menstruation, during sexual intercourse, or during urination)
   (2) *two gastrointestinal symptoms:* a history of at least two gastrointestinal symptoms other than pain (eg, nausea, bloating, vomiting, other than during pregnancy, diarrhea, or intolerance of several different foods)
   (3) *one sexual symptom:* a history of at least one sexual or reproductive symptom other than pain (eg, sexual indifference, erectile or ejaculatory dysfunction, irregular menses, excessive menstrual bleeding, vomiting throughout pregnancy)
   (4) *one pseudoneurological symptom:* a history of at least one symptom or deficit suggesting a neurological condition not limited to pain (conversion symptoms such as impaired coordination or balance, paralysis or localized weakness, difficulty swallowing or lump in throat, aphonia, urinary retention, hallucinations, loss of touch or pain sensation, double vision, blindness, deafness, seizures; dissociative symptoms such as amnesia; or loss of consciousness other than fainting)
C. Either (1) or (2):
   (1) after appropriate investigation, each of the symptoms in Criterion B cannot be fully explained by a known general medical condition or the direct effects of a substance (eg, a drug of abuse, a medication)
   (2) when there is a related general medical condition, the physical complaints or resulting social or occupational impairment are in excess of what would be expected from the history, physical examination, or laboratory findings
D. The symptoms are not intentionally produced or feigned (as in factitious disorder or malingering).

Undifferentiated Somatization Disorder

A. One or more physical complaints (eg, fatigue, loss of appetite, gastrointestinal complaints).
B. Either (1) or (2):
   (1) after appropriate investigation, each of the symptoms in Criterion B cannot be fully explained by a known general medical condition or the direct effects of a substance (eg, a drug of abuse, a medication)
   (2) when there is a related general medical condition, the physical complaints or resulting social or occupational impairment are in excess of what would be expected from the history, physical examination, or laboratory findings
C. The symptoms cause clinically significant distress or impairment in social, occupational, or other important areas of functioning.
D. The duration of the disturbance is at least 6 months.

E. The disturbance is not better accounted for by another mental disorder (eg, another somatoform disorder, sexual dysfunction, mood disorder, anxiety disorder, sleep disorder, or psychotic disorder).

F. The symptom or deficit is not intentionally produced or feigned (as in factitious disorder or malingering).

Reprinted, with permission, from *Diagnostic and Statistical Manual of Mental Disorders,* 4th ed. Copyright 1994 American Psychiatric Association.

General Considerations

A. Major Etiologic Theories: There are no well-accepted theories as to the etiology of somatization disorder. Patients with this disorder often come from chaotic, unstable, and dysfunctional families in which alcohol was abused. These patients often use physical symptoms as a coping mechanism. The high rate of psychiatric comorbidity associated with somatization disorder suggests that the disorder may represent a common final symptomatic pathway for different psychiatric problems, particularly major depression and personality disorder.

B. Epidemiology: Reports of the incidence of somatization disorder in the general population vary widely, depending on the populations studied and the techniques used. According to the Epidemiologic Catchment Area (ECA) studies, the incidence of somatization disorder is 0.1–0.4%. However, in one investigation of an academic family practice, 5% of patients met criteria for somatization disorder. A similarly high incidence has been demonstrated for hospitalized medical or surgical patients. Of note, most patients with somatization disorder are not diagnosed as such, and because of their "doctor-shopping" behavior they see multiple physicians, often simultaneously. The prevalence of undifferentiated somatization disorder (the subsyndromal form of the disorder) is much higher than that of somatization disorder and may affect as much as 4–11% of the general population. Individuals who meet the full criteria for somatization disorder tend to be female, unmarried, nonwhite, poorly educated, and from rural areas.

C. Genetics: The evidence for a genetic influence in the development of somatization disorder is limited but suggestive of a common genetic tendency associated with criminality. Women are more likely to express this genetic tendency as somatization disorder, and men more likely to express it as antisocial personality disorder. It is difficult to delineate precise genetic mechanisms in the face of massive environmental influences.

Clinical Findings

A. Signs & Symptoms: Patients with somatization disorder, by definition, present to physicians with multiple unexplained physical symptoms. These pre-

sentations are often accompanied by a sense of urgency. Thus these patients are subjected to numerous invasive diagnostic or treatment procedures. Symptoms are multisystemic in nature and frequently involve chronic pelvic pain, atypical facial pain, and nonspecific subjective complaints such as dizziness. Medical care costs for these patients may run as high as 2 to 8 times that of age-matched control subjects. Patients with somatization disorder also have a number of psychological symptoms, including depression, anxiety, suicidal gestures, and substance abuse. They may be addicted to prescribed medications, and at times they may exhibit drug-seeking behaviors.

B. Psychological Testing: There are no specific psychological tests for somatization disorder, but patients with this disorder usually score high on MMPI scales 1 (hypochondriasis) and 3 (hysteria) and on the somatization scale of the Hopkins Symptom Check List-90.

C. Laboratory Findings & Imaging: There are no specific laboratory findings for somatization disorder. The diagnosis is based on a lack of objective evidence to substantiate physical disease. Neuroimaging studies have not been reported.

Differential Diagnosis & Comorbidity

Organic physical disease is always part of the differential diagnosis for these multisymptomatic patients who often carry poorly documented diagnoses of systemic diseases (eg, systemic lupus erythematosus). Many of these patients have received one or more "fashionable diagnosis" such as fibromyalgia, dysautonomia, chronic fatigue syndrome, or total allergy syndrome. Few physicians have the means or the energy to make complete reviews of these patients' medical records, but such reviews generally fail to demonstrate objective evidence for any of these diagnoses.

Patients with somatization disorder almost always have one or more comorbid Axis I psychiatric diagnosis and almost always meet criteria for at least one personality disorder. Despite the multiplicity of psychiatric signs and symptoms, and a medical history of multiple unexplained physical complaints, patients with somatization disorder are often unrecognized.

Treatment

Patients with somatization disorder perceive themselves as being medically ill and are unlikely to seek psychiatric care for their distress. They may resent any implication that their problems are psychogenic and may reject referrals for psychiatric treatment. Thus the primary management of these patients falls on the primary care physician and his or her capability to coordinate care with multiple medical specialists.

A. Management Principles: Primary care physicians can use several simple management techniques to significantly lower medical care utilization by patients with somatization disorder. These principles include the following: (1) schedule frequent appointments without requiring development of a new symptom; (2) avoid statements that the symptoms are "all in your head;" (3) undertake invasive diagnostic or therapeutic procedures only if objective signs or symptoms are present; and (4) prescribe all medications and coordinate medical care.

B. Treatment of Comorbid Disorders: As noted earlier in this chapter, patients with somatization disorder usually have one or more comorbid psychiatric disorder that requires treatment (eg, major depression, panic disorder, drug dependence).

C. Group Therapy: Patients with somatization disorder frequently experience a high degree of psychosocial distress but have relatively little social support. The provision of group experiences, particularly those that are supportive rather than insight oriented, may significantly reduce medical care utilization. Group support allows these patients to feel socially connected and reduces their need to reach out to the medical system for assistance.

Complications & Adverse Outcomes of Treatment

Patients with somatization disorder are at risk for iatrogenic complications of invasive or therapeutic procedures (eg, peritoneal adhesions resulting from multiple abdominal operations). Habituation to prescribed analgesics or anxiolytics also occurs frequently. Clinicians must exercise caution when prescribing any potentially lethal medication for these patients because they are prone to impulsive acting-out behaviors including suicide attempts. Conversely, an approach that is too confrontational about the basic psychological issues underlying the medical care–seeking behaviors may motivate these patients to find a physician who is less psychologically minded and more accommodating to requests for medications and operations.

Prognosis & Course of Illness

Somatization disorder is a chronic problem that continues throughout the patient's life. Management principles are aimed at reducing symptoms and containing medical care costs, not at cure. These patients frequently experience iatrogenic complications from medications and surgical procedures; however, one long-term study found no evidence of reduced longevity, which suggests that these patients do not have any underlying biological disease.

Bhrir K, Hotopf M: Somatization disorder. Br J Hosp Med 1997;58:145.

Ford CV: Somatization and fashionable diagnoses. Scand J Work Environ Health 1997;23(Suppl 3):7.

Smith GR Jr, Monson RA, Ray DC: Psychiatric consultation in somatization disorder: a randomized, controlled study. N Engl J Med 1986;314:1407.

HYPOCHONDRIASIS

DSM-IV Diagnostic Criteria

A. Preoccupation with fears of having, or the idea that one has, a serious disease based on the person's misinterpretation of bodily symptoms.

B. The preoccupation persists despite appropriate medical evaluation and reassurance.

C. The belief in Criterion A is not of delusional intensity (as in delusional disorder, somatic type) and is not restricted to a circumscribed concern about appearance (as in body dysmorphic disorder).

D. The symptoms cause clinically significant distress or impairment in social, occupational, or other important areas of functioning.

E. The duration of the disturbance is at least 6 months.

F. The preoccupation is not better accounted for by generalized anxiety disorder, obsessive-compulsive disorder, panic disorder, a major depressive episode, separation anxiety, or another somatoform disorder.

Specify if:

With poor insight: if, for most of the time during the current episode, the person does not recognize that the concern about having a serious illness is excessive or unreasonable.

Reprinted, with permission, from *Diagnostic and Statistical Manual of Mental Disorders,* 4th ed. Copyright 1994 American Psychiatric Association.

General Considerations

A. Major Etiologic Theories: Hypochondriasis has been interpreted from a psychodynamic perspective as the turning inward of unacceptable feelings of anger. An alternative explanation is that hypochondriasis is learned behavior resulting from a childhood in which family members were excessively preoccupied with illness and bodily functions. Other proposed etiologies include the view that hypochondriasis is a form of depression or obsessive-compulsive disorder, with a symptomatic focus on bodily function. Hypochondriasis is likely a multidetermined disorder.

B. Epidemiology: The incidence of hypochondriasis in the general population is not known. Between 4% and 6% of the patients in one internal medicine clinic met DSM-IV criteria for hypochondriasis. The typical age at onset is young adulthood, and the disorder occurs with an approximately equal frequency in men and women. Contrary to popular belief, it is not more prevalent among the elderly. Transient hypochondriasis frequently follows acute illness or injury and may be viewed as a normal hypervigilant scanning of bodily functions for detection of further injury.

C. Genetics: Hypochondriasis is a familial disorder, but there is no direct evidence of genetic input. The increased incidence in family members can be explained on the basis of learned behavior or the indirect influence of psychiatric disorders that do have genetic input (eg, major depression) and that occur in both the patient and family members.

Clinical Findings

A. Signs & Symptoms: The hypochondriacal patient typically presents with fear and concern about disease rather than with dramatic symptoms. The fears may emanate from the misinterpretation of normal bodily sensations. Sensations regarded as normal aches and pains by most people are interpreted by the hypochondriacal patient as evidence of serious disease. The hypochondriacal patient characteristically relates his or her history in an obsessively detailed manner, often with relatively little affect. These patients tend to be emotionally constricted and are limited in their social, occupational, and sexual functions. Many hypochondriacal patients keep their own personal medical records. They often own the *Physicians' Desk Reference* or the *Merck Manual.* They feel transient relief when reassured that they do not have serious disease but, within hours or days, begin to obsessively doubt that assurance and may return for another visit.

B. Psychological Testing: Psychological testing (eg, using the MMPI) generally demonstrates a preoccupation with somatic symptoms in association with underlying depression and anxiety.

C. Laboratory Findings & Imaging: No laboratory findings are diagnostic of hypochondriasis. The diagnosis is often made by exclusion when all tests for physical diseases are normal. Neuroimaging studies for hypochondriasis have not been reported.

Differential Diagnosis & Comorbidity

The hypochondriacal patient must be reevaluated continually for the possibility that physical disease may underlie each new symptomatic complaint. Hypochondriacal patients may have concurrent relatively benign polysymptomatic illnesses (eg, irritable bowel syndrome) that they interpret as evidence of more severe disease. They also have a higher prevalence of major depression, panic disorder, and obsessive-compulsive disorder than is expected for the general population. These patients may interpret as evidence of disease the physiologic symptoms of major depression or panic disorder.

Treatment

Treatment of hypochondriasis falls predominantly to the primary care physician to whom these patients repeatedly return; hypochondriacal patients see their problems as medical, not psychiatric. Although some patients ultimately accept referral to a psychiatrist, premature referral may destroy rapport and make management more difficult. Within the primary care setting, patients should be seen at regularly scheduled intervals. Each new complaint or worry should be accompanied by a limited evaluation to ensure that it does not represent the development of organic disease. Invasive procedures should not be undertaken without clear indication. The doctor-patient relationship should be warm, trusting, and empathetic and should gradually enable these patients to express their emotional feelings more openly.

A. Treatment of Comorbid Disorders: Hypochondriasis is often accompanied by depression, anxiety, or obsessive-compulsive disorder. When one or more of these disorders is present, appropriate treatment should be initiated. Hypochondriacal patients tend to be inordinately sensitive to medication side effects. They continually scan their bodies in a hypervigilant fashion for bodily sensations. It is often necessary to initiate pharmacologic treatment with very low dosages—while encouraging the patient to tolerate side effects—and then to gradually increase the dosage into the therapeutic range as tolerated.

B. Psychotherapeutic Approaches: Hypochondriacal patients are usually not good candidates for traditional insight-oriented psychotherapy because they tend to be alexithymic (unable to express feelings in words). However, a recently developed psychotherapeutic approach appears to hold promise. The approach is based on the provision of new information, discussion, and exercises intended to modulate the sensations of benign bodily discomfort that are due to normal physiology and to help patients reattribute these sensations to their appropriate cause rather than to fears of serious illness. This combined behavioral intervention can be used by the primary care physician or by staff working within the medical setting.

Group therapy techniques can also meet these patients' needs for relationships and can be a vehicle by which cognitive-behavioral approaches are used to modify these patients' illness behavior.

Complications & Adverse Outcomes of Treatment

Failure to recognize hypochondriasis may result in needless expense due to exhaustive medical evaluation. Purely medical management may reinforce the symptoms, and iatrogenic complications may result from unneeded invasive procedures.

Prognosis & Course of Illness

Hypochondriasis is characterized by a chronic fluctuating course. With few exceptions, cure is not to be anticipated for these long-term patients. Patients whose hypochondriasis is related to a defined depressive episode or to panic disorder often experience a significant relief of hypochondriacal symptoms when the comorbid condition is treated effectively. A few patients with more severe chronic comorbid depression or obsessive-compulsive disorder will deteriorate. Patients with good premorbid psychological health who demonstrate transient hypochondriasis in response to acute illness or life stress have a good prognosis and may show complete remission of symptoms.

Barsky AJ: Hypochondriasis: medical management and psychiatric treatment. Psychosomatics 1996;37:48.

BODY DYSMORPHIC DISORDER

DSM-IV Diagnostic Criteria

A. Preoccupation with an imagined defect in appearance. If a slight physical anomaly is present, the person's concern is markedly excessive.
B. The preoccupation causes clinically significant distress or impairment in social, occupational, or other important areas of functioning.
C. The preoccupation is not better accounted for by another mental disorder (eg, dissatisfaction with body shape and size in anorexia nervosa).

Reprinted, with permission, from *Diagnostic and Statistical Manual of Mental Disorders,* 4th ed. Copyright 1994 American Psychiatric Association.

General Considerations

A. Major Etiologic Theories: Theories of the etiology of body dysmorphic disorder (BDD) are closely tied to issues of comorbidity (see later section). Many clinicians believe that BDD is the somatic expression of obsessive-compulsive disorder or, on occasion, a delusion reflecting an underlying psychotic process. Cultural values that emphasize personal appearance may also contribute to the development of BDD.

B. Epidemiology: The incidence of BDD, first described in DSM-III-R in 1987, is not known. Patients with BDD are most often seen by dermatologists and plastic surgeons. Despite opinions that the disorder is rare, one study of college students determined that a significant minority of both women and men met DSM-III-R criteria for BDD. Certainly, many adolescents are preoccupied with their appearance, and there is probably a dimensional rather than a categorical quality to BDD that ranges from relatively normal concern with one's body (in a society preoccupied with appearance) to a delusional intensity to the preoccupation that becomes totally incapacitating.

Of those individuals who present for clinical attention, there is a roughly equal distribution between men and women. Most patients are 20–40 years old. A high percentage of these patients have never married or are unemployed.

C. Genetics: No studies have reported evidence for a genetic influence in the development of BDD.

Clinical Findings

A. Signs & Symptoms: Patients with BDD are most commonly preoccupied with hair or facial features such as the shape of the nose. Other parts of the body such as breasts or genitalia can also be the source of preoccupation. For example, a man may become preoccupied with the size of his penis. Patients may spend hours each day gazing in a mirror or other reflective surfaces. Fears of humiliation, because of the imagined defect, may cause these patients to become housebound, unable to use public transportation or attend social functions or work. These patients may visit physicians multiple times seeking treatment, particularly surgical intervention to correct defects that are imperceptible to the normal observer.

B. Psychological Testing: Psychological testing can help determine the presence of comorbid disorders. Tests may indicate depression, obsessive-compulsive disorder, social phobia, or an underlying psychotic process.

C. Laboratory Findings & Imaging: No specific laboratory findings establish a diagnosis of BDD, and no neuroimaging studies of BDD have been reported.

Differential Diagnosis & Comorbidity

The differential diagnosis of BDD includes delusional disorder, somatic type, in which the patient has a clear-cut noninsightful distortion of reality; anorexia nervosa, in which the patient has a distorted body image and refuses to maintain body weight at or above a minimally normal weight for age and height; and gender identity disorder, in the which the patient is preoccupied with his or her body, thinking that it reflects the wrong gender (ie, transsexualism).

A controversial issue is whether obsessive-compulsive disorder with a somatic preoccupation is different from BDD. Some clinicians believe that BDD is obsessive-compulsive disorder that has taken the form of preoccupation with a body part. Monosymptomatic hypochondriacal psychosis is closely related to BDD and to delusional disorder, somatic type. In this disorder the patient has the conviction (delusion) that he or she is ugly, misshapen, emits a foul odor (bromosis), or is infested with parasites (parasitosis).

Most patients with BDD have a comorbid psychiatric disorder, most commonly major depression, social phobia, psychotic disorders, obsessive-compulsive disorder, or substance abuse disorders.

Treatment

BDD can best be conceptualized as a syndrome of heterogeneous etiology rather than as a specific entity. As such, one must keep in mind the high incidence of psychiatric comorbidity and the various underlying psychiatric disorders that are manifested as a preoccupation with appearance. Treatment must be flexible and based on the needs of the patient. Many of these patients seek surgery, and the psychiatrist may be asked to render an opinion as to whether surgery is contraindicated. Although surgery has been beneficial in some instances, this is the exception rather than the rule. Many patients do not experience relief of symptoms after surgical intervention and may experience a worsening of symptoms or a psychotic response.

A. Treatment of Comorbid Conditions: Comorbid psychiatric conditions such as major depression should be treated. A selective serotonin reuptake inhibitor (SSRI) should be the first choice as an antidepressant medication because SSRIs are also effective in treating obsessive-compulsive disorder, which is believed by some to underlie many, if not most, cases of BDD. A positive response to SSRIs has also been reported in patients whose symptoms have a delusional intensity, lending further credence to the opinion that BDD is a variant of OCD. For other patients whose somatic beliefs have a delusional component (eg, monosymptomatic hypochondriasis), pimozide (1.0–10.0 mg daily) has been reported to be effective; however, this medication must be used with caution because of potential cardiotoxicity.

B. Psychotherapy: Psychotherapy has not been useful in treating symptoms specifically associated with BDD; however, it may help these patients with associated interpersonal issues such as social phobia. Behavioral therapy using exposure with a response-prevention technique has been reported to be helpful.

Complications & Adverse Outcomes of Treatment

It is important to recognize the intensity of the BDD patient's distress. These patients are at risk for suicide or the development of psychosis.

Prognosis & Course of Illness

The long-term outcome of BDD is unknown. Diagnostic criteria for the disorder have been formulated only recently, and data are preliminary. Earlier reports on dysmorphophobia (an earlier described syndrome that is similar to BDD) suggest that a significant proportion of these patients develop psychotic processes and that most are severely disabled from their disorder. Recent reports of success in treating BDD with SSRIs may portend a more favorable long-term prognosis.

Phillips KA, Kim JM, Hudson JL: Body image disturbance in body dysmorphic disorder and eating disorders: obsessions or delusions? Psychiatr Clin N Am 1995;18:317.
Phillips KA et al: Body dysmorphic disorder: 30 cases of imagined ugliness. Am J Psychiatry 1993;150:302.

PAIN DISORDER

DSM-IV Diagnostic Criteria

A. Pain in one or more anatomical sites is the predominant focus of the clinical presentation and is of sufficient severity to warrant clinical attention.
B. The pain causes clinically significant distress or impairment in social, occupational, or other important areas of functioning.
C. Psychological factors are judged to have an important role in the onset, severity, exacerbation, or maintenance of the pain.
D. The symptom or deficit is not intentionally produced or feigned (as in factitious disorder or malingering).
E. The pain is not better accounted for by a mood, anxiety, or psychotic disorder and does not meet criteria for dyspareunia.

Specify if:

> *Acute:* duration of less than 6 months.
> *Chronic:* duration of 6 months or longer.

General Considerations

Pain syndromes are categorized based on whether they are associated primarily with (1) psychological factors, (2) a general medical condition, or (3) psychological factors and a general medical condition. The second categorization is not considered to be a mental disorder but is related to the differential diagnosis. This classification of pain appears to be superior to previous systems because it takes into account underlying physical disease to which the patient may be reacting in an exaggerated form. Thus the clinician can avoid the either-or dualism that prevailed earlier. Most patients probably have some degree of physical disease that initiates painful sensations, and it is the response to these sensations that constitutes abnormal illness behavior.

A. Major Etiologic Theories: Pain is a heterogeneous disorder. No single etiologic factor is likely to apply to all patients. Among the proposed etiologies are psychodynamic formulations that pain represents an unconsciously determined punishment to expiate guilt or for aggressive feelings or an effort to maintain a relationship with a lost object. Consistent with psychodynamic theories, some patients with pain syndromes demonstrate masochistic, self-defeating personality characteristics.

Another etiologic theory proposes that pain represents learned behavior. It is hypothesized that the patient's previous experiences of personal pain have led to changes in other persons' behavior, thereby reinforcing the experience of pain and pain behaviors. Consistent with this theory are observations that some pain patients have experienced medical illnesses or injuries associated with pain or lived in childhood homes where disease, illness, and pain were present. It has also been proposed that pain represents a somatic expression of depression. There is a high incidence of depression in pain patients and among their family members.

Because pain is a subjective symptom, it is easy to simulate. A substantial percentage of litigants who claim pain have been shown to exaggerate or outright malinger the symptom.

B. Epidemiology: Pain is the most common complaint with which patients present to physicians. According to one study, 14% of internal medicine private patients had chronic pain. Those who seek medical care for chronic pain may be a subgroup of those who experience it. Epidemiologic studies have found that recurrent or persistent pain has a prevalence of one third to one half of the general population of adults.

C. Genetics: No studies have related genetic factors to pain disorder.

Clinical Findings

A. Signs & Symptoms: Patients who repetitively seek treatment for pain may represent a subset of individuals with pain but who have certain patterns of illness behavior, rather than reflecting psychological characteristics of all persons who have pain per se. Pain syndromes include atypical facial pain, chronic pelvic pain, chronic low back pain, recurrent or persistent headaches, and so on. These patients' descriptions of pain are often dramatic and include vivid descriptions such as "stabbing back pain" or "a fire in my belly."

No common symptoms or psychological features describe all pain patients. Despite this heterogeneity, pain patients share some features. Pain patients tend to focus on their pain as an explanation for all their problems; they deny psychological problems and interpersonal problems, except as they relate to pain. These patients frequently describe themselves as independent, yet observations of them suggest that they are dependent on others. They frequently demand that the doctor remove the pain, and they are willing to accept surgical procedures in their search for pain relief. "Doctor shopping" is common. Family dynamics are altered in a manner that makes the pain patient the focus of the family's life.

Pain patients often see themselves as disabled and unable to work or perform usual self-care activities. They demand, and often receive, a large number of medications, particularly habituating sedatives and analgesics. The pain persists despite chronic and often excessive use of these medications, on which these patients may become both psychologically and physiologically dependent.

B. Psychological Testing: Psychological tests such as the MMPI are often used to evaluate pain patients. Common findings include somatic preoccupation, underlying depression or anxiety, and a tendency to deny psychological symptoms. The McGill Pain Questionnaire, a patient self-report test, frequently discloses that the patient uses idiosyncratic and colorful words to describe his or her pain experience.

C. Laboratory Findings & Imaging: In experimental settings, pain disorder patients often have a lower threshold for pain than do normal subjects. It is difficult to determine if this greater sensitivity is the result of physiologic or psychological differences.

Differential Diagnosis & Comorbidity

The differential diagnosis of pain disorder inevitably involves underlying disease processes that may cause the pain. The coexistence, however, of such disease does not rule out the diagnosis of pain disorder if psychological factors are believed to exacerbate or intensify the pain experience. Patients with chronic pain have a high frequency of comorbid psychiatric disorders, including depressive spectrum disorders, anxiety disorders, conversion disorder, and substance abuse disorders. Many of these patients meet diagnostic criteria for a personality disorder, most commonly dependent, passive-aggressive, or histrionic personality disorders.

Treatment

The treatment of acute pain disorder is generally aimed at reducing the patient's underlying anxiety and the acute environmental stressors that exacerbate the patient's personal distress. Psychiatrists are much more likely to be involved in the evaluation than in the treatment of chronic pain syndromes. Psychiatrists may see patients with these syndromes on referral or as a part of a multidisciplinary pain treatment team. Because patients with chronic pain often resent implications that their pain has psychological causes, psychiatrists are usually most effective when serving as consultants to other health care providers. Chronic pain characteristically leads to changes in behavior that are reinforced by environmental factors. These patients have often assumed an identity as a chronically disabled person and have taken a passive stance toward life. The major objectives for treatment must be to make the patient an active participant in the rehabilitation process, to reduce the patient's doctor shopping, and to identify and reduce reinforcers of the patient's pain behaviors.

A. Treatment of Comorbid Disorders: Treatment of the symptom of pain often involves attention to coexisting or secondary psychiatric disorders. Major depression should be treated pharmacologically, and anxiety disorders should be treated as indicated with relaxation techniques, behavioral therapy, or pharmacotherapy. Substance abuse problems frequently require detoxification and appropriate rehabilitation techniques to maintain abstinence. Patients whose pain appears to be related to symptoms of posttraumatic stress disorder may require treatment for that disorder. Specialized treatment programs for the survivors of violent crimes or sexual abuse may be indicated.

B. Psychotherapy: Insight-oriented psychotherapy may be helpful for the few patients who have identified unconscious conflictual issues. However, the vast majority of patients with chronic pain are not psychologically oriented, and insight psychotherapy is not efficacious. Supportive psychotherapy may be helpful in reassuring and encouraging these patients and in improving their compliance with other aspects of the treatment program. As a general rule, behavioral therapy is the most effective type of psychotherapy in the treatment of pain disorders. Both operant conditioning and cognitive-behavioral therapy are widely used (see Chapter 2).

Operant conditioning is based on the concept that certain learned behaviors develop in response to environmental cues. Thus the patient has learned a variety of pain behaviors that are elicited in certain situations. Patients often communicate their pain to others (eg, by grimacing) to elicit responses. Behavioral analysis identifies both the stimuli and the response-altering reinforcements to these behaviors. The behavioral therapist works to substitute new behaviors for previously learned pain behaviors. Patients are praised for increasing their activity and are not rewarded for pain. Behavioral techniques are most useful when the patient's family is included in the overall treatment program, so that pain behavior is not reinforced when the patient returns home.

Cognitive-behavioral therapy techniques focus on identifying and correcting the patient's distorted attitudes, beliefs, and expectations. One variety of this treatment involves teaching the patient how to relax or refocus thinking and behavior away from the preoccupation of pain.

C. Pharmacotherapy: Patients with chronic pain have generally received prescriptions for multiple analgesics, often including opiate medications. These patients may demand increasingly larger dosages of medication if they have become dependent, and they may exhibit considerable resistance to discontinuing or decreasing medications. Clinicians must explain to these patients that medications have not been successful in relieving pain and that other techniques are indicated. Medications may play a limited role as part of the overall treatment. As a general rule, nonsteroidal anti-inflammatory agents rather than opiates should be the first choice in medication. When more potent analgesics are indicated, they should be prescribed on a fixed-dosage schedule rather than on a variable-dosage schedule. Patients who are prescribed medication on an as-needed basis are much more likely to engage in pain behaviors to indicate the need for medication. The use of a fixed-

dosage schedule enables the extinction of pain behaviors as a means of communicating the need for more medication. Patients who have been prescribed opiates either over a long period of time or in high dosages may require a detoxification program rather than abrupt discontinuation.

Antidepressant medications (eg, amitriptyline, 25–100 mg at bedtime) are often helpful to pain patients, particularly when symptoms of major depression are present. Some reports indicate that the tricyclic antidepressants are effective in reducing pain, in dosages below those usually considered to be effective for antidepressant activity. If the patient has anxiety symptoms, the clinician should avoid prescribing medications that have potential for habituation (eg, benzodiazepines). A sedating tricyclic antidepressant may be a better choice for such patients.

D. Pain Clinics & Centers: Chronic pain patients are often disabled and receive fragmented medical care from multiple specialists. A pain clinic provides comprehensive integrated medical care. These clinics seem to work best when a strong behavioral therapy component is associated with a comprehensive evaluation and when treatment interventions include the patient's spouse, family, and when applicable, employer. The therapeutic focus of pain clinics is to transfer the patient's sense of responsibility for treatment from physicians and medications to the patient himself or herself and to work actively within a rehabilitation program to restore self-care and social and occupational functioning. The focus is on rehabilitation more than it is on pain relief. The message provided is that the patient must learn how to "play hurt." These techniques are often useful for short-term improvement in function. Limited data are available regarding long-term outcome.

Complications & Adverse Outcomes of Treatment

Pain disorder patients are at risk for iatrogenic addiction to opiate compounds or benzodiazepines. These patients often sabotage their treatment programs, proclaim that psychiatric treatment was not successful, and then use this as proof that their pain has a physical cause.

Prognosis & Course of Illness

Surprisingly little information is available concerning prognosis. Clinicians may see patients who have complained of chronic pain for many years, even decades, and who, in the interim, have been subjected to multiple surgical procedures and have experienced iatrogenic complications. Factors known to be of poor prognostic significance include ongoing litigation related to the pain (eg, when the illness or accident that caused the pain was associated with a potentially compensable injury), unemployment, loss of sexual interest, or a history of somatization prior to the onset of chronic pain.

Eisendrath SJ: Psychiatric aspects of chronic pain. Neurology 1995;45(Suppl A):S26.

Fishbain DA et al: Chronic pain–associated depression: antecedent or consequences of chronic pain? A review. Clin J Pain 1997;13:116.

SOMATOFORM DISORDER NOT OTHERWISE SPECIFIED

The diagnostic category of somatoform disorder not otherwise specified consists of a widely varied group of disorders that mimic physical disease or have an uncertain psychological relationship to physical disease. Included among these disorders are false pregnancy, psychogenic urinary retention, and mass psychogenic illness (so-called mass hysteria).

GENERAL PRINCIPLES FOR THE TREATMENT OF SOMATIZING PATIENTS

As noted earlier in this chapter, the somatizing disorders display considerable phenomenological overlap and fluidity of symptomatic expression over time. Relatively few somatizing patients fit clearly into one of the somatoform disorder categories described in this chapter. Table 25–3 provides general guidelines for the management of somatization disorders.

Table 25–3. General guidelines for the treatment of somatization disorders.

1. The clinician must remain vigilant to the possibility that the patient has covert physical disease and may develop physical disease during the course of treatment for his or her somatization.
2. A patient with somatization should not be conceptualized from an either-or perspective. Most somatizing patients have some degree of concurrent physical disease.
3. To the greatest extent possible, medical or surgical care should be coordinated by one primary care physician. Psychiatric consultation, however, is often valuable in helping the primary care physician formulate a treatment plan for the patient.
4. The somatizing patient frequently has a comorbid psychiatric disorder. When identified, such disorders should be treated because the somatization may represent the symptomatic expression of one of these disorders.
5. The somatizing patient should not be told that his or her symptoms are psychogenic or "all in your head." Such comments are almost inevitably rejected and destroy therapeutic rapport, and they may be inaccurate.
6. Invasive diagnostic or therapeutic procedures for the somatizing patient should be initiated only for objective signs and symptoms, not for subjective complaints.
7. The acute onset of a somatoform disorder may be associated with an acute stressor in the patient's life (eg, physical or sexual abuse).
8. Chronic somatization is rarely responsive to traditional insight-oriented psychotherapy, but behavioral modification techniques are often useful in modifying the patient's illness behavior.
9. The treatment of somatization disorders generally requires multiple treatment techniques provided by a multidisciplinary treatment team.
10. Somatization is often a chronic condition (ie, "illness as a way of life"), and cure is improbable. Somatizing patients require ongoing management using techniques that reduce the risk of iatrogenic complications.

Factitious Disorders & Malingering

Charles V. Ford, MD

FACTITIOUS DISORDERS

DSM-IV Diagnostic Criteria

A. Intentional production or feigning of physical or psychological signs or symptoms.

B. The motivation for the behavior is to assume the sick role.

C. External incentives for the behavior (such as economic gain, avoiding legal responsibility, or improving physical well-being, as in malingering) are absent.

Factitious disorders are consciously determined surreptitious simulations or productions of diseases. Factitious illness behavior is relatively uncommon, but when present it consumes large amounts of professional time and medical costs. The Munchausen syndrome by proxy is a particularly malignant form of child abuse that physicians must identify and manage in order the save the health or lives of children.

DSM-IV lists four diagnostic subtypes of factitious disorder:

A. Factitious Disorder With Predominantly Psychological Signs & Symptoms: Patients with factitious disorders may simulate psychological conditions and psychiatric disorders. For example, a patient may feign bereavement by reporting that someone to whom he or she was close has died or been killed in an accident. Patients may simulate symptoms of posttraumatic stress disorder or provide false reports of previous trauma (eg, a civilian accident or combat experience). Closely related to factitious posttraumatic stress disorder is the false victimization syndrome, in which the patient falsely claims some type of abuse. For example, a woman may falsely report that she had been raped. Other simulated psychological disorders include various forms of dementia, amnesia, or fugue; multiple personality disorder; and more rarely, schizophrenia.

B. Factitious Disorder With Predominantly Physical Signs & Symptoms: The production of physical symptoms or disease is probably the most common form of factitious disorder. Essentially all medical diseases and symptoms have been either simulated or artificially produced at one time or another. Among the most common of these disorders are factitious hypoglycemia, factitious anemia, factitious gastrointestinal bleeding, pseudoseizures, simulation of brain tumors, simulation of renal colic, and more recently, simulation of AIDS.

C. Factitious Disorder With Combined Psychological & Physical Signs & Symptoms: A patient may be admitted to the hospital with factitious physical symptoms and, in the course of hospitalization, perhaps in an attempt to obtain more sympathy or interest, may report or simulate a variety of psychological symptoms such as having experienced the recent loss of a close relative or friend or having been raped in the past.

D. Factitious Disorder Not Otherwise Specified: This category is reserved for forms of factitious disorder that do not fit one of the other categories. It includes the Munchausen syndrome by proxy, in which one person surreptitiously induces disease or reports disease in another person. Most commonly this is the behavior of a mother in reference to a young child.

General Considerations

A. Major Etiologic Theories: Explanations for the apparently nonsensical and bizarre illness behavior of factitious disorder are largely speculative. Underlying motivations for this behavior are probably heterogeneous and multidetermined. The following explanations have been suggested:

1. The search for nurturance—Individuals in the sick role are characteristically excused from societal obligations and cared for by others. When alternative sources of care, support, and nurturance are lacking, a person may deliberately induce illness as a way of seeking such support. Many patients with factitious disorder are themselves caretakers. Factitious illness behavior allows for a reversal of roles: instead of caring for others, the patient assumes the dependent cared-for role.

2. Secondary gains—Patients with factitious disorders sometimes use illness to obtain disability benefits or release from usual obligations such as working. Their illnesses may elicit from family members attention that might not otherwise be forthcoming. When litigation is involved, the boundary between factitious disorder and malingering becomes blurred or disappears.

3. The need for power & superiority—A person who successfully perpetuates a ruse may have a feeling of superiority in his or her capacity to fool others. This has been described as "putting one over" or "duping delight." Thus the individual can experience a transformation from feeling weak and impotent to feeling clever and powerful over others. Simultaneously the individual may devalue others whom he or she regards as stupid or foolish because they have been deceived.

4. To obtain drugs—Some patients have used factitious illness to obtain drugs. Even those patients who have sought controlled substances appear to have done so more for the thrill of fooling the physician than because of addiction.

5. To create a sense of identity—A patient with severe characterological defects may have a poor sense of self. The creation of the sick role and the associated pseudologia fantastica (pathologic lying) may provide the patient with a role by which his or her personal identity is established. Such a person is no longer faceless but rather the star player in high drama.

6. To defend against severe anxiety or psychosis—A patient with overwhelming anxiety due to fears of abandonment or powerlessness may use a factitious illness to defend against psychological decompensation. Through the perpetuation of a successful fraud and the simultaneous gratification of dependency needs, the patient feels powerful, in control, and cared for.

B. Epidemiology: The incidence of factitious illness behavior is unknown but is probably more common than is recognized. One Canadian study estimated that approximately 1 in 1000 hospital admissions is for factitious disease. However, another investigation of an entirely different type determined that approximately 3.5% of renal stones submitted for chemical analysis were bogus and represented apparent attempts to deceive the physician. A study of patients referred with fever of unknown origin to the National Institutes of Health found that almost 10% had a factitious fever. One can conclude that the incidence of factitious disorder, except in certain specialized

clinical settings, is relatively uncommon but may be more frequent than is recognized.

Age and gender distribution varies according to the clinical syndromes described in the next section. Patients with the full-blown Munchausen syndrome are most frequently unmarried middle-aged men who are estranged from their families. Patients with simple factitious disorder are most likely to be unmarried women in their 20s or 30s who work in health-service jobs such as nursing. Perpetrators of the Munchausen syndrome by proxy are most often mothers of small children who themselves may have previously engaged in factitious disease behavior or meet the criteria for somatization disorder.

C. Genetics: No information is available regarding a relationship between factitious disorders and heredity.

Clinical Findings

A. Signs & Symptoms: DSM-IV diagnostic criteria do not adequately describe the different clinical syndromes of persons who present with factitious disorder. Three major syndromes have been identified, although some overlap may exist.

1. Munchausen syndrome (peregrinating factitious disorder)—The original Munchausen syndrome, as described by Asher, consists of the simulation of disease, pseudologia fantastica, and peregrination (wandering). Some patients with this disorder have achieved great notoriety. These patients typically present to emergency rooms at night or on the weekends when they are more likely to encounter inexperienced clinicians and when insurance offices are more likely to be closed. Their symptoms are often dramatic and indicate the need for immediate hospitalization. Once hospitalized they become "star patients" because of their dramatic symptoms, the rarity of their apparent diagnosis (eg, intermittent Mediterranean fever), or because of the stories that they tell about themselves (eg, tales of being a foreign university president or a former major league baseball player). These patients confuse physicians because of inconsistencies in their physical and laboratory findings and because of their failure to respond to standard therapeutic measures. They rarely receive visitors, and it is difficult to obtain information concerning prior hospitalizations; their frequent use of aliases makes it difficult to track them. When confronted with their factitious illness behavior, they often become angry, threaten to sue, and sign out of the hospital against medical advice. They then travel to another hospital, where they once again perpetuate their ruses.

Personal historical information about Munchausen syndrome patients is limited because they are unreliable historians and are reluctant to divulge accurate personal information. What is known may be somewhat selective in that it is derived from a subgroup of patients who have allowed themselves to be studied.

These individuals often come from chaotic, stressful childhood homes. They sometimes report that they were institutionalized or hospitalized during childhood, experiences that were not regarded as frightening but rather were considered a reprieve from stress at home. Childhood neuropathic traits (eg, lying or fire setting) are often reported. Many of these patients have worked in health-related fields (eg, as a hospital corpsman in the military). Many have a history of psychiatric hospitalization and legal difficulties.

2. Simple factitious disorder (non-peregrinating)—The most common form of factitious disorder is simple factitious disorder. Disease presentations may involve dermatologic conditions from self-inflicted injuries or infections, blood dyscrasia from the surreptitious use of dicumarol or self-phlebotomy, hypoglycemia from the surreptitious use of insulin, and other diseases. The patient generally has one primary symptom or finding (eg, anemia) and is characteristically hospitalized on multiple occasions, but the physician or hospital staff never learns the true nature of the underlying "disease." In the process of their hospitalizations these patients become the object of considerable concern from physicians, colleagues, and family members, with whom they typically have conflicted relationships.

Patients with simple factitious disorder often lie, exaggerate, and distort the truth but not to the same extent, or with the degree of fantasy, as those with the Munchausen syndrome. Patients with simple factitious disorder may perpetuate the ruse for years before being discovered. Unmasked, these patients typically react with hostility, eliciting angry disbelief from treating physicians, nurses, and other staff. Even in the face of incontrovertible evidence, these patients often continue to deny the true nature of their problems.

Patients with simple factitious disorder typically come from dysfunctional families and exhibit histrionic or borderline personality characteristics.

3. Munchausen syndrome by proxy—This invidious disorder, in which a mother produces disease in her child, was first described in 1978. Subsequently, hundreds of case reports from all over the world have confirmed this form of child abuse. Every major children's hospital will see several cases per year.

In the Munchausen syndrome by proxy, the perpetrator (usually the mother) presents a child (usually an infant) for medical treatment of either simulated or factitiously produced disease. For example, the child may have collapsed after the mother surreptitiously administered laxatives or other medications, or the child may have experienced repeated attacks of apnea secondary to suffocation (eg, by pinching the nostrils). After the child has been hospitalized, the mother is intensely involved in her child's care and with the ward staff. Interestingly, the mother is surprisingly willing to sign consent forms for invasive diagnostic procedures or treatment. The child may inexplicably improve when the mother is out of the hospital for a period of time. The child's father is usually uninvolved or absent.

When the mother is confronted with suspicions (or proof) that she has caused the child's illness, she often reacts with angry denial and hospital staff may also express disbelief. Reasonable suspicion of Munchausen syndrome by proxy mandates reporting, as a form of child abuse, to the appropriate child protective services. Children who have been victims of Munchausen syndrome by proxy have a high mortality rate (almost 10% die before reaching adulthood). Studies of their siblings show a similarly high mortality rate because this disease-producing behavior may be perpetrated on subsequent children. These children may need to be placed outside the home (eg, with other relatives or in a foster-care setting).

B. Psychological Testing: Psychological test results of Munchausen syndrome patients reflect severe characterological problems often of the sociopathic, narcissistic, or histrionic type. Approximately 30% of Munchausen syndrome patients have some form of cerebral dysfunction. This dysfunction is most commonly demonstrated by the patient's verbal IQ score being significantly greater than his or her performance IQ score, a finding possibly related to pseudologia fantastica.

Test results of patients with simple factitious disorder are consistent with histrionic or borderline personality traits, somatic preoccupation, and conflicts about sexuality.

Test results of patients with Munchausen syndrome by proxy reflect personality disorders (eg, narcissistic) and concurrent Axis I disorders (eg, major depression). Frequently they demonstrate no clear-cut abnormality.

C. Laboratory Findings & Imaging: Laboratory testing may disclose inconsistent findings, not typical of known physical diseases (eg, the pattern of hypokalemia that occurs with surreptitious ingestion of diuretics). The presence of toxins or medications, the use of which the patient denies, may establish the diagnosis of factitious disease behavior. For example, phenolphthalein may be present in the stool of a baby who is experiencing diarrhea as a result of Munchausen syndrome by proxy.

No neuroimaging studies have been reported for factitious disorder.

Differential Diagnosis & Comorbidity

As with all somatizing disorders, the diagnosis of factitious disorders involves ruling out the presence of a genuine disease process. Patients with factitious disorder often have physical disease, but the disease is the result of deliberate and surreptitious behavior such as self-phlebotomy. Occasionally a patient with a genuine physical disease (eg, diabetes mellitus) will learn how to manipulate symptoms and findings in such a way as to create a combination of physical disease and factitious disorder. In such cases both the disease process and the behavior will require therapeutic attention.

Factitious disorder must also be distinguished from malingering; the difference here is one of motivation. The person with malingering has a definable external goal that motivates the behavior, such as disability payments from an insurance company, whereas with factitious disorders, the patient's goal is to seek the sick role for the psychological needs it fulfills. Malingering and factitious disorders often overlap.

Patients with factitious disorders may also meet the criteria for other somatoform disorders, particularly somatization disorder or other Axis I disorders such as major depression or, more rarely, schizophrenia. Most patients with factitious disorders are comorbid for one of the cluster B personality disorders (ie, antisocial, borderline, histrionic, narcissistic).

Management & Treatment

Therapeutic approaches to factitious disorder must be different from those used to treat specific disease states. A factitious disorder represents disordered behavior that is determined by widely varied and often multiple motivations. The clinician must evaluate and develop a separate treatment plan for each patient. Further, because factitious behavior is often associated with severe personality disorders the clinician must avoid splitting and other manipulative behaviors by the patient. Thus a multidisciplinary management strategy involving attorneys, nurses, social workers, and other professionals is essential. Unfortunately for many patients with factitious disorder, the goal must be to contain symptoms and avoid unnecessary and expensive medical care rather than to effect a cure.

A. Staff Meetings: When factitious disorder is suspected, the treating physician must recruit a multidisciplinary task force to assist with ethics and management. Such a task force, and associated staff meetings, educate all health care personnel as to the nature of the disorder, facilitate communication in such a manner as to defuse attempts by the patient to split staff, and ensure a united front for treatment. The multidisciplinary task force might include hospital administrators, the hospital attorney, a chaplain or ethicist, the patient's primary physician, a psychiatrist, and representatives from the nursing staff. Although this degree of involvement may seem like overkill, it is necessary in order to anticipate medico-legal complications.

B. Confrontation: When factitious disorder is suspected or has been confirmed, the medical staff must confront the patient. Such confrontation is generally best accomplished with several of the multidisciplinary staff members present. The staff should communicate to the patient that they know he or she has been surreptitiously producing or simulating the

disease and that such behavior is indicative of internal distress. The staff should suggest to the patient that it is time to reformulate the illness from a physical disease to a psychological disorder. The patient should be told that the treatment team is concerned and that appropriate help and treatment can be made available. Despite such a supportive approach, many patients will continue to deny that they have contributed to their illness and will angrily reject any referral for psychological help.

C. Treatment of Comorbid Disorders: Patients must be evaluated carefully for comorbid psychiatric disorders such as major depression or schizophrenia. The presence of another Axis I disorder is relatively uncommon but when present must be treated before proceeding with psychotherapy and other management.

D. Psychotherapeutic Techniques: The overwhelming majority of patients with factitious illness have severe underlying personality disorder. Despite their superficial confidence and, at times, braggadocio, these patients are quite fragile. They are not candidates for confrontative insight-oriented psychotherapy and may decompensate in such treatment. The techniques described in this section are suggested for use by either psychiatrists or other members of the medical treatment team as indicated. Many patients completely reject any psychiatric treatment, and therapeutic efforts must be made by nonpsychiatric personnel.

1. Individual psychotherapy—Psychotherapy needs to be supportive, empathic, and nonconfrontative. At times just "being there" and allowing the patient to talk, even if much of the talk consists of pseudologia fantastica, provides sufficient support for the patient to no longer feel the need to engage in factitious illness behavior. Such treatment is not curative but helps prevent further iatrogenic complications and high medical utilization.

2. Face-saving opportunities—At times the patient will discard the symptom if he or she does not need to admit the behavior. For example, the patient may be told that the problem will resolve with physical therapy, medications, or other treatment techniques. The patient may use such an opportunity to discard symptoms in a face-saving manner and behavior without ever overtly acknowledging culpability for factitious illness behavior.

3. Inexact interpretations—Insight-oriented psychotherapy is almost always contraindicated. However, it may be useful to make interpretations without direct confrontation. For example, a patient whose factitious illness behavior is tied to losses or separation might be told in a very general way that it seems that he or she has difficulty in dealing with disappointments in life.

4. Therapeutic double-binds—The patient who is suspected of factitious illness behavior might be told that such suspicions exist—and that if symptoms fail to respond to a proposed treatment then such a failure would be confirmation of factitious illness. Although this technique may be symptomatically effective, there are obvious questions as to its ethical appropriateness. For example, is it ethical to lie to a lying patient in order to effect change?

5. Family therapy—Patients with simple factitious disorder often come from dysfunctional families and are experiencing current conflicted interpersonal relationships. The patient's factitious illness behavior may be a way of controlling or manipulating the family in order to obtain a sense of power or gratification of dependency needs. Family therapy may be one way to address distorted communications in the family and provide for the more appropriate expression of needs.

Treatment Issues in Munchausen Syndrome by Proxy

When the victim of Munchausen syndrome by proxy is a child, it may be necessary to place the child in foster care in order to protect his or her health and life. The child will require supportive psychological assistance to deal with separation from the parent and changes in his or her environment.

Perpetrators of Munchausen syndrome by proxy, usually mothers, generally have severe personality disorders, which are very difficult to treat. This is especially true when the perpetrator continues to deny her behavior. Many psychiatrists believe that return of the child to the mother must depend on the mother's acknowledgment of her behavior, the requirement that she stop it, and her recognition of the needs and rights of the child. These mothers may have severe narcissistic personality disorder, in which others are seen merely as objects to be manipulated rather than as separate persons with feelings, needs, and rights. When there is a history of an unexplained death of a sibling, extra care must be taken to ensure the safety of the child.

Ethical & Medico-Legal Issues

Many ethical and medico-legal issues are raised in treating factitious disorders. Some physicians may believe that because patients with these disorders are liars, they can treat them in a cavalier manner. The following discussion demonstrates that this is not the case.

A. Confidentiality: Because a patient with factitious disorder has presented himself or herself to the physician fraudulently, violating the traditional doctor-patient relationship, a legitimate question can be raised as to whether this invalidates the physician's obligation of confidentiality. To what extent should such an individual be allowed to perpetuate fraud, as it may affect family members, friends, and other physicians? This question is not easily answered, but from a medico-legal standpoint any violation of confidentiality must be in the interest of protecting the patient's health or significantly reducing the damage

to others. Such violations should not occur capriciously but only after careful consideration and consultation with the multidisciplinary task force.

B. Surreptitious Room Searches: The medical literature on factitious disorders contains multiple descriptions of searches of patients' rooms after they have been sent off for testing or for other reasons. Syringes and other paraphernalia may have been found, thereby confirming the diagnosis. Such searches, however, violate patients' civil rights and should be undertaken only after careful consideration and consultation with the multidisciplinary task force.

C. Withdrawal of Medical Care: The physician who finds that he or she has been the object of the fraudulent seeking of medical care is likely to react with anger and possibly rejection. The expenditure of professional time and the use of scarce medical supplies for patients with factitious disorders may be questioned. However, an analogy can be drawn to the question of whether medical care should be withdrawn from a patient with liver cirrhosis who continues to drink alcohol or from a patient with emphysema who continues to smoke cigarettes. The point at which one starts to enter the "slippery slope" is always an issue for debate. Medical care should be withdrawn only after careful consideration of the medico-legal ramifications.

D. Involuntary Psychiatric Treatment: Many patients with factitious disorder engage in self-injurious behavior that could permanently affect body function or cause death. Involuntary psychiatric treatment has been suggested but is generally rejected by the courts. In one case, a judge provided an "outpatient commitment" for a patient and ordered that all of her (publicly funded) medical care be coordinated by a guardian. Such an approach seems eminently reasonable, but it may be difficult to effect in many states, especially if the patient is covered by private insurance.

E. Malpractice Lawsuits: On the surface, one might ask how or why a patient might ever initiate a malpractice lawsuit against a physician when the patient is responsible for the medical illness. Such lawsuits, however, have occurred and can emerge in one of two different forms. One form of lawsuit can occur because many of these patients have severe borderline personality disorder. Such individuals are likely to idealize a physician initially and then later devalue him or her. With such devaluation comes rage and a resort to malpractice suits as a way of inflicting injury. The lay people who comprise juries are not knowledgeable about factitious disorders and may side with the patient.

Another form of lawsuit can occur when the patient admits factitious disorder and sues the physician for failure to recognize it. In other words, "I was lying to you, but this is a recognized medical illness, and you were incompetent not to have recognized my fraudulent behavior." One such lawsuit was settled out of court with a payment to the patient.

F. Reporting Requirements: If the health of another individual is involved (particularly that of a child), the clinician is legally required to report his or her suspicions to the appropriate authorities. In the case of children, this is a legal requirement equivalent to that of reporting any suspected child abuse. Insofar as the report is made in good faith, the physician is exempt from prosecution for the violation of confidentiality.

Complications & Adverse Outcomes of Treatment

Patients with factitious disorder have a remarkable ability to obtain hospitalization and to be treated with invasive procedures. As a result, these patients often experience unnecessary operations such as nephrectomies and even pancreatectomies. They are at risk for a number of iatrogenic complications, and physicians may contribute to drug dependence. Hundreds of thousands of dollars, millions in some cases, may be spent in the diagnosis and treatment of surreptitious and self-induced illness. The physician is also at risk. When angered, patients with these disorders may initiate lawsuits and, at the very least, will generally create disarray and dissension among their medical caretakers.

For the victim of the Munchausen syndrome by proxy, the clinician's failure to recognize the disorder or to take decisive action may result in continued medical treatment, medical complications, or even death.

Prognosis & Course of Illness

Relatively little is known about the long-term outcome of factitious disorder. Some patients die as a result of their factitious illness behavior, and others experience severe medical complications including the loss of organs (eg, pancreas or kidney) or limbs. If the factitious disorder is the outgrowth of, for example, a psychotic depression, the prognosis is better than if the factitious illness results from severe personality disorder, as is usually the case. Although there are reports of successful psychotherapeutic intervention with some patients, there is no evidence of continued remission on follow-up. Munchausen syndrome appears to be relatively refractory to treatment, although the ultimate outcome for most of these patients is unknown. When confronted, some patients with simple factitious disorder enter psychotherapy and appear to improve and demonstrate fewer symptoms. Some patients deny their illness and merely change physicians, continuing their factitious illness behavior elsewhere; other patients deny their illness but apparently cease their behavior after being confronted with it.

The long-term prognosis of Munchausen syndrome by proxy is not encouraging. Victims have a high mortality rate during childhood, and those who survive childhood may develop somatoform disorders or factitious disorders upon reaching adulthood. Because this is a recently recognized disorder, long-term follow-up information is not yet available.

Asher R: Munchausen syndrome. Lancet 1951;1:339.

Feldman MD, Eisendrath SJ (editors): *The Spectrum of Factitious Disorders.* American Psychiatric Press, 1996.

Feldman MD, Ford CV: *Patients or Pretenders?: The Strange World of Factitious Disorders.* John Wiley & Sons, 1994.

Souid AK, Keith DV, Cunningham AS: Munchausen syndrome by proxy. Clin Pediatr 1998;37:497.

MALINGERING

General Considerations

Malingering differs from factitious disorder in that it is a deliberate disease simulation with a specific goal (eg, to obtain opiates). Malingering is underdiagnosed, often because of the physician's fear of making false accusations. However, covert surveillance has indicated that as many as 20% of pain clinic patients misrepresent the extent of their disability.

Malingering may include the deliberate production of disease or the exaggeration, elaboration, or false report of symptoms. The essential diagnostic issue for malingering is the determination that the person is willfully simulating disease for a defined purpose. But no physician is a mind-reader. Thus conscious intent must be inferred from other behaviors and psychological testing.

Malingering is not a psychiatric diagnosis but rather a situation in which someone is deliberately using a bogus illness to obtain a recognizable goal. The goal may be deferment from military service, escape from incarceration (eg, not guilty by reason of insanity), procurement of controlled substances, or monetary compensation in a personal injury lawsuit.

A. Major Etiologic Theories: Malingering, by definition, is determined by a person's willful behavior to use illness for an external goal. It has been proposed, however, that malingering is one extreme of a continuum of conscious-unconscious motivation that is anchored at the other extreme by conversion symptoms. Many simulated symptoms lie somewhere between these extremes and have both conscious and unconscious components.

Patients with antisocial personality disorder are believed to be more inclined to malinger, using physical symptoms as one of their means to manipulate or defraud others. All personality types, however, have been described in association with malingering, and it can be viewed as a coping mechanism when other coping strategies are ineffective. For example, a malingered symptom may be one mechanism for an exploited laborer to get out of an intolerable work situation.

B. Epidemiology: Malingering is most frequently seen in settings in which there may be an advantage to being sick (eg, in the military or in front of worker's compensation review boards). The prevalence of malingering is not known, but it is probably underdiagnosed.

Clinical Findings

A. Signs & Symptoms: Malingering may involve either exaggeration or elaboration of genuine illness for secondary gain (eg, continued disability after a mild industrial injury) or the simulation of disease (eg, faked injuries after a contrived automobile accident). It may be inferred in persons who behave differently and demonstrate different function when they think they are not being observed. For example, insurance companies may covertly videotape "disabled workers" who water ski on weekends.

B. Psychological Testing: Malingered psychological symptoms can often be detected from psychological testing. The validity scales of the Minnesota Multiphasic Personality Inventory (MMPI) may demonstrate changes indicative of false reporting. Further, significant differences between the obvious and subtle subscales of the MMPI clinical scales (eg, on the scale for depression) are correlated with deliberate misrepresentation. Mental status examinations and psychological testing may reveal findings that are inconsistent with, or clearly not typical of, the simulated disorder.

Differential Diagnosis

The differential diagnosis of malingering includes physical disease; factitious disorder (ie, with no discernible motive); somatoform disorders, particularly conversion disorder (in which the motive is unconscious); and pseudo-malingering. In the latter situation the patient believes that he or she is in conscious control of a symptom but actually has a disease (eg, a person who is psychotic pretends to be psychotic in order to hide from himself the fact that he is not in control of his mental processes).

Management & Treatment

"Treatment" of malingering is, in a sense, a contradiction in terms because the "patient" does not want to be well until the desired goal (eg, financial compensation) is achieved. The physician must be alert in order to avoid becoming an accomplice in the malingerer's manipulations. At times, subtle hints to the malingerer that the ruse has been detected will motivate the malingerer to drop the malingered symptom in a face-saving manner.

Complications & Adverse Outcomes of Treatment

It is commonly believed that malingered symptoms disappear when the malingering has achieved the patient's goal. In the process of the illness, the malingerer may experience iatrogenic complications of diagnostic or therapeutic procedures. A psychological complication occurs when, after years of litigation, the malingerer has come to believe in the illness (ie, through learned behavior) and does not relinquish the symptom after successful resolution of the lawsuit.

Prognosis & Course of Illness

Little is known about the prognosis of malingering. Persons who are successful at perpetuating disease simulations do not come to medical attention. The judgment of the morality of malingering is largely a matter of the observer and circumstances. Most people would regard the defraudment of an insurance company, through a false injury, as an antisocial act. In contrast, the malingering of a prisoner of war who is attempting to manipulate his or her captors would be seen by most compatriots as a skillful coping mechanism.

Kay NR, Morris-Jones H: Pain clinic management of medico-legal litigants. Injury 1998;29:305.

Pankratz L: *Patients Who Deceive: Assessment and Management of Risk in Providing Health Care and Financial Benefits.* Charles C Thomas, 1998.

Weintraub MI (guest editor): Neurologic clinics: malingering and conversion. Reactions 1995;13:229.

GENERAL REFERENCES

Eisendrath SJ: Factitious disorders and malingering. Pages 1803–1818 in Gabbard GO (editor): *Treatments of Psychiatric Disorders.* Vol 2, 2nd ed. American Psychiatric Press, 1995.

Ford CV: *Lies! Lies!! Lies!!!: The Psychology of Deceit.* American Psychiatric Press, 1996.

Dissociative Disorders

27

Barry Nurcombe, MD

General Considerations

The cardinal feature of the dissociative disorders is an acute or gradual, transient or persistent, disruption of consciousness, perception, memory or awareness, not associated with physical disease or organic brain dysfunction, and severe enough to cause distress or impairment. Four types are described in DSM-IV, and there is a miscellaneous fifth group (Table 27–1). The distinction between these types may be blurred, particularly when patients exhibit symptoms from more than one type.

A. Major Etiologic Theories: Normal dissociation is an adaptive defense used to cope with overwhelming psychic trauma. It is commonly encountered during and after civilian disasters, criminal assault, sudden loss, and war. In normal dissociation, the individual's perception of the traumatic experience is temporarily dulled or dispelled from consciousness. Normal dissociation prevents other vital psychological functions from being overwhelmed by the traumatic experience. The capacity to dissociate, as evidenced by susceptibility to hypnosis, is widely distributed among normal people. However, it is unclear whether pathologic dissociation is an extreme or more enduring form of normal dissociation (ie, whether there is a continuum of dissociation between

Table 27–1. Types of dissociative disorders.

Dissociative amnesia
Dissociative fugue
Dissociative identity disorder
Depersonalization disorder
Dissociative disorder not otherwise specified:
    Dissociative hallucinosis
    Dissociation following torture or political indoctrination
    Somnambulism
    "Out-of-body" experiences
    Dissociative trances that are culturally sanctioned
    Culture-bound "possession" states
    Ganser syndrome

normal and abnormal) or whether the pathologic form is distinctive. Recent studies of trauma subjects have found only a low correlation between hypnotizability and measures of dissociation. Theories concerning the basis of pathologic dissociation can be classified as psychological, neurocognitive, traumagenic, and psychosocial.

1. Psychological theories—Janet postulated that some people have a constitutional "psychological insufficiency" that renders them prone to dissociate in the face of frightening experiences. At that time, memories associated with "vehement emotions" become separated or dissociated from awareness in the form of subconscious fixed ideas, which are not integrated into memory. Rather, they remain latent and are prone to return to consciousness as **psychological automatisms** such as hysterical paralyses, anesthesias, and somnambulisms (trance states).

Breuer and Freud suggested that hysterical patients experience inadmissible ideational "complexes" resulting in a splitting of the mind and the emergence of abnormal (hypnoid) states of consciousness. Pathologic associations formed during the hypnoid state fail to decay like ordinary memories but reemerge to disrupt somatic processes in the form of hysterical sensorimotor symptoms or disturbances of consciousness. Breuer and Freud disputed Janet's concept that dissociation is a passive process reflecting a hereditary degeneracy. They introduced the concept of an active defensive process that energetically deflects the conscious mind from disruptive ideas. Out of this theory emerged the later psychoanalytic concepts of repression and ego defense.

Dissociative amnesia and dissociative fugue characteristically arise in a setting of overwhelming stress, particularly in time of war or civilian catastrophe. Murderers, for example, often claim amnesia for the crime long after it would be legally advantageous to do so. Money problems, the impending disclosure of a sexual misdemeanor, marital conflict, or the death of a spouse are the usual precipitants of amnesia and fugue. Sometimes, the dissociative state is precipitated by an intolerable mood, such as severe depression with intense guilt. Dissociation blots out the unendurable memory, and the fugue represents an attempt to get away and start a new life.

It is unclear whether depersonalization represents a minor variant of global dissociation or a different process. In depersonalization, affect and the sense of being connected is split off from the individual's sense of self and perception of the outside world, giving rise to the feeling of being like a robot or in a dream. Depersonalization may be the subjective component of a biological mechanism that allows an animal to function in a terrifying situation, whereas dissociation is represented by the freezing behavior that enables hunted animals to escape detection. These extreme survival maneuvers are subject to overload. Learned helplessness in animals, for example, may represent a breakdown of those neural circuits that modulate the sensitivity of the brain to incoming stimuli.

2. Neurocognitive theories—Episodic memory is a form of explicit memory involving the storage of events that then have access to conscious awareness. Episodic memory is usually recounted in words, as a narrative. If significant enough, episodic memories become part of **autobiographical memory,** the history of the self. The medial temporal lobe, particularly the hippocampus, is essential to the encoding, storage, and retrieval of episodic memory. Dissociation may represent an interference with the encoding, storage, or retrieval in narrative form of traumatic episodic memories.

The locus coeruleus is an important source of noradrenergic fibers that project to the cerebral cortex, hypothalamus, hippocampus, and amygdala. The amygdala and orbitofrontal cortex select out those stimuli that have been primary reinforcers in the past. The amygdala projects to the hippocampus (via the entorhinal cortex), to the sensory association cortex, and to the hypothalamus and brain stem, coordinating a central alarm apparatus that scans the sensory input for stimuli that the animal has learned to fear, and sounds an alert when such stimuli are encountered. Evidence indicates that serotonin acts postsynaptically in the amygdala to provoke the synthesis of enkephalins, which modulate or dampen the affect associated with fearful experience and may interfere with the consolidation of traumatic memories. If the amygdaloid alarm system becomes overloaded and breaks down, the animal will be at the mercy of raw fear. Thus, whenever reminders of trauma are perceived in the environment, or whenever fragments of traumatic episodic memory threaten to emerge into awareness, an alarm is sounded and the fail-safe, last-resort defense of dissociation must be invoked.

Traumatic memories are stored in two systems: (1) the hippocampal explicit episodic memory system and (2) the amygdaloid implicit alarm system. The amygdaloid system can disrupt storage and retrieval via the hippocampal system. Research suggests that immature animals exposed to early inescapable stress or gross deprivation of cospecies contact are particularly vulnerable to subsequent trauma. In primates, morphine decreases (and naloxone increases) the amount of affiliative calling of an animal separated from its mother, whereas diazepam reduces freezing and hostile gestures in reaction to direct threat, probably through the prefrontal cortex. Animal research has suggested that high circulating corticosteroid levels in stressed juveniles are associated with a reduction in the population of glucocorticoid receptors in the hippocampus. Furthermore, neuroimaging studies of veterans with chronic posttraumatic stress disorder have demonstrated an apparent shrinkage in hippocampal volume.

3. Traumagenic theories—Clinical evidence for the linkage between emotional trauma and dissociation is derived from the following observations: (1) the high prevalence of histories of childhood trauma reported by patients with dissociative disorder, (2) elevated levels of dissociation in people who report child abuse, (3) elevated levels of dissociation in combat veterans with posttraumatic stress disorder, (4) the prevalence of acute dissociative reactions in war or disaster, and (5) the observation that marked dissociation during a traumatic experience predicts subsequent posttraumatic stress disorder. Almost all adults with dissociative identity disorder report significant trauma in childhood, particularly incest, physical abuse, and emotional abuse. These patients commonly report repeated abuse, often of an extremely sadistic, bizarre nature.

4. Psychosocial theories—The difficulty of corroborating retrospective accounts of abuse has provoked much controversy. Are these reports false, unwittingly created by clinical interest and the recent explosion of coverage in the media? The possibility of iatrogenic facilitation cannot be excluded. The more dramatic forms of dissociative disorder—particularly fugue and multiple identity—may represent, at least in part, forms of abnormal illness behavior, distorted attempts by emotionally needy patients to elicit care and protection from therapist-parent surrogates, or bids to retain the interest of therapists in the context of an intense transference relationship. Traumagenic and psychosocial theories are not necessarily mutually exclusive.

B. Epidemiology: Epidemiologic data on dissociative disorders are patchy. Studies of combat soldiers have found a prevalence of dissociative amnesia of 5–8%. There are no reliable data on dissociative fugue. The prevalence of dissociative identity disorder is disputed but probably low. Case reports suggest a female-to-male ratio of at least 5:1. This ratio might be exaggerated, because males with dissociative disorder, who are likely to be episodically violent, are likely to be directed to the correctional system. Dissociative identity disorder is found in all ethnic groups, though mainly in whites, and in all socioeconomic groups. Depersonalization is a frequent concomitant of anxiety disorders, posttraumatic stress disorder, and severe depression. Up to one half of college students claim to have experienced depersonalization at some time in their lives. It has been reported that 80% of psychiatric inpatients suffer from depersonalization, but in only 12% is the symptom long lasting, and in no case is it the only symptom. The sex ratio is equal.

DISSOCIATIVE AMNESIA & DISSOCIATIVE FUGUE

DSM-IV Diagnostic Criteria

Dissociative Amnesia

A. The predominant disturbance is one or more episodes of inability to recall important personal information, usually of a traumatic or stressful nature, that is too extensive to be explained by ordinary forgetfulness.

B. The disturbance does not occur exclusively during the course of dissociative identity disorder, dissociative fugue, posttraumatic stress disorder, acute stress disorder, or somatization disorder and is not due to the direct physiological effects of a substance (eg, a drug of abuse, a medication) or a neurological or other general medical condition (eg, amnestic disorder due to head trauma).

C. The symptoms cause clinically significant distress or impairment in social, occupational, or other important areas of functioning.

Dissociative Fugue

A. The predominant disturbance is sudden, unexpected travel away from home or one's customary place of work, with inability to recall one's past.

B. Confusion about personal identity or assumption of a new identity (partial or complete).

C. The disturbance does not occur exclusively during the course of dissociative identity disorder and is not due to the direct physiological effects of a substance (eg, a drug of abuse, a medication) or a general medical condition (eg, temporal lobe epilepsy).

D. The symptoms cause clinically significant distress or impairment in social, occupational, or other important areas of functioning.

Reprinted, with permission, from *Diagnostic and Statistical Manual of Mental Disorders,* 4th ed. Copyright 1994 American Psychiatric Association.

Clinical Findings

A. Signs & Symptoms: The amnesia for distressing events can be localized (ie, complete amnesia for events during a circumscribed period of time), selective (ie, failure to remember some but not all events during a circumscribed period of time), generalized (ie, affecting an entire life), or continuous (ie, failure to remember anything after a particular date). Patchy amnesia is prevalent among people exposed to military or civilian trauma. A common sequence is for the patient to progress from a first stage, characterized by an acute altered state of consciousness (mental confusion, headache, and preoccupation with a single idea or emotion), to a second stage in which he or she loses the sense of personal identity. At this point the patient may be found wandering in a fugue state, unable to give an account of himself or herself. Rarely, the patient enters a third stage in which he or she assumes a new identity, usually one more gregarious and uninhibited than previously. The diagnostic separation of amnesia from fugue may be illusory, because the two conditions are probably on a continuum. During the first stage of confusion and altered consciousness, some patients report audiovisual hallucinations and a preoccupation with quasidelusional ideas. This condition, originally known as hysterical twilight state, lacks the disorganization of thought processes and affective incongruity found in schizophrenia. The patient operates at a higher level of consciousness than is associated with epilepsy or other organic brain dysfunctions.

B. Psychological Testing: Table 27–2 lists tests that are useful screens in the diagnosis of dissociative disorders.

Differential Diagnosis & Comorbidity

Dissociative amnesia and dissociative fugue must be differentiated from delirium or dementia. The clinician must exclude amnestic disorders due to such medical conditions as vitamin deficiency, head trauma, carbon monoxide poisoning, and herpes encephalitis as well as amnestic disorders secondary to alcoholism (Korsakoff's syndrome); to anxiolytic, anticonvulsant, sedative, and hypnotic drugs; and to steroids, lithium, or β-blockers. The clinician must also distinguish other organic disorders such as the retrograde amnesia of head injury, seizure disorder (particularly the dreamy state of temporal lobe epilepsy), and transient global amnesia due to cerebral vascular insufficiency.

Differential diagnosis is based on a full history, a detailed mental status examination, physical and neurologic examination, and when appropriate, special investigations such as a toxicology screen, laboratory testing, electroencephalography, brain imaging, and neuropsychological testing. The most difficult diagnostic problems arise when dissociation is superimposed on organic disease (eg, pseudoseizures coexisting with epilepsy). The differentiation of dissociative disorders from malingering is discussed later in this chapter.

Table 27–2. Screening tests for dissociative disorders.

Test	Description
Dissociative Disorders Interview Schedule (DDIS)	A structured interview that examines for dissociative disorder, somatoform disorder, depression, borderline personality disorder, substance abuse, and physical and sexual abuse
Structured Clinical Interview for the DSM-IV Dissociative Disorders (SCID-D)	A semistructured interview derived from the SCID
Dissociative Experiences Scale (DES)	A 28-item self-report questionnaire that screens for dissociative symptoms in adults (age 18 years and older)
Adolescent Dissociative Experiences Scale (A-DES)	A 30-item self-report screening questionnaire for adolescents (age 12–20 years)
Child Dissociative Checklist (CDC)	A 20-item screening checklist to be completed on children (age 5–12 years) by a parent or adult observer
Structured Interview for Reported Symptoms (SIRS)	A structured interview designed to detect the malingering of psychosis

Treatment

Patience and the expectation that memory loss will soon clear are usually enough to help the amnestic patient recover. The key to treatment is a safe environment (eg, hospitalization) removed from the source of stress and a trusting therapeutic relationship. Hypnotherapy or narcoanalysis (eg, using amobarbital, benzodiazepines, or methylamphetamine) are sometimes required to facilitate recall.

Prognosis & Course of Illness

Dissociative amnesia and dissociative fugue are usually short lived; however, after restoration of memory and identity, the patient must deal with the source of the problem.

DISSOCIATIVE IDENTITY DISORDER

DSM-IV Diagnostic Criteria

A. The presence of two or more distinct identities or personality states (each with its own relatively enduring pattern of perceiving, relating to, and thinking about the environment and self).
B. At least two of these identities or personality states recurrently take control of the person's behavior.
C. Inability to recall important personal information that is too extensive to be explained by ordinary forgetfulness.
D. The disturbance is not due to the direct physiological effects of a substance (eg, blackouts or chaotic behavior during alcohol intoxication) or a general medical condition (eg, complex partial seizures).

Note: In children: the symptoms are not attributable to imaginary playmates or other fantasy play.

Reprinted, with permission, from the *Diagnostic and Statistical Manual of Mental Disorders,* 4th ed. Copyright 1994 American Psychiatric Association.

Clinical Findings

A. Signs & Symptoms: Dissociative identity disorder (DID) is usually not diagnosed until patients are in their late 20s, but retrospective evidence indicates that it begins much earlier, usually in childhood. Thus patients with DID are likely to have had years of treatment before the correct diagnosis is made. These patients commonly exhibit transient depression, mood swings, sleep disturbance, nightmares, and suicidal behavior. They are often self-injurious and exhibit a host of dissociative symptoms including amnesia, episodes of "lost time" (episodes of amnesia varying from several minutes to several days), depersonalization, fugue, and hallucinations. Anxiety and its somatic concomitants (eg, dyspnea, palpitations, chest pain, choking sensations, faintness, tremors) commonly herald a switch of alter personalities. Quasineurologic symptoms such as headache, syncope, pseudoseizures, numbness, paresthesia, diplopia, tunnel vision, and motor weakness are sometimes encountered. Symptoms referable to the cardiorespiratory or gastrointestinal systems or to the reproductive tract may dominate the clinical presentation.

Questioning will reveal that most patients have audiovisual hallucinations and quasidelusions. The auditory hallucinations may be fragments of conversations heard during traumatic experiences or may be metaphoric expressions of self-disgust in the form of hostile voices that revile and derogate the patient or command him or her to self-injury, to commit suicide, or to attack others. Other voices may be conversations between people about the patient, people offering solace, and the weeping and crying of distressed children. Some patients report a sense of being controlled, alterations in their body image, or the conviction that they are being followed or that their lives are threatened by shadowy enemies (eg, the former perpetrators of alleged "ritual abuse"). Discontinuities of thought and occasional thought "slippages" may be the result of alter switching or the intrusion of traumatic themes into the stream of thought, in the form of microdissociations.

As mentioned earlier in this chapter, these patients have often had many medical and neurologic investigations. Many have been treated for mood disorder, anxiety disorder, or schizophrenia. Many wander from job to job, place to place, and doctor to doctor. Many are prone to repeated victimization by virtue of their poor choice of occupation or consorts.

The cardinal feature of DID is multiple personalities, two or more entities, each of which has a characteristic and separate personality, history, affect, values, and function. The number of alters is usually about ten, though it may be many more. Typically, the alters are somewhat two-dimensional in quality and include such entities as the host personality; a variety of child personalities (eg, innocent child, traumatized child, "Pollyanna"); a persecutor; a cross-sex alter; an internal helper; a brazen, promiscuous "hussy;" a variety of demons; and "no one." These entities usually first emerge during childhood in the form of imaginary protectors or companions that help the child cope with recurrent experiences of abuse and fear. The alter personalities often switch abruptly, producing a bewildering change in demeanor, sometimes with anxiety and apparent disorganization of thought. Sometimes one alter or several alters will be unaware of the other alters. Often alters will communicate with each other. The complete dramatis personae usually emerge only after therapy.

It can be difficult to elicit alter personalities. The clinician must have a reasonable suspicion that DID is present (eg, in a patient who exhibits abrupt changes in demeanor, "lost time," total amnesia for childhood, and many physical symptoms). The exploration of puzzling events or lost time will often elicit an alter. Sometimes the clinician must ask directly to speak to "that part of you" that did something or experienced something.

B. Psychological Testing: See discussion of dissociative amnesia and dissociative fugue.

Differential Diagnosis & Comorbidity

DID is most likely to be confused with the following conditions: partial complex seizures, schizophrenia, bipolar disorder, major depression with psychotic features, Munchausen syndrome, Munchausen syndrome by proxy, and malingering. Partial complex seizures, which usually last no more than a few seconds, may be confused with alter switching; however, other cardinal signs of DID are not seen in epilepsy. Occasionally, telemetry is required.

Patients with DID frequently report the following phenomena: quasidelusions; ideas of being externally controlled; auditory hallucinations involving conversations; comments about the patient cast in the third person; commands; and ideas of thought loss. Together with the disruption of thinking coincident with alter switching or microdissociation, it is not surprising that

patients with DID have often been mistakenly diagnosed as having schizophrenia. DID should be differentiated from schizophrenia by the lack of emotional incongruity; the dramatic, care-eliciting presentation; the history of severe trauma; the alter personalities; and high scores on dissociation scales. Hypnosis is sometimes helpful in distinguishing DID from schizophrenia.

Rapid-cycling bipolar disorder is sometimes confused with the apparent mood swings caused by alter switching in DID. However, the term "rapid-cycling" refers to brief intervals between episodes of mania or depression, not to the brevity of the episodes themselves.

Major depression with psychotic features can be confused with DID if only a superficial diagnostic evaluation has been completed, particularly because many patients with DID have an associated depressive mood. In major depression with psychotic features, the auditory hallucinations and delusions are consistent with the prevailing depressive mood. For example, the patient hears voices derogating him or her for being a bad person, and is convinced that he or she has committed an unpardonable sin, is impoverished, is being hounded by tax officials, or is rotting inside. In DID, the hallucinations are often derogatory, but they convey the theme of helpless victimization and command patients to hurt others or themselves.

In some cases of Munchausen syndrome, the pseudopatient has presented himself or herself for medical attention with the symptoms of DID. In some cases of Munchausen syndrome by proxy, a mother has presented her child with symptoms of DID. The imposture is deliberate, but the gain obscure. Satisfaction is apparently obtained from being the center of medical investigations and therapeutic attention or from being the parent of a child with dramatic psychopathology. In malingering, the gain is less enigmatic: The pseudopatient is usually a criminal defendant seeking exculpation on the grounds of insanity.

Treatment

The treatment of DID is the subject of much controversy. It must be understood that a powerful body of opinion questions the validity of this diagnosis and questions therapeutic approaches that seek to integrate alters. Kluft describes four approaches to treatment: (1) integrate the alters; (2) seek harmony between the alters; (3) leave the alters alone and focus on improving adaptation to the here-and-now; and (4) regard the alters as artifacts, ignoring them and treating other symptoms (eg, depression).

The last of these approaches is adopted by those who believe that DID is a fictitious condition generated or reinforced by the clinicians who treat it. The first three approaches are not mutually exclusive and are adopted in accordance with the patient's capacity to tolerate the stress of integrating the alter personalities.

Excessively rapid movement in the assessment or treatment of DID will generate resistance. Once DID is identified and the diagnosis communicated, the patient will experience anxiety. Patients with DID tend to be profoundly distrustful of others and may themselves be deceptive. Patients are likely to be hypersensitive to deceit, impatience, or authoritarianism. Clinicians must be able to tolerate uncertainty, normalize any anomalous experiences that patients divulge, and eschew premature reassurance.

Many patients report complete amnesia for early and middle childhood. Most are also confused about current experience and are able to report the past in only piecemeal fashion. Clinicians should inquire about instances of lost time, depersonalization, out-of-body experiences, flashbacks, and hallucinations. Most patients with DID are able to suppress alter switching during brief contact, but they are likely to manifest the phenomenon if the interview session extends over an hour.

Hypnosis can be useful when rapid diagnosis is required, although it may be preferable to allow the alters to emerge spontaneously. The clinician should explore each alter with regard to the following information: name, age, and sex; developmental origin; dominant affect and perceptual style; survival functions; and unique symptoms and dysfunctions. The clinician should ask to speak to a particular alter identified by name or behavior and should ask for a signal (eg, a lifted finger) as a signal of the alter's willingness to appear. Rapport must be developed with each alter. After conducting the appropriate interview, the clinician should ask the alter to resubmerge. Although initially the clinician must treat each alter as if he or she is a separate person, it is important to convey the understanding that each alter is but a dissociated element of the client as a whole.

It can be useful to draw maps, diagrams, or family trees of the internal system of alters, identifying the components by name, age, and sex. These maps must be revised regularly throughout treatment. When a particular alter acknowledges lost time, another alter may have been internally active during that period. The internal helper alter may be the most reliable informant in the clinician's attempt to conceptualize the structure of personality fragments.

Treatment is either supportive or integrative. Integrative therapy is likely to be more complex and concomitantly more risky. A number of issues should be considered before embarking on integrative therapy. Table 27–3 lists situations in which integrative therapy is contraindicated.

If supportive therapy is pursued because the patient has a limited potential for integration, the clinician attempts to rehabilitate the patient by strengthening the ego of the host personality and by helping the patient to cope with reality. The emphasis is on stabilization, control of affect and impulse, increased responsibility in everyday behavior, and palliation of distress.

Table 27–3. Contraindications for integrative therapy.

Severe ego defect related to early neglect and trauma, and a lifelong reliance upon dissociative defenses.

Severe, pervasive comorbid pathology, particularly borderline personality disorder, histrionic personality disorder, depression, substance abuse, and eating disorder.

Poor environmental support. If the patient is involved in dysfunctional and nonsupportive relationships, retraumatization is likely to occur. There must be at least a moderate level of environmental stability and support.

The incapacity of the clinician to tolerate devaluation, acting-out behavior, suicidality, self-injury, and deceptiveness.

The inability of patient and clinician to establish and maintain a therapeutic alliance. The therapist must provide a flexible balance between support and interpretation, and maintain stable boundaries in interaction with the patient. The patient is likely to test the limits by acting out, seduction, failing to appear for appointments, or devaluing the clinician.

If prognostic factors are favorable, integrative therapy can be attempted. Integrative therapy aims to uncover dissociated and repressed traumatic experiences, integrate personality functioning, and replace dissociation with other defenses. Whenever the patient is overwhelmed in the course of therapy, the clinician must revert to supportive therapy. Whether the treatment is supportive or integrative, attention must be given to the shame and low self-esteem associated with sexual victimization.

Alters should be directed toward verbal and creative affective expression instead of impulsive, destructive, self-defeating acting out. Each alter represents the expression of a fixed idea: images, thoughts, or associations related to a particular traumatic experience that retains a pristine emotional charge because it has been sequestered from the normal processes of memory decay. The therapist must relate effectively to each of these internal fragments, seeking to improve the contribution of each fragment to overall functioning. The superordinate aim of integrative therapy is to promote the confluence of the entire system, not to strengthen dissociation between alters. The amount of time devoted to the development of greater general ego strength should exceed the amount of time spent in strengthening separate alters.

Persecutory and malevolent alters are best dealt with by patient rechanneling of hostile impulses in more appropriate directions, particularly by expressing rage in words or artistic productions rather than in deeds. Malevolent alters should be confronted gently with the identity confusion that leads them to consider themselves as part of the abuser rather than as part of the patient.

The internal helper alter is a useful ally in treatment and can serve as a consultant to the therapist, providing information about the total system. The ultimate aim of integrative therapy is to reverse the pervasive attachment disruption and splitting that have accompanied abuse. As the patient improves, he or she may begin to grieve for a lost childhood and for normal attachment experiences that were lost or never provided.

The therapist should help the patient develop effective coping skills, using a gentle, educative approach, modeling accurate perception, management of affect, containment of impulse, and the consideration of alternative responses to stress. Inhibited, withdrawn alters will benefit from the encouragement of self-expression and self-assertion. Shame-based alters require the supportive resolution of shame. As the patient becomes more aware of different traumata, a dialogue may occur between the different alters. The therapist should emphasize the need for cooperation. The aim is toward increased dialogue and mutual cooperation.

The **abreaction of emotion** is an essential component of therapy and is aimed at resolving dissociation and restoring integration. The important component of abreaction may be not so much the catharsis of feeling as the subsequent reformulation of traumatic memories. Some patients revert to dissociative trances when they are about to remember and disclose particular traumatic experiences, and spontaneous abreaction may be triggered by reminders of trauma such as anniversaries. However, abreaction without reformulation is unproductive. During abreaction, the therapist's task is to keep the patient safe, nudge him or her toward reality, and keep him or her in the abreaction until it is concluded. Abreaction is followed by debriefing and exploration of the meaning of the experience. Successful abreaction requires full experience of the affect associated with the event, not just a disembodied memory. Premature initiation of abreaction, or the induction of abreaction in patients who cannot tolerate it, is counterproductive. Table 27–4 summarizes the sequential stages in psychotherapy with these patients.

Late in the therapy, the spontaneous fusing of alters signals readiness for personality unification. Usually this proceeds as two or more alters combine at a time. The therapist must be patient and not press for premature fusion. Full integration involves (1) reduced

Table 27–4. Stages in the integrative psychotherapy of dissociative identity disorder.

1. Establish a working alliance.
2. Make the diagnosis, inform the patient, and maintain the therapeutic alliance.
3. Make contact with the different alters.
4. Explore the structure of the system of alters.
5. Understand the particular "fixed idea" behind each alter.
6. Work with the problems of particular alter states.
7. Help the patient develop increasing cooperation between alter states.
8. Help the patient develop nondissociative coping skills.
9. Confront dissociation and support the patient's integration of memory, affect, and identity via the abreaction of traumatic experience.
10. Help the patient develop and consolidate a new identity.

reliance on the dissociative segregation of experience, (2) absence of the signs of DID, (3) the blending of alters into a single nondissociative personality, and (4) the harmonious coexistence of different aspects of the patient's personality. Integration is relative. Some patients are able to tolerate complete fusion and unification. Others are not capable of full unification but benefit from improved functional integration.

Prognosis & Course of Illness

DID is a chronic condition that does not remit. It usually begins in childhood as a form of dissociative hallucinosis (see "Miscellaneous Types of Dissociation" section later in this chapter), but the full syndrome does not coalesce until adolescence. Some patients develop histrionic or borderline personalities, with a stormy adulthood. Others are introverted, depressed, and socially avoidant. Males are more likely to have a history of episodic violence with legal involvement. Many people with DID manage to conceal their symptoms for years.

DEPERSONALIZATION DISORDER

DSM-IV Diagnostic Criteria

A. Persistent or recurrent experiences of feeling detached from, and as if one is an outside observer of, one's mental processes or body (eg, feeling like one is in a dream).
B. During the depersonalization experience, reality testing remains intact.
C. The depersonalization causes clinically significant distress or impairment in social, occupational, or other important areas of functioning.
D. The depersonalization experience does not occur exclusively during the course of another mental disorder, such as schizophrenia, panic disorder, acute stress disorder, or another dissociative disorder, and is not due to the direct physiological effects of a substance (eg, a drug of abuse, a medication) or a general medical condition (eg, temporal lobe epilepsy).

Reprinted, with permission, from the *Diagnostic and Statistical Manual of Mental Disorders,* 4th ed. Copyright 1994 American Psychiatric Association.

Clinical Findings

A. Signs & Symptoms: The onset of depersonalization disorder is usually sudden and typically occurs in a setting of anxiety. Derealization is commonly associated with depersonalization. Patients feel numb and out of touch with their feelings, bodies, and surroundings. Sometimes they feel as if they are observing themselves or as though they are automatons in a dream. Depersonalization is difficult to describe, and patients may express concern about "going crazy," particularly if the condition is accompanied by déjà vu experiences and distortions in sense of time. Depression and anxiety are commonly associated with depersonalization.

B. Psychological Testing: See discussion of dissociative amnesia and dissociative fugue.

Differential Diagnosis & Comorbidity

Dissociative disorders in which depersonalization is the cardinal symptom probably merge imperceptibly with other disorders in which depersonalization is a subsidiary symptom. For example, depersonalization is likely to be elicited from patients with anxiety disorders (particularly panic disorder), other dissociative disorders, depressive disorder, and borderline personality disorder. Depersonalization has been reported in 11–42% of schizophrenic patients. In schizophrenia, depersonalization tends to become incorporated into the prevailing delusional system. Depersonalization may also be encountered in substance abuse, particularly with alcohol, marijuana, hallucinogens, cocaine, phenylcyclidine, methylamphetamine, narcotics, and sedatives. Depersonalization has also been reported after medication with indomethacin, fenfluramine, and haloperidol.

In epilepsy, particularly temporal lobe epilepsy, depersonalization may be encountered as an aura, as part of the seizure itself, or between seizures. Depersonalization in epilepsy is more likely to be associated with stereotypic movements (eg, lip smacking), senseless words or phrases, and loss of consciousness than in dissociative disorders, in which it is likely to be more highly elaborated. Depersonalization may also be evident in postconcussive disorder, Meniere's disease, cerebral atherosclerosis, and Korsakoff's syndrome.

Treatment

If depersonalization is a subsidiary symptom, the primary disorder should be treated. There have been no controlled studies of treatment for depersonalization disorder proper. The relative effectiveness of supportive psychotherapy, hypnosis, exploratory psychotherapy, family therapy, and cognitive-behavioral therapy is not known. Psychotherapy focuses on the recovery of the traumatic experience from which the pathologic dissociation is thought to have arisen. Hypnosis may help in this regard. Cognitive-behavioral desensitization, flooding, and exposure have also been recommended.

Prognosis & Course of Illness

Some depersonalization syndromes, particularly after acute stress, are transient. However, depersonalization can evolve into a chronic, intractable, disabling disorder.

DISSOCIATIVE DISORDER NOT OTHERWISE SPECIFIED

Diagnostic Criteria

A. Includes dissociative symptomatology that does not fit all the criteria for the other four types of dissociative disorder.

B. Includes dissociative hallucinosis, dissociative states following torture or political indoctrination, somnambulism, "out-of-body" experiences, dissociative trances that are part of culturally sanctioned rituals, culture-bound "possession" states (eg, amok), and the Ganser syndrome (hysterical pseudodementia).

Clinical Findings

A. Signs & Symptoms: Dissociative hallucinosis is a form of posttraumatic stress disorder commonly encountered in sexually or physically abused adolescents, particularly in inpatient settings. Patients, usually female, experience recurrent, dramatic episodes of audiovisual hallucinosis, dissociative trances, autohypnoid states, suicidal behavior, and self-injury (eg, wrist cutting). Male patients with this condition are often subject to intermittent explosive outbursts during which they are assaultive or self-injurious (eg, by punching their fists against a wall) and are apparently out of touch with their surroundings. The dissociative episodes are usually precipitated by experiences that reactivate traumatic memories of sexual coercion, helplessness, humiliation, or rejection.

Dissociative trances may be part of the rituals of some religions. Culture-bound syndromes such as amok, latah, malgri, and koro are usually preceded by intense emotion (eg, fear, humiliation), associated with the conviction of being possessed by a demon or spirit, and accompanied by dissociated, out-of-control behavior.

The **Ganser syndrome** (hysterical pseudodementia) is a condition in which the patient exhibits symptoms of an apparent dementia or psychosis that are too exaggerated or inconsistent to fit such a diagnosis. For example, the patient may exhibit **vorbeireden,** a phenomenon in which the patient's incorrect answers imply knowledge of the correct answer (eg, Question: "How many legs has a cow?" Answer: "Five."). Several of Ganser's original cases probably had delirium. Vorbeireden can also occur in organic brain disease such as stroke or cerebral tumor. The psychogenic variety is most often encountered in a legal setting and must be differentiated from malingering. It is usually associated with global amnesia for a crime and a dissociative shut-down of intellectual processes, producing apparent dementia.

B. Psychological Testing: See discussion of dissociative amnesia and dissociative fugue.

Differential Diagnosis & Comorbidity

Dissociative hallucinosis, with its dramatic, recurrent audiovisual hallucinosis, fear of attack, explosive violence, suicidality, and self-injurious behavior must be differentiated from schizophrenia, substance-induced psychosis, major depression with psychotic features, and epilepsy.

Treatment

In many adolescents with dissociative hallucinosis, rudimentary or nascent forms of DID may be noted. In such cases, clinicians should avoid reinforcing the development of alters and relate to the patient as a whole. Hospitalization may be necessary in order to provide safety, prevent suicide and self-injury, and contain episodic dyscontrol. Individual, group, and family therapy are helpful. Pharmacotherapy, judiciously prescribed, can be a useful adjunct to treatment.

Prognosis & Course of Illness

The prognosis for acute episodes of dissociative hallucinosis is good. However, the long-term outlook depends on the quality of family support and the patient's personality.

PHARMACOTHERAPY IN DISSOCIATIVE DISORDERS

Pharmacotherapy is adjunctive in the treatment of dissociative disorders. Neuroleptic medication is contraindicated: Not only is it ineffective, but it aggravates dissociation. Antidepressant medication, particularly heterocyclic agents or serotonin reuptake inhibitors, can be helpful in counteracting insomnia, impulsiveness, depersonalization, and comorbid depression. Benzodiazepines can be helpful in acute dissociation and panic but should be used cautiously in the long term because of the danger of addiction.

DISSOCIATION FOLLOWING ACUTE TRAUMA

Following acute trauma, such as that associated with a civilian catastrophe or criminal assault, dissociation is commonly encountered as a part of a posttraumatic stress disorder (see Chapter 23). Treatment involves a safe environment, individual psychotherapy, and when required, group therapy. When children are involved, following a civilian catastrophe, preventive intervention can be provided in schools.

Hornstein NL, Putnam FW: Clinical phenomenology of child and adolescent dissociative disorders. J Am Acad Child Adolesc Psychiatry 1992;31:1077.

Kluft RP, Fine CG (editors): *Clinical Perspectives on Multiple Personality Disorder.* American Psychiatric Press, 1993.

Lowenstein RJ: Psychogenic amnesia and psychogenic fugue. Pages 189–222 in Tasman A, Goldfinger SM (editors): *Review of Psychiatry.* Vol 10. American Psychiatric Press, 1991.

McHugh PR, Putnam FW: Resolved: multiple personality is an individually and socially created artifact. J Am Acad Child Adolesc Psychiatry 1995;34:957.

Michelson LK, Ray WJ: *Handbook of Dissociation: Theoretical, Empirical and Clinical Perspectives.* Plenum Publishing Corp, 1996.

Nurcombe B: Dissociative hallucinosis and allied conditions. Pages 107–128 in Volkmar F (editor): *Psychoses of Childhood & Adolescence.* American Psychiatric Press, 1996.

Putnam FW: The process of dissociation. In: Peterson G (chair): *Dissociative Disorders in Children and Adolescents.* Institute VII, Annual Conference of the American Academy of Child and Adolescent Psychiatry, New York, 1994.

Putnam FW: *Dissociation in Children and Adolescents.* Guilford Press, 1997.

Steinberg M: The spectrum of depersonalization: Assessment and treatment. Pages 223–247 in Tasman A, Goldfinger SM (editors): *Review of Psychiatry.* Vol 10. American Psychiatric Press, 1991.

28

Sexual Dysfunctions & Paraphilias

Jonathan E. May, PhD

SEXUAL DYSFUNCTIONS

The human sexual response cycle begins with sexual desire and moves through a physiologic process that for purposes of this discussion may be divided into three phases: arousal/excitement, orgasm, and resolution. Sexual dysfunction is defined as a disturbance in sexual desire or in the physiologic processes that underlie the sexual response cycle, or as pain associated with penetration and sexual intercourse. There are no specifically identified dysfunctions associated with the resolution phase, during which the anatomic structures involved in sexual response return to a baseline state, although some patients do report emotional distress related to events that occur during this phase. In order to meet *Diagnostic and Statistical Manual of Mental Disorders,* 4th edition (DSM-IV) criteria, the disturbance or pain must be "persistent or recurrent" and must cause "marked distress or interpersonal difficulty." Occasional, episodic, difficulties with sexual function are common and are not diagnosed. Sexual dysfunction, a disturbance in process, is quite distinct from paraphilias, which are defined by the nature of the persons, objects, or activities that serve as the focus for sexual desire and arousal.

In order to successfully treat sexual disorders, providers must remain aware that they are working in an arena in which symptoms and patients' reports are influenced in a highly interactive manner by multiple and complex psychological, physiologic, social, and interpersonal variables. Patients with sexual problems may be affected strongly by shame, guilt, embarrassment, or anxiety. Information important to accurate diagnosis may involve secrets that have been hidden from sexual partners or remote emotional trauma that has not been discussed with anyone. Lack of information, misinformation, and highly charged emotions relating to sexuality are common in both lay and professional communities. Practitioners must always approach patients in a respectful and open-minded manner, with the awareness that it may be difficult for patients to discuss or accurately describe their sexual difficulties, and that the information initially presented to them may be inaccurate or distorted.

The question of etiology in sexual dysfunction is complex. Most of the dysfunctions have multiple potential etiologies, ranging from predominantly organic to predominantly psychological, and there are many possible contributing factors in both the organic and the psychological domains. Etiology in a particular case often involves a combination of factors from both domains. Many of the causal factors are nonspecific, that is, they may be found in the history of patients with different dysfunctions or persons with no dysfunction. The specific dysfunction that becomes manifest in a particular patient is the result of a complex interplay between the patient's life history and psychosocial etiologic factors as well as preexisting biological and psychological predispositions.

Any of the sexual dysfunction diagnoses may be qualified by the following specifiers: *lifelong type* or *acquired type, generalized type* or *situational type,* and *due to psychological factors* or *due to combined factors.* These specifiers have etiologic and therefore prognostic and treatment significance. Lifelong disorders are likely to be caused by congenital organic factors or by influences from the early stages of psychosocial development. Acquired disorders are more likely related to psychosocial influences from later in the life span, to drug or medication effects, to physical trauma, or to illness that became significant later in life. Situational disorders occur with particular partners, and not others, or under particular circumstances, and the etiology can often be found in issues that are specific to a particular relationship or a particular sexual activity. Generalized disorders have a more global impact and often have more complex or more deeply rooted causation. If a medical condition plays a significant causal role the disorder is usually generalized.

The sexual dysfunctions are discussed in this chapter in the order in which they become manifest in the sexual response cycle.

DESIRE PHASE DISORDERS

1. HYPOACTIVE SEXUAL DESIRE DISORDER

DSM-IV Diagnostic Criteria

A. Persistently or recurrently deficient (or absent) sexual fantasies and desire for sexual activity. The judgment of deficiency or absence is made by the clinician, taking into account factors that affect sexual functioning, such as age and the context of the person's life.
B. The disturbance causes marked distress or interpersonal difficulty.
C. The sexual dysfunction is not better accounted for by another Axis I disorder (except another sexual dysfunction) and is not due exclusively to the direct physiological effects of a substance (eg, a drug of abuse, a medication) or a general medical condition.

Reprinted, with permission, from *Diagnostic and Statistical Manual of Mental Disorders,* 4th ed. Copyright 1994 American Psychiatric Association.

General Considerations

Hypoactive sexual desire disorder is also commonly referred to as inhibited sexual desire disorder. The decision as to what level of sexual interest is deficient, hypoactive, or inhibited is a clinical judgment made with reference to factors in a particular person's life relevant to sexual function (eg, physical health, age). Hypoactive sexual desire disorder does not necessarily imply an inability to respond and function sexually.

Although some patients with this disorder seek treatment on their own initiative, most are brought or led to treatment as a result of relationship dissatisfaction by a partner with a higher level of sexual desire. Care must be taken to distinguish hypoactive sexual desire from discrepant levels of sexual interest within a couple, which can also lead to relationship distress and dissatisfaction but should be treated differently. Relationship issues or information that has been concealed from the sexual partner may play a role in shaping the presenting problem. For example, a wife having an active sexual affair but no longer interested in her husband may be brought to treatment by the unknowing husband for sexual desire problems. These possibilities should be assessed carefully.

A. Major Etiologic Theories: There are multiple possible etiologies for hypoactive sexual desire disorder. Numerous medical, psychological, social, and interpersonal factors, singly or in combination, can result in the loss of sexual desire.

1. Psychological factors—If the predominant causal factors are psychological (the term here including social and interpersonal factors), or a combination of psychological and medical, the diagnosis is simply hypoactive sexual desire disorder. The experience of frequent "failures" in sexual interaction due to arousal or orgasm phase sexual dysfunction, accompanied by significant negative affect, will often result in a suppression of sexual desire. Painful intercourse can create the same dynamic. Lack of interest in or attraction to one's regular sexual partner, based on either physical or psychological factors, can lead to loss of sexual desire. Lack of attraction on a psychological basis may occur as a result of one or both partners having a separately diagnosed mental disorder, including personality disorders, which can seriously exacerbate marital conflict or place one or the other spouse in a prolonged caretaking role. Loss of libido is one of the prominent symptoms of depression, and depression should always be considered in any evaluation of the etiology of hypoactive sexual desire disorder (see Chapter 21). Persistent, strong, negative affect in a marital relationship can also lead to the disorder. Frequently this negative affect is anger, secondary to marital conflict; occasionally it may be guilt secondary to a previous or active extramarital affair or simply attraction to another person. Fear of pregnancy or sexually transmitted disease is sometimes causal. The inculcation of antisexual attitudes in childhood is a frequent though more remote etiologic factor. The residual effects of sexual trauma in childhood may adversely affect sexual desire, as may the occurrence of sexual trauma in adult life. Persistent pressure for sexual performance, which may result if there is an imbalance in sexual interest between the members of a couple, may result in hypoactive sexual desire disorder. An interesting special case arising from performance pressure is the loss of desire that sometimes occurs as a result of infertility treatment programs and the performance demands such programs often create on certain fertile days. Increasingly today people are leading lives associated with chronic high stress and fatigue, often secondary to career demands; this too can be a causal factor in the loss of sexual interest. Compulsive, pleasure-denying personality styles have also been observed in such patients. This list provides a flavor of the many psychosocial factors often found to be active in the etiology of hypoactive sexual desire disorder.

2. Medical factors—If hypoactive sexual desire disorder is judged to be exclusively the result of a specified medical condition the diagnosis is male or female hypoactive sexual desire disorder due to a medical condition (with the condition specified). In many cases, however, loss of desire is due to a combination of medical and psychological factors. Loss of interest in sex can often result simply from the debilitating effects of chronic illness and pain. As might be imagined, the number of medical conditions that can affect sexual interest in this manner is huge and includes chronic rheumatologic and pulmonary conditions, degenerative neurologic conditions, advanced malignancies, and cardiovascular, renal, orthopedic, and thyroid conditions. Any urologic or gynecologic condition that causes pain during intercourse can also result indirectly in loss of desire. Estrogen deficiency can be an indirect cause of loss of sexual interest in women as a result of changes in the female genitalia that make intercourse painful. Conditions causing hyperprolactinemia will result in a loss of sexual interest in both men and women. Testosterone plays a major role in the genesis of sexual desire in both sexes, and any medical condition that results in a substantial decrease in available testosterone in either gender will usually result in a loss of sexual interest and eventually a loss of function. Such conditions include traumatic injury to the testes, testicular atrophy, Klinefelter's syndrome, chemotherapy, pelvic radiation, bilateral oophorectomy, adrenalectomy, and Addison's disease. Although it is well established that androgens are a critical part of the physical substrate of sexual interest for both men and women, the very different normal ranges of circulating testosterone for men and women should be kept in mind for both diagnostic and treatment purposes.

3. Pharmacologic factors—Numerous medications and drugs used for recreation have the side effect of reducing sexual interest. If the loss of sexual desire can be explained fully by substance or medication use it will be diagnosed as substance-induced sexual dysfunction with impaired desire. Agents with clear antiandrogenic effects (eg, medroxyprogesterone acetate, cyproterone acetate) are sometimes used to decrease sex drive in sex offenders. Agents prescribed for other purposes (eg, flutamide, leuprolide acetate, and cytotoxic chemotherapeutic agents) can have similar effects. Among the antidepressants the selective serotonin reuptake inhibitors (SSRIs), tricyclic antidepressants (TCAs), and monoamine oxidase inhibitors (MAOIs) have all shown some negative impact on sexual interest, although in the case of depression, it is important diagnostically to separate the primary impact of depression in lowering libido from the possible effects of antidepressant agents. Some agents have what appear to be paradoxical dosage-related effects, in which low dosages tend to cause an increase in sexual interest whereas high dosages or chronic use will result in a loss of interest. These agents include alcohol, benzodiazepines, barbiturates, and stimulants such as cocaine or amphetamines. Narcotics appear to have a consistently negative effect on sexual desire. Many antihypertensive agents and β-blockers are frequently associated with decrements in sexual interest, and loss of interest has also been reported in association with many neuroleptics.

B. Epidemiology: There are no reliable data on the occurrence of hypoactive sexual desire disorder in the general population. It is clear, however, that it occurs with a significant frequency and that since the mid-1980s an increasing proportion of patients presenting for treatment of sexual dysfunction present with hypoactive sexual desire disorder. According to one estimate, approximately one third of patients presenting for such help had desire-related problems; the same author suggested that the incidence was likely to increase as the population aged.

C. Genetics: With the exception of infrequent syndromes in which genetic influences might result in endocrine dysregulation, genetic etiologies are not common in hypoactive sexual desire disorder.

Clinical Findings

A. Signs & Symptoms: Hypoactive sexual desire disorder is in many respects a subjectively defined entity. Usually the primary presenting feature is individual or couple dissatisfaction with the frequency of sexual activity. Relationship difficulties secondary to this dissatisfaction may also be apparent.

B. Psychological Testing: There appears to be little relationship between other psychopathology and hypoactive sexual desire disorder other than the observation that people with serious psychopathology often have a reduced frequency of sexual activity. Traditional psychological assessment is useful only in that it may uncover preexisting psychopathology (eg, serious depression, thought disorder, personality disorders) that could complicate treatment.

C. Laboratory Findings: Endocrine workups are useful in identifying those patients whose hypoactive sexual desire disorder has a hormonal etiology. The following battery may be useful: testosterone, bioavailable testosterone, prolactin, total estrogens, luteinizing hormone, follicle-stimulating hormone, and a thyroid profile (estradiol is substituted for estrogens in women).

Differential Diagnosis

The most important issues in the differential diagnosis are separating hypoactive sexual desire disorder with a psychogenic etiology from substance-induced hypoactive sexual desire disorder and hypoactive sexual desire disorder due to general medical conditions. These diagnoses indicate very different treatment approaches. These differentials are not simple, and combined etiologies are common. History can sometimes be definitive, as is often the case in situational loss of desire, but in many cases of global dysfunction endocrine factors must be ruled out through specific testing.

Treatment

Treatment must be grounded firmly in an understanding of etiology (Table 28–1). Hypoactive sexual desire disorder with an endocrine etiology is often treated successfully through hormone supplementation. The use of testosterone to treat the disorder in

Table 28–1. Treatment of hypoactive sexual desire disorder.

Etiology	Treatment
Psychological	Sex, couples, or individual psychotherapy, as indicated. Referral after medical factors have been ruled out or optimally treated.
Medical	Evaluation and appropriate treatment of any endocrine, urologic, or gynecologic factors related to decreased desire or coital pain. Optimal treatment of any generally debilitating medical condition.
Pharmacologic	Termination or adjustment of, or substitution for, any contributing pharmacologic agents. Abstinence from alcohol or other contributing nonprescription drugs.

patients with laboratory values clearly in the normal range is not generally recommended, although it may be useful for patients with values at the lower end of the range. In some situations, the medical condition that creates an endocrine imbalance can be treated successfully.

Hypoactive sexual desire disorder with a psychogenic or combined etiology is often amenable to psychotherapy with a therapist who is experienced and well trained in the treatment of sexual dysfunction. The precise direction of such treatment must be informed by an understanding of the specific causal factors in each case. The involvement of both members of a couple in treatment is often crucial; however, when childhood trauma or abuse, or even trauma later in life, is important in the etiology individual treatment may be necessary before couples therapy can proceed productively. Causal factors in desire phase disorders tend to be more complex and resistance to treatment more prominent than in arousal or orgasm phase disorders; treatment therefore tends to be longer and more difficult.

Sildenafil (Viagra) is expected to be of only marginal use in the treatment of male hypoactive sexual desire disorder, as it facilitates the physiologic process of erection in the presence of interest and desire but not desire itself. It may be of some benefit in selected cases in which the loss of desire is secondary to the emotional trauma of repeated erectile failure.

Complications, Comorbidity, & Adverse Outcomes

The administration of supplemental testosterone may carry some medical risks, particularly in men who have a history of certain carcinomas, and contraindications should be evaluated carefully. In psychotherapy, there is the risk of aggravating relationship or individual problems, particularly if one or both partners is emotionally fragile or has a personality disorder or other individual psychopathology.

Prognosis & Course of Illness

Prognosis and course are highly variable and dependent on the history and causal factors in each specific case. With appropriate treatment hormonally caused hypoactive sexual desire disorder has a favorable prognosis. Situational and acquired hypoactive sexual desire disorder tend to have a more favorable prognosis. Although generalized and lifelong subtypes can also be treated successfully, therapy tends to be more lengthy and complex. With couples in stable, committed relationships the nature of the relationship between the partners will have a significant impact on the prognosis and difficulty of therapy.

Crenshaw TL, Goldberg JP: *Sexual Pharmacology: Drugs That Affect Sexual Functioning.* WW Norton, 1996.
Kaplan HS: *The Sexual Desire Disorders: Dysfunctional Regulation of Sexual Motivation.* Brunner/Mazel, 1995.
Kolodny RC, Masters WH, Johnson VE: *Textbook of Sexual Medicine.* Little, Brown, 1979.
Leiblum SR, Rosen RC (editors): *Sexual Desire Disorders.* Guilford Press, 1988.
Wincze JP, Carey MP: *Sexual Dysfunction: A Guide for Assessment and Treatment.* Guilford Press, 1991.

2. SEXUAL AVERSION DISORDER

DSM-IV Diagnostic Criteria

A. Persistent or recurrent extreme aversion to, and avoidance of, all (or almost all) genital sexual contact with a sexual partner.

B. The disturbance causes marked distress or interpersonal difficulty.

C. The sexual dysfunction is not better accounted for by another Axis I disorder (except another sexual dysfunction).

Reprinted, with permission, from *Diagnostic and Statistical Manual of Mental Disorders,* 4th ed. Copyright 1994 American Psychiatric Association.

General Considerations

Whereas the defining feature of hypoactive sexual desire disorder is lack of sexual desire, the defining feature of sexual aversion disorder is aversion to and active avoidance of sexual situations, with accompanying fear and anxiety. The anxiety may be moderate to severe. The aversion may be to all sexual contact with a partner or to a particular aspect of sexual interaction (eg, kissing, touching and caressing, genital secretions, penetration, orgasm). It may be to a particular partner or all partners. Persons with sexual aversion disorder do not necessarily lack all sexual desire, although in many cases they do. If the aversion is directed toward a particular sexual experience, desire for other forms of sexual activity may remain. Patients with this disorder frequently develop an extensive array of avoidance behaviors to reduce the likelihood that they will be trapped into engaging in the feared sexual activity.

A. Major Etiologic Theories: Many of the same psychosocial factors active in the etiology of hypoactive sexual desire disorder have also been implicated in the etiology of sexual aversion disorder. Remote causal factors may include a rigid upbringing with strong antisexual messages from parents or significant subcultural groups, or sexual trauma in childhood. Sexual trauma later in life may also be a factor. Situational aversion, focused on particular forms of sexual activity or particular partners, can often be related to specific traumatic events. Sexual aversion disorder can be acquired during a relationship when a person with hypoactive sexual desire disorder or just relatively lower sexual interest is persistently pressured to perform sexually. It can also result when intercourse becomes associated with pain, either through one particularly powerful episode or when a person continues to have intercourse repeatedly despite significant pain. On some occasions the association of significant emotional pain (eg, guilt, embarrassment, humiliation) with intercourse can result in sexual aversion disorder. Chronic, unresolved anger in a relationship is a frequent causal factor.

No psychopharmacologic agents or general medical conditions are involved directly in the etiology of sexual aversion disorder, although any condition that contributes to hypoactive sexual desire disorder or painful intercourse could be involved indirectly. There is speculation that some people are biologically predisposed to high levels of anxiety and panic and that this predisposition in interaction with life experience (eg, instances of trauma) may be a major etiologic factor.

B. Epidemiology: There is little good information available about the epidemiology of sexual aversion disorder.

C. Genetics: Other than the involvement of genetic influences in a possible biological predisposition to high levels of anxiety and panic, there is little evidence for genetic involvement in the etiology of this disorder.

Clinical Findings

A. Signs & Symptoms: Avoidance of sexual behavior; associated extreme anxiety, even panic; and reports of fear and disgust relating to sexual behavior are symptoms of this disorder.

B. Psychological Testing: Traditional psychological testing is generally not useful in making this diagnosis, although it can be helpful in identifying co-existing psychopathology.

C. Laboratory Findings: Laboratory work is generally not useful in the diagnosis of this disorder.

Differential Diagnosis

If sexual aversion disorder is secondary to another Axis I disorder (eg, posttraumatic stress disorder) the diagnosis of sexual aversion disorder is not made unless the sexual problem is an independent focus of clinical attention. The disorder may coexist with and sometimes be secondary to other sexual dysfunctions (eg, female sexual arousal disorder), in which case both diagnoses are made. A thorough history provides the primary vehicle for the accurate diagnosis of this disorder.

Treatment

The optimal treatment for this disorder is generally psychotherapy with a therapist experienced and skilled in treating sexual dysfunction (Table 28–2). Care should be taken to evaluate and treat any medical condition that could be contributing to pain or discomfort during intercourse. If the patient is in a stable relationship, therapy will almost always involve both members of the couple at some point. Depending on the specific etiologic factors, some degree of individual treatment may be necessary before couples therapy can be productive. The therapy process almost always includes significant elements of psychosexual education and gradual in vivo exposure, in an anxiety-reducing context, to the specific feared objects or behaviors. The exposure process must be calibrated carefully. Some therapists have found antianxiety agents useful as a adjunctive tool in this phase of therapy.

Complications, Comorbidity, & Adverse Outcomes

There is some evidence that other anxiety disorders occur at a higher rate in patients diagnosed with sexual aversion disorder than in the general population. This makes intuitive sense if a biological predisposition to anxiety plays a causal role. It is important to tailor treatment to the individual, so as not to expose patients to situations that create counter-therapeutically high levels of anxiety or not to use arousal-enhancing techniques that are culturally or morally unacceptable to the patient.

Prognosis & Course of Illness

From a learning-theory perspective, sexual aversion disorder can be seen as a very stable disorder in that it is self-reinforcing; the avoidant behavior reduces anx-

Table 28–2. Treatment of sexual aversion disorder.

Etiology	Treatment
Psychological	Sex, couples, or individual psychotherapy, as indicated.
Medical	Appropriate treatment of any medical condition that could contribute to coital pain or discomfort or to decreased desire.
Pharmacologic	Termination or adjustment of, or substitution for, any prescription or nonprescription drugs that could contribute to coital pain or discomfort or to decreased desire.

iety and is therefore reinforced. There are no good data on the natural course of this disorder in the general population, but anecdotal evidence suggests that it can be quite resistant to change without intervention. With treatment the prognosis is good for the amelioration of the aversive and acute anxiety symptoms and less positive for the greater therapeutic success of movement toward positive sexual interest. Prognosis depends heavily on the specific causal factors involved in a particular case and on the nature of the patient's relationship with his or her sexual partner (if any). Without treatment this disorder can disrupt marital relationships and can lead to lives of social isolation and loneliness for those who are not married.

Kolodny RC, Masters WH, Johnson VE: *Textbook of Sexual Medicine.* Little, Brown, 1979.

Masters WH, Johnson VE: *Human Sexual Inadequacy.* Little, Brown, 1970.

SEXUAL AROUSAL DISORDERS

1. FEMALE SEXUAL AROUSAL DISORDER

DSM-IV Diagnostic Criteria

A. Persistent or recurrent inability to attain, or to maintain until completion of the sexual activity, an adequate lubrication-swelling response of sexual excitement.

B. The disturbance causes marked distress or interpersonal difficulty.

C. The sexual dysfunction is not better accounted for by another Axis I disorder (except another sexual dysfunction) and is not due exclusively to the direct physiological effects of a substance (eg, a drug of abuse, a medication) or a general medical condition.

Reprinted, with permission, from *Diagnostic and Statistical Manual of Mental Disorders,* 4th ed. Copyright 1994 American Psychiatric Association.

General Considerations

Female sexual arousal disorder is less studied and less well understood than its male counterpart, erectile disorder (described in the next section). The boundary between female sexual arousal disorder and female hypoactive sexual desire disorder can be somewhat blurred. Some authors suggest that women in general are less dramatically reactive to this disorder than men are to erectile failure, which many men view as catastrophic. In many settings, women still tend to be less subject to performance pressure than men are and manage this disorder through a variety of behaviors from sexual avoidance to the use of lubricants. However, women who persist in having intercourse with little arousal, particularly if intercourse becomes associated with pain because of inadequate lubrication, run the risk of progressing to hypoactive

sexual desire disorder or even sexual aversion disorder.

A. Major Etiologic Theories: Many psychological factors, medical conditions, and pharmacologic agents may contribute, either alone or in interaction, to the etiology of female sexual arousal disorder.

1. Psychological factors—If female sexual arousal disorder is judged to be due to psychological factors, or to the combined effects of psychological and organic factors, it is diagnosed simply as female sexual arousal disorder. Numerous psychosocial factors may be implicated in the etiology of this condition. In fact, any factor that produces strong negative affect in consistent association with efforts at sexual interaction will have a negative impact on arousal. One set of such factors may be related to a patient's current relationship. These include lack of sexual attraction and interest in the partner, anger and hostility toward the partner, and lack of sexual knowledge and/or poor sexual communication on the part of the couple, leading to stimulation that is not adequate to produce arousal. Chronic difficulty in achieving orgasm accompanied by strong negative affect can lead to arousal difficulty. Major depression can clearly impact female sexual arousal. More remote factors include those previously mentioned for hypoactive sexual desire disorder and sexual aversion disorder: a history of sexual abuse or trauma in childhood or adulthood and a rigid upbringing with strong antisexual messages.

Despite the number of medical conditions and pharmacologic agents described in the next two sections, the general consensus is that female arousal is more robust to the impact of such factors than is arousal (erection) in the male and that most cases of female sexual arousal disorder have a psychogenic etiology.

2. Medical factors—If the arousal disorder is judged to be explained fully by a medical condition, it is referred to as other female sexual dysfunction due to a medical condition (with the condition specified). Comparatively little is known about the etiologic role of pharmacologic agents and medical conditions in female sexual arousal disorder. Any condition that causes chronic general debility and fatigue could play an indirect causal role. Any condition that results in atrophic vaginitis and associated coital pain could also be an indirect causal factor. Most commonly such vaginitis would result from an estrogen-deficiency state that could be secondary to menopause, lactation, surgical removal of the ovaries, chemotherapy, or radiation. Androgen-deficiency states, which also have multiple possible causes, can impair arousal, desire, and orgasm in women. Medical conditions that affect the neurologic substrate of sexual function and impair arousal in males may have a similar effect in women. These conditions include diabetes, multiple sclerosis, alcoholic neuropathy, head trauma or cerebrovascular accident affecting the areas of the brain important to sexual function, and other disorders affecting the spinal cord. Vascular conditions resulting in occlusion of the pelvic blood vessels could play a role.

3. Pharmacologic factors—If the arousal disorder is judged to be explained fully by substance use, it is referred to as substance-induced sexual dysfunction with impaired arousal. Antihistamines, ephedrine, anticholinergic drugs, and some antipsychotics may affect female arousal by lessening lubrication. Antihypertensives may have an impact, as may any agent that reduces androgens. Recreational drugs implicated in loss of sexual desire may also have a primary or indirect impact on sexual arousal. Chemotherapy administered as treatment for malignancy may also lead to difficulty with sexual arousal.

B. Epidemiology: There is little good epidemiologic information regarding female sexual arousal disorder, which for many years was grouped for research purposes with female hypoactive sexual desire disorder or anorgasmia.

C. Genetics: Except for rather rare genetically influenced disease states that affect endocrine function, genetic factors appear to play little role in female sexual arousal disorder.

Clinical Findings

A. Signs & Symptoms: The diagnosis is based primarily on the subjective report of lack of sexual arousal in a seemingly conducive setting. Centers with the equipment necessary to directly measure female sexual arousal are rare.

B. Psychological Testing: The diagnosis of female sexual arousal disorder does not imply the existence of any other psychopathology. Psychological testing is not useful in establishing the diagnosis but may play a role in identifying coexisting psychopathology that could affect treatment.

C. Laboratory Findings: Any laboratory testing to establish the diagnosis of a causally related medical condition is useful. The endocrine workup described in the discussion of hypoactive sexual desire disorder would be helpful in identifying cases in which hormonal factors are etiologically important.

Differential Diagnosis

Separating disorders of female sexual arousal due to medical conditions or pharmacologic agents exclusively from those due primarily to psychological factors or a combined etiology is important because of treatment implications. In the design of a treatment program an understanding of the roles of hypoactive sexual desire disorder, female sexual arousal disorder, and anorgasmia is important. These disorders may coexist and may be causally related. In most cases, this differential can be established by history.

Treatment

If a general medical condition is implicated as a primary factor in the etiology, treatment of that condition

Table 28–3. Treatment of femal sexual arousal disorder.

Etiology	Treatment
Psychological	Sex, couples, or individual psychotherapy, as indicated.
Medical	Appropriate treatment of any medical condition that could contribute to coital discomfort, decreased desire, or impaired vasocongestion or lubrication. Treatment may include hormone supplementation or vaginal creams or lubricants.
Pharmacologic	Termination or adjustment of, or substitution for, any prescription or nonprescription drugs that could contribute to coital discomfort, decreased desire, or impaired vasocongestion or lubrication.

should be the primary focus (Table 28–3). Fortunately, estrogen-deficiency states can often be treated effectively, either through systemic hormone replacement or through the local application of estrogen-containing creams or suppositories. If estrogen is absolutely contraindicated, other vaginal creams and lubricants may be helpful. Androgen can also be replaced if needed. If the disorder is substance induced, discontinuation of the suspected agent if possible, or switching to an alternative agent if a medication is part of a necessary treatment program, can often be helpful.

Psychotherapy with a therapist experienced and well trained in the treatment of sexual dysfunction is the approach of choice for disorders with primarily psychogenic or combined etiology. If the patient is in a committed relationship, therapy will at some point involve both members of the couple. Therapeutic techniques may involve exploratory therapy to identify and work through reactions to traumatic events, psychosexual education, arousal-enhancing imagery and fantasy, masturbatory exercises, and anxiety-reducing sensate focus exercises as suggested by Masters and Johnson and Kaplan.

Since the 1998 release of sildenafil as a treatment of male sexual arousal problems there has been speculation about its effectiveness as a treatment for arousal problems in women. Ongoing research is examining this question, but as of this writing no definitive results have been released.

Complications, Comorbidity, & Adverse Outcomes

There are few common comorbidities with female sexual arousal disorder except for those physical conditions that are responsible etiologically for some presenting cases (see "Major Etiologic Theories" section). Other sexual dysfunctions (eg, anorgasmia, hypoactive sexual desire disorder) may coexist with female sexual arousal disorder. Lack of caution in the use of estrogen replacement could lead to an increased risk of cancer in the estrogen-sensitive organs. With psychotherapy, there is always some risk of exacerbating relationship problems or preexisting individual psychopathology.

Prognosis & Course of Illness

There is little information as to the natural course of untreated female sexual arousal disorder in the general population. Experience suggests that it is highly variable, with remission occurring in some patients, a constant but rather benign course in others, and a progression to hypoactive sexual desire disorder or sexual aversion disorder occurring in still others, particularly when persistent pressure for sexual activity is present. The latter course may be accompanied by disturbance in marital or other sexual relationships.

Crenshaw TL, Goldberg JP: *Sexual Pharmacology: Drugs That Affect Sexual Functioning.* WW Norton, 1996.

Tollison CD, Adams HE: *Sexual Disorders: Treatment, Theory, Research.* Gardner, 1979.

2. MALE ERECTILE DISORDER

DSM-IV Diagnostic Criteria

A. Persistent or recurrent inability to attain, or to maintain until completion of the sexual activity, an adequate erection.

B. The disturbance causes marked distress or interpersonal difficulty.

C. The sexual dysfunction is not better accounted for by another Axis I disorder (except another sexual dysfunction) and is not due exclusively to the direct physiological effects of a substance (eg, a drug of abuse, a medication) or a general medical condition.

Reprinted, with permission, from *Diagnostic and Statistical Manual of Mental Disorders,* 4th ed. Copyright 1994 American Psychiatric Association.

General Considerations

Male erectile disorder is the male counterpart of female sexual arousal disorder. Other terms for this disorder are erectile dysfunction, erectile incompetence, and impotence. The latter term is preferentially used by urologists but carries a pejorative connotation that has led the mental health field in the direction of other terminology. There is wide variation in the presentation of male erectile disorder. At one extreme are men who report never, under any circumstances, having attained an erection sufficient for intercourse. This dysfunction would be described with the specifiers *generalized* and *lifelong* and would suggest a difficult treatment course. At the other extreme are men who have a history of globally good function but now cannot function with a particular sexual partner, although they perform well in all other circumstances. This dysfunction is described as *acquired* and *situational;*

the cause is probably to be found in the circumstances surrounding the problematic relationship. Some men experience a gradual onset of erectile difficulty, whereas others experience a sudden onset, with a well-remembered traumatic experience. Some can attain erections and function well during masturbation but cannot become erect in the presence of an intended partner. Some do achieve erections with their partners, but lose them before penetration or during thrusting before orgasm. Each of these particular patterns has etiologic, prognostic, and treatment significance.

In modern American culture, as in many others, men experience a strong demand for sexual performance. Sexual function, usually seen as synonymous with erection, is a critical element in the male cultural role. Perhaps because of this, men in general have a tendency to react with strong negative affect to instances of erectile failure. The emotions and thoughts men have described include anger, depression, anxiety, embarrassment, humiliation, feelings of worthlessness, focused anxiety about failure and sexual performance, and even suicidal ideation. This strong emotional reaction often complicates the clinical picture and may be instrumental in converting a single episode of erectile difficulty into a chronic disorder.

Male erectile disorder is probably the most thoroughly researched of all the sexual dysfunctions.

A. Major Etiologic Theories: When sexual dysfunction first became the subject of widespread clinical and scientific interest in the early 1970s, following the publication of Masters and Johnson's pioneering work, it was assumed, but with little good evidence, that approximately 90% of all erectile disorders had a psychogenic etiology. Since that time great strides have been made in understanding the anatomy and physiology underlying the erectile response. Now the contrary assumption is made, that most erectile disorders have an organic etiology, but there is still little good population incidence data to support either position on this issue. The typical case of male erectile disorder may involve a complex of two or more psychological, medical, pharmacologic, or situational factors in an interactive etiology.

1. Psychological factors—If the etiology of the male erectile disorder is judged to be predominantly psychogenic, or due to an interaction of psychogenic and organic factors, it is diagnosed as male erectile disorder. Numerous psychosocial and situational factors (eg, anger at a partner, stress, fatigue, excessive alcohol consumption) can lead to an occasional episode of erectile failure. Psychogenic male erectile disorder develops when the erectile failure becomes persistent and recurrent. This usually occurs when isolated episodes of failure lead to a generalized loss of confidence in sexual performance and an expectation of failure.

In many men, the negative affect associated with the inability to attain an erection in a sexual situation is so strong that this expectation of failure leads to a persistent performance anxiety associated with any demand for sexual function. This anxiety, through mechanisms not entirely understood, interferes repeatedly with effective erectile function, leading to a self-reinforcing cycle of failure, performance anxiety, and failure. Performance anxiety is almost universally the proximal cause in psychogenic male erectile disorder; however, there are several layers of potential casual factors.

The immediate psychosocial and situational factors associated with the initial failures that began the pattern may be quite varied, and their identification, if possible, is important for treatment purposes. Relationship issues and a couple's style of communication about sexual issues and expectations may play an important role in creating or maintaining psychogenic male erectile disorder. In addition, developmental factors in childhood or later sexually related trauma can play a role in creating a vulnerability for the onset of psychogenic male erectile disorder in the context of particular life events. These factors are too numerous to list exhaustively and may include most of those discussed in relation to other sexual dysfunctions. A few of the possible more remote, causal factors include extremely negative and restrictive attitudes toward sexuality inculcated at an early age, a history of childhood sexual abuse or trauma, fear of personal intimacy, and a primarily homoerotic or paraphilic sexual orientation. These remote causes are often best conceptualized within a cognitive-behavioral or psychodynamic framework.

2. Medical factors—If the disorder is judged to be explained fully by the effects of a medical condition, the diagnosis will be male erectile disorder due to a medical condition (with the condition specified). Multiple organic conditions can interfere with effective erectile function. Endocrine imbalance (eg, testosterone deficiency, severe hyperprolactinemia) can be an important factor but accounts for only a small proportion of cases. Vascular and neurologic etiologies are much more common. On one level, erection is a hemodynamic phenomenon. Any condition that impairs arterial flow into the penis, or seriously enhances venous flow out of the penis, can play a role. Arteriosclerosis affecting the central pelvic arteries or the finer arteries providing blood to the penis directly is a common causal factor. Excessive outflow of blood from the penis through an imprecisely understood process referred to as "venous leak" can interfere with the maintenance of erection, even if arterial flow is sufficient.

Any factor that impairs neurologic control over the structures involved in the erectile process can also cause male erectile disorder. Neurogenic causes can exist at the level of the cerebral hemispheres, the spinal cord, or the peripheral nervous system. Stroke, multiple sclerosis, traumatic nervous system injury, and peripheral neuropathy are potential neurogenic

causal factors. Diabetes is one of the medical conditions most commonly implicated in the etiology of male erectile disorder. It probably impairs erectile function through two mechanisms: peripheral neuropathy and vascular deterioration.

3. Pharmacologic factors—If the dysfunction is explained fully by substance use the diagnosis is substance-induced sexual dysfunction with impaired arousal. Numerous agents have an effect on erectile function. Both acute and chronic alcohol use have negative effects. With acute use, although the user may initially report an enhanced ability to become aroused with increasing blood levels, there is a clear, dose-related, negative impact on erectile function. Chronic use leads to an increased incidence of male erectile disorder, probably through the mechanisms of peripheral neuropathy and impaired endocrine function. The reversibility of these effects is unclear. Nicotine is a vasoconstrictor that has a negative impact on erectile function. Narcotic addiction is associated with an increased incidence of male erectile disorder. Cocaine and amphetamine use acutely and in the initial stages are reported to serve as sexual stimulants but at increased dosages are associated with male erectile disorder. The disorder is a potential side effect of many antihypertensive agents, but this effect is highly variable and individual, and it may be difficult to determine if a particular agent is the responsible factor in a specific patient.

Cimetidine has a well-established association with male erectile disorder. In the realm of psychoactive agents, a number of antipsychotics have been associated with male erectile disorder, probably through the mechanism of dopamine blockade; however, other agents (eg, haloperidol) are infrequently associated with such problems. Lithium has a more frequently reported association with male erectile disorder than does carbamazepine. Although particular agents differ significantly in the reported frequency of male erectile disorder as a side effect, there is an association between male erectile disorder and both the TCAs and the MAOIs. There have been reports of an increased incidence of male erectile disorder with SSRI use, but the effects of this class of agents are much more dramatic in other areas of sexual function. Trazodone has peculiar effects. It has been reported to increase sexual interest and to enhance erection; its most common serious sexual side effect is priapism (prolonged erection), as opposed to male erectile disorder.

B. Epidemiology: A cursory review of a newspaper in any major metropolitan area will reveal a plethora of advertisements for "Impotence Treatment Centers," suggesting that the problem is ubiquitous. As with most sexual problems, the collection of accurate population data is fraught with difficulty, and estimates of the prevalence of male erectile disorder vary widely. It is generally accepted that the prevalence increases with age, not so much as a result of normal aging but secondary to the concomitantly increasing incidence of medical conditions and psychosocial factors that affect erectile function. A prevalence of 4–9% has been reported from community surveys. It has been reliably reported that male erectile disorder is the most frequent presenting complaint at sex therapy clinics, with the proportion ranging from 35% to 53%. Up to 50% of men might experience significant erectile difficulty, either transient or persistent, at some point in their lives. Acquired male erectile disorder is far more common than is the lifelong type. Lifelong male erectile disorder is usually of psychogenic etiology, but it can also result from congenital medical conditions, usually those involving serious endocrine disturbance.

C. Genetics: Except in the case of relatively rare disease states that affect endocrine function, genetic factors play little direct role in the etiology of male erectile disorder. Hypothetically, genetic factors influencing more general affective tendencies, particularly any such factors leading to enhanced general levels of anxiety, could play an indirect etiologic role.

Clinical Findings

A. Signs & Symptoms: The diagnosis is based primarily on the patient's or his partner's report of lack of adequate erectile function in a seemingly conducive setting.

B. Psychological Testing: A diagnosis of male erectile disorder does not imply the existence of any other psychopathology. Traditional psychological testing is not useful in establishing the diagnosis but may be helpful in identifying any coexisting psychopathology that could affect treatment.

C. Laboratory Findings: Multiple assessment techniques have been developed that can be useful in investigating possible etiologies. Hormone levels including serum testosterone, luteinizing hormone, and prolactin and thyroid function tests are useful in detecting the small proportion of erectile disorders due to endocrine abnormalities. Screening for diabetes will help detect the small number of patients for whom erectile dysfunction is the initial presenting symptom of that illness.

Further laboratory assessment becomes increasingly complex and expensive. Nocturnal penile tumescence measurement can be useful in differentiating organic and psychogenic etiologies but to be done properly requires referral to a fully equipped sleep laboratory. A number of procedures can be used to evaluate vascular function including trial injections of vasodilators (eg, papaverine), Doppler ultrasound, and penile cavernosography. There are no neurologic tests currently available to evaluate the innervation of the penile corpora, but other neurologic assessment techniques to evaluate the innervation of the pelvic, bladder, and genital areas can contribute useful information. Some of these evaluation procedures can be expensive; they should be used judiciously and are best performed by a specialist (eg, urologist, vascular surgeon, neurologist) who has an interest in the assessment and treatment of erectile dysfunction.

Differential Diagnosis

The differential between male erectile disorder that is primarily psychogenic, primarily due to a general medical condition, or primarily due to substance use is important in that it has significant treatment implications. For example, it is unwise to use an irreversible invasive treatment in a patient with a primarily psychogenic problem, unless the problem is recalcitrant to less invasive procedures. Often a thorough psychosexual and medical history is sufficient to establish etiology. For example, a relatively young, healthy man who is capable of a good erection in nondemanding situations but cannot attain one when attempting intercourse almost certainly has a psychogenic problem. Similarly, a man with insulin-dependent diabetes mellitus diagnosed 20 years earlier who has experienced a gradual decline in erectile function over 10 years almost certainly has male erectile disorder due to medical factors. If history alone is not sufficient some of the laboratory procedures referred to in the "Laboratory Findings" section may be useful. It is also important to assess for the presence of other sexual dysfunctions, as the performance anxiety that usually underlies psychogenic male erectile disorder can be secondary to repeated sexual distress due to premature ejaculation or inhibited ejaculation, or to sexual pressures exerted on a man with hypoactive sexual desire disorder. Coexisting mental disorders (eg, severe depression, personality disorder), which could have causal implications or significantly affect treatment, should also be assessed.

Treatment

Since its introduction in the spring of 1998, sildenafil has become a major treatment option for erectile dysfunction (Table 28–4). Sildenafil works by inhibiting the action of the enzyme phosphodiesterase-5 (PDE5), which itself breaks down guanosine monophosphate, critical to the enhancement of penile blood flow during erection. By exerting its influence so selectively on a step of the natural process, sildenafil enhances erection under conditions of sexual interest, arousal, and stimulation and allows the erection to detumesce when the conditions have resolved. Sildenafil appears to be most effective in men with mild to moderate psychogenic erectile disorder, in whom no organic etiology has been demonstrated, but it is clearly also effective in some cases of erectile disorder with organic etiology. In contrast, sildenafil does not enhance sexual desire, and it obviously does not resolve complex relational difficulties, which are important in maintaining some cases of erectile disorder.

Despite the "breakthrough" success of sildenafil, it is not the treatment of choice or the sole treatment for all cases of erectile disorder. Appropriate treatment

Table 28–4. Treatment of male erectile disorder.

Etiology	Treatment
Psychological	Trial of sildenafil. Sex, couples, or individual psychotherapy, as indicated.
Medical	
Endocrine	Hormone regulation.
Other treatable medical causes	Appropriate treatment of contributing medical conditions. Trial of sildenafil.
Medical etiology not responsive to other treatments	Vacuum devices, vasodilators (injection or suppository), or penile prosthesis implantation.
Pharmacologic	Termination or adjustment of any contributing prescription medications. Trial of sildenafil if not contraindicated. Abstinence from contributing over-the-counter or nonprescription drugs.

still flows from accurate diagnosis; all patients with erectile disorder should receive an evaluation for treatable causes. For many patients a thorough history is adequate; for others some of the evaluation procedures described in the preceding sections may be necessary.

Endocrine abnormalities can often be treated adequately with hormone replacement. If male erectile disorder is a result of substance abuse, that problem should be the initial focus of treatment. If the cause is a prescription drug, the first treatment approach should be an attempt to find substitute agents with the necessary therapeutic effect but without sexual side effects. Unfortunately, this is not possible in many cases (eg, severe hypertension treated with multiple agents).

Some medical conditions that lead to male erectile disorder can be treated directly with a resulting positive affect on sexual function, but again, in many cases organic changes are irreversible, and normal erectile function cannot be restored. Several treatment options are available for men with irreversible male erectile disorder, caused by medical problems or necessary pharmacologic agents, that does not respond to a trial of sildenafil. Externally applied vacuum devices create erections by using a pressure differential to pull blood into the penis and trap it there temporarily with a constriction ring. The self-injection of vasodilating drugs into the corpora cavernosa, at a properly titrated dose, will create a temporary erection in patients whose vascular systems are not severely compromised. Papaverine, phentolamine, and prostaglandin E, alone or in combination, are the agents most commonly used for this purpose.

A system with a similar mechanism, which delivers the active agents through a urethral suppository, has come on the market. The implantation of penile prostheses, which hold the penis sufficiently rigid for intercourse, is among the most invasive of treatments for male erectile disorder. There are several varieties of prostheses, ranging from relatively simple semi-

rigid rods to complex systems involving reservoirs of saline solution, a pump in the scrotum, and inflatable cylinders in the corpora. These surgical approaches are best accessed by referral to a urologist who has an interest in the treatment of male erectile disorder; none of them should be first-line treatments for male erectile disorder with a psychogenic etiology, in view of the success rates achieved by both sildenafil and psychological treatment. Revascularization procedures to restore blood supply to the penis in patients in whom this has been seriously compromised, and procedures to correct problems with venous leakage, have been attempted more often. The success rates for these procedures are unclear.

When the etiology is psychogenic or psychogenic factors play a major role in a combined etiology, short-term use of sildenafil may alleviate performance anxiety sufficiently to completely resolve the erectile disorder. In other such cases, psychotherapy with a therapist well-trained and experienced in the treatment of sexual dysfunction remains useful. Patients with moderate to severe erectile disorder that do not respond successfully to sildenafil may respond to an appropriate course of psychotherapy or to psychotherapy combined with sildenafil. In other patients sildenafil may immediately relieve the erectile dysfunction, but normal function without medication remains problematic. In such patients psychotherapy may be useful in moving to successful, medication-free sexual function.

In still other patients, difficult relationship issues, treatable by therapy but not medication, may be a major obstacle to the resumption of satisfactory erectile function. When possible, therapy will involve both members of a committed couple. The major task of therapy is to help the couple create an emotional context for their sexual interaction that does not involve pressure, expectation of failure, or performance anxiety. The sensate focus procedures initially elaborated by Masters and Johnson, and later by Kaplan and others, are almost always part of the treatment process.

Relationship or individual intrapsychic issues that must be addressed before sexual function can be confidently restored are integrated into the process to the degree necessary to achieve treatment goals. Couples therapy, cognitive-behavioral therapy, and psychodynamic modalities may be used in addressing such issues.

The good news today for patients with male erectile disorder is that a multitude of treatment approaches are available and that most cases can be treated successfully if the patient is persistent and strongly motivated.

Complications, Comorbidity, & Adverse Outcomes

Frequent comorbidities with male erectile disorder are the general medical conditions that can contribute to its etiology, for example, diabetes, vascular disease, neuropathy, and much more rarely endocrine dysfunction. From the psychological perspective, depression, loss of self-esteem, and relationship disruption often coexist with erectile disorder.

Sildenafil may lead to significant loss of blood pressure in men taking nitroglycerin and should not be prescribed for such patients.

Patients whose erectile disorder is treated with medical-surgical procedures are subject to multiple potential complications. We discuss a few of the more common ones here. Even the vacuum device, which is quite benign, can lead to hematoma; the injection process by some reports to Peyronie's disease and certainly to priapism if dosage limits are not observed; and the surgical procedures to infection and, if the more complex prostheses are implanted, to device failure.

Psychotherapy also has the potential for adverse outcome. In this format relationship problems or pre-existing individual psychopathology could be exacerbated.

Prognosis & Course of Illness

The natural course of untreated male erectile disorder in the general population will be variable because of the heterogeneity of its etiology. Although there is little good research on untreated outcomes, it is likely that some cases of psychogenic male erectile disorder will spontaneously remit, whereas others will become more deep seated and well established, but the relevant proportions are unknown. Erectile disorder with organic etiology is less likely to show spontaneous remission.

Crenshaw TL, Goldberg JP: *Sexual Pharmacology: Drugs That Affect Sexual Functioning.* WW Norton, 1996.

Masters WH, Johnson VE: *Human Sexual Inadequacy.* Little, Brown, 1970.

Rosen RC, Leiblum SR (editors): *Erectile Disorders: Assessment and Treatment.* Guilford Press, 1992.

Wincze JP, Carey MP: *Sexual Dysfunction: A Guide for Assessment and Treatment.* Guilford Press, 1991.

ORGASMIC DISORDERS

1. FEMALE ORGASMIC DISORDER

DSM-IV Diagnostic Criteria

A. Persistent or recurrent delay in, or absence of, orgasm following a normal sexual excitement phase. Women exhibit wide variability in the type or intensity of stimulation that triggers orgasm. The diagnosis of female orgasmic disorder should be based on the clinician's judgment that the woman's orgasmic capacity is less than would be reasonable for her age, sexual experience, and the adequacy of sexual stimulation she receives.
B. The disturbance causes marked distress or interpersonal difficulty.
C. The orgasmic dysfunction is not better accounted for by another Axis I disorder (except another sexual dysfunction) and is not due exclusively to the direct physiological effects of a substance (eg, a drug of abuse, a medication) or a general medical condition.

Reprinted, with permission, from *Diagnostic and Statistical Manual of Mental Disorders,* 4th ed. Copyright 1994 American Psychiatric Association.

General Considerations

Female orgasmic disorder has previously been referred to as inhibited female orgasm, anorgasmia, and frigidity. It may be lifelong or acquired, generalized or situational. The lifelong type is usually generalized, whereas the acquired type may be either generalized or situational. There are many women who are not orgasmic with the penile thrusting of intercourse alone but are orgasmic under other circumstances. These women, in general, do not meet the criteria for this diagnosis; it is assumed that either for reasons of anatomical arrangement or because of sexual behavior patterns, they do not receive the stimulation needed to reach orgasm through intercourse. Nonetheless, women or couples with this problem, also known as coital anorgasmia, may be helped to achieve orgasm during intercourse through sex therapy, if that is a significant goal.

A. Major Etiologic Theories: Etiologic considerations may be grouped into psychological, medical, and pharmacologic categories.

1. Psychological factors—If female orgasmic disorder is judged to be due to psychological factors, or to the combined effects of psychological and organic factors, it is diagnosed simply as female orgasmic disorder. There are few clearly demonstrated connections between historical psychosocial events and female orgasmic disorder; however, the same psychosocial factors found in the histories of women with other sexual dysfunctions tend to be found in the histories of these women but to a milder extent. A common immediate psychological factor is obsessive self-observation while trying to achieve orgasm. Another common cause is the failure, perhaps through lack of knowledge or experience, to receive adequate clitoral stimulation. A personality style with strong needs for control and difficulty in "letting go" is often found in anorgasmic women. Serious psychological problems such as major depression may also negatively affect female orgasm.

2. Medical factors—If the orgasmic disorder is determined to be due exclusively to the effects of a medical condition, the diagnosis would be other female sexual dysfunction due to a medical condition (with the condition specified). Organically based orgasm disorders are rare in healthy women, and almost all lifelong disorders appear to be psychogenic; however, a number of injuries and illness—including neurologic disorders affecting the spinal cord or peripheral pelvic innervation (eg, alcoholic neuropathy, multiple sclerosis, diabetes mellitus, severe malnutrition and vitamin deficiency, amyotrophic lateral sclerosis, and polio)—can impair female orgasm. Traumatic or surgical injuries to the spinal cord or peripheral nerves can cause similar problems. Liver and renal disease appear to negatively affect female orgasm, as do endocrine disorders resulting in testosterone deficiency and thyroid deficiency.

3. Pharmacologic factors—If the disorder is judged to be explained fully by substance use it is referred to as substance-induced sexual dysfunction with impaired orgasm. A number of street drugs and prescription medications have the potential to impair female orgasm. Although low doses of alcohol are associated with positive sexual feelings, a higher rate of orgasmic dysfunction has been associated reliably with chronic heavy usage. High doses of opiates, barbiturates, and benzodiazepines may inhibit female orgasm, whereas more normal usage will not. TCAs and MAOIs are clearly related to impaired female orgasm, and orgasmic delay is one of the more commonly known side effects of the SSRIs. A reduced orgasmic response has also been reliably reported in association with some neuroleptics and antihypertensives (but not the diuretics).

B. Epidemiology: As with all of the sexual dysfunctions, accurate population data are difficult to acquire. Female orgasmic disorder is generally reported to be the most common of the disorders occurring among women presenting at sex therapy centers for treatment. A number of community studies have suggested a rate of 5–10% for lifelong female orgasmic disorder in the general population.

C. Genetics: Except for relatively rare genetically influenced disease states that affect endocrine function or pelvic anatomy, genetic factors appear to play little role in female orgasmic disorder.

Clinical Findings

A. Signs & Symptoms: The diagnosis is based primarily on the subjective report of recurrent absence of orgasm in a context in which the clinician would judge stimulation to be adequate.

B. Psychological Testing: Female orgasmic disorder does not imply the existence of any other psychopathology. Psychological testing is not useful in establishing the diagnosis but may play a role in identifying coexisting psychopathology that could affect treatment.

C. Laboratory Findings: A variety of laboratory tests may be useful in establishing the existence of a causally related medical condition. Such conditions are usually either neurologic or endocrine. Evaluation of possible testosterone or thyroid deficiency states is important.

Differential Diagnosis

It is important to separate cases of female orgasmic disorder with a primarily medical or pharmacologic etiology from the majority of cases with a psychogenic etiology. It is also important to be aware of the possibility of coexisting sexual dysfunctions. A woman who becomes increasingly frustrated and upset because of a lack of orgasm may develop female sexual arousal disorder or hypoactive sexual desire disorder, which would need to be considered in treatment planning. In some patients, lack of orgasm may be best accounted for by another Axis I disorder (eg, major depression), in which case the diagnosis of female orgasmic disorder is usually not made and the depression should be the initial focus of treatment. Again, a careful history is critical for accurate diagnosis.

Treatment

If female orgasmic disorder is due to a medical condition, that condition should be the initial focus of treatment (Table 28–5). Education of the patient about the sexual impact of the illness is useful. If lack of orgasm is secondary to prescription medications, equally efficacious substitutes should be sought, because sexual side effects, if not addressed, often lead to noncompliance. If the problem is due to ongoing drug or alcohol abuse, that problem area should be the initial focus of treatment.

Psychogenic female orgasmic disorder is best treated through referral to a psychotherapist who is

Table 28–5. Treatment of female orgasmic disorder.

Etiology	Treatment
Psychological	Sex, couples, or individual psychotherapy, as indicated.
Medical	Appropriate treatment of contributing medical conditions. Education regarding the impact of relevant medical conditions on sexuality. Hormone regulation, if indicated.
Pharmacologic	Termination or adjustment of any contributing prescription medications. Abstinence from alcohol or other contributing nonprescription drugs.

well trained and experienced in the treatment of sexual dysfunction. If the disorder is lifelong, the treatment of choice usually involves psychosexual education and guided masturbatory practice. The success rate is very good under these circumstances (80–90%). Self-help manuals are useful supplements to this process. If the orgasmic disorder is acquired or situational, and is not due to a medical problem or pharmacologic agent, the causal factors probably involve relationship issues or recent sexual trauma. Therapy would involve both members of the affected couple, if possible, and would utilize dynamic, cognitive-behavioral, or systems approaches, as well as directed sensate focus exercises to decrease sexually related anxiety. The success rate in treating the acquired type, while still good, is not as high as for the lifelong type. Couples therapy is also useful as a part of the treatment of the lifelong type, helping integrate the orgasmic response into the couple's sexual repertoire once it has been achieved initially through masturbatory practice.

Complications, Comorbidity, & Adverse Outcomes

Female orgasmic disorder can lead to marital dissatisfaction. In some women, the frustration of repeated arousal with no orgasmic release eventually results in secondary female sexual arousal disorder or hypoactive sexual desire disorder. Psychotherapy can have adverse outcomes, usually the exacerbation of either preexisting individual psychopathology or marital distress. The patient may reject the suggestion of masturbatory exercises, if consideration has not been given to the congruence of this procedure with the patient's preestablished sexual value system.

Prognosis & Course of Illness

As with most of the sexual dysfunctions, little data are available regarding the natural course of untreated female orgasmic disorder. It seems likely that some cases of the acquired type would remit spontaneously and that fewer cases of the lifelong type would also. The lifelong type has an excellent prognosis with treatment but an uncertain prognosis without.

Crenshaw TL, Goldberg JP: *Sexual Pharmacology: Drugs That Affect Sexual Functioning.* WW Norton, 1996.

Heiman JR, LoPiccolo J: *Becoming Orgasmic: A Sexual and Personal Growth Program for Women,* revised and expanded ed. Simon & Schuster, 1988.

Kaplan HS (editor): *The Evaluation of Sexual Disorders: Psychological and Medical Aspects.* Brunner/Mazel, 1983.

2. MALE ORGASMIC DISORDER

DSM-IV Diagnostic Criteria

A. Persistent or recurrent delay in, or absence of, orgasm following a normal sexual excitement phase during sexual activity that the clinician, taking into account the person's age, judges to be adequate in focus, intensity, and duration.

B. The disturbance causes marked distress or interpersonal difficulty.

C. The orgasmic dysfunction is not better accounted for by another Axis I disorder (except another sexual dysfunction) and is not due exclusively to the direct physiological effects of a substance (eg, a drug of abuse, a medication) or a general medical condition.

Reprinted, with permission, from *Diagnostic and Statistical Manual of Mental Disorders,* 4th ed. Copyright 1994 American Psychiatric Association.

General Considerations

Male orgasmic disorder has previously been referred to as retarded ejaculation, ejaculatory incompetence, ejaculatory inhibition, and inhibited orgasm. As with the other sexual dysfunctions it is subject to the specifiers *lifelong* or *acquired, generalized* or *situational,* and *due to psychological factors* or *due to combined factors.* Patients with male orgasmic disorder are typically able to have firm erections and to achieve penetration. They then often report periods of intercourse sometimes extending into hours, without orgasm. They may report a high sex drive. These patients often come to treatment because of a frustrated desire for pregnancy on their own or their partner's part. Some patients have concealed the lack of orgasm from their sexual partner. Occasionally the female partner has even become the object of infertility evaluation and treatment. This may result in significant marital distress when the truth is revealed. Such cases tend to occur in populations in which access to information about sexuality has been restricted for religious or cultural reasons. Many men with male orgasmic disorder can achieve orgasm through oral or manual partner stimulation but not through intercourse. Others cannot reach orgasm through partner stimulation at all but can through masturbation. Only a very few experience orgasm solely through nocturnal emission, and fewer still absolutely no orgasm at all. The latter condition suggests an organic etiology.

A. Major Etiologic Theories: Patients with this condition present for treatment relatively infrequently. Perhaps consequently, there is no universally accepted mechanism for psychogenic causation, although it is believed that almost all cases of the lifelong type (exceptions being rare congenital disorders) are psychogenic, as are a fair proportion of the acquired type.

1. Psychological factors—If the etiology of orgasmic disorder is judged to be predominantly psychogenic, or due to an interaction of psychogenic and organic factors, the diagnosis is simply male orgasmic disorder. One view suggests that the primary immediate psychological cause of orgasmic failure may be obsessive self-observation focused on the issue of climax. This either prevents the patient from reaching the level of arousal necessary for orgasm or creates anxiety that through some unknown mechanism blocks the orgasmic response. The substrate that triggers orgasm is distinct from that underlying erection. Relationship or intrapsychic issues may serve as more remote factors in the causal process; these might include almost all of the issues involved in the remote causation of other male sexual dysfunctions. For this disorder, Kaplan (1983, p. 218) suggested that issues of ambivalence and anger toward women, and "fears of intimacy, commitment, and pleasure," may be particularly common. A contrasting view is that the patient does not receive adequate stimulation to achieve orgasm during intercourse because he has an erotic preference for his own touch (masturbation) as opposed to sex with a partner. Others have noted more superficially straightforward causes including fear of pregnancy, repeated use of ejaculatory delay as a contraceptive method, and lack of adequate stimulation in the simple sense. Acquired, psychogenic, male orgasmic disorder can result from a serious psychosexual trauma or from relationship problems. Any psychological condition that reduces sexual interest (eg, depression) may also impair orgasmic function.

2. Medical factors—If this dysfunction can be explained entirely by a medical condition the diagnosis is other male sexual dysfunction due to a medical condition (with the condition specified). Although the prevalence of impaired orgasm secondary to medical conditions is relatively low, a number of medical conditions can lead to such an outcome. Traumatic or surgically caused injury to the spinal cord and disease or tumor of the spinal cord affecting the pathways that mediate ejaculation, neuropathy, or surgical or traumatic injury of the peripheral nerves underlying orgasm may all result in male orgasmic disorder. Multiple sclerosis, diabetes, alcoholism, and Parkinson's disease are other disease states that could be implicated. Neurologic conditions that impair sensation in the penis could also be involved, as could severe endocrine abnormalities.

3. Pharmacologic factors—If the orgasmic impairment is entirely due to substance abuse the diagnosis is substance-induced sexual dysfunction with impaired orgasm. A number of recreational drugs and prescription medications can interfere with male orgasm. The SSRIs are a recent and flagrant example, but the MAOIs and TCAs also may have this side effect. Alcohol and opioids can clearly delay male orgasm, as can some neuroleptics and antihypertensives.

B. Epidemiology: It is generally agreed that male orgasmic disorder is the sexual dysfunction least encountered in clinical practice. Masters and Johnson reported that 17 out of the 448 cases of male sexual disorder treated at their clinic involved this disorder, a rate of approximately 3.8%. Estimates of prevalence in the general population range from 4% to 10%,

but the data suffer from the usual problems surrounding surveys of sexual behavior (ie, people tend to respond inaccurately to questions about sexual behavior and function or dysfunction, because the area is so highly private, personal, and strongly connected to self-esteem), and some authorities suggest the incidence is higher.

C. Genetics: Except for those cases in which male orgasmic disorder is secondary to a rare and severe congenital endocrine disorder, genetic factors have little direct role in the etiology of this dysfunction.

Clinical Findings

A. Signs & Symptoms: The diagnosis is based primarily on the patient's or his sexual partner's report of absence of ejaculation during coitus.

B. Psychological Testing: The diagnosis of male orgasmic disorder does not imply the existence of other psychopathology. Traditional psychological testing is not useful in establishing the diagnosis but may be helpful in identifying coexisting psychopathology that could affect treatment.

C. Laboratory Findings: The primary medical factors that could result in this condition are endocrine or neurologic. Hormone levels may identify those rare patients whose ejaculatory impairment is the result of an endocrine condition. Neurologic evaluation would be that appropriate for the suspected condition. It is useful to examine the patient for sensation in the pelvic and genital area and to question him about bowel and bladder control.

Differential Diagnosis

For treatment purposes, it is important to obtain a clear history, so as to accurately delineate both the characteristics of the disorder (eg, lifelong versus acquired) and the circumstances under which orgasm does occur. Male orgasmic disorder resulting from psychological or combined factors, for purposes of treatment, must be differentiated from that secondary to medical conditions or substance use. Several related disorders should be differentiated (eg, ejaculation without pleasurable sensation, orgasm with no discharge of semen, orgasm with leakage, or emission of semen but no forceful ejaculation). These disorders would be diagnosed as sexual dysfunction not otherwise specified.

Another condition to be differentiated from male orgasmic disorder is retrograde ejaculation. This occurs when the function of the internal urinary sphincter has been disrupted. During orgasm the ejaculate travels back into the bladder instead of being propelled through and out of the penis; the result is usually a sensation of orgasm without any seminal discharge. The causes of retrograde ejaculation are always organic, rarely diabetic neuropathy, but more usually as a side effect of thioridazine use or as a complication of prostate surgery.

Treatment

Male orgasmic disorder caused entirely by a medical condition can rarely be reversed, unless the causal condition is an infrequent endocrine disorder (Table 28–6). If the causal factor is a prescription medication, the situation should be discussed with the patient and alternative therapeutic agents sought. If the cause is drug or alcohol abuse the problem of abuse or dependence must be addressed first and any residual sexual dysfunction treated after the resolution of the primary problem. If the condition is due to psychogenic or combined factors, referral to a psychotherapist well trained and experienced in the treatment of sexual dysfunction is indicated. In cases of lifelong, psychogenic male orgasmic disorder of mild to moderate severity, the prognosis with treatment is excellent.

Treatment is far more likely to succeed if both members of a couple can be involved. The usual treatment approach involves starting with whatever sexual activity currently results in orgasm for the male, and from that point gradually involving the partner on an in vivo basis in graded exercises successively approximating orgasm inside the vagina. Severe cases may involve more therapeutic work on intrapsychic issues with dynamic or cognitive-behavioral approaches as well as the in vivo process; the outcome is also less clear. Acquired psychogenic male orgasmic disorder may also require a more complex treatment, involving more focus on current couple issues or the need to deal with the aftereffects of serious psychosexual trauma.

Complications, Comorbidity, & Adverse Outcomes

A common consequence of male orgasmic disorder, if left untreated, is marital distress. This may result from a desire to have children, which is obviously impaired by this disorder, or from the female partner's interpretation of the symptom. Some women will interpret the lack of male orgasm as a hostile withholding, others as a sign that they are not physically attractive to their partner or that the lack of orgasm is

Table 28–6. Treatment of male orgasmic disorder.

Etiology	Treatment
Psychological	Sex, couples, or individual psychotherapy, as indicated.
Medical	Appropriate treatment of contributing medical conditions. Education regarding the impact of relevant medical conditions on sexuality. Hormone regulation, if indicated.
Pharmacologic	Termination or adjustment of any contributing prescription medications. Abstinence from alcohol or other contributing nonprescription drugs.

due to a deficit in their sexual performance. If sexuality becomes a major issue within the couple, or for the individual man, secondary male erectile disorder or hypoactive sexual desire disorder may develop. Psychotherapy has potentially adverse outcomes. As this form of treatment typically involves couples therapy these adverse outcomes may include the exacerbation of marital or couple distress as well as the exacerbation of preexisting individual psychopathology.

Prognosis & Course of Illness

Little information is available about the natural course of untreated male orgasmic disorder. The prognosis, with treatment, is generally good for cases with a psychogenic etiology, poor for cases with a medical etiology.

Crenshaw TL, Goldberg JP: *Sexual Pharmacology: Drugs That Affect Sexual Functioning.* WW Norton, 1996.

Kaplan HS (editor): *The Evaluation of Sexual Disorders: Psychological and Medical Aspects.* Brunner/Mazel, 1983.

Kolodny RC, Masters WH, Johnson VE: *Textbook of Sexual Medicine.* Little, Brown, 1979.

Leiblum SR, Rosen RC (editors): *Principles and Practice of Sex Therapy: Update for the 1990s,* 2nd ed. Guilford Press, 1989.

Masters WH, Johnson VE: *Human Sexual Inadequacy.* Little, Brown, 1970.

3. PREMATURE EJACULATION

DSM-IV Diagnostic Criteria

A. Persistent or recurrent ejaculation with minimal sexual stimulation before, on, or shortly after penetration and before the person wishes it. The clinician must take into account factors that affect duration of the excitement phase, such as age, novelty of the sexual partner or situation, and recent frequency of sexual activity.

B. The disturbance causes marked distress or interpersonal difficulty.

C. The premature ejaculation is not due exclusively to the direct effects of a substance (eg, withdrawal from opioids).

Reprinted, with permission, from *Diagnostic and Statistical Manual of Mental Disorders,* 4th ed. Copyright 1994 American Psychiatric Association.

General Considerations

The diagnosis of premature ejaculation may be qualified by the specifiers of *lifelong* or *acquired, generalized* or *situational,* and *due to psychological factors* or *due to combined factors.* Although premature ejaculation may occur episodically for many men, in practice true situational-type premature ejaculation, with rapid ejaculation occurring involuntarily and consistently under a particular set of circumstances, or with a particular partner, and not under other circumstances or with other partners, is exceedingly rare. The most common pattern is generalized, lifelong, and psychogenic; the acquired type beginning later in life is less frequent and requires careful attention to potential organic factors. Even in the most common pattern, most men will agree that they have more ejaculatory control during masturbation than when attempting intercourse.

With the question of "How long is long enough," the definitional boundaries of this condition sometimes become unclear. A number of issues must be considered, including the man's subjective sense of control and the length of coital connection needed for the female partner to achieve orgasm. Men have been known to seek treatment for premature ejaculation, with concomitant feelings of inadequacy about their performance (because their partners were unable to reach orgasm), although they could sustain intercourse for up to 45 minutes. Further question about whether premature ejaculation is a disorder in the normative sense arise from the finding that 75% of a sample of over 6000 men ejaculated within 2 minutes of penetration. The range commonly encountered in clinical practice includes men who ejaculate at the very beginning of the process of penetration to men who can withhold orgasm for 1–5 minutes. Definitional problems aside, premature ejaculation causes significant distress for large numbers of men and women, and its treatment is worthy of discussion.

A. Major Etiologic Theories:

1. Psychological factors—If premature ejaculation is due entirely to psychological factors, or to a combination of psychological and medical factors, the diagnosis is simply premature ejaculation. Almost all cases of lifelong, generalized, premature ejaculation are believed to be of psychogenic etiology. This said, there is little agreement on a unified theory of psychogenic causation. Older formulations that pointed to anger and hostility toward women as causal factors have generally been discredited. A rather interesting view holds that premature ejaculation has a reproductive advantage and thus has been selected for over the course of evolution. Masters and Johnson observed that many of their patients with premature ejaculation had a history of hurried early sexual encounters (eg, in automobiles, in the homes of parents, or with prostitutes interested in rapid turnover). These circumstances would encourage early sexual release. Premature ejaculation could thus be viewed as a habit pattern, resistant to change, established early in a man's sexual history.

From another perspective, ejaculatory control has been described as a learned process, in which awareness of the rising levels of sexual arousal leading to orgasm is critical. Men, who for some reason (eg, distraction, anxiety, overconcern with partner satisfaction) do not learn to discriminate the levels of arousal immediately preceding orgasm do not learn ejacula-tory control. In this case, the immediate psychological causal factor has been characterized as lack of sexual sensory awareness. There appears to be a well-established inverse relationship between frequency of ejaculation and ejaculatory control. There has been speculation that men ejaculate in response to a range of levels of sexual arousal and that men with premature ejaculation have an innately low threshold. This theory has yet to receive widespread empirical support. Despite the lack of an accepted causal mechanism, the excellent response of the majority of cases of premature ejaculation to psychotherapeutic treatment is taken as support of psychological causation. Although acquired premature ejaculation is more likely to be related to medical factors, it can also be secondary to psychosocial factors such as a low frequency of intercourse, sex with a new partner, sexually focused anxiety, and relationship issues.

2. Medical factors—If premature ejaculation is explained entirely by medical causes, the diagnosis would be other male sexual dysfunction due to a medical condition (with the condition specified). There are only a few congenital conditions involving damage to the urinary tract or spinal cord that can result in lifelong premature ejaculation, the most common of which is spina bifida. In such rare cases other signs of neurologic impairment would also be expected.

Secondary or acquired premature ejaculation is much less frequent than is the lifelong type and is more likely to be related to organic factors. Acquired premature ejaculation often develops secondary to progressive organic erectile impairment, in response to efforts to ejaculate rapidly before loss of erection. Some spinal cord disorders and surgical procedures can cause acquired premature ejaculation more directly by impairing the neural substrate underlying the ejaculatory reflex. A patient presenting with acquired premature ejaculation, therefore, should receive a careful physical workup, especially if he does not report any unusual psychosexual stressors or trauma.

3. Pharmacologic factors—No pharmacologic agents have a clear causal association with premature ejaculation; however, there seems to be an association between opioid withdrawal and premature ejaculation. If this is judged to be the sole cause the diagnosis would be substance-induced sexual dysfunction with impaired orgasm.

B. Epidemiology: Although the usual problems exist with prevalence data in regard to premature ejaculation, it is generally accepted that premature ejaculation is the most common of the male sexual dysfunctions in the general population. It is particularly common among young males, the majority of whom experience premature ejaculation in their early attempts at intercourse. Some estimates suggest a prevalence in the general male population of greater than 33%. Because the ejaculatory response tends to slow down with age, prevalence would decrease in older age groups.

C. Genetics: With the exception of genetic contributions to the rare congenital disorders associated with lifelong premature ejaculation, or the progressive neurologic disorders sometimes associated with acquired premature ejaculation, there is no clearly established genetic influence on this disorder.

Clinical Findings

A. Signs & Symptoms: The diagnosis is based primarily on the patient's or his sexual partner's report of rapid ejaculation during attempts at coitus.

B. Psychological Testing: The diagnosis of premature ejaculation does not imply the existence of any other psychopathology. Traditional psychological testing is not useful in establishing the diagnosis but may be helpful in identifying coexisting psychopathology that could affect treatment.

C. Laboratory Findings: Laboratory tests play little role in the diagnosis of premature ejaculation. In cases of acquired premature ejaculation, laboratory work may be useful in evaluating the possible existence of a progressive organically based erectile disorder or one of the progressive neurologic conditions sometimes associated with acquired premature ejaculation.

Differential Diagnosis

In general, diagnosis is not difficult. Care should be taken to evaluate the possibility of a progressive organic erectile disorder or an underlying neurologic condition in cases of acquired premature ejaculation.

Treatment

If a medical condition is involved in the etiology of premature ejaculation, that condition should be the initial focus of treatment, and the capacity for control of ejaculation once the medical condition is treated optimally should be evaluated and discussed with the couple (Table 28–7). Such cases will be rare. The vast majority of cases have a psychogenic etiology, and referral to a psychotherapist with training and experience in the treatment of sexual dysfunction leads to optimal treatment. Some good self-help manuals exist, but there has been no thorough evaluation of the outcome of treatment through use of manuals alone. They are helpful as adjuncts to a more comprehensive treatment program.

Table 28–7. Treatment of premature ejaculation.

Etiology	Treatment
Psychological	Sex, couples, or individual psychotherapy, as indicated.
Medical	Appropriate treatment of contributing medical conditions. Education regarding the impact of relevant medical conditions on sexuality.
Pharmacologic (rare)	Education concerning the effect of opioid withdrawal on ejaculation.

Psychotherapeutic treatment of premature ejaculation is highly successful; the best success rate is achieved when treatment is done in the context of a committed couple. The core of the treatment process is to gradually, through successive approximation, acclimate the patient to higher and more extended periods of sexual arousal without ejaculation. The female partner is involved in stimulating the male, at first manually and later during controlled intromission. Either the "stop-start" or "squeeze" techniques may be used effectively. Both of these techniques involve a period of stimulation followed by a pause prior to the point of ejaculatory inevitability, with this cycle repeated a number of times in each "homework" session. The squeeze technique involves a squeeze applied to the head of the penis to lower arousal at the time of each pause. As these techniques are practiced, the man learns to tolerate increasing intervals and an increased intensity of stimulation without ejaculation, and he learns the use of pausing and changing patterns of motion in delaying orgasm. If this treatment process is pursued with persistence, the success rate is above 90%.

Couples therapy will also include psychosexual education and will address other relationship issues on an as-needed basis. Treatment of men without partners is more problematic because of the difficulty in transferring learning (of ejaculatory control) to an in vivo context. Treatment in such cases usually involves psychosexual and social education, particularly in regard to developing relationships, coupled with a training program involving masturbatory conditioning, fantasy, and relaxation training.

Recently some efforts have been made to treat premature ejaculation through the use of SSRIs, which have a well-known side effect of orgasmic delay in both men and women. These efforts have met with reasonable success, but further research is needed, and the use of a systemic pharmacologic agent in the long-term treatment of a chronic condition for which other effective treatments exist must be weighed.

Complications, Comorbidity, & Adverse Outcomes

For young men without partners, premature ejaculation can result in heightened sexual and social anxiety and can impair the development of relationships, leading some men in the long term to isolation and even depression. For some men, the repeated frustration and embarrassment of not being able to satisfy their sexual partners leads to a secondary male erectile disorder or hypoactive sexual desire disorder. Premature ejaculation can also contribute to chronic anger and distress within a couple, depending in part on the sexual partner's reaction to and interpretation of the symptom. Psychotherapeutic treatment can have adverse outcomes. In the case of couples therapy these outcomes may include the exacerbation of preexisting couple-related issues or individual psychopathology.

Prognosis & Course of Illness

Although numerous young men experience episodes of rapid ejaculation early in their sexual history, and eventually learn ejaculatory control, well-established cases of premature ejaculation seem to be quite resistant to change without therapeutic intervention. Ejaculatory urgency declines with age, and many cases may gradually remit over a span of decades secondary to the aging process. The prognosis with treatment in a couples context is excellent.

Kaplan HS: PE: *How to Overcome Premature Ejaculation.* Brunner/Mazel, 1989.

Kinsey AC, Pomeroy WB, Martin CE: *Sexual Behavior in the Human Male.* WB Saunders, 1948.

Kolodny RC, Masters WH, Johnson VE: *Textbook of Sexual Medicine.* Little, Brown, 1979.

Masters WH, Johnson VE: *Human Sexual Inadequacy.* Little, Brown, 1970.

SEXUAL PAIN DISORDERS

1. DYSPAREUNIA

DSM-IV Diagnostic Criteria

A. Recurrent or persistent genital pain associated with sexual intercourse in either a male or female.

B. The disturbance causes marked distress or interpersonal difficulty.

C. The disturbance is not caused exclusively by vaginismus or lack of lubrication, is not better accounted for by another Axis I disorder (except another sexual dysfunction), and is not due exclusively to the direct physiological effects of a substance (eg, a drug of abuse, a medication) or a general medical condition.

General Considerations

The pain of dyspareunia may be experienced before, during, or after intercourse, although it is most common during. It may be associated particularly with orgasm. In women, the pain may be superficial, or it may be experienced as deep pain during penile thrusting. The diagnosis is subject to the specifiers *lifelong* or *acquired, generalized* or *situational,* and *due to psychological factors* or *due to combined factors.* The diagnosis may be made in conjunction with other sexual dysfunction diagnoses with the exception of vaginismus, which is in itself a cause of coital pain. The diagnosis is not made if any other Axis I disorder better accounts for the symptoms.

A. Major Etiologic Theories: Many medical conditions can result in dyspareunia in women and men. Even when an initial medical evaluation is negative, subtle, difficult-to-detect pathology may exist as the causal factor. Nevertheless, some dyspareunia is predominantly psychogenic in nature, and in many cases psychogenic and organic factors coexist.

1. Psychological factors—Lazarus's tripartite categorization of psychogenic causal factors is useful:

Developmental factors include the transmission of misinformation about sexuality that creates sexual anxiety and an upbringing in the context of a rigid antisexual morality that leads to guilt and shame about sexuality.

Table 28–8. Possible medical causes of dyspareunia.

Men	Women
Acquired or congenital abnormalities of the penis	Anorectal disease
Infectious urethritis or chemical irritation of the urethra (possibly by contraceptive agents)	Atrophic vaginitis, either postmenopausal or secondary to estrogen deficiency
Lesion on the shaft of the penis	Bartholin's and Skene's gland abnormalities
Lesion, infection, or irritation affecting the foreskin (particularly in uncircumcised men)	Broad ligament lesions
Infection of the bladder, prostate, or epididymis	Chemical irritation
Inguinal hernia	Chemical or traumatic irritation or pathologic lesions of the clitoris
Postorgasmic headache	Congenital shortening of the vagina
Spasm of the cremaster muscles	Endometriosis
	Fixed uterine retroversion
	Inadequate lubrication
	Intact or rigid hymen or irritated hymenal remnants
	Pelvic inflammatory disease
	Penile deformation in the partner secondary to Peyronie's disease
	Postorgasmic headache
	Sexually transmitted diseases
	Surgical scarring
	Urethritis
	Vulvar vestibulitis
	Vulvitis from numerous possible infectious agents

Traumatic factors include sexual abuse in childhood, rape, or other sexual assault.

Relational factors involve the person's current relationship and the numerous difficulties that can potentially arise there: resentment, hostility, distrust, sexual clumsiness or lack of experience, insufficient foreplay, or lack of sexual attraction to the partner.

According to Lazarus, almost 50% of his cases of psychogenic female dyspareunia had causal factors from the relational category.

2. Medical factors—If the pain is judged to be due entirely to a medical condition the appropriate diagnosis is male or female dyspareunia due to a medical condition (with the condition specified). Numerous medical conditions can result in dyspareunia. Table 28–8 lists the most common conditions.

3. Pharmacologic factors—If the pain is judged to be due entirely to a pharmacologic agent the appropriate diagnosis is substance-induced sexual dysfunction with sexual pain. Antihistamines or other agents that may reduce vaginal secretions are associated with dyspareunia in women. There is otherwise little information available about the role of pharmacologic agents in this dysfunction.

B. Epidemiology: Dyspareunia is an infrequent presenting complaint to clinics specializing in the treatment of sexual dysfunction. Community studies, however, suggest that it is much more common in women in the general population than among those presenting to such specialized clinics; some estimates suggest a prevalence of 33%. It is a more common complaint in the offices of general practitioners and gynecologists. Data in this area are notoriously vague, but the incidence of dyspareunia appears to be much lower in men than in women, and a primarily psychogenic etiology is less likely in men than in women.

C. Genetics: Genetic influences certainly play a role in some of the congenital conditions associated with dyspareunia, but there is no evidence that genetic factors have a more direct causal role in psychogenic dyspareunia.

Clinical Findings

A. Signs & Symptoms: The diagnosis is based primarily on the patient's self-report of pain associated with intercourse. Numerous signs and symptoms are associated specifically with the multiple medical conditions that can be involved in the etiology.

B. Psychological Testing: The diagnosis of dyspareunia does not imply the existence of any other psychopathology. Traditional psychological testing is not useful in establishing the diagnosis but may be helpful in identifying coexisting psychopathology that could affect treatment.

C. Laboratory Findings: Laboratory work is useful in the evaluation of the multiple possible medical conditions that could result in dyspareunia. The laboratory values of interest would be specific to each condition and are too numerous to mention here.

Differential Diagnosis

Accurate diagnosis is critical in the treatment of dyspareunia. Much time, money, and emotional effort can be wasted in misdirected attempts to treat biologically based dyspareunia with psychotherapy. The evaluation of possible medical etiologies is complex and will be accomplished optimally only through referral to a urologist or gynecologist who has an interest in sexual function in a holistic sense, including the subjective component as well as the adequate functioning of the reproductive system. Many potential medical causes of dyspareunia are subtle and easily missed. Situational conditions are more likely to be psychogenic, but the symptoms of some medical conditions (eg, endometriosis) will fluctuate over time. Pain in specific areas that can be reproduced during examination is almost certainly of a biological origin; precise specification of the location, type of pain, and circumstances of its occurrence greatly facilitates diagnosis.

Treatment

If a medical condition is implicated in the etiology of dyspareunia that condition should be the initial focus of treatment. At times the pain can be alleviated entirely, sometimes with a treatment as simple as the routine use of a lubricant (Table 28–9). At other times psychotherapy may be needed as well as treatment of the causal medical condition, to deal with the psychological overlay that may develop secondary to an organically based dyspareunia.

Psychogenic dyspareunia is best treated through referral to a psychotherapist well trained and experienced in the treatment of sexual dysfunction. Treatment approaches will be varied and based on a clear understanding of the psychological causal factors. If the patient is in a committed relationship, the sexual partner will almost always be involved in therapy at some point. If the causal factors are predominantly

Table 28–9. Treatment of dyspareunia.

Etiology	Treatment
Psychological	Sex, couples, or individual psychotherapy, as indicated. Referral to be made only after a thorough medical evaluation for causes of coital pain.
Medical	Thorough gynecologic or urologic evaluation for causes of coital pain. Appropriate treatment of contributing medical conditions. Referral for psychological treatment as above if a significant psychological overlay remains after the resolution of medical problems.
Pharmacologic	Termination or adjustment of, or substitution for, any contributing pharmacologic agents.

developmental or traumatic, considerable individual treatment may be necessary initially. If the causal factors are relational, a more broadly based couples therapy may be appropriate. If the primary immediate cause is anxiety about penetration due to misinformation, a treatment approach similar to that to be described for vaginismus may be appropriate (see later in this chapter).

Complications, Comorbidity, & Adverse Outcomes

By decreasing the frequency of coitus and creating stress, anxiety, and avoidance in relation to sexual activity, dyspareunia can impair the formation of relationships for people without partners, or it can interfere with the stability of ongoing relationships. This can lead to marital distress, social and sexual avoidance and isolation, social withdrawal, loneliness, and depression. Continuing attempts at painful intercourse can lead to vaginismus, sexual arousal disorders, hypoactive sexual desire disorder, and sexual aversion disorder. Clinical reports suggest that in many cases, dyspareunia exists in patients with a history of sexual abuse and trauma. This possibility should be investigated appropriately and the residual effects treated if indicated. Psychotherapeutic treatment has the potential for adverse outcome, including the exacerbation of both individual psychopathology and relationship issues.

Prognosis & Course of Illness

Little information is available about the natural course of dyspareunia in the general population, but the information that is available suggests the disorder may become chronic or may remit spontaneously in roughly equivalent proportions of those with the disorder. Little empirical information is available on treatment outcome.

Kaplan HS (editor): *The Evaluation of Sexual Disorders: Psychological and Medical Aspects.* Brunner/Mazel, 1983.
Lazarus AA: Dyspareunia: a multimodal psychotherapeutic perspective. In: Leiblum SR, Rosen RC (editors): *Principles and Practice of Sex Therapy: Update for the 1990s,* 2nd ed. Guilford Press, 1989.

2. VAGINISMUS

DSM-IV Diagnostic Criteria

A. Recurrent or persistent involuntary spasm of the musculature of the outer third of the vagina that interferes with sexual intercourse.
B. The disturbance causes marked distress or interpersonal difficulty.
C. The disturbance is not better accounted for by another Axis I disorder (eg, somatization disorder) and is not due exclusively to the direct physiological effects of a general medical condition.

General Considerations

The muscle spasms of vaginismus usually occur in sexual situations before or during attempts at penetration. The spasms may be so intense that penetration is impossible, or less intense, so that penetration may be forced with the usual unfortunate consequence of painful intercourse. Women with vaginismus will have varying degrees of phobic anxiety about vaginal penetration with accompanying avoidance behavior. Many women with vaginismus are otherwise sexually responsive, able to experience sexual arousal and even orgasm. Some women with vaginismus are unable to tolerate the insertion of any object into the vagina, whereas in other women the muscle spasms are specific to coitus and even gynecologic examination may be tolerated. The diagnosis of vaginismus may be qualified by the specifiers *lifelong* or *acquired, generalized* or *situational,* and *due to psychological factors* or *due to combined factors.* In some cases the motivation of women seeking treatment for vaginismus may be more influenced by a desire to have children, or to deflect a spouse's negative affect, than by an innate interest in experiencing pleasurable sexual intercourse. Vaginismus may be diagnosed in conjunction with other sexual dysfunctions except dyspareunia.

A. Major Etiologic Theories: Vaginismus often develops after a history of repeated episodes or even a single incident of painful intercourse. In this circumstance, vaginismus can be considered a classically conditioned response that serves the purpose of pain avoidance.

1. Medical factors—When vaginismus is judged to be explained entirely as the effect of a general medical condition, it is diagnosed as other female sexual dysfunction due to a medical condition (with the condition specified). In many cases the cause of the pain is a general medical condition. Multiple medical conditions can result in coital pain (see Table 28–8). Clinicians should be aware that any of these conditions could be causally implicated in vaginismus. In some cases the symptom of vaginismus will remain long after the underlying disorder that caused the pain has resolved, in which case the dysfunction could be seen as being maintained by psychological mechanisms although the original etiology was medical. Repeated attempts at intercourse that are painful because of inadequate lubrication secondary to a sexual arousal disorder may also lead to vaginismus.

2. Psychological factors—The etiologic mechanism of psychogenic vaginismus is poorly understood, yet clinical experience suggests that a variety of psychosocial factors may be implicated in the etiology. These include a rigid upbringing in a family that transmitted strongly negative moral messages about sexuality, a prior sexual trauma, fear of pregnancy, sexual dysfunction in the male partner, uncertainty over sexual orientation, and fear of injury or sexually transmitted disease. As discussed in the preceding section, the association of vaginal penetration with any source of physical pain or psychologically painful affect may be causal, although at times the source of the psychological distress may be difficult to identify.

3. Pharmacologic factors—There is no evidence that any pharmacologic agent has a direct causal relationship to vaginismus, although any agent that contributes to discomfort during intercourse could play an indirect role.

B. Epidemiology: There are no data reflecting the prevalence of vaginismus in the general population. In the United States and Western Europe it is one of the less frequent presenting complaints at sexual dysfunction clinics, although anecdotal evidence suggests that its prevalence in the general population is not insignificant. There may be important cultural differences in prevalence.

C. Genetics: Genetic factors may play a role in some of the medical conditions related to coital pain; otherwise, there is no evidence for a direct genetic role in the etiology of vaginismus.

Clinical Findings

A. Signs & Symptoms: The initial diagnosis is based on a patient's, or her sexual partner's, report of vaginal muscle spasm interfering with intercourse. The diagnosis is confirmed if such a response is elicited on gynecologic examination, although clinicians must be aware that this will not happen if the response is specific to coitus. If vaginismus is related to a medical condition, signs and symptoms specific to that condition may be present.

B. Psychological Testing: The diagnosis of vaginismus does not imply the existence of any other psychopathology. Traditional psychological testing is not useful in establishing the diagnosis but may be helpful in identifying coexisting psychopathology that could affect treatment.

C. Laboratory Findings: No laboratory findings are specific to vaginismus. Laboratory work is useful in the evaluation of the multiple possible medical conditions that could result in coital pain and thus vaginismus. The laboratory values of interest would be specific to each medical condition and are too numerous to review here.

Differential Diagnosis

Gynecologic evaluation is crucial in the diagnosis of vaginismus. The symptom does not always occur in the context of the examination, but if it does occur the diagnosis is confirmed. The most important differential is between vaginismus due to psychological causes and vaginismus due to combined causes or resulting entirely from a general medical condition; the gynecologic examination is critical in establishing this differential. Occasionally careful history taking is required to distinguish vaginismus from problems due to a male partner's inadequate erection, as the two dysfunctions may coexist.

Treatment

If vaginismus is due to combined factors or secondary to a general medical cause of coital pain, the medical condition should be the initial focus of treatment. However, the symptom may remain after the resolution of the medical condition. Referral to a psychotherapist trained and experienced in the treatment of sexual dysfunction is appropriate in these cases and in cases in which the causal factors are clearly psychological (Table 28–10). Treatment always involves a component of psychosexual education for the woman and her sexual partner if she is in a committed relationship. The core of the treatment process involves the gradual deconditioning of any phobic anxiety and associated avoidance behavior related to the thought or anticipation of vaginal penetration as well as deconditioning of the vaginal muscle spasms themselves. Careful evaluation of the woman's sexual value system and her attitudes toward masturbation and touching her own genitals are required in individually tailoring the treatment program.

In general, the initial phases of the treatment program will be done by the woman alone, unless she has a supportive sexual partner and desires his presence. The woman will be given homework assignments that involve examining her own genitalia, and then, at her own pace and under her control, gradually inserting progressively larger objects into her vagina, coupled with appropriate fantasy and relaxation exercises. The objects used may be a set of graduated dilators, or the patient's and the sexual partner's fingers, depending on what is most acceptable to the patient. The woman is encouraged to insert the smallest object first (eg, smallest dilator, little finger) and, as comfort develops, to gradually move to larger objects (eg, large

Table 28–10. Treatment of vaginismus.

Etiology	Treatment
Psychological	Sex, couples, or individual psychotherapy, as indicated. Referral to be made only after a thorough medical evaluation for causes of coital pain.
Medical	Thorough gynecologic evaluation for causes of coital pain. Appropriate treatment of contributing medical conditions. Referral for psychological treatment as above if vaginismus persists after the resolution of the cause of pain.
Pharmacologic	Termination or adjustment of, or substitution for, any contributing pharmacologic agents.

dilator, larger fingers, two fingers) until a phallic-sized object can be tolerated comfortably. The sexual partner's involvement is encouraged gradually, so that the woman may begin inserting (again at her own pace and under her control) her partner's fingers and eventually his erect penis. Major factors influencing the success of therapy appear to be a positive and supportive relationship with the partner, and positive rapport with the therapist, both of which help the patient tolerate and defuse the anxiety generated by the treatment process. Treatment will involve broader couple issues as necessary.

Complications, Comorbidity, & Adverse Outcomes

Vaginismus is believed to be a major causal factor in unconsummated marriage. By interfering with sexual intercourse it can lead to marital conflict and particularly distress related to the desire to have children. A woman with lifelong, generalized vaginismus will find it difficult to form and maintain heterosexual relationships. Heightened sexual and social anxiety, social isolation, loneliness, and depression may result. Repeated, painful attempts at intercourse may lead to sexual arousal or desire disorders. A common complication is the development of a male erectile disorder in the male sexual partner. Psychotherapeutic treatment has the potential for adverse outcomes such as the exacerbation of the couple's distress or of preexisting individual psychopathology.

Prognosis & Course of Illness

With appropriate treatment the prognosis for vaginismus is excellent. Little information is available about the natural history of untreated vaginismus in the general population.

Wincze JP, Carey MP: *Sexual Dysfunction: A Guide for Assessment and Treatment.* Guilford Press, 1991.

PARAPHILIAS

In general less is known about the paraphilias than about the sexual dysfunctions. Much of the information available is relevant to the paraphilias in general. Comments about etiology, the value of psychological testing, and so on are more likely to be relevant to the broad category rather than to one specific diagnosis. For that reason we initially review these disorders as a broad category and then provide a brief discussion of individual diagnoses.

Diagnostic Criteria

A. Recurrent, intense sexually arousing fantasies, sexual urges, or behaviors—generally involving (1) nonhuman objects, (2) the suffering or humil-

iation of oneself or one's partner, or (3) children or other nonconsenting persons—that occur over a period of at least 6 months (American Psychiatric Association 1994, pp. 522–523).

B. The diagnosis is not made unless the fantasies, sexual urges, or behaviors cause clinically significant distress or impairment in social, occupational, or other important areas of function.

General Considerations

The separate paraphilic diagnoses are characterized by the different objects, behaviors, and so on that serve as the focus for arousal. As varied and creative as human behavior is, there are many potential paraphilic foci. A number of named paraphilias (eg, klismaphilia, formicophilia) are not denoted specifically in DSM-IV. These are diagnosed as paraphilia not otherwise specified.

Paraphilic behavior may or may not involve a victim (ie, a coerced partner). Fetishism, in which sexual arousal and masturbation is focused on a nonhuman object, is victimless; whereas pedophilia, which entails sexual behavior between an adult and a child, does involve a victim. Society has a strong interest in the management of paraphilias that involve victims; this powerfully affects the process of assessment and treatment for these disorders. Paraphilic individuals whose behavior involves victims usually present for treatment as a result of contact with the legal system. Their motivation for treatment may be questionable and their truthfulness modulated by a concern for legal consequences. Victimless paraphilic individuals rarely present for treatment unless their disorder has caused disruption in a significant relationship and the other person, usually a spouse or concerned parent, has brought them for treatment.

For some individuals with these disorders the paraphilic object or behavior, or related fantasy, is a prerequisite for sexual arousal, whereas others are able to function sexually without paraphilic stimuli. For many individuals, the paraphilic thoughts and behavior are ego-syntonic, and the paraphilic behavior may be vigorously defended intellectually. Others may feel guilty and shameful about their paraphilic urges and behaviors. Paraphilic urges are often perceived as strong compulsions. A commonly reported pattern begins with a gradual buildup of paraphilic thoughts, fantasies, and urges, which are resisted successfully at first. Eventually the urges reach a level perceived as overwhelming and uncontrollable, and behavioral acting-out occurs. Some patients report falling into a trance-like state at this time. Following a period of paraphilic behavior, the individual often experiences guilt and self-recrimination and vows not to act out again; this sets the stage for the cycle to begin anew. Such patients subjectively perceive their paraphilic sexuality as uncontrollable.

Because of the difficulty and uncertain effectiveness of treatment, the optimal treatment approach in situations in which the paraphilia causes little harm to the patient and poses no danger to others may be to work with the patient to manage the paraphilia, that is, to limit the negative impact of the paraphilia on the patient's life and on the lives of those close to the patient. More aggressive approaches are indicated, and often legally mandated, when the patient's behavior poses a risk of harm to other members of the community.

A. Major Etiologic Theories: There is no generally accepted and clearly understood etiologic mechanism for the paraphilias. According to Money, some form of biological vulnerability, perhaps related to temporal lobe or limbic epilepsy, interacts with repressive sexual experiences during childhood to produce a paraphilic "lovemap." He points to the years of childhood sexual play as the vulnerable developmental period.

Others find little evidence to support a biological predisposition. Most investigators who seek primarily psychosocial explanations, whether from the analytic or behavioral school, also look to a vulnerable period in childhood as formative. Numerous psychoanalytic theories interpret specific paraphilic symptomatology as symbolically expressive of psychological conflicts originating in childhood.

Cognitive-behavioral therapists view the paraphilias as the product of a faulty childhood learning environment. For one of many possible reasons, a paraphilic object or behavior becomes associated with sexual arousal. This association is subsequently reinforced by sexual arousal, masturbation, and orgasm in the presence of the paraphilic focus, either in fantasy or in vivo. Such histories can be clearly discerned in the reports of some, but not all, paraphilic patients. An example would be a patient who was left at home alone frequently between the ages of 8 and 12. He began playing with and dressing in his sister's clothing taken clandestinely from her drawers, and his first masturbatory experiences occurred while dressed in her clothes. His entire subsequent sexual history was colored with powerful elements of transvestic fetishism.

In many cases the initial exposure to sexual arousal in an atypical context may seem almost incidental, whereas other cases (eg, involving sexual abuse) may seem more psychologically salient. The role of repeated reinforcement through masturbation and orgasm in a paraphilic context (either in vivo or in fantasy) is viewed as critically important. Other elements that appear commonly in the developmental history of paraphilic individuals and may play a role in etiology include a poor understanding of human sexuality, lack of consistent parenting, poor self-esteem, and lack of social confidence.

Exposure to a paraphilic situation at a vulnerable developmental period and the obstacles to the development of a normal sexual arousal pattern posed by poor self-confidence and social skills may interactively result in a persistent paraphilic arousal pattern. In many cases the same individual will exhibit more than one paraphilic pattern (eg, diagnoses of both frotteurism and voyeurism may be applicable).

B. Epidemiology: There are no reliable data on the prevalence of the paraphilias in the general population. People with these diagnoses rarely present spontaneously for treatment. In clinics specializing in the treatment of these disorders the most common presenting complaints are pedophilia, voyeurism, and exhibitionism, but this may merely indicate that these are the paraphilic behaviors that most often come to the attention of the legal system. The ready availability of paraphilic pornography and the proliferation of self-help and support groups for self-designated "sex addicts," transvestites, and transsexuals suggests a significant frequency of occurrence. Paraphilias are rarely diagnosed in women, with the exception of sexual masochism, in which the female-to-male ratio is 1:20. Anecdotal reports and case studies indicate that paraphilias do occur occasionally in women.

C. Genetics: There is no evidence of a direct causal role for genetic factors in the paraphilias.

Clinical Findings

A. Signs & Symptoms: Paraphilic diagnoses are based primarily on reports of behavior by the patient and others. The presence of feminine articles of clothing may provide clues for the diagnosis of transvestic fetishism. An overly intense indulgence in sexual masochism may leave visible physical sequelae.

B. Psychological Testing: There are no psychological tests that will diagnose paraphilias definitively, but such tests may be useful in identifying coexisting areas of psychopathology that could affect treatment.

C. Laboratory Findings: Psychophysiological assessment of sexual arousal utilizing a penile plethysmograph while exposing the patient to an array of sexual stimuli has been used to assess sexual arousal patterns. Although this process has some clinical utility, its validity and reliability has been questioned, as it may be possible to manipulate the results through the use of internal mental imagery.

Differential Diagnosis

A diagnostic issue related to the paraphilias is the definition of the boundary between pathology and normality. The range of human sexual behavior and fantasy is wide, and the realm of socially acceptable behavior may vary significantly across different cultural and ethnic groups. It is particularly important to remember the diagnostic criterion requiring clinically significant distress or impairment in making paraphilic diagnoses. To this might be added concerns relating to the manipulation or abuse of others.

It may sometimes seem difficult to distinguish fetishism (in which the erotic object is often an article of female clothing) from transvestic fetishism (in which sexual arousal comes from the act of cross-dressing) and gender identity disorder (in which cross-dressing represents dissatisfaction with one's gender and is not done primarily for sexual arousal).

Atypical sexual behavior may result from other causes (ie, poor judgment or poor impulse control secondary to other psychopathology, cognitive deterioration, or intoxication). Such behavior will be associated with dementia, substance abuse or intoxication, an acute episode of schizophrenia, or a manic episode, and will not represent a long-lasting, recurrent, and persistent pattern for the particular individual.

Treatment

A. Cognitive-Behavioral Approaches: The paraphilias are notoriously resistant to treatment. Many patients are brought to treatment by legal or social forces and at least initially have little innate motivation. Nonetheless, since the early 1970s a number of cognitive-behavioral approaches have been developed that show some promise. Most of these approaches involve a multifaceted treatment program with components designed to reduce socially unacceptable sexual arousal patterns; increase socially acceptable arousal patterns; provide assertiveness, social, and sexual skills training; challenge distorted cognition; provide training in coping with anxiety, depression, and other negative affect; and provide training in relapse prevention. A number of aversion procedures, some of them dramatically unpleasant, have been developed over the years to reduce unacceptable arousal patterns.

Today more humane, covert sensitization procedures, orgasmic satiation, and training in victim awareness and stimulus control are utilized. Masturbatory orgasmic reconditioning procedures can be used to enhance appropriate arousal patterns. Paraphilic acting-out often occurs in the context of emotional distress; the teaching of skills for coping with negative emotions can help to improve behavioral control under these circumstances. There is now some evidence that such comprehensive treatment programs reduce the recidivism rates for sex offenders who have been incarcerated for rape and pedophilic or exhibitionistic behavior. Shame aversion therapy has shown some promise in reducing exhibitionistic behavior.

B. Pharmacologic Approaches: Since 1970 there has been increasing acceptance of the use of pharmacologic agents (eg, antiandrogens) in the treatment of paraphilias that present a danger to others. In the United States the primary agent used has been medroxyprogesterone acetate; in Europe, cyproterone acetate has been used for similar purposes. In theory these agents will reduce the activity of testosterone, lower sex drive, and decrease all aspects of sexual function including fantasy, erection, masturbation, and orgasm. These agents are generally used as a component of a comprehensive treatment program and the results have been promising.

C. Long-Term Treatment & Relapse Prevention: None of the treatments are cures. Long-term treatment and relapse prevention strategies are important considerations. Paraphilic urges and fantasy are not eliminated but reduced in frequency and intensity, while the patient is helped to gain control over his own behavior. The treatment process remains a difficult one for both the patient (who is being asked to give up a highly rewarding behavior under coercive circumstances) and the therapist (who is usually entangled to some degree in the legal system and morally worried about the harm that his or her patients might do to others).

Complications, Comorbidity, & Adverse Outcomes

Even victimless paraphilias that are practiced in secret may have a negative psychosocial impact on the individual. Such practices have a tendency to be compulsively consuming of one's emotional energy and time and thus may adversely affect occupational function and the individual's ability to form interpersonal relationships. The revelation of such behavior may threaten the stability of relationships and result in marital distress, social isolation and withdrawal, loneliness, and depression. Paraphilias involving victims may lead to conflict with the legal system, incarceration, social ostracism, and other major life disruption in addition to the complications described above. Frequent, unprotected and indiscriminate sexual activity is likely to lead to the acquisition or the spreading of sexually transmitted disease. Overly intense sadistic or masochistic behavior may lead to traumatic injury, which can be severe.

Any treatment program for paraphilic disorders carries with it a significant failure rate and the assurance that some of one's patients will offend against the public. Medical treatment approaches carry the risk of pharmacologic side effects. Weight gain commonly occurs, and medroxyprogesterone acetate may elevate blood glucose levels. Psychotherapy always carries some risk of adverse outcome, including the exacerbation of preexisting individual psychopathology or, in couples therapy, the exacerbation of relationship distress.

Prognosis & Course of Illness

There is no reliable information on the natural course of untreated paraphilic disorders in the general population, but from what is known of these disorders in clinical and legal settings, it can be assumed that they are chronic and resistant to change. Paraphilic urges and fantasy likely decline in frequency and intensity in the latter decades in a manner analogous to the decline in frequency and urgency of more typical forms of sexuality. The prognosis is improved with treatment, but the treatment failure rate is still high.

PARAPHILIC DIAGNOSES

The descriptions in the sections that follow are based on DSM-IV diagnostic criteria.

Exhibitionism

Exhibitionism involves recurrent, intense, sexually arousing fantasies, sexual urges, or behaviors involving the exposure of one's genitals to an unsuspecting stranger. The exhibitionist may or may not masturbate coincidentally with the exposure of his genitals. The victim's reaction, or the exhibitionist's fantasy of that reaction, plays a major role in his sexual satisfaction. Exhibitionistic behavior is often ritualized, with the same behavioral patterns repeated during each episode.

Fetishism

Fetishism involves recurrent, intense, sexually arousing fantasies, sexual urges, or behaviors involving nonliving objects, often articles of women's clothing. These objects are not limited to articles of women's clothing used in cross-dressing or to devices designed for the purpose of sexual stimulation.

The fetish object is frequently used for arousal during masturbation, and sexual arousal may be impossible in the absence of the object. If there is a sexual partner, the partner may be asked to wear or in some way use the fetish object during sexual activity.

Frotteurism

Frotteurism involves recurrent, intense, sexually arousing fantasies, sexual urges, or behaviors involving touching and rubbing against a nonconsenting person. This behavior frequently occurs in crowded public places, which afford the perpetrator a reasonable opportunity for escape.

Pedophilia

Pedophilia involves recurrent, intense, sexually arousing fantasies, sexual urges, or behaviors involving sexual activity with a prepubescent child or children (generally age 13 years or younger). A person must be at least 16 years of age and at least 5 years older than the child or children affected for the diagnosis to be made. Individuals in late adolescence involved in an ongoing sexual relationship with a 12 or 13 year old are excluded.

Individuals with this disorder tend to focus on children in a specific age range. Some have exclusively heterosexual interests (eg, focusing on girls age 8–11 years), others have exclusively homosexual interests (eg, focusing on boys age 9–12 years), whereas still others are attracted to either sex. The behavior may range from looking, to fondling, masturbation, and various degrees of penetration and coercion. Pedophiles may confine their behavior to their own children, their extended family, or strangers. Individuals with pedophilia often use elaborate intellectual rationalization to justify their behavior and may have well-developed and practiced manipulative techniques to entice children into sexual interaction. In many cases, this is an extremely chronic disorder with strong compulsive elements. Some individuals who focus on strangers have molested hundreds of children. This is one of the paraphilias that creates the most intense social approbation and is likely to lead to extensive entanglement in the legal system and incarceration.

Sexual Masochism

Sexual masochism involves recurrent, intense, sexually arousing fantasies, sexual urges, or behaviors involving the act (real, not simulated) of being humiliated, beaten, bound, or otherwise made to suffer.

Pornography related to sadomasochistic themes is widely available, but the implications of this availability for the prevalence of such disorders in the population are unclear. Some individuals confine their masochistic urges to fantasy, some act on these urges alone accompanied by masturbation, and others involve partners. Some prostitutes develop flourishing practices serving the needs of men with this disorder for domination. Some individuals need to escalate the intensity of their masochistic behavior over time, which on occasion results in severe injury or death.

Sexual Sadism

Sexual sadism involves recurrent, intense, sexually arousing fantasies, sexual urges, or behaviors involving acts (real, not simulated) in which the psychological or physical suffering (including humiliation) of a victim is sexually exciting to the person.

Some individuals with sexual sadism confine their sadism to fantasy, others team up with a consenting partner (often with sexual masochism), and still others inflict sexual pain on unwilling victims. The latter individuals have a tendency to continue to act out until apprehended and often escalate the severity of their sadistic behavior until they may present a true danger of death or serious injury to their victims. Sadistic sexual fantasies often begin in childhood, and the disorder has a chronic course.

Transvestic Fetishism

Transvestic fetishism involves recurrent, intense, sexually arousing fantasies, sexual urges, or behaviors involving cross-dressing. The diagnosis may be qualified by the specifier *with gender dysphoria,* if the patient has persistent discomfort with his assigned gender role.

In this disorder cross-dressing is done for purposes of sexual arousal and is usually accompanied by masturbation. Men with this disorder may take pleasure in wearing concealed articles of female clothing throughout the day. Cross-dressing behavior often takes on elements of increasing risk over time, beginning with cross-dressing alone in the privacy of the home and progressing to going out in public completely cross-dressed. At times the risk of discovery seems to contribute to the individual's sexual arousal.

This disorder is sometimes accompanied by gender dysphoria but is not diagnosed if the cross-dressing occurs only in the context of gender dysphoria without the element of sexual arousal. There is an extensive transvestic subculture with published magazines and a national organization of support groups. Episodes of cross-dressing may be accompanied by varying degrees of dissociation. The disorder tends to be chronic. Transvestic fetishism is not necessarily associated with a homosexual sexual object preference.

Voyeurism

Voyeurism involves recurrent, intense, sexually arousing fantasies, sexual urges, or behaviors involving the act of observing an unsuspecting person who is naked, in the process of disrobing or engaging in sexual activity.

In general, for individuals with this disorder the act of looking is the source of sexual arousal, and although it may be fantasized, no sexual contact with the person observed is sought. Occasionally, however, an individual may place himself in a compromising position in order to observe and may contact and even harm the victim in order to escape discovery. Although it is clearly infrequent, there have been reports of chronic voyeurism evolving into rape.

Paraphilia Not Otherwise Specified

This category includes the numerous paraphilic foci that are not included in the preceding categories.

American Psychiatric Association: Pages 522–532 in *Diagnostic and Statistical Manual of Mental Disorders,* 4th ed. American Psychiatric Association, 1994.

Marshall WL, Laws DR, Barbaree HE (editors): *Handbook of Sexual Assault: Issues, Theories, and Treatment of the Offender.* Plenum Publishing Corp, 1990.

Money J: *Gay, Straight and In-Between: The Sexology of Erotic Orientation.* Oxford University Press, 1988.

Eating Disorders

29

Harry E. Gwirtsman, MD, & Michael H. Ebert, MD

The eating disorders, anorexia nervosa and bulimia nervosa, may be classified as true psychosomatic illnesses, inasmuch as an underlying biological vulnerability interacts with a particular cultural stress in order to produce behavioral and psychological symptoms. For example, anorexia and bulimia nervosa are more prevalent in industrialized societies, where there is an overabundance of food and where attractiveness in women is linked with being thin, than in agriculturally based societies. Immigrants from cultures in which anorexia nervosa is rare are more likely to develop the illness as they assimilate the ideals of a thin body appearance.

ANOREXIA NERVOSA

DSM-IV Diagnostic Criteria

A. Refusal to maintain body weight over a minimally normal weight for age and height (eg, weight loss leading to maintenance of body weight less than 85% of that expected; or failure to make expected weight gain during a period of growth, leading to body weight less than 85% of that expected).

B. Intense fear of gaining weight or becoming fat, even though underweight.

C. Disturbance in the way in which one's body weight or shape is experienced, undue influence of body weight or shape on self-evaluation, or denial of the seriousness of the current low body weight.

D. In postmenarcheal females, amenorrhea, ie, the absence of at least three consecutive menstrual cycles. (A woman is considered to have amenorrhea if her periods occur only following hormone, eg, estrogen, administration.)

Specify type:

Restricting type: during the current episode of anorexia nervosa, the person has not regularly engaged in binge-eating or purging behavior (ie, self-induced vomiting or the misuse of laxatives, diuretics, or enemas).

Binge-eating/purging type: during the current episode of anorexia nervosa, the person has regularly engaged in binge-eating or purging behavior (ie, self-induced vomiting or the misuse of laxatives, diuretics, or enemas).

General Considerations

In some ways, the term anorexia nervosa is a misnomer, because the affected individual's appetite and craving for food are usually preserved. Nevertheless, the individual will actively counter the feelings of hunger with disordered thinking, leading to self-imposed starvation. The threshold for defining the amount of weight loss considered to be serious enough to qualify for the diagnosis of anorexia nervosa is computed on the basis of the Metropolitan Life Insurance tables or pediatric growth charts. A body mass index less than or equal to 17.5 kg/m^2 (calculated as weight in kilograms/height in meters^2) represents an alternative guideline accepted by many researchers. Nevertheless, these standards are only suggested guidelines, and clinicians should also consider the individual's body build and weight history.

A. Major Etiologic Theories: The incidence and prevalence of eating disorders have increased greatly in the latter half of the 20th century. This increase is due in part to cultural pressures in industrialized societies (placed largely on women), including an overemphasis on a slim female figure with an almost prepubescent shape. This emphasis is depicted in magazines, the entertainment industry, and beauty contests. Nevertheless, anorexia nervosa cannot be completely culturally based, because it appears to have been described almost 300 years ago, when cultural pressures were different. Consequently, part of the etiology of eating disorders must be biological, with the degree of phenotypic expression determined by cultural factors. Disturbances in central nervous system monoamines, particularly norepinephrine and serotonin, and in certain neuropeptides have been reported in the acute phase of anorexia nervosa. Few of these abnormalities persist into the weight-restored phase of the illness, and those that do may be at least partially related to the state of malnutrition.

B. Epidemiology: Lifetime prevalence rates for anorexia nervosa in females are approximately 0.5–1.0, or 1 in 100–200 individuals. Many more individuals exhibit symptoms that do not meet the criteria for the disorder (ie, eating disorder not otherwise specified; see later in this chapter), but this is an area for continued research. More than 90% of affected individuals are female, and data concerning the prevalence of the illness in males are scant. Worldwide, the disorder appears to be most common in the United States, Canada, Europe, Australia, Japan, New Zealand, and South Africa; but few systematic studies of the illness have been conducted in other countries.

The onset of illness is bimodal: One peak occurs in early adolescence (age 12–15 years) and another in late adolescence and early adulthood (age 17–21 years); the mean age at onset is approximately 17 years. It rarely appears de novo before puberty or after age 40 years. Often an associated life event, such as moving away from home, precedes the first episode of anorexia nervosa.

C. Genetics: Concordance rates for monozygotic twins with anorexia nervosa are higher than those for dizygotic twins. Among first-degree biological relatives, there is an increased risk for anorexia nervosa and for mood disorder, the latter found particularly among the relatives of individuals with the binge-eating/purging type.

Clinical Findings

A. Signs & Symptoms: Weight loss is frequently accomplished by reduction in total food intake and also involves the exclusion of highly caloric foods, leading to an extremely restricted diet. Patients may lose weight by purging (via either self-induced vomiting or misuse of laxatives and diuretics) or by exercising excessively. As weight continues to decline, the patient's fear of becoming fat may increase, as do feelings of being overweight. The body image distortion that these individuals experience has a wide range, from the fervently held belief that one is globally overweight, to a realization that one is thin but that certain body parts such as the abdomen, buttocks, or thighs are too big. Such disturbed self-perceptions may be modified by cultural factors and may not present prominently. Instead the patient may complain of a distaste for food or epigastric discomfort as the expressed motivation for food restriction.

Self-esteem in patients with anorexia nervosa is overly dependent on body shape and weight, and these patients seem obsessed with employing a wide variety of techniques to estimate body size, including frequent weighing, measuring of body parts, and looking in the mirror for perceived fat. Losing weight is judged to be an admirable achievement of unusual self-discipline, whereas weight gain is regarded as an unacceptable failure of self-control. Meanwhile, patients typically deny the serious medical implications of malnutrition.

Most patients with anorexia nervosa have food-related obsessions. They frequently hoard food or collect recipes and may be involved in food preparation for the family or in food-related professions (eg, waitress, cook, dietitian, nutritionist). They may also have fears of eating in public. Such obsessions have also been observed in other forms of starvation, including experimental starvation.

Signs of starvation account for most of the physical findings in anorexia nervosa. These signs include emaciation; significant hypotension, especially orthostatic; bradycardia; hypothermia; skin dryness and flakiness; Lanugo, or the presence of downy body hair on trunks or extremities; peripheral edema, especially ankle edema; petechiae on extremities; sallow complexion; salivary gland hypertrophy, particularly of the parotid gland; dental enamel erosion; and Russell's sign, or scars and calluses on the back of the hand. Amenorrhea may precede the onset of appreciable diminished weight, because it may be related to the loss of body fat stores rather than decrease of body mass. Menarche may be delayed in prepubertal females.

Among patients who frequently engage in purging behaviors, many do not binge eat. Instead they regularly vomit after consuming small meals.

B. Psychological Testing: Although extensive psychological testing is not used in the diagnosis of anorexia nervosa, screening tests can be extremely valuable in identifying eating psychopathology in community samples. Two such tests are the Eating Disorders Inventory and the Eating Attitudes Test. These tests are also useful in documenting improvement during treatment. It is also important to assess coexisting Axis I and Axis II psychiatric illness with relevant instruments such as the Structured Clinical Interview for the DSM-IV or the Beck Depression Inventory.

C. Laboratory Findings & Imaging: Most organ systems are affected by malnutrition, and a variety of physical disturbances can be noted (Table 29–1). Coexisting dehydration may be indicated by an elevated blood urea nitrogen. If induced vomiting is part of the clinical picture, then metabolic alkalosis may ensue, with elevated serum bicarbonate, hypochloremia, and hypokalemia. Laxative abuse may cause metabolic acidosis and a positive stool for occult blood. Neuroendocrine abnormalities are also common.

Amenorrhea is the result of abnormally low levels of estrogen secretion, which is due to a diminution of pituitary release of follicle-stimulating hormone and luteinizing hormone.

Differential Diagnosis

General medical conditions such as chronic inflammatory bowel disease, hyperthyroidism, malignan-

Table 29–1. Laboratory abnormalities in anorexia nervosa.

Category	Common	Uncommon/Rare
Hematology	Leukopenia Mild anemia	Thrombocytopenia
Chemistry	Abnormal luteinizing hormone (LH) release Elevated blood urea nitrogen Elevated cortisol Elevated liver functions Elevated serum bicarbonate Hypercarotenemia Hypercholesterolemia Hypochloremia Hypokalemia Low estrogen (females) Low normal thyroxine (T_4) Low triiodothyronine (T_3)	Hyperamylasemia Hypomagnesemia Hypophosphatemia Hypozincemia Low testosterone (males) Metabolic acidosis
Miscellaneous	Positive stool for occult blood	
Electrocardiogram	Sinus bradycardia	Arrhythmias
Electroencephalogram	Diffuse abnormalities	
Resting energy expenditure	Significantly reduced	
Brain imaging	Increased ventricular/brain ratio Widened cortical sulci	

cies, and AIDS can cause serious weight loss; however, it is rare for patients with these disorders to have a distorted body image, a fear of becoming obese, or a desire for further weight loss. Such medical conditions are also usually not associated with increased exercise and activity, except for hyperthyroidism. Superior mesenteric artery syndrome, a disorder characterized by postprandial vomiting secondary to intermittent gastric outlet obstruction, may precede or occur concurrently with anorexia nervosa when significant emaciation is present.

Coexisting major depressive disorder may present a difficult differential diagnosis. Most individuals with uncomplicated major depression do not have an excessive fear of gaining weight; however, even after weight restoration, anorexic patients may experience episodes of depression that require intervention. Individuals with schizophrenia may present with fluctuating weight patterns and bizarre beliefs related to food, but rarely demonstrate the body image disturbance and fear of fat associated with anorexia nervosa.

Because the diagnostic criteria for social phobia, obsessive-compulsive disorder, and body dysmorphic disorder overlap with those of anorexia nervosa, additional diagnoses of these disorders should be made only if individuals with anorexia nervosa have fears, obsessions, or body distortions unrelated to eating, food, or body shape and size.

Treatment

Anorexic individuals seldom seek professional assistance on their own, but instead are persuaded or coerced by family members to be evaluated for treatment. These individuals rarely complain about the weight loss per se but rather will describe the somatic or psychological distress related to the consequences of starvation, such as cold intolerance, muscle weakness or loss of stamina, constipation, abdominal pain, and mental depression. Frequently patients deny the core problem, and the history obtained from such patients is unreliable. Consequently it is advisable for the clinician to obtain information from family members or other outside sources to accurately evaluate features of the illness, such as the degree of weight loss.

A multidisciplinary approach is essential in treating anorexia nervosa. Patients may require acute intensive medical intervention to correct fluid and electrolyte imbalances, cardiac problems, and organ failure. The advent of behavior therapies has reduced markedly the morbidity and mortality of the illness; these therapies are now the centerpiece of most inpatient therapeutic programs. There is general agreement that weight restoration should be a central goal for the seriously underweight patient, and most of these patients will require inpatient management, during which controlled conditions can be achieved. In such an environment, patients are encouraged to consume increased numbers of calories in order to earn specific privileges, such as increased activity, decreased need for staff supervision, visits from relatives, and therapeutic sessions. During this phase, patients must be engaged in individual and family therapy in order to secure their cooperation and alliance with the treatment program.

Careful attention must be paid to caloric intake, so that these patients are not fed too quickly, but they must receive enough food to overcome their metabolic resistance, both during and immediately after the weight-gaining phase. Pharmacologic agents, such as antidepressants, neuroleptics, cyproheptadine, and lithium, may be helpful adjuncts, especially for patients who have coexisting depressive or psychotic features. No specific psychopharmacologic agent has been discovered that can induce an anorexic patient to eat and gain weight outside of a structured behaviorally oriented program.

Complications, Comorbidity, & Adverse Outcomes of Treatment

Medical complications of anorexia nervosa are common, especially if the disease has been present for 5 years or more. Complications include anemia, which is usually normochromic and normocytic (ie, with normal erythrocyte indices); impaired renal function, which is associated with chronic dehydration and hypokalemia, or the direct toxicity of laxatives; cardiovascular complications such as arrhythmias and hypotension; osteoporosis, resulting from diminished dietary calcium, increased cortisol, and decreased estrogen secretion; and dental decay.

Many patients with anorexia nervosa exhibit symptoms of depressed mood, social withdrawal, irritability, insomnia, and diminished interest in sex. Almost 50% meet criteria for major depressive disorder, but these features may be complications of starvation rather than a truly comorbid condition. Such depressive symptoms should be reassessed after weight restoration, because they persist in a subset of patients. Patients with the bulimic type of anorexia nervosa are more likely to abuse alcohol or other drugs, exhibit labile mood, be sexually active, and have other impulse-control problems. If anorexia nervosa develops prior to puberty, it may be associated with more severe comorbid mental disturbances.

Obsessive-compulsive symptoms unrelated to food, body shape, or weight may be present and may warrant a diagnosis of obsessive-compulsive disorder. Other psychological symptoms, such as feelings of ineffectiveness, a need to control one's environment, inflexible thinking, limited social spontaneity, and overly restrained initiative and emotional expression, may also be observed during the course of the illness (Table 29–2).

Prognosis & Course of Illness

Reviews of follow-up studies show that about 45% of patients have an overall good outcome, about 30% have an intermediate outcome (ie, still having considerable difficulty with the symptoms of the illness), and about 25% have poor outcome and rarely achieve a normal weight. Between 5% and 10% of patients with anorexia nervosa die as a result of complications. Patients who have had the illness chronically or intermittently for 12 years or more have death rates as high as 20%. Most commonly death results from the con-

Table 29–2. Comorbidity of anorexia nervosa.

Disorder	Percentage
Anxiety disorders	60–65
Phobia	40–61
Obsessive-compulsive disorder	26–48
Mood disorders	36–68
Substance abuse	23–35
Personality disorders	23–35
Cluster A	<5
Cluster B	15–55
Cluster C	15–60

sequences of starvation, suicide, or electrolyte imbalance. Approximately 40% of patients are able to give up the peculiarities related to food consumption acquired during the anorexic episode, such as binge eating, laxative abuse, or other obsessive food rituals. Only about 25% will be able to give up the weight phobias and distorted body image associated with the disorder. These observations indicate that the psychological sequelae of anorexia nervosa are perhaps the most enduring and resistant to treatment. Some research suggests that an onset during early adolescence (ie, age 13–15 years) may be associated with a better prognosis.

BULIMIA NERVOSA

DSM-IV Diagnostic Criteria

A. Recurrent episodes of binge eating. An episode of binge eating is characterized by both of the following:

  (1) eating, in a discrete period of time (eg, within any 2-hour period), an amount of food that is definitely larger than most people would eat during a similar period of time and under similar circumstances

  (2) a sense of lack of control over eating during the episode (eg, a feeling that one cannot stop eating or control what or how much one is eating)

B. Recurrent inappropriate compensatory behavior in order to prevent weight gain, such as self-induced vomiting; misuse of laxatives, diuretics, enemas, or other medications; fasting; or excessive exercise.

C. The binge eating and inappropriate compensatory behaviors both occur, on average, at least twice a week for 3 months.

D. Self-evaluation is unduly influenced by body shape and weight.

E. The disturbance does not occur exclusively during episodes of anorexia nervosa.

Specify type:

Purging type: during the current episode of bulimia nervosa, the person has regularly engaged in self-induced vomiting or the misuse of laxatives, diuretics, or enemas.

Nonpurging type: during the current episode of bulimia nervosa, the person has used other inappropriate compensatory behaviors, such as fasting or excessive exercise, but has not regularly engaged in self-induced vomiting or the misuse of laxatives, diuretics, or enemas.

Reprinted, with permission, from *Diagnostic and Statistical Manual of Mental Disorders,* 4th ed. Copyright 1994 American Psychiatric Association.

General Considerations

The term bulimia has a Greek derivation meaning "ox hunger" and connotes a state in which an individual repetitively consumes a feast-like quantity of food. For this condition to be classified as a psychiatric disorder, some emotional distress must be associated with the habit of binge eating. More recently, the subjective quality of a feeling of loss of control over the eating has become integrally associated with the illness.

The modern definition of bulimia first appeared in DSM-III, which relied on a series of descriptive criteria to characterize the disorder. Many of the descriptors were mostly accurate, such as "inconspicuous eating" and "frequent weight fluctuations." However, the criteria lacked specificity because no measure of the severity or frequency of binge eating had been set. Additionally, a poorly formulated conceptualization of comorbidity mandated the presence of depressed mood and excluded the possibility of an association with anorexia nervosa. Many binge eaters do not necessarily have concomitant depression, and a number

of patients with food-restrictive anorexia nervosa eventually develop bulimic behaviors. Consequently, an enormous overlap exists between anorexia and bulimia nervosa, approaching 50% of patients with anorexia.

The revised diagnostic criteria (DSM-IV) have provided solutions to many of these problems. First, the disorder was renamed bulimia nervosa, distinguishing it from the activity of binge eating. The severity criterion now requires at least two binge-eating episodes for a period of 2 months or more. Additionally, a previous history or concurrent diagnosis of anorexia nervosa does not exclude the diagnosis of bulimia nervosa. Finally, the symptom of purging one's food has been incorporated as a required criterion.

This classification method set up an interesting dilemma: How does one diagnose repetitive binge eating that is out of control in patients who do not purge their food? DSM-IV has proposed research diagnostic criteria for binge-eating disorder (Table 29–3). The new definition has incorporated a severity criterion (Criterion C) of two binge-eating episodes per week for a 6-month period of time. The characteristics of binge-eating disorder bear a striking resemblance to those of bulimia in DSM-III. To add more specificity to the diagnosis, the concurrent appearance of frequent purging behavior, as seen in bulimia nervosa, and diet pill abuse are exclusionary criteria.

A. Major Etiologic Theories: The cultural pressures described previously for anorexia nervosa also operate in the etiology of bulimia nervosa, namely the excessive idealization of thinness and the prejudice against obesity. These pressures are particularly evident when career choices involve public display of the body, such as in dancing, fashion modeling, acting, and so on. Bulimic symptomatology is especially prevalent in women who have chosen such careers.

Preexistent trauma such as sexual or physical abuse may be a risk factor for eating disorders; however, a recent review of the literature was unable to find a

Table 29–3. DSM-IV research diagnostic criteria for binge-eating disorder.[1]

A. Recurrent episodes of binge eating. An episode of binge eating is characterized by both of the following:
  (1) eating, in a discrete period of time (eg, within any 2-hour period), an amount of food that is definitely larger than most people would eat in a similar period of time under similar circumstances
  (2) a sense of lack of control over eating during the episode (eg, a feeling that one cannot stop eating or control what or how much one is eating)
B. The binge-eating episodes are associated with three (or more) of the following:
  (1) eating much more rapidly than normal
  (2) eating until feeling uncomfortably full
  (3) eating large amounts of food when not feeling physically hungry
  (4) eating alone because of being embarrassed by how much one is eating
  (5) feeling disgusted with oneself, depressed, or very guilty after overeating
C. Marked distress regarding binge eating is present.
D. The binge eating occurs, on average, at least 2 days a week for 6 months.
E. The binge eating is not associated with the regular use of inappropriate compensatory behaviors (eg, purging, fasting, excessive exercise) and does not occur during the course of anorexia nervosa or bulimia nervosa.

[1] Reprinted, with permission, from *Diagnostic and Statistical Manual of Mental Disorders,* 4th ed. Copyright 1994 American Psychiatric Association, pp. 729–731.

specific causal relationship between early abuse experiences and bulimia nervosa.

As with anorexia nervosa, some research has linked aberrant central nervous system monoamine metabolism with bulimia nervosa, particularly serotonin deficiency. Whether these biological abnormalities are the cause or consequence of the binge-purge behaviors has yet to be determined. However, it is of interest that fluoxetine, a pharmacologic agent that presumably makes more serotonin available at the synapse, has demonstrated efficacy in this disorder.

B. Epidemiology: Prevalence rate estimates for bulimia are based predominantly on surveys carried out in high school and college populations. Table 29–4 summarizes the results of 22 studies of approximately 18,000 high school and college individuals. The behavior of binge eating was found to be extremely common, appearing in 36% of respondents across studies. This prevalence rate declines as progressively restrictive definitions are applied. Only 1–3% of respondents engaged in binge-purge behavior so severe that it met the criteria for a psychiatric illness as defined in DSM-IV. Nevertheless, as Table 29–4 illustrates clearly, the reservoir of individuals who engage in binge-eating behavior is quite large. This provides a population of susceptible candidates whose behaviors may intensify, provided that current cultural stressors, such as the overvaluation of an excessively thin appearance, continue unabated.

The Epidemiologic Catchment Area study, the largest survey of psychiatric disorders in the United States to date, was carried out before the criteria for bulimia or bulimia nervosa were available and, therefore, was unable to assess the prevalence of this disorder. However, at a prevalence rate of 1–3%, bulimia nervosa is at least as common in the female population as other major psychiatric disorders such as schizophrenia (1.5%) and major depressive disorder (1.3%). Furthermore, available evidence indicates that the incidence of eating disorders and particularly bulimia nervosa has continued to increase.

Table 29–4. Prevalence rate estimates for bulimia.[1]

	Mean	Range
Binge eating	36%	7–75%
Weekly binge eating	16%	5–39%
DSM-III bulimia	9%	3–19%
DSM-III-R bulimia nervosa	2%	1–3%

[1] Modified and reproduced, with permission, from Devlin MJ et al: Is there another binge eating disorder? A review of the literature on overeating in the absence of bulimia nervosa. Int J Eating Dis 1992;11:333; Fairburn CG, Beglin SJ: Studies of the epidemiology of bulimia nervosa. Am J Psychiatry 1990;147:401; and from Mitchell JE: *Bulimia Nervosa.* University of Minnesota Press, 1990.

Most surveys that have examined the sex ratio of patients with bulimia or bulimia nervosa have found the overwhelming preponderance (98–100%) to be female. The average age at onset of the disorder is 18–20 years, and most patients are seen for psychiatric consultation after 3–5 years. Thus epidemiologic research demonstrates complete unanimity in reporting that bulimia, like anorexia nervosa, is almost exclusively a disorder of young women.

Although, as mentioned earlier in this chapter, the female population in the industrialized world yearns to emulate the slimmest appearing models, in reality an extremely high proportion of women are overweight. Over 18 million women (27.1%) in the United States are overweight, and over 7 million (10.8%) are severely overweight (Table 29–5). Furthermore, obesity appears to be most prevalent in minorities, especially in African Americans and Hispanics. A field study of binge-eating disorder has found that this is an extremely prevalent problem. Two percent of individuals in a community sample identified themselves as having had the disorder. Furthermore, the prevalence rate of binge-eating disorder is 30% among obese individuals involved in weight loss programs and is as high as 70% in self-help groups such as Overeaters Anonymous. According to available studies, 60–75% of patients with binge-eating disorder are female.

C. Genetics: Studies have reported an increased risk of substance abuse, alcoholism, and mood disorders in the first-degree relatives of patients with bulimia nervosa. A large study has found a higher concordance rate for bulimia nervosa in monozygotic than dizygotic female twin pairs. It is less well established that there is an increased frequency of obesity in first-degree relatives of bulimic individuals. The D_2 dopamine receptor has emerged as a possible candidate gene meriting further study, but the field currently lacks animal models that might illuminate further genetic and biological research.

Clinical Findings

A. Signs & Symptoms: It is very important to be able to differentiate a clinically defined binge from what would normally be considered a feast during holidays such as Thanksgiving. In one study, bulimic patients were asked to engage in binge-eating and purging behavior while in a controlled hospital environment. Bulimic subjects consumed over 3000 calories during each binge, and this food was ingested in less than 40 minutes, followed by a purge. Frequently, individuals with bulimia nervosa will engage in repetitive binge-purge activity. Typically bulimic individuals will consume high-caloric, easily ingested foods such as ice cream or cake, but this is not always the case.

Vomiting is by far the most widely used compensatory behavior to control weight, probably because it is also the most efficient means of preventing weight

Table 29–5. Estimated prevalence of overweight and severe overweight for persons age 20–74 in the United States.[1]

	Men		Women	
	Overweight	**Severely Overweight**	**Overweight**	**Severely Overweight**
White	24.4%	7.8%	24.6%	9.6%
Black	6.3%	10.4%	45.1%	19.7%
Mexican	31.2%	10.8%	41.5%	16.7%
Total	24.2%	8.0%	27.1%	10.8%
	15.4 million	5.1 million	18.6 million	7.4 million

[1] Adapted, with permission, from the National Health and Nutrition Examination Survey (1976–1980). Kuczmarski RJ: Prevalence of overweight and weight gain in the United States. Am J Clin Nutr 1992;55:495S.

gain. Vomiting is used by 80–90% of bulimic individuals. Approximately one third of patients with bulimia nervosa abuse laxatives; enemas and diuretics are used much less frequently.

Self-esteem in patients with bulimia nervosa is inordinately dependent on body shape and weight but not to the degree observed in patients with anorexia nervosa. Although bulimic patients generally feel that they cannot control the binge-purge behavior, they are frequently able to engage in the behavior only surreptitiously, and plan binges around important daily activities such as work and school.

B. Psychological Testing: As with anorexia nervosa, the diagnosis of bulimia nervosa does not depend on the results of psychological tests, although the tests mentioned in the discussion of anorexia nervosa are useful for screening purposes and for monitoring treatment response. The Eating Disorders Examination is perhaps the most extensively used comprehensive interview-based assessment instrument for the clinical characterization of an eating disorder. As with anorexia nervosa, it is helpful to use the appropriate psychological tests to characterize and quantify comorbid depression, anxiety, or Axis II disorders.

C. Laboratory Findings & Imaging: Vomiting leads to a loss of gastric hydrochloric acid, which results in hypochloremia and, via renal compensatory mechanisms, hypokalemia. Serum electrolytes frequently demonstrate metabolic alkalosis, with elevations in serum bicarbonate. Serum amylase has also been mildly elevated, predominantly the S amylase fraction, derived from the salivary glands. Hypomagnesemia is another common finding in the purging type of bulimia. In bulimic individuals who abuse laxatives, chronic diarrhea may lead to metabolic acidosis and hyponatremia.

Differential Diagnosis

Few medical syndromes mimic the major features of bulimia nervosa. Most of these syndromes are rare neurologic illnesses such as the Kluver-Bucy syndrome, the Kleine-Levin syndrome, or brain tumors originating near or invading the hypothalamic area. Occasionally patients develop bulimic symptoms in the context of certain types of epilepsy or in the course of progressive dementias. None of these syndromes is associated with the overconcern with body shape and weight characteristic of bulimia.

DSM-IV rules out the diagnosis of bulimia nervosa if patients meet the weight criterion for anorexia nervosa; however, the course of an eating disorder may exhibit sequential episodes of both disorders. Patients with major depression often exhibit atypical features, including overeating during the wintertime; however, such patients rarely engage in compensatory behaviors in order to control weight. The eating disorder most commonly seen in an office-based practice is eating disorder not otherwise specified (see later in this chapter). This disorder presents a challenge to clinicians who are unfamiliar with the specific criteria for bulimia nervosa. These criteria must all be met before the patient can be diagnosed with a particular form of bulimia nervosa.

Treatment

Treatment of bulimia nervosa is currently accomplished by a variety of approaches. Patients who demonstrate major electrolyte disturbance, who have depression with suicidal ideation, or who have not responded to outpatient management are candidates for inpatient treatment. Hospitalization is rarely required for uncomplicated bulimia nervosa. Many psychosocial approaches have value in the treatment of this disorder, and current research emphasizes the short-term effectiveness of cognitive-behavioral and interpersonal psychotherapy. Group psychotherapy has also been found to be a superior form of treatment. Antidepressants of every class, including tricyclics, monoamine oxidase inhibitors, trazodone, and selective serotonin reuptake inhibitors, have demonstrated efficacy in reducing bulimic symptoms. Several medication trials are sometimes required to establish the proper medication for a given patient. Approximately 15–20% of patients may require only a pharmacologic agent to achieve a response.

Table 29–6. Medical complications of bulimia nervosa.

Cardiovascular Cardiomyopathy (with ipecac abuse) Electrocardiogram changes and arrhythmias Orthostatic hypotension **Dehydration and electrolyte abnormalities** Hypokalemia Hyponatremia (with laxative abuse) Metabolic alkalosis **Dental** Increased caries Upper incisor erosions **Dermatologic** Hand abrasions (Russell's sign) Petechial hemorrhages	**Endocrine** Abnormal dexamethasone suppression test Irregular menses and amenorrhea **Gastrointestinal** Cathartic colon (with laxative abuse) Constipation Esophageal/gastric perforations (Mallory-Weiss syndrome) Esophagitis/gastritis Gastrointestinal bleeding Salivary gland hypertrophy **Neurologic** Increased seizure frequency Reversible cerebral atrophy

Complications, Comorbidity, & Adverse Outcomes of Treatment

Binge eating is a dangerous behavior pattern, and it becomes even more hazardous when coupled with purging. Complications may affect almost every bodily system ranging from the integument to glandular regulation by the neuroendocrine system (Table 29–6). Even so, many bulimic individuals are able to continue their aberrant eating behaviors for many years before seeking treatment. Frequently the appearance of a medical complication, such as gastrointestinal bleeding, dental caries, or loss of dental enamel from the lingual surfaces of the incisors, initiates the process of psychiatric referral and treatment. By the time bulimic individuals become patients, however, their metabolic disturbances are quite advanced. Investigations have revealed that more than 50% of patients with diagnosed bulimia nervosa exhibited signs of dehydration and an electrolyte abnormality, 25% had metabolic alkalosis and diminished serum chloride, and 14% had demonstrable hypokalemia. Such metabolic abnormalities are usually associated with muscle fatigue and general malaise and can also be responsible for the pathogenesis of dangerous cardiac tachyarrhythmias. Though not common, patients with bulimia nervosa may develop potentially fatal complications such as cardiac arrhythmias, orthostatic hypotension, seizures, or gastric rupture.

A frequently noted physical sign is the chipmunk appearance of the face, caused by marked hypertrophy of the salivary glands. Another hallmark of the illness is Russell's sign, consisting of abrasions, calluses, or scars on the back of the hand used to manually induce vomiting. In general, medical complications are more common in patients with the purging type of bulimia than in those with the nonpurging type.

Patients with bulimia nervosa have high rates of coexisting psychopathology (Table 29–7). Rates of mood disorder range from 24% to 88%, although the symptoms of major depression with melancholic features are observed less frequently. Concomitant personality disorder may also complicate bulimia nervosa, with rather low rates of the cluster A (schizoid, schizotypal, paranoid) subtypes but significantly higher rates of comorbid cluster B (histrionic, borderline, narcissistic, antisocial) and cluster C (avoidant, obsessive-compulsive, dependent, passive-aggressive) forms. Obsessive-compulsive disorder is also noted, but studies show considerable variation in reports of coprevalence rates, ranging from 3% to 80%. Rates of other anxiety disorders (eg, generalized anxiety, phobias, panic disorder) are lower, ranging from 2% to 31%.

Accumulating evidence indicates that patients with binge-eating disorder have increased psychopathology compared to obese control subjects who do not engage in binge eating. The disorders most frequently associated with binge-eating disorder appear to be major depression, panic disorder, bulimia nervosa, borderline personality disorder, and avoidant personality disorder.

Prognosis & Course of Illness

Little is known about the natural history or long-term outcome of bulimia nervosa. Approximately 70% of those who complete treatment programs report substantial reduction of bulimic symptoms. Of the seven follow-up studies that have relevant data, four are based on retrospective data (Table 29–8). The

Table 29–7. Comorbidity of bulimia nervosa.

Disorder	Percentage
Mood disorders	24–88
Anxiety	2–3
Obsessive-compulsive disorder	3–80
Substance abuse	9–55
Personality disorders	
Cluster A	<10
Cluster B	2–75
Cluster C	16–80

Table 29–8. Outcome studies of bulimia nervosa.[1]

Study (Population Size)	Number of Studies	Design[2]	Follow-up Interval (Range)	Rate of Recovery (Range)
Outpatients ($N = 200$)	5	R = 3, P = 2	2.2 years (1–6 years)	46% (29–71%)
Inpatients ($N = 280$)	2	R = 1, P = 1	2.2 years (2–5 years)	38% (13–41%)

[1] Adapted, with permission, from Herzog DB et al: The course and outcome of bulimia nervosa. J Clin Psychiatry 1991;52(Suppl):4.
[2] R, retrospective; P, prospective.

studies are split between inpatient and outpatient samples, with a mean follow-up period of 2.2 years (range 1–6 years). Overall, the rates of recovery are disappointing, with only 46% of outpatients and 38% of inpatients meeting the criteria for recovery. The term "recovery" has not yet been fully defined for bulimic disorders, and it varies from study to study. Nevertheless, the data thus far argue strongly that treatment for bulimia nervosa is only partially effective and that relapse is quite common. Patients with bulimia nervosa may require more prolonged therapy in order to experience a sustained remission.

No information is available yet on the outcome of binge-eating disorder, although it is well known that obesity in general has an extremely poor long-term outcome.

EATING DISORDER NOT OTHERWISE SPECIFIED (NOS)

DSM-IV Diagnostic Criteria

The eating disorder not otherwise specified category is for disorders of eating that do not meet the criteria for a specific eating disorder. Examples include:

1. For females, all of the criteria for anorexia nervosa are met except that the individual has regular menses.
2. All of the criteria for anorexia nervosa are met except that, despite significant weight loss, the individual's current weight is in the normal range.
3. All of the criteria for bulimia nervosa are met except that the binge eating and inappropriate compensatory mechanisms occur at a frequency of less than twice a week or for a duration of less than 3 months.

4. The regular use of inappropriate compensatory behavior by an individual of normal body weight after eating small amounts of food (eg, self-induced vomiting after the consumption of two cookies).
5. Repeatedly chewing and spitting out, but not swallowing, large amounts of food.
6. Binge-eating disorder: recurrent episodes of binge eating in the absence of the regular use of compensatory behaviors characteristic of bulimia nervosa (see Table 29–3).

Reprinted, with permission, from *Diagnostic and Statistical Manual of Mental Disorders,* 4th ed. Copyright 1994 American Psychiatric Association.

American Psychiatric Association: Practice guidelines for eating disorders. Am J Psychiatry 1993;150:212.

Anderson AE: *Practical Comprehensive Treatment of Anorexia Nervosa and Bulimia.* Johns Hopkins University Press, 1985.

Brownell KD, Fairburn CG (editors): *Eating Disorders and Obesity: A Comprehensive Textbook.* Guilford Press, 1995.

Fairburn CG, Wilson GT (editors): *Binge Eating: Nature, Assessment, and Treatment.* Guilford Press, 1993.

Garner DM, Garfinkel PE (editors): *Handbook of Treatment for Eating Disorders,* 2nd ed. Guilford Press, 1997.

Halmi K (editor): *Psychobiology and Treatment of Anorexia Nervosa and Bulimia.* American Psychiatric Press, 1992.

Kaye WH, Gwirtsman HE (editors): *A Comprehensive Approach to the Treatment of Normal Weight Bulimia.* American Psychiatric Press, 1985.

Mitchell JE: *Bulimia Nervosa.* University of Minnesota Press, 1990.

Pope HG, Hudson JI: Is childhood sexual abuse a risk factor for bulimia nervosa? Am J Psychiatry 1992;149:455.

Yager J, Gwirtsman HE, Edelstein CK (editors): *Special Problems in Managing Eating Disorders.* American Psychiatric Press, 1992.

30

Sleep Disorders

Camellia P. Clark, MD, Polly J. Moore, PhD, RPsgT, Tahir I. Bhatti, MD,
Erich Seifritz, MD, & J. Christian Gillin, MD

GENERAL APPROACH TO THE PATIENT

OFFICE EVALUATION

Clinicians should always include a few screening questions about sleep and wakefulness in the review of systems. Most doctors neglect to ask about sleep and wakefulness; most patients with sleep-wake disorders do not bring these complaints to the attention of their physicians unless specifically questioned about sleep-wake symptoms. In particular, it is important to ask about the quantity and quality of sleep, excessive fatigue and daytime sleepiness, use of sedatives and stimulants (including coffee), timing of sleep and wakefulness throughout the 24-hour day, and unusual behaviors during sleep, including snoring, gasping, dyspnea, orthopnea, or unusual movements.

A thorough sleep history will lay the foundation for accurate diagnosis and effective treatment of any sleep disorder (Table 30–1). Patients' sleep complaints will usually fall into four general categories: complaints of difficulty initiating sleep or staying asleep (insomnia), difficulty staying awake during the day (hypersomnia), having abnormal movements or behaviors during sleep (parasomnias), timing of the sleep-wake cycle at undesired or inappropriate times over a 24-hour day (circadian rhythm disorders), or a combination of any of the above.

During the evaluation of a patient who has a sleep complaint, the patient's bed partner and other informants might be included. The sleep evaluation for sleep apnea, periodic limb movements during sleep, or excessive daytime sleepiness is often initiated by the bed partner because the patient is frequently unaware of his or her sleep and wakefulness difficulties. The disorder may disturb household members. This is the case particularly for patients who have unusual sleep-related behaviors (eg, night terrors in children) or loud snoring or leg kicking during sleep.

A key element in the sleep history is the sleep diary, a log the patient keeps on a daily basis to track his or her sleep patterns, usually over a period of about 2 weeks. This log can be given to the patient during the initial visit and assesses sleep onset, time of awakening in the morning, time spent in bed, time spent out of bed during the night, and number of awakenings. It also assesses other factors affecting sleep such as caffeine, alcohol, or medication use; naps during the day; levels of stress during the day; and other symptoms or illnesses.

As with evaluation of any specific complaint, the clinician should obtain a thorough history of all pertinent medical and psychiatric problems, family history, review of medications, review of relationship and environmental stressors, review of systems as well as a complete physical examination including a thorough neurologic exam. Specific questions that lead to diagnosis are outlined in Figure 30–1.

SLEEP LABORATORY EVALUATION

Most sleep complaints can be managed by the nonspecialist, with the motivation and cooperation of the patient, through behavioral modification, treatment of underlying and comorbid diagnoses, and appropriate use of medications for symptomatic relief of sleep-related symptoms. For some conditions, such as sleep apnea, periodic limb movements during sleep, narcolepsy, parasomnias with potential for serious injury, or intractable insomnia, referral to a sleep disorder center should be considered. To gain maximal diagnostic value from the sleep recording, patients may be asked to maintain a regular sleep-wake schedule prior to the recording and to abstain from drugs or medications that may affect sleep. In some cases, toxicology screens may be obtained prior to sleep study.

Nocturnal polysomnography (PSG) involves recording the patient's sleep overnight in the sleep laboratory. Ideally, polygraphic sleep recordings are obtained at

Table 30–1. Office evaluation of chronic sleep complaints.[1]

1. Detailed history and review of the sleep complaint, as well as predisposing, precipitating, and perpetuating factors
2. Review of the difficulties falling asleep, maintaining sleep, and awakening early
3. Timing of sleep and wakefulness over the 24-hour day
4. Evidence of excessive daytime sleepiness and fatigue
5. Bedtime routines, sleep setting, preoccupations, anxiety, beliefs about sleep and sleep loss, fears about consequences of sleep loss, nightmares, enuresis, and sleepwalking
6. Medical and neurologic history and examination and routine laboratory examinations
7. Review of use of prescription and nonprescription medications, hypnotics, alcohol, and stimulants
8. Evidence of sleep-related breathing disorders: snoring; orthopnea; dyspnea; headaches; falling out of bed; nocturia; obesity; short, fat neck; enlarged tonsils; narrow upper oral airway; and foreshortened jaw (retrognathia)
9. Abnormal movements during sleep: "jerky legs," leg movements, myoclonus, "restless legs," leg cramps, and cold feet
10. Psychiatric history and examination
11. Social and occupational history, marital status, living conditions, financial and security concerns, and physical activity
12. Sleep-wake diary for 2 weeks
13. Interview with bed partners or persons who observe the patient during sleep
14. Tape recording of respiratory sounds during sleep to screen for sleep apnea

[1] From Gillin JC, Ancoli-Israel S: The impact of age on sleep and sleep disorders. Chapter 10 in Salzman C (editor): *Clinical Geriatric Psychopharmacology,* 2nd ed. Williams & Wilkins, 1992. With permission.

night, during daytime naps, or both, in a consistently quiet, dark, and comfortable laboratory environment on a multichannel electroencephalogram (EEG) or polygraph machine. Surface electrodes are affixed to the skin to monitor brain wave activity or EEG, bilateral eye movement activity or electrooculogram (EOG), and muscle tonus or electromyogram (EMG) recorded from the chin musculature. From these tracings, the stage of sleep for each 30- or 60-second period can be determined by visual scanning. The most common EEG leads used in sleep recordings are central (C3, C4) and occipital (O1, O2) sites and are often referenced to contralateral preauricular electrode sites.

Changes in the EEG frequencies discriminate the waking and NREM (or non–rapid eye movement) sleep stages; the concurrent presence of eye movements in the EOG, the dramatic decrease in muscle tone in the EMG, and a desynchronized EEG distinguish REM (rapid eye movement) sleep. During waking, the EEG **alpha wave** (8–13 Hz) is most prominent in the occipital leads; as sleep onset occurs, this frequency tends to drop out of the tracing. The EOG at sleep onset may also reveal slow, rolling eye movements. Filter settings appropriate for each channel maximize signal quality and readability and minimize intrusion of nonphysiologic sources of artifact into the recording. Table 30–2 defines terms commonly used in sleep studies.

OVERVIEW OF SLEEP

SLEEP STAGES & ARCHITECTURE

Normal sleep consists of two major states: REM sleep and NREM sleep (see Table 30–3 for a comparison). **REM sleep** is also sometimes called either dreaming sleep (because it is associated with dream-

ing) or paradoxical sleep (because the brain seems paradoxically to be activated during this state). **NREM sleep** conforms to traditional concepts of sleep as a time of decreased physiologic and psychological activity and is further divided into four sleep stages on the basis of visually scored EEG patterns.

Sleep normally begins with stage 1, a brief transitional phase, before progressing successively into stages 2 through 4, during which the EEG continues to synchronize or decline in frequency and increase in amplitude. Stage 2 sleep is defined by the presence of sleep spindles and K complexes in the EEG. Stages 3 and 4 sleep, also called **delta sleep** or slow-wave sleep, are defined by the presence of **delta waves** (0.5–2 Hz) in moderate (25–50%) and large (over 50%) proportions of an **epoch** (30- to 60-minute period) of sleep, respectively. Delta sleep is typically most intense in the first NREM period of the night, and the amount of delta sleep declines with each successive NREM period (Figure 30–2).

REM sleep is characterized by an activated (high-frequency and low-amplitude) desynchronized EEG, loss of tone in the major antigravity muscles, and periodic bursts of binocularly synchronous rapid eye movements. In the normal young adult, the first REM period usually begins about 70–100 minutes after the onset of sleep, a term referred to as **REM latency** (the elapsed time between the onset of sleep and the first REM period). REM latency may be significantly shorter in some patients with depression, eating disorders, borderline personality disorder, schizophrenia, alcohol-related disorders, or other psychiatric disorders. Thereafter, NREM and REM sleep oscillate with a cycle length of roughly 90 minutes. The first REM period usually lasts about 15 minutes; successive REM periods in young people increase in length throughout the night to about 25–40 minutes.

In a standard, complete polysomnographic workup, additional physiologic monitoring would entail various cardiorespiratory measures such as respiratory ef-

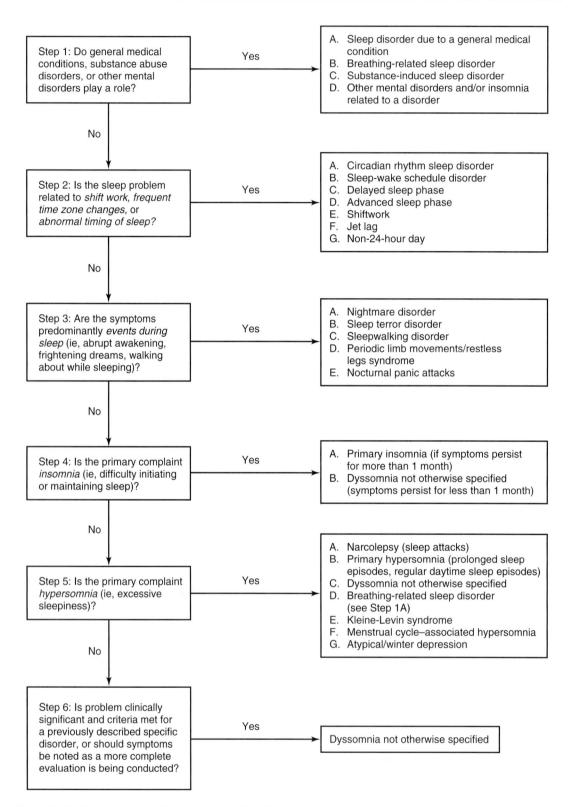

Figure 30–1. Steps for a sleep disturbance algorithm. (Reproduced, with permission, from Gillin JC, Ancoli-Israel S, Erman M: Sleep and sleep-wake disorders. Pages 1217–1248 in Tasman A, Kay J, Lieberman JA [editors]: *Psychiatry 2.* Saunders, 1996.)

Table 30–2. Glossary: terms commonly used in sleep studies.

Term	Definition
Alpha wave	8- to 12-Hz EEG wave characteristic of relaxed wakefulness; especially prominent in occipital EEG leads
Delta wave	EEG wave ≥75 microvolts amplitude and ≤2-Hz frequency; amplitude tends to decrease with age
REM sleep	Rapid eye movement sleep, characterized by bursts of rapid eye movements, low-voltage fast EEG, and atonia; associated with dreaming
NREM sleep	Non–rapid eye movement sleep; consists of four stages
Total sleep time	NREM sleep + REM sleep
Stage 1	A transitional state of lighter sleep between wakefulness and full sleep; characterized by low-voltage, mixed-frequency EEG and rolling eye movements
Stage 2	Sleep characterized by K complexes and spindles (short bursts of 12- to 14-Hz EEG activity); usually about 45–75% of total sleep time
Stage 3	Sleep characterized by 20–50% delta waves per *epoch* (30–60 seconds)
Stage 4	Sleep characterized by ≥50% delta waves per epoch
Delta sleep	Stages 3 and 4, also known as slow-wave sleep; declines with normal aging, depression, alcoholism, and other conditions
Sleep latency	Time from "lights out" to sleep onset
REM latency	Time from sleep onset to REM sleep onset; normally varies from about 70–100 minutes (in young adults) to 55–70 minutes (in elderly); may be abnormally short in narcolepsy, depression, and other conditions
REM density	A measure of eye movement frequency during REM sleep; often increased in depression
Sleep efficiency	Time asleep divided by total time in bed (usually expressed as a percentage); normally ≥90% in young adults; decreases somewhat with age
Wakefulness after sleep onset	Time awake after sleep onset
Respiratory disturbance index	Respiratory events (apneas + hypopneas) per hour of sleep (RDI); also known as apnea-hypopnea index (AHI)
Hypopnea	A reduction ≥50% in depth of respiration lasting ≥10 seconds
Multiple Sleep Latency Test (MSLT)	Objective measure of excessive daytime sleepiness in which sleep latency and REM latency are measured at four to five 20-minute nap opportunities spaced 2 hours apart throughout the day
PLMS index	Leg kicks per hour of sleep, also known as myoclonus index; normally ≤5; PLMS, periodic limb movements during sleep

Table 30–3. Comparison of NREM and REM sleep.[1]

Characteristic	NREM Sleep	REM Sleep
EEG	Spindles, K complexes, delta waves, synchronized	Low-voltage, mixed-frequency, saw-tooth waves, activated
EOG	Quiescent or slow movements	Bursts of fast movements
EMG	Partial relaxation	Atonia of antigravity muscles
Intercostal muscles	Partial relaxation	Atonia
Genioglossus	Partial relaxation	Hypotonic
Blood pressure	Decreased, steady	Variable
Heart rate	Decreased, steady	Variable
Cardiac output	Decreased	Decreased
Cerebral glucose metabolism	Decreased	Unchanged or increased
Brain temperature	Decreased	Increased
Respiratory rate	Decreased	Variable
Ventilatory response to CO_2	Intact	Partially impaired
Genitalia	Infrequent tumescence	Tumescence
Mentation	Conceptual, abstract, infrequent dreaming	Perceptual, frequent dreaming
Pathology	Night terrors, somnambulism, panic attacks	Nightmares, REM sleep behavior disorder

[1] From Gillin JC, Zoltoski RK, Salin-Pascual R: Basic science of sleep. Chapter 1.9 in Kaplan HI, Sadock BJ (editors): *Comprehensive Textbook of Psychiatry/VI,* 6th ed. Williams & Wilkins, 1995. With permission.

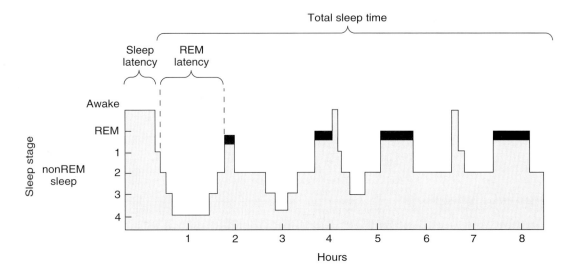

Figure 30–2. Hypnogram of normal sleep. (Reproduced, with permission, from Gillin JC, Ancoli-Israel S: The impact of age on sleep and sleep disorders. Chapter 10 in Salzman C [editor]: *Clinical Geriatric Psychopharmacology,* 2nd ed. Williams & Wilkins, 1992.)

fort monitoring at the chest and abdominal levels, plus an airflow measure such as end tidal CO_2 or nasal or oral thermistor, blood O_2 saturation, and an electrocardiographic reading. These measures are used to quantify the extent of sleep-related cardiac and breathing disturbances. Respiratory effort monitors include inductive plethysmography, strain gauges, and intercostal EMG. Esophageal pressure transducers also have been used, in the diagnosis of upper airway resistance syndrome.

Periodic limb movements during sleep (PLMS) are monitored with surface EMG electrodes adhered to the shins or the forearms. To aid in screening for nocturnal epilepsy, supplemental EEG leads may be added to the montage. Nocturnal penile tumescence monitoring is also helpful in discriminating psychogenic versus physiogenic impotence.

The multiple sleep latency test (MSLT) may be conducted on the day after the nocturnal polysomnogram and is an objective measure of propensity to fall asleep. The patient is given four or five opportunities to nap, each spaced 2 hours apart (eg, 10 A.M., 12 noon, 2 P.M., 4 P.M., 6 P.M.). Elapsed time to onset of any sleep stage in each nap is averaged over all naps. (If no sleep onset occurs, the "nap" is terminated after 20 minutes.) An average sleep latency of less than 5 minutes on the MSLT is considered indicative of pathologic sleepiness but is not in itself diagnostic of any specific disorder. However, the MSLT can be particularly useful in evaluating narcolepsy; the occurrence of REM sleep in two or more of the nap trials is considered diagnostic.

Ambulatory sleep recording devices are being developed to facilitate sleep measurement of patients in their own homes overnight. Though full of promise, at the present time the status of ambulatory recording remains tentative because of technical drawbacks and the possibility of false-negative evaluations. Ambulatory devices are presently considered a supplementary or lower-cost prescreening tool to augment a formal sleep evaluation but cannot substitute for it. Online PSG by trained technicians is still considered the gold standard for sleep evaluation: Technician observations provide not only high-quality recordings and valuable diagnostic information (eg, documenting the appearance of sleep behaviors such as those in REM behavior disorder) but also an additional measure of safety (eg, ability to obtain immediate medical care should serious dysrhythmias occur).

NEUROBIOLOGY OF SLEEP

The neurophysiologic underpinnings of sleep and wakefulness remain incompletely understood. Components of REM sleep itself—that is, periodic episodes of REM and muscle atonia—are generated within the brain stem. In contrast, NREM sleep is partially controlled by brain regions some of which are more rostral such as the basal forebrain, thalamus, hypothalamus, and perhaps the brain stem area near the nucleus solitarius. No specific neuroanatomic "sleep center" has yet been identified with certainty for the entire constellation of either REM or NREM sleep, although components of sleep appear to depend on specific areas.

No specific "sleep neurotransmitter" has yet been accepted by the majority of investigators (Table

Table 30–4. Neurotransmitters and neuromodulators that may regulate sleep-wake states.[1,2]

Substance	Possible Roles in the Regulation of Sleep-Wakefulness
Serotonin	L-Tryptophan has hypnotic effects, increases delta sleep. Serotonergic neurons in DRN cease firing in REM sleep and may inhibit cholinergic neurons in LDT-PPT, PGO waves, and REM sleep.
Norepinephrine	Noradrenergic neurons in LC cease firing in REM sleep and, together with the basal forebrain, inhibit cortical EEG synchronization through influence on the thalamus.
Dopamine	Dopamine mediates alerting effects of amphetamine and cocaine and sedating effects of antipsychotics. Sleepiness of narcolepsy may be related to decreased dopamine turnover.
Gamma aminobutyric acid (GABA)	Hypnotic and other effects of benzodiazepines may be mediated through enhancement of GABA.
Adenosine	Adenosine appears to promote sleep. Alerting effects of caffeine may be mediated by blockade of adenosine receptors.
Interleukins and other immune modulators	Interleukins promote slow-wave sleep in animals, and immune modulators may be increased in plasma at sleep onset in normal control subjects. NREM sleep measures may correlate with natural killer-cell activity in humans.
Prostaglandins	Prostaglandins D_2 and E_2 increase sleep and wakefulness, respectively, in animals.
Endogenous sleep factors	Putative hypnotoxins include DSIP, uridine, arginine vasotocin, and muramyl peptides.

[1] From Gillin JC, Zoltoski RK, Salin-Pascual R: Basic science of sleep. Chapter 1.9 in Kaplan HI, Sadock BJ (editors): *Comprehensive Textbook of Psychiatry/VI,* 6th ed. Williams & Wilkins, 1995. With permission.
[2] DRN, dorsal raphe nucleus; DSIP, delta-sleep-inducing peptide; EEG, electroencephalogram; LC, locus coeruleus; LDT-PPT, laterodorsal tegmental and pedunculopontine tegmental nuclei; NREM, non–rapid eye movement; PGO, pontine-geniculate-occipital; REM, rapid eye movement.

30–4). Perhaps the greatest consensus is that cholinergic neurons, with their cell bodies in the laterodorsal tegmental nucleus and the pedunculopontine tegmental groups in the dorsal tegmentum, are crucial for the initiation and maintenance of REM sleep. Serotonergic neurons and noradrenergic neurons originating in the dorsal raphe and locus coeruleus, respectively, apparently inhibit REM sleep or components of it. Histaminergic neurons, originating in the posterior hypothalamus, send neurons to cerebral cortex that apparently help maintain arousal. Although some cholinergic neurons originating in the basal forebrain maintain cortical EEG arousal, other neurons (for which chemical identity has not yet been established) fire selectively during NREM sleep and may play an important role in the maintenance of this stage of sleep. Finally, a number of **sleep factors,** or endogenous sleep-inducing compounds, have been postulated. These factors include delta-sleep-inducing peptide (DSIP), interleukin-1, tumor necrosis factor (TNF), adenosine, prostaglandin D_2, and a variety of other substances.

SLEEP & CIRCADIAN RHYTHMS

The sleep-wake cycle is an example of a circadian rhythm in humans. The rhythm of sleep and wakefulness is governed by one or more internal biological "clocks" (called oscillators), environmental stimuli, and a host of processes that promote or inhibit arousal.

In the absence of cues about the time of day (**Zeitgebers** or time-givers), humans tend to self-select a sleep-wake cycle of about 25 hours—that is, the average elapsed duration between wake-up times is about 25 hours. For example, if a person lives in an experimental environment free of time cues and is allowed to go to bed and arise at will, that person will tend to go to sleep about an hour later each "night" and to wake up about an hour later each "morning." For this reason, shifts in the cycle of rest and activity are usually easier when the cycle is lengthened rather than shortened—in traveling west rather than east, for example—or when rotating from an afternoon to an evening work shift, rather than from an afternoon to a morning work shift.

Under normal conditions, however, the circadian oscillator is entrained to our 24-hour environment by Zeitgebers such as social activities, meals, and especially by environmental light. Information about light reaching the retina is conveyed to the suprachiasmatic nucleus in the anterior hypothalamus. The suprachiasmatic nucleus is an important oscillator that maintains the circadian rhythm of sleep-wakefulness. Lesions of the suprachiasmatic nucleus in rats, hamsters, and monkeys eliminate the normal 24-hour sleep-wake cycle. In these experimental animals, sleep and wakefulness occur in short bouts evenly distributed over the 24-hour day.

In addition to synchronizing the circadian oscillator with the environment, the timing of light exposure can also shift the phase position of the oscillator (ie, the temporal relationship between rhythms or between one rhythm and the environment). Bright light (1500 lux) in the evening hours (6 P.M. to 9 P.M.) coupled with darkness from 9 P.M. to 9 A.M. tends to cause a phase delay in sleep-wake and other biological oscillators (ie, one would go to bed later and wake up later). In contrast, exposure to bright light in the early morning hours (5 A.M. to 7 A.M.) coupled with darkness in the evening tends to advance the phase position of the oscillator (ie, one would go to bed earlier and wake up earlier). Furthermore, bright light during daylight hours can enhance the amplitude of the circadian rhythm, thereby demarcating the periods of both nocturnal sleep and daytime wakefulness.

Other effects of light have also been described. Exposure to bright light during the nocturnal hours inhibits the synthesis and release of melatonin, which is normally secreted by the pineal gland during this time. Although the precise function of melatonin in humans is not known, some investigators believe it may synchronize circadian rhythms and may have mild hypnotic properties. In addition, bright light may have intrinsic alerting and mood-elevating effects. Bright light has been reported to have antidepressant effects in seasonal depressions occurring in the winter and in some patients with major depressive disorder or premenstrual depression.

SLEEP CHANGES WITH DEVELOPMENT & AGING

Sleep-wake states change dramatically across the life span, not only with regard to the amount of sleep, but also to ultradian and circadian timing (Figure 30–3). The newborn human infant may average about 16 hours of sleep a day, of which about 50% is REM sleep. The duration of the REM-sleep cycle in infancy is relatively short compared to that of adults, and the sleep-wakefulness cycle is polyphasic, with numerous short bouts of sleep and wakefulness occurring across the 24-hour period.

During the first months of life, sleep-wake cycles gradually change as sleep at night and wakefulness by day become consolidated, although napping may continue into childhood. By 3 or 4 years of age, a child's REM-sleep levels will have fallen to adult levels of about 20–25% and will stay in this range for the remainder of the life span. With advancing age, REM latency tends to decrease and the length of the first REM period tends to increase.

The amount of time spent in delta (stages 3 and 4) sleep each night peaks in early adolescence and gradually shortens with age until it nearly disappears around the sixth decade of life. Young adults typically spend about 15–20% of total sleep time in delta sleep.

Sleep tends to be shallow, fragmented, and shorter in duration in middle-aged and elderly adults compared to young adults. In addition, daytime sleepiness increases. The relative amount of stages 1 and 2 sleep tends to increase and of stages 3 and 4 sleep to decrease. Men tend to lose delta sleep at an earlier age than do women.

This loss of delta sleep results from a reduction in overall EEG amplitude rather than a reduction in the number of waves in the delta frequency range.

After the age of 65, about one in three women and one in five men report that they take over 30 minutes to fall asleep. Wake time after sleep onset (WASO) and number of arousals increase with age; this increase may be due at least in part to the greater incidence of sleep-related breathing disorders, PLMS, and other physical conditions in these age groups. WASO may also increase with age because older people are more easily roused by either internal or external stimuli.

Changes in the circadian rhythm may lead to increased daytime fatigue and napping and to poor nocturnal sleep. Time isolation studies of the circadian temperature rhythm in the elderly have shown a phase advance of their daily temperature minimum (about 1–2 hours before that of younger individuals) and a decrease in the amplitude of their temperature rhythm. As people age, they tend to choose an "early-to-bed, early-to-rise" pattern of sleep-wakefulness (consistent with a phase-advanced rhythm as compared to younger adults).

Besides the biological changes, psychosocial alterations may partially disrupt or weaken the role of Zeitgebers such as social activities, meal times, and light. Napping also increases with age, although it rarely accounts for a large proportion of total sleep time in healthy individuals. It has also been suggested that the total sleep amount per 24 hours does not change with aging.

Some researchers have noted similarities between age-related changes in sleep and circadian rhythm and those seen in depression; however, the REM-sleep abnormalities seen in depression are usually not present in normal aging.

Diagnostic Classification Steering Committee; Thorpy MJ (chair): *The International Classification of Sleep Disorders: Diagnostic and Coding Manual.* American Sleep Disorders Association, 1990.

Ferber R, Kryger MH (editors): *Principles and Practice of Sleep Medicine in the Child.* Saunders, 1995.

Kryger MH, Roth T, Dement WC (editors): *Principles and Practice of Sleep Medicine,* 2nd ed. Saunders, 1994.

Mistlberger RE et al: Recovery sleep following sleep deprivation in intact and suprachiasmatic nuclei-lesioned rats. Sleep 1983;6:217.

Rechtschaffen A, Kales A (editors): *A Manual of Standardized Terminology, Techniques, and Scoring System for Stages of Human Subjects.* US Government Printing Office, 1968.

CLINICAL SYNDROMES

This section follows the system put forth in the *International Classification of Sleep Disorders* (ICSD), which groups sleep complaints by primary sympto-

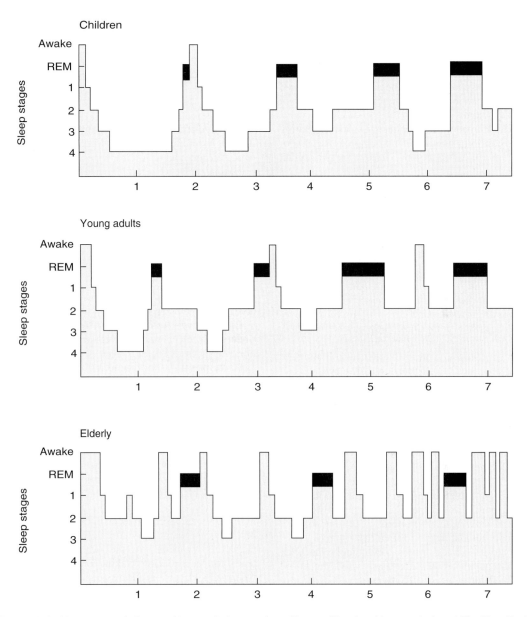

Figure 30–3. Hypnogram of changes in normal sleep cycles with age. (Reprinted by permission of *The New England Journal of Medicine* from Kales A, Kales D: Sleep disorders: recent findings in the diagnosis and treatment of disturbed sleep. N Engl J Med 1974;290:487. Copyright 1974 Massachusetts Medical Society.)

matology: insomnia, or disorders of initiating and maintaining sleep; hypersomnia, or disorders of excessive daytime sleepiness; parasomnias; and circadian rhythm disorders. This section is followed by a brief discussion of sleep alterations associated with psychiatric disorders, substance use, and medical-surgical conditions.

INSOMNIA

DSM-IV Diagnostic Criteria

A. The predominant complaint is difficulty initiating or maintaining sleep, or nonrestorative sleep, for at least 1 month.

B. The sleep disturbance (or associated daytime fatigue) causes clinically significant distress or impairment in social, occupational, or other important areas of functioning.

C. The sleep disturbance does not occur exclusively during the course of narcolepsy, breathing-related sleep disorder, circadian rhythm sleep disorder, or a parasomnia.

D. The disturbance does not occur exclusively during the course of another mental disorder (eg, major depressive disorder, generalized anxiety disorder, a delirium).

Reprinted, with permission, from *Diagnostic and Statistical Manual of Mental Disorders,* 4th ed. Copyright 1994 American Psychiatric Association.

General Considerations

Transient difficulty sleeping is a vastly more common phenomenon than is chronic insomnia. Particularly when the onset of the complaint is coincident with a recent stressful life event, such as bereavement, the short-term administration of mild sedative-hypnotics such as benzodiazepines may be indicated.

The diagnosis of chronic insomnia is based on the subjective complaint of difficulty in initiating or maintaining sleep or of nonrestorative sleep (not feeling well-rested after sleep that is apparently adequate in amount) for a duration of 1 month. Insomnia is more common in women than in men; is more common with age; and is often associated with medical and psychiatric disorders or with abuse of alcohol, drugs, and medications. Because chronic insomnia most often occurs as a comorbid diagnosis with other disorders, the clinician should look carefully for other conditions and treat the primary disorder. In fact, primary insomnia in its "pure" form apparently comprises only a very small proportion of the population of patients complaining of difficulty sleeping.

Chronic insomnia can be a very complex disorder, perhaps a multitude of disorders, and there is great need for clarification of and specificity in the patient's symptoms and in his or her sleep patterns and habits. For example, complaints of insomnia in early morning may indicate a depressive disorder; complaints of insomnia in the first part of the night may suggest a circadian disorder. The degree of consequent daytime impairment should also be established when evaluating a complaint of insomnia. To add to the complexity, sleep-wake disturbance can be an undesired effect of the administration or discontinuation of numerous medications.

Perhaps somewhat surprisingly, many of the primary sleep disorders associated with a complaint of insomnia also overlap with the disorders of excessive daytime sleepiness.

Clinical Findings

A. Insomnia Associated With Behavioral or Psychophysiologic Disorders: Acute stress is probably the most common cause of transient and short-term insomnia. These patients may not come to the attention of a clinician because the condition is self-limited and usually resolves without intervention. Polysomnographic abnormalities have been documented in acute bereavement; however, persistent insomnia over months should raise the consideration of depression, adjustment disorder, and other disorders in the differential diagnosis.

B. Psychophysiologic Insomnia: Psychophysiologic insomnia is defined as a "disorder of somatized tension and learned sleep-preventing associations that result in a complaint of insomnia" (ICSD 1990, p. 28). All patients with chronic insomnia probably develop some learned sleep-preventing associations, such as marked overconcern with their inability to sleep. The frustration, anger, and anxiety associated with trying to sleep or maintain sleep serve only to arouse them as they try to go to sleep or maintain sleep. These patients may acquire aversive associations with their bedrooms and often sleep better in other places such as in front of the television set, in a hotel, or in the sleep laboratory.

C. Insomnia Associated With Psychiatric Disorders: See "Sleep and Psychiatric Disorders" section later in this chapter.

D. Insomnia Associated With Sleep-Induced Respiratory Impairment: Complaints of insomnia occur in patients with central-type sleep apnea and can be found in obstructive-type sleep apnea, in which brief awakenings follow termination of apneic events. These disorders are discussed further in the "Hypersomnias" section later in this chapter.

E. Insomnia Associated With Sleep-Related Movement Disorders: Restless leg syndrome (RLS) and PLMS are often discussed together because of the clinical overlap in presentation and symptoms. RLS has often been described as an uncomfortable "creeping, crawling" sensation or "pins and needles feeling" in the limbs, especially in the lower extremities. RLS tends to occur during waking and at sleep onset, whereas PLMS occurs during sleep. Patients with RLS sometimes also have PLMS, but patients with PLMS often do not have RLS. For most patients with RLS, being recumbent increases the discomfort in the legs and leads to difficulty sleeping. Further sleep disruption may occur if movement of the affected limb becomes the only way to relieve the dysesthesia, as has been reported anecdotally. Patients with RLS or PLMS may present with either of two very different primary complaints: insomnia or hypersomnia.

The movements in PLMS are involuntary, rhythmic, periodic contractions of the anterior tibial muscle with dorsiflexion of the ankle. The twitches or contractions themselves are about 0.5–5 seconds in duration, usually occurring roughly every 20–40 seconds over periods that can last from minutes to hours. Each movement may lead to a brief arousal from sleep, although the degree of disruption can vary greatly from patient to patient and even between nights for a given patient. PLMS may thus provoke tremendous fragmentation of sleep throughout an entire night, a disruption of which the patient is commonly not consciously aware. The incidence of PLMS increases with advancing age: Patients aged 30–50 years have a slight chance of developing PLMS; the chance increases to 30% over the age of 50 years and to almost 50% over the age of 65 years. Polysomnographic evaluation confirms and quantifies severity of PLMS and resultant sleep disruption.

Differential diagnosis is an important issue here. Other medical causes should be ruled out, including peripheral neuropathies, myelopathies, anemia, chronic pulmonary disease, uremia, rheumatoid arthritis, vitamin or mineral deficiencies, or malignancy. Medications such as tricyclic antidepressants or lithium (or withdrawal from other medications) can precipitate RLS and PLMS. Other motor disorders such as akathisia, hypnic jerks, or nocturnal leg cramps should also be ruled out.

Treatment of RLS and PLMS has been controversial and remains an active area of research. Most treatments reduce either the muscle activity or the sleep disruption. Most pharmacologic treatment has been directed at PLMS and generally involves one of three drug categories: dopaminergic agents (L-dopa, bromocriptine); gamma amino butyric acid (GABA)-ergic agents (eg, baclofen, carbamazepine, and benzodiazepines, especially clonazepam); and opioids such as codeine and propoxyphene.

F. Insomnia Associated With Neurologic Disorders: See "Sleep and Medical Conditions" section later in this chapter.

Treatment

A. Nonpharmacologic Approaches:

1. Doctor-patient relationship—The doctor-patient relationship is often important not only for its positive benefits but also for preventing secondary complications of insomnia, such as psychological dependence and misuse of hypnotics, alcohol abuse, and circadian disturbances.

2. Counseling & psychotherapy—Some authorities advocate psychotherapy because they believe that insomnia results from anxiety, depression, obsessive rumination, internalization of emotions, and other cognitive and emotional arousal processes.

3. Sleep hygiene—Stimulus-control treatment approaches (Table 30–5) have been shown in some studies to be effective, usually with young patients who have relatively mild insomnia.

4. Behavioral & biofeedback techniques—These techniques include autogenic training, progressive muscle relaxation, EMG biofeedback, and EEG feedback. Although these techniques appear to be safe, their effectiveness and indications are not well established.

5. Sleep restriction therapy—Because many patients with chronic insomnia both underestimate

Table 30–5. Stimulus-control treatment.

Keep bedtimes and awakening times constant, even on the weekends.
Do not use the bed for watching television, reading, or working. If sleep does not begin within a period of time, say, 30 minutes, leave the bed and do not return until drowsy.
Avoid napping.
Exercise regularly (three to four times per week), but try to avoid exercising in the evening if this tends to interfere with sleep.
Discontinue or reduce alcohol, caffeine, cigarettes, and other substances that may interfere with sleep.
"Wind down" before bed with quiet or relaxing activities.
Maintain a cool, comfortable, and quiet sleeping environment.

their actual sleep time and have poor sleep efficiency, it has been proposed that patients limit the time they spend in bed to the estimated duration of total sleep. For example, if the patient reports sleeping 6 hours per night, he or she is required to limit time in bed to 6 hours or slightly more. This simple maneuver usually produces mild sleep deprivation, shortens sleep latency, and increases sleep efficiency. As sleep becomes more consolidated, the patient is allowed to gradually increase time in bed.

B. Pharmacologic Approaches:

1. Over-the-counter sleeping pills—The effectiveness of these drugs is not well documented. They have potential side effects because they often contain scopolamine, diphenhydramine, or salicylate and many unidentified compounds. Elderly patients may be particularly vulnerable to anticholinergic side effects of antihistamines.

2. Sedative-hypnotics—The most widely used sedative-hypnotics are benzodiazepines. They usually have characteristic effects on sleep, including shortening of sleep latency, improvement of sleep continuity, elevation of stage 2 sleep (with increased spindles), decreased slow-wave sleep, and decreased REM sleep. Long-term administration can lead to tolerance and the need for larger doses. Benzodiazepines are generally not overused in the United States. Recreational use of benzodiazepines is rare. Abuse is more often associated with simultaneous use, for example, with alcohol and stimulants. Short-term use of benzodiazepines to treat insomnia and long-term use to treat anxiety disorders are usually not associated with serious clinical problems. Benzodiazepines are safer than barbiturates, making them a better treatment choice (Table 30–6).

Although the beneficial effects of the nonbenzodiazepine hypnotics zolpidem and zopiclone, which also allosterically bind at the $GABA_A$ receptor complex, are well established and are essentially identical to those of benzodiazepines, their dependence liability has not been investigated sufficiently. Generally, the same precautions applied to benzodiazepine use should be applied to these medications.

Table 30–6. Comparison of benzodiazepines with short and long elimination half-lives.[1]

Characteristic	Elimination Half-life[2]	
	Short	Long
Accumulation with repeated use	0	++++
Next-day hangover effects, sedation	+	+++
Tolerance	+++	+
Anterograde insomnia	+++	+
Risk of rebound insomnia	+++	0
Risk of early morning insomnia	+	0
Risk of daytime anxiety	+	0
Anxiolytic effects the next day	0	++
Full benefits on the first night	+++	++

[1] From Gillin JC: Clinical sleep-wake disorders in psychiatric practice: dyssomnias. Pages 373–380 in Dunner DL (editor): *Current Psychiatric Therapy.* W.B. Saunders, 1992. With permission.
[2] 0, absent; +, minimal; ++, mild; +++, moderate; ++++, severe.

3. Sedating antidepressants—Relatively small doses of some antidepressants such as amitriptyline and trazodone have been helpful in treating insomnia in some patients who don't have depression. Recent anecdotal evidence suggests that nefazodone may also be useful in this regard.

Potential Treatment Complications

Withdrawal from prolonged administration of high-dose benzodiazepines is associated with insomnia, anxiety, seizures, psychosis, delirium tremens, and hyperpyrexia and may be fatal if clinical management is inappropriate. Withdrawal insomnia, the so-called **rebound insomnia,** occurs after administration of short-half-life benzodiazepines at usual doses and is characterized by difficulties falling asleep or maintaining sleep, rebound of REM sleep, and nightmares. These symptoms may be reduced by carefully tapering the dose in an asymptotic manner (ie, with decreasing steps of dose-reduction as withdrawal progresses). Finally, the patient should be kept on a very low dose (25% of initial dose) for some days to weeks before complete discontinuation. Withdrawal symptoms may be treated with β-blockers such as propranolol, with α_2 agonists such as clonidine, or with anticonvulsants such as carbamazepine.

Obermeyer WH, Benca RM: Effects of drugs on sleep. Neurol Clin 1996;14:827.

HYPERSOMNIAS

DSM-IV Diagnostic Criteria

Primary Hypersomnia

A. The predominant complaint is excessive sleepiness for at least 1 month (or less if recurrent) as evidenced by either prolonged sleep episodes or daytime sleep episodes that occur almost daily.
B. The excessive sleepiness causes clinically signifi-
cant distress or impairment in social, occupational, or other important areas of functioning.
C. The excessive sleepiness is not better accounted for by insomnia and does not occur exclusively during the course of another sleep disorder and cannot be accounted for by an inadequate amount of sleep.
D. The disturbance does not occur exclusively during the course of another mental disorder.
E. The disturbance is not due to the direct physiological effects of a substance or a general medical condition.

Narcolepsy

A. Irresistible attacks of refreshing sleep that occur daily for at least 3 months.
B. The presence of one or both of the following:
   (1) cataplexy (ie, brief episodes of sudden bilateral loss of muscle tone, most often in association with intense emotion)
   (2) recurrent intrusions of elements of rapid eye movement sleep into the transition between sleep and wakefulness, as manifested by either hypnopompic or hypnagogic hallucinations or sleep paralysis at the beginning or end of sleep episodes
C. The disturbance is not due to the direct physiological effects of a substance or another general medical condition.

Breathing-Related Sleep Disorder

A. Sleep disruption, leading to excessive sleepiness or insomnia, that is judged to be due to a sleep-related breathing condition (eg, obstructive or central sleep apnea syndrome or central alveolar hypoventilation syndrome).
B. The disturbance is not better accounted for by another mental disorder and is not due to the direct physiological effects of a substance or another general medical condition (other than a breathing-related disorder).

Reprinted, with permission, from *Diagnostic and Statistical Manual of Mental Disorders,* 4th ed. Copyright 1994 American Psychiatric Association.

General Considerations

Hypersomnia can take on many forms, from the patient with atypical depression who sleeps 14 hours a day to the patient with narcolepsy who falls asleep abruptly while riding a bicycle. It is important to differentiate between fatigue, or general tiredness, and excessive daytime sleepiness (EDS). EDS is defined as a pathologic propensity to sleep excessively or to fall asleep too easily or in inappropriate situations.

As in any sleep history but particularly with this type of complaint, it is important to obtain a careful accounting of the patient's nocturnal sleep habits. Perhaps the most common cause of EDS in the general population today is a chronic lack of sleep, frequently caused by social and work demands of society. Furthermore, patients with conditions that are not technically classified as hypersomnias (such as PLMS and obstructive sleep apnea) may often present with a chief complaint of EDS as a result of the disturbance in nocturnal sleep.

Clinical Findings

A. Sleep Apnea: Sleep apnea is characterized by interrupted breathing during sleep and may be classified as central, obstructive, or mixed. Diagnosis is confirmed by a **respiratory disturbance index** (respiratory events per hour; also known as the apnea-hypopnea index) of greater than 10 events per hour.

In central sleep apnea, respiratory drive governed by the brain stem "shuts off" during sleep. This condition may occur in a variety of neurologic and cardiovascular disorders and may also occur in insomnia. Treatment is generally supportive. Theophylline, medroxyprogesterone, and some antidepressants have been recommended as respiratory stimulants.

Obstructive sleep apnea (OSA) is caused by intermittent obstruction of the upper airway during sleep. This is probably the most common disease causing excessive daytime sleepiness and is one of the more prevalent diseases (estimated at 1–2% of the general population). Patients may complain of EDS, snoring, headaches, dry mouth on awakening, or gasping during sleep. PSG may also reveal tachycardias, bradycardias, or other dysrhythmias; decreased oxygen saturation (as measurable by pulse oximetry); frequent arousals; and hypertension as well as short sleep latency on the MSLT. In addition to the general risks associated with EDS (eg, fatigue-related accidents or injuries, or impaired judgment due to sleepiness), patients are at increased risk of pulmonary hypertension, right-sided heart failure, stroke, myocardial infarction, and sudden death. They also may experience impotence, cognitive problems, and a depression-like syndrome that generally remits with treatment.

Although OSA is most common in overweight, middle-aged men, it can occur in any age group (including children) and gender. It may be associated with hypothyroidism, anatomic abnormalities such as tonsillomegaly, or craniofacial anomalies (which may be quite subtle) such as retrognathia.

B. Snoring: Snoring may disrupt sleep and lead to EDS (manifested as polysomnographic arousal) in the absence of measurable apnea. The upper airway resistance syndrome (UARS) entails nonocclusive airway collapse associated with negative intrathoracic pressure; unfortunately, the esophageal pressure transducer essential to making the diagnosis is not used in all sleep laboratories. Epidemiology and prognosis are unknown. Although control of snoring with laser-assisted uvulo-palatoplasty (LAUP) has been reported, many clinicians are concerned about the indiscriminate use of LAUP without appropriate sleep

workup. For example, it is possible for an patient with undiagnosed OSA to think he is cured after LAUP resolves his snoring, but the silent apneas remaining unresolved will continue to disrupt sleep and lead to persistent EDS.

C. Narcolepsy: Narcolepsy is a disorder classically associated with uncontrollable sleep attacks in which the patient abruptly falls asleep in inappropriate (eg, while eating), embarrassing (eg, during intercourse), and even dangerous (eg, while driving) situations. Although sleep attacks have been described as brief (eg, lasting 15–20 minutes) and refreshing, this is not always true. Most narcoleptics experience related symptoms, including **cataplexy** (a sudden loss of muscle tone), **hypnagogic hallucinations** (dreamlike experiences while falling asleep but not yet asleep), and **sleep paralysis** (brief paralysis associated with the onset of sleep or wakefulness). However, only 10–15% of narcoleptic patients will have all four major symptoms (the classic tetrad). Many narcoleptic patients also report having performed complex behaviors (such as walking from one place to another or writing) without recalling them.

Even in the absence of serious consequences, these symptoms can be frightening for patients and vexing for family members, coworkers, and others. The symptoms can be misinterpreted or misidentified by lay people and unwary clinicians alike. For example, milder episodes of cataplexy (dropping a cup upon hearing a joke) may be attributed to carelessness or clumsiness. Alternatively, a patient may be misdiagnosed as psychotic if his or her doctor mistakenly assumes the hypnagogic hallucinations occur during full wakefulness or have the same significance as waking hallucinations.

Narcolepsy is believed to result from defective REM sleep regulation. Cataplexy and sleep paralysis can be thought of as atonia without REM, whereas hypnagogic hallucinations and sleep attacks have been likened to REM intrusion. Narcolepsy has a prevalence of roughly 0.1%. It generally begins in adolescence and occurs equally in males and females. Empiric evidence of increased incidence associated with positive family history and histocompatibility locus antigen (HLA)-typing studies are consistent with a genetic contribution. The antigens HLA-DR2 and DQw are highly prevalent in narcolepsy, although this statement requires some qualifications: First, antigen prevalence may vary in different ethnic groups such as African Americans. Second, advances in HLA typing may result in reclassification or renaming of the antigens involved.

Diagnosis of narcolepsy is confirmed in the sleep laboratory by a sleep-onset REM period (on all-night PSG) or a positive MSLT (eg, REM onset during two of the daytime nap opportunities).

D. Idiopathic CNS Hypersomnia: Idiopathic CNS hypersomnia is a relatively rare disorder of unpredictable, prolonged sleep periods, usually beginning gradually before age 25. These patients do not complain of cataplexy, sleep paralysis, or hypnagogic hallucinations or show sleep-onset REM periods.

E. Idiopathic Recurrent Stupor: Idiopathic recurrent stupor is a disease of unknown etiology, in which the patient experiences recurring stuporous, unresponsive states that resemble drunkenness or grogginess and that may last for a few hours to a few days. These patients may show sleep apnea events without significant desaturation upon PSG or a diffuse fast (14- to 16-Hz) activity upon EEG. Blood and cerebrospinal fluid levels of endozepine-4, an endogenous benzodiazepine, are unusually high during these stuporous states; successful treatment has been reported with flumazenil, a benzodiazepine-receptor antagonist.

F. Recurrent Hypersomnia (Kleine-Levin syndrome): Recurrent hypersomnia is characterized by infrequent (usually once or twice a year) episodes of sleeping 18 or more hours per day for at least 3 days at a time. Episodes may also be associated with hyperphagia, hypersexuality, irritability, and confusion, with normal interepisode functioning. It occurs most commonly in adolescent males.

Treatment of Hypersomnia

Treatment of hypersomnia depends in large part on the specific diagnosis. When possible, treatment should attempt to correct some aspect of the pathophysiology itself. For example, treatment of OSA generally consists of nasal continuous positive airway pressure (NCPAP) or bilevel positive airway pressure (BiPAP) delivered through a nasal or oronasal mask (BiPAP provides different pressures for inhalation and exhalation). This treatment "props" open the airway with room air delivered at low pressures (typically 5–15 cm H_2O). Obese patients should be encouraged to lose weight; weight loss, even if much less than that required to reach ideal weight, can be very helpful. A variety of dental devices have been developed to hold the tongue forward and the airway open. Multiple surgical procedures have been developed, including the uvulo-palatopharyngoplasty (UPPP), which enlarges the upper airway by removing soft tissue.

Treatment of narcolepsy is based on the individual patient's specific target symptoms, the severity of the symptoms, and lifestyle considerations unique to the patient. Although some patients with narcolepsy are able to achieve reasonable control of their sleep attacks by structuring their days with scheduled naps, many patients require stimulants (eg, methylphenidate, amphetamines, pemoline) for EDS. More recently, modafinil has shown considerable promise in preventing sleep attacks and appears to be well tolerated. Treatment of cataplexy and other cardinal symptoms is based on inhibition of REM sleep by antidepressants such as protriptyline or monoamine oxidase inhibitors.

Treating other causes of hypersomnia tends to be more difficult than managing narcolepsy; however, similar use of stimulants has been partially successful.

Aldrich MS: Diagnostic aspects of narcolepsy. Neurology 1998;50(Suppl 1):S2.

Fry JM: Treatment modalities for narcolepsy. Neurology 1998;50(Suppl 1):S43.

Kadotani H, Faraco J, Mignot E: Genetic studies in the sleep disorder narcolepsy. Genome Res 1998;8:427.

Tinuper P et al: Idiopathic recurring stupor. Neurology 1994;44:621.

US Modafinil in Narcolepsy Multicenter Study Group: Randomized trial of modafinil for the treatment of pathological somnolence in narcolepsy. Ann Neurol 1998;43:88.

PARASOMNIAS

DSM-IV Diagnostic Criteria

Nightmare Disorder

A. Repeated awakenings from the major sleep period or naps with detailed recall of extended and extremely frightening dreams, usually involving threats to survival, security, or self-esteem. The awakenings generally occur during the second half of the sleep period.

B. On awakening from the frightening dreams, the person rapidly becomes oriented and alert (in contrast to the confusion and disorientation seen in sleep terror disorder and some forms of epilepsy).

C. The dream experience, or the sleep disturbance resulting from the awakening, causes clinically significant distress or impairment in social, occupational, or other important areas of functioning.

D. The nightmares do not occur exclusively during the course of another mental disorder and are not due to the direct physiological effect of a substance or a general medical condition.

Sleep Terror Disorder

A. Recurrent episodes of abrupt awakening from sleep, usually occurring during the first third of the major sleep episode and beginning with a panicky scream.

B. Intense fear and signs of autonomic arousal, such as tachycardia, rapid breathing, and sweating, during each episode.

C. Relative unresponsiveness to efforts of others to comfort the person during the episode.

D. No detailed dream is recalled, and there is amnesia for the episode.

E. The episodes cause clinically significant distress or impairment in social, occupational, or other important areas of functioning.

F. The disturbance is not due to the direct physiological effect of a substance or a general medical condition.

Sleepwalking Disorder

A. Repeated episodes of rising from bed during sleep and walking about, usually occurring during the first third of the major sleep episode.

B. While sleepwalking, the person has a blank, staring face, is relatively unresponsive to the efforts of others to communicate with him or her, and can be awakened only with great difficulty.

C. On awakening (either from the sleepwalking episode or the next morning), the person has amnesia for the episode.

D. Within several minutes after awakening from the sleepwalking episode, there is no impairment of mental activity or behavior (although there may initially be a short period of confusion or disorientation).

E. The sleepwalking causes clinically significant distress or impairment in social, occupational, or other important areas of functioning.

F. The disturbance is not due to the direct physiological effect of a substance or a general medical condition.

Reprinted, with permission, from *Diagnostic and Statistical Manual of Mental Disorders*, 4th ed. Copyright 1994 American Psychiatric Association.

General Considerations

Parasomnias are sleep-related disorders characterized by unusual events or behaviors occurring either during sleep or during sleep-wake transitions. These events are considered normal physiologic behaviors during conditions of wakefulness, but during sleep they may be injurious to the patient and disruptive and distressing to family and friends. A parasomnia can be classified according to the stage of sleep in which it occurs. During NREM sleep, the following parasomnias occur: sleep terrors, sleepwalking, sleep bruxism,

sleep starts, rhythmic movement disorder, sleep-related abnormal swallowing, and confusional arousals. These NREM-related parasomnias are more often associated with what seems to be an incomplete arousal from sleep, especially deep slow-wave sleep. Presumed to be related at least in part to the cortical desynchrony of slow-wave sleep, these parasomnias are associated with being difficult to arouse, being confused upon awakening, and having little memory for the event. Parasomnias associated with REM sleep include nightmares, REM sleep behavior disorder, sleep paralysis, and REM sleep–related sinus arrest. The next section discusses parasomnias that are similar in their initial presentation (Table 30–7).

Clinical Findings

A. Nightmare Disorder: Nightmare disorder (formerly known as dream anxiety disorder) occurs during REM sleep and can be contrasted with the NREM-associated sleep terror disorder (formerly called night terrors). Awakening, becoming alert, and being able to recall the nightmare are typical with this disorder, in contrast to a NREM-related sleep terror. Sleep terrors are associated with being difficult to arouse and being confused and disoriented on awakening. A sleep terror typically begins with screaming and multiple signs of autonomic activation, seemingly provoked by a dream, although these patients rarely if ever report dream content. After the event subsides the patient retains little or no memory of the event. Usually the family of the sleep terror patient will ask for the evaluation, but the nightmare sufferer will usually be self-referred.

Table 30–7. A comparison of parasomnias by symptoms and findings.[1]

Characteristic	Nightmare Disorder	Sleep Terror Disorder	REM Sleep Behavior Disorder	Sleepwalking Disorder
Sleep stage	REM	NREM	REM	NREM
Dream recall	Yes	No	Yes	No
Motor activity	No	Screaming, motoric agitation	Yes	Yes
On awakening	Alert	Confused, disoriented	Alert	Confused, disoriented
Time of night	Last third of night	First third of night	Second half of night	First half of night
Prevalence	Children, 20%; adults, 5–10%	Children, 5%; adults, <1%	Unknown	Children, 1–20%; adults, <1%
Autonomic activation	Slight, secondary to fear	Extreme, with sweating and vocalizations	Associated with REM and motor activity	Not present
Danger to self	No	No	Patient acts out dream	Patient walks anywhere
Treatment	Monitor; symptoms usually decrease with age; if severe consider psychotherapy	Monitor; symptoms usually decrease with age; if severe consider low-dose tricyclic or benzodiazepine	Clonazepam, 0.5–1.0 mg at bedtime; secure environment	Maintain a safe environment and monitor symptoms

[1] From Gillin JC, Ancoli-Israel S: The impact of age on sleep and sleep disorders. Chapter 10 in Salzman C (editor): *Clinical Geriatric Psychopharmacology,* 2nd ed. Williams & Wilkins, 1992. With permission.

B. Sleepwalking: In sleepwalking disorder (also called somnambulism), the patient will have repeated episodes of complex motor behaviors, again, associated with an incomplete arousal from NREM sleep. Like in sleep terrors, the patient is difficult to awaken, is confused upon arousal, and exhibits reduced alertness and moderate unresponsiveness to attempts at communication.

C. REM Sleep Behavior Disorder: In REM sleep behavior disorder, the muscle atonia characteristic of REM sleep does not occur, enabling patients to "act out" their dreams. These behaviors can entail elaborate and purposeful movements such as running, jumping, and hitting. The patient usually has vivid dream recall upon awakening. Dreams seem to have a heightened aggressive or physical quality to them. Like sleepwalking, this disorder may lead to serious injury to the patient (and bed partner).

Other parasomnias are listed in Table 30–8. For a more in-depth discussion of the parasomnias, please refer to ICSD.

Treatment of Parasomnias

Treatment of parasomnias may include minimizing the problem behavior itself (eg, using dental appliances for bruxism or behavioral measures for enuretic children) or treating the cause or precipitant (eg, modification of psychosocial stressors or psychotherapy for nightmare disorders). In other cases, it may be more practical to minimize consequences of the disorder; for example, reassurance that children do not suffer during sleep terrors or recall them afterward may be very helpful for the families. Finally, safety (to the patient and others) is crucial in the treatment of REM sleep behavior disorder or sleepwalking. For example, patients and families should be counseled to remove or modify environmental hazards by padding sharp pieces of furniture, putting safety gates at the top of stairs (if the patient sleeps in an upstairs bedroom), and so on.

It is helpful to remember which disorders are associated with REM and NREM sleep; for example, severe nightmare disorder, nightmares associated with posttraumatic stress disorder, and REM sleep behavior disorder have been treated with REM-suppressing medications such as monoamine oxidase inhibitors. Good sleep hygiene is also important; for example, slow-wave sleep rebound resulting from sleep deprivation might worsen sleepwalking and other parasomnias that occur during slow-wave sleep. NREM parasomnias have been treated, with variable success, with benzodiazepines or low-dose tricyclic antidepressants (which suppress slow-wave sleep to some extent).

CIRCADIAN RHYTHM DISORDERS

DSM-IV Diagnostic Criteria

A. A persistent or recurrent pattern of sleep disruption leading to excessive sleepiness or insomnia that is due to a mismatch between the sleep-wake schedule required by a person's environment and his or her circadian sleep-wake pattern.
B. The sleep disturbance causes clinically significant distress or impairment in social, occupational, or other important areas of functioning.
C. The disturbance does not occur exclusively during the course of another sleep disorder or other mental disorder.
D. The disturbance is not due to the direct physiological effect of a substance or a general medical condition.

Adapted, with permission, from *Diagnostic and Statistical Manual of Mental Disorders,* 4th ed. Copyright 1994 American Psychiatric Association.

General Considerations

In disturbances of circadian rhythms, there is a misalignment between the timing of sleep-wake patterns and the desired or normal pattern. These patients may complain of either insomnia or hypersomnia. Again, careful questioning of the patient coupled with the sleep diary will be useful in diagnosing these disorders (see Table 30–9 for a list of terms commonly used in the study of circadian rhythms).

Two processes appear to mediate an individual's propensity to sleep: a homeostatic process by which the propensity to sleep is related directly to the duration of prior wakefulness, and a circadian process that regulates the propensity to sleep across a 24-hour day. In persons living on a normal sleep schedule, the circadian sleep propensity is greatest at night and in midafternoon.

Circadian rhythm disorders illustrate the dissociation of an apparently intact sleep-wake system from its circadian mooring and demonstrate the potential ease with which a patient can become desynchronized with his or her surroundings. Inadequate exposure to natural sunlight is believed by some investigators to

Table 30–8. Other parasomnias.

Serious
Nocturnal paroxysmal dystonia
REM sleep–related sinus arrest
Rhythmic movement disorder (formerly called jactatio capitas nocturna, or head banging)
Sudden infant death syndrome
Sudden unexplained nocturnal death syndrome

Benign
Bruxism (tooth grinding)
Confusional arousals
Enuresis
Nocturnal leg cramps
Primary snoring
Sleep paralysis
Sleep starts
Sleep talking (somniloquism)
Sleep-related abnormal swallowing syndrome
Sleep-related painful erections

Table 30–9. Glossary: terms commonly used in the study of circadian rhythms.[1]

Term	Definition
Chronobiology	The study of circadian rhythms
Circadian rhythm	Refers to biological rhythms having a cycle length of about 24 hours. Derived from Latin: *circa dies,* "about 1 day." Examples include the sleep-wake cycle in humans and temperature, cortisol, and psychological variation over the 24-hour day. Characterized by exact cycle length, amplitude, and phase position.
Phase position	Temporal relationship between rhythms or between one rhythm and the environment. For example, the maximum daily temperature peak usually occurs in the late afternoon.
Phase-advanced rhythm	Patient retires and arises early.
Phase-delayed rhythm	Patient retires and arises late.
Zeitgebers	Time cues such as social activities, meals, and bright lights.

[1] From Gillin JC, Ancoli-Israel S: The impact of age on sleep and sleep disorders. Chapter 10 in Salzman C (editor): *Clinical Geriatric Psychopharmacology,* 2nd ed. Williams & Wilkins, 1992. With permission.

result in **seasonal affective disorder,** a depressive disorder found especially in patients residing in northern latitudes that experience a dramatic seasonal shortening of the day length and, correspondingly, of the period of light. For many of these patients, treatment with bright light can be an effective antidepressant therapy. In this way, theoretically, conditions in which a patient's exposure to natural light is minimal, such as during hospitalization or institutionalization, might provoke the increased occurrence of circadian rhythm desynchronization.

Clinical Findings

A. Jet Lag (Time Zone Change) Syndrome: Jet lag is characterized by varying degrees of insomnia, EDS, impaired performance, and gastrointestinal or other symptoms that follow rapid travel across multiple time zones. Individuals differ in susceptibility to jet lag. Resolution involves realigning the circadian clock with the new light-dark cycle. As mentioned earlier, eastward travel (entailing a phase advance of the biological clock) usually takes longer to adjust to than does westward travel (which entails a phase delay).

B. Shift Work Sleep Disorder: Shift work sleep disorder involves symptoms of insomnia, hypersomnia, or both, at inappropriate times, in relationship to certain work schedules (eg, rotating or permanent shift work, or irregular work hours). Complications include gastrointestinal symptoms, possibly cardiovascular symptoms, increased abuse of alcohol, disruption of family and social life, low morale and productivity, and high absenteeism. Many individuals never adjust completely to the work schedule because they try to revert back to a normal sleep-wake schedule on weekends and holidays in order to participate in family and social activities.

C. Delayed Sleep Phase Syndrome: In delayed sleep phase syndrome, the major sleep period is delayed by several hours in relation to the desired clock time. The major symptom is difficulty in waking up at the desired time in the morning, as well as prolonged sleep latency at night. It is most prevalent in adolescence. A standard method of treatment is to phase-delay the onset of bedtime and arousal by 2–3 hours per day each day, thereby eventually cycling the sleep period around the clock after a period of several days and bringing it to the desired time. Once the desired schedule is achieved, a key element in maintenance is enforcing a consistent wake-up time.

D. Advanced Sleep Phase Syndrome: In advanced sleep phase syndrome, the major sleep period is advanced in relation to the desired bedtime, resulting in complaints of early evening sleepiness, early sleep onset, and early morning awakening. Because normal aging tends to be associated with this pattern, this syndrome is probably more common in the elderly than in the young. Exposure to evening light may be helpful.

E. Non-24-hr Sleep-Wake Syndrome: Non-24-hr sleep-wake syndrome is a chronic disorder in which the individual shows daily delays of 30 minutes to 2 hours in both sleep onset and wake times under normal environmental conditions. It is as though these patients are experiencing a temporal-isolation environment without normal time cues (like the experimental isolation described earlier in this chapter) and are living on an approximately 25-hour, free-running rest-activity cycle that is continuously shifting in and out of phase with real-world time. This disorder appears to be rare in the general population but may occur in as many as 40% of blind individuals. It may result from entrainment cues not properly synchronizing the suprachiasmatic nucleus with the environment, but personality disorders may also be involved (eg, individuals who willfully or unconsciously disregard environmental cues).

Treatment

A. General Principles: First, an attempt should be made to synchronize sleep and wakefulness to the underlying phase position of the circadian clock. Second, because the natural cycle length of the circadian clock is longer than 24 hours, it is usually easier to phase-delay than to phase-advance the clock. Shift workers, for example, tend to do better when shifting in a "clockwise direction" (ie, from day to evening to night work schedules) than when shifting in a counterclockwise direction. Third, appropriate time cues (eg, entrainment of a consistent sleep-wake period or timed exposure to bright light) should be used to move and establish the phase position of the biological clock.

B. Bright Light: The efficacy of bright light in the treatment of sleep disturbances is not yet established. In patients who have sleep disturbances that are associated with circadian dysregulations (eg, jet lag), seasonal affective disorder, or possibly dementia, bright light may be beneficial in readjusting and synchronizing the sleep-wake rhythm and the internal clock. Appropriate use of zeitgebers such as social events, meals, and well-defined daily schedules may also be helpful.

C. Melatonin: Although not yet proven or approved by the FDA, melatonin might become beneficial in the treatment of circadian sleep disturbances. Treatment with both bright light and melatonin would need to be carefully timed, because the sensitivity of the biological clock undergoes a circadian variation.

Arendt J, Deacon S: Treatment of circadian rhythm disorders—melatonin. Chronobiol Int 1997;14:185.

SLEEP & OTHER DISORDERS

SLEEP & PSYCHIATRIC DISORDERS

Many psychiatric disorders and substance use disorders are associated with subjective and objective sleep abnormalities. Psychotropic medications frequently have effects on sleep and sleepiness. The high prevalence of comorbid psychiatric and substance use disorders mandate careful attention to diagnosis in every case.

1. MOOD DISORDERS

Effect of the Disorders

Sleep alterations are characteristic of depression and mania and may be present in hypomania, dysthymia, and cyclothymia (see Chapter 21). Polysomnographic abnormalities have also been reported in patients with borderline personality disorder, which has comorbidity and symptomatic overlap with affective disorders.

REM abnormalities found in studies of major depression include shortened REM latency, increased duration of first REM period, and increased **REM density** (a measure of eye movements during REM sleep) compared to nondepressed, healthy sleepers. Other polysomnographic abnormalities are increased sleep latency, reduced sleep efficiency, and decreased slow-wave sleep. Approximately 70% of depressed patients complain of insomnia, although hypersomnia with increased total sleep time also occurs, particularly in patients with bipolar disorder, in young patients with unipolar depression, and in patients with atypical depression.

Mania is characterized by diminished total sleep time and other abnormalities on PSG. Insomnia is often an early symptom and must be treated aggressively in patients with bipolar disorder, preferably before full-blown mania develops. In many patients with bipolar disorder, mania can be precipitated by seemingly minor amounts of sleep deprivation or by jet lag. Some of the benzodiazepines are particularly useful for attempting to prevent or abort mania, especially clonazepam, which is said to have antimanic properties beyond its sedative-hypnotic effects. However, by the time many patients with bipolar disorder present for treatment, clonazepam alone will not be sufficient treatment.

Medications Used to Treat the Disorders

A. Antidepressants: Various types of sleep deprivation, including total (full night), partial (early or late), and selective REM sleep deprivation, have shown antidepressant effects, although these effects are transient, and practical limitations preclude performing sleep deprivation routinely in clinical practice. Antidepressants were initially thought to act by suppressing REM sleep, but several antidepressants (eg, trimipramine, buproprion, nefazodone) do not suppress REM.

Clinical experience advocates the use of sedating antidepressants in treating depression associated with severe insomnia and the use of activating antidepressants for treating hypersomnic or atypical depressions; however, few polysomnographic or clinical studies have tested this notion. Exceptions certainly exist: for example, fluoxetine is considered to be an activating antidepressant, yet in some cases insomnia improves as the patient's depression improves. Moreover, some patients complain of daytime sedation while taking fluoxetine (possibly caused by sedative properties of its metabolite norfluoxetine). Still others benefit from fluoxetine yet require concurrent medications (short-term benzodiazepines or long-term augmentation with sedating antidepressants such as trazodone) to control insomnia.

B. Tricyclic Antidepressants: In general, tertiary amines are more sedating than are secondary amines.

C. Monoamine Oxidase Inhibitors: Monoamine oxidase inhibitors are associated with complaints of insomnia and thus should generally be given earlier in the day.

D. Miscellaneous Antidepressants: Maprotiline and amoxapine are considered moderately sedating; venlafaxine is reported to cause occasional insomnia. Concern about orthostatic side effects and priapism has limited the enthusiasm researchers have had for trazodone. Its congener, nefazodone, with its limited α blockade, is virtually free of these effects and thus may be more useful as a primary antidepressant or as an augmentation to other treatments of depression associated with insomnia.

E. Mood Stabilizers: Carbamazepine and valproic acid are anticonvulsants and can cause EDS, especially in combination with other medications. In polysomnographic studies, lithium has improved multiple sleep variables in patients with acute mania (although it is difficult to tell how much of the improvement in sleep was related to general improvement).

2. ANXIETY DISORDERS

Effect of the Disorders

Polysomnographic abnormalities have been documented in generalized anxiety disorder, panic disorder, posttraumatic stress disorder (PTSD), and obsessive-compulsive disorder (OCD) (see Chapters 22, 23, and 24); in addition, patients with these disorders commonly complain of difficulty initiating or maintaining sleep, or of disrupted, nonrestorative sleep. In OCD, some of the sleep disruptions may be secondary to the anxiety symptoms (eg, rituals become so time-consuming that sleep time is limited, or initial insomnia occurs as a result of worrying about the obsessions). Nightmares are common in PTSD. Some patients who have panic disorder experience sleep panic attacks (during slow-wave sleep). Though simple phobia per se has little, if any, effect on sleep, it is easy to see how the PTSD patient with nightmares or the patient with nocturnal panic attacks could develop a phobic avoidance of sleeping (particularly if the patient mistakes the panic attacks for dangerous cardiac events, for example).

Medications Used to Treat the Disorders

Treatment for anxiety disorders may include benzodiazepines, in which case selection of a particular agent depends on the type of anxiety and the pharmacologic properties of the agent. For example, a patient whose anxiety is manifest primarily as insomnia might benefit from a relatively short-acting hypnotic at bedtime; patients with severe daytime anxiety may benefit from daytime sedation (see Table 30–6). Liability for tolerance, withdrawal, and abuse must be considered for all the benzodiazepines.

Antidepressants are also useful for treating some types of anxiety. For example, selective serotonin re-uptake inhibitors (SSRIs) or clomipramine can be used to treat OCD, and SSRIs can be used to treat panic disorder. Buspirone is a nonsedating, nonbenzodiazepine anxiolytic that is not likely to be associated with dependence and is beneficial for treating some types of anxiety (eg, generalized anxiety disorder) or as an augmenting agent in the treatment of OCD. It has not been shown to be helpful for panic symptoms. Because of its slow onset of action, buspirone is frequently given with a brief initial course of benzodiazepines until it takes effect.

3. DEMENTIA

Effect of the Disorder

Dementia is one of the most common health problems in older populations, and Alzheimer's disease is the most common type of dementia. The waking EEG in Alzheimer's patients typically shows a diffuse slowing and decrease of predominant alpha waves and an increase in the occurrence of delta and theta waves. Some studies suggest that the amount of slow waves in the waking EEG is related positively to the degree of dementia, and that the occurrence of theta waves is one of the most sensitive signs of the progression of Alzheimer's disease. Because patients with dementia exhibit delta and theta waves during waking, polygraphic measures may not be helpful in discriminating between waking and sleep. Behavioral observations often must be used.

Polysomnographic features include sleep fragmentation; prolonged sleep latency; lowered sleep efficiency; and decreased total sleep time, delta sleep, and NREM sleep. EEG sleep of dementia patients is also often disturbed by respiratory disturbances and PLMS. In moderate to severe forms of Alzheimer's disease and other dementias, disturbed sleep at night and excessive sleepiness by day, night wandering, disorientation and confusion (called sundowning), and problems of behavioral management are common reasons for institutionalization and for disruption in the lives of family caregivers (see Chapter 17).

The neurobiological underpinnings of the changes of REM sleep in dementia are of particular scientific interest. As mentioned earlier, the onset and offset of REM sleep appears to be controlled by cholinergic, serotonergic, and noradrenergic neurons. Alzheimer's disease is associated with a decrease in cholinergic activity, and one might predict reduced REM in these patients. Several studies have reported such findings.

Because REM sleep tends to be decreased in dementia and increased in depression, some investigators believe this measure distinguishes memory dysfunction in dementia and depression; however, this research is not yet ready to be applied in clinical practice. In nursing homes, sleep disorders represent a major medical and social problem. It has been reported that the severity of dementia is highly correlated with sleep apnea, and it has been suggested that sleep apnea with possible hypoxic damage to the brain coupled with daytime sleepiness might accelerate the dementing process and influence the psycho(social)motoric performance of these patients. In addition, sleep apnea increases the risk of mortality in this population. Nursing home patients also have been shown to spend more time in bed throughout the 24-hour day, and they exhibit poor sleep efficiency and pronounced sleep fragmentation.

Medications Used to Treat the Disorder

Many classes of psychotropic medications have been tried for treating the behavioral problems associated with dementia. Both insomnia and excessive sleepiness have occurred following administration of tacrine; the effects of donepezil on sleep-wake behavior are not known.

4. PSYCHOTIC DISORDERS

Effect of the Disorders

Most of the sleep-related studies on psychotic disorders have focused on schizophrenia, and early theories attempted to find a REM-sleep connection or abnormality. Subjectively positive symptoms showed a significant correlation with dream mentation during the night; however, NREM sleep phenomena have been among the most consistent findings in schizophrenia, in the form of a decrease in the amount of NREM stages 3 and 4 sleep.

Objectively measured sleep disturbance in schizophrenia can be recorded, especially at the onset of the acute psychotic state. A reversal of the sleep-wake cycle often occurs with positive symptoms. Increased insomnia (ie, a significantly increased sleep onset latency) is associated with periods of increased agitation.

There is a high incidence of comorbid sleep disorders in schizophrenia. Such disorders can include sleep disturbance caused by medications, substance abuse, sleep apnea, or other medical or psychiatric disorders. Although narcolepsy is associated with hallucinations and increased EDS, as is schizophrenia, the narcoleptic patient will also have symptoms of cataplexy and sleep paralysis and the hallucinations are most commonly associated with sleep onset. These features will aid in the differential diagnosis of the two disorders (see Chapter 19).

Sleep problems found in schizoaffective disorders are similar to those found in delusional depression (see Chapter 20). These patients tend to have fragmented sleep and many of the same sleep abnormalities as in affective disorders.

Medications Used to Treat the Disorders

For the conventional antipsychotics, sedation generally increases with decreasing potency. Risperidone

has been associated with rare reports of EDS. Clozapine can be quite sedating and is associated with enuresis and excessive drooling during sleep.

5. SOMATOFORM & RELATED DISORDERS

Symptom overlap between chronic fatigue syndrome (CFS) and primary fibromyalgia syndrome (PFS) includes loss of energy, severe fatigue, tiredness, and easy fatigability. In PFS, pain may be the predominant symptom; in CFS, fatigue and cognitive impairment are the predominant symptoms. Both disorders have a high comorbidity with depression; however, the sleep abnormalities observed in CFS or PFS are distinct from those observed in major depression. See Chapter 25 for more information on these disorders.

Patients who have PFS may experience a nonrestorative sleep syndrome in which alpha-frequency (ie, waking) EEG waves intrude into NREM sleep patterns; however, this abnormality may be found in other chronic pain disorders.

6. FACTITIOUS DISORDER OR MALINGERING

It may be difficult to ascertain the veracity of a patient's sleep complaints. Underestimating the amount of time spent asleep and exaggerating the amount of waking time in the night is common, and this phenomenon may be exacerbated in insomnia. Some insomniac patients may experience a phenomenon known as "sleep state misperception." These patients subjectively experience wakefulness throughout the night, even though objective sleep measures indicate apparent continuous normal sleep. Sleep state misperceivers are thought to comprise a fairly small percentage of the number of patients with insomnia; however, clinicians should evaluate with care possible secondary gain from a complaint of insomnia. See Chapter 26 for more information on factitious disorders and malingering.

Clinicians should be alert to the possibility of patients feigning narcolepsy in order to obtain prescription stimulants. Although some individuals may be knowledgeable about narcoleptic symptomatology and may even attempt to produce rapid eye movements during sleep laboratory testing in an effort to simulate sleep-onset REM periods, narcoleptic polysomnographic findings are considered very difficult to fake in the absence of the disorder.

REM behavior disorder is believed to be impossible to simulate on PSG. Other parasomnias may be somewhat more difficult to confirm with a sleep study because the occurrence of these events is usually less frequent than nightly and may not be likely to be captured on a particular night of study. Some sleep laboratories have had success in eliciting parasomnias or other NREM sleep–related behaviors with the use of sound stimulation presented during delta sleep.

With regard to sleep disorders, at least one case of Munchausen syndrome by proxy has been documented. In this case, a parent complained of sleep-related apneic spells in an infant, which the parent was found to be producing or simulating by smothering the child with a pillow.

7. EATING DISORDERS

Even subjective sleep complaints in patients who have eating disorders such as anorexia and bulimia are inconsistent (see Chapter 29). Anorexic patients may report a reduced need for sleep, although complaints of insomnia are rare. Bulimic patients may tend to complain of increased amounts of sleep following binge-eating episodes.

Objective findings of abnormal sleep in patients who have eating disorders have also been inconsistent. Some studies have suggested trends toward reduced sleep efficiency, reduced total sleep time, and reduced slow-wave sleep. REM latency may be reduced, as sometimes occurs in major depression, but REM density may be decreased from normal (rather than being enhanced from normal, as it is in depression).

Clinicians should also be aware of the existence of a sleep-related binge-eating disorder, which has all the earmarks of a classic delta sleep–related parasomnia (ie, automatic behaviors occur during delta sleep, the level of arousal is incomplete during the event, and later there is no memory for the event).

Ballenger JC et al: Consensus statement on panic disorder from the International Consensus Group on Depression and Anxiety. J Clin Psychiatry 1998;59(Suppl 8):47.

Benca RM: Sleep in psychiatric disorders. Neurol Clin 1996;14:739.

Bottai T et al: Clonazepam in acute mania: time-blind evaluation of clinical response and concentrations in plasma. J Affect Disord 1995;36:21.

Casey DE: Side effect profiles of new antipsychotic agents. J Clin Psychiatry 1996;57(Suppl 11):40.

Rush AJ et al: Comparative effects of nefazodone and fluoxetine on sleep in outpatients with major depressive disorder. Biol Psychiatry 1998;44:3.

Sharpley AL, Cowen PJ. Effect of pharmacologic treatments on the sleep of depressed patients. Biol Psychiatry 1995;37:85.

SLEEP & SUBSTANCE USE

Use of any psychoactive compound will generally affect sleep, particularly in the setting of pathologic use, abuse, or dependence (see Chapter 18). Drug effects on sleep are multifaceted and are determined by drug type, frequency, dosage and duration of (chronic or acute) use, degree of intoxication, and comorbidity with medical or psychiatric disorders as well as by possible gradual changes in the brain in response to the drug(s). A systematic description of sleep disturbances associated with substance abuse is rather complex because polysubstance abuse is common and might include drugs with different and sometimes opposite effects on sleep.

Here we review the sleep alterations associated with the most commonly misused drugs such as alcohol, stimulants, opioids, nicotine, caffeine, and anxiolytics. However, some practical guidelines for the clinical management of sleep disturbances associated with substance abuse should be considered. The diagnosis of substance abuse is often difficult to assess and may be missed unless a rigorous examination is carried out. The same patient often uses stimulating and sedating drugs simultaneously; therefore, a consistent textbook-like clinical picture is often absent. Dual-diagnosis psychiatric disorders (such as depression, schizophrenia, anxiety disorders, or personality disorders) combined with misuse of drugs—are often encountered in clinical practice. It is clinically useful to determine, if possible, which disorder is the primary one and which is the secondary one. This determination will facilitate the clinical treatment and management of the disorders and improve preventive measures.

1. ALCOHOL

Acute Effects

Alcohol is often self-prescribed for insomnia, anxiety, stress, and other disturbances. The acute use of alcohol initially increases slow-wave sleep and decreases REM sleep and may be experienced as helpful in insomnia. However, acute alcohol-induced sleep may also be characterized by fragmentation, early awakening, and hangover symptoms the next day. Alcohol may also induce sleepiness during the day, particularly if used in combination with other sedating compounds.

Chronic Effects

Sustained misuse of alcohol for its hypnotic effects induces adaptive changes that lead to restlessness, arousals, sweating, dry mouth, and bad dreams during nocturnal sleep. Alcohol may also exacerbate sleep-related respiratory disorders, essentially by potentiating sleep-related atonia during sleep.

Between 6% and 50% of the general psychiatric patient population meet criteria for alcoholism. Heavy alcohol dependence is commonly associated with chronic insomnia, even if patients are drinking at bedtime. Alcohol-induced sleep is usually characterized by shortened and fragmented sleep at the end of the night. Because of initial REM suppression, REM sleep will increase in the second part of the night. In severe cases, alcohol abuse may result in a polyphasic sleep-wake pattern, in which sleep and wakefulness occur in short bouts irregularly distributed throughout the 24-hour day.

Withdrawal

Acute withdrawal is initially associated with insomnia characterized by a loss of NREM sleep and by REM sleep disturbances. During intermediate withdrawal, patients exhibit a prolongation of sleep latency, a loss of slow-wave sleep, increased amount of arousals and stage 1 sleep, and reduced total sleep time. In addition, REM density is usually increased during subacute withdrawal. These sleep disturbances may last as long as 2 years. Recent research has also suggested that sleep disturbances, particularly REM sleep disturbances, at the beginning of a withdrawal program are associated with a greater likelihood of relapse.

Other Sleep Problems

Alcoholic patients may also experience hypersomnia, which may occur as a result of alcohol intoxication, during brief periods of abstinence, and after a delirium tremens. Alcoholic patients often experience parasomnias such as bedwetting, sleep terrors, nightmares, sleepwalking, snoring, or apnea.

Treatment

Treatment of alcohol-related insomnia includes withdrawal, the resolution of possible underlying disorders, psychotherapy, sleep hygiene, sleep restriction therapy, and pharmacotherapy. The latter has to be considered carefully, and the pros and cons of hypnotic drugs must be evaluated. Benzodiazepines exhibit cross-tolerance with alcohol, bear the risk of abuse, and are not likely to be helpful on a long-term basis. Sedating antidepressants such as trimipramine, doxepin, trazodone, and amitriptyline might be administered in low dosages; however, their therapeutic value has not been evaluated. Another possibility is treatment with carbamazepine or chloral hydrate, which could also be beneficial in preventing seizures; however, the efficacy of these drugs for treatment of other symptoms is uncertain.

2. STIMULANTS

Amphetamine, methylphenidate, fenfluramine, and pemoline have beneficial effects in the treatment of narcolepsy and may have therapeutic effects in the management of hypersomnia associated with this condition. Intoxication with stimulants—such as cocaine, methamphetamine, phenmetrazine, methylenedioxymethamphetamine (MDA), and 3,4-methylenedioxymethamphetamine (MDMA; also called "ecstasy"), propylhexedrine (the active ingredient of

nasal decongestants), fenfluramine, pemoline, and even caffeine—is usually associated with sleep loss, often for several days. Amphetamines and cocaine stimulate the dopaminergic arousal system and fenfluramine the release of serotonin. Withdrawal after bouts of heavy use of these compounds may be followed by hypersomnia.

Chronic stimulant use may be associated with tolerance and with abuse of sedating drugs such as alcohol, benzodiazepines, or barbiturates. These sedating drugs are used as a self-treatment for insomnia and anxiety. Withdrawal is usually characterized by depression, hypersomnia, hyperphagia, and anhedonia. Sleep during the first week or so shows increased total sleep time and REM sleep and a shortened REM latency. During subacute withdrawal, patients usually experience poor sleep with decreased amounts of slow-wave sleep. Treatment of acute and subacute withdrawal is symptomatic; long-term treatment includes careful and comprehensive psychotherapeutic management.

3. OPIOIDS

Somewhat paradoxically, the acute administration of morphine, heroin, and other opioids to normal subjects reduces total sleep time, sleep efficiency, slow-wave sleep, and REM sleep but may improve sleep in patients with painful conditions. If tolerance for opiates develops, these sleep disturbances may disappear. Withdrawal is usually accompanied by acute insomnia among other symptoms; however, these symptoms usually last only for a few days. Fortunately, methadone seems not to have a negative impact on sleep.

4. NICOTINE

Little is known about the effects of chronic nicotine abuse on sleep. Withdrawal may be associated with initial difficulties falling asleep or with hypersomnia; however, these symptoms are generally minor compared to other withdrawal symptoms. Treatment with nicotine patches might be considered, but patches have been associated with increased dreaming and insomnia.

5. CAFFEINE

There are large interindividual differences regarding the effects of caffeine on sleep. Caffeine intoxication usually is associated with insomnia. Caffeine may trigger panic attacks and the sleep disturbances associated with panic. The acute administration of caffeine decreases sleep EEG intensity in the low frequencies, probably because it blocks adenosine receptors. Acute withdrawal is usually associated with hypersomnia. Paradoxically, caffeine may have hypnotic effects in geriatric patients, probably because of alterations of brain perfusion.

Benca RM: Sleep in psychiatric disorders. Neurol Clin 1996;14:739.

Obermeyer WH, Benca RM: Effects of drugs on sleep. Neurol Clin 1996;14:827.

SLEEP & MEDICAL-SURGICAL CONDITIONS

Sleep complaints are often encountered in a variety of medical-surgical conditions, especially in the hospital. Virtually any type of pain, anxiety, or discomfort can cause insomnia, as can restriction of normal movement (eg, traction), disruption of normal circadian zeitgebers in the intensive care unit, noisy monitors, round-the-clock neurologic checks, and so on.

1. MEDICAL CONDITIONS

Epilepsy

Approximately 80% of epileptic patients have seizures predominantly during sleep or on arousal from sleep. REM sleep has some protective effect against seizures. In addition, sleep deprivation can trigger seizure activity. The various anticonvulsants in common use have differing effects on sleep.

Headache

Migraines and cluster headaches tend to occur in sleep in susceptible individuals. In addition, sleep deprivation may trigger migraines in some patients.

Trauma

Serious brain injuries are associated with profound disruption of the sleep-wake cycle that may persist long after the initial insult. Even less serious head injuries (eg, concussions) may be followed by sleep disturbance.

Movement Disorder & Neuromuscular Disorders

Movement disorders and neuromuscular disorders may interfere with sleep.

Cardiovascular Disorders

Cardiovascular disorders may disturb sleep via pain, palpitations, or other discomforts (eg, orthopnea or paroxysmal nocturnal dyspnea in congestive heart failure). Resting ischemic pain is generally considered an ominous sign. Sleep-associated autonomic changes may trigger dysrhythmias and variations in blood pressure. There is a clear circadian rhythm for propensity to myocardial infarction and sudden cardiac death; both occur more frequently during morning hours, when the propensity to REM sleep is relatively high.

Respiratory Disorders

Respiratory disorders frequently disrupt sleep because of patient discomfort (see "Sleep Apnea" section earlier in this chapter).

Gastrointestinal Disorders

Gastrointestinal disorders frequently disturb sleep because of nocturnal gastric acid production in combination with pathology such as peptic ulcer or gastroesophageal reflux. In severe cases the acid reflux may result in aspiration and pulmonary complications.

Other Disorders

Chronic hemodialysis patients commonly experience severe PLMS. Other endocrinopathies (eg, hyperthyroidism) and toxic or metabolic derangements (eg, hyperammonemia) are also associated with sleep disorders.

2. MEDICATIONS

Clinicians must consider medication effects (singly or as drug interactions) in the differential diagnosis of sleep complaints in medical conditions. Medications may exert their effects through direct effects on sleep stages (eg, pindolol-associated nightmares), through effects on sleep disorders (eg, worsening of PLMS caused by the dopamine antagonist metoclopramide), and through seemingly unrelated physiologic effects (eg, diuretic medication leading to nocturia). Patients with sleep apnea or heavy snoring must not be given medications that depress respiration.

Although some classes of medications are more widely known for causing sleep complaints than are others, virtually any class of medication may be involved. Anecdotal reports and small case series may not be reflected in the *Physicians' Desk Reference.*

3. SLEEP & THE REPRODUCTIVE CYCLE

Sleep Problems During the Menstrual Cycle

Episodic hypersomnia associated with the menstrual cycle has been reported. Several psychiatric disorders that may themselves be associated with sleep symptoms may temporarily worsen premenstrually. In addition, insomnia may occur in connection with premenstrual dysphoric disorder.

Sleep Problems During Pregnancy

The first trimester is generally associated with increased daytime sleepiness, possibly as a result of the sedating effects of progesterone; however, physical discomfort may disrupt sleep at any stage of gestation. Evidence suggests that insomnia and daytime fatigue due to pain and discomfort peak in the third trimester.

In addition to the normal sleep effects of pregnancy, many gravid women develop onset or worsening of PLMS. Mechanical, physiologic, and hormonal effects of pregnancy are also associated with increased incidence and severity of snoring, and obstructive sleep apnea develops in some cases.

Sleep Problems Postpartum

The sleep-disrupting effects of babies are well known; however, the postpartum period is a time of potential risk for more serious conditions (eg, affective disorders and psychosis) that may include insomnia. Little research has attempted to separate the physical and hormonal effects of lactation on sleep or to examine the implications of sleeping arrangements (eg, infant cosleeping) on the mother's sleep.

Sleep Problems During Menopause

Physical discomfort (eg, hot flashes resulting from vasomotor instability) can disrupt sleep. Polysomnographic studies have shown diminished REM and total sleep time and increased sleep latency in menopausal women.

Harding SM: Sleep in fibromyalgia patients: subjective and objective findings. Am J Med Sci 1998;315:367.

Obermeyer WH, Benca RM: Effects of drugs on sleep. Neurol Clin 1996;14:827.

Impulse-Control Disorders

31

John W. Thompson, Jr., MD, & Daniel K. Winstead, MD

INTERMITTENT EXPLOSIVE DISORDER

DSM-IV Diagnostic Criteria

A. Several discrete episodes of failure to resist aggressive impulses that result in serious assaultive acts or destruction of property.
B. The degree of aggressiveness expressed during the episodes is grossly out of proportion to any precipitating psychosocial stressors.
C. The aggressive episodes are not better accounted for by another mental disorder (eg, antisocial personality disorder, borderline personality disorder, a psychotic disorder, a manic episode, conduct disorder, or attention-deficit/hyperactivity disorder) and are not due to the direct physiological effects of a substance (eg, a drug of abuse, a medication) or a general medical condition (eg, head trauma, Alzheimer's disease).

Reprinted, with permission, from *Diagnostic and Statistical Manual of Mental Disorders,* 4th ed. Copyright 1994 American Psychiatric Association.

General Considerations

A. Major Etiologic Theories: The outbursts associated with intermittent explosive disorder (sometimes referred to as episodic dyscontrol) were initially viewed as the result of limbic system discharge or dysfunction or even as interictal phenomena. *Diagnostic and Statistical Manual of Mental Disorders,* 4th edition (DSM-IV) would now exclude those patients in whom an aggressive episode was thought to be related to a general medical condition (eg, temporal lobe seizures, delirium) or to the direct psychological effects of a substance, whether a drug of abuse or a prescribed medication. Disorders that can be identified as resulting from neurologic insult or a seizure disorder are now classified elsewhere. Nevertheless, neurologic soft signs, nonspecific electroencephalogram (EEG) changes, or mild abnormalities on neuropsychological testing have been noted in patients given this diagnosis.

Psychodynamic explanations have also been proposed. Childhood abuse is thought to be a risk factor for the development of this disorder. Others postulate narcissistic vulnerability as a possible mechanism that triggers these attacks. Thus one can conceptualize the assaultive episodes as perhaps resulting from a real or perceived insult to one's self-esteem or as a reaction to a perceived threat of rejection or abandonment.

B. Epidemiology: Little is known about the incidence or prevalence of intermittent explosive disorder. Although the general consensus is that this is a rare disorder, several authors have speculated that it might be more common than previously thought.

C. Genetics: Little is known about the genetics of intermittent explosive disorder. Family studies of individuals with this disorder have shown high rates of mood and substance use disorders in first-degree relatives.

Clinical Findings

A. Signs & Symptoms: Aggressive outbursts occur in discrete episodes and are grossly out of proportion to any precipitating event. Furthermore, there is often a lack of rational motivation or clear-cut gain to be realized from the aggressive act itself. The patient expresses embarrassment, guilt, and remorse after the act and is often genuinely perplexed as to why he or she behaved in such a manner. Some patients have described periods of exhaustion and sleepiness immediately after these acts of violence.

B. Psychological Testing: Neuropsychological testing may reveal minor cognitive difficulties such as letter reversals. A careful history may reveal developmental difficulties such as delayed speech or poor coordination. A history of febrile seizures in childhood, episodes of unconsciousness, or head injury may be reported.

C. Laboratory Findings: Laboratory findings are nonspecific. Nonspecific EEG findings may be noted. Several research projects have found signs of altered serotonin metabolism in cerebrospinal fluid or platelet models.

Differential Diagnosis

If the behavior can be better explained by an underlying neurologic insult, then the correct diagnosis would be personality change due to [general medical condition], aggressive type. The clinician must decide whether the aggressive or erratic behavior would be better explained as a result of a specific personality disorder or conduct disorder. Purposeful behavior with subsequent attempts to malinger must be distinguished from intermittent explosive disorder. Recent studies suggest a high rate of combined lifetime mood and substance use disorders in patients with this disorder.

Treatment

Both psychotherapy and pharmacotherapy have been described as treatments for intermittent explosive disorder; however, no double-blind, randomized, controlled trials have been conducted. There are case reports or open trials of the use of anticonvulsants, antipsychotics, antidepressants, benzodiazepines, β-blockers, lithium carbonate, stimulants, and opioid antagonists. Novel anxiolytics such as buspirone have been efficacious in individual cases. Current scientific data are insufficient and inconclusive regarding treatment of the disorder; therefore, clinicians must proceed with individualized treatment plans based on their best clinical judgment.

Complications, Comorbidity & Adverse Outcomes of Treatment

Intermittent explosive disorder can be complicated by legal difficulties, job loss, difficulties with interpersonal relationships, and divorce. Although patients may have been prone to lose their temper repeatedly over a long period of time, they may not seek medical attention until a major life disruption has resulted from one of these outbursts.

Adverse outcomes of treatment are related to the side effects of particular medications used to treat this disorder.

Prognosis & Course of Illness

Intermittent explosive disorder is thought to have its onset in adolescence or young adulthood and to run its course by the end of the third decade of life. Here again, the data for such conclusions are quite limited.

Kim SW: Opioid antagonists in the treatment of impulse-control disorders. J Clin Psychol 1998;59:159.
McElroy SL, Soutullo CA, Beckman DA, et al: DSM-IV intermittent explosive disorder: a report of 27 cases. J Clin Psychol 1998;59:203.

KLEPTOMANIA

DSM-IV Diagnostic Criteria

A. Recurrent failure to resist impulses to steal objects that are not needed for personal use or for their monetary value.

B. Increasing sense of tension immediately before committing the theft.

C. Pleasure, gratification, or relief at the time of committing the theft.

D. The stealing is not committed to express anger or vengeance and is not in response to a delusion or a hallucination.

E. The stealing is not better accounted for by conduct disorder, a manic episode, or antisocial personality disorder.

General Considerations

Although kleptomania has been recognized, since the early 19th century, as an ego-dystonic impulse to steal, little systematic study has been undertaken to better understand this disorder. The individual with kleptomania often feels guilty and fears apprehension and prosecution. Several psychiatric disorders have been linked to kleptomania; the most recent studies point to eating disorders and compulsive spending.

A. Major Etiologic Theories: The etiology of kleptomania is unknown. It may represent a symptom rather than a disorder.

B. Epidemiology: Because most shoplifters steal for profit, fewer than 5% of shoplifters meet criteria for kleptomania. It is a rare disorder of unknown prevalence, although the disorder may be more common than thought. Kleptomania is more common in women than in men.

C. Genetics: Little is known about the genetics of kleptomania. Family studies have demonstrated high rates of mood, substance use, and anxiety disorders in first-degree relatives.

Clinical Findings

A. Signs & Symptoms: The hallmark of kleptomania is the failure to resist the impulse to steal useless objects that have little monetary value. This behavior is not usually purposeful but is performed to relieve a sense of inner tension. There is often a sense of relief upon completion of the theft. The theft usually occurs in retail stores or work locations or from family members. Some patients report feeling high or euphoric while stealing. Most feel guilty after the act and may donate stolen items to charity, return items to the location from which they were stolen, or pay for the stolen items.

A comprehensive history may reveal other compulsive behavior that does not meet full criteria for obsessive-compulsive disorder (OCD). Symptoms of mood disorders, substance use disorders, anxiety disorders, and eating disorders may also be common in this population.

B. Psychological Testing & Laboratory Findings: Neuropsychological testing and laboratory data are nonspecific.

Differential Diagnosis

The diagnosis of kleptomania should not be given if the patient's behavior is better accounted for by antisocial personality disorder, bipolar disorder, or conduct disorder or if stealing occurs as a result of anger or vengeance or as the result of a hallucination or delusional belief. Other important diagnoses to consider include major depression, anxiety disorder, and substance use disorders.

Treatment

Psychotherapy and pharmacotherapy have been useful in single reports. Selective serotonin reuptake inhibitors (SSRIs) and lithium are the agents used most frequently to treat kleptomania. Response rates are confounded by the high rates of comorbid mood and eating disorders.

Complications, Comorbidity, & Adverse Outcomes of Treatment

The majority of patients with kleptomania have a lifetime diagnosis of major mood disorder. Anxiety disorder is also common, as are substance use and eating disorders. Complications include apprehension, arrest, and conviction for stealing as well as shame and embarrassment to the patient, friends, and family members. Other risks might include self-destructive behavior associated with major mood disorders and substance use.

Adverse outcomes of treatment are related to side effects of medication and failure to recognize comorbid conditions that may be treated easily.

Prognosis & Course of Illness

Kleptomania is thought to begin in adolescence and can continue into the third or fourth decades of life. The course is not well studied and includes a spectrum from brief episodic symptoms to chronic stealing behavior.

Black DW: Compulsive buying: a review. J Clin Psychol 1996;57(Suppl 8):50.
McElroy SL, Keck PE Jr., Phillips KA: Kleptomania, compulsive buying, and binge-eating disorder. J Clin Psychol 1995;56(Suppl 4):14.

PYROMANIA

DSM-IV Diagnostic Criteria

A. Deliberate and purposeful fire setting on more than one occasion.
B. Tension or affective arousal before the act.
C. Fascination with, interest in, curiosity about, or attraction to fire and its situational contexts (eg, paraphernalia, uses, consequences).
D. Pleasure, gratification, or relief when setting fires,

or when witnessing or participating in their aftermath.
E. The fire setting is not done for monetary gain, as an expression of sociopolitical ideology, to conceal criminal activity, to express anger or vengeance, to improve one's living circumstances, in response to a delusion or hallucination, or as a result of impaired judgment (eg, in dementia, mental retardation, substance intoxication).
F. The fire setting is not better accounted for by conduct disorder, a manic episode, or antisocial personality disorder.

Reprinted, with permission, from *Diagnostic and Statistical Manual of Mental Disorders,* 4th ed. Copyright 1994 American Psychiatric Association.

General Considerations

Pyromania strikes fear in the hearts of mental health professionals, because there is a serious potential for harm to the patient and to society. The therapist must balance carefully the issues surrounding confidentiality and the duty to protect third parties from the danger presented by these patients.

A. Major Etiologic Theories: The etiology of pyromania is not well understood. There is little research to support any hypotheses.

B. Epidemiology: The epidemiology of pyromania is unclear. After other causes of fire setting are ruled out, only a small population of pyromaniac individuals remains. Pyromania is thought to be rare. In clinical populations, however, fire-setters are not uncommon. Between 2% and 15% of psychiatric inpatients are fire-setters. The peak age of fire-setters is 13 years, and 90% of fire-setters are male. Many are from emotionally and economically deprived families.

C. Genetics: Little is known about the genetics of pyromania.

Clinical Findings

A. Signs & Symptoms: The signs and symptoms of true pyromania may be indistinguishable from other forms of fire setting. Diagnosis is by exclusion. Most fire setting cannot be classified as an impulse-control disorder, but impairment in the ability to control impulses is recognized in most cases of arson. Patients are usually identified after legal charges have been filed.

B. Psychological Testing: Psychological testing of fire-setters reveals a significant amount of psychiatric comorbidity; however, studies on pure populations of pyromaniacs are not available. Among fire-setters, suicidal behaviors have been reported. Screening for suicide is warranted for this population.

C. Laboratory Findings: Lower cerebrospinal fluid concentrations of 3-methoxy-4-hydroxyphenylglycol and 5-hydroxyindoleacetic acid have been reported in fire-setters as compared to control subjects.

Differential Diagnosis

The diagnosis of pyromania should not be given if fire setting can be accounted for more appropriately by motives of profit, crime concealment, or revenge or as a symptom of another psychiatric disorder. Fire setting has been found in over half of children with conduct disorder. It may be a harbinger of adult antisocial personality disorder.

Treatment

Early intervention programs with adolescent fire-setters have reported success in deterring fire setting. Other comorbid psychiatric disorders such as schizophrenia and bipolar disorder should be treated aggressively.

Complications, Comorbidity, & Adverse Outcomes of Treatment

A significant number of fire-setters will repeat this behavior. While they are working with such patients, therapists must be constantly aware of the potential for harm to third parties.

Little is known about the comorbidity of pyromania with other psychiatric disorders. Fire setting is quite common among psychiatric inpatients: The most common associations are psychotic disorders, mood disorders, and severe personality disorder. Female fire-setters have a high degree of psychiatric comorbidity, as high as 92% in one study.

Prognosis & Course of Illness

The prognosis and course of illness are unclear. Early detection and the treatment of comorbid psychiatric disorders are recommended.

Barnett W, Richter P, Sigmund D, et al: Recidivism and concomitant criminality in pathological firesetters. J Forensic Sci 1997;42:879.

Geller JL: Arson in review. From profit to pathology. Psychiatr Clin N Am 1992;15:623.

Puri BK, Baxter R, Cordess CC: Characteristics of firesetters. A study and proposed multiaxial psychiatric classification. Br J Psychiatry 1995;166:393.

PATHOLOGIC GAMBLING

DSM-IV Diagnostic Criteria

A. Persistent and recurrent maladaptive gambling behavior as indicated by five (or more) of the following:

   (1) is preoccupied with gambling (eg, preoccupied with reliving past gambling experiences, handicapping or planning the next venture, or thinking of ways to get money with which to gamble)

   (2) needs to gamble with increasing amounts of money in order to achieve the desired excitement

   (3) has repeated unsuccessful efforts to control, cut back, or stop gambling

   (4) is restless or irritable when attempting to cut down or stop gambling

   (5) gambles as a way of escaping from problems or of relieving a dysphoric mood (eg, feelings of helplessness, guilt, anxiety, depression)

   (6) after losing money gambling, often returns another day to get even ("chasing" one's losses)

   (7) lies to family members, therapist, or others to conceal the extent of involvement with gambling

   (8) has committed illegal acts such as forgery, fraud, theft, or embezzlement to finance gambling

   (9) has jeopardized or lost a significant relationship, job, or educational or career opportunity because of gambling

   (10) relies on others to provide money to relieve a desperate financial situation caused by gambling

B. The gambling behavior is not better accounted for by a manic episode.

Reprinted, with permission, from *Diagnostic and Statistical Manual of Mental Disorders,* 4th ed. Copyright 1994 American Psychiatric Association.

General Considerations

A. Major Etiologic Theories: The etiology of pathologic gambling is unknown. Biochemical, behavioral, psychodynamic, and addiction-based theories have been proposed.

B. Epidemiology: Pathologic gambling is the only impulse-control disorder that is not rare. The prevalence has been estimated at 0.2–3.3%, varying with the number of gaming venues available. Roughly two thirds of gamblers are male. Pathologic gambling is a growing problem in adolescent and elderly populations.

C. Genetics: Family studies of pathologic gamblers reveal higher rates of pathologic gambling in first-degree relatives than in the general population. The rates of mood disorder and substance use disorder in first-degree relatives are many times that of the general population.

Clinical Findings

A. Signs & Symptoms: Pathologic gamblers spend excessive amounts of time at gaming establishments or obtaining money to gamble. They deplete family bank accounts, borrow money from family members, lie about their gambling, and attempt to recoup their losses with large bets. They repeatedly promise to cut back on their gambling and make unsuccessful attempts to do so.

Pathologic gamblers usually present to mental

health professionals after they have been forced into treatment because of illegal activity to obtain funds. For example, they write bad checks and embezzle money or engage in insurance fraud. Up to 75% of the members of Gamblers Anonymous admit to engaging in illegal activity.

The gambler's spouse is likely to be significantly depressed. Some studies have reported higher rates of child abuse by the gambler and particularly by the spouse. This is more likely to occur when the spouse confronts the gambler about depletion of family resources. The clinician often should interview the extended family to understand the full extent of the patient's borrowing. The clinician also should take a careful history of mood symptoms and suicidal ideation, because 20% of individuals in treatment for pathologic gambling have reported attempting suicide.

Differential Diagnosis

Pathologic gambling must be separated from social gambling. Social gambling usually occurs with friends, and the amount of money to be spent is determined before gambling starts. Social gambling is time limited and does not cause significant financial constraints on the family. Professional gambling, in contrast to pathologic gambling, involves calculated bets without significant attempts to recoup losses (called "chasing losses"). Other differential diagnoses include manic episodes and antisocial personality disorder. Many gamblers appear to be hypomanic while gambling and depressed when on a losing streak, thus making bipolar II disorder particularly difficult to differentiate.

Prognosis & Course of Illness

The typical pathologic gambler goes through several phases before coming to the attention of mental health professionals. Onset is usually in adolescence or early adulthood. The winning phase begins after the patient has a large windfall that equals half of a normal year's salary. The gambler then starts betting regularly, feeling euphoric as he or she does so, seeking more and more "action." At first, many gamblers are adept at winning money.

The losing phase usually begins as a streak of bad luck (referred to by Gamblers Anonymous populations as the "bad beat"). Losing begins a cycle of chasing losses with foolish bets that plunge the gambler further and further into debt. As the bets become more and more risky, the gambler enters a phase of desperation when illegal sources of money are considered. Desperation usually occurs after the family bank account and retirement savings are depleted. The gambler may contemplate or attempt suicide at this point.

Another clinical presentation of gambling has been described as "the escape artist." The escape artist gambles to pass time and avoid boredom. Women and the elderly are overrepresented in this group.

Treatment

Several treatment approaches are available, from Gamblers Anonymous to inpatient psychiatric treatment. Some programs involve a multidisciplinary 12-step addiction-based model designed specifically for the pathologic gambler. The gambler must take responsibility for his or her debt, cut up credit cards, and allow someone else to handle his or her money. Medication management can be helpful if comorbid psychiatric disorders are present. SSRIs have been recommended, but no controlled studies are available to date.

Complications, Comorbidity, & Adverse Outcomes of Treatment

Complications of treatment include continued gambling, side effects of medication, and suicide. Comorbid conditions include substance use disorder, depression, bipolar disorder, and attention-deficit/hyperactivity disorder. Antisocial and narcissistic personality disorders may be present. Outcomes vary depending on the population studied and the method used. Some surveys report a 55% response rate at 1 year after inpatient treatment. Surveys of Gamblers Anonymous groups show lower response rates, in the 10% range at 1-year follow-up.

DeCaria CM, Hollander E, Grossman R, et al: Diagnosis, neurobiology, and treatment of pathological gambling. J Clin Psychol 1996;57(Suppl 8):80.

Lesieur HR, Rosenthal RJ: Pathological gambling: a review of the literature. Journal of Gambling Studies 1991;7:5.

TRICHOTILLOMANIA

DSM-IV Diagnostic Criteria

A. Recurrent pulling out of one's hair resulting in noticeable hair loss.

B. An increasing sense of tension immediately before pulling out the hair or when attempting to resist the behavior.

C. Pleasure, gratification, or relief when puling out the hair.

D. The disturbance is not better accounted for by another mental disorder and is not due to a general medical condition (eg, a dermatological condition).

E. The disturbance causes clinically significant distress or impairment in social, occupational, or other important areas of functioning.

Reprinted, with permission, from *Diagnostic and Statistical Manual of Mental Disorders*, 4th ed. Copyright 1994 American Psychiatric Association.

General Considerations

A. Major Etiologic Theories: The etiology of trichotillomania is unknown; however, various theories have been proposed about the pathogenesis of this complex disorder. Psychoanalytic theory views pathologic hair pulling as a manifestation of disrupted psychosexual development, often due to pathologic family constellations. In contrast, behavioral theory conceptualizes hair pulling as a learned habit similar to nail biting or thumb sucking. More recently, a biological theory has been postulated as several researchers have proposed a serotonergic abnormality in trichotillomania and have suggested that this disorder may be a pathologic variant of species-typical grooming behaviors. Neuropsychological abnormalities, treatment response to some antidepressants, and frequent comorbidity with OCD have led to speculations regarding a neurobiological etiology, perhaps involving frontal lobe or basal ganglia dysfunction.

B. Epidemiology: The incidence of trichotillomania in the general population is unknown, but estimates have placed its prevalence in the United States as high as 8 million people. A recent survey of 2579 college freshmen indicated that 0.6% would have met criteria for trichotillomania at some point in their lifetimes. Trichotillomania appears to be more prevalent in females (although males may predominate in patients under age 6 years).

C. Genetics: Family studies are suggestive of a genetic predisposition for trichotillomania but may reflect environmental learning and are inconclusive.

Clinical Findings

A. Signs & Symptoms: Patients, particularly young ones, frequently deny that they pull their hair intentionally. Others typically describe pulling their hair when alone, but they may pull it openly in front of immediate family members. These episodes tend to occur during sedentary activities such as watching television, reading, studying, lying in bed, or talking on the telephone, and they may be more frequent during periods of stress. Patients may be unaware that they are pulling their hair until they are in the middle of an episode. Some patients report being in a trance-like state when they pull their hair. These episodes may last a few minutes or a few hours. Patients may pull a few hairs or many hairs per episode. Many patients do not feel pain when the hair is pulled; some patients report that it feels good.

Patients frequently engage in oral manipulation of the hair once it is pulled including nibbling on the roots or swallowing the hair. The later behavior can lead to a rare but serious complication, namely a trichobezoar (hair ball) in the gastrointestinal tract. Consequences of a trichobezoar can be life threatening and include obstruction, bleeding, perforation, pancreatitis, and obstructive jaundice.

Patients typically pull hair from their scalp, and objective assessment may reveal diffuse hair thinning to virtual baldness. The typical patient demonstrates patchy areas of alopecia without inflammation that spare the periphery. Many patients are adapt at hiding areas of hair loss by judicious hair styling but may ultimately resort to hairpieces and wigs when the areas become too large or too numerous to hide. Patients may also pull hair from other parts of their body, including eyelashes, eyebrows, pubic hair, or hairs from their face, trunk, extremities, or underarms.

B. Psychological Testing & Laboratory Findings: Although psychological testing may not be useful in confirming a diagnosis of trichotillomania, a punch biopsy may be of some help in this regard. The biopsy results typically reveal increased catagen hairs along with melanin pigment casts and granules in the upper follicles and infundibulum.

Differential Diagnosis

According to DSM-IV diagnostic criteria, a diagnosis of trichotillomania is not warranted if the condition can be better accounted for by another mental disorder and is not due to a general medical condition. For example, if a patient has another significant Axis I psychiatric disorder (eg, a condition with delusions or hallucinations) that might account for the hair pulling, then the diagnosis of trichotillomania would not be warranted. When patients deny that they pull their hair intentionally, dermatologic consultation may be required to rule out other causes of hair loss. Most notable among these conditions is alopecia areata, but tinea capitis, traction alopecia, androgenic alopecia, monilethrix, and other dermatologic conditions must be considered. A punch biopsy may be indicated particularly when one of these disorders is suspected.

Treatment

An initial double-blind cross-over trial compared clomipramine to desipramine in 13 patients with trichotillomania screened to rule out neurologic disorder, mental retardation, primary affective disorder, psychosis, and OCD. Clomipramine produced improvement in clinical symptoms (33–53% reduction in severity scores) on each of three rating scales designed to assess trichotillomania symptomatology and clinical improvement; scores on two of the three scales were statistically significant. Two subsequent placebo-controlled, double-blind cross-over studies failed to show efficacy for fluoxetine.

Relatively little rigorous research has been conducted concerning differential effectiveness of treatments for trichotillomania. Clomipramine and behavior therapy probably constitute the current treatments of choice, but this conclusion is tempered by the paucity of treatment outcome studies. Trichotillomania occurs with variable levels of severity in terms of hair pulling and comorbid psychopathology. As a result, response to treatment is highly variable and rather unpredictable.

Complications, Comorbidity, & Adverse Outcomes of Treatment

Although the hair loss in these patients is self-induced, they are often particularly sensitive to comments about their appearance and go to great lengths to hide their disfigurement. These patients are often fearful that their shameful "secret" will be discovered and that they will be ridiculed in public. If the disorder is protracted, the patient's self-esteem can suffer drastically. Some individuals develop avoidant behavior and become socially withdrawn in order to avoid exposure.

Little is known about the comorbidity of trichotillomania. Aside from the possibility that the disorder may be related to anxiety or mood disorders, there has been much speculation that it may be a variant of OCD. Some research lends support to this hypothesis; however, the studies that failed to show efficacy for fluoxetine would possibly argue against such a relationship.

Trichotillomania in preadolescents (particularly in those under age 6 years) is thought to be associated with little psychopathology. In adolescent and adult patients, however, association with other mental disorders has been demonstrated. In a study of 60 adult chronic hair-pullers (50 of whom met strict criteria for trichotillomania), only 18% did not demonstrate a current or past diagnosis of an Axis I psychiatric disorder other than trichotillomania. The lifetime prevalence of mood disorders was 65%, and 23% met criteria for current major depressive episode. Lifetime prevalence of anxiety disorders was 57%, and 10% demonstrated a current diagnosis of OCD and 5% a history of OCD. Another 18% endorsed present or past obsessions and compulsions not meeting the full criteria for OCD. Lifetime prevalence of panic disorder with or without agoraphobia was 18%, generalized anxiety disorder 27%, simple phobia 32%, eating disorder 20%, and substance abuse disorder 22%.

A smaller study that used standardized assessment techniques found that 45% of the trichotillomania patients studied met criteria for current or past major depression, 45% had generalized anxiety disorder, 10% had panic disorder, and 35% had alcohol or substance abuse. Unfortunately, patients with OCD were excluded from the study.

Adverse outcomes of treatment are limited to the usual side effects experienced with clomipramine or other antidepressants. Although there might be adverse consequences of psychodynamic psychotherapy or a behavioral treatment approach, such adverse outcomes are generally thought to be rare and unpredictable at best.

Prognosis & Course of Illness

The prognosis and course of illness generally can be predicted from the age at onset. Trichotillomania begins most often in childhood or young adolescence. Hair pulling in very young children is frequently mild and may remit spontaneously. Patients with a later age at onset tend to have more severe symptoms that run a chronic course. These patients are thought to have a higher incidence of comorbid anxiety and depressive disorders.

Keuthen NJ, O'Sullivan RL, Goodchild P, et al: Retrospective review of treatment outcome for 63 patients with trichotillomania. Am J Psychiatry 1998;155:560.

Minichiello WE, O'Sullivan RL, Osgood-Hynes D, et al: Trichotillomania: clinical aspects and treatment strategies. Harv Rev Psychiatry 1994;1:336.

IMPULSE-CONTROL DISORDERS NOT OTHERWISE SPECIFIED

The diagnosis of impulse-control disorders not otherwise specified (NOS) is given to patients who exhibit an impulse-control problem that does not fit into one of the other five categories or is not listed elsewhere in DSM-IV (eg, substance abuse, a paraphilia). Common examples of impulse-control disorders NOS are face picking, sexual behaviors, compulsive shopping, or repetitive self-mutilation.

McElroy SL, Hudson JI, Pope HG Jr., et al: The DSM-III-R impulse control disorders not elsewhere classified: clinical characteristics and relationship to other psychiatric disorders. Am J Psychiatry 1992;149:318.

32

Adjustment Disorders

Ronald M. Salomon, MD, & Lucy Salomon, MD

DSM-IV Diagnostic Criteria

A. The development of emotional or behavioral symptoms in response to an identifiable stressor(s) occurring within 3 months of the onset of the stressor(s).

B. These symptoms or behaviors are clinically significant as evidenced by either of the following:
   (1) marked distress that is in excess of what would be expected from exposure to the stressor
   (2) significant impairment in social or occupational (academic) functioning

C. The stress-related disturbance does not meet the criteria for another specific Axis I disorder and is not merely an exacerbation of a preexisting Axis I or Axis II disorder.

D. The symptoms do not represent bereavement.

E. Once the stressor (or its consequences) has terminated, the symptoms do not persist for more than an additional 6 months.

Reprinted, with permission, from *Diagnostic and Statistical Manual of Mental Disorders,* 4th ed. Copyright 1994 American Psychiatric Association.

General Considerations

A. Major Etiologic Theories: Normal challenges of life are usually taken in stride, with socially and culturally prescribed ranges of expected responses. Commonly encountered events may disrupt an unusually crucial part of a self-view (Table 32–1). Stressors leading to adjustment disorders are often termed "problems in coping." Among adolescents, adjustment disorders frequently occur following disappointment(s) in relationships with family members or friends. Complex difficulties may be encountered among homosexual teens. An adjustment disorder may be present in a posthospitalization reaction, after treatment for another, otherwise unrelated disorder. For example, after being hospitalized for severe obsessive-compulsive disorder (OCD), a patient may express a behavioral conduct disturbance that is otherwise atypical for OCD. It may then be appropriate to add an adjustment disorder diagnosis. Exceptionally severe or extreme stressors may precipitate maladaptive responses. Retirement and aging may bring feelings of loss, passed health and vigor, and fear of the future. When the symptoms are less than those required for acute stress disorder, the diagnosis of adjustment disorder may be appropriate.

Challenging diagnostic situations can arise when the stressor is in some way subtle, for example, in a change of a previously stable life situation without any obvious tragic occurrence. The clinician may inadvertently overlook adjustment disorder as a diagnosis if the stressor is not clear. Adaptation difficulties in a marriage, pregnancy, or childbirth provoke feelings of guilt because the occurrence "should" be welcomed not shunned. Natural preferences for lifestyle stability may be difficult to reconcile with goals requiring change. For example, a stably married individual unexpectedly facing parenthood also faces a difficult role change, increased responsibility, and loss of freedom. Improved coping may result from an understanding of the individual's long-standing fear that he or she could be thrust into the role of single parent, as may have happened in his or her own family.

B. Risk Factors: Major early risk factors include prior stress exposure, stressful early childhood experiences, and a history of affective or eating disorder. Family unity disruptions or frequent family relocations predispose children to adjustment disorders. The incidence of adjustment disorders is greater in children of divorced families following a subsequent, independent stressor. Death of a parent also predisposes children to adjustment disorders, and a high suicide risk has been reported, especially after the loss of the father. Adjustments to living with extended family (eg, in-laws, step-parents) are additional predisposing factors. The outlet of symptom expression—be it depressed mood, conduct disturbance, or anxiety—may be determined by individual prior experiences or biological constitutional factors. Prior exposure to war, without meeting criteria for posttraumatic stress disorder (PTSD; see Chapter 23), is another risk factor for adjustment disorders. As in PTSD, neurobiologi-

Table 32–1. Commonly observed precipitants for adjustment disorders.

College or university adjustments
Conscription into military service
Death of parent or companion
Natural disaster
New marriage or cohabitation
Pregnancy
Recent or anticipated combat
Recent or anticipated loss
Retirement
Terminal illness in self, parent, or companion

cal characteristics (eg, elevated corticosteroid in response to stress) have been associated with the development of adjustment disorders.

Immigrant populations are at risk for adjustment disorders. It is overly simplistic to label the entire immigration process as a precipitant; rather, precipitant stressors should be identified separately. For example, among new immigrants to Israel, stress responses to missile attacks during the Gulf War could be predicted by the immigrants' adaptation prior to the attacks. Laotian Hmong immigrants in Minnesota were the focus of highly informative investigations that showed the need for studies of preventive interventions. Acculturation is similar to other novel situations in many ways, but it also presents individuals with a large number of unique difficulties, all at the same time (Table 32–2). Any or all of these factors may require attention in treatment.

Factors that increase susceptibility in one situation may decrease it in another. For example, a high educational level may protect an individual when facing one stressor but may pose a risk factor for adjustment disorders in another context. Small-town life may predispose by providing too much shelter from stress and limited support networks.

Chronic illness increases the need for medical contacts and may constitute a major challenge to usual coping. Illness appears to be more of a precipitating factor than a predisposing factor. Evidence suggests that adjustment disorders are not found more fre-

Table 32–2. Stressors among immigrant populations.[1]

Isolation from family and ethnic supports
Longing for familiar environments, all the while teaching hosts about the culture
Novel cognitive styles, task expectations
Reordering of developmental sequences, social expectations, and milestone assessments
Social and language challenges
Trauma of the journey for self and immigrant cohort
Unfamiliar time concepts and spatial orientation

[1] Reprinted, with permission, from Zipstein D, Hanegbi R, Taus R: An Israeli experience with Falasha refugees. In: Williams CL, Westermeyer J (editors): *Refugee Mental Health in Resettlement Countries.* Hemisphere, 1986.

quently among those with medical illnesses. In contrast, should an adjustment disorder occur it will often affect the clinical course of a somatic illness. The course of asthma, chronic obstructive pulmonary disease, diabetes mellitus, end-stage renal disease, systemic lupus erythematosus, stroke, coronary artery disease, HIV/AIDS, chronic pain or headache, or cancer may be affected by the individual's adjustment. Illness behavior, the give and take between the patient and caregivers, and secondary gain affect assessments of adjustment. Lifestyle versus coping style and the setting of expectations for treatment compliance require skilled clinical judgment. For example, the asthmatic adolescent who occasionally rebels by skipping a scheduled inhaler dose may not need as rigid a guideline as a patient with insulin-dependent "brittle" (ie, extremely volatile) diabetes who skips insulin shots.

C. Epidemiology: In the United States, adjustment disorder diagnoses are quite common. Among psychiatric admissions, one estimate suggests that 7.1% of adults and 34.4% of adolescents had adjustment disorders. Many of these individuals merit substance abuse and conduct disorder diagnoses. Among university students receiving psychiatric assessments, a very high proportion were diagnosed as having adjustment disorders. Large population studies such as the Epidemiologic Catchment Area study have not assessed adjustment disorders because of a lack of sensitivity in the instrument used, the Diagnostic Interview Schedule. Further studies are needed to better understand cultural influences on population rates for adjustment disorders.

D. Genetics: Other than a global suggestion that a family history of psychiatric disorder is a risk factor for adjustment disorders, little is known about genetic inheritance or determinants of adjustment disorders. This is not surprising given the heterogeneity of a disorder defined by stressors rather than specific symptoms.

al-Ansari A, Matar AM: Recent stressful life events among Bahraini adolescents with adjustment disorder. Adolescence 1993;28:339.

Leigh H: Physical factors affecting psychiatric condition. Gen Hosp Psychiatry 1993;15:155.

Newcorn JH, Strain J: Adjustment disorder in children and adolescents. J Am Acad Child Adolesc Psychiatry 1992; 31:318.

Strain J et al: The problem of coping as a reason for psychiatric consultation. Gen Hosp Psychiatry 1993;15:1.

Clinical Findings

A. Signs & Symptoms: In a primary care setting, distress reported by individuals, friends, or family members must be assessed carefully. Individual distress is variably reported and interpreted. Adjustment disorder diagnoses derive solely from expressed emotional and behavioral symptoms that may not be verbalized clearly by the patient and may be minimized, masking severe distress. Symptoms themselves may contribute further to the individual's loss of confidence and disrupted sense of safety and well-being. Maladaptive behavior, fears, and uncertainties arise from losing control as customary defenses fail. The gravity of the stressor is interpreted in a context of past encounters with similar events and cannot be evaluated solely by the therapist's or society's standards. Stress must be evaluated in terms of the individual's subjective perceptions, giving these perceptions some degree of validity. Adjustment will be facilitated when the therapist shows flexibility and acceptance of the individual's needs and distress. This requires careful listening and sensitivity because, with its paucity of somatic symptoms, individuals with adjustment disorders can masquerade as healthy and fairly stable, hiding high fragility and possibly even suicidal risk. Clinicians may not appreciate the importance of a seemingly minor stressor, but they must always give utmost respect to the individual, scheduling an interview period that is long enough to understand the patient's subjective perceptions.

The distress experienced with adjustment disorders may include dissimilar emotions and behaviors simultaneously. Such distress is beyond the expected response to the identified stressor, which may be identified on Axis IV. Any suspicion of heightened severity, intensity (eg, suicidal risks), or duration—beyond that manageable by the primary care clinician—or failure of a sufficient supportive intervention indicates a need for professional psychiatric assessment and treatment. Symptoms may be delayed, especially in women, and may change over time. Chronic stress may elicit chronic adjustment disorders. Clinical observations of the course of adjustment disorders reveal a strong association with suicidality, personality disorders, and drug use. A lack of suicide attempts in a first episode does not protect from risk of future attempts. Completed suicide appears to be more frequent after an earlier attempt. The severity and lethality of suicide attempts often increase over time. Individuals with adjustment disorders should not be viewed as less of a suicide risk than those with major depressive disorder.

B. Psychological Testing: Psychological testing (eg, using the Minnesota Multiphasic Personality Inventory) has documented adjustment disorder risk factors (see "General Considerations" section earlier in this chapter) and comorbidity with Type A personality style and other personality disorders (especially cluster B). Psychological testing can help the clinician to identify suicidal individuals, the degree of depression, and the level of hopelessness. Testing suggests that adjustment disorders are more likely among individuals with a socially prescribed perfectionism—a tendency toward exaggerated perceptions that others have inordinately high expectations of them. No impairment on neuropsychological testing is observed in patients with adjustment disorders; impairments are found in patients with depression and other disorders.

C. Laboratory Findings: Pathophysiologic studies of adjustment disorders show little evidence of somatic involvement, although different mechanisms may be involved among different symptom groups. Patients with adjustment disorders resemble normal control subjects in most physiologic studies, with the nonspecific exception of elevated cortisol response to stress and decrease in delta sleep (eg, following marital separation or soon after divorce). In comparison to patients with adjustment disorders and control subjects, individuals with major depressive episodes exhibit more physiologic markers of change (eg, event-related potentials, decreased heart rate, and cortisol and ACTH suppression following dexamethasone).

Diagnostic Considerations

Lacking clear behavioral or emotional symptom criteria, the purpose of diagnostic labeling in adjustment disorders is sometimes questioned. Diagnostic recording allows communication with patients, insurers, and other clinicians. It assists in disease control by focusing research and guiding therapeutic selection. Contemporary knowledge of phenomenology: differential diagnosis, prognosis, course, and future risks may be illuminated by naming a disorder. Even though more studies are needed, the adjustment disorder diagnosis fulfills these expectations. The therapist will find criteria easily met, defensible, and practical. However, the adjustment disorder diagnosis must not become a conciliatory label to avoid controversies. A diagnostic label cannot reconcile societal and individual standards of response to a stressor. Examples include the societal acceptance of requests for death, euthanasia, or "rational suicide;" the differentiation between biological and functional (purely psychological) disorders; or other similar contemporary issues. They must remain foci of controversy rather than indications of underlying psychopathology. When used with relatively poor specificity or to evade controversy, the adjustment disorder diagnosis effectively minimizes organic relationships and diminishes the credibility of psychiatric nosology.

Adjustment disorder diagnoses are useful when the psychological stress of a physical illness causes psychiatric symptoms. In a way, adjustment disorder is the converse of psychological factors affecting physical illness, in which a defensive coping style (eg, repression) might worsen a systemic problem (eg, peptic ulcer). It may be appropriate to give both diagnoses.

Clinical use of the adjustment disorder diagnosis may be less prevalent in other countries, even though true prevalence may be similar. The description of these symptoms in *International Classification of Diseases,* 10th edition, (ICD-10) largely overlaps with *Diagnostic and Statistical Manual of Mental Disorders,* 4th edition (DSM-IV). In ICD-9, the term "adjustment reaction" was used for disturbances lasting weeks to months, and symptoms lasting hours to days were labeled "acute reaction to stress." This system required a retrospective view because duration could not be established at the onset of symptoms. There are other possible reasons for intercultural differences in the use of the adjustment disorder diagnosis. In some European countries, reimbursement for treatment does not cover extensive care for minor conditions. Culture-specific syndromes, such as the Latino *ataque de nervios,* apply to a variety of symptom presentations, many of which do not come to psychiatric attention. Appendix I of DSM-IV is devoted to cultural syndromes. In addition, substance abuse and alcoholism diagnoses are often comorbid in patients with adjustment disorders. Because thresholds for the diagnosis of substance abuse are interpreted differently from one country to the next, international standardization of adjustment disorder diagnosis may be difficult to achieve.

Greenberg WM, Rosenfeld DN, Ortega EA: Adjustment disorder as an admission diagnosis. Am J Psychiatry 1995;152:459.

Oquendo MA: Differential diagnosis of *ataque de nervios.* Am J Orthopsychiatry 1995;65:60.

World Health Organization: *International Classification of Diseases,* 4th ed., 9th rev. U.S. Department of Health and Human Services, 1991.

World Health Organization: *International Statistical Classification of Diseases and Related Health Problems,* 10th rev. World Health Organization, 1992.

Differential Diagnosis

The diagnosis of adjustment disorder is relatively straightforward, provided the clinician considers a wide range of stressors and other Axis I diagnoses. The clinician should exclude any specified symptom complex that meets diagnostic criteria for another Axis I disorder that may be related to a specific stressor. Other Axis I diagnoses should be recorded if criteria are met, and adjustment disorders rarely add to the diagnostic description. However, if a discrete recent stressor is identified, an adjustment disorder diagnosis may be more appropriate than, for example, anxiety disorder not otherwise specified or depressive disorder not otherwise specified.

When symptoms do not resolve quickly and therapy reveals other psychopathology or personality disorder, initial diagnoses of adjustment disorder are often revised. Where the diagnosis is uncertain, a provisional diagnosis accommodates individuals who may otherwise resist treatment because of preconceived expectations or who may fear the stigma of psychiatric labels. They may accept more readily a temporary and minimal diagnosis, one that permits further assessment. It is often appealing to initially view a new patient as healthy, with a milder diagnosis. The temporary and relatively vague nature of the adjustment disorder diagnostic category allows for changes in the primary admitting diagnosis. Emergency room diagnoses of adjustment disorder are often changed to conduct disorder or substance abuse. This broadly inclusive diagnosis allows symptoms to be addressed while relatively mild, before a major syndrome develops, such as a major depressive episode. Given these properties, one must anticipate some vagueness and ambiguity.

The diagnosis of PTSD differs from adjustment disorder in accordance with the extreme severity of the stressor. In PTSD, the stressor is usually beyond the normal range of experience and leads to symptoms that are more specific, severe, enduring, and handicapping (see Chapter 23).

Acute stress disorder also follows an extreme stressor, more severe than stressors in adjustment disorder, and is associated with specific, severe symptoms (see Chapter 23). Acute stress disorder differs from PTSD in that the former remits after 1 month. The adjustment disorder diagnosis differs from both stress disorders in that it is applicable to a wider range of presentations than these very specific and severe disorders. Again, the emotional and behavioral responses in adjustment disorders are out of proportion to the stressor.

General medical conditions may cause psychiatric symptoms physiologically (and not psychologically as in adjustment disorders) and should be reported as such (eg, mood disorder due to general medical condition). Individuals with chronic medical conditions may merit a second diagnosis of psychological factors affecting physical condition, reflecting both directions of the mind-body interaction. In the impulse-control disorders, specifically intermittent explosive disorder, the precipitant stressor is minute in significance.

Normal grief reactions or bereavement may show cultural variability and may be difficult to differentiate from adjustment disorders. Suicide risks may be present in any of these individuals, no matter which diagnosis is ultimately given. If the reaction to the stressor is within expectable and culturally acceptable norms, nonpathologic reaction to stress should be recorded.

The constant flow of symptoms in cluster B personality disorders often overlap with adjustment disorder symptoms, so that an adjustment disorder diagnosis is redundant in most cases. By definition, behavioral and emotional disturbances are excessive in personality disorders; these individuals would almost all be diagnosed as having adjustment disorder. However, according to DSM-IV, adjustment disorders should be specified under circumstances in which the observed adjustment disorder is atypical for that personality disorder type.

Other, often comorbid, diagnoses that need to be assessed include psychological factors affecting medical condition, substance or alcohol abuse or dependence, somatoform and factitious disorders, and psychosexual disorders.

Treatment

Individuals who have adjustment disorders will often appear to be relatively healthy compared to other diagnostic populations, sometimes deceptively so. Although overall successful treatment rates are greater than 70% in adjustment disorders, about one third of patients do not fare well. Timely intervention can prevent later, more serious problems and may point to underlying weaknesses that may be a focus of treatment. According to the patient's capacities, various therapeutic techniques can be chosen that may challenge erroneous beliefs and help the patient develop a psychological understanding of the problem. Adjustment difficulties worsen in the face of novel stressors when strong emotions are harbored but are poorly recognized or awkwardly expressed. Early intervention is probably more critical than is a specific therapeutic approach. As in other disorders, the building of an alliance in the course of diagnostic interviewing is critical to the success of future therapy. The careful interviewer will patiently avoid judgmental inflection and allow the individual wide latitude for emotional expression. An expeditious identification of the stressor in a permissive environment, allowing open expression of the fears and perceived helplessness, helps build an alliance focused on management of emotions resulting from the stressor. Table 32–3 summarizes psychotherapeutic and pharmacologic approaches to the treatment of adjustment disorders.

A. Psychoanalytic & Psychodynamic Approaches: There are numerous viewpoints from which psychological disturbances can be modeled in the effort to create treatment approaches. Historically, psychoanalytic and psychodynamic approaches have taken a leading role in the interpretation of behavior and emotion. In this view, individuals with adjustment disorders struggle unsuccessfully with effects of a stressor that most would manage more adaptively. Different forms of stress, difficult as they are to quantify, affect individuals in markedly different ways. Each individual has coping skills and mechanisms, some of which are used out of habit. Patients accommodate more easily to currently unmanageable stress when a history of similar difficulties is brought to light. Such a history can be examined in the transference, where perceptions of the relationship between the patient and the therapist are contaminated by attributes from prior relationships even though the therapist has remained neutral. As therapy unfolds, the therapist becomes a target for misdirected anger and resentment, which is pointed out and examined as a means of exploring the problem. The work of therapy is to help the patient recognize and understand the unconscious struggle that arises when the pursuit of pleasure and relief from irritants (the pleasure principle) stands in the way of grasping reality (the reality principle), as pursued within the transference relationship.

Trauma or loss may be perceived as an assault on a strongly developed self-perception, too noxious to be accessible to grief-coping mechanisms. Inflated perceptions of the self and subsequent unreasonable expectations are usually strongly guarded secrets. In an analytic treatment, transference may contain the perception that the therapist is a harbinger of these demands. The overburdening super-ego (internal conscience) can then be revealed as the true aggressor, alleviating the exaggerated sense of depth in the loss. Although the loss remains a reality, its importance then diminishes to a more expected and acceptable level. Being able to project the cause of discomfort away from inappropriate self-blame onto a realistic outside agent will relieve the patient's sense of responsibility for the loss. For example, irrational guilt can arise over having been away on a needed errand when a parent dies of cancer. The patient, after expressing a feeling that even the therapist blames him or her, is able to examine the need to accept the cancer as the cause of the loss.

Other briefer types of therapies are also used and are encouraged in the current managed care environment. Although good comparison studies are lacking, certain individuals will probably do as well with these "more efficient" approaches. Brief psychodynamic, crisis-focused, time-limited psychotherapies require careful patient selection based on finding strong past interpersonal relationships, high premorbid functioning, and an absence of Axis II personality disorder. Some authors limit the use of these more confrontational techniques to situations in which there is a circumscribed focus, high motivation and capacity for insight, and a strong degree of involvement in the interview. The time-structure of this technique is set out clearly at the beginning, with planned termination emphasized and deliberately placed as a new stressor

Table 32–3. Treatment of adjustment disorders.

Treatment Approach	Primary Method	Secondary Methods
Behavioral	Psychodynamic psychotherapy	Cognitive-behavioral, interpersonal, or supportive psychotherapy
Pharmacologic	Antidepressant (eg, sertraline, 25–75 mg daily)	*Only if patient has no history of alcohol abuse*: hypnotics (eg, zolpidem, 5–10 mg at bedtime for 10 days) or anxiolytics (eg, clonazepam, 0.5 mg at bedtime for 10 days)

to be managed throughout the treatment. Goals must be defined clearly. For example, self-deprecating patients may perceive parents as simultaneously ideal and unreproachable and yet harsh and overly demanding. Such patients may have recurrent, severe (but brief) emotional disturbances after any confrontation with their bosses. They may benefit from a better understanding of emotional similarities to maladaptive but customary rules of relationships from childhood. Such therapy allows a recognition of relationship patterns without focusing primarily on the transference.

B. Cognitive-Behavioral Approaches: Cognitive-behavioral therapy provides the patient with tools for recognition and modification of maladaptive beliefs regarding the stressor and the patient's ability to cope with it. Adjustment disorders can be addressed effectively in this way because the importance of the stressor is often unrealistically overestimated in the patient's perception. In a cognitive-behavioral therapy the patient learns to recognize connections between emotions and maladaptive perceptions or beliefs, and then learns to challenge those beliefs.

C. Interpersonal Therapy: Some clinicians prefer an interpersonal therapy stance, especially for patients who have chronic medical illness or HIV infection. Many patients with severe medical illness will shun intrapsychic introspection and benefit more from a psychoeducational approach. The discussion remains in a here-and-now framework about the sick role, which is a complicated balance of needs, independence, and becoming a more or less willing target for the caring of other individuals. Open discussions ensue about who does what for whom in which way, and about how the illness and its consequences will affect the self and others. Modeling of coping mechanisms can be helpful. Even humor can be effective, if introduced carefully. Death and dying may become more approachable. These individuals often latch on eagerly to a reframing of problems from this interpersonal perspective and welcome discussions of ways to change dysfunctional behavior patterns in receiving care. The therapist may be able to address issues inaccessible to the medical-surgical team. The patient may be reluctant to seem ungrateful—or, worse, is fearful of losing the relationship with the primary care physician—and is vigilant to preserve a view of the medical caregiver's goal as the one whose sole task is to provide medical treatment.

D. Supportive Therapy: Supportive therapy is erroneously written off as hand-holding and comforting, whereas "real therapy" is said to demand more confrontation, analysis, and intellectualization. Supportive therapy should involve specific strategies and careful planning. Interventions are conceived with the goal of shoring up inadequate defense mechanisms. The intervention gently guides the individual to a verbalization of emotions regarding the stress. Communication, relaxation, and anger control (eg, counting to ten) are emphasized. In an acute crisis involving loss, or in medical settings where new information brings acute distress, a skilled supportive intervention can be eminently appropriate and effective.

E. Family Therapy: Family therapy is often recommended and can be among the most effective approaches to alleviating adjustment disorders by identifying the role the family plays in promoting a maladaptive coping response. However, many families are ill-prepared to participate in treatment for the "identified" patient. In family sessions, lines of support can be examined and reestablished by skillful work to minimize distortions, blame, and isolation.

F. Pharmacotherapy: Pharmacotherapy is often used to treat adjustment disorders and may be useful when specific symptoms merit a medication trial. Drug selection is based on the symptoms, for example, a short course of a benzodiazepine for adjustment disorder with anxious mood. The treatment goal is rapid symptom relief and prevention of a chronic disorder, such as generalized anxiety disorder. Antidepressants are used frequently. Selective serotonin reuptake inhibitors are generally well-tolerated and appear to be beneficial for some patients (according to case studies), but double-blind, placebo-controlled studies are lacking. Short-term trials of benzodiazepines and alprazolam are often prescribed, for example, for adjustment disorder involving anticipatory anxiety prior to chemotherapy. Hypnotics, such as zolpidem, should be considered for short-term use. The use of herbal preparations, such as St. John's Wort, merits further study.

G. Nontraditional Approaches: In association with other treatments, nontraditional approaches can provide added benefit. Relaxation techniques and yoga, massage, and progressive muscle relaxation have been reported as helpful. Guided exposure or guided imagery can help with anticipatory stressors. Acupuncture has been used to treat adjustment disorders; the results lack sharp definition. Supervised sleep deprivation, also effective in treating endogenous and reactive depressions, may be useful in treating adjustment disorders.

The financing of treatment for adjustment disorders will depend increasingly on the recognition that treatment improves outcome and quality of life, prevents more serious reactions from developing, and reduces the risk of recurrences. There is little to be gained by waiting for the occurrence of disorders that are difficult to treat. An adjustment disorder should receive a complete treatment, assuring restored premorbid functioning. Even so, briefer and equally effective therapies will need to be used. To justify treatment, third-party payers typically require information about symptoms that indicate risk, treatment goals, and therapeutic methods to be used.

Rickel AU, Allen L: *Preventing Maladjustment from Infancy Through Adolescence.* Sage, 1987.

Schatzberg AF: Anxiety and adjustment disorder: a treatment approach. J Clin Psychiatry 1990;51(Suppl 11):20.

Speer DC: Can treatment research inform decision makers? Nonexperimental method issues and examples among older outpatients. J Consult Clin Psychol 1994;62:560.

Complications, Comorbidity, & Adverse Outcomes

Recovery from adjustment disorders can be complicated by a variety of poor outcomes. Although risk factors are intuitively evident when reading thoughtfully, it is all too easy to overlook them in the clinical setting. For example, persistent denial of the importance of the stressor may result in masked or displaced anger with a strong risk of suicidality. The denial will sometimes justify, in the patient's distorted view, deceit in order to conceal issues such as physical safety and suicidality. Highly ambivalent, mixed emotional struggles (eg, terminal illness in an unfaithful spouse) require the clinician to be extra attentive and cautious.

In the presence of a comorbid cluster B personality disorder, adjustment disorder episodes frequently reoccur, to the point where diagnosing them separately is not necessary. However, it is still necessary to treat the adjustment disorder in this common context. According to one study, 15% of individuals with an adjustment disorder also met criteria for one of the cluster B personality disorders (ie, antisocial, histrionic, borderline, or narcissistic personality disorders). A personality disorder diagnosis predicts poor acute outcome and chronically impaired social support among individuals with an adjustment disorder. Comorbid substance abuse is common in individuals with a primary diagnosis of adjustment disorder. Although in the view of French investigators alcoholism may "protect" from stress (cf, discussion of cultural norms, earlier in this chapter), it clearly diminishes coping skills, promotes social isolation, and adds a suicide risk factor.

Some adverse outcomes are iatrogenic. Although helpful for some patients, the risks of somatic treatments must be explained carefully. Medications carry side effects and other risks (eg, suicide by overdose of tricyclic antidepressants), and for these disorders the potential for benefit has not been demonstrated against placebo. Hypomanic or manic switches occur occasionally even with modern antidepressants, and individual risk for this response cannot be predicted reliably. Movement disorder has been reported after single doses of neuroleptics. Benzodiazepines may impair judgment and pose risks of abuse and dependence.

Prognosis & Course of Illness

Symptoms of adjustment disorders usually resolve quickly, with or without resolution of the stressors. Generally, inpatient stays are shorter for adjustment disorders than for depression. Long-term outcome surveys suggest cautious optimism in the prognosis for treated children as well as adults. Adjustment disorders may reoccur in children and adolescents with greater frequency than in adults. Clearly this is a period fraught with many somatic changes and social adjustment requirements. For a first-time diagnosis, the majority of adults will fare very well after suicide risks abate. Adjustment disorders in children and adolescents predict future episodes of adjustment disorders but do not predict future affective episodes. Recovery is not affected by comorbidity; the prognosis of an adjustment disorder alone is the same as for an adjustment disorder with comorbid diagnoses.

These findings suggest that, although short-term prognosis is quite good, there may be an increased frequency of Axis I or Axis II diagnoses in the longer term. Further research is needed to identify individual prognostic factors and appropriate treatments.

Chess S, Thomas A: *Origins and Evolution of Behavior Disorders.* Brunner/Mazel, 1984.

Greenberg WM, Rosenfeld DN, Ortega EA: Adjustment disorder as an admission diagnosis. Am J Psychiatry 1995;152:459.

Kovacs M et al: A controlled prospective study of DSM-III adjustment disorder in childhood. Short-term prognosis and long-term predictive validity. Arch Gen Psychiatry 1994;51:535.

Personality Disorders

33

Leslie C. Morey, PhD, & John R. Hubbard, MD, PhD

PERSONALITY DISORDERS IN GENERAL

DSM-IV Diagnostic Criteria for a Personality Disorder

A. An enduring pattern of inner experience and behavior that deviates markedly from the expectations of the individual's culture. This pattern is manifested in two (or more) of the following areas:
1. cognition (ie, ways of perceiving and interpreting self, other people, and events)
2. affectivity (ie, the range, intensity, lability, and appropriateness of emotional response)
3. interpersonal functioning
4. impulse control

B. The enduring pattern is inflexible and pervasive across a broad range of personal and social situations.

C. The enduring pattern leads to clinically significant distress or impairment in social, occupational, or other important areas of functioning.

D. The pattern is stable and of long duration and its onset can be traced back at least to adolescence or early adulthood.

E. The enduring pattern is not better accounted for as a manifestation of another mental disorder.

F. The enduring pattern is not due to the direct physiological effects of a substance (eg, a drug of abuse, a medication) or a general medical condition (eg, head trauma).

Reprinted with permission from *Diagnostic and Statistical Manual of Mental Disorders,* 4th ed. Copyright 1994 American Psychiatric Association.

General Considerations

A personality disorder is diagnosed when a pattern of personality traits is characteristically inflexible and maladaptive and causes significant impairment or personal distress to the patient. Because traits are enduring patterns of perceiving and relating to the environment and to oneself, personality disorders tend to be long-term conditions that are difficult to change. These disorders are coded on Axis II of the *Diagnostic and Statistical Manual of Mental Disorders,* 4th edition (DSM-IV). The disorders are not mutually exclusive; the majority of patients meeting criteria for one personality disorder will meet criteria for other personality disorders. When this occurs, the clinician should diagnose all relevant disorders and list them in order of importance.

The personality disorders are grouped into three different clusters: cluster A (paranoid, schizoid, schizotypal), which includes individuals who are odd or eccentric; cluster B (antisocial, borderline, histrionic, narcissistic), which includes individuals with dramatic, acting-out behaviors and who have problems with empathy; and cluster C (avoidant, dependent, obsessive-compulsive), which includes personality styles marked by prominent anxiety and novelty avoidance. Cooccurrence among personality disorders within a cluster is particularly common, and typically a patient meeting criteria for a particular disorder will also exhibit some features of other disorders within the same cluster. In addition to these 10 specific disorders, DSM-IV includes criteria for two additional personality disorders in an appendix: passive-aggressive personality disorder and depressive personality disorder.

A. Major Etiologic Theories: The causes of personality disorders are not well understood, and as with essentially every other type of psychiatric disorder, they probably involve various combinations of biopsychosocial etiologies. Developmental and environmental problems have been a major focus of concern in this area because onset occurs early in life and is frequently associated with reported disruptive childhood (real or perceived) experiences.

Of particular interest has been the extremely high rate of reported neglect and childhood sexual, physical, or emotional abuse in patients with certain personality disorders, especially borderline personality disorder. Childhood abuse, particularly by relatives and other caregivers, is likely to contribute to problems in self-image, mood stability, intimacy, and trust. It is also possible that excessive attention (ie, pampering) can lead to poorly developed coping skills similar to that which occur as a result of neglect. For example, an excessive sense of entitlement could be enhanced by neglect of a child's normal needs or by overindulgence to the point of distorting healthy expectations.

Freud theorized that certain personality types developed from fixation at different stages of development. For example, developmental fixation at the oral stage may lead to dependent and demanding personalities; at the anal stage, to enhanced obsessive-compulsive behaviors and emotional distance; and at the phallic stage, to superficial relationships and histrionic behaviors.

Although psychodynamic and environmental factors appear to greatly influence the development of personality disorders, some studies indicate that a genetic contribution to the etiology of Axis II disorders may exist. For example, adoption and other family studies suggest a significant genetic component to antisocial personality and borderline personality disorders. Risk of developing antisocial personality disorder is particularly enhanced when the patient has a father with antisocial personality disorder or alcoholism, even when the patient is adopted away from the biological father. Interestingly, antisocial personality disorder is reportedly not associated with living in high crime communities. Twin, adoption, and family investigations also indicate that patients with schizotypal personality disorder have a genetic association with schizophrenia. The possible neurochemical and genetic contributions to the development of these disorders may help explain why some people in very similar situations (such as abuse) develop a personality disorder whereas others do not. We discuss additional etiologic concepts in the sections on each individual personality disorder.

B. Epidemiology: The prevalence of personality disorders has been estimated at 5–20% in the community. The rate is higher in clinical settings, with as many as 50% of psychiatric patients meeting criteria for at least one Axis II disorder. Mildly problematic personality traits are even more prevalent, occurring in about 20–30% of the general population.

Personality disorders frequently have comorbid Axis I disorders of nearly all types; mood, anxiety, and substance abuse disorders are common correlates. For example, it has been reported that over 50% of patients hospitalized with major depressive disorder also have a diagnosable personality disorder. In many cases the personality disorder is thought to predispose the individual to the recurrence of Axis I problems. The presence of an Axis I problem can complicate the process of establishing a personality disorder diagnosis, because common indicators of personality disorders (eg, interpersonal withdrawal or dependency) can be influenced considerably by mood state. Careful inquiry may be needed to establish that particular problems persist as part of an enduring personality pattern

that reflects a true long-standing personality disorder diagnosis.

The personality disorder diagnoses have frequently been criticized for being misapplied as a function of gender bias. Some personality disorders are diagnosed more frequently in men, whereas others are identified more often in women. For example, borderline personality disorder appears to be far more common in women, and antisocial personality disorder predominates in men. Some researchers have speculated that the two personality disorders are the same illness but tend to manifest differently by gender. Studies using standardized diagnostic techniques tend to show gender differences that are less sizable than clinical observation. Clinicians should be cautious not to misdiagnose personality disorders because of stereotypes about typical gender roles.

Clinical Findings

A. Signs & Symptoms: As a group, the personality disorders may be one of the most complicated mental disorders to diagnose and treat. Diagnosis is difficult partly because of the nature of the difficulties themselves and because the disorders tend to be poorly differentiated and the boundary between normality and a disorder less distinct. Treatment of these disorders is difficult because, almost by definition, they are well-established behaviors or ways of thinking that are not altered easily.

Some manifestations of personality disorders are evident early in life. Signs of these disorders are typically recognizable by adolescence, although caution is warranted in using these diagnoses in children or adolescents because the fixedness of these traits is unknown in early years. Although some behaviors in children (such as aggressiveness and stealing) can predict later personality problems, others (such as social isolation) seem to be of little predictive value and should not automatically be assumed to reflect enduring characteristics.

Manifestations of personality disorders are also stable over time and across situations. An individual with a so-called normal personality has the capacity to adapt to the demands of different situations and to life changes. The individual with a personality disorder has a very limited or possibly no adaptive capacity. Certain core personality traits are particularly enduring (including the predisposition to experience anxiety, be introverted, lack conscientiousness, be interpersonally disagreeable, and be open to new experiences), and individuals with personality disorders often exhibit the extremes of these traits. Thus individuals with personality disorders and those with so-called normal personalities differ primarily in degree rather than kind. This implies that having a personality disorder is not an either-or distinction; rather, personality issues can play a role for an individual to a greater or a lesser extent, and prominent personality traits can be important in planning treatment for the psychiatric patient who does not have a formal personality disorder. DSM-IV explicitly recommends that such traits also be noted on Axis II.

Personality disorders are also distinct in that they are largely ego-syntonic. The early psychoanalytic writers assumed that personality disorders involved character traits that were an essential part of the personality, rather than being symptoms experienced by the person as alien. This distinction is of clear utility in distinguishing certain Axis I and Axis II disorders, such as obsessive-compulsive disorder from obsessive personality disorder (see later in this chapter). However, because the key problems in personality disorders are experienced as a fundamental part of the personality rather than as a distressing symptom, the person often has limited insight into the nature of his or her difficulties. For example, the presenting complaint in many patients with personality disorders is likely to involve marked depression, anxiety, or interpersonal conflict—such patients rarely will complain of identity diffusion or lack of empathy. People with personality disorders are likely to present for treatment only during times of crisis, even though their core deficits are present much of the time. Thus in identifying these disorders it is essential to pay careful attention to indicators of character, which can sometimes be overlooked in the context of an immediate crisis.

Personality disorders are largely interpersonal in nature. Most personality disorder diagnoses are based on reports or observations by others of an individual's interpersonal behavior, and these patients are dysfunctional primarily through their expression in the social milieu. These disorders are disturbances in the sense that the individual's behaviors are disturbing to someone else, and in many cases any experienced distress is the result of the social consequences (eg, divorce, job loss, arrest) of the disorder rather than of the disorder itself. In many cases the assessment process can be facilitated greatly by the presence of an informant (eg, spouse, family member) who can give his or her perspective on the nature of the patient's difficulties.

B. Psychological Testing: A number of psychological tests have been developed to help assess patients for possible personality traits and disorders. Of particular usefulness are the Millon Clinical Multiaxial Inventory (MCMI), the Personality Assessment Inventory (PAI), and the Minnesota Multiphasic Personality Inventory (MMPI).

The MCMI is a 175-question, self-administered, true-false inventory that provides information on personality style, significant personality patterns, and clinical disorders. The self-administered PAI was developed not only to aid in assessment but also to provide guidance in treatment planning. It includes 344 items, grouped into 22 overlapping full scales. These scales consist of 4 validity scales, 11 clinical scales, 5 treatment issue scales, and 2 interpersonal scales. The MMPI was developed to help in diagnosis of mental disorders but is more often used to describe the patient. It consists of over 500 items and includes nine basic clinical scales (hypochondriasis, depression, hysteria, psychopathic deviance, masculinity/femininity, paranoia, anxiety, schizophrenia, and mania). Validity scales and special scales are also included. Other assessment instruments have been developed, and various semistructured interview protocols, such as the Structured Clinical Interview for the DSM-IV, can also be used.

C. Laboratory Findings: As indicated earlier in this chapter, personality disorders appear to have a biological or genetic component. There are no biological markers for personality disorders; however, certain associations have been reported. For example, low platelet monoamine oxidase activity has been found in patients who have schizotypal personality disorder. Low 5-hydroxyindoleacetic acid in the cerebrospinal fluid of patients who have borderline personality disorder has been negatively associated with suicide attempts and aggressive behavior. In addition, abnormal dexamethasone suppression tests are less likely to be found in personality disorder patients with depression than in patients with major depressive disorder that is not associated with an Axis II diagnosis. This finding may suggest less of a biological component or possibly a different neurochemical nature to depression in patients with personality disorders, as compared to patients with major depressive disorder who do not have Axis II pathology.

At least subtle electroencephalographic disturbances have been observed in patients with certain personality disorders such as antisocial or borderline personality disorders. An increase in slow-wave sleep activity has been reported most frequently. Overall, these changes suggest that a possible mild central nervous system injury or developmental defect may be associated with certain Axis II psychiatric disorders.

Treatment

A. Medical Approaches: In general, no single pharmacologic treatment is effective in the treatment of a particular personality disorder. Certain medications may be of use in reducing certain features of the disorders, but they are generally limited and are typically ineffective in alleviating other symptoms. Because of the enduring nature of the problems associated with these disorders, symptoms that have responded to pharmacologic treatment often return when the medication is stopped. The effect of somatic treatments may be limited as a result of the large psychosocial component of Axis II pathology.

B. Social Approaches: Socially based treatments, such as group therapy, are often thought to be of particular use with personality disorders because so many of them are distinctly interpersonal in nature. Furthermore, the feedback of peers often is an advantage because of the long history of difficulty with authority that these patients manifest and because of their frequently poor insight into their condition.

C. Psychological Approaches: Patients with personality disorders tend to be challenging to therapists. The fixedness and duration of their problems makes these problems difficult to alter in a brief treatment. Many of the disorder subtypes are also very taxing to treat. The patient is often angry, manipulative, demanding, defensive, or angry. Significant transference and countertransference reactions are common. Specific therapy techniques (eg, behavioral, cognitive, interpersonal) may work differentially with the different personality disorders; however, across the different techniques the alliance between therapist and patient is critical. A stance of collaboration, rather than control or rescue, is necessary if one is to avoid some of the difficulties in working with these patients. Many of these patients appear to benefit from supportive and cognitive therapy that is focused more on current life issues than on past concerns (eg, reported instances of victimization).

Prognosis

By definition, a personality disorder is an enduring pattern of behaving and thinking that is reasonably stable over time. Thus in the absence of intervention the condition will likely remain stable for many years, with the individual's level of functional impairment being relatively constant. Although the limited evidence confirms that certain personality disorder diagnoses are stable over time, it is not clear that this represents stability of traits within the diagnosis, because some features of the disorder may be replaced by others as the patient ages. The personality disorders characterized by impulsivity and anger (eg, borderline and antisocial personality disorders) tend to show some reduction in these features as the individual reaches middle age, but other impairments are likely to remain intact. Because of the enduring nature of their problems, patients with personality disorders tend to be less responsive to nearly any form of treatment than are psychiatric patients who do not have such disorders.

INDIVIDUAL PERSONALITY DISORDERS

CLUSTER A PERSONALITY DISORDERS

1. PARANOID PERSONALITY DISORDER

DSM-IV Diagnostic Criteria

A. A pervasive distrust and suspiciousness of others such that their motives are interpreted as malevo-

lent, beginning by early adulthood and present in a variety of contexts, as indicated by four (or more) of the following:
   (1) suspects, without sufficient basis, that others are exploiting, harming, or deceiving him or her
   (2) is preoccupied with unjustified doubts about the loyalty or trustworthiness of friends or associates
   (3) is reluctant to confide in others because of unwarranted fear that the information will be used maliciously against him or her
   (4) reads hidden demeaning or threatening meanings into benign remarks or events
   (5) persistently bears grudges, ie, is unforgiving of insults, injuries, or slights
   (6) perceives attacks on his or her character or reputation that are not apparent to others and is quick to react angrily or to counterattack
   (7) has recurrent suspicions, without justification, regarding fidelity of spouse or sexual partner
B. Does not occur exclusively during the course of schizophrenia, a mood disorder with psychotic features, or another psychotic disorder and is not due to the direct physiological effects of a general medical condition.

General Considerations

A. Major Etiologic Theories: Although the etiology of paranoid personality disorder is unknown, both genetic and environmental aspects likely play a role. For example, the risk of developing the disorder is enhanced in families with a history of schizophrenia and delusional disorders. Environmentally, the risk for this disorder appears to be increased if the individual's parents exhibited irrational outbursts of anger. In such instances, the frequent fear the individual experienced as a child may be projected onto others later.

B. Epidemiology: The prevalence of paranoid personality disorder has been estimated at 0.5–2.5% in the general population. It is relatively common in clinical settings, particularly among psychiatric inpatients. These individuals typically do not seek treatment on their own but are referred by family members or employers. There is some evidence that the disorder is more common among individuals with a family history of schizophrenia or delusional disorder, persecutory type. The disorder may be slightly more common in men than in women. Caution should be used in applying the diagnosis to members of ethnic or cultural minorities or to recent immigrants, because a guarded attitude or mistrust concerning the evaluation process can be a reaction to the assessment context in such individuals, or it may be appropriate to the patient's country of origin rather than being a more generalized personality pattern.

Clinical Findings

The cardinal feature of paranoid personality disorder is generalized distrust or suspiciousness. Individuals with this disorder feel that they have been treated unfairly by others, are resentful of this mistreatment, and bear long-lasting grudges against those who have slighted them in some way. They place a high premium on autonomy and react in a hostile manner to others who seek to control them. These patients are unsuccessful in intimate relationships because of their suspiciousness and aloofness. The disorder may be contrasted with Axis I disorders—such as delusional disorder, persecutory type, or schizophrenia, paranoid type—by the absence in the former of delusions, hallucinations, and defective reality testing.

On clinical interview, patients who have paranoid personality disorder are formal, businesslike, skeptical, and mistrustful. These patients may be quite tense in this context, exhibiting poor or fixated eye contact. Interviews with such individuals tend to be uncomfortable and leave the clinician feeling uneasy. These patients will frequently question the interviewer about the purpose or utility of a particular query. They consistently project blame for their difficulties onto others, externalizing their own emotions while paying keen attention to the emotions and attitudes of others. Underlying their formal and at times moralistic presentation is considerable hostility and resentment.

The disorder often appears in combination with schizotypal personality disorder, although this is because of the shared feature of paranoid ideation. Other common cooccurrences include borderline and narcissistic personality disorders. When paranoid personality disorder is comorbid with narcissistic personality disorder, the paranoid features serve to justify the patient's self-importance: The obstructions of others are seen as evidence of the merit of the patient's overvalued ideas.

Treatment

A. Medical Approaches: There have been little data to suggest that pharmacologic interventions are of significant benefit. Low-dose antipsychotic medications may decrease the patient's paranoia and anxiety. Under situations of stress, some patients decompensate, and the paranoid ideation reaches delusional proportions, in which case antipsychotic medication can be of more benefit.

B. Social Approaches: Group therapy can be quite difficult with these patients, as their lack of basic trust prevents them from being integrated fully into the group. Their wariness and suspiciousness may become self-fulfilling, as their hostility makes other members uncomfortable and rejecting. These patients have particular difficulty in groups in which

other patients are healthier. They sometimes present in couples or family therapy, and working with them in this context is also delicate. Such patients often feel that the therapist and family members are colluding against them; a co-therapist can be helpful to prevent or diffuse such feelings.

C. Psychological Approaches: Patients with paranoid personality disorder represent a unique challenge to the psychotherapist. They have difficulty relinquishing control, which is required in directive therapy, and may not tolerate the ambiguity associated with less directive interventions. Regardless of technique, the clinician should take particular care to be straightforward and respectful. Among behavioral techniques, social-skills role playing, particularly involving appropriate expression of assertiveness, can help such patients overcome their tendency to withdraw sullenly from situations in which they feel they have been treated unfairly. Cognitive techniques focus on the patient's overgeneralizations (eg, "That person didn't talk to me; therefore, he hates me.") and propensity to dichotomize the social world into trustworthy and hostile. In dynamic and interpersonal approaches, interpretations should be used sparingly; treatment should focus on the gradual recognition of the origins and negative consequences of the patient's mistrust. This approach should result in the increasing acceptance that many of the patient's problems are internal rather than the product of external sources.

Prognosis

Little is known about the long-term outcome of paranoid personality disorder. Although the disorder is difficult to treat, patients with the disorder appear to have a greater adaptive capacity than do patients who have personality disorders associated with severe social detachment (eg, schizoid personality disorder). However, under stress, patients with paranoid personality disorder withdraw and avoid attachments, thus perpetuating their mistrust.

2. SCHIZOID PERSONALITY DISORDER

DSM-IV Diagnostic Criteria

A. A pervasive pattern of detachment from social relationships and a restricted range of expression of emotions in interpersonal settings, beginning by early adulthood and present in a variety of contexts, as indicated by four (or more) of the following:
  (1) neither desires nor enjoys close relationships, including being part of a family
  (2) almost always chooses solitary activities
  (3) has little, if any, interest in having sexual experiences with another person
  (4) takes pleasure in few, if any, activities
  (5) lacks close friends or confidants other than first-degree relatives

(6) appears indifferent to the praise or criticism of others

(7) shows emotional coldness, detachment, or flattened affectivity

B. Does not occur exclusively during the course of schizophrenia, a mood disorder with psychotic features, another psychotic disorder, or a pervasive developmental disorder and is not due to the direct physiological effects of a general medical condition.

Reprinted, with permission, from *Diagnostic and Statistical Manual of Mental Disorders,* 4th ed. Copyright 1994 American Psychiatric Association.

General Considerations

A. Major Etiologic Theories: The causes of schizoid personality disorder are not understood. Genetic factors are suspected to be involved, and some reports suggest that patients with this disorder often come from environments that are deficient in emotional nurturing.

B. Epidemiology: Estimates of the prevalence of schizoid personality disorder in the general population vary with the criteria used, ranging from 0.5% to 7%. Individuals with this disorder are relatively uncommon in clinical settings. The features of the disorder rarely distress the individuals who have it, and their general withdrawal means that they rarely disturb others. The disorder may be slightly more common, or more likely to cause impairment, in men than in women. The symptoms of schizoid personality disorder resemble the negative symptoms of schizophrenia and are associated with increased heritability in the latter disorder. Thus an increased prevalence of schizoid personality disorder among individuals with a family history of schizophrenia might be expected, although the available data are equivocal.

Clinical Findings

The life history of patients with schizoid personality disorder is typically characterized by a preference for solitary pursuits. These individuals may have no intimate relationships and little apparent interest in them, outside of internal fantasy. The social detachment and affective constriction of these patients make them appear aloof, distant, and difficult to engage in a clinical interview. These patients are more likely to demonstrate interest when describing abstract pursuits that require no personal involvement. Although reality testing is generally intact in these patients, their lack of social contact precludes the correction of their somewhat idiosyncratic interpretations of social transactions. Patients with schizoid personality disorder can be distinguished from those with avoidant personality disorder by the former group's indifference and lack of interest in others. In contrast to the schizotypal personality, the schizoid personality is effectively flat and unresponsive, rather than behav-

iorally eccentric, although the disorders cooccur with some frequency.

Treatment

A. Medical Approaches: Little is known about effective treatment of schizoid personality disorder. Thus far, effective pharmacotherapy has not been demonstrated.

B. Social Approaches: Often individuals with schizoid personality disorder come to treatment at the request of family members. In some cases, family-based intervention might help clarify for the patient the family's expectations and perhaps address any intolerance and invasiveness on the part of the family that could be worsening the patient's withdrawal. Group therapy can also be helpful as a source of directed feedback from others that would otherwise be missed or ignored. Such settings also allow for the modeling and acquisition of needed social skills. The initial participation of the patient with schizoid personality disorder will invariably be minimal, and the therapist may need to act to prevent the patient from being the target of other group members. Forced intimacy may also precipitate a breakdown.

C. Psychological Approaches: Psychotherapeutic interventions tend to be difficult, because patients with schizoid personality disorder are often not psychologically minded and typically experience no distress. An alliance is often impeded by the low value that these individuals place on relationships. More cognitively based treatment approaches may receive greater initial acceptance, and distorted expectancies and perceptions about the importance and usefulness of relationships with others can be explored. The tendency of these patients to intellectualize and distance themselves from emotional experience can restrict the impact of these techniques.

Prognosis

The prognosis is poor. Patients with schizoid personality disorder display problems at an earlier age than do patients with other personality disorders, and they have more severe problems after initial treatment. Social disinterest tends to self-perpetuate isolation, and flattened affect does nothing to encourage others to interact. However, relative to patients with other personality disorders, those with schizoid personality disorder are less likely to manifest anxiety or depression, particularly if the patients are not in occupational situations that tax their limited social skills.

3. SCHIZOTYPAL PERSONALITY DISORDER

DSM-IV Diagnostic Criteria

A. A pervasive pattern of social and interpersonal deficits marked by acute discomfort with, and reduced capacity for, close relationships as well as by cognitive or perceptual distortions and eccentricities of behavior, beginning by early adulthood and present in a variety of contexts, as indicated by five (or more) of the following:

(1) ideas of reference (excluding delusions of reference)

(2) odd beliefs or magical thinking that influences behavior or is inconsistent with subcultural norms (eg, superstitiousness, belief in clairvoyance, telepathy, or "sixth sense"; in children and adolescents, bizarre fantasies or preoccupations)

(3) unusual perceptual experiences (including bodily illusions)

(4) odd thinking and speech (eg, vague, circumstantial, metaphorical, overelaborate, or stereotyped)

(5) suspiciousness or paranoid ideation

(6) inappropriate or constricted affect

(7) behavior or appearance that is odd, eccentric, or peculiar

(8) lack of close friends or confidants other than first-degree relatives

B. Does not occur exclusively during the course of schizophrenia, a mood disorder with psychotic features, another psychotic disorder, or a pervasive developmental disorder.

Reprinted, with permission, from *Diagnostic and Statistical Manual of Mental Disorders,* 4th ed. Copyright 1994 American Psychiatric Association.

General Considerations

A. Major Etiologic Theories: Schizotypal personality disorder occurs more frequently among the biological relatives of schizophrenic individuals than in the general population. This finding, together with twin studies, suggests a genetic component to this illness; however, the precise causes of the disorder are unknown.

B. Epidemiology: The prevalence rate of schizotypal personality disorder has been estimated at approximately 3%, and the disorder is slightly more prevalent in male patients. The disorder may be manifested during childhood or adolescence as social isolation and peculiar behavior or language. These children are often teased. Although the features of the disorder resemble schizophrenia, rates of depressive and anxiety disorders are quite high among such patients. These features often constitute the presenting complaint, rather than the cognitive anomalies that are more striking to the objective observer.

Clinical Findings

A concept originating in the writings of Sandor Rado, schizotypal personality disorder was first officially included in DSM-III, where it was separated from borderline personality disorder in an effort to distinguish two forms of what had been referred to as borderline schizophrenia. This distinction separated effectively unstable individuals (ie, those with borderline personality disorder) from those with cognitive aberrations (ie, those with schizotypal personality disorder). Schizotypal personality disorder is considered by some researchers to reflect a schizophrenia spectrum disorder, and the DSM-IV criteria reflect a level of adaptation between schizoid personality and schizophrenia. The disorder resembles the residual phase of chronic schizophrenia, distinguished primarily by a past episode of active schizophrenia. However, the relatives of schizophrenic patients who display schizotypal personality disorder tend to exhibit social isolation and poor rapport rather than the psychotic-like symptoms of referential ideation or perceptual distortion. Thus, although the disorder appears with greater than expected frequency in the relatives of schizophrenic patients, it is not merely a milder form of schizophrenia. The disorder can also be distinguished from schizoid personality disorder by the degree of affective constriction in the latter disorder, in contrast to the marked social anxiety and cognitive distortions associated with the former.

Treatment

A. Medical Approaches: Low-dose neuroleptic medication is helpful in the treatment of cognitive peculiarities, depression, odd speech, anxiety, and impulsivity in patients with schizotypal personality disorder. These medications are particularly useful in patients with moderately severe schizotypal symptoms and mild, transient psychotic episodes. It is unknown whether antipsychotic medications have a prophylactic benefit in preventing worsening of this disorder.

B. Social Approaches: Group therapy can help patients with schizotypal personality disorder to address social anxiety and awkwardness and also to draw support in knowing that others have insecurities as well. Patients with more severe symptoms may prove disruptive, particularly if prominent paranoid ideation is present. Patients with overtly eccentric behavior may make other group members uncomfortable and become a scapegoat of group process.

C. Psychological Approaches: Patients with schizotypal personality disorder are poorly suited for traditional psychoanalytic treatments because of a propensity to decompensate under unstructured conditions. A supportive approach, with an emphasis on reality testing and attention to interpersonal boundaries is probably best suited to the early stages of treatment. Directive approaches focused on problematic behavior (eg, social-skills training) can be useful. Attempts should also be made to address cognitive distortions such as referential, paranoid, or magical thinking. This can be accomplished through educative interventions that teach patients to corroborate their thoughts with environmental evidence rather than with personal feelings.

Prognosis

Estimates of the proportion of patients with schizotypal personality disorder who go on to develop schizophrenia are variable. This proportion is generally thought to be low, but some estimates are as high as 20–25%. Paranoid ideation, social isolation, and magical thinking seem to be most predictive of the later development of schizophrenia. These symptoms are also most associated with a poor prognosis and more chronic outcome and with a course resembling that of chronic schizophrenia with milder levels of impairment.

CLUSTER B
PERSONALITY DISORDERS

1. ANTISOCIAL PERSONALITY DISORDER

DSM-IV Diagnostic Criteria

A. There is a pervasive pattern of disregard for and violation of the rights of others occurring since age 15 years, as indicated by three (or more) of the following:
  (1) failure to conform to social norms with respect to lawful behaviors as indicated by repeatedly performing acts that are grounds for arrest
  (2) deceitfulness, as indicated by repeated lying, use of aliases, or conning others for personal profit or pleasure
  (3) impulsivity or failure to plan ahead
  (4) irritability and aggressiveness, as indicated by repeated physical fights or assaults
  (5) reckless disregard for safety of self or others
  (6) consistent irresponsibility, as indicated by repeated failure to sustain consistent work behavior or honor financial obligations
  (7) lack of remorse, as indicated by being indifferent to or rationalizing having hurt, mistreated, or stolen from another
B. The individual is at least age 18 years.
C. There is evidence of conduct disorder with onset before age 15 years.
D. The occurrence of antisocial behavior is not exclusively during the course of schizophrenia or a manic episode.

Reprinted, with permission, from *Diagnostic and Statistical Manual of Mental Disorders,* 4th ed. Copyright 1994 American Psychiatric Association.

General Considerations

A. Major Etiologic Theories: There is considerable interest in determining the causes of antisocial personality disorder, and it appears that both biological and environmental factors are involved. Individuals are at increased risk for this disorder if they had an antisocial or alcoholic father (even if they were not raised by that person). Twin studies also support a genetic component to the etiology of antisocial personality disorder. The primary environmental deficient appears to be the lack of a consistent person to give emotional and loving support as a young child. Surprisingly, merely living in a high crime area does not in and of itself increase the risk of antisocial personality disorder.

Antisocial personality disorder appears to be reasonably common in the general population (the rate is estimated at 3% in males). However, such patients rarely seek treatment voluntarily, appearing with greater frequency when interventions are mandated, such as in substance abuse treatment or correctional settings. The disorder is diagnosed roughly three times more frequently in men than in women. By definition, the disruptive behavioral features of the disorder are observed early, during adolescence or even childhood. These features tend to remit as the individual reaches middle age, particularly after age 40 years.

Clinical Findings

The critical feature of antisocial personality disorder is a disregard for the rights and feelings of others, a shortcoming that leads to a variety of antisocial behaviors first noted during adolescence or even childhood. In clinical settings, the antisocial person is not as anxious or dysphoric as would be expected. These individuals are frequently brought to treatment against their will or agree to treatment to avoid a less-desirable alternative such as prison. On interview, these patients may seem quite normal, ingratiating, or even charming, but their history will reveal a long record of failures in meeting social role obligations. Their intimate relationships are casual and short-lived, and substance abuse is common.

Patients with antisocial personality disorder tend to be easily bored and impulsive. They constantly seek novelty in their relationships and surroundings. They are most likely to be alert to the possibilities of reward and seem unable to avoid behavior that has a high probability of punishment. They also appear to be less responsive to emotionally arousing situations than most individuals, which helps to differentiate them from those with borderline personality disorder. The latter patients may engage in manipulative behavior to ensure that their needs are met; patients with antisocial personality disorder may exploit others solely for personal benefit or at times for no apparent motivation. A lack of empathy leads those with antisocial personality disorder to believe that others are fully as eager to exploit them as they are to exploit others, and they often rationalize their antisocial behavior as defensive.

Treatment

A. Medical Approaches: Some evidence suggests that impulsive, aggressive behaviors in personality disorders are associated with reduced central 5-hydroxytryptamine function. Preliminary evidence suggests that selective serotonin reuptake inhibitors

(SSRIs) are effective in reducing aggression. Lithium, carbamazepine, and possibly propranolol may also be used to reduce impulsive aggression in some patients. Medication should be monitored closely because of the heightened risk for abuse.

B. Social Approaches: Socially based interventions, particularly with others of similar temperament, are often considered to be the treatment of choice. In social contexts, rationalization and evasion can be confronted by others who recognize these patterns. Group membership and caring for others allows patients with antisocial personality disorder to experience feelings of belonging that many never received from their families. Therapeutic communities that emphasize responsibilities toward others are often used. One socially based approach for adolescents is a wilderness program that stresses group cooperation in overcoming difficult or dangerous tasks. Other milieu-based treatment that requires patient interdependence can also be helpful. Family therapy may be useful when the family system is contributing to or perpetuating the antisocial behavior; however, family therapy often devolves into supporting beleaguered relatives, which need not be done in conjoint sessions.

C. Psychological Approaches: The theoretical literature views the psychotherapy of antisocial personality disorder with considerable pessimism. In behavioral treatments utilizing contingency management, patients with this disorder will respond to conditions of reward, but such behaviors rarely generalize beyond the specific contingency. Punishment-based techniques are typically ineffective. Traditional psychotherapy is impeded by the patient's interpersonal indifference, which hinders the formation of a true alliance. Dropout rates from therapy are as high as 70%. Cognitive approaches involve addressing distortions that are typically self-serving or that minimize the future consequences of the individual's behavior, but the efficacy of these approaches is largely unknown.

Prognosis

Little is known about the prognosis of antisocial personality disorder. The disorder is thought to be among the most treatment refractory of the personality disorders. The behavioral problems associated with the disorder tend to peak in late adolescence and early adulthood, and 30–40% of patients may show great improvement by the time they reach their fourth decade. During later years these individuals are at risk for chronic alcoholism and late-onset depressions.

2. BORDERLINE PERSONALITY DISORDER

DSM-IV Diagnostic Criteria

A. A pervasive pattern of instability of interpersonal relationships, self-image, and affects, and marked impulsivity beginning by early adulthood and present in a variety of contexts, as indicated by five (or more) of the following:
  (1) frantic efforts to avoid real or imagined abandonment.

Note: Do not include suicidal or self-mutilating behavior covered in criterion 5.

  (2) a pattern of unstable and intense interpersonal relationships characterized by alternating between extremes of idealization and devaluation
  (3) identity disturbance: markedly and persistently unstable self-image or sense of self
  (4) impulsivity in at least two areas that are potentially self-damaging (eg, spending, sex, substance abuse, reckless driving, binge eating)

Note: Do not include suicidal or self-mutilating behavior covered in criterion 5.

  (5) recurrent suicidal behavior, gestures, or threats, or self-mutilating behavior
  (6) affective instability due to a marked reactivity of mood (eg, intense episodic dysphoria, irritability, or anxiety usually lasting a few hours and only rarely more than a few days)
  (7) chronic feelings of emptiness
  (8) inappropriate and intense anger or difficulty controlling anger (eg, frequent displays of temper, constant anger, recurrent physical fights)
  (9) transient, stress-related paranoid ideation or severe dissociative symptoms

Reprinted, with permission, from *Diagnostic and Statistical Manual of Mental Disorders,* 4th ed. Copyright 1994 American Psychiatric Association.

General Considerations

The earliest references to borderline conditions in psychiatry concerned forms of behavior that were seemingly between normality and insanity. For example, Kraepelin's influential writings made references to types of "psychopathic conditions" that were on the border between pronounced pathologic states and mere personality eccentricities. However, the modern interest in borderline conditions originated with the psychoanalytic movement. Freud's distinction between transference neuroses and narcissistic neuroses delineated those patients suitable for psychoanalysis from those who were not; the former were amenable to analytic interventions whereas the latter could not form the transferential relationship that was a theoretical prerequisite to analysis. As the popularity of psychoanalytic treatments grew, so too did the recognition of the vast number of patients who seemed to be at the margins of analytic suitability. These marginal cases served as the impetus for increasing discussions of the analyzability of so-called borderline cases. Thus for the psychoanalytic writers the border in question was one between psychosis and neurosis, as opposed to one between normality and psychopathology. Knight emphasized that such patients often overtly displayed neurotic symptoms that represented a superficial "holding operation" serving to obscure severe regression and weakening of ego functions such as realistic planning, maintenance of object relationships, and defenses against primitive impulses.

These early uses of the term borderline were made in reference to conditions related in some way to severe psychiatric disorders such as schizophrenia or affective disorder. Initially, this use of the concept referred to schizophrenia spectrum disorders that alternatively have been described as latent schizophrenia, ambulatory schizophrenia, pseudoneurotic schizophrenia, or preschizophrenia. However, research conducted in preparing DSM-III was influential in separating this pattern from the borderline concept. This separation was incorporated into DSM-III, and the borderline schizophrenia concept was named schizotypal personality disorder.

The DSM conceptualization presents the concept of borderline personality disorder as a categorical psychopathologic entity. An alternative viewpoint, taken by theorists such as Kernberg and Millon, is that borderline refers to a severely dysfunctional level of personality organization. For Kernberg, the term borderline describes a region of psychic functioning between the neurotic and psychotic ranges, consistent with the traditional psychoanalytic view. In contrast, Millon views borderline personality as representing the most severe range of personality disorder, an endpoint to which other personality types may deteriorate under stress.

A. Major Etiologic Theories: Borderline personality disorder is rather common, typically accounting for one third or more of personality disorder diagnoses. The causes of the disorder are uncertain. Psychoanalytical work commonly focuses on disturbance in the normal separation-individuation phase of development between the child and the mother. This problem is thought to leave the child with problems of separation and self-identity. For example, the normal turmoil of breaking up a dating relationship may lead to extreme feelings of rejection and cause severe emotional lability and even self-injury.

Other environmental influences are also suspected. A major area of concern is that the vast majority of patients with borderline personality disorder report childhood sexual, physical, or emotional abuse. In some cases borderline personality disorder could be related closely to posttraumatic stress disorder. These patients often also report sexual, physical, or emotional abuse by many other people in their adult life and commonly complain of being victimized in various ways by health care workers or other people in authority. These observations complicate the understanding of these patients' allegations of abuse, and each accusation must be considered on an individual basis. Dissociation, splitting, repression, mood lability, identity problems, and other symptoms may result if abuse has occurred.

Other forms of inconsistent parenting such as neglect or poor expression of affection may be a part of the etiology. Some patients may be from turbulent or broken homes, and mental illness or substance abuse problems in one or both parents can disrupt effective parenting. Some researchers speculate that overindulgence can also lead to immature coping styles similar to those that often occur in association with insufficient nurturing.

The possible genetic influences are not well-understood for borderline personality disorder. Some investigators have speculated that a genetic problem leads to enhanced anxiety and emotional lability. A genetic component to the illness could help explain why some people develop this disorder and others do not under similar circumstances.

B. Epidemiology: The prevalence of borderline personality disorder is about 2–4% in the general population. The disorder is particularly common among psychiatric inpatients; as many as 20% of such patients meet criteria for the disorder. Borderline personality disorder is identified more commonly in women than in men, although evidence suggests that it may be underidentified in men. The features of the disorder are more common among young adults, and the more disruptive behavioral features of the disorder seem to diminish during middle age. Although identity confusion and moodiness are common in the teenage years, other features of the disorder can be identified reliably in later adolescence.

Clinical Findings

Borderline personality disorder is characterized by a poorly established self-image that is heavily dependent on relationships, in combination with an expectation of mistreatment or exploitation. This combination of features makes those with the disorder concerned about close relationships and highly sensitive to changes in these relationships. These patients tend to react to interpersonal conflicts with dramatic emotional changes and impulsive self-destructiveness. They often meet criteria for a mood disorder such as dysthymic disorder or major depression, but their mood is very reactive to external events and will often switch between rage, despair, and anxiety over the course of a single day. Multiple suicidal gestures and self-mutilation are among the most striking behaviors of patients with borderline personality disorder. Such behavior is noted primarily after interpersonal turmoil, often rejection by an intimate. Suicidal gestures tend to increase in lethality as they recur, and completed suicide occurs in nearly 10% of these patients.

The assessment of borderline personality disorder is complicated by the cognitive style these patients manifest. Patients with this disorder view their world in extreme ways. Although positive elements can be found, patients' evaluations of themselves and their surroundings tend to be negative in the extreme. This cognitive style, at interview, leads to a very negative portrayal of the patient's mental state and life circumstances. The patient may admit to a wide variety of negative symptomatology, including severe depression and anxiety, psychotic features, paranoid ideation, or somatic concerns. The clinical picture may be more pathologic than would be reported by an objective observer. This is not to say that these patients malinger their symptoms; rather, their proclivity to evaluate their mental status negatively leads to self-reported clinical pictures that are more pathologic than are outwardly apparent. These patients may appear more impaired on unstructured as opposed to structured assessment techniques, although this is also a function of the affective content of the assessment. For example, cognitive assessments of patients with borderline personality disorder arouse little emotional turmoil; hence, little impairment is evident on these tasks.

Treatment

A. Medical Approaches: Patients with borderline personality disorder tend to experience crises that necessitate short-term hospitalization, typically involving acute stabilization of suicidal ideation. Some of these patients quickly become dissatisfied with the hospital and wish to leave against medical advice, whereas others seem to become attached to the hospital and are very reluctant to leave. It is not uncommon for a patient with this disorder to make numerous complaints about a hospital while doing everything he or she can to prolong the stay.

There is currently no single drug treatment of choice for borderline personality disorder. Acute treatments directed at affective dysregulation, impulsivity, perceptual distortion, and anxiety may make these patients more amenable to psychosocial treatment, but maintenance medication trials generally show limited efficacy. Acute treatment with low-dose neuroleptics may be tried to reduce mild psychotic features. Lithium and anticonvulsants (such as carbamazepine and valproic acid) have been used for mood swings and impulsive behaviors. SSRIs, tricyclic antidepressants (TCAs), and monoamine oxidase inhibitor (MAOI) antidepressants may be prescribed for depression. SSRIs are often selected to reduce risk of overdose.

Some reports suggest that some patients with borderline personality disorder appear to do worse on some anxiolytic medications, particularly benzodiazepines, than on placebo. For example, alprazolam has been reported to exacerbate anger problems and behavioral dyscontrol in some patients.

Finally, any medication should be monitored carefully and prescribed cautiously because of enhanced risks for noncompliance, substance abuse, and use in suicide attempts or gestures.

B. Social Approaches: Group therapy can be a useful forum in which to work with the interpersonal problems of these patients. In such settings, these patients can form attachments to several group members, rather than to a single individual who will eventually be viewed as untrustworthy. Having other peers available to mediate inevitable conflicts with other group members is also helpful. Family therapy can be helpful, but care must be taken to maintain the goal of assisting the patients to achieve autonomy, rather than to succumb to repeated efforts at placing blame for patients' difficulties.

C. Psychological Approaches: Psychotherapy with these patients is made difficult by the severity and nature of the pathology and by the strong reactions evoked in the therapist. A solid alliance is fundamental to the success of any form of therapy. In the initial stages of treatment, a supportive approach can be helpful in establishing this alliance. Often a hierarchy of treatment priorities must be followed, with suicidality receiving highest priority, followed by threats to the treatment and behaviors that interfere with quality of life. Only then can therapy focus on other issues such as attempting to increase specific behavioral skills (eg, emotional regulation, self-management). As part of the treatment process, patients must recognize the pattern of self-destruction and victimization that has characterized their lives and understand its origin. Patients should also explore their rigid, discrete good-versus-bad view of others, recognizing that others' motivations (like their own) are more complex than they appear, and that their sensitivity to others' untrustworthiness is often a distortion arising out of experience.

Prognosis

Patients with borderline personality disorder repeatedly engage in self-destructive behaviors and will sometimes sabotage treatment when it seems to be going well. Their behavior tends to become even more dramatic and dangerous as others around them reject them or habituate to their constant demands and crises. As a result, long-term prognosis is poor, and suicide rates are as high as 8.5%. The degree of impairment and suicide risk peak during early adulthood. Impulsive behaviors seem to diminish as patients reach middle age, but the interpersonal deficits that mark the disorder persist into late adulthood.

3. HISTRIONIC PERSONALITY DISORDER

DSM-IV Diagnostic Criteria

A. A pervasive pattern of excessive emotionality and attention seeking, beginning by early adulthood and present in a variety of contexts, as indicated by five (or more) of the following:
   (1) is uncomfortable in situations in which he or she is not the center of attention
   (2) interaction with others is often characterized by inappropriate sexually seductive or provocative behavior

(3) displays rapidly shifting and shallow expression of emotions

(4) consistently uses physical appearance to draw attention to self

(5) has a style of speech that is excessively impressionistic and lacking in detail

(6) shows self-dramatization, theatricality, and exaggerated expression of emotion

(7) is suggestible, ie, easily influenced by others or circumstances

(8) considers relationships to be more intimate than they actually are

Reprinted, with permission, from *Diagnostic and Statistical Manual of Mental Disorders,* 4th ed. Copyright 1994 American Psychiatric Association.

General Considerations

A. Major Etiologic Theories: The etiology of histrionic personality disorder is not well understood. Some researchers speculate that a frequent problem in parent-child relationships leads to low self-esteem. Dramatic behavior and other means to superficially impress others may be linked to the individual's self-concept that he or she is not worthy of attention without special behaviors. There also appears to be a family association between histrionic and antisocial personality disorders and, as with borderline personality disorder, these disorders could be gender-related expressions of the same illness.

B. Epidemiology: The prevalence rate of histrionic personality disorder has been estimated at 2–3% in the general population. Rates of the disorder are much higher in psychiatric and general medical settings because such patients actively pursue treatment, in comparison with those who have other personality disorders. Histrionic personality tends to be diagnosed more frequently in women, and the disorder may be overlooked in men. Epidemiologic studies suggest that the gender difference is either slight or nonexistent.

Clinical Findings

The cardinal feature of histrionic personality disorder is the deliberate use of excessive, superficial emotionality to draw attention, evade unpleasant responsibilities, and control others. Such patients feel best when they are the center of attention and will become disappointed or petulant should the attention shift. Their emotions are labile, and they may exhibit temper tantrums, tearful outbursts, or dramatic accusations. These displays are often used to provoke a reaction from those around them, such as guilt, sympathy, or acquiescence.

Patients with this disorder are often quite concerned with physical appearance and attractiveness and may dress and carry themselves in a seductive or provocative manner. The clinical interview may be dominated by flirtatious banter, interspersed with dramatic anecdotes about the patient's life circumstances. Unlike in many other personality disorders, the patient with histrionic personality disorder places a premium on interpersonal relationships, and the quality of these relationships (at least their superficial quality) is quite important to him or her. However, the patient's anecdotes reveal a pattern of unsuccessful relationships, with a seemingly capricious flight from relationship to relationship. Although such descriptions may be passionate and colorful, they tend to be imprecise and lack detail, and the information obtained will be more impressionistic than specific. Also prominent in the patient with histrionic personality disorder is the repression of anger and other disturbing affects; anger tends to be expressed either fleetingly or indirectly. More comfortable with the expression of physical rather than psychological symptoms, these patients may present with somatoform disorders such as somatization or conversion disorder. Substance abuse disorders are common, as are other cluster B personality disorders.

Treatment

A. Medical Approaches: There is little or no evidence that pharmacologic treatment is effective for histrionic personality disorder. Patients with this disorder often present with major depressive disorder. The need for antidepressants should be evaluated carefully to determine whether the symptoms are primarily a means of securing medical attention. In some patients MAOIs have been reported to be useful. Because these patients are likely to misuse prescription medication, caution is warranted when prescribing such medications.

B. Social Approaches: Patients with histrionic personality disorder may derive particular benefit from group therapy, particularly from groups comprised of similar patients. Such groups provide these patients with a mirror of their own behavior and confront shallow or diverting emotional displays rather than accepting them. Moreover, these patients have considerable need for approval from others, and thus will be more likely to accept confrontations in order to avoid being rejected by other members. These patients can be challenging to work with in couples therapy; their commitment to the marital relationship is often tenuous, or they are unwilling to risk relinquishing the degree of control they maintain in the relationship. Role-reversal techniques provide an opportunity for the mirroring described earlier in this section.

C. Psychological Approaches: Given the degree of emotional display that characterizes histrionic personality disorder, patients with the disorder have remarkably little insight, and most psychotherapeutic techniques used are insight oriented. The tumultuous relationship history of the patient is likely to repeat itself within the therapy relationship, because provocative behavior masks exceptionally strong needs for nurturing. Identification of the patient's true feelings engendered in the therapy relationship and the delineation of the self-perpetuating quality of these emotions are important strategies. A focus on the links between thoughts and feelings can also increase the patient's capacity for reflection, in turn decreasing the likelihood of impulsive behavior.

Prognosis

In the absence of comorbid personality disorders (particularly those from cluster B), the prognosis for histrionic personality disorder is relatively good. These patients tend to be reasonably effective in social contexts, which can allow them to be the beneficiaries of social feedback. In the face of abandonment, they are vulnerable to depression, but as with many of their other complaints the dysphoria is short lived and highly reactive to external circumstances. The prognosis is considerably more guarded if the patient meets criteria for other cluster B personality disorders (as is often the case).

4. NARCISSISTIC PERSONALITY DISORDER

DSM-IV Diagnostic Criteria

A. A pervasive pattern of grandiosity (in fantasy or behavior), need for admiration, and lack of empathy, beginning by early adulthood and present in a variety of contexts, as indicated by five (or more) of the following:

   (1) has a grandiose sense of self-importance (eg, exaggerates achievements and talents, expects to be recognized as superior without commensurate achievements

   (2) is preoccupied with fantasies of unlimited success, power, brilliance, beauty, or ideal love

   (3) believes that he or she is "special" and unique and can only be understood by, or should associate with, other special or high-status people (or institutions)

   (4) requires excessive admiration

   (5) has a sense of entitlement, ie, unreasonable expectations of especially favorable treatment or automatic compliance with his or her expectations

   (6) is interpersonally exploitative, ie, takes advantage of others to achieve his or her own ends

   (7) lacks empathy: is unwilling to recognize or identify with the feelings and needs of others

   (8) is often envious of others or believes that others are envious of him or her

   (9) shows arrogant, haughty behaviors or attitudes

Reprinted, with permission, from *Diagnostic and Statistical Manual of Mental Disorders,* 4th ed. Copyright 1994 American Psychiatric Association.

General Considerations

A. Major Etiologic Theories: The cause of narcissistic personality disorder is unknown. The lack of clear parental appreciation of the child's accomplishments may be involved. This deficiency (or possibly excess attention to accomplishments in some cases) could lead the child to continually seek adoration.

B. Epidemiology: The prevalence of the disorder is estimated to be less than 1% in the general population but more frequent in clinical samples (2–16%). The disorder is somewhat more common in men than women. Adolescents are normally self-focused, and such attitudes may be developmental rather than a harbinger of personality disorder. Individuals with narcissistic personality disorder dislike growing old and may become more depressed and demanding during the fourth or fifth decades of life.

Clinical Findings

Patients with narcissistic personality disorder lack empathy and concern for others. At first contact, such individuals may demand to see the person in charge, feeling that the uniqueness of their problems necessitates intervention by the highest status clinician available. Such patients readily attribute the source of their problem to people who do not appreciate, support, or defer to them. Because of their vulnerability to criticism, any suggestion to the contrary provokes anger or disdain. Narcissism can be confused with hypomania because of the grandiosity common to both disorders; however, patients with narcissistic personality disorder have a haughty and arrogant bearing. Also, rather than being overly involved in a whirl of activities, these individuals are more selective, participating only in those impressive tasks that merit their special talents and unique abilities.

Narcissistic personality disorder is commonly associated with antisocial personality disorder. Some researchers have suggested that the former is merely a less aggressive version of the latter. The patient with narcissistic personality disorder is also less likely to be thrill-seeking and impulsive than is the individual with antisocial personality disorder. Narcissistic personality disorder can be distinguished from borderline personality disorder by the professed independence and desire for interpersonal control associated with the former disorder in contrast to the neediness of patients with the latter disorder. Mood disorders are relatively common in these patients. In some individuals the inflated self-esteem is thought to compensate for self-criticism and doubt. These individuals are particularly vulnerable to depressive episodes and social withdrawal following injury to their self-image. Other patients react to similar events by becoming enraged, sometimes with acute paranoid ideation and marked deterioration in judgment.

Treatment

A. Medical Approaches: These patients rarely seek treatment or understand the need for change.

There is little or no evidence to suggest that pharmacotherapy is effective in the treatment of narcissistic personality disorder.

B. Social Approaches: Patients with narcissistic personality disorder can be disruptive in a heterogeneous group if criticism by other group members precipitates rage or withdrawal. The therapist must ensure that some support for the patient is provided in order to render the inevitable confrontations more palatable to the patient. Treatment in a homogeneous group can help these patients to increase their empathic understanding through mirroring of their own maladaptive patterns.

Patients with narcissistic personality disorder present to couples therapy with some frequency, and the therapist must guard against blaming them for the disruptions in the relationship. Often the behavior patterns of the couple are complementary and self-sustaining. In such cases role-play and role-reversal techniques may be particularly useful.

C. Psychological Approaches: Psychotherapy with these patients is challenging. The therapist must avoid the two extremes of joining the patient in his or her self-admiration, or of criticizing the patient (which will likely lead to termination of treatment). Although confronting the patient is necessary, it should be carefully timed and presented with a tone of support and empathic acceptance. Cognitive interventions can be directed at the evaluative distortions of self and other that are typical in these patients. These distortions often involve a magnification of the differences between the patient and other people: If the difference favors the patient, others are viewed with contempt; if the difference favors another, the patient feels worthless and humiliated. This situation can be addressed by modifying the patient's standards and goals to an internal frame of reference, rather than a comparison with others.

Prognosis

Little is known about the long-term outcome of narcissistic personality disorder. In the absence of treatment, the features of the disorder are unlikely to diminish. Indeed, they may worsen during middle age. The features of the disorder tend to self-perpetuate, with the patient's devaluation of others eventually driving away those who might have provided the expected admiration. The depression resulting from such rejections is typically resolved by a defensive self-aggrandizement that repeats the cycle.

CLUSTER C
PERSONALITY DISORDERS

1. AVOIDANT PERSONALITY DISORDER

DSM-IV Diagnostic Criteria

A. A pervasive pattern of social inhibition, feelings of inadequacy, and hypersensitivity to negative evaluation, beginning by early adulthood and present in a variety of contexts, as indicated by four (or more) of the following:

(1) avoids occupational activities that involve significant interpersonal contact, because of fears of criticism, disapproval, or rejection

(2) is unwilling to get involved with people unless certain of being liked

(3) shows restraint within intimate relationships because of a fear of being shamed or ridiculed

(4) is preoccupied with being criticized or rejected in social situations

(5) is inhibited in new interpersonal situations because of feelings of inadequacy

(6) views self as socially inept, personally unappealing, or inferior to others

(7) is unusually reluctant to take personal risks or to engage in any new activities because they may prove embarrassing

Reprinted, with permission, from *Diagnostic and Statistical Manual of Mental Disorders,* 4th ed. Copyright 1994 American Psychiatric Association.

General Considerations

A. Major Etiologic Theories: The etiology of avoidant personality disorder is unknown. Because shyness and fear of strangers is a normal component of certain developmental stages it would appear that patients with this disorder may be stagnated in their emotional growth in this regard. It also suggests caution in diagnosing this disorder in children or adolescents.

B. Epidemiology: The prevalence of avoidant personality disorder has been estimated at 0.5–1.0%, with comparable numbers of men and women. The disorder overlaps a great deal with generalized social phobia, to the extent that the two diagnoses may be alternative names for the same condition. The primary distinction lies in the enduring nature of the personality disorder, with characteristics such as low self-esteem and intense desire for acceptance reflecting an enduring part of the personality rather than a situational concern.

Clinical Findings

In interviewing patients with avoidant personality disorder, the clinician will note the marked anxiety and discomfort these patients experience in discussing their problems. Their excessive concern with evaluation by others will be particularly apparent in the clinical interview, during which they may interpret innocuous questions as criticism. The social anxiety associated with the disorder leads to interpersonal withdrawal and avoidance of any unfamiliar or novel social situations, primarily because of fears of rejection rather than disinterest in others. In those relationships that are maintained, patients tend to adopt a passive, submissive role, as they are particularly uncomfortable in situations in which there is a great deal of public scrutiny and failures are likely to be widely known.

Treatment

A. Medical Approaches: There is some support in the literature for the use of SSRIs, MAOIs, and β-blockers for controlling the symptoms of social phobia, suggesting that these medications may also be helpful in treating avoidant personality disorder. The medication may facilitate early efforts at increasing social risk-taking and allow the patient some success experiences that could be built on in other forms of treatment. Other forms of anxiolytic medication may also be helpful for this purpose.

B. Social Approaches: Group therapy may be of particular use in obliging patients with this disorder to have contact with strangers within a generally accepting and supportive environment. The apprehensions that invariably emerge can assist such patients in understanding the effect that their rejection sensitivity has on others. Active participation in the group should not be forced immediately; patients should be given some time to acclimate to the group process. Family or couples therapy may be of particular benefit for patients who are involved in an environment that perpetuates avoidant behavior by undermining self-esteem.

C. Psychological Approaches: Patients with avoidant personality disorder often seek psychotherapy for assistance with their difficulties. Such patients are reluctant to disclose personal information out of fear of rejection and humiliation, and early efforts are typically directed at establishing trust through provision of support and reassurance. Subsequent efforts may be directed at encouraging assertive behavior and exploring distorted thoughts and attitudes that maintain withdrawal. Gradual exposure to social tasks of increasing potential for provoking anxiety can lead to success experiences that enable these patients to tolerate risk-taking in the future.

Prognosis

Little is known about the natural course and outcome of avoidant personality disorder. The social anxiety and withdrawal associated with this disorder is longstanding and generalized, suggesting that it is refractory to change; however, many patients with this disorder manage some form of adaptation to their problems and show little impairment in favorable interpersonal and occupational settings. The prognosis tends to be poorer if other personality disorders are also present or if the patient is in a fixed, unsupportive environment that may maintain the avoidance behaviors.

2. DEPENDENT PERSONALITY DISORDER

DSM-IV Diagnostic Criteria

A. A pervasive and excessive need to be taken care of that leads to submissive and clinging behavior and

fears of separation, beginning by early adulthood and present in a variety of contexts, as indicated by five (or more) of the following:

(1) has difficulty making everyday decisions without an excessive amount of advice and reassurance from others

(2) needs others to assume responsibility for most major areas of his or her life

(3) has difficulty expressing disagreement with others because of fear of loss of support or approval.

Note: Do not include realistic fears of retribution.

(4) has difficulty initiating projects or doing things on his or her own (because of a lack of self-confidence in judgment or abilities rather than a lack of motivation or energy)

(5) goes to excessive lengths to obtain nurturance and support from others, to the point of volunteering to do things that are unpleasant

(6) feels uncomfortable or helpless when alone because of exaggerated fears of being unable to care for himself or herself

(7) urgently seeks another relationship as a source of care and support when a close relationship ends

(8) is unrealistically preoccupied with fears of being left to take care of himself or herself

Reprinted, with permission, from *Diagnostic and Statistical Manual of Mental Disorders,* 4th ed. Copyright 1994 American Psychiatric Association.

General Considerations

A. Major Etiologic Theories: Theories about the cause of dependent personality disorder often suggest a childhood environment in which dependent behaviors were directly or indirectly rewarded and independent activities were discouraged. Increasing evidence (eg, from twin studies) also suggests possible, but poorly defined, genetic influences.

B. Epidemiology: The prevalence of dependent personality disorder has been estimated at 2–3% in the general population. The disorder is heavily represented in mental health treatment settings because of the general propensity that patients with the disorder have for help-seeking behavior. Although the disorder is slightly more common in women than in men in clinical settings, the gender distribution in the community is roughly equivalent. Generally, the diagnosis is not used with children or adolescents, whose dependent behavior is developmentally appropriate.

Clinical Findings

The hallmark of dependent personality disorder is a lifelong interpersonal submissiveness. This submissiveness can be in reference to a particular relationship, but more commonly it is a generalized style of relating to others. The dependency arises from poor self-esteem and feelings of inadequacy that drive those afflicted to rely entirely on others to get their needs met. Because abandonment is so greatly feared, any expression of displeasure or anger is inhibited so as not to endanger relationships. As with borderline personality disorder, patients with dependent personality disorder submerge their identity within the context of a dependency relationship. However, the dependent patient lacks the history of turbulent relationships that characterizes borderline personality disorder, and the rage and manipulativeness of the latter disorder contrast with the appeasement that typifies the dependent individual. Nonetheless, some patients meet criteria for both disorders.

Many individuals who have Axis I disorders, particularly mood and anxiety disorders, or general medical disorders can appear quite dependent and present with low self-esteem. In these individuals the features may be limited to the duration of the disorder and do not reflect a long-standing personality pattern. Queries about premorbid personality directed to the patient or family members can clarify this issue. Dependent personality disorder commonly cooccurs with many Axis I and Axis II disorders and when present with cluster B personality disorders can reduce the likelihood of acting-out behaviors.

Treatment

A. Medical Approaches: Patients who have dependent personality disorder often experience fatigue, malaise, and vague anxiety. Such symptoms may lead these patients to delay efforts at establishing independence, and antidepressant or antianxiety therapy can be useful. Anxiolytic medication may also be useful during crises that emerge after efforts at establishing autonomy, because fears of abandonment and separation (imagined or real) may be exacerbated during these times. Such interventions should be time limited and focused on specific target symptoms, because these patients are at increased risk of addiction.

B. Social Approaches: Patients with this disorder often derive considerable benefit from group therapy, as it offers an opportunity for the development of supportive peer relations with low risk for abandonment. Group members will typically reinforce the patient's efforts at establishing autonomy and provide a protected arena in which to try out new and more constructive interpersonal behaviors. Family or couples therapy can also be helpful but often present the challenge of working within a system in which the patient's dependency may play an important functional role. It is critical to enlist the support of other family members for the patient's efforts at autonomy, lest the patient be undermined or meet with rejection or withdrawal that would only perpetuate the dependency cycle.

C. Psychological Approaches: Patients with dependent personality disorder are generally receptive to treatment as part of a more general pattern of seeking assistance and support from others. The primary goal of such interventions is to make the patient more autonomous and self-reliant. Low self-esteem is a fundamental issue that typically arises from distorted appraisals of the abilities of self and others. It can be useful to break down the treatment process into clear but manageable goals, allowing the patient to experience early success. Assertiveness training is a typical component of treatment; role-playing focusing on communication skills (particularly of negative feelings) allows the patient to practice assertive behaviors. Exploration of past separations and their impact on current behaviors, as well as exploration of the current long-term effects of dependent behavior, can help the patient arrive at a greater understanding of his or her difficulties, with the self-discovery reflecting another step toward autonomy.

Prognosis

The prognosis of dependent personality disorder in the absence of comorbid diagnoses is generally good. Individuals with this disorder are likely to have had at least one supportive relationship in the past and generally have a capacity for empathy and trust exceeding that observed in most other personality disorders. The primary obstacles involve the exacerbation of anxieties as efforts toward establishing autonomy are made and the emergence of severe depression should the patient's desperate clinging behaviors ultimately lead to the rejection that is so greatly feared.

3. OBSESSIVE-COMPULSIVE PERSONALITY DISORDER

DSM-IV Diagnostic Criteria

A. A pervasive pattern of preoccupation with orderliness, perfectionism, and mental and interpersonal control, at the expense of flexibility, openness, and efficiency, beginning by early adulthood and present in a variety of contexts, as indicated by four (or more) of the following:

  (1) is preoccupied with details, rules, lists, order, organization, or schedules to the extent that the major point of the activity is lost

  (2) shows perfectionism that interferes with task completion (eg, is unable to complete a project because his or her own overly strict standards are not met)

  (3) is excessively devoted to work and productivity to the exclusion of leisure activities and friendships (not accounted for by obvious economic necessity)

  (4) is overconscientious, scrupulous, and inflexible about matters of morality, ethics, or values (not accounted for by cultural or religious identification)

  (5) is unable to discard worn-out or worthless objects even when they have no sentimental value

(6) is reluctant to delegate tasks or to work with others unless they submit to exactly his or her way of doing things

(7) adopts a miserly spending style toward both self and others; money is viewed as something to be hoarded for future catastrophes

(8) shows rigidity and stubbornness

Reprinted, with permission, from *Diagnostic and Statistical Manual of Mental Disorders,* 4th ed. Copyright 1994 American Psychiatric Association.

General Considerations

A. Major Etiologic Theories: Psychoanalytical theories suggest a stagnation in the anal stages of development in patients with obsessive-compulsive personality disorder. It is still uncertain whether overly controlling parenting has an influence on this disorder. Genetic components to this disorder are still uncertain.

B. Epidemiology: The prevalence of obsessive-compulsive personality disorder has been estimated at roughly 1% in the general population. Although it is more common in clinical settings than in the general population, it is seen less often than many other personality disorders because people with this disorder view the traits in question as desirable rather than problematic. The disorder appears to be more common in men than in women.

Clinical Findings

Obsessive-compulsive personality disorder is characterized by rigidity and affective constriction. The disorder differs from the Axis I manifestation of obsessive-compulsive disorder in that the latter involves intrusive obsessions and compulsions that are experienced as ego-alien, whereas the personality disorder involves traits that are ego-syntonic. Thus the two disorders involve problems in significantly different spheres. For example, the Axis I disorder is typically associated with marked distress concerning obsessions or compulsions, whereas the patient with obsessive-compulsive personality disorder may admit to no such distress aside from a tendency to worry. Indeed, the patient with this disorder typically views his or her preoccupation with order and perfectionism as a positive characteristic that makes him or her superior to others. As a result, the relationship between the Axis I and Axis II disorders is imperfect at best, and the available evidence suggests that fewer than half of the patients with the Axis I disorder display the obsessive-compulsive personality style, other personality disorders being just as common.

Patients with obsessive-compulsive personality disorder tend to have difficulty in personal relationships because they do not like to submit to others' ways of doing things. This can lead to occupational problems, because these individuals often will simply refuse to work with others. They are not interested in the affec-

tive quality of relationships and have a formal and somewhat stilted style of relating. In the clinical interview, they will describe their life in a solemn, intellectualized way, as though describing a casual acquaintance. Their emotional tone is likely to be muted, but they will take the interview very seriously, providing exceptionally detailed responses to questions, complete with precise dates and numbers. They will generally defer to the authority of the interviewer but may attempt to control the course of the interview by compartmentalizing topics or correcting the clinician's imprecise comments.

Treatment

A. Medical Approaches: Pharmacotherapy has not been demonstrated to be very effective in the treatment of obsessive-compulsive personality disorder. Although serotonergic drugs such as clomipramine and SSRIs have been shown to be of use in the treatment of Axis I obsessive-compulsive disorder, the association between these two disorders is not strong and the target symptoms of improvement for the medication are not typically noted in the personality disorder. Medication may be useful as an adjunct to other forms of therapy during crises in which anxiety and depression are prominent.

B. Social Approaches: Group therapy is difficult with these patients. They typically attempt to ally themselves with the therapist in treating the other group members who have the "real" problems. One advantage of treatment in this forum is that the intellectualized explanations offered by the patient are interrupted frequently, which increases their anxiety but leaves them more open to new experiences. In family or couples therapy, a major challenge will involve having the patient relinquish control over other family members. This process can be assisted by prescribing homework tasks in which various roles (including decision making) are reassigned within the family. The patient's desire to conform to the authority of the therapist can be used to facilitate the loosening of control over others as well as himself or herself.

C. Psychological Approaches: The individual with obsessive-compulsive personality disorder desires to perform well as a patient, consistent with his or her general pattern of perfectionism in other life areas. However, the general constriction and distrust of affective expression creates a number of resistances for the therapist. Patients may be highly critical of themselves or of the therapy, demanding justification for every intervention offered. A central part of the treatment will involve exploring the source and the unreasonable nature of the harsh and rigid standards the patient has set for both self and others. Given the rationalizing and intellectualizing nature of these patients, cognitive interventions are often well received. Such efforts focus on the inaccuracy of key assumptions held by these patients (eg, "I must be perfectly in control of my environment." "Any failure is intolerable."), with the consequences of such beliefs explored and the ways to refute these beliefs discussed.

Prognosis

Little is known about the prognosis of obsessive-compulsive personality disorder. In the absence of cooccurring disorders, the outlook is probably favorable relative to other personality disorders, because the patient's capacity for self-discipline and order precludes many of the problems typical of personality disorders. A minority of these patients go on to develop Axis I anxiety disorders (including obsessive-compulsive disorder). The self-criticism and barren emotional life of these patients leave them particularly vulnerable to late-onset depression.

OTHER PERSONALITY DISORDERS

Two personality disorders are described in an appendix to DSM-IV: passive-aggressive (negativistic) personality disorder and depressive personality disorder. Although officially classified as personality disorders not otherwise specified, passive-aggressive personality disorder has been in the nomenclature for many years, and depressive personality disorder has been the focus of considerable research.

In DSM-IV, passive-aggressive personality disorder has been relegated to an appendix titled "Criteria sets provided for further study." This disorder is characterized by passive resistance and negativistic attitudes toward others who place demands on the person with the disorder. These demands are resented and opposed indirectly, through procrastination, stubbornness, intentional inefficiency, and memory lapses. Such individuals tend to be sullen, irritable, and cynical, and they chronically complain of being underappreciated and cheated. Interest in attachment relationships is typically low, as such people tend to be unsuccessful in interpersonal relationships because of their capacity to evoke hostility and negative responses from others.

Depressive personality disorder is characterized by enduring depressive cognitions and behaviors. Some researchers have proposed that this is essentially the same concept as dysthymic disorder. These individuals are gloomy and their self-esteem is habitually low. They are harsh on themselves and tend to be judgmental of others. They are pessimistic about the future and remorseful about the past. They tend to be quiet, passive, and unassertive. The disorder can be distinguished from major depression by its chronicity and by the absence of somatic signs of depression such as sleep or appetite disturbance.

Andreasen NC, Black DW: *Introductory Textbook of Psychiatry,* 2nd ed. American Psychiatric Press, 1995.

Benjamin LS: *Interpersonal Diagnosis and Treatment of Personality Disorders.* Guilford Press, 1993.

Coccaro EF: Psychopharmacologic studies in patients with personality disorders: review and perspective. J Personal Disord 1993;7(Suppl):181.

Hubbard JR, Saathoff GB, Barnett BL Jr.: Recognizing borderline personality disorder in the family practice setting. Am Fam Phys 1995;52:908.

Livesley WJ: *The DSM-IV Personality Disorders.* Guilford Press, 1995.

Millon T: *Disorders of Personality: DSM-IV and Beyond.* John Wiley & Sons, 1996.

Morey LC: *An Interpretative Guide to the Personality Assessment Inventory (PAI).* Psychology Resources, 1996.

Waldinger RJ: *Psychiatry for Medical Students,* 3rd ed. American Psychiatric Press, 1997.

Section IV.
Techniques & Settings in Child & Adolescent Psychiatry

Diagnostic Encounter

34

Barry Nurcombe, MD, William Bernet, MD, & Vernon H. Sharp, MD

I. INTERVIEWING PARENTS

Barry Nurcombe, MD

INITIAL CONTACT

Children are usually referred to psychiatrists by their parents or caregivers. Parents should be made aware that a collaborative approach to diagnosis and treatment is essential and that their children over the age of 3 years should be prepared for the diagnostic encounter. The initial contact is usually made over the telephone by the parent or referring agent. The importance of the impression made at that first contact cannot be underestimated. The initial intake staff member gathers identifying information and a brief history of the presenting complaint. Emergency situations must be dealt with at once and urgent situations within 24 hours. Table 34–1 lists situations, roughly in the order of frequency, that require immediate evaluation.

SEQUENCE OF INTERVIEWS

If the initial interview is prompted by a crisis, or if the family has come a long distance, the clinician should see the whole family together. Even if there is no crisis, some clinicians still favor interviewing the whole family first whereas others prefer interviewing the parents first, before interviewing the child or adolescent at a separate later interview. Even if the parents are separated or divorced, it is preferable to interview both parents, unless the tension between them would be unmanageable. Other clinicians prefer to interview an adolescent first, before interviewing the parents. In any case, the clinician should try to avoid having the child wait outside while lengthy parent interviews are conducted. At some point, the parents will need to be interviewed to obtain a detailed history (see "Interviewing Parents" section) and the family interviewed together to throw light on family dynamics (see "Interviewing Families" section).

INTAKE QUESTIONNAIRES & CHECKLISTS

Important data can be collected even before the first interview. For example, the parent can complete a Child Behavior Checklist and a developmental history form. Teacher versions of the Child Behavior Checklist can also be obtained if the child's behavior in school is an important issue. Previous mental health evaluations, medical records, and school records are also available in some cases. Thus the clinician can focus during the parent interview on the developmental issues and symptom patterns that emerge from the preliminary data.

PURPOSE OF THE PARENT INTERVIEW

The initial parent interview serves several purposes. Most important, it helps the clinician to form an alliance with the parents, and it helps the parents prepare the child for the next interview. The clinician can use the parent interview to obtain a formal history of the child's presenting problem, medical history, early development, school progress, and peer relations as well as information on the child's recreational activities and interests, home and family environment, and family history. The clinician can also gather from this interview information about parent-child relations and communi-

Table 34–1. Situations requiring immediate evaluation.

Suicidality
Homicidal impulses
Dangerous assaultiveness
Dangerous risk-taking (eg, running away from home)
Drug or alcohol intoxication
Psychotic thought disorder (eg, hallucinations, delusions)
Impending parental breakdown related to the child's disruptive behavior
Recent trauma (eg, as a result of rape or civilian catastrophe)
Recent loss with abnormal grief reaction
Acute school refusal
Suspension or expulsion from school
Police involvement
Physical deterioration in a patient known to have an eating disorder

cation, the parents' child-rearing techniques and methods of discipline used, and the family's values and aspirations. The clinician can gather information on the parents' current marital relationship and its development and can ascertain how the parents comprehend the child's problem and the kind of help they are seeking.

SEQUENCE OF THE PARENT INTERVIEW

The parent interview proceeds through four key stages: (1) inception, (2) reconnaissance, (3) detailed inquiry, and (4) termination.

Inception

The interviewer begins by greeting the parents in the waiting room and ushering them into the office, indicating where they should sit. The interviewer then tells the parents what he or she already knows and invites them to tell their story.

Reconnaissance

The interviewer should let the parents proceed at their own pace without interruption other than to facilitate the flow of associations or clarify issues. As the story unfolds, the interaction between them is observed. Do they support each other? Does one parent do most of the talking? Do they interrupt or contradict each other? Which issues evoke the most emotion from them? Do they express warmth, humor, coolness, detachment, remoteness, tension, irritation, or hostility? If one parent becomes upset, how does the other respond?

Detailed Inquiry

After the parents have finished their story, the areas listed in the next several sections are explored. These areas should be surveyed in a standard diagnostic inquiry, and particular areas should be explored in depth according to the diagnostic hypotheses triggered by the clinical pattern that is emerging.

A. The Problem: When did the problem first appear? Did its onset coincide with a physical or psychosocial stressor? What has been the evolution of the problem? Is the problem persistent or intermittent? If intermittent, do exacerbations coincide with vicissitudes in physical health or the environment (eg, family, school, peer relations)? What have the parents done about it? Are there any other problems in the child's behavior at home, at school, with siblings, or with peers?

B. Referral: Who referred the parents? Why do they come now? How do they feel about it? Have they sought help before? If so, from whom, and how effective was the help? What kind of help do they expect now?

C. Medical History: Has the child had any significant physical illness, physical disability, surgery, accidents, or hospitalizations? If so, at what age, what was the duration, and did any adverse psychological reactions occur? Has the child sustained any head injuries or had seizures, syncope, headaches, eye symptoms, abdominal or limb pains, nausea or vomiting, or prolonged or frequent absences from school? Has the child had previous psychological disturbances? If so, what were the cause, treatment, and outcome? Is the child currently taking any medication? Does he or she have significant allergies?

D. Developmental History:

1. Pregnancy—What were the circumstances surrounding conception of the child (eg, motivation, acceptance, convenience, emotional turmoil, reaction of in-laws)? How was the marital relationship during pregnancy? How was the mother's physical and emotional health during pregnancy? Did she have toxemia, eclampsia, kidney disorder, hypertension, or febrile illness? Did she have any x-rays taken during pregnancy? Did she take prescribed or over-the-counter medications, tobacco, drugs, or alcohol during pregnancy, and if so, how much and how often? Did she experience excessive nausea, vomiting, or vaginal bleeding during pregnancy? How was she prepared for labor? Did the parents have a sex preference?

2. Delivery—Did the mother have a normal confinement? Was the child born at term? How long did labor last? What was the nature of the delivery? Did any complications occur? How soon did the mother see the infant after delivery? What were the mother's initial thoughts on seeing the infant?

3. Neonatal status—What was the infant's birth weight, maturity, and physical condition? Was the infant in intensive care? If so, for how long? What was the method of feeding? How well did the infant gain weight as a neonate? Did the infant have problems with asphyxia, cyanosis, jaundice, convulsions, vomiting, rigidity, or respiratory disorder?

4. Feeding—Was the child breastfed? If so, for how long? Was formula used? When were solids introduced? How well did the child gain weight? Did the child have problems with vomiting, diarrhea, constipation, colic, food allergies, or eczema? Did later conflicts over eating occur (eg, refusal to eat, bulimia, hoarding)? What are the child's current eating habits?

5. Motor development—At what age (in months) did the child first hold his or her head erect, sit alone, stand, and walk alone? How is the child's coordination (gross and fine)? Is the child right- or left-handed? Does the child have repetitive motor habits?

6. Speech development—When did the child first use single words, two- and three-word phrases, and sentences? Did the child have trouble with faulty articulation or stammering? How is the child's current language, vocabulary, and syntax?

7. Sphincter control—When did the child first learn to control his or her bladder and bowels? What method of training was used? How did the child respond (eg, with resistance or acceptance)? Did the child regress during training? Has the child had problems with enuresis or encopresis?

8. Sleep—Has the child had previous sleep problems? What are the child's current sleep habits (eg, is the child a deep sleeper, restless, or insomniac)? Does the child have fears of the dark or of being alone? Does the child sleepwalk, have nightmares or night terrors, or resist going to bed?

9. Sexual development—Did the child display early sexual curiosity or sex play? Has the child received sex education? Has the child experienced menarche, masturbation, or nocturnal emissions? What is the child's gender-role identification? Is he or she interested in the opposite sex? Has the child experienced any sexual trauma?

E. Educational Progress:

1. Academics & activities—What schools has the child attended? What grade is the child in now? Who are the child's teachers? How is the child's current academic performance? Does the child have any learning problems or any need for special education or tutoring? Does the child participate in school sports and activities?

2. Behavior—How are the child's relationships with peers and teachers? How does the child respond to school rules? What is the child's capacity to concentrate? Does the child have problems with truancy, fear of going to school, or school refusal? What is the child's attitude toward homework? Does the child exhibit any antisocial behavior at school? Does the child have any history of drug or alcohol use or abuse?

3. Ambitions & involvement—What are the child's ambitions? Is the child involved in social and recreational activities?

F. Home Environment:

1. Physical arrangement—Where is the home located? What is the neighborhood like? What are the neighbors like? How is the home laid out? What are the sleeping arrangements? Does the home have inside and outside spaces for play? Are the parents satisfied with the domestic arrangements?

2. Schedule—What is the child's typical weekday and weekend schedule, from rising to retiring?

G. Parent-Child Relationships:

1. Child's behavior—How was the child's early temperament (ie, easy or difficult)? Has this changed with age? What is the child's general mood? What is the child's capacity for affection, tolerance for frustration, and proneness to tantrums? Is the child aggressive, resentful, fearful, or timid; depressed; sociable; and accepting of limits, rules, and discipline? How does the child respond to punishment (ie, by being stubborn or compliant)?

2. Parenting methods—What methods do the parents use to set limits and discipline the child? Are these methods applied with consistency? How much time does the family spend together (ie, father-child, mother-child, entire family)?

3. Attitudes & conflicts—What are the child's attitudes toward each parent (eg, closeness, mutual understanding)? Do conflicts about dependence and independence exist between the child and parents?

H. Social Relationships:

1. Siblings & peers—How are the child's relationships with siblings and peers? Does the child tend to be a leader, a follower, or a protector? Is the child overly dependent?

2. Games—Is the child able to win or lose at games? What are the child's favorite games?

3. Social behavior—Does the child exhibit any antisocial behavior? How are the child's relationships with authority figures?

I. Family Background:

1. Parents—What is each parent's age, occupation, and physical and mental health? What is each parent's drug and alcohol intake? What are the age, health, and occupations of both sets of grandparents? What are each parent's family, educational, and occupational backgrounds? Pay particular attention to the emotional climate of each parent's family of origin, the relationship between the parents and their parents, the parents' schooling, and their occupational histories. What is the family history of psychiatric disorders, mental retardation, learning problems, substance abuse, antisocial behavior, or physical illness?

2. Marital history—Were the parents married previously? How did they meet, and what was their courtship like? Where they both accepted by their in-laws? What were the early years of marriage like (eg, sexual adjustment, division of labor, management of money, method of settling interparental disputes)? Is there a history of competition, unfulfilled needs, hostility, abuse, or separations? How good are each parent's parenting ability and capacity for affection? What is their motivation for childcare and childrearing?

3. Siblings—How old is each of the child's siblings? What is the current health of each sibling? How does each sibling do in school or in his or her occupation? What is each sibling's overall personality? How does each sibling relate to the child?

4. Family values—What is the family's ethnic or sociocultural background? Is there a relative emphasis on conformity or independence, authority or freedom, warmth or coolness, control or expression? What are the family's religion and moral and esthetic values? Does the family put an emphasis on education, money, success, prestige, or gender differentiation?

5. Family & community—How involved is the family in school activities, religious organizations, cultural bodies, and civic affairs?

Termination

At the end of the parent interview (usually one or two 2-hour interviews), the information gathered is summarized. The parents should be invited to add anything they think is important and to correct any misinformation. The interviewer should then tell them when he or she wants to see the child and the family again.

Nurcombe B: The diagnostic encounter in child psychiatry: data gathering. Pages 460–506 in Nurcombe B, Gallagher RM (editors): *The Clinical Process in Psychiatry.* Cambridge University Press, 1986.
Simmons JE: *Psychiatric Examination of Children,* 2nd ed. Lea & Febiger, 1974.

II. EVALUATING INFANTS

Barry Nurcombe, MD

PURPOSE OF THE INFANT EVALUATION

The psychiatric evaluation of infants and their parents is designed to yield information concerning the following: the nature and development of the problem perceived by the parents; the child's developmental history; the parent's history (eg, early relationships, prior experience with children, knowledge of child development, marital relationship, and medical and psychiatric history); parent-child interaction; infant development and attachment; and the parents' perception of the infant.

Information on these matters is gathered by interviewing the parent, observing the infant, observing the interaction between parent and infant, and if necessary, conducting standardized assessments.

INTERVIEWING THE INFANT'S PARENTS

Infants and their parents are usually referred by a pediatrician because of disturbances in regulation (eg, insomnia, excessive crying, feeding problems, head banging), social disturbances (eg, interactional apathy or negativism, traumatic separation, excessive separation anxiety), psychophysiologic disturbances (eg, failure to thrive, vomiting), or developmental delay.

It is debatable whether, at the first interview, the parents should be interviewed alone or together with the infant. The infant's presence is likely to generate historical information from the parents that might otherwise be missed. However, a number of interviews will be required, observation of parent-child interactions will always be necessary, and the aim of the interview will not be achieved unless a working alliance is formed.

The interview begins with introductory questions about family structure and dates of birth and quickly proceeds to a history of the problem. The following questions could be asked: When did the problem begin? How has it evolved? What is the problem now? What have the parents done about it? How do they account for it? Why do they come for help now? What do they want from the clinician?

Next, the clinician elicits the infant's developmental history, including the circumstances surrounding, and the reaction of both parents to, conception, pregnancy, delivery, and early infant care. The child's medical history will also be gathered.

As the alliance deepens, the clinician elicits information about the parents' relationships with their own parents and siblings, their prior experience of childcare, their knowledge of child development, their preconceptions about being a parent, and their expectations about the baby (and whether these expectations have been borne out). The history and current status of the marital relationship will also be explored. If other individuals provide a significant amount of the infant's care, they should also be interviewed.

The clinician seeks to identify critical dynamic sequences of behavioral interaction (eg, the mother becomes anxious, disorganized, and angry if the baby refuses to eat), looking for connections between present emotional interactions and past significant relationships and events.

OBSERVING THE PARENT-INFANT INTERACTION

During the interview, parents should be encouraged to attend to the infant's needs, for example, consoling, changing, or feeding the infant, if necessary. Parents will also be asked to play with the child. Parent-child dyads can then be observed with regard to the quality of attachment, the vigilance of the parents concerning the infant's safety, the parents' attunement to and effectiveness in responding to the infant's need states, the quality of parent-child play, parental teaching ability, parental control, the affective tone of the interaction, and infant temperament. The clinician should remember that he or she is observing only brief samples of dyadic behavior. By seeking a working alliance and putting the parents at ease, the clinician can try to ensure that the samples of behavior seen are representative.

The next several sections describe specific observations about the parent-child interaction that the clinician can make during the infant evaluation.

A. Attachment: How close is each dyad? Are they, for example, detached or clinging, or able to separate sufficiently to allow the infant to explore? Does the infant seek body or eye contact with the parent? Does contact with the parent reassure the child, or is the infant inconsolable? Does the infant explore the surroundings recklessly, confidently, cautiously, or not at all? Does the infant get pleasure from the exploration? How does he or she respond to separation? How does the parent feel about it?

B. Protection: Is the parent vigilant, overprotective, or careless in regard to the infant's reckless, cautious, or confident exploration? Or does the parent strike a good balance, given the infant's apparent temperament? How does the parent feel about the infant's exploration?

C. Regulation of Need States: Is the parent attuned to the infant's needs concerning hunger, discomfort, pain, or stimulation? Does the parent know when to stimulate the infant, when to back off, and when and how to console the infant? Does the parent make effective use of eye contact, soothing voice, smiling, facial movement, wrapping, touching, holding, rocking, nursing, and dorsal patting or rubbing in stimulating or consoling the infant? How does the infant respond to the parent's ministrations?

D. Play: Do parent and infant play together in a manner appropriate to the infant's developmental level? Do parent and infant enjoy the playful interaction?

E. Teaching: If the infant is old enough, ask the parent to teach him or her to stack blocks or solve a puzzle. Does the parent make effective use of modeling and language? Does the infant imitate the parent? Does the parent allow the infant sufficient opportunity for trial and error to solve a problem independently?

F. Control: Does each parent maintain calm, confident control of the infant, or is the parent helpless, passive, inconsistent, disorganized, explosive, punitive, or overly controlling? How effectively does the parent communicate in words? How does the infant respond? In response to the parent's attempts to control his or her behavior, is the infant heedless, provocative, negativistic, passive, disorganized, or biddable?

G. Emotion: What is the affective tone of the interaction? Is the infant generally happy, angry, sad, neutral, or affectively "empty," or unresponsive? What is each parent's emotional state? Are the members of the dyads attuned to each other? If the infant becomes upset, is he or she able to regain equanimity in a reasonable time?

H. Temperament: Temperament refers to relatively enduring characteristics of the infant's behavioral response to the internal and external environments. Despite potential limitations in the duration and representativeness of the behavioral sample elicited, the clinician may be able to make observations concerning the infant's activity level, tendency to approach or withdraw from people, adaptability to new situations, affective intensity, mood, persistence with tasks or play, sensory threshold, and distractibility.

STANDARDIZED TESTING

Through standardized testing, the clinician can explore hypotheses generated from the history and observation of parent-infant interaction. Tests are available, for example, with regard to infant psychomotor development, parent-infant interaction, infant attachment, quality of the home environment, infant temperament, and the parent's working model of the infant. Although some of these tests are best regarded as research instruments, several may have clinical utility. Furthermore, parents can be involved in the data-gathering process of many of these tests, with potentially great educational benefit.

A. Developmental Level: Tests of infant development have only modest predictive validity with regard to tested intelligence in later childhood. There is increasing evidence that intellectual development is characterized by individual differences and discontinuity rather than a smooth progression. Possibly, early infant development tests must be applied too soon to tap those elements of intelligence (eg, language-based cognitive skills) that are highly responsive to the home environment. Nevertheless, if the infant tests very low in some or all developmental domains, the clinician should be concerned.

1. Brazelton Neonatal Behavioral Assessment Scale—The Brazelton Neonatal Behavioral Assessment Scale (NBAS) was designed for use with the full-term neonate, but it has also been modified to apply to high-risk infants. The NBAS is usually administered 3 and 9 days after birth. It surveys reflexes and behavioral responses in such a way as to yield a profile of social interactiveness, state control, motoric behavior, and physiologic response to stress. It has modest predictive power with regard to later developmental measures.

2. Bayley Scales of Infant Development (2–30 months)—The Bayley Scales assess development in three domains: mental (perception, memory, problem solving, communication), psychomotor (gross and fine motor), and behavior (the affective responses of the infant). This test uses a structured play approach.

3. Infant Muller Scales of Early Learning (0–38 months)—The Infant Muller Scales of Early Learning assess gross motor development, visual reception, visual expression, language reception, and language expression. It is useful in following the progress of children who are thought to have specific areas of developmental delay.

4. Other instruments—The Transdisciplinary Play-Based Assessment and the Connecticut Infant-Toddler Developmental Assessment Program involve the parents with the clinical team in the collection of data on different domains of development.

B. Parent-Child Interaction: The Greenspan-Lieberman Observation System for Assessment of Caregiver Interaction During Semistructured Play and the Parent-Child Early Relationship Assessment rate interactive behavior from videotaped samples of free or semistructured play. Parental detachment, emotional negativity, lack of vocal contact, lack of visual contact, and inconsistency, for example, can be detected, along with infant detachment, negative affect, inattention, and defects in motor and communication skills.

C. Infant Attachment: The best known measure of infant attachment is the Strange Situation (12–24 months). In this technique, the infant-parent dyad is exposed to a series of brief episodes involving gradually increasing stress, as the parent stays with the child, leaves, returns, and leaves; a stranger joins the child; and the parent finally returns. The child's behavior during the two reunion episodes is classified as secure, insecure-avoidant, insecure-resistant, or disorganized. Disorganized behavior is particularly likely to be associated with serious environmental pathology and poor outcome.

D. Home Environment: The Home Observation for Measurement of the Environment (two versions: 0–3 years, 3–6 years) assesses the quality of intellectual stimulation in the home by rating the parent's involvement with and responsiveness to the child, the organization of the home environment, and the provision of a variety of play materials.

E. Infant Temperament: The Revised Infant Temperament Questionnaire asks the parent to rate the infant in nine domains of temperament and allows the infant to be categorized as easy, slow to warm up, difficult, intermediate low, or intermediate high. This instrument is a measure of parental perception of the infant and is influenced by the parent's personality.

F. The Parent's Working Model of the Child: The Working Model of the Child Interview is a research instrument with potential clinical applicability. It is a structured interview that explores topics such as the child's development, the parent's perception of the child's personality and behavior, and the parent-child relationship. The parent's responses are rated on a number of scales (eg, coherence, richness, flexibility,

intensity), and the parental model of the child is classified as balanced, disengaged, or distorted.

DIAGNOSTIC FORMULATION & TREATMENT PLANNING

The diagnostic hypotheses generated during the parent interview are tested and refined during the observation of parent-infant interaction, and when required, through the use of standardized tests. If no pediatric examination has been completed, or if specialized pediatric consultation is required, this will be requested. The current problem is classified, for example, according to the NCCIP scheme (Table 34–2). Next a diagnostic formulation is completed and a treatment plan designed (see Chapter 36), and the diagnosis and plan are discussed with the parents as the clinician seeks to consolidate the working alliance preparatory to the treatment phase.

Clark R, Paulsen A, Conlin S: Assessment of developmental status and parent-infant relationships. Pages 191–209 in Zeanah CH (editor): *Handbook of Infant Mental Health.* Guilford Press, 1993.

Hirshberg LM: Clinical interviews with infants and their families. Pages 173–190 in Zeanah CH (editor): *Handbook of Infant Mental Health.* Guilford Press, 1993.

Lamb ME et al: Infancy. Pages 241–270 in Lewis M (editor): *Child and Adolescent Psychiatry.* Williams & Wilkins, 1996.

Mayes LC: Infant assessment. Pages 431–439 in Lewis M (editor): *Child and Adolescent Psychiatry.* Williams & Wilkins, 1996.

National Center for Clinical Infant Programs: *Diagnostic Classification Study Manual.* NCCIP, 1991.

Table 34–2. The NCCIP classification of infant disorders.

Disorder of social development and communication
  Autism
  Atypical pervasive developmental disorder
Psychic trauma disorder
  Acute, single event
  Chronic, repeated
Regulatory disorder
  Hypersensitivity type
  Under-reactive type
  Active-aggressive type
  Mixed type
  Regulatory-based sleep disorder
  Regulatory-based eating disorder
Disorders of affect
  Anxiety disorder
  Mood disorder
    Prolonged bereavement
    Depression
    Labile mood disorder
    Mixed disorder of emotional expressiveness
    Deprivation syndrome
Adjustment reaction disorders

III. INTERVIEWING CHILDREN

Barry Nurcombe, MD

PURPOSE OF THE CHILD INTERVIEW

Depending on the child and the clinical circumstances, an interview with a child of 4–11 years of age has a number of possible purposes. The interview can help the clinician ascertain how the child feels about being interviewed and what the child believes to be the purpose of the interview. It can also help to correct misapprehension and orient the child to the interview. The interview can be used to determine whether the child recognizes that a problem exists and, if so, what accounts for it. In terms of aiding the diagnosis, the interview can be used to complete a mental status examination; to explore the child's self-concept and perceptions of the key figures in his or her world (eg, family, friends, authorities); to assess the child's emotional, social, and moral development; and to gauge the effectiveness of the child's coping mechanisms. Finally, the interview can be used to establish a working alliance and to assess the child's capacity to benefit from treatment.

FACTORS AFFECTING THE CHILD INTERVIEW

Although the primary purpose of the interview is diagnostic, it is artificial to separate diagnosis from treatment. Adverse impressions formed early can impede or obstruct therapy; in contrast, if an alliance is formed early, the child will be more willing to return for treatment.

The type of interview that evolves depends on the child's developmental level, personality, and expectations; the environment in which the interview takes place; the interviewer's personality and interactive style; and the goals of the interview. For example, a preschool child is likely to express ideas and feelings through actions rather than words. In contrast, a mature 11-year-old child may be able to converse throughout the interview. Most children mix play with conversation. The clinician must therefore combine observation, play, and conversation in different degrees with children of different maturity levels.

The well-adjusted child is likely to be reticent about sharing very personal matters with a stranger, unless he or she accepts the need to do so. The psychologically disturbed child is even more inhibited; initially, such children may express fantasies, secrets, or private fears indirectly. In contrast, some disorganized, emotionally needy younger children have such poor defenses that they release a torrent of psychopathologic material before they have established a trusting relationship with the examiner.

The child's expectation of the interview greatly influences its course. Children seldom come to a psychiatrist of their own accord, and the individuals who bring them may not have prepared them well. Children may enter the interview hostile, fearful, bewildered, apathetic, or even eager for help. Younger children commonly fear bodily invasion (eg, receiving injections) or are concerned that the physician will expose their secret inferiorities or shameful memories. These children may be afraid that they will be induced to talk about matters so frightening that they have never talked about them before. Adolescents universally have a fear of being rendered helpless. Children with a history of antisocial behavior may expect a tricky cross-examination. Children with learning problems may be afraid of being exposed as dunces. The experienced interviewer can often anticipate these fears and deal with them early in the interview.

Office Environment

Although an experienced clinician can be surprisingly effective in unpromising surroundings, adequate space and equipment are helpful. Some clinicians have access to separate playrooms with extensive equipment and fittings, but most must arrange their own offices to interview children.

An ideal room will be large enough to have a carpeted section for seated interviewing, a section with linoleum-tiled surface for play, and a small table and chairs. Play equipment should be stored in a lockable cupboard that has additional space for materials associated with particular patients who are in therapy. Otherwise, the equipment is communal. An inquisitive child can be told that the play material belongs to the office and may not be taken away.

With regard to play equipment, it is preferable to err on the side of frugality. Clinicians should remember that equipment is a means to the development of a relationship and the expression of thoughts and feelings. The less clutter, the more the child must draw from inside. A list of basic equipment would include the following: easel, newsprint paper and felt pens, blocks, assorted toy wild and domestic animals, matchbox cars, dolls (representing parents, brother, sister, baby, grandparents, together with nurse and doctor), one or two stuffed animals, a rubber ball, a pack of playing cards, and a set of checkers. Clinicians can add to this list other items (eg, puppets, toy pistols, board games, dolls' house furniture, plastic construction models), guided by their interest and what seems to work best for them. Clinicians should avoid games that preclude fantasy, such as chess or Scrabble. Finger paints, poster colors, and Play-Doh are suitable only for fully equipped playrooms, but clinicians may wish to keep a soccer ball, a football, and a baseball and glove for outdoor play.

Clinicians should not be anchored to the office. An occasional visit to a soda fountain, outdoor construction site, nursery, or gymnasium can be very useful, especially with highly active youngsters who find a restricted environment tedious.

Style of the Interview

The goals of the interview shape its style to some degree. Sometimes it is essential to obtain from the child a detailed account of a past event, especially in medico-legal situations. Such situations are much less common than those in which clinicians can allow the interview to evolve as the interaction dictates.

Two polar interviewing styles are exemplified by the relatively **unstructured approach** and the highly **structured interview.** Structured interviewing may be valuable for research purposes, but it is not recommended for regular clinical interviewing.

A **semi-structured interview** involves the application of a flexibly and sensitively applied systematic approach. The interview should be organized in accordance with a hypothetico-deductive strategy, but it should not compromise a positive relationship for the sake of extracting information. In most cases, two or three 1-hour interviews are required in order to gather enough information to reach a reliable diagnosis.

Clinicians who wish to work with children should enjoy being with children. They should be sufficiently in touch with the past to be able to recapture and empathize with the sadness, anger, frustration, bewilderment, and enthusiasms of childhood. Clinicians should be warm, accepting, and supportive but neither overly identified with the child nor intolerant of children's natural messiness. Some interviewers are active, engaging, and direct. Some are very quiet, saying no more than is necessary to keep the child's conversation flowing. Some use humor to relax the anxious child. All should be unhurried, with no axe to grind; children are very perceptive of intolerance or irritation cloaked by a falsely bright exterior. The best interviewer is a kind of catalyst—able to attend when the child is freely associating or playing, able to interpolate a comment or question to get a stalled interview started, able to get down on the floor and play with the child when it is appropriate to do so, but capable of setting reasonable limits. Skillful clinicians inject only as much of themselves into the situation as necessary to allay the child's anxiety and promote his or her self-expression.

Clinicians should reflect on their personal responses to each patient. When these responses are dominant, inexorable, and overly generalized, they disrupt the empathic acceptance required for effective interviewing. They can vary from intellectualization and boredom when confronted by an inarticulate child, to the need to rescue a troubled child from what

are perceived as villainous parents. The rescuer is likely to set up an unproductive tug-of-war with parents. Others are prone to reductionistic thinking, avoiding close contact with the child and withdrawing into their particular theoretical preference (eg, neurobiology, systems theory, psychoanalytic theory, cognitive-behavioral theory).

CONDUCTING THE CHILD INTERVIEW

Guidelines

The interviewer should not wear a white coat; it signals needles to some children. Clothing should enable the interviewer to sit on the floor if needed. The interviewer should not whisper to the parents about the child in the child's presence. He or she should speak openly, or leave comments to a later time.

The interviewer should try to avoid taking notes during the interview. A few key phrases may be jotted down to provide reminders of the sequence of events. The interviewer then may dictate his or her memory of the interview as soon as it is finished.

Special Considerations

The cardinal aim of the first interview is to help the child relax with the interviewer and to lay the foundation of trust. Nothing should be allowed to compromise this aim, because without trust little can be achieved. If trust does develop, the interviewer will be able to clarify the purpose of the interview, ascertain whether the child perceives problems in his or her life, evaluate the child's affect and capacity to relate to the interviewer, and catch a glimpse of his or her family life. Further specific features of the child's history and mental status can often wait for a second or third interview, unless the child is especially cooperative at the initial interview, or unless the matter is urgent.

The mere expression of feeling during play, without reflection or understanding, is not helpful. The child who breaks things or attacks the interviewer is likely to be terrified or overcome with remorse. In any case, he or she will be reluctant to return. The following rule may bear repeating to the child: "You may say or do what you want, but you must stay with me for the allotted time, and I will not allow you to break things or hurt yourself or other people." This precaution needs to be stated only if the child seems likely to infringe on the implicit rule.

At the start of the interview, the interviewer should go into the waiting room and greet the parents and child. He or she should sit beside the child and offer an introduction. The interviewer should tell the child that together they will talk, draw, and play for about an hour and then should invite the child into the interview room. If the child is resistant, the interviewer should wait briefly to see if the parents can reassure the child. If this does not work, the parents may be asked to bring the child into the room, indicating that they will be leaving when the child is comfortable. Usually, the parents can leave after a short time, at a signal from the interviewer. If not, it is seldom necessary for the parents to be present for more than one or two interviews.

For the younger child, the interviewer will have set out suitable play materials in the interview room. The child of 9 or 10 years of age can be ushered to an appropriate chair. The interviewer can begin by asking older children why their parents asked them to come and how they feel about it. If the child cannot say, the interviewer should tell the child what he or she already knows and ask for the child's personal reaction to this information. If the child is younger, he or she may be invited to use the play equipment. The interviewer should not push the child. The play theme should emerge on its own. The interviewer may then gently test the child to see whether he or she is prepared to talk.

Questions to Ask

If the child is comfortable conversing with the interviewer, the topics listed in Table 34–3 can be touched on. These topics flow in a natural sequence from neutral to personal. The first seven topics, though informative, are essentially ice-breakers. The last four topics require reflection and are likely to be more difficult for the child. However, the list should not be followed rigidly; rather, the topics can be explored in a discretionary manner. One child may be disposed to give a detailed account of peer and family relations, another will provide little on anything beyond neutral topics, and a third will prefer to play with toys and to converse intermittently about them.

Children are relatively more concrete and egocentric about the world than are adolescents. They have difficulty understanding abstractions, taking an objective view of themselves, and accurately timing past events. Questions should not be framed in a leading or suggestive manner (a caution that applies particularly in medico-legal situations). Children are confused by

Table 34–3. Issues covered during the child interview.

Content Category	Issues Covered
Attendance	Reason for and feelings about attendance.
School	School, class, teacher. Best and least liked teachers. Reasons? Best and least liked subjects. Reasons? School grades and homework. Liking for other school activities. Reasons? Changes of school? Reasons?
Neighborhood	Neighborhood, social groups, clubs.
Recreation	Hobbies, talents. Best liked activity. Reasons? Sports.
Social relationships	Best friend. Reason best friend is liked? Enemies. Reasons enemies are disliked? Experiences of persecution or scapegoating.
Leadership/ambitions	Opportunities and aspirations for leadership. Ambition with regard to occupation, marriage, and family.
Illness	Recent illnesses, experiences of hospitalization.
Domestic arrangements	House: layout, yard space, bedroom. Chores. Parents, siblings, pets. Family activities most enjoyed. Relationship between parents, alliances within the family, and conflicts within the family.
Fantasy	Dreams, good and bad. Three wishes. What would the child do with $1,000,000? Mutual story-telling. Drawings: of the family doing something together, of a person, of "something nice" and "something nasty."
Symptoms	Fears, anxiety, obsessions, compulsions, dissociative phenomena, depression, depersonalization. If indicated, hallucinations, ideas of reference, delusions, concerns about death, suicidal ideation, difficulty controlling anger, and antisocial behavior.
Insight	Understanding of the reason for attendance. Understanding of the nature of the problem. Desire for help.

complex or compound questions: One idea to one question is best. The interviewer should avoid asking children "Why?" because it puts them on the defensive. Consider the following example:

Patient: The other kids pick on me.
Clinician: Why?
Patient: I don't know. They're mean.

The clinician might have asked the following questions: What do they say? What do they do? How do you feel about it? What do you do about it? When a child uses an unusual word or phrase, particularly if it has an "adult" quality, do not assume it has the same meaning for the child that it has for you. Inquire further.

The interviewer should avoid trying to ferret out the truth from a child who has been involved in antisocial behavior. Instead he or she should try to get in touch with the child's feelings about the situation and what led up to it. It can sometimes be useful to gently point out discrepancies or inconsistencies to an older child who is apparently fabricating a story.

When the interviewer introduces matters that have an anxiety-laden connotation, especially if they seem to imply that the child is "weird" or unique, it can be helpful to associate the issue with the difficulties of other children in similar circumstances. These are known as **buffer comments.** Consider the following example:

Clinician: I see a lot of kids here who have problems after their parents get divorced. Some of them can't help blaming somebody. I wonder if you ever felt like that.

Ending the Interview

At the end of the interview, the clinician should recapitulate with the child what they have both learned about the child's reasons for being seen and how he or she feels about it. If another interview is planned, the interviewer should indicate when it will be. Children should not be asked if they would like to return for another visit. The child may be taken back to the parents in the waiting room. Whispered hallway consultations with the parents should be avoided. If urgent consultation with the parents is needed at that time, the interviewer should conduct the discussion briefly in the interview room, preferably with the child present.

INTERPRETING CHILDHOOD FANTASY

The interpretation of childhood play and fantasy is a specialized skill requiring theoretical knowledge and supervised practical experience. It is important to know the normative fantasies of children of different ages. For example, 4-year-old children often have fantasy themes concerning omnipotence, loss of approval,

bodily injury, and curiosity about body differences and functions. By 5–6 years of age, children have an emerging capacity for guilt following transgressions. The polarities of love and hate, kindness and cruelty, death and rebirth are often expressed in fantasy. By 7–8 years of age, children have a fear of injury, particularly in competitive interaction with peers. There are emerging fears of inferiority in comparative strength, speed, beauty, or intelligence, and a concern with rules and conformity. Gender-role differences are also important. By 9–10 years of age, children have a capacity for guilt and internal conflict, but morality tends to be black and white. Children may be normally preoccupied with the themes of television shows and cartoons, particularly those themes having to do with invulnerability, pursuit and rescue, transgression and punishment. Gender-role differences become more imperative as adolescence approaches.

The clinician should not be surprised if an 8-year-old child prefers to draw with paper and pencil than with poster colors or finger paints. No particular importance should be attached to the observation that a 4 year old enjoys constructing towers and knocking them over or that a 6 year old recounts episodes of "Spiderman." The trick is to recognize deviations from, distortions of, or immaturity in, the normative phase–related themes discussed in this section. Children struggling to cope with unresolved inner conflicts concerning self-control, dependence and independence, activity and passivity, recklessness and injury, male and female, transgression and punishment, invulnerability and helplessness, and dominance and submission are likely to express these themes in play over and over again. It is the idiosyncratic details; the repetitiousness; and the distorted, deviant, or grossly immature theme that should alert the interviewer to fantasy material of diagnostic importance.

Lewis M: Psychiatric assessment of infants, children, and adolescents. Pages 440–456 in Lewis M (editor): *Child and Adolescent Psychiatry: A Comprehensive Textbook.* Williams & Wilkins, 1996.
Simmons JE: *Psychiatric Examination of Children,* 3rd ed. Lea & Febiger, 1981.

IV. INTERVIEWING ADOLESCENTS

William Bernet, MD

PURPOSE OF THE ADOLESCENT INTERVIEW

The initial psychiatric interview of an adolescent has three general purposes: (1) establishing the possible diagnoses, (2) providing therapeutic intervention, and (3) creating a foundation for psychiatric treatment. The first purpose is to establish the possible diagnoses. The interview of the adolescent is only one part—perhaps the most important part—of the full diagnostic process, which also includes interviewing the parents and may include psychological testing, laboratory tests, a physical examination, and the gathering of information from outside sources.

The second purpose for the initial interview is to provide some form of therapeutic intervention. After a single conversation this intervention is not likely to constitute a cure but may simply be a sense of relief for the adolescent to get something off his or her chest. The youngster may leave the appointment with a sense of satisfaction that somebody is making an effort to listen to his or her grievances or with a sense of hope that there will be a way to solve a particular problem over a period of time.

The third purpose of the initial interview is to create a foundation for a continuing course of psychiatric treatment. It is the time to start negotiating the alliance between the therapist and the adolescent. That is, the interviewer communicates that he or she will try to understand the youngster's point of view, even if he or she doesn't agree with it. The interviewer will promote the interests of the patient in both the short term (eg, resolving an immediate impasse or conflict) and the long term (eg, defining and encouraging goals and aspirations). At the same time the interviewer will help the adolescent acknowledge and accept his or her responsibilities to family and community.

FACTORS AFFECTING THE ADOLESCENT INTERVIEW

Although the diagnostic process can be both productive and enjoyable, it is frequently a difficult experience for both the interviewer and the interviewee. A physician who feels perfectly comfortable and competent in dealing with an adult patient may become frustrated and tongue-tied when he or she tries to develop a conversation with a 14-year-old adolescent. It is almost always possible to establish rapport and collect information from adolescents, despite the tension and suspicion that may be sensed by both parties.

The physical setting of the interview is important. The office does not need to be fancy, but it should be comfortable and pleasant, relatively soundproof, and located far enough from the waiting room to create a sense of privacy.

Style of the Interview

The general manner in talking with adolescents should be relaxed and informal. It is good to have a sense of humor. Stuffiness creates distance; arrogance invites sarcasm; authoritarianism invites defiance. Being informal and friendly does not mean that the interviewer should become chummy and ingratiating. Teenagers want some degree of social distance between themselves and adults.

Should the interviewer initially meet with the parents, with the teenager, or with the entire family together? It depends on the presenting problem and the circumstances of the interview, but the most common format is for the interviewer to go to the waiting room, introduce himself or herself to both the patient and the parents, ask the patient to come with him or her to the office, and indicate that he or she will meet with the parents in a little while. The purpose, of course, is to communicate to the teenager that this meeting is for the teenager. It is helpful to know the parents' primary concerns ahead of time, which can be learned at the time the appointment is set up or perhaps through an intake questionnaire.

Some adolescents are cooperative, talkative, and quite aware of the purpose of the meeting. In that case, the patient may be perfectly willing to launch into a discussion of the reason for the evaluation. Other youngsters are embarrassed, guilty, or defensive. In that case, it is usually preferable initially to avoid the topics that are most difficult and to spend some time talking about subjects that are important but not as threatening. This part of the interview is an opportunity to take an interest in the patient's general life experience, not just in the immediate problem area. By the end of the meeting, the interviewer should know about the teenager's assets and successes as well as his or her problems.

Asking direct questions may not be the best way to elicit information. Teenagers become defensive almost automatically when they hear questions like "Where did you go?" and "Why did you do it?" Instead of asking, "Why did you steal that car?" the interviewer might say, "Tell me what you were you thinking about when you were driving the car."

The interviewer may wish to propose other forms of communication, in addition to the usual dialogue. It might be helpful to ask the youngster to draw a picture of what happened or what he or she observed. The teenager may be able to communicate through dolls or puppets. Young adolescents may be more comfortable with play materials that are typically used with younger children. However, the interviewer should be careful not to insult a more mature teenager by suggesting that he or she use the dolls that are in the office.

Interviews Are Like Poetry

The communications of teenagers and all patients can be considered on several levels. The **content** refers to the actual meaning of the words involved. For example, a youngster may relate a significant fact, that he is failing the ninth grade for the second time. The **form** of the communication refers to the manner in which the statement is made. The statement may be anything from quite coherent to very illogical, simple or convoluted, accompanied or not by inappropriate affect. For example, the boy who was failing the ninth grade repeatedly may announce it with undue bravado, rather than with the contrition one would expect. The **meaning** of the statement may go beyond the conscious, literal words of the content. For example, the meaning of failing the ninth grade twice may be a terrible feeling of pessimism and hopelessness. Finally, communication may be considered from the point of view of **transference.** That is, the youngster may assume that the interviewer will berate him for failure in the same way that his parents did.

Countertransference

The interviewer should examine his or her own feelings toward the patient and the patient's family. These feelings, called **countertransference,** can promote or impede the progress of the evaluation. For instance, the clinician investigating a case of alleged child abuse may be horrified at the youngster's suffering and outraged at the father who allegedly caused it. The interviewer's outrage may interfere with his or her objectivity.

Barker P: *Clinical Interviews with Children and Adolescents.* WW Norton & Company, 1990.

Bernet W: Humor in evaluating and treating children and adolescents. J Psychother Pract Res 1993;2:307.

Katz P: Establishing the therapeutic alliance. Adolescent Psychiatry 1998;23:89.

Meeks J, Bernet W: *The Fragile Alliance.* Krieger Publishing, 1990.

CONDUCTING THE ADOLESCENT INTERVIEW

It is advisable for the interviewer to develop and follow a fairly consistent format in interviewing adolescents. Such a format helps the interviewer remember to touch on a number of important areas in addition to the topic that is of most immediate interest. The interviewer should follow a regular format but be flexible and ready to improvise. As the interviewer moves from one topic to the next, he or she should use transitions and keep the youngster informed about why a particular subject is being discussed. For example, the interviewer could say, "Now I want to ask you some questions about your family, so that I know who everybody is."

Starting the Interview

One way to start the interview is to ask the youngster whose idea it was to come for the appointment. That may lead to a discussion of the chief complaint and the present illness.

If the patient is defensive, the interviewer can invite the patient to tell about school, which is usually a nonthreatening subject. The patient can describe his or her schedule, comment on specific subjects studied, and talk about what he or she thinks is the best part and the worst part of school. A discussion of the patient's ideas about what he or she will be doing after high school graduation gives an indication of the patient's level of optimism and his or her ability to engage in long-range planning.

Collecting Information

The interviewer might ask whether other children in the patient's school get in trouble and what happens to them, which is an opportunity for the youngster to talk about the various bad things that a child might do without necessarily attributing any of it to himself or herself. The discussion of other children in school leads naturally to the topic of peer relationships. Most teenagers can relate what they enjoy doing with friends and also what they may like to do by themselves.

Talking about enjoyable activities gives the adolescent an opportunity to tell about special interests, abilities, hobbies, music, and television. The interviewer can ask about the television shows that the youngster enjoys and ask whether he or she can relate what happened during specific episodes. Not only does this test the patient's memory and ability to organize a narrative, but the youngster may project his or her own issues and concerns onto favorite television shows.

Another useful topic is the youngster's version of his or her health history, because he or she may have interesting and unusual notions about illnesses and operations he or she has had. The health history leads to other areas, such as substance abuse. The interviewer should ask specifically about use of tobacco, alcohol, marijuana, cocaine, hallucinogens, and inhalants. The health history also leads to a discussion of sexual activities and related issues, such as sexually transmitted diseases.

It is always important for the youngster to tell about his or her family: the names of family members, their ages, what kind of work they do, whether they have had serious illness or problems. It might be useful to ask what the parents do when the youngster has been particularly good or particularly bad. The interviewer could ask if the parents are unusually strict, which leads to questions about emotional abuse and physical abuse.

Incorporating the Mental Status Examination

One way to blend the history and the mental status examination is to take an **inventory of affects.** The interviewer may ask the patient to tell about a time when he or she was particularly happy, a time he or she was worried, a time he or she was frustrated, and so on. The interviewer may ask about a time that something funny or silly happened or ask the patient to relate a favorite joke.

If the patient has been depressed, the examiner should ask about suicidal thoughts and behaviors, which are not unusual among adolescents (see Chapter 39). Sometimes it is preferable to be indirect, using questions such as, "Have you ever known anybody who was suicidal?" "Did your friend ever do anything to actually hurt himself?" or "Did anything like that ever happen to you?" Teenagers should be encouraged to tell a parent or other adult if they have persistent or serious suicidal thoughts. If suicidality is a serious concern, this would be a good time to tell the youngster about both confidentiality and the exceptions to confidentiality. Most youngsters find it reassuring (rather than threatening) to learn that the new doctor will keep them safe by discussing dangerous or risky impulses with their parents.

Depending on the differential diagnoses that the interviewer is considering, it may be appropriate to ask the patient about psychotic processes such as delusions, hallucinations, thought insertion and removal, and ideas of reference. Because many adolescents like to demonstrate what they know about psychological phenomena, it is possible to ask a series of questions such as, "Do you know what a hallucination is?" "Can you give me an example of a hallucination?" "Have you ever known anybody who hallucinated?" and "Does that ever happen to you?"

Getting to the Point of the Interview

The interview should not end without addressing the issue or the behavior that led to the referral in the first place. Almost always, that topic will come up at some point during the interview—at the outset of the interview; during the discussion of the patient's school activities, friends, medical history, and family; or through questions related to mental status. Occasionally the patient is so defensive, embarrassed, or simply lacking in insight that he or she seems to avoid the basic reason for the evaluation. Perhaps the parents have brought the youngster because of their concerns about inappropriate sexual behaviors, bizarre obsessive preoccupations, or persistent antisocial conduct. In such cases, the patient may be strongly motivated to keep the interviewer busy discussing other topics. If the youngster seems to be avoiding the subject, the interviewer can bring it up by saying, for example, "Your mom told me on the phone that you have been taking three or four showers every day. Can you tell me about that?" The interviewer can explain that he or she needs to hear the whole story, including the adolescent's side of the story, in order to be of help.

Ending the Interview

After collecting this information, the clinician may want to summarize his or her understanding of the most significant topics. This summary communicates to the patient that the interviewer has tried to understand the situation from the patient's point of view and also allows the patient to make additions or corrections.

It is good to end the initial interview on a positive note. For example, the interviewer can comment positively on the youngster's plans for the future, make specific suggestions regarding the patient's presenting problems, or simply say that the interviewer has enjoyed the meeting.

The end of the initial interview is also an appropriate time to touch on the subject of confidentiality. Because the interviewer is about to meet with the patient's parents, he or she might say, "We have talked about a lot of things today. Is there anything you said that I should not discuss with your folks?" This is a concrete way of communicating that the material discussed in therapy is generally confidential. The patient's answer may tell a lot about his or her relationship with the parents, and it also protects the therapist from making some blunder with the parents early in the relationship with the family. The interviewer can add that he or she would need to tell the parents if the patient appeared to be at risk for self-harm or for harming another person.

American Academy of Child and Adolescent Psychiatry: Practice parameters for the psychiatric assessment of children and adolescents. J Am Acad Child Adolesc Psychiatry 1997;36:4S.

Kalogerakis MG: Emergency evaluation of adolescents. Hosp Commun Psychiatry 1992;43:617.

STRUCTURED DIAGNOSTIC PROCEDURES

Clinical information regarding adolescents may also be collected through structured interviews and standardized inventories. These tools are commonly used in clinical research and epidemiologic studies, but they may be useful in clinical practice in some circumstances. These structured procedures are not required for a satisfactory diagnostic interview of an adolescent but may increase the sensitivity of the evaluation in some cases. See Chapter 35 for more information on structured interviews. Another instrument is the Child Behavior Checklist, a questionnaire regarding symptoms and behaviors that may be completed independently by the father, mother, and adolescent. The responses are compared to normative data, and the patient is scored along internalizing and externalizing symptom clusters.

Weist MD, Baker-Sinclair ME: Use of structured assessment tools in clinical practice. Adolescent Psychiatry 1997;21:235.

V. INTERVIEWING FAMILIES

Vernon H. Sharp, MD

IMPORTANCE OF THE FAMILY INTERVIEW

The family (considered in its broadest sense to include the combined nuclear and extended family system) is the developmental matrix for every child's behavior: normal and symptomatic. This universal principle is the foundation for family interviewing. The family interview provides a rapid and cost-effective method of diagnosis and treatment in child and adolescent psychiatry.

Family diagnosis is concerned with the prevailing condition of the family. Family assessment is the process of gathering information about that condition. Although the clinician endeavors to understand each individual, assessment in family interviewing concerns the patterns of interaction of those individuals.

The symptomatic behavior of the child or adolescent may not be the source of the family's problems, but rather its result. In children and adolescents, symptoms are shaped by the family matrix in which they start and are perpetuated. Symptoms in young people develop as their hereditary endowment is shaped by their experiences in the family environment. Pathologic behavior can be interpreted as a strategy for survival in a maladaptive family system.

These concepts are embodied in family systemic thinking in four ways: (1) Symptoms reflect family relationship disturbances and not simply deviant behavior; (2) if the patient is approached as the exclusive repository of pathology, much diagnostic and therapeutic leverage is lost; (3) functional psychopathology can be fully understood only in context of the family matrix; and (4) if the dysfunctional family matrix can be changed, the child's or adolescent's symptoms will change.

There is currently much debate in the field of family therapy concerning a reliable classification of family psychopathology. A discussion of the various approaches is beyond the scope of this chapter.

PURPOSE OF THE FAMILY INTERVIEW

The family interview can provide important interactional data not available from individual interviews and contribute to efficient and cost-effective assessment and treatment planning. The goals of the family interview are as follows: to gather a comprehensive history of the present illness, to observe and assess pathogenic family interactions, to determine whether functional illness stems from pathologic family interactions, to formulate a family diagnosis and design a treatment plan, to promote the family's understanding and motivation for treatment, and to negotiate a therapeutic alliance concerning the diagnosis and treatment plan.

CONTENT OF THE FAMILY INTERVIEW

Table 34–4 lists the topics commonly covered in a family interview. Steirlin et al consider it desirable that all members of the family be present at the first interview. Clinicians may find this unfamiliar, but it is surprisingly easy to accomplish. Frequently a sibling will provide the key to a therapeutic dilemma, saving hours of diagnostic time. In the first interview the various functions of each child for the parents and for each other usually become clear. Table 34–5 lists the aspects of family interaction that can be observed in a family interview.

The parents and the clinician often have a justifiable concern that children should not be unnecessarily burdened with the problems of marital discord; however, such problems are already part of the children's experience. Siblings are part of the family and are consciously or unconsciously aware of their parents' or siblings' difficulties. Because the family's problems are never discussed in a way that leads to solution and reconciliation, they tend to nourish unhealthy fantasy or promote unexpressed feelings of insecurity. Indeed, the first interview with the whole family may offer a chance for relief. At last, long-concealed doubts, anger, and differences can be discussed, and children's fears that they are the cause of their parents' difficulties are allayed.

Children can offer crucial help to the clinician in his or her efforts to establish contact with the family. Younger children, especially, are relatively untouched by convention and social inhibitions and can become the therapist's ally. While fearful and guilt-laden parents often find it hard to be open about their differences, small children are often quick to come to the central problem. Take, for example, a family with two boys, aged 5 and 7. The older child has various physical symptoms and is physically immature and severely hyperkinetic. The parents complain vigorously about their son, but when questioned about what makes the symptoms better or worse, their answers are vague. Further, they appear guarded about their relationship and the family's emotional climate. Tactful questioning is to no avail. As the parents attempt to

Table 34–4. Issues covered during the family interview.

Content Category	Issues Covered
Explicit information	What are the chief complaints of the family and the patient? ("Patient" denotes the identified patient; however, the symptomatic child often turns out to be quite adaptable and is the symptom bearer for an even more disturbed family system.) How do family members understand the present problem? How does the patient see it? Have organic factors been considered (hereafter, it will be assumed that these have been ruled out)? Why does the family come in at this time? What is the background of the problem? How has the family attempted to solve this problem in the past? What are the family's expectations of the interview? What are their motivations and resistances?
Background information	Perinatal and childhood development Current medical problems and medications Past medical and psychiatric illnesses and hospitalizations Family medical and psychiatric history Family demographics Family's employment, educational, housing, and financial status Legal problems of family and patient, past and present
The patient's relationships	With peers (Is the patient gregarious? Popular? Friendly? A loner? Combative?) With teachers and school personnel (Is the patient an academic success or failure? Compliant? Oppositional?) With siblings (Is the patient cooperative? Antagonistic?) With parents and extended family (Are family relationships close? Harmonious? Frictional? Distant? Hostile?) Are supportive aunts, uncles, or grandparents available?
Family's relationships	With the community, such as church and school (Is the family connected? Participative? Isolated? Aloof?) With extended family (Is the family cordial? Warm? Welcoming? Distant? Cold? Rejecting?) With friendship networks (Is the family rewarding? Congenial? Conflictual? Isolated?)

sustain a bland facade, the younger child suddenly says, "But you're always fighting!" Thereafter, it develops that the patient's symptoms are worst in the evenings and over the weekends when the parents are together and quarreling. In this family, marital conflict was the heart of the problem. In subsequent therapeutic sessions, if the conflict can be dealt with constructively, the parents will communicate better and the child's hyperactivity is likely to improve.

It is appropriate to honor legitimate wishes for privacy. For example, when parents want to discuss sexual problems, the children may be asked to wait in a playroom. Similarly, the wish for an individual interview, as might be requested by an adolescent, can be legitimate.

Table 34–5. Aspects of family interaction observed in the family interview.

Aspects of Family Interaction	Questions to Consider
Overall family communication	Are family members harmonious? Cooperative? Irritable? Immature?
Parental interaction	Are the parents close? Encouraging independence? Responsible? Congenial? Remote? Unstable? Frictional?
Parent-child interaction	Are the parents appreciative? Accepting? Supportive? Respectful of privacy? Critical? Neglectful? Discouraging independence? Intrusive? Do exclusive alliances exist (eg, overly close mother and overly dependent child, excluding father)?
Sibling interaction	Interviews that include the patient's siblings can provide crucial data. Is the patient treated as the perfect child? Is the patient being scapegoated (ie, blamed for the family's problems)? Do the siblings accept the blaming or try to defend the patient?
Extended family interaction	Does the patient have a supportive aunt, uncle, or grandparent who resists the pathogenic atmosphere of the nuclear family? Is the mother so attached to her own mother that she is more like a child herself? Is the father's anger toward a family member taken out on one of the children?

CONDUCTING THE FAMILY INTERVIEW

Haley has proposed four stages for the initial interview: (1) introduction, (2) problem identification, (3) family interaction, and (4) conclusion.

Introduction

In the introduction, the clinician greets the family members, learns their names, and sets them at ease. The clinician gives recognition and status to every family member through direct interaction with each of them. He or she explains the rationale for involving all members of the family, for example, by saying, "The more members of the family I see, the more they can help me to help Billy. Besides, I can get much more information more quickly." The clinician acknowledges family members' apprehensions and provides support. He or she avoids guilt-inducing statements by reframing the problem, for example: "Society is sometimes critical of these problems, but I can see you've done the best you could in the face of many difficulties." Finally, he or she observes the patterns of power and affiliation as they are revealed, for example, in where family members sit and who speaks out.

Problem Identification

In the problem identification stage, the clinician elicits a statement of the problem from each member of the family. Labels attached to people are transformed into relationship questions (eg, the statement "She's spoiled" elicits from the clinician, "I see, who spoils her the most?"). Statements that are too long or too short are controlled (eg, with responses such as "Excuse me. I need to interrupt you Mary, so I can hear what Tom has to say" or "I'm surprised Mr. Smith. You must have noticed more than that."). At the end of this stage, the clinician elicits from a family member a summary of the problem (eg, "Mr. Smith would you summarize the problem as we've been discussing it?").

Family Interaction

In the family interaction stage, the clinician has two members talk with each other about the problem (eg, "Talk directly to your wife about this, instead of telling me."). The discussion may be interrupted to bring other family members into the conversation (eg, "They seem to be stuck. Why don't you help them out?"). The seating arrangement may be changed in order to alter interactive patterns (eg, "Mom, I'd like you to sit by Dad and give Billy a bit more space on the sofa."). The interviewer may reframe the family views of reality, for example, by emphasizing a family member's good intentions or recasting symptoms as having a positive function in the family (eg, "What do you think might happen if they didn't have you to worry about?").

Conclusion

In the conclusion, the clinician provides a summary in such a way as to engender hope (eg, "Most families have some periods of difficulty with their teenagers, and they get past them."). The clinician provides encouragement so as to increase motivation for treatment. Humor may be useful. The clinician invites questions to increase understanding, outlines a treatment plan, and arranges further sessions with key family members, as necessary.

A CASE STUDY

The identified patient, Billy, has been referred because of school refusal in second grade. He is 6 years old and is accompanied by his parents and two older siblings.

Billy's symptoms, which began shortly after his father lost a middle management job as a result of corporate downsizing, have worsened over an 8-month period, despite efforts to help him by family and school. After Billy's father lost his job, the parents began to quarrel. Billy is most likely to refuse to go to school when parental friction is greatest.

Early in the history-taking part of the interview, the parents begin to argue about the facts. Billy leaves his chair, huddles under his mother's arm, starts to suck his thumb, and distracts the parents. The father then turns his anger on Billy, yelling, "Stop bothering your mother and get back to your chair!" Billy looks stunned and starts to cry. At this point, the mother, pampering Billy, angrily criticizes the father for being too harsh. The father, wounded, withdraws into sullen silence, drawing the two older children into the confusion. Billy's older brother supports the father. His sister supports her mother. The parents are heartened by their children's support and relax. Billy goes back to his chair. Calm is restored. The interview resumes, but the same pattern recurs three more times in the course of the interview.

Family Assessment

Family assessment elucidates the family's relationship patterns. Billy's family responds to its distress with a blindly repetitive pattern. The pattern fails to relieve the distress. Assessment leads to treatments aimed at pathogenic interaction patterns, in order to change the problematic behavior.

A. Explicit Information: The family's complaint is Billy's school refusal, which is seen as Billy's problem. Because Billy's symptoms clearly began at a time of family stress (ie, father's job loss), an organic cause is unlikely. The family comes in now because

Billy's symptoms have become worse. Their goal is to relieve Billy's symptoms.

B. Background Information: A history of unremarkable childhood development is obtained. Billy had the usual childhood diseases without hospitalizations. There are no current medical problems. The family medical and psychiatric history is unremarkable.

C. Family Demographics: This is an educated, middle-class family. Its finances are threatened because of the father's unemployed status. There are no legal problems.

D. Patient's Relationships: The patient's relationships with peers and teachers are limited by his school refusal. He is immaturely attached to his mother, distant from his father, and detached from his siblings.

E. Observational Data: The emotional climate in this family is conflictual and immature. The parental interactions are hostile and childlike, with incessant squabbling. The mother's interactions with the patient are smothering and infantilizing, excluding the father. The father displaces his anger at his wife onto Billy. Billy responds to his parents' quarreling with intrusive, protective, self-defeating behavior, showing little evidence of comfortable distance or a respect for privacy in the family. The older siblings take sides in ways that split the family and encourage the parents to abdicate their responsibilities as parents. The oldest son's alliance with his father sets him against his mother. The daughter's alliance with her mother sets her against her father. At the first sign of friction between his parents, Billy steps in and distracts them but remains "caught in the middle" throughout the interview. Repeatedly, and at considerable cost to himself, he absorbs the painful, angry tension between his parents, each time restoring the family to a temporary balance.

Family Diagnosis

Although Billy is the youngest, he is the pivotal family member, as he has been given the power to regulate the expression of his parents' unresolved conflicts. Parental conflicts are detoured through him, overwhelming him and leaving him little emotional energy to cope with school. Although the parents behave in stereotyped, immature ways, the children can be seen as taking care of them. Their caretaking puts them in parental roles toward their parents, reversing the normal generational hierarchy. Rather than settling differences in healthy ways, Billy's parents rely on their children for support and protection. Rewarded by his parents for soaking up their pain, Billy is predisposed to future self-defeating behavior. Moreover, his normal maturation is blocked. As things stand, should he extricate himself from his key peacekeeping position, his parents would suffer. Billy's school refusal is greatest when the parental friction is greatest. He unwittingly stays home to protect his parents from hurting each other.

As the identified patient, Billy plays a vital role in his family. His symptoms stabilize the transactions between his parents. By focusing on his problems, his parents avoid their own. While the other family members are stuck in unchanging roles, Billy maintains a delicate balance between going to school and staying home to protect his parents from themselves. In this way, he signals not only his own distress but the family's as well and is instrumental in getting help for the whole system.

Family Treatment

Family treatment often seeks to restructure pathogenic family relationships, thus eliminating the need for the identified patient's role. In this case, Billy's parents lack relationship skills and cannot cope with the family crisis. After establishing rapport and trust, the clinician could refer the family to family therapy. The goal of family therapy would be to help the parents resolve their marital issues with a more appropriate caretaker (ie, the therapist). The children could then be excused from the treatment and from their dysfunctional supportive roles. As Billy's parents stop drawing him into their conflicts, his school refusal would probably abate within a few weeks, without further medical intervention.

Beavers WR, Hampson RB: *Successful Families: Assessment and Intervention.* WW Norton & Company, 1990.

Glick ID, Clarkin JF, Kessler DR: *Marital and Family Therapy,* 3rd ed. Grune & Stratton, 1987.

Gurman AS, Kniskern DP: *Handbook of Family Therapy.* Vol 2. Brunner/Mazel, 1991.

Kerr M, Bowen M: *Family Evaluation.* Norton, 1988.

Ravenscroft R: Family therapy. In: Lewis M (editor): *Child and Adolescent Psychiatry: A Comprehensive Textbook.* Williams & Wilkins, 1996.

35

Diagnostic Evaluation

Barry Nurcombe, MD, Michael Tramontana, PhD, & Joseph D. LaBarbera, PhD

Based on the diagnostic hypotheses (generated, tested, and refined during history taking), the mental status examination, and the observation of family interaction, the inquiry plan proceeds to physical examination and, if required, to laboratory testing, special investigations, consultations, and psychological testing.

Figure 35–1 summarizes the flow of clinical reasoning from history taking, mental status examination, the generation of diagnostic hypotheses, through physical examination and special investigations, the refinement of the clinical pattern, secondary diagnostic hypotheses, psychological testing, and the diagnostic conclusion, to the diagnostic formulation and treatment plan.

I. CHILD MENTAL STATUS EXAMINATION

Barry Nurcombe, MD
& Michael Tramontana, PhD

PURPOSE OF THE CHILD MENTAL STATUS EXAMINATION

The child mental status examination is a set of systematic observations and assessments that provide a detailed description of the child's behavior during the diagnostic interview. Combined with the history and physical assessment, the mental status examination yields evidence that helps the clinician to refine, delete, or accept the diagnostic hypotheses generated during the diagnostic encounter (see Chapter 34), and to decide whether special investigations are needed in order to test particular diagnostic hypotheses. Thus the mental status examination is an integral part of the inquiry plan. In accordance with the diagnostic hypotheses and the inquiry plan, the mental status examination may be brief or comprehensive, but it always incorporates both standard and discretionary probes.

The mental status examination of the adolescent is similar to that of the adult (see Chapter 8). However, the examination of children is sufficiently different to warrant separate discussion. Many of the observations required to complete the mental status examination are made in the course of the semistructured interview with the child (see Chapter 34). Other observations, such as the clinical tests that screen cognitive functions, are part of a standardized set of questions.

AREAS ADDRESSED BY THE MENTAL STATUS EXAMINATION

Table 35–1 lists the areas covered by the mental status examination. For the most part, the first five areas are noted as the interview proceeds, whereas the last five require special questions.

Appearance
Note the following: height, weight, nutritional status; precocious or delayed physical maturation or secondary sexual characteristics; abnormalities of the skin, head, facies, neck, or general physique; personal hygiene and grooming; and style and appropriateness of dress.

Motor Behavior
Observe the following: general level of physical activity (eg, hyperkinesis, hypokinesis, bradykinesis), in comparison with others of the same age; abnormalities of gait, balance, posture, tone, power, and fine and gross motor coordination; abnormal movements (eg, tremor, twitching, shivering, tics, fidgeting, choreiform movements, athetoid movements, motor overflow); mannerisms, rituals, echopraxia, or stereotyped movements; motor impersistence; or pronounced startle response.

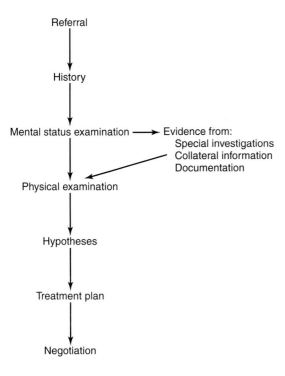

Referral

↓

History

↓

Mental status examination ⟶ Evidence from:
Special investigations
Collateral information
Documentation

↓

Physical examination

↓

Hypotheses

↓

Treatment plan

↓

Negotiation

Figure 35–1. The process of clinical reasoning.

Voice, Speech, & Language

Listen for the following: accent; abnormality in pitch, tone, volume, phonation, or prosody (eg, squawking, shouting, whispering, monotony, hoarseness, scanning, high-pitched voice); abnormality in the amount of speech (eg, mute, impoverished, voluble, loquacious) or its tempo (eg, slowed, accelerated); abnormal rhythm (eg, stuttering); abnormal articulation (eg, dyslalia); unusual or inappropriate use of words (eg, idioglossia, profanity); echolalia; abnormal syntax; and impairment in expressive or receptive language.

Interaction With the Examiner

Note the patient's eye contact (eg, eyes averted, unfocussed, staring). Is the child friendly and cooperative, or resistant, oppositional, shy, or withdrawn? Is

Table 35–1. Areas covered by the mental status examination.

Appearance
Motor behavior
Voice, speech, and language
Interaction with the examiner
Mood and affect
Cognitive functions
Thought processes
Thought content
Fantasy
Insight

he or she assertive, aggressive, impudent, sarcastic, cynical, fearful, clinging, inhibited, indifferent, clowning, invasive, coy, or seductive? Is the child a reliable informant?

Mood & Affect

In demeanor and conversation, does the patient show evidence of a persistent abnormality of mood or of poor emotional regulation? For example, is there evidence of anxiety, tension, rage, depression, elevation of mood, silliness, apathy, or anhedonia? Is the child emotionally labile, or conversely, does he or she exhibit a restricted range of affect? Which topics evoke the most intense emotion?

Cognitive Functions

Cognitive screening tests do not replace formal psychological testing. They serve as rapid clinical screens to determine whether formal testing is required. The following areas should be tested: attention, orientation, memory (immediate, recent, remote), judgment, abstraction, and intelligence (see Panels I–VI). Do not proceed with the tests described in the accompanying panels unless the patient has demonstrated a basic familiarity with numbers, letters, and words (see Table 35–2).

Thought Processes

Is there evidence of abnormal tempo, with flight of ideas or acceleration, slowing, or poverty of thought processes? Does the stream of thought lack clear goal direction, with vagueness, incoherence, circumstantiality, tangential thinking, derailment, or clang associations? Is the normal continuity of associations disrupted by perseveration, circumlocution, circumstantiality, distractibility, or blocking? Is there evidence of impairment in logical or metaphorical thinking, for example, in a blurring of conceptual boundaries or excessively concrete thinking?

Thought Content

From the history given by the parents, the intake questionnaires and checklists, and free discussion with the child, the clinician will have generated hypotheses that can be tested by direct probes concerning clinical phenomenology. The following symptoms may not be routinely checked unless there are good hypothetico-deductive reasons for doing so: anxiety, separation anxiety, school refusal, panic attacks, phobias, obsessions, compulsions, impulsions, delusions, hallucina-

Table 35–2. Prescreening questions for cognitive testing.

Area	Ask Patient To
Numbers	Count from 1 to 20
Letters	Recite the alphabet
Words	Point to his or her nose, mouth, chin, neck, and knees

I. ASSESSMENT OF ATTENTION

Clinician: "Listen carefully. I'm going to say some numbers, but sometimes I'll say a letter instead. Say Yes! each time you hear me say a letter instead of a number."
Recite the following at the rate of one item per second:

1 2 3 D 9 8 A 4 E Z 6 1 5 9 T 3 B 8 2 Q 7 3 2 J L 4 8 2 C

Evaluation:
Record number of errors of omission: _____
Record number of errors of commission: _____
Total: _____

Clinician: "Listen again. This time I'm going to say some letters, but sometimes I'll say a number instead. Say Yes! each time you hear me say a number instead of a letter."
Recite the following at the rate of one item per second:

B K L 4 O(oh) 6 P M 9 C N F O(oh) P 6 S 1(one) E G 3 J H U 0(zero) 9 6 W T 5

Evaluation:
Record number of errors of omission: _____
Record number of errors of commission: _____
Total: _____

Serial sevens. *Clinician:* "Can you subtract 7 from 100? What is 100 minus 7?" *If correct, say:* "Good. I want you to count backwards, taking 7 from 100, then 7 from 93, as far back as you can." *(Record response)*

Correct answer: 93, 86, 79, 72, 65, 58, 51, 44, 37, 30, 23, 16, 9, 2

Evaluation:
Record time (seconds) taken to reach final number: _____
Record number of errors: _____

If the subject cannot subtract 7 from 100, try serial threes.

Serial threes. *Clinician:* "Can you subtract 3 from 20? What is 20 minus 3?" *If correct, say:* "Good. I want you to count backwards, taking 3 from 20, then 3 from 17, as far back as you can." *(Record response).*

Correct answer: 17, 14, 11, 8, 5, 2

Evaluation:
Record time (seconds) taken to reach final number: _____
Record number of errors: _____

II. ASSESSMENT OF ORIENTATION

Ask the patient the following questions:

Time:

"What is the day of the week?"
"What is the date?"
"What season is it?"
"What time is it?"
"How long have we been talking here?"

Place:

"What is this place?"
"What kind of place is this?"
"How did you get here?"
"How far is this place from your home?"

Person:

"Tell me your name."
"What school do you go to?"
"What grade are you in at school?"
"Who am I?"
"What is my job?"
"Why have you come to see me?"

Evaluation:

Record number of accurate responses: _____

III. ASSESSMENT OF MEMORY

Recent Memory

Clinician: "Now I will give you three things to remember, and in a few minutes I will ask you to recall what they are. John Smith, 500 Kings Highway, Green." *After a few minutes, say:* "Please repeat those three things."

Evaluation (choose one):

Accurate
Needs prompting
Cannot repeat any
Refused

Clinician: "Now keep those things in your mind until I ask you for them again."

(continued)

III. ASSESSMENT OF MEMORY *(continued)*

Immediate Memory

Clinician: "I want you to listen carefully and repeat these numbers after me." *Speak at the rate of one number per second. Continue upward until the patient fails. Record the last accurate repetition.*

> 8
> 4 3
> 3 9 6
> 4 2 1 9
> 8 5 1 9 2
> 9 3 5 2 8 6
> 7 5 8 3 9 2 4

Evaluation (record number):
> Unable
> Refused

Clinician: "Now please repeat these numbers backward." *Continue upward until the patient fails. Record the last accurate repetition.*

> 3
> 9 1
> 4 7 3
> 5 8 2 9

Evaluation (record number):
> Unable
> Refused

Clinician: "Now, what were those three things I asked you to remember?"

Correct answer: John Smith, 500 Kings Highway, Green

Evaluation (choose one):
> Refused
> None correct
> Parts of A *or* B correct, only
> Parts of both A *and* B correct
> C correct, only
> Two fully correct, only
> Two out of three correct
> Three correct

Remote Memory

Clinician:
> "What is your address?"
> "What is your telephone number?"
> "Where were you born?"
> "What is the date of your birthday?"
> "What is your mother's name?"
> "Where was she born?"
> "What is the date of your mother's birthday?"
> "What is your father's name?"
> "Where was he born?"
> "What is the date of your father's birthday?"

Evaluation:
> Record number of accurate responses: _____

IV. ASSESSMENT OF JUDGMENT

Clinician: "Suppose the teacher had her back to the class and someone else flicked a rubber band at you. What would you do?"

Wait for spontaneous answer and record it.

If no answer is given, offer the following prompts:
"Ignore it?"
"Raise your hand to tell the teacher?"
"Go after the one that threw it?"

Clinician: "Suppose you were out walking and you saw smoke pouring out of the roof of a house on your street. What would you do?"

Wait for spontaneous answer and record it.

If no answer is given, offer the following prompts:
"Arouse someone in the house and tell them?"
"Ring a fire alarm?"
"Run home and tell your mother?"
"Ignore it?"

Clinician: "Imagine you were walking home from school and a girl in front of you dropped her purse without knowing it. What would you do?"

Wait for spontaneous answer and record it.

If no answer is given, offer the following prompts:
"Tell her or give it back?"
"Ignore it?"
"Look inside?"
"Keep it?"

V. ASSESSMENT OF ABSTRACTION

Clinician: "Tell me how these two things are alike:"

wood and coal
apple and peach
ship and automobile
iron and silver
baseball and orange
airplane and kite
ocean and river
penny and quarter

Clinician: "Do you know what a proverb is?" *(If not, discontinue.)*
"Good. Tell me, in your own words, what these proverbs mean."

A stitch in time saves nine.
People in glass houses should not throw stones.
A rolling stone gathers no moss.

VI. ASSESSMENT OF VOCABULARY

Clinician: "Tell me the meaning of the following words:" *Read out loud, ceasing after five consecutive items are incorrect:*

orange   roar   juggler
envelope   scorch   brunette
straw   muzzle   peculiarity
puddle   haste   priceless
tap   lecture   regard
gown   mars   disproportionate
eyelash   skill   shrewd
     tolerate

Evaluation:

Number Correct	Vocabulary Age
5	6 years
6	6 years 8 months
7	7 years 4 months
8	8 years
9	8 years 8 months
10	9 years 4 months
11	10 years
12	10 years 8 months
13	11 years 4 months
14	12 years
15	13 years 3 months
16	14 years
17	14 years 3 months
18	14 years 6 months
19	14 years 9 months
20	Average adult

VII. ASSESSMENT OF DRAWING

Clinician: Use a No. 2 pencil with eraser on 8 × 11 blank paper. Instruct the patient as follows: "On this piece of paper, I would like you to draw a whole person. It can be any kind of person, just make sure it's a whole person and not a stick figure or a cartoon figure." *For a young child who does not understand "person":* "You may draw a man or woman, a boy or girl." *(There is no time limit.)*

Evaluation: One point (3 months) is given for each item. Multiply the total number of correct items by 3. This is the patient's "drawing age" in months. Quote drawing age in years and months. Calculate the patient's "drawing quotient" as follows:

$$\frac{\text{Drawing age}}{\text{Chronological age}} \times 100$$

Each feature present:

Head	Ear	Shoulders	Leg
Eye	Hair	Arm	Foot
Nose	Neck	Hand	Heel
Mouth	Trunk	Finger	Clothing

Details:

Pupil	Nostrils	Hands distinct from arms
Eyebrow	Two-dimensional nose	Arm joints
Eyelash	Hair more than on crown	Leg joints

Correct number of features:

Two eyes	Ten toes
Two ears	Two articles of clothing
Two hands	Four articles of clothing
Ten fingers	Costume complete

Relatively correct location:

Symmetrical features	Legs attached to trunk
Ears in correct position	Opposition of thumb
Neck continuous with head	Joints shown
Arms from shoulders	

Proportional size:

Head more than circle	Fingers longer than wide
Eye longer than high	Arms in proportion
Body longer than head	Legs in proportion

In profile:

Eyes glance to front
Forehead shown
Chin projection shown
Profile
Correct profile

tions, ideas of reference, ideas of influence, thought alienation, thought broadcasting, depersonalization, déjà vu, derealization, suicidal ideation, impulses to injure the self or others, preoccupation with somatic functioning, somatic symptoms, stealing, fire setting, truancy, and fighting. In contrast, suicidal ideation, self-injury, assaultive impulses, substance abuse, physical or sexual abuse, risk taking, and antisocial behavior must always be inquired about when diagnostic evaluations are undertaken with adolescents.

Fantasy

The child's fantasy is elicited through play, drawing, and storytelling. By his or her unobtrusive interest, the clinician can facilitate the child's fantasy and encourage the child to express it. Table 35–3 lists a variety of techniques that can be used to elicit fantasy.

Insight

Is the child aware that he or she has a problem? If so, how is the problem conceptualized? Does the child want help for the problem?

STRUCTURED INTERVIEWING

Semistructured playroom interviews with children 7–12 years of age have been found to have a test-retest reliability of .84 and an interrater reliability of

.74, with regard to the detection of abnormality. However, interviewers who are unaware of the parents' perception of the child's problems tend to underestimate abnormality in comparison with parent reports of child behavior.

In order to compensate for the potential unreliability of unstructured or semistructured interviewing, a number of structured interviews have been introduced. As a rule, these interviews are too cumbersome for everyday clinical work; however, they are widely used to standardize subject selection in research studies. Arguably, semistructured and structured interviewing complement each other: The semistructured interview yields information mainly about the child's perception of the environment and itself, whereas the structured interview focuses on symptomatology. When reliable diagnostic categorization is the overriding consideration, structured interviews, such as those described in this section, are clearly preferable. It should be remembered, however, that with children younger than 10–12 years of age, the reliability of direct questions concerning symptomatology is affected by the fact that children are limited in their capacity to be objective about themselves. Furthermore, emotionally disturbed preadolescents tire if exposed to long, tedious interviews and may become careless in their answers. Table 35–4 provides more detailed information on these instruments.

A. Diagnostic Interview for Children and Adolescents (DICA): DICA is a semistructured interview that uses a modular technique, organized by diagnostic

---

Table 35–3. Techniques to elicit fantasy.

After the child has drawn a person, ask him or her the following types of questions:
Is that person a man or a woman, a boy or a girl?
How old is (he/she)?
What is (he/she) doing in that picture?
What is (he/she) thinking about?
How does (he/she) feel about it?
What makes (him/her) happy?
What makes (him/her) sad?
What makes (him/her) mad?
What makes (him/her) scared?
What does (he/she) need most?
What's the (best/worst) thing about (him/her)?
Tell me about (his/her) family?
What will (he/she) do next?

Use the Kinetic Family Drawing Test:
 a. Ask the child to draw his or her family doing something together.
 b. Note who the child puts in the family; the proximity of the figures; the coherence of or separations between group members; the relative importance and power of the family members; and their apparent emotions, attachments, rivalries, and so on.
 c. Ask the child to explain the drawing, saying what the family members are doing, thinking, and feeling, and what the outcome will be. Base your questions, in part, on discretionary probes derived from the dynamic hypotheses you have generated.

Ask the child to draw "something nice" and "something nasty." Consider using the following questions as icebreakers:
What would you do if you had a million dollars?
If you had three wishes, what would they be?
If you were wrecked on a desert island, who (and what) would you like to have with you?
Ask the child to tell you about (good/bad) dreams he or she has had recently.
Ask the child for the earliest thing he or she can remember, and for his or her earliest memory about his or her family.

Table 35–4. Structured interviews in child and adolescent psychiatry.

Instrument	Target Age (years)	Time Needed (minutes)	Reliability
Diagnostic Interview for Children & Adolescents (DICA)	6–17	60–90	Interrater and test-retest reliabilities are acceptable Parent-child agreement: 0–.87 on specific items (κ = .76–1.00 for anxiety and conduct disorders)
Diagnostic Interview Schedule for Children (DISC)	9–17	60–90	Interrater reliability: .94–1 for symptoms Test-retest reliability for parents: .9 (symptoms), .76 (syndromes); for children aged 14–18: .81 (symptoms), .36 (syndromes) Parent-child agreement: .27 (greatest for disruptive symptoms, less for depression or anxiety)
Schedule for Affective Disorders and Schizophrenia for School-Age Children (K-SADS)	6–18	180	Interrater reliability: .65–.96 (syndromes) Test-retest reliability: variable, .09–.89 (symptoms), .24–.7 (syndromes) Parent-child agreement: .08–1.00 (symptoms)
Child Assessment Schedule (CAS)	7–17	45–75	Interrater reliability: .73 (for content, less for diagnosis); higher for hyperactivity and aggression (.8), less for anxiety (.6)
Interview Schedule for Children (ISC)	8–17	90–120	Interrater reliability: .64–1.0 Parent-child agreement: .2–.95 (symptoms), .32–.86 (syndromes), lowest for subjective symptoms
Child & Adolescent Psychiatric Assessment (CAPA)	8–18	90–120	Not available

syndrome. Parent, child, and adolescent versions are available. Clinical judgment is required at several decision points; otherwise, lay interviewers can administer DICA. A computerized version is available for recording and scoring results. DICA has reasonable validity comparing pediatric and psychiatric referrals (especially in academic and relationship problems).

B. Diagnostic Interview Schedule for Children (DISC): DISC is a highly structured interview that is organized by topic and is closer to a natural free-flowing interview. It is mainly epidemiologic in purpose. Parent and child versions are available, and clinical judgment is not required. DISC has reasonable validity comparing pediatric and psychiatric referrals. Diagnoses are generated by computer algorithm.

C. Schedule for Affective Disorders and Schizophrenia for School-Age Children (K-SADS): K-SADS is a semistructured instrument that is used extensively in child psychiatry research. Parent, child, and epidemiologic versions are available. Clinical judgment is required. The same clinician interviews the parent and the child and attempts to resolve discrepancies in their reports. This interview was originally developed to identify children with affective disorder and now emphasizes affective, anxiety, and schizophrenic disorders. It is scored manually, and diagnosis is reached from summary ratings. Pilot validity data come from follow-up, treatment change, and biological correlate studies.

D. Child Assessment Schedule (CAS): CAS is a semistructured interview that has been used with both children and adolescents. Parent and child versions are

available. Interviewer training is required. Interview items are grouped by topic (eg, school, peers, family), not syndrome. CAS does not cover posttraumatic stress disorder, dissociative disorder, or adolescent schizophrenia. Its pilot validity was estimated by comparing inpatients, outpatients, and normal subjects.

E. Interview Schedule for Children (ISC): ISC was designed originally for a longitudinal study of depressed children and may be most useful for the diagnosis of depression. Parent and child versions are available. ISC requires clinical skill, judgment, and training.

F. Child and Adolescent Psychiatric Assessment (CAPA): CAPA is intended for use in both clinical and epidemiologic settings. Parent and child versions are available. It starts with an unstructured discussion and proceeds to a systematic inquiry into a broad range of symptoms for which an extensive glossary is available. It contains psychosocial and family functioning sections. Lay or clinician interviewers can administer it, and it is scored by computer algorithm.

Angold A: Clinical interviewing with children and adolescents. Pages 51–63 in Rutter M, Taylor E, Hersov L (editors): *Child and Adolescent Psychiatry,* 3rd ed. Blackwell Scientific, 1994.

Costello AJ: Structured interviewing. Pages 457–464 in Lewis M (editor): *Child and Adolescent Psychiatry.* Williams & Wilkins, 1996.

Lewis M: Psychiatric assessment of infants, children, and adolescents. Pages 440–456 in Lewis M (editor): *Child and Adolescent Psychiatry: A Comprehensive Textbook,* 2nd ed. Williams & Wilkins, 1996.

Simmons JE: *Psychiatric Examination of Children,* 3rd ed. Lea & Febiger, 1981.

II. PHYSICAL EXAMINATION, LABORATORY TESTING, & SPECIAL INVESTIGATIONS

Barry Nurcombe, MD

PHYSICAL EXAMINATION

Usually, a physical examination has already been completed by the child's pediatrician. If not, the clinician should refer the family to the primary physician. In some circumstances, however, it is important that the child psychiatrist complete the physical examination. Table 35–5 lists aspects of the physical examination to which the clinician should pay particular attention.

Table 35–6 lists symptoms that could be referable to the central nervous system and indicate the need for a neurologic examination. The psychiatrist can perform a brief, routine neurologic screen during the interview by observing the child's speech, gait, posture, balance, gross and fine motor tone, power and coordination, facial symmetry, and ocular movements and by checking for tics, tremor, clonus, or choreiform movements of the fingers and hands. Table 35–7 lists extensions to the routine screen that can be implemented by baring the child's feet and forearms.

Some child psychiatrists avoid physical examination. The clinician may worry that an upsetting physical examination will impede a positive relationship or tilt the spontaneous development of the child's transference. There may be some point to these considerations, but the potential benefits of a nonintrusive physical examination outweigh its disadvantages.

Table 35–5. Physical examination items deserving special attention.

Growth parameters: height, weight, and head circumference plotted on standard curves
Minor physical anomalies (associated with developmental problems such as hyperactivity):
  Abnormally small or large head
  "Electric" hair (fine, dry hair standing upright from the scalp)
  Epicanthic folds (skin folds in the upper internal eyelid)
  Hypertelorism (eyes deep-set and widely separated)
  Low-set, malformed, asymmetrical ears with adherent earlobes
  High palate
  Furrowed tongue
  In-curved little finger
  Long third toe
  Syndactyly
  Gap between first and second toes
Other head, face, or body dysplasias that might indicate a congenital disorder (eg, signs of fetal alcohol syndrome)

Table 35–6. Symptoms that indicate the need for neurologic examination.

Headache
Visual impairment
Deafness
Tinnitus
Poor balance
Episodic disruption of consciousness
Memory defects
Intermittent confusion
Anesthesia
Paresthesia
Motor weakness
Impaired coordination
Abnormal movements
Recent loss of sphincter control

Soft or nonfocal signs are phenomena thought to have no clear locus or origin, to be developmentally normal up to a certain age, and to reflect uneven neurologic maturation in older children. Table 35–8 lists commonly identified neurologic soft signs. Can these signs be consensually identified and elicited in a standard manner? Do they have significant test-retest and interrater reliability? Do they occur frequently enough in an at-risk population to make them worth eliciting? Are they singly or in clusters associated with disorders such as learning disability, attention-deficit/hyperactivity disorder, or schizophrenia? Do they predict which hyperkinetic children will respond to stimulant medication? For none of these questions is there a clear answer.

Table 35–7. Extension of the neurologic examination.

Domain	Functions or Abnormalities
Cranial nerves	Movement of eyes, face, and tongue Pupillary reflexes Visual fields Hearing
Motor power and tone	Shoulder Elbow Wrist Hand Knee Ankle
Reflexes	Biceps Triceps Supinator Patellar Ankle Plantar
Fundi	Papilledema Anterio-venous abnormalities Abnormal pigmentation

Note: Leave the examination of the reflexes and fundi to the end.

Table 35–8. Neurologic soft signs.

Choreiform or athetoid movements, especially of the out-stretched fingers and hands
Dysdiadochokinesia (difficulty performing rapid alternating movements)
Dysgraphesthesia (difficulty interpreting a figure traced on the palm of the hand)
General clumsiness
Synkinesis (the tendency for other parts of the body to move in unison when one part is moving)

Pincus J: The neurological meaning of soft signs. Pages 479–483 in Lewis M (editor): *Child and Adolescent Psychiatry.* Williams & Wilkins, 1991.

SPECIAL INVESTIGATIONS

The routine use of special investigations for all referred adolescents is not justified. Before ordering a consultation, test, or special investigation, the clinician should consider whether it is a screen inquiry that has a reasonable chance of yielding important information in the clinical population in question (eg, routine drug or pregnancy testing for hospitalized adolescents) or, in the case of a discretionary probe, whether the particular inquiry could conceivably rule out (or help to rule in) a diagnostic hypothesis. Table 35–9 lists the types of consultations and special investigations often used in child and adolescent psychiatry.

CLINICAL SITUATIONS LIKELY TO REQUIRE SPECIAL INVESTIGATIONS

The clinician must rule out physical disease, by the judicious ordering of specific consultations, tests, or investigations for several clinical situations. Table

Table 35–9. Common consultations and special investigations.

Consultations
Pediatric consultation
Neurologic consultation
Other specialist consultations (eg, speech pathology)
Special investigations
Laboratory testing (eg, blood, urinalysis, electrolytes, liver function, thyroid function, urine drug screening, genetic screening)
Acoustic and ophthalmologic examination
Electroencephalography
Neuroimaging
Psychological testing

35–10 lists the clinical situations in which organic causes must be ruled out.

Acute or Subacute Disintegration of Behavior and Development

After a period of normal or relatively normal development, the child may fail to make developmental progress and lose recently acquired skills such as sphincter control, coordination, dexterity, attention and concentration, memory, language, capacity for problem solving, school performance, emotional control, and social competence. In some cases, the child may demonstrate abnormal motor patterns, hallucinations, delusions, and disorganization of thinking. Table 35–11 lists organic causes that must be excluded.

Acute Psychotic Episode

The child or adolescent may become mentally disorganized, socially inappropriate, emotionally incongruent, or emotionally labile and may report audiovisual hallucinations, illusions, ideas of reference, and delusions of persecution or grandeur. Sometimes the patient becomes mute, immobile, posturing and apparently self-absorbed, assuming odd postures of the arms, head, and trunk. The following disorders must be excluded: substance-induced psychotic disorder (using urine and blood toxicology) and psychotic disorder due to general medical condition, which requires pediatric consultation and tests specific to hypothesized medical condition (eg, anorexia, hyperthyroidism, hypersteroidism, neurologic disorder).

Anorexia or Weight Loss

The child or adolescent may lose weight markedly as a result of voluntary restriction of food intake. The following conditions should be ruled out: chronic systemic infection (especially tuberculosis); systemic malignancy (especially pancreatic, mediastinal, retroperitoneal, pulmonary, lymphatic, or leukemic malignancy); hypothalamic or pituitary tumor (using skull x-rays, computed tomography [CT] scan, tomogram of sella turcica, or MRI [magnetic resonance imaging]); diabetes mellitus (using urinalysis and glucose tolerance testing); hyperthyroidism (using thyroid function tests); and drug addiction (using toxicology screens).

Attention-Deficit, Hyperactivity, and Impulsivity

Before or after starting school, the child may demonstrate poor concentration, distractibility, and a tendency to impulsiveness, with or without hyperactivity and learning problems. Table 35–12 lists organic causes that must be excluded.

Delay in Speech and Language Development

The child may manifest a relative delay in comprehending speech or in expressing and correctly enunci-

Table 35–10. Clinical situations likely to require special investigation.

Acute or subacute disintegration of development and behavior, with loss of previously attained developmental milestones, deterioration in school performance, and the emergence of erratic aggressive behavior, clinging dependency, or confusion
Acute psychotic episode
Anorexia or weight loss
Attention-deficit, hyperactivity, and impulsivity, especially if of recent or sudden origin
Delay in speech and language development, loss of previously acquired speech and language, or the recent emergence of deviant speech or language
Depression, especially if associated with slowed thinking, deterioration of concentration, vagueness, and fatigue
Episodic or progressive lapses or deterioration of awareness with dreaminess; obtundation; defect in the sensorium; and perhaps, subjective depersonalization, derealization, and hallucinosis
Episodic violence out of proportion to the apparent precipitant, often with memory gaps or amnesia for the episode
General or specific learning problems (eg, in reading, writing, or calculation)
Localized or generalized abnormal movements that may be associated with vocal abnormalities
Pervasive developmental impairment (especially if associated with an uneven profile of abilities)
Sleep disturbance or excessive drowsiness
Somatoform symptoms of recent onset that mimic a physical disorder but are not consistent with the typical pattern of physical disorder

ating words, phrases, and sentences. Table 35–13 lists organic causes that must be excluded.

Depression

The child or adolescent may become underactive or overactive; insomniac or hypersomniac; impaired in thought tempo, concentration, and energy; readily provoked to tantrum or weeping; socially withdrawn; or preoccupied with thoughts of low self-esteem, guilt, and loss. The differential diagnosis includes virtually any physical disorder that could sap energy, impair thinking, and disrupt the capacity to cope.

The following general systemic diseases should be excluded: malignancy, chronic infectious disease, viral infection (eg, influenza, infectious hepatitis, infectious mononucleosis), hypothyroidism, hypoadrenalism, chronic anemia, and subnutrition (eg, anorexia nervosa). Chronic intoxication with anticonvulsants

Table 35–11. Excluding organic causes of disintegration of behavior and development.

Possible Organic Cause	Special Investigations
General systemic disease	
Thyroid disorder	Thyroid function tests
Adrenal insufficiency	Adrenal function tests
Porphyria	Examination for urinary porphyrins
Disseminated lupus erythematosus (LE)	Examination for LE cells
Wilson's disease	Serum ceruloplasmin
Toxic factors	
Delirium due to systemic infection, electrolyte abnormality, or physiologic toxins	Electroencephalography; specific biochemical, bacteriologic, or virologic tests
Drugs (eg, intoxication with sympathomimetic drugs, anticholinergic drugs, hallucinogens, or anticonvulsants; withdrawal from sedatives)	Urine drug screen, blood toxicology
Central nervous system disease	
Seizure disorder	Electroencephalography with nasopharyngeal electrodes, telemetry
Space-occupying lesion	Skull x-ray, CT scan, MRI
Herpes encephalitis	Electroencephalography, examination of cerebrospinal fluid, immunologic testing
Metabolic or subacute viral encephalitis	Electroencephalography, examination of cerebrospinal fluid, immunologic testing
Degenerative diseases	Urine amino acids, electroencephalography, MRI, biopsy
Demyelinating disease	MRI
Leukemic infiltration of central nervous system	Examination of blood and cerebrospinal fluid

Table 35–12. Excluding organic causes of attention-deficit, hyperactivity, and impulsivity.

Possible Organic Cause	Special Investigations
Hyperthyroidism	Thyroid function tests (if there is other evidence of hyperdynamic cardiovascular function and sympathetic overactivity)
Plumbism	Urine lead levels, examination of blood for stippled cells, x-rays of long bones
Seizure disorder	Electroencephalography with nasopharyngeal leads
Sleep apnea	Otorhinolaryngologic examination, sleep electroencephalography and observation
Sydenham's chorea	Blood antistreptolysin-O antibody titer

or sedatives must be excluded (using urine drug screens and blood levels), as must degenerative central nervous disease (using central nervous system examination, specific tests for the systemic diseases being excluded, CT scan, or MRI).

It is often difficult to determine to what degree a child's depression is part of a pathophysiologic process or to what degree it represents a secondary psychological reaction to loss of function, hospitalization, restriction of freedom, lack of stimulation, or loneliness.

Episodic or Progressive Lapses or Deterioration of Awareness

The patient, usually an adolescent, may experience recurrent episodes during which he or she has a sense of being abruptly altered, different, or unreal and of observing the self as a spectator. The adolescent may perceive that the world is unreal and different or that conversations and scenes have been experienced previously in precisely the same manner. The following organic causes must be excluded: seizure disorder (using electroencephalography), cardiac arrhythmia (using electrocardiology), narcolepsy (using electroencephalography), migraine, and hallucinogenic drug use (using urine drug screen).

Episodic Violence

The child or adolescent may periodically lose control, assault others, or destroy property. The behaviors may be unheralded but usually arise from an emotional context of tension with or without alcohol or drug intake and are disproportionate to the apparent provocation. The individual may or may not have a conduct disorder. The following disorders must be excluded: temporal lobe seizures (using electroencephalography with nasopharyngeal leads), herpes encephalitis (using electroencephalography, immunologic study, and examination of cerebrospinal fluid for viral culture and immunology), drug effects (eg, alcohol, phencyclidine, hallucinogens, amphetamine) (using urine drug screen), and idiosyncratic reaction to alcohol (using patient's history).

General or Specific Learning Problems

The child or adolescent may manifest a general or specific difficulty in learning, particularly in reading, writing, written expression, calculation, or spatial skills. Table 35–14 lists organic causes that must be excluded.

Localized or Generalized Abnormal Movements

The child or adolescent may manifest repetitive movements that may or may not be partly or wholly under control. The following disorders must be excluded: attention-deficit/hyperactivity disorder, tic disorder, Sydenham's chorea (using antistreptolysin-O titer), Huntington's disease, Wilson's disease, paroxysmal choreoathetosis, dystonia musculorum deformans, cerebellar tumor or degeneration, and drug effects (eg, caffeinism, extrapyramidal side effects of neuroleptic medication).

Table 35–13. Excluding organic causes of speech and language development delay.

Possible Organic Cause	Special Investigations
Deafness	Acoustic testing
Palatal abnormality	Physical examination
Cerebral palsy	Neurologic examination
Mental retardation	Physical examination, psychological testing
Seizure disorder	Electroencephalography
Aphasia	Consult with speech pathology, neuropsychological testing
Developmental articulatory dyspraxia	Consult with speech pathology and pediatric neurology
Pervasive developmental disorder	See Table 35–11

Table 35–14. Excluding organic causes of learning problems.

Possible Organic Cause	Special Investigations
Visual defect	Test visual acuity and visual fields; ophthalmoscopy
Deafness	Acoustic testing
Cerebral palsy	Neurologic examination
Mental retardation	Physical examination, psychological testing
Seizure disorder	Electroencephalography
Dementia due to intracranial space–occupying lesion or cerebral degeneration	Neurologic examination: skull x-rays, CT scan, MRI
Inability to pay attention in class because of debilitating illness, fatigue, hunger, pain, or drug use	None

Pervasive Developmental Impairment

During infancy or afterward, the child may manifest a severe arrest or retardation of language, intellect, and social development. Additional features may include unexplained episodes of panic or rage, marked resistance to environmental change, hyperactivity, repetitive motor phenomena, and deviant speech and language. The onset may be in early infancy (before 30 months) or afterward (up to about 7 years). Sometimes the child regresses from a state of relatively normal development to a state of developmental impairment. More often, the child's abnormal development becomes evident gradually. Several organic causes must be excluded (Table 35–15).

Sleep Disturbance or Excessive Drowsiness

The child may present with hypersomnia, insomnia, nightmares, night terrors, restless sleep, or sleepwalking. Table 35–16 lists organic causes that must be excluded.

Somatoform Symptoms

The child or adolescent may develop a set of symptoms that mimic physical disorder. Common conversion symptoms are loss of consciousness, loss of phonation, motor impairment, abnormal movements, seizures, special sensory defect, anesthesia, pain, loss of balance, bizarre gait, or gastrointestinal complaints such as vomiting and abdominal pain. Conversion disorder can mimic many physical conditions. The inquiry plan should both exclude the hypothetical physical disorder and establish positive criteria for conversion (ie, emotional trauma coinciding with onset; pattern of symptoms representing the patient's naive idea of pathology; contact with a model for the disease; pattern of symptoms fulfilling a communicative purpose; secondary gain for the patient in the sense of nurturance, security, or avoidance of difficulty; and pattern of symptoms and signs inconsistent with physical disease). Table 35–17 lists the physical disorders especially likely to be mistaken for a conversion disorder.

Bailey A: Physical examination and medical investigations. Pages 79–93 in Rutter M, Taylor E, Hersov L (editors): *Child and Adolescent Psychiatry,* 3rd ed. Blackwell Scientific, 1994.

Gillberg C: Part III: Assessment. Pages 295–322 in Gillberg C (editor): *Clinical Child Neuropsychiatry.* Cambridge University Press, 1995.

Table 35–15. Excluding organic causes of pervasive developmental impairment.

Possible Organic Cause	Special Investigations
Hearing impairment	Acoustic testing
Aphasia	Speech pathology consultation, language testing
Seizure disorder	Electroencephalography
Chromosomal anomaly	Chromosome analysis (especially if the child looks dysplastic)
Metabolic disorder	Tests for amino acids in the urine (especially phenylketonuria)
Intracranial lesion	Skull x-ray, CT scan, MRI (only if an intracranial space–occupying lesion or demyelinating disease is suspected)
Herpes encephalitis	Virologic studies of the cerebrospinal fluid, immunologic testing (if there has been an acute or subacute regression), electroencephalography

Table 35–16. Excluding organic causes of sleep disturbance or excessive drowsiness.

Possible Organic Cause	Special Investigations
Seizure disorder	Electroencephalography (including polysomnography)
Delirium (eg, in acute febrile illness or toxic states)	Electroencephalography
Narcolepsy	Electroencephalography
Intoxication with or withdrawal from sedative, opiate, anticonvulsant, neuroleptic, or antidepressant drugs	Urinary drug screen
Hypoglycemia	Blood sugar (eg, insulinoma)
Sleep apnea	Polysomnography, otorhinolaryngologic examination
Any debilitating disease, especially disease associated with chronic hypoxia (eg, congenital heart disease, pulmonary insufficiency, anemia)	None

III. PERSONALITY EVALUATION

Joseph D. LaBarbera, PhD

PURPOSE OF THE PERSONALITY EVALUATION

Questions that come to the attention of clinicians often relate to differential diagnosis (ie, whether a pa-

tient is more appropriately assigned one DSM-IV diagnosis as opposed to another). However, even in this age of managed care and associated limitations on testing, psychologists are still occasionally asked to perform evaluations that characterize the patient beyond this reductionistic level and that describe the patient's resources and liabilities, underlying conflicts, stress tolerance, and so on. Indeed, many psychologists take the position that in order to effectively assign a specific diagnostic label it is frequently necessary to understand the functioning of the whole person.

Table 35–17. Excluding disorders likely to be mistaken for conversion disorder.

Possible Organic Cause	Special Investigations
General systemic disease	
Disseminated lupus erythematosus (LE)	Examination for LE cells
Hypocalcemia	Blood calcium
Hypoglycemia	Blood sugar (eg, insulinoma)
Porphyria	Urinary porphyrins
Central nervous system disease	
Multiple sclerosis	Neurologic examination, MRI
Movement disorders (chorea, dystonia musculorum deformans, Tourette's syndrome, Wilson's disease)	None
Spinal cord tumor	Neurologic examination, radiography, MRI
Intracranial space–occupying lesion (especially in brain stem, cerebellum, frontal lobe, or parietotemporal cortex)	Neurologic examination, skull radiography, CT scan, MRI
Seizure disorder	Electroencephalography
Migraine	None
Dystonic reactions produced by neuroleptic drugs	None

TYPES OF PERSONALITY EVALUATIONS

Personality evaluation can be divided into three main areas. These include behavior rating scales used to assess a patient's overt behavior and, by extension, psychological functioning; projective tests ordinarily used to describe a patient's underlying concerns, issues, perceptions of other people, and self-attributions (the "content" of the mind, if you will); and structural tests used to characterize the patient's psychological structure, including coping resources, typical defensive tactics, capacity for intimacy, and reasoning capacity (the "form" of the mind). A fourth group of scales is used to assess the patient's functioning with respect to a specific diagnosis, such as depression. Table 35–18 summarizes these scales.

Behavior Rating Scales

Behavior rating scales are used both by psychologists and by clinicians, including child psychiatrists. They describe a patient's functioning in everyday life, as a step toward understanding the patient. Perhaps the most well-known of such scales is Achenbach's Child Behavior Check List. This scale requires a parent to respond to questions related to the child's social functioning and behavioral problems. On the basis of these responses, the child is rated on a number of symptom groupings, or factors, that can be divided into two categories: those that reflect internalizing psychopathology (eg, sadness, withdrawal, anxiety) and those that reflect externalizing psychopathology (eg, temper outbursts, demandingness, stubbornness). Such rating scales, although perhaps limited in the amount of information obtained from the respondent, are useful in that they provide psychologists with data derived from a careful observer, namely the parent.

Projective Tests

Projective measures assume that a subject projects unconscious issues, themes, and expectancies onto an ambiguous external stimulus, thereby providing the diagnostician with meaningful clinical data. Traditionally, such techniques have been organized on the basis of their assumed depth of exploration. For example, the Incomplete Sentences Test, which requires a patient to complete sentence stems such as "I like" or "My mother," is assumed to gather information of which the patient is reasonably conscious or aware. Alternatively, the Thematic Apperception Test may evoke material that is deeper and less obvious in meaning to the patient. However, the latter task is hampered by the fact that such information is generally quite symbolic in nature and hence is open to misinterpretation on the part of the examiner. Moreover, data derived from projective testing often has limited connection to the specific question being posed by the referral source, which often relates to distinguishing between competing diagnostic possibilities or characterizing a patient's psychological assets and liabilities.

The reader may note that in discussing projective measures, we have yet to describe the Rorschach Inkblot Test. During the past 15 years or so, there has been much discussion of the nature of the Rorschach task. Various authors have noted that, in fact, there are two essential Rorschach functions. First, the Rorschach may serve as a projective measure, evoking material that leads us to define a person's idiosyncratic or specific concerns, fears, conflicts, or interests. For example, an abused teenage girl may provide the response "two men killing a little girl," emphasizing the degree to which this particular person fears or anticipates that aggressive males may victimize her.

Second, various authors have said that the real strength of the Rorschach task lies not in its projective function but in its use as a means of evoking behavior that can illuminate the patient's personality structure. For example, regardless of the particular content of a given protocol, one might assess the degree to which the outlines of a patient's perceptions match the outlines of the test stimuli, based on a consensus of others. Weakness in this regard may be interpreted as an impairment in perceptual accuracy or reality interpre-

Table 35–18. Types of personality evaluation.

Evaluation Type	Function	Examples
Behavior rating scales	Describe an individual's functioning in everyday life	Achenbach's Child Behavior Check List
Projective tests	Characterize an individual's underlying concerns	Incomplete Sentences Test Thematic Apperception Test
Structural tests	Depict a person's personality	Rorschach Inkblot Test Minnesota Multiphasic Psychiatric Inventory-A (MMPI-A) Millon Adolescent Personality Inventory
Specific diagnosis scales	Assess an individual's functioning with respect to a specific diagnosis	Children's Depression Inventory Revised Child Manifest Anxiety Scale

tation. Likewise, responses may be assessed with respect to unrealistic reasoning (eg, "looks like a bat because it's green"). In general, most contemporary research and clinical work on the Rorschach relates to this use as a perceptual-cognitive task, as opposed to a stimulus to fantasy.

Structural Tests

The Rorschach may be viewed as a structural task in the above-described manner. That is, information provided on this measure can be used to paint a picture of an individual quite apart from his or her worries, concerns, or problematic issues. In addition to the Rorschach, the Minnesota Multiphasic Personality Inventory-Adolescent (MMPI-A) is frequently administered to young patients. A revision of the MMPI-2 for adolescents, this scale involves the original set of basic scales, which assess functioning along dimensions such as depression, hypochondriasis, rebelliousness, and social introversion. The test is published with information permitting scoring on various subscales that compose the basic scales. Finally, content scales are provided that are, for the most part, rationally derived groupings of items relating to matters such as obsessiveness, family problems, and school problems. MMPI-A administration and interpretation proceeds much like the relevant scale for adults. The patient is asked to complete almost 500 questions, and responses are then interpreted based on patterns of scale elevations.

The MMPI-A cannot be administered to children under the age of 13 years. Instead, an MMPI-like technique, the Personality Inventory for Children, may be administered. This test requires a knowledgeable adult, preferably the primary caregiver, to characterize the child by answering over 400 questions. The responses can be scored to provide information in areas such as depression, somatic problems, delinquency, withdrawal, and so on. Both the MMPI-A and the Personality Inventory for Children contain validity scales to evaluate the respondent's response set (ie, attempts to provide an unrealistically positive or negative impression).

The Millon Clinical Multiaxial Inventory was originally published as an alternative to the MMPI, which was considered to be weak in several areas. For example, the MMPI has been considered excessively Axis I oriented, neglecting factors such as personality styles and disorders that may lay the groundwork for the development of Axis I features, such as affective disorders, anxiety disorders, and so on. Millon's tests also offer a different definition of scale elevations. Millon has made the point that, in view of the differing base rates for different forms of psychopathology, the traditional mode of interpreting personality scales is insufficient. The Millon Adolescent Clinical Inventory provides more of a focus on Axis II disorders.

Specific Diagnostic Scales

In this era of managed care, an emphasis has been placed on the definition of very specific questions for the psychologist to address. Thus scales assessing specific clinical entities are becoming used much more frequently than before. Traditional measures (eg, the Beck Depression Inventory) are often used. So too are versions adapted for younger patients such as the Children's Depression Inventory. The Revised Child Manifest Anxiety Scale is also used frequently.

Archer RP: *MMPI-A: Assessing Adolescent Psychopathology.* Lawrence Erlbaum Associates, 1992.

Exner JE: *The Rorschach: A Comprehensive System.* John Wiley & Sons, 1993.

Millon T: *Toward a New Personology.* John Wiley & Sons, 1990.

36

Diagnostic Formulation, Treatment Planning, & Modes of Treatment

Barry Nurcombe, MD

DIMENSIONS OF THE DIAGNOSTIC FORMULATION

The diagnostic formulation summarizes and integrates relevant issues from the biopsychosocial, developmental, and temporal axes. The **biopsychosocial axis** refers to multiple systems, from molecular to sociocultural, that interact constantly and are manifest in current objective behavior and subjective experience. The **developmental axis** is applied to different levels of the biopsychosocial axis in order to determine whether each level is developmentally normal, delayed, advanced, or deviant. The **temporal axis** refers to the ontogenesis of the individual from his or her origins to the present and beyond.

Biopsychosocial Axis

Current functioning is the expression of multiple biopsychosocial levels within the patient, as he or she interacts with the physical, family, sociocultural, occupational and economic environment. In order to evaluate present functioning, the clinician examines the levels and systems described in Table 36–1.

Developmental Axis

Each level of the biopsychosocial axis can be assessed with regard to what would be expected for that age. Some of these assessments (eg, height, weight, head circumference) are very accurate. For others (eg, intelligence), although a number of assessment instruments are available, existing measures represent a composite of skills potentially affected by extraneous factors (eg, social class, motivation). For still others (eg, ego defenses, working models of attachment), measurement techniques are relatively crude and the norms subjective.

Nevertheless, during interviewing and mental status examination, the clinician will scan the levels shown

in Table 36–2 for delay, precocity, or deviation from the normal and, when appropriate, order formal special investigations.

Temporal Axis

All of us have come from somewhere, exist where we are now, and are headed somewhere. Using the temporal axis, the clinician explores the unfolding of a problem up to the present time and attempts to predict where the patient is headed. The mileposts in this evolution can be classified, somewhat arbitrarily, in the following sequence: (1) predisposition, (2) precipitation, (3) presentation, (4) pattern, (5) perpetuation, (6) potentials, and (7) prognosis.

1. Predisposition: What early biological or psychosocial factors have stunted or deflected normal development, or rendered the patient vulnerable to stress? Table 36–3 lists several examples.

Given the current state of knowledge, it is often dif-

Table 36–1. The biopsychosocial axis.

Level	Systems Assessed
Physical level	Peripheral organ systems Immune system Autonomic system Neuroendocrine system Sensorimotor system
Psychological level	Information-processing systems Communication systems Social competence Internal working models of the self and others Unconscious conflicts, ego defenses, and coping style Patterns of psychopathology
Social level	Physical environment Family system (nuclear and extended) Sociocultural systems (peers, adults, school)

Table 36–2. The developmental axis.

Level	Systems Assessed	Assessment Method
Physical level	Peripheral organ systems (eg, height, weight, head circumference)	Growth charts
	Sensorimotor system	Developmental assessment, neuropsychological testing
Psychological level	Information processing	Intelligence testing, special testing for memory and other cognitive functions, educational attainment testing, neuropsychological testing
	Communication	Speech and language assessment, neuropsychological testing
	Social competence	Behavioral observation, psychological testing
	Internal working models	Interviewing, personality testing
	Conflicts, defenses, coping style	Interviewing, behavioral observation, personality testing
	Symptom patterns	Interviewing, checklists, structured interviews
Social level	Family system, peer relations, school functioning	Family interviews, observations, checklists

ficult or impossible to reconstruct these factors and their effects on the growing organism, particularly with regard to inherited vulnerability or propensity (eg, as hypothesized for depressive disorder). However, postnatal deprivation or trauma may be recorded, for example, in the patient's medical record.

2. Precipitation: A precipitant is a physical or psychosocial stressor that challenges the individual's coping capacity and causes him or her to exhibit the symptoms and signs of psychological maladjustment. Table 36–4 lists several examples. A temporal relationship exists between the precipitant and the onset of symptoms. Sometimes the precipitant (eg, interparental conflict) later becomes a perpetuating factor. Sometimes the precipitant is a reminder of a previous traumatic experience. Sometimes the precipitant ceases, and the patient returns to normal coping. Sometimes the precipitant ceases, but maladaptive coping persists or even worsens. In that case, perpetuating factors must be sought (see below).

Not all current patterns of psychopathology have precipitants. Some psychopathologies (eg, early infantile autism) have evolved continuously since infancy or early childhood. The clinician should look for a precipitant when normal functioning is succeeded by the onset of psychopathology.

3. Presentation: The clinician should consider why the family is presenting at this time. Is it, for example, that the child's behavior worries them or disrupts family functioning? Has the family's capacity to tolerate the child's behavior deteriorated? If so, why?

4. Pattern: The current pattern represents the current biopsychosocial axis. The clinician should evaluate the patient's current physical, psychological, and social functioning. To the extent that abnormalities in physical functioning (eg, somatoform symptoms), information processing (eg, amnesia), communication (eg, mutism), internal models (eg, self-hatred), coping style (eg, compulsive risk-taking), and social competence (eg, social withdrawal) can be defined as psychopathologic phenomena, the clinician will assemble configurations of symptoms and signs

Table 36–3. Predisposing biological and psychosocial factors.

Genetic vulnerability or propensity
Chromosomal abnormality
Intrauterine insult or deprivation
Perinatal physical insult
Postnatal malnutrition, exposure to toxins, or physical trauma
Physical illness
Neglect or maltreatment
Parental loss, separation, or divorce
Exposure to psychological trauma

Table 36–4. Examples of precipitating factors.

Physical
  Physical illness
  Surgery
  Accidental injury
Psychosocial
  Civilian catastrophe
  War
  Parental conflict, separation, or divorce
  Loss of a loved one
  Rejection
  Academic stress
  Hospitalization

Table 36–5. Factors involved in the quality of family interactions.

The quality of communication about important matters between family members. Do they express their messages clearly and do they listen to and hear each other?

The capacity of family members to share positive and negative emotion. Are they able to praise and encourage each other? Can they express love? If they are angry with one another, can they say so without losing control?

The sensitivity of family members to each other's feelings. Are they aware when other family members are sad, upset, hurt, enthusiastic, or happy, and do they respond accordingly?

The capacity of the family to set rules and control behavior. Are they clear about rules and consistent in their following up of whether the rules are followed? If children must be disciplined, are penalties appropriate and timely?

The appropriateness and flexibility of family roles. Is it clear who does what in the family? If one family member is absent or indisposed, can other family members fill in?

The capacity of the family to solve problems and cope with crises. When the family is confronted with a problem, can family members work together to solve it?

that form categorical syndromes (eg, residual posttraumatic stress disorder) and dynamic patterns (eg, traumatophilia, introversion of aggression, unassimilated conflict about past trauma).

The clinician also evaluates the family, and the social, school, cultural, and economic environment in which the family lives. Table 36–5 lists the issues to consider in evaluating the quality of family interactions.

5. Perpetuation: If the precipitating stress (eg, parental conflict) does not dissipate, the child's maladaptation is likely to continue. If the stress is removed, the child is likely to spring back to normality. If not, the clinician must ask why not. The reason could be either within or outside the child.

Internal perpetuating factors can be biological or psychological. For example, overwhelming psychic trauma can trigger a train of unreversed biochemical derangements, involving catecholamines, corticosteroids, and endogenous opiates, that cause the numbing and hyperarousal associated with the traumatic state. Unresolved psychic trauma can also produce a personality that seeks compulsively to reenter traumatic situations, thus reexposing the self to victimization and further trauma.

External perpetuating factors include the reinforcement of child psychopathology that occurs in dysfunctional family systems, for example, the protective parent who shields a delinquent child from punishment, or the anxious, enmeshed parent who reinforces a child's separation anxiety and school refusal.

6. Potentials: In addition to addressing psychopathology and defects, the clinician should consider the child's physical, psychological, and social strengths. A child with a learning problem may be talented at sports or be physically attractive, or he or she may have a supportive family. In treatment planning, the clinician must consider how strengths can be harnessed in order to circumvent or compensate for defects or problems.

7. Prognosis: The clinician should predict what is likely to happen with or without treatment, remembering that it is impossible to anticipate all the unfortunate and fortuitous happenstance that can block, divert, or facilitate a particular life trajectory.

THE DIAGNOSTIC FORMULATION: AN EXAMPLE

The clinician should summarize the diagnostic formulation in a succinct manner. Consider the following example:

Susan is a 14-year-old adolescent who has a 2-month history of the following symptoms, which were precipitated by her observation of a house fire in which the 4-year-old brother she was babysitting perished: traumatic nightmares, intrusive memories, frequent reminders, emotional numbing, avoidance of situations that remind her of the event, startle responses, irritability, depressive mood, social withdrawal, guilt, and suicidal ideation. She has acute posttraumatic stress disorder with complicated bereavement and secondary depression precipitated by psychic trauma.

Susan's physical health is good and her sensorimotor functioning intact. She is of low average intelligence and approximately 2 years retarded in reading, language, and mathematical attainment. She has very low self-esteem, views herself as the family drudge, and is resentful of her alcoholic father's domination of her mother and her siblings. She has a close relationship with a married sister.

Susan's symptoms are reinforced by her mother's bereavement and the family's emotional insensitivity and poor communication. This is a large family, in which Susan has played the role of parentified child, supporting the mother and taking responsibility for much of the housekeeping and child care. Susan was predisposed to develop a depressive trauma reaction by her longstanding (but suppressed) resentment at being the family drudge and at being the frequent target of her father's emotional abuse.

Susan has the following strengths and potentials: She has supportive friends; her older married sister is very helpful; and she enjoys child care.

Without treatment, the current posttraumatic stress disorder is likely to continue. There is a risk of suicide.

GOAL-DIRECTED TREATMENT PLANNING

The purpose of treatment can range from short-term crisis management to long-term rehabilitation, remediation, or reconstruction. For that reason, the goals of treatment will vary according to the level of care the patient is receiving. The following levels of care are provided in child and adolescent mental health services: very brief hospitalization, brief hospitalization, brief partial hospitalization, extended day programs, residential treatment, intensive outpatient care, and outpatient care (see Chapter 16). Very brief hospitalization (1–14 days) is suited to crisis alleviation. Brief hospitalization (2–4 weeks) aims at stabilization, as do brief partial hospitalization programs. Residential treatment programs, extended partial hospitalization programs, and outpatient treatment programs have more ambitious goals related to remediation, reconstruction, or rehabilitation.

COMPONENTS OF GOAL-DIRECTED TREATMENT PLANNING

The essence of goal-directed planning is the extraction of treatment foci from the diagnostic formulation and the expression of the foci as goals and objectives, with predictions of the time required for goal attainment. Based on the goals, treatment methods can be selected. Based on the objectives, goal attainment (ie, treatment effectiveness) can be monitored until the goal is attained and treatment terminated (see Figure 36–1).

Foci

Those problems, defects, and strengths that can be addressed, given the resources and time available, should be extracted from the diagnostic formulation.

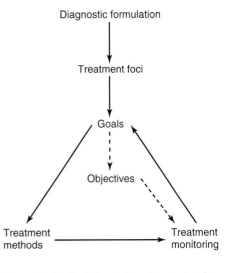

Figure 36–1. Goal-directed treatment planning.

The clinician should not merely list behaviors in an unintegrated "laundry list." Pivotal foci, those internal or external factors that activate, reinforce, or perpetuate psychopathology, are especially important. For example, mother-child enmeshment may be the key to a problem of separation anxiety. A behavioral program for separation anxiety applied in the school setting will fail unless the clinician addresses the mother's involvement in her child's fear of leaving home.

Goals

Goals indicate what the clinician or clinical team aims to achieve, at the given level of care, on the patient's behalf (Table 36–6). A goal is a focus preceded by a verb. The focus "depressive mood," for example, becomes "Alleviate depressive mood" when rewritten as a goal. As described in the introduction to this section, goals are categorized according to whether they promote crisis alleviation, stabilization, reconstruction, remediation, rehabilitation, or compensation. Crisis alleviation, stabilization, reconstruction, and remediation foci are preceded by verbs such as "alle-

Table 36–6. Categorization of treatment goals.

Category	Example
Behavioral	Reduce the frequency and intensity of aggressive outbursts.
Educational	Remediate reading deficit.
Familial	Enhance quality of communication and emotional sensitivity between father and patient.
Medical	Stabilize diabetes mellitus.
Physical	Increase weight.
Psychological	Alleviate unresolved conflict concerning past physical abuse.
Social	Reduce the intensity and frequency of provocative behavior toward authority figures.

viate," "ameliorate," "remediate," "eliminate," "reduce the intensity of," "reduce the frequency of," "stabilize," or "counteract." Rehabilitation and compensation goals are preceded, for example, by "enhance," "augment," "facilitate," or "increase the intensity/frequency of." Behavioral goals are best suited to crisis alleviation and stabilization settings (eg, inpatient hospitalization).

Objectives

Goals assert what the clinician aims to do. Objectives indicate what the patient will (be able to) do, say, or exhibit at the end of that stage of treatment. Objectives should always be stated in behavioral terms. Goals and objectives may be intermediate (eg, at the point of discharge from hospital) or terminal (eg, at the end of outpatient treatment). Goals and objectives may be ambitious (eg, "Resolve internal conflict regarding punitive father figure" or "The patient will be able to cooperate approximately with his superior at work in the performance of his assigned tasks") or advisedly limited (eg, "Gain weight. At the end of hospitalization, the patient will weigh 79 pounds").

Whereas goals take the long, abstract view, objectives indicate when enough is enough, making the clinician or the team accountable and alerting them when treatment is not progressing as well as predicted.

Target Date

For each set of goals and objectives, a time is predicted. For example, the goal "Alleviate depressive mood and suicidal ideation" may have the objective "The patient will express no suicidal ideation spontaneously or during mental status examination for a period of 1 week." The clinician may predict that such a stabilization objective will be attained, for example, in 3 weeks.

Therapy

For each goal, the clinician selects a therapy or set of therapies, according to the following criteria: most empirical support, resource availability (ie, clinical resources, time, finances), least risk, greatest economy (ie, time, expense), and appropriateness to family values and interaction style.

The modes of therapy are discussed in the next section of this chapter. Do not confuse the term "objective" with a therapeutic strategy or tactic. An objective is the behaviorally stated endpoint of a phase of treatment. Treatment strategies or tactics (eg, "Encourage father to attend patient's baseball games") represent the means of getting to the endpoint, that is, the adaptation of a particular intervention to the needs of the patient and family.

Treatment Monitoring

Objectives are the key to monitoring both the patient's progress and the treatment plan's effectiveness. Progress can be assessed by periodic milieu observa-

tions, mental status examinations, measurement of vital signs or other physical parameters, laboratory testing, standard questionnaires, rating scales, or psychological testing. To the extent that an objective can be measured, the measure should be stated (eg, "The patient's score will drop to below 12 on the Conners Parent-Teacher Questionnaire"). Not all objectives can be measured numerically, and for some, subjective, qualitative monitoring is required. The clinician should not fall into the trap of deleting objectives that cannot be measured objectively. Some pivotal goals and objectives, particularly those related to psychodynamic or family systems issues, require qualitative monitoring; and ingenious assessments of dynamic issues can sometimes be planned. For example, the goal "Resolve conflict about past sexual abuse" could be monitored, for a particular patient, in terms of the frequency, duration, and acuity of dissociative episodes.

Revision

If progress stalls, the patient deteriorates, or unforeseen complications arise, the clinician or team will be alerted by the treatment monitors. Then a decision must be made. Continue? Change the goals? Modify the objectives? Reconsider the therapy? Periodic treatment monitoring (eg, monthly for outpatient treatment, daily for inpatient or partial hospitalization) keeps the clinician or team accountable and prevents therapeutic drift.

Termination

When the objectives are reached, the patient is ready to either move on to the next phase or level of treatment or terminate the treatment.

THE DISADVANTAGES & ADVANTAGES OF GOAL-DIRECTED TREATMENT PLANNING

Goal-directed treatment planning must be learned. It does not build on the naturalistic process of treatment planning (which usually starts from treatments rather than goals). It requires the clinician to be explicit about matters that are customarily avoided or blurred (eg, target dates). Imposed on uncomprehending or resistant clinicians, goal-directed treatment plans may be relegated to the status of irrelevant paperwork or to a mindless printout from a computerized treatment planning menu.

Goal direction has numerous advantages, however. It provides a common intellectual scaffolding with which a clinical team can plan. It serves notice to clinicians to monitor progress and review their plans if they are ineffective. It provides a useful basis for negotiating with families, obtaining truly informed consent, and facilitating or consolidating the treatment alliance. Finally, it is a potentially useful tool for utilization review and outcome research.

Nurcombe B: Goal-directed treatment planning and the principles of brief hospitalization. J Am Acad Child Adolesc Psychiatry 1989;27:26.

Nurcombe B, Gallagher RM: *The Clinical Process in Psychiatry.* Cambridge University Press, 1986.

TYPES OF TREATMENT

A sophisticated, multifaceted, individually designed management plan requires a comprehensive biopsychosocial, temporal, and developmental diagnostic formulation. The diagnostic formulation should be shared with the patient and parents at a special interview, and the parents' and patient's collaboration sought in following the goal-directed treatment plan.

In almost every case, a combination of techniques will be used in child and adolescent psychiatry because the biopsychosocial needs of patients demand a multifaceted treatment plan. For example, an adolescent hospitalized for anorexia nervosa is likely to require a combination of the following forms of therapy: (1) pediatric treatment to correct subnutrition and fluid and electrolyte imbalance, follow nutritional progress, and treat medical complications; (2) behavior modification to counteract voluntary restriction of food intake; (3) nutritional education; (4) individual expressive psychotherapy to provide insight and promote conflict resolution; and (5) family therapy to help the family undo the parent-child enmeshment and hidden interparental conflict that are commonly associated with this disorder.

There are three broad modes of treatment in child and adolescent psychiatry: *physical, psychological,* and *social.* Within each mode there are modalities (eg, medication); within each modality there are techniques or classes (eg, tricyclic antidepressant medication); and within each technique there are specific subtechniques, therapies, or agents (eg, imipramine). Research into the treatment of child and adolescent psychiatric disorders has far to go. Even though few if any specific treatments have been established, evidence is gathering that some empirical treatments (eg, clomipramine in obsessive-compulsive disorder) work better than placebo. Until more evidence is at hand, many of the indications for treatment described in the sections that follow are based on clinical experience rather than controlled experimentation. This chapter introduces readers to the broad range of modalities available. Subsequent chapters relate the details of treatment for particular conditions.

PHYSICAL TREATMENT

Electroconvulsive treatment is not used in child and adolescent psychiatry except perhaps in rare cases of adolescent catatonic schizophrenia unresponsive to antipsychotic medication. The only physical treatment of significance is psychopharmacology.

1. GENERAL PRINCIPLES OF PSYCHOPHARMACOLOGY

1. Before commencing pharmacotherapy, the clinician should obtain from the patient a full psychiatric and medical history, a medication history, and a history of allergic reactions; ascertain what other drugs the patient is currently taking; and ask whether the patient is using illicit drugs.
2. Psychopharmacologic treatment should always be part of a broader treatment plan derived from a diagnostic formulation.
3. Parents and child should be involved in the treatment plan; informed consent for pharmacologic treatment must be obtained; and parents and child should be educated about the nature, side effects, risks, and benefits of the medication proposed (and of the alternative treatments, if any).
4. Psychopharmacologic treatment targets symptoms, not disorders.
5. The clinician should ask the parents and child about misconceptions they may have of drug treatment in general or the particular pharmaceutical agent prescribed. For example, parents may be afraid that drug treatment will lead to addiction, whereas children may feel inferior if they must take drugs ("crazy pills") at school.
6. The clinician should seek a working alliance with responsible, informed parents and an educated patient.
7. When necessary, after getting permission, the clinician should form a working alliance with the school.
8. A medical examination, appropriate special investigations, and laboratory tests (including pregnancy testing in female patients) are required in order to rule out contraindicated conditions.
9. The clinician should quantify the targeted baseline symptom(s) and monitor progress with appropriate checklists or rating scales.
10. The clinician should select an appropriate drug according to the following criteria: least known risk and best evidence of efficacy. If possible, the clinician should follow FDA guidelines, but if not, he or she should make a rational choice based on available scientific evidence. If the choice is nonstandard, the clinician must document a risk-benefit analysis and ask for a consultation from a colleague.
11. It is advisable to start with a low dosage and increase it gradually until the symptoms remit, no further improvement accrues, the upper recommended dosage is reached, or complications occur. Treatment should be maintained at the lowest effective dosage.

12. The clinician should monitor side effects regularly.
13. Side effects (eg, the sedative effect of imipramine) can sometimes be used to treat other symptoms.
14. The clinician should monitor serum levels if he or she is unsure whether the patient is receiving an adequate dose, or if there is a possibility that a toxic level of drug has been reached.
15. The clinician should prescribe medication for as short a period as possible. When medication is an adjunctive part of treatment, for example, it may be possible to discontinue it when psychosocial therapies are in place. "Drug holidays" are sometimes appropriate (eg, when the child is out of school).
16. Polypharmacy should be avoided. The clinician should use drug combinations only after single appropriate drugs have been given an adequate trial and found ineffective.
17. When withdrawing medication, the clinician should taper the dosage.

2. CLASSES OF PSYCHOPHARMACOLOGIC AGENTS

The following classes of medication are used in child and adolescent psychiatry: psychostimulants, adrenergic agents, antidepressants, antipsychotics, lithium, anxiolytics, anticonvulsants, and miscellaneous agents.

Psychostimulants

The best-known psychostimulants are methylphenidate, dextroamphetamine sulfate, and magnesium pemoline. They are the drugs of choice for treating attention-deficit/hyperactivity disorder and narcolepsy in childhood and adolescence, and possibly in preschool children. They should be used with caution if the patient or family members have a history of substance abuse or antisocial behavior; if the patient has tic disorder, psychosis, liver impairment, growth failure, or a cardiac abnormality; or if the patient is pregnant. They should be used with caution if the patient is taking a monoamine oxidase inhibitor (MAOI). Common side effects are insomnia, irritability, anorexia, nausea, abdominal pain, and increased hyperactivity. Less common side effects are depression, social withdrawal, psychosis, tics, growth retardation, and hepatitis (pemoline). Psychostimulants should be monitored carefully if used in combination with anticoagulants, anticonvulsants, guanethidine, phenylbutazone, heterocyclic antidepressants (eg, imipramine), sympathomimetics, or MAOIs. Patients taking psychostimulants should be monitored for involuntary movements, heart rate, and growth rate.

Adrenergic Agents

The most commonly prescribed adrenergic agents are clonidine and guanfacine. Both are often used in combination with methylphenidate in treating attention-deficit/hyperactivity disorder. Clonidine targets impulsivity and hyperactivity and has also been used in treating Tourette's syndrome, opioid withdrawal, nicotine withdrawal, anxiety disorder, agitation, bipolar disorder, and posttraumatic stress disorder. Guanfacine targets inattention, impulsivity, and hyperactivity in attention-deficit/hyperactivity disorder. Clonidine should be used with caution if depression, a cardiovascular or renal disorder, or diabetes mellitus is present. Its main side effects are sedation, hypotension, headache, dizziness, gastrointestinal symptoms, and depression. Guanfacine, though less sedating, has similar side effects. Both drugs have a potential for augmenting the sedating effects of other central nervous system (CNS) depressants and for a hypertensive rebound after abrupt discontinuation.

Antidepressants

The antidepressants most often used in child and adolescent psychopharmacology are tricyclic antidepressants (TCAs) and selective serotonin reuptake inhibitors (SSRIs).

A. Tricyclic Antidepressants: The most commonly prescribed TCAs are imipramine, amitriptyline, desipramine, nortriptyline, and clomipramine. These drugs are used to treat depression, enuresis, attention-deficit/hyperactivity disorder, separation anxiety disorder, and posttraumatic stress disorder. Clomipramine is the drug of choice in treating obsessive-compulsive disorder and has also been used to treat trichotillomania. The TCAs are contraindicated if the patient is pregnant, has had a hypersensitivity reaction, or is taking an MAOI. They should be used with caution if the patient has schizophrenia or an epileptic, cardiac, or thyroid disorder. Side effects include increased pulse rate, cardiac conduction slowing, arrhythmia, and heart block; anticholinergic symptoms; anxiety, psychosis, mania, and confusion; seizures; insomnia; tics, tremor, and incoordination; skin rash; and photosensitivity. Sudden death has been associated with high dosages of imipramine and desipramine, possibly because of cardiac conduction abnormalities. A baseline electrocardiogram (ECG) is indicated, and ECG monitoring is required at intervals as the dosage is increased. A complete blood count, differential diagnosis, pregnancy testing, and substance abuse history should be obtained, because when TCAs are taken along with marijuana and nicotine, their cardiac side effects may be aggravated. Plasma levels should be drawn 1 week after the last dosage increase. TCAs must be tapered when being discontinued.

B. Selective Serotonin Reuptake Inhibitors: The three members of the SSRI class currently prescribed in the United States are fluoxetine, sertraline, and paroxetine. They are indicated for the treatment of depression, attention-deficit/hyperactivity disorder, obsessive-compulsive disorder, trichotillomania, anxiety disorder, eating disorder, posttraumatic stress disorder, drug craving, and self-injurious behavior. They are contraindicated if the patient has been taking MAOI drugs within the past 5 weeks, if the patient is pregnant, or if the patient has liver disease. There is no evidence that fluoxetine precipitates suicidal behavior. Common side effects are gastrointestinal symptoms, nervousness, restlessness, insomnia, intensified dreaming, dry mouth, and sexual dysfunction. Less common side effects are excitability, mania, rash, hair loss, and seizures. The SSRIs interact with MAOIs, TCAs, lithium, and tryptophan and should not be prescribed with benzodiazepines or buspirone. Before administering an SSRI, the clinician should record the patient's vital signs, height, weight, and liver function, and should test for pregnancy. Patients should be monitored at each visit for the emergence of mania and excitation, and every 3 months for height and weight. A medication trial of 6–8 weeks is required. SSRIs may be discontinued without tapering.

C. Trazodone: Trazodone is a second- or third-line antidepressant with sedative side-effects. The indications for trazodone use in children and adolescents have not been established; but it has been used to treat depression associated with marked insomnia.

D. Bupropion: Bupropion is a second- or third-line drug for treatment of major depressive disorder and possibly attention-deficit/hyperactivity disorder. Indications have not been established for children and adolescents.

E. Monoamine Oxidase Inhibitors: The best-known members of the MAOI class are tranylcypromine, phenelzine, isocarboxyzid, and moclobemide. Because of their potentially dangerous interaction with dietary tyramine and with a variety of other drugs, MAOIs are not recommended for treatment of disorders in children and adolescents. MAOIs are described in more detail in Chapter 21.

Antipsychotics

The most commonly prescribed antipsychotics are the phenothiazines, thioxanthenes, diphenylbutylpiperidines, butyrophenones, dibenzoxazepines, and indolic compounds. They are indicated for the treatment of schizophrenia, delirium, and Tourette's syndrome. They have also been used to alleviate self-injury and aggressiveness in pervasive developmental disorder and for nonspecific agitation. They are contraindicated if the patient has a history of hypersensitivity, agranulocytosis, or neuroleptic malignant syndrome. They should be used with caution in pregnant patients, in patients who are in a coma, and in patients who are also taking CNS depressants. Antipsychotic agents are described in more detail in Chapter 19.

Lithium

Lithium is indicated in the treatment of bipolar disorder in adolescents, and it has been used in the treatment of bipolar disorder in children (to augment TCAs). It has also been used to treat bulimia and attention-deficit/hyperactivity disorder and to alleviate violent behavior. Bipolar disorder can be difficult to distinguish from schizophrenia, schizoaffective disorder, and schizophreniform disorder. Adolescent patients who exhibit psychosis should be monitored carefully for mood disorders, and a trial of lithium should be considered. In adult psychotic patients, lithium potentiates neuroleptic medication and stabilizes mood. Lithium in combination with haloperidol alleviates explosive aggression in patients with conduct disorder. Lithium has been used to treat intractable attention-deficit/hyperactivity disorder, but its effectiveness is uncertain. Lithium may be useful, perhaps in combination with fluoxetine, in treating bulimia. Lithium is contraindicated if the patient has had a previous allergic reaction to the drug. It should be used with caution in pregnant patients and in patients who have severe dehydration; renal, cardiovascular, or thyroid disease; or diabetes mellitus. Lithium mobilizes calcium and may affect bone growth. Lithium is described in more detail in Chapter 21.

Anxiolytics

The anxiolytics most commonly prescribed in child and adolescent psychiatry are benzodiazepines, antihistamines, and azaspirones (buspirone). Antidepressant drugs and the β-blocker propranolol also have antianxiety effects.

The benzodiazepines most often used in child and adolescent psychiatry are diazepam, chlordiazepoxide, oxazepam, clonazepam, alprazolam, lorazepam, midazolam, triazolam, and flurazepam. The chief antihistamines are diphenhydramine, hydroxyzine, and promethazine.

Partly because of diagnostic confusion in the field of juvenile anxiety disorders and partly because of the paucity of controlled studies, knowledge concerning the indications for anxiolytics is patchy. Anxiolytics have been used to treat panic disorder, separation anxiety disorder, generalized anxiety disorder, posttraumatic stress disorder, insomnia, sleepwalking, night terrors, and acute violent behavior. Anxiolytics are described in more detail in Chapter 22.

The high-potency anxiolytics alprazolam and clonazepam may be useful in treating panic disorder and agoraphobia. Lorazepam and oxazepam can be useful in the short-term treatment of agitation or acute violence. Buspirone causes less sedation and has less abuse potential than do benzodiazepines and may be useful in treating generalized anxiety disorder and obsessive-compulsive disorder. Benzodiazepines should be used to treat insomnia only for relatively brief periods of time and only if the immediate benefits outweigh the risks of hangover and rebound insomnia.

Propranolol has been used with aggressive patients and in treating performance anxiety, generalized anxiety disorder, panic disorder, hyperventilation, posttraumatic stress disorder, withdrawal from alcohol, neuroleptic-induced akathisia, and lithium tremor.

Anticonvulsants

The anticonvulsants most often used in child and adolescent psychopharmacology are carbamazepine, valproic acid, and phenytoin. They have been used to treat alcohol withdrawal, trigeminal neuralgia, bipolar disorder, major depression, intermittent explosive disorder, attention-deficit/hyperactivity disorder, psychosis, enuresis, and night terrors. Carbamazepine and valproic acid may be used to supplement lithium in treating refractory mania and as an adjunct to neuroleptic medication in the treatment of psychosis. Carbamazepine is a second-line drug in the treatment of depression. There is a need for controlled studies of the effectiveness of these three drugs in intermittent explosive disorder and conduct disorder. Carbamazepine is a drug of last resort in treating attention-deficit/hyperactivity disorder. Anticonvulsant medication is contraindicated in patients with known hypersensitivity, bone marrow depression, liver disease, or renal disease; in pregnant patients; and in patients concurrently taking MAOIs. Anticonvulsants are described in more detail in Chapter 21.

Miscellaneous Agents

Opiate antagonists (eg, naloxone, naltrexone) have been used to counteract self-injurious behavior in mentally retarded children and in children with early infantile autism. There are conflicting reports concerning the long-term benefit of naltrexone in these conditions. Triiodothyronine has been used to augment TCAs in treating adult major depression. There are no controlled studies of its use in juveniles. Despite initially promising data, the usefulness of fenfluramine in treating autistic disorder has not been confirmed.

Green WH: *Child and Adolescent Clinical Pharmacology,* 2nd ed. Williams & Wilkins, 1994.

Green WH: Principles of Psychopharmacology and Specific Drug Treatments. Pages 772–807 in Lewis M (editor): *Child and Adolescent Psychiatry: A Comprehensive Textbook,* 2nd ed. Williams & Wilkins, 1996.

Kutcher SP: *Child and Adolescent Psychopharmacology.* WB Saunders, 1997.

Rosenberg DR, Holttum J, Gershon S: *Textbook of Pharmacology for Child and Adolescent Psychiatric Disorders.* Brunner/Mazel, 1994.

PSYCHOLOGICAL TREATMENT

Psychological treatments include a variety of techniques in four main groups: (1) individual psychotherapy, (2) behavior modification, (3) social and cognitive-behavioral therapy, and (4) remedial therapies and education.

1. INDIVIDUAL PSYCHOTHERAPY

The different forms of individual psychotherapy vary in accordance with four dimensions: (1) brief versus protracted; (2) supportive, directive, and reality-oriented versus expressive, exploratory, and oriented to unconscious material; (3) structured, interpretive versus unstructured, client-centered; and (4) play-oriented versus verbally-oriented.

Supportive Psychotherapy

Supportive psychotherapy represents a loose collection of techniques without distinctive theoretical basis derived broadly from humanistic understanding and personal experience.

A. Aims: The aims of supportive psychotherapy are to (1) establish a close relationship; (2) define current problems; (3) consider and implement problem solutions; (4) avoid ego-alien, unconscious material; and (5) restore preexistent ego defenses.

B. Indications: Supportive psychotherapy is indicated for the treatment of adjustment disorders, temporary emotional crises due to situational stress, remitted psychotic disorders when the patient is in need of rehabilitative help, and substance use disorders.

C. Contraindications: Supportive psychotherapy should not be used to treat severe disorders that require more specific or more extensive therapy.

D. Dangers: Supportive psychotherapy is relatively safe except for the possibility of excessive dependency on the therapist. The development of an undesirably intense relationship with the therapist is a potential problem with any therapeutic technique, but it is more likely in intensive psychotherapy.

Client-Centered Therapy

Client-centered therapy is a form of play therapy or verbal psychotherapy in which the patient (client) is gently encouraged to explore personal feelings and attitudes. In client-centered therapy the therapist empathically reflects the feelings, explicit or implicit, in the patient's play and verbal or nonverbal communications. The pace of therapy is determined by the patient. Therapy is usually brief to intermediate in duration.

A. Aims: The aims of client-centered therapy are to (1) establish an empathic, accepting relationship and (2) to encourage self-exploration by judicious reflection of feeling.

B. Indications: Client-centered therapy is indicated for the treatment of adjustment reactions and mild anxiety disorders in children and adolescents. It is also useful for treating problems of adolescence that involve career choice, academic commitment, or mild identity confusion.

C. Contraindications: Client-centered therapy should not be used to treat severe disorders, especially psychosis or prepsychosis, conduct disorder, and borderline personality.

D. Dangers: Client-centered therapy could lead to excessive or unresolved dependence in some cases. Otherwise, it is relatively safe.

Exploratory Psychotherapy

Exploratory psychotherapy is a form of play therapy or verbal psychotherapy in which the patient's unconscious conflicts, usually in a specified area, are resolved by interpretations based on the patient's play or verbal and nonverbal behavior. It is usually extended in duration (6–12 months) and moderately intensive (1–2 times per week).

A. Aims: The aims of exploratory psychotherapy are to (1) establish a relationship, (2) recognize transference feelings, (3) help the patient to become aware of unconscious wishes and defenses by judicious interpretation, and (4) terminate the relationship.

B. Indications: Exploratory psychotherapy is indicated for treatment of anxiety, somatoform, and dissociative disorders; personality disorders and interpersonal difficulties related to neurotic conflict; and trauma spectrum disorders.

C. Contraindications: Exploratory psychotherapy is contraindicated if the patient's ego strength is too fragile to cope with the emergence of traumatic material in the context of a close therapeutic relationship, or if the patient has a psychotic or prepsychotic disorder.

D. Dangers: Exploratory psychotherapy could cause an intense transference reaction with severe emotional turmoil.

Child & Adolescent Psychoanalysis

Child and adolescent psychoanalysis is an extensive (eg, 1–5 years) and intensive (eg, 3–5 times per week) form of exploratory therapy in which a radical resolution of unconscious conflicts is sought through the exploration of a transference relationship between patient and analyst.

A. Aims: The aims of child and adolescent psychoanalysis are to (1) establish a relationship, (2) encourage spontaneous expression of thoughts and emotions (through play and conversation), (3) aid resolution of unconscious conflict by interpreting unconscious wishes and ego defenses, (4) support the patient in working through personal solutions to problems that have been rendered conscious in analysis, and (5) terminate the relationship.

B. Indications: Child and adolescent psychoanalysis is indicated for treatment of anxiety disorders, somatoform disorders, trauma spectrum disorders, and borderline personality disorder (if not severe).

C. Contraindications: Child and adolescent psychoanalysis should not be used to treat psychotic disorders, pervasive developmental disorder, conduct disorders, severe personality disorders, or other disorders in patients who cannot tolerate intimacy.

If this form of therapy is to succeed, the patient must have reasonable capacity to tolerate tension and intimacy, the ability to express emotions in words, the motivation to seek help, and considerable economic resources.

D. Dangers: The dangers of child and adolescent psychotherapy are similar to those associated with exploratory psychotherapy.

2. BEHAVIOR MODIFICATION

Behavior modification represents a group of loosely associated therapeutic techniques derived from the principles of learning.

A. Aims:

1. Systematic desensitization—Exposing the patient to progressively more anxiety-provoking stimuli, while at the same time teaching him or her to relax, or pairing the phobic stimuli with a pleasant activity (such as eating), or associating the phobic stimuli with pleasant fantasy.

2. Reinforcement of coping responses—Rewarding responses that counteract, or are incompatible with, the problem behavior.

3. Exposure—Forced entry into the phobic situation and the prevention of avoidance.

4. Shaping—Rewarding progressive approximations to desired responses, especially in habit training.

5. Token reinforcement—Poker chips, stars on a calendar, and the like can be exchanged at stipulated times for reward (eg, money, privileges). The tokens are used for immediate reinforcement of desirable behavior.

6. Aversion—Interrupting undesirable behavior (eg, self-destructive head banging) by applying a noxious stimulus (eg, an electric shock) whenever the undesirable behavior is expressed.

7. Time-out—Deprivation of anticipated reinforcement (eg, attention) by consistently isolating the child when the undesirable behavior (eg, tantrums) is expressed.

8. Massed practice—Multiple repetitions of an undesired behavior (eg, a habit spasm) in order to weaken its association with an underlying emotional state (eg, anxiety).

9. Substitution—Replacing an undesirable behavior (eg, smoking) with a neutral one (eg, chewing).

B. Indications: Behavioral therapy is indicated for treatment of phobic disorders, eating disorders, oppositional defiant disorder, and preschool management problems (eg, tantrums) as well as for habit training (eg, functional enuresis or encopresis).

C. Contraindications: Behavioral therapy should not be used to treat psychosis or in situations in which the patient has transference fears of, or is resistant to, being controlled.

D. Dangers: Behavioral therapy could lead to deterioration or aggravation of the psychiatric condition (reported after implosion) or to the appearance of new undesirable behavior (eg, if desensitization is too limited in scope).

3. SOCIAL & COGNITIVE-BEHAVIORAL THERAPY

Social and cognitive-behavioral therapy is a group of techniques that focus on intermediate cognitive responses as the primary target for intervention, with the aim of changing behavior.

A. Aims:

1. Participant modeling—Combining the observation of a model who behaves in a desired way with the opportunity to practice the desirable behavior.

2. Interpersonal problem-solving—Teaching the patient to infer the causes and consequences of interpersonal events and actions, and to consider alternative solutions to interpersonal dilemmas.

3. Cognitive-behavioral therapy—Helping the patient to define and alter the self-defeating expectations and attitudes that underlie maladaptive behavior.

4. Self-instruction training—Teaching the patient to reflect upon a problem rather than act impulsively.

B. Indications: Social and cognitive-behavioral therapy is used to encourage behavior that will counteract a phobia, to overcome social impulsiveness or inhibition, to counteract the pessimism that predisposes an adolescent to depression, to replace motor impulsiveness with reflectiveness, or to counteract obsessive-compulsive behavior.

C. Contraindications: Social and cognitive-behavioral therapy should not be used to treat psychosis.

D. Dangers: Social and cognitive-behavioral therapy could lead to deterioration or aggravation of the psychiatric condition or to the appearance of new undesirable behavior if the therapy is too limited in scope.

4. REMEDIAL THERAPIES & EDUCATION

Remedial therapies and education represent a large group of remedial or rehabilitative programs designed to help the child or adolescent overcome chronic physical, educational, or social handicap, or make the most of talents and potential strengths.

A. Aims: Remedial therapies and technologies have been developed for a variety of disabilities, including cerebral palsy, orthopedic handicap, blindness, deafness, aphasia, and learning disability.

These therapies may be provided in a separate institution (eg, a school for the hearing impaired) or incorporated in a regular school program (ie, in the case of mainstreaming). The current trend is toward mainstreaming whenever possible.

B. Dangers: The child may be labeled and discriminated against in a separate (categorical) program, a disabled child's needs may overwhelm teacher and classmates in a mainstream program, or the child may not be accepted by unimpaired classmates.

SOCIAL TREATMENT

Group Therapy

In group therapy, groups of six to eight children or adolescents, with a group leader, meet anywhere from daily to once per week. Groups for preschool children emphasize social stimulation. Activity groups for latency-age children emphasize socialization. Groups for adolescents focus on mutual support and the sharing of common problems. Group therapy is often used as an adjunct to other forms of therapy (eg, during hospitalization).

A. Aims: The aims of group therapy are to (1) provide social experience, (2) allow expression of feeling in an accepting environment, (3) foster awareness of common experience and allow the group to consider solutions to common problems, and (4) promote group cohesiveness (eg, during hospitalization).

B. Indications: Group therapy is indicated during hospitalization of latency-age children or adolescents. It is useful for treating problems with social isolation and for helping adolescents who share the same problem (eg, divorce, physical handicap, substance abuse).

C. Contraindications: Group therapy should not be used to treat disorders in patients who are disturbed by forced intimacy.

D. Dangers: Preferably, though it is not always possible, the group should be balanced, with a judicious combination of aggressive "instigators," compulsive "neutralizers," and dependent "followers." If there are too many aggressive children, the group will explode. If there are too many neutralizers or followers, group process gets bogged down.

Role Play

Role play is a subtechnique of group therapy, commonly used in hospital treatment, in which a recent social incident is reenacted. The role players usually are not the individuals who were involved in the incident, but those who were involved will help with the reenactment.

Role playing is used to help patients develop insight and consider common problems and alternative solutions. It can be used as a medium for cognitive-behavioral therapy.

Casework for Parents

Casework varies from intermittent contact with the patient's parents (in order to keep them informed about progress) to intensive therapy, for example, in regard to marital problems, child management, or health care.

A. Aims: Casework may be used to provide information, promote more consistent child management or health care, institute a behavior modification program at home, resolve marital problems, or prepare one or both parents for referral to another therapist.

B. Indications: Casework is indicated whenever the child is in intensive individual therapy, in order to keep parents aware and involved; and to facilitate behavior modification in the natural environment by enlisting the parents as agents of the therapeutic plan.

C. Contraindications: If parents are mutually antagonistic, they may need to be interviewed separately.

Conjoint Family Therapy

Conjoint family therapy is a form of group therapy in which the patient's whole family receives treatment. The family members meet with a family therapist (sometimes with male or female cotherapists) for intensive brief therapy (in order to promote crisis resolution) or for more extended periods of time (if radical changes in family interaction are proposed).

A. Aims: Conjoint family therapy is used to resolve family crises; to promote a common understanding of family problems; to consider alternative solutions to common problems, especially when the family has reached an impasse; to foster a common awareness of previously unexpressed family rules, roles, and expectations; and to alter long-standing maladaptive interaction patterns (eg, coalitions, rifts, scapegoating, enmeshment, or skewing), abnormal patterns of communication, and emotional insensitivity between family members.

B. Indications: Conjoint family therapy is indicated when the patient is recovering following hospitalization for severe mental illness and whenever the patient's problems are perpetuated by deleterious family interaction patterns.

C. Contraindications: Conjoint family therapy should be used with caution in the following situations: (1) when family members are excessively hostile or intrusive toward the patient, (2) when the parents are on the verge of separating, or (3) when the patient needs to become independent of the family system.

D. Dangers: Conjoint family therapy could result in the problem shifting to another family member, as the homeostasis of the family is changed when the designated patient improves. It also could accentuate a preexistent rift between the parents.

Psychiatric Hospitalization

Psychiatric hospitalization involves the placement of a severely disturbed child or adolescent in a psychiatric inpatient unit that has special programs and a therapeutic milieu designed for children or adolescents. The special program coordinates psychiatric, pediatric, psychological, nursing, educational, and oc-

cupational care and therapies. The placement may be brief (eg, 1–2 weeks), intermediate (2–4 weeks), or extended (longer than 1 month) depending on the patient's needs.

A. Aims: Psychiatric hospitalization aims to temporarily separate a disturbed patient from the family; to stabilize suicidal, self-injurious, aggressive, or disorganized psychotic behavior; or to institute treatment programs that require complex coordination and intensive monitoring.

B. Indications: Psychiatric hospitalization is warranted when suicidal, aggressive, or disruptive behavior is beyond the control of the family and is caused by treatable mental illness (especially schizophreniform, schizophrenia, and severe mood disorders). It is also warranted when the child's severe emotional disorder is perpetuated by complex family interaction pathology or when comprehensive diagnostic evaluation of a complex case is needed, especially for cases that require the coordination of a number of specialties (eg, an adolescent who has a chronic physical illness associated with a serious psychiatric disorder and family interaction problems).

Specific disorders warranting hospitalization include the following: depressed mood and suicidality secondary to emotional stress; severe anxiety, somatoform, and dissociative disorders; severe eating disorder; substance use disorder; organic mental disorder (eg, substance-induced delirium or hallucinosis); and pervasive developmental disorder (for diagnosis, behavioral analysis, and management planning in aggressive or self-injurious patients).

C. Contraindications: Psychiatric hospitalization should not be used to treat conduct disorder of the undersocialized, aggressive type without treatable comorbid psychiatric disorder or in some cases of personality disorder (especially of borderline type) in which there is a danger of reinforcing a patient's chronic sick role. Furthermore, it is contraindicated if hospitalization could cause alienation between the patient and his or her family.

D. Dangers: Psychiatric hospitalization may accentuate dependency and inadvertently train the child or adolescent to be a "patient." It may lead to scapegoating and permanent extrusion by an alienated family. Also, excessive pressure on inexperienced inpatient unit staff could lead to communication breakdown and deleterious effects on all patients. These dangers can be averted if the safeguards listed in Table 36–7 are implemented.

Specialized Partial Hospitalization or Residential Units

Residential programs are based usually on an educational or behavioral (rather than a medical) model, with programs designed for children or adolescents who have special problems. Partial hospitalization programs are based on a psychiatric inpatient model, except that the patient returns home each night. In all

Table 36–7. Safeguards against the dangers of hospitalization.

Clear but nonautocratic psychiatric leadership
Staff selected for defined but overlapping roles
Clarity of general aims and individual treatment goals
Good coordination of, and communication between, staff
A plan for postdischarge disposition
Family involvement in admission, diagnosis, management planning, and continuing treatment
An environment that, as far as possible, approximates that of the average child of that age (in schooling, social opportunity, and recreation) and that deemphasizes chronic invalidism
Partial hospitalization for less severely disturbed patients
Planned discharge to outpatient or partial hospital care as soon as possible
Good coordination between regional inpatient unit and community mental health agencies and clinicians

Table 36–8. Examples of partial hospitalization programs.

Pediatric hospital units for infants and children who have experienced physical neglect or abuse affecting physical health
Preschool daycare programs for children with special physical, educational, or psychological needs (eg, culturally disadvantaged children or children with pervasive developmental disorders)
Residential units for children and adolescents with severe physical handicaps or disorders
Residential units for adolescents with substance dependence (usually emphasizing behavior control)
Residential units for adolescents with conduct disorder (usually emphasizing behavior control)
Residential units for the mentally retarded
Boarding schools for adolescents with learning and emotional problems

cases, the child's or adolescent's problems are more severe or complex than can be dealt with in conventional outpatient treatment. Examples are given in Table 36–8.

Other Placements Away From Home

Other placements may involve temporary or permanent placement of a child or adolescent in a foster or group home. Options include (1) foster placement as a temporary expedient, while the parents and child are in treatment, preparatory to the return of the child; (2) permanent foster placement, with or without view to adoption, after disintegration of the home of origin or when the parents are unable to provide adequate care; (3) group home placement for children and adolescents who are emotionally too overreactive to cope with the emotional vicissitudes of foster home placement; and (4) community group homes designed to promote independent-living skills for mentally retarded adolescents or adolescents with pervasive developmental disorders.

Lewis M: Treatment. Sect 7, Pages 765–934 in Lewis M (editor): *Child and Adolescent Psychiatry: A Comprehensive Textbook,* 2nd ed. Williams & Wilkins, 1996.

Section V.
Syndromes & Their Treatments in Child & Adolescent Psychiatry

Disorders Usually Presenting in Infancy or Early Childhood (0–5 years)

37

Barry Nurcombe, MD, Mark L. Wolraich,MD, Michael Tramontana, PhD, & Wendy Stone, PhD

I. DEVELOPMENTAL DISORDERS OF ATTACHMENT, FEEDING, ELIMINATION, & SLEEPING

Barry Nurcombe, MD

Normal infants are born with the capacity to attach to their parents and to elicit care from them. Defects in the infant's capacity to attach or elicit care, and deficiencies or disruption in the response of the caregiver, can be associated with a number of conditions such as reactive attachment disorder, rumination disorder of infancy, nonorganic failure to thrive, and psychosocial dwarfism. These conditions commence in infancy and, if not corrected, distort later social and intellectual development. Sleep problems often commence in the first 2 years of age. Pica and elimination disorders are usually first diagnosed between 2 and 5 years of age.

DISORDERS OF ATTACHMENT

DSM-IV Diagnostic Criteria

Reactive Attachment Disorder

A. Markedly disturbed and developmentally inappropriate social relatedness in most contexts, beginning before age 5 years, as evidenced by either (1) or (2):

(1) persistent failure to initiate or respond in a developmentally appropriate fashion to most social interactions, as manifest by excessively inhibited, hypervigilant, or highly ambivalent and contradictory responses (eg, the child may respond to caregivers with a mixture of approach, avoidance, and resistance to comforting, or may exhibit frozen watchfulness)

(2) diffuse attachments as manifest by indiscriminate sociability with marked inability to exhibit appropriate selective attachments (eg, excessive familiarity with relative strangers or lack of selectivity in choice of attachment figures)

B. The disturbance in Criterion A is not accounted for solely by developmental delay (as in mental retardation) and does not meet criteria for a pervasive developmental disorder.

C. Pathogenic care as evidenced by at least one of the following:

(1) persistent disregard of the child's basic emotional needs for comfort, stimulation, and affection

(2) persistent disregard of the child's basic physical needs

(3) repeated changes of primary caregiver that prevent formation of stable attachments (eg, frequent changes of foster care)

D. There is a presumption that the care in Criterion C is responsible for the disturbed behavior in Criterion A (eg, the disturbances in Criterion A began following the pathogenic care in Criterion C).

533

Reprinted, with permission, from *Diagnostic and Statistical Manual of Mental Disorders,* 4th ed. Copyright 1994 American Psychiatric Association.

General Considerations

Major Etiologic Theories: Bowlby conceptualized attachment as the biologically based tendency for infants to elicit care from and maintain proximity to their mothers. Babies elicit care by crying, vocalizing, reaching, sucking, making eye contact, and smiling. They maintain proximity first by clinging and following and later by using their mother as a secure base from which to explore the world. The mother, in turn, ministers to the infant's physical, emotional, and social needs and protects the infant from danger. Both mother and infant monitor proximity in the second year, so that the child's exploration is curtailed when danger is perceived by one or both attachment partners.

The infant who perceives the mother as consistently sensitive and responsive to his or her needs develops a secure relationship. In contrast, if the mother's availability is perceived as unpredictable, the child will develop a sense of insecurity. A loss or severing of the attachment relationship leads to a condition interpreted as the early equivalent of grief.

By 12 months of age, the normal infant has developed a primary attachment figure, the caregiver to whom the child preferentially seeks proximity when threatened or insecure. Infants also have one or more secondary attachment figures to whom they will go if the primary figure is unavailable. Through multiple transactions involving the dual-attachment system of mother and infant, the child constructs working models of attachment—internal representations of the self in relation to others, with perceptual, mnemonic, affective, and behavioral components. These structures have profound implications for later social relationships and for the child's capacity to trust other people. The child's working models of attachment may be associated with a sense of predictability, reliability, affection, and well-being, or with inconsistency, ambivalence, rejection, loss, rage, anxiety, or sadness.

Disordered attachment is characterized by the capacity for attachment to a primary figure; however, the attachment relationship is pervaded by excessive inhibition, heedlessness, or role reversal. In **disrupted attachment,** the mother-infant relationship has been severed, and the infant reacts with developmental arrest, disturbances of eating and sleep, loss of interest in surroundings and play, social withdrawal, and apparent depression.

Severe disturbances or disruptions of the attachment relationship are likely to disrupt or impair one or more of the following aspects of development: (1) relationships with and interest in other people; (2) the capacity to explore the world; (3) cognitive development; (4) the regulation of activity, sleep, feeding, and elimination; or (5) physical growth.

By the end of the first year of life, mother-infant attachment relationships can be characterized as secure, avoidant, resistant, or disorganized. Upon reunion with the mother after a brief separation, the infant will greet the mother and seek proximity (secure), avoid the mother (avoidant), resist the mother with irritation and ambivalence (resistant), or demonstrate freezing, confusion, stereotyped movements, and incoherent, contradictory behavior (disorganized). Disorganized attachment predicts later disruptive behavior disorder. Table 37–1 describes the factors that cause disorders of attachment.

The mother's working models of attachment, developed from her own early attachment experiences, affect her capacity to respond to the infant's attachment needs. If the mother's working models of self-other attachment are suffused with ambivalence, rage, sadness, or emptiness, and her representation of an attachment figure is characterized by rejection, sadism, explosiveness, inconsistency, or remoteness, a similar pattern of behavior is likely to be repeated with the infant. Thus when unresolved parental conflicts are reactivated by the demands of infant care, "ghosts in the nursery" can disrupt or preclude good mothering.

Clinical Findings

A. Reactive Attachment Disorder: Reactive attachment disorder represents a failure of the infant to develop a normal attachment relationship to a primary

---

Table 37–1. Factors that cause disorders of attachment.

A relative incapacity of the mother or primary caregiver to provide consistent affection, to minister to the child's physical needs, or to convey to the child that he or she will be protected from danger

A relative insensitivity or lack of attunement by the mother to the infant's affective states, with a corresponding failure to respond promptly and appropriately to the infant's needs and to provide adequate tactile stimulation

A deficiency in the infant's capacity to elicit care from the mother or to attach to her

Extremes of infant temperament—either marked sluggishness and withdrawal or excessive irritability, hypersensitivity, aversion from touch, and lack of adaptability

A combination of a lack of maternal capacity, sensitivity, or interest and a defect in the infant's capacity for attachment or self-regulation

A severance of the attachment relationship as a result of loss or separation, particularly if the infant's environment subsequently fails to provide adequate surrogate care

The exposure of the infant to multiple, changing caregivers, particularly if the care provided is perfunctory and lacking in affection

attachment figure. The infant demonstrates one of two types of reaction: (1) socially withdrawn, emotionally constricted, anergic, and apparently unable to derive pleasure from social contact or play; or (2) socially indiscriminate and emotionally shallow. Both types of reactive attachment disorder are associated with parental neglect or maltreatment or institutional child-rearing with multiple caregivers. Infants exposed to early maltreatment demonstrate disorganized attachment as toddlers and grow into socially withdrawn or aggressive, disruptive children.

B. Disordered Attachment: In disordered attachment, the infant has a primary attachment figure, but the attachment relationship is pathologic, with an imbalance between proximity seeking and exploration. There are three types: (1) disordered attachment with inhibition, (2) disordered attachment with self-endangerment, and (3) disordered attachment with role reversal.

In **disordered attachment with inhibition,** the infant is emotionally constricted, lacking in vitality, socially avoidant, and loath to explore the environment even when it is apparently safe to do so. The child clings persistently to the mother or avoids contact with her.

Children who demonstrate **disordered attachment with self-endangerment** are reckless, heedless, and accident prone. Even when hurt, they rebuff their mother's attempts to comfort them. Sometimes they are self-injurious, banging their heads or biting themselves. When anxious, they are more likely to run away than to seek contact comfort from their parents.

In **disordered attachment with role reversal,** the child exhibits a precocious, overdeveloped solicitousness to the mother, alternating with punitive, bossy, controlling behavior.

C. Disrupted Attachment: Infants older than 6 months (the age at which the primary attachment figure is first recognized) react to separation from or loss of the attachment figure with the following sequence of behavior: (1) protest, (2) depression, and (3) detachment. Children in the stage of protest cry, demand that the parent return, and reject the attempts of others to comfort them. Depression and detachment are associated with sad facies, anergia, insomnia, anorexia, loss of interest in surroundings, social withdrawal, "empty" clinging, and developmental arrest or regression. The child reacts to reminders of the primary attachment figure by ignoring or rejecting them or with a reactivation of protest.

Differential Diagnosis

Attachment disorders should be distinguished from pervasive developmental disorder, mental retardation, and language disorder. Pervasive developmental disorder, particularly infantile autism, is characterized by delay and deviance in the development of social relationships, language, and intellect. The impairment of social relationships in autism is profound and not re-versible by effective parenting. Furthermore, a history of parental failure, maltreatment, or loss is not usually encountered, and autism is associated with characteristic peculiarities of movement, language, and intellectual patterning.

Mental retardation aggravated by parental neglect or maltreatment presents a difficult differential diagnosis. Attachment relationships are intact in uncomplicated cases of mental retardation, other than in the profoundly retarded. Similarly, children with developmental language disorders do not demonstrate attachment pathology unless the language delay is associated with parental neglect.

Treatment

In the most egregious circumstances, parental rights must be terminated and early adoption sought. In most cases, however, remedial treatment will be appropriate.

The assessment of the family, and particularly of the parent-child interaction, has therapeutic implications, as described in Chapter 34. Parent-infant psychotherapy addresses (1) parental problems that impair care-giving, (2) the constitutional or temperamental factors in the infant that impede attachment, and (3) the match between the infant's needs and temperament and the parent's style of nurturance. Parenting problems could be related to current psychopathology (eg, depression); unresolved conflict related to past trauma, abuse, rejection, or neglect; or inexperience and lack of flexibility. Other, more experienced parents in mutual support groups can offer helpful advice concerning feeding, daily care, methods of consolation, and play. Nurse home visitors can work with parents to improve the quality of the match between the infant's needs and temperament and the parent's sensitivity and responsiveness, and to help parents enjoy their children.

Comorbidity

Reactive attachment disorder is a serious biopsychosocial condition. Older studies reported significant mortality and severe psychosocial morbidity associated with this disorder. However, the negative outcomes of these studies are compounded by the very poor quality of the institutions in which the studied children were housed. A number of investigations have compared the outcome of higher quality institutional rearing with that of early adoption or placement in foster care. Children raised initially in institutions tend to become more restless, distractible, disobedient, oppositional, and irritable than do control subjects. Children adopted early from institutions are better attached to their adoptive parents and siblings than are those who have been reunited with their families of origin.

For maximum benefit to intellectual development, children should probably be placed well before 4½ years of age. However, this question remains: Is there a watershed age beyond which the effects of early adoption are irreversible? In any case, a radical change of circumstances is required to remedy reactive attachment disorder and, despite the likelihood of individual differences in the capacity to benefit from environmental enrichment, it would be prudent to place children as early as possible.

Prognosis & Course of Illness

The prognosis of reactive attachment disorder and disordered and disrupted attachment has not been studied thoroughly. Insecure and, particularly, disorganized attachment during infancy have been found to predict disruptive behavior, impulse-control problems, peer relationship problems, oppositional behavior, low self-esteem, and lower social competence in preschool and school-aged children.

Lieberman AF, Zeanah CH: Disorders of attachment in infancy. Child Adolesc Psychiatr Clin N Am 1995;4:571.

FEEDING & EATING DISORDERS OF INFANCY OR EARLY CHILDHOOD

PICA

DSM-IV Diagnostic Criteria

A. Persistent eating of nonnutritive substances for a period of at least 1 month.
B. The eating of nonnutritive substances is inappropriate to the developmental level.
C. The eating behavior is not part of a culturally sanctioned practice.
D. If the eating behavior occurs exclusively during the course of another mental disorder (eg, mental retardation, pervasive developmental disorder, schizophrenia), it is sufficiently severe to warrant independent clinical attention.

Reprinted, with permission, from *Diagnostic and Statistical Manual of Mental Disorders,* 4th ed. Copyright 1994 American Psychiatric Association.

General Considerations

A. Major Etiologic Theories: The cause of pica is not known. Several theories have been proposed. The nutritional theory relates pica to iron deficiency and an appetite for minerals. However, it is uncertain whether iron deficiency, which is often found in association with pica, is primary or secondary. Another theory suggests that pica, a normal phenomenon in infancy when the mouth is used as a perceptual organ, is a manifestation of delayed development; that is, it represents the retention of developmentally immature behavior, particularly in socially disadvantaged and mentally retarded children. Yet another theory, which

applies to pregnant women who chew starch or clay, emphasizes the role of cultural beliefs and custom.

B. Epidemiology: The prevalence of pica varies widely. It is much more common among rural pregnant black women and among institutionalized mentally retarded patients.

Clinical Findings

Children with pica eat dirt, stones, ice, paint, burned match heads, starch, feces, hair, and so on. Laboratory studies are needed to rule out lead poisoning. Aside from lead poisoning, pica can lead to excessive weight gain, malnutrition, intestinal blockage, intestinal perforation, and malabsorption.

Treatment

The proper treatment of pica is unclear. Behavioral techniques have been recommended. Ferrous sulfate therapy has been recommended on the theory that the condition is caused by iron deficiency.

Lacey EP: Phenomenology of pica. Child Adolesc Psychiatr Clin N Am 1993;2:75.

RUMINATION DISORDER

DSM-IV Diagnostic Criteria

A. Repeated regurgitation and rechewing of food for a period of at least 1 month following a period of normal functioning.
B. The behavior is not due to an associated gastrointestinal or other general medical condition (eg, esophageal reflux).
C. The behavior does not occur exclusively during the course of anorexia nervosa or bulimia nervosa. If the symptoms occur exclusively during the course of mental retardation or a pervasive developmental disorder, they are sufficiently severe to warrant independent clinical attention.

Reprinted, with permission, from *Diagnostic and Statistical Manual of Mental Disorders,* 4th ed. Copyright 1994 American Psychiatric Association.

General Considerations

A. Major Etiologic Theories: In infants, rumination is thought to be associated with deprivation of maternal attention or neglect. In older, mentally retarded patients, rumination has been ascribed to self-stimulation and is most often encountered in a setting of institutional neglect. Gastroesophageal reflux, hiatus hernia, or esophageal spasm may be diagnosed, but the significance of these conditions is not clear, and it should not be assumed that, even if present, they cause rumination. Rumination has been interpreted as a complex, learned behavior reinforced by maternal attention or oral sensory gratification.

B. Epidemiology: The incidence of rumination in the general population of infants is unknown. Rumination among the mentally retarded occurs more commonly in males, particularly among the profoundly retarded. The prevalence in institutional populations is 6–10%.

Clinical Findings

Ruminators stimulate their gag reflexes manually or adopt postures that facilitate regurgitation. The frequency can vary from several times per minute to once per hour. Regurgitated food fills the cheeks and may be stirred about by the tongue before being reswallowed or spit out. Ruminators can sometimes be diverted from the practice temporarily, if they are offered interesting things to do after eating.

Differential Diagnosis

Rumination should be differentiated from other causes of vomiting and gastroesophageal reflux.

Treatment

In infants, it may be enough to provide consistent, noncontingent, contact comfort, with holding, rocking, eye contact, and soothing vocalizations. In older children (eg, in those who are mentally retarded), or in infants for whom adequate nurturance has been insufficient to eliminate the condition, behavioral treatment will be required. The design of the specific treatment plan depends on a detailed behavioral analysis of the antecedents, the behavior, and its consequences. Usually reinforcement techniques are applied first, and aversive techniques are held in reserve in case reinforcement alone is insufficient. When the perpetuating reinforcer is intrinsic (eg, self-stimulation in older patients) rather than extrinsic (eg, operant vomiting reinforced by parental attention), treatment may need to be prolonged. The feeding of satiating quantities of high-caloric food is sometimes useful as a preliminary treatment in underweight patients. The provision of a substitute oral stimulant, such as chewing gum, after meals can also be helpful.

Prognosis & Course of Illness

Rumination has a serious prognosis. Unless treated successfully, it could lead to inanition and death.

Johnson JM: Phenomenology and treatment of rumination. Child Adolesc Psychiatr Clin N Am 1993;2:75.

FEEDING DISORDER OF INFANCY OR EARLY CHILDHOOD (NONORGANIC FAILURE TO THRIVE)

DSM-IV Diagnostic Criteria

A. Feeding disturbance as manifested by persistent failure to eat adequately with significant failure to gain weight or significant loss of weight over at least 1 month.

B. The disturbance is not due to an associated gastrointestinal or other general medical condition (eg, esophageal reflux).
C. The disturbance is not better accounted for by another mental disorder (eg, rumination disorder) or by lack of available food.
D. The onset is before age 6 years.

Reprinted, with permission, from *Diagnostic and Statistical Manual of Mental Disorders,* 4th ed. Copyright 1994 American Psychiatric Association.

General Considerations

A. Major Etiologic Theories: Organic and nonorganic failure to thrive are not distinguished sharply. Aside from the 10% of cases of failure to thrive that are caused by clear-cut physical disease, subtle constitutional or temperamental factors in the infant often interact with a relative impairment of parenting capacity to cause this condition. However, all cases have the same final common pathway: insufficient food intake.

Among the subtle constitutional factors that interact with or trigger environmental failure are the following: hypotonic lips; poor sucking; tongue dysfunction; oral-motor impairment; poor coordination of sucking and swallowing; gastroesophageal reflux; minor forms of cerebral palsy; Sandifer's syndrome (involving tension spasm and esophageal reflux); sleep apnea; and the aftermath of nasogastric, parenteral, or gastrostomy feeding. In some cases, feeding difficulties disrupt the mother-infant interaction, engendering a vicious cycle.

Early studies implicated maltreatment and neglect as the cause of nonorganic failure to thrive. Better controlled studies have cast doubt on the universality of this theory; however, follow-up studies of these children have demonstrated an increased risk of subsequent maltreatment and neglect.

Controlled studies of maternal characteristics have produced conflicting results. Some studies suggest an increased prevalence of depression, personality disorder, and substance abuse. Controlled observations of the mother-infant interaction have demonstrated in mothers less reciprocity, less sensitivity to the infant's cues, greater conflict over control issues, and more negative affect; whereas infants with nonorganic failure to thrive are relatively more inhibited, less cooperative, and more likely to avert their gaze from their mothers.

B. Epidemiology: Nonorganic failure to thrive has been found to occur in 2–5% of admissions to pediatric hospitals. It appears to be equally common in both sexes. English studies that followed birth cohorts in a socially disadvantaged London health district identified 3.5–4.6% as having nonorganic failure to thrive by 12 months of age. Most of these children had never been referred for pediatric evaluation. About 20% of families living in a socially disadvantaged inner city area will have at least one child who fails to thrive. Late birth order in a large, closely spaced family is a risk factor.

Clinical Findings

Nonorganic failure to thrive is usually noticed in the first year of life. The infant is cachectic and prone to infection. Developmental delay is the rule, but the severity of the delay is variable. These children are listless and hypotonic, exhibiting abnormal postures and intense gaze. They prefer inanimate objects to people, and they are prone to self-stimulation. They look sad and are irritable, withdrawn, or hypervigilant.

Although in clinical studies the mothers of children with nonorganic failure to thrive have seemed to demonstrate psychopathology, controlled studies have yielded inconsistent findings. One such study demonstrated increased rates of depression, substance abuse, and personality disorder. High rates of insecure and disorganized attachment were noted in the children.

Differential Diagnosis

Nonorganic failure to thrive and psychosocial dwarfism (discussed later in this chapter) must be distinguished from organic causes of failure to thrive and short stature, such as hereditary short stature, chromosomal abnormality (eg, 46 X0, trisomy 23), dysmorphic short stature (eg, Noonan's syndrome, Russell-Silver syndrome), skeletal dysplasia (eg, achondroplasia, hypochondroplasia), endocrinopathy (eg, growth hormone deficiency, growth hormone resistance, hypothyroidism, hypercortisolism, congenital adrenal hyperplasia), other causes of malnutrition, or systemic disease (eg, chronic pulmonary disease, congenital heart disease, malabsorption syndrome, renal disease, chronic anemia). Children with nonorganic failure to thrive or psychosocial dwarfism were usually of normal size at birth.

Treatment

If the child's survival is in question, he or she must be removed from the home and hospitalized or placed into foster care. In extreme circumstances, parental rights must be terminated.

A variety of behavioral techniques have been used to counteract or remediate abnormal feeding behavior in infants. These techniques are used in tandem with individual psychotherapy aimed to enhance maternal consistency and sense of competence and to decrease maternal stress. If the mother has a diagnosable psychiatric disorder (eg, depression or substance use disorder), it should be treated. Casework can be provided in the home by a trained social worker or nurse, with attention given to financial, marital, or employment problems. Dyadic therapy involving both infant and mother is recommended when unresolved issues related to pathogenic maternal working models of attachment impede adequate child care. It is unclear whether or when supportive casework is preferable to dyadic therapy.

Prognosis & Course of Illness

Most children with nonorganic failure to thrive do not become psychosocial dwarfs. Psychosocial dwarfism is potentially reversible, if the child is removed from the noxious home environment. However, if the child is returned to an adverse situation, developmental failure will recur. The later the onset, the better the prognosis for intellectual and language functioning.

PSYCHOSOCIAL DWARFISM

Diagnostic Criteria

- Growth failure (marked linear growth retardation and delayed epiphyseal maturation)
- Neuroendocrine dysfunction (reversible hypopituitarism)
- Bizarre eating and drinking behavior (eg, polyphagia, polydipsia, hoarding)
- Dramatic weight gain after hospitalization but reversion to growth failure after return to family

General Considerations

A. Major Etiologic Theories: Psychosocial dwarfism is caused by dysfunctional growth hormone secretion which reverses when the child is hospitalized and provided with effective parental care. The condition is usually associated with severe neglect and maltreatment. It is not clear why some children respond to a noxious environment in this manner and others do not.

B. Epidemiology: The incidence of psychosocial dwarfism in the general population of infants is unknown.

Clinical Findings

Psychosocial dwarfism is usually diagnosed between 18 months and 7 years of age. Severe growth retardation with cognitive and language delays is sometimes preceded by feeding problems in infancy. The child exhibits polyphagia, food hoarding, pica, and insomnia, sometimes wandering at night apparently to look for food. Food fads, enuresis, encopresis, and self-induced vomiting are commonly associated with psychosocial dwarfism. Mental retardation or borderline intelligence is also a concomitant. The symptoms of psychosocial dwarfism have been associated with disorders of biological rhythms, self-regulation, mood, and social relationships. Sleep, appetite, and satiety are disturbed, and these children have a deficiency in the normally pulsed release of growth hormone into the bloodstream. Sometimes these children are destructive, urinating or defecating in inappropriate places. The condition is potentially reversible, at least in part, if the child is provided with adequate, nurturant surrogate care.

Differential Diagnosis

Psychosocial dwarfism should be distinguished from short stature due to endocrine disorder, constitutional factors, or stress.

Treatment

When children with psychosocial dwarfism are provided with adequate surrogate parental care, physical and mental growth occurs within a few weeks, and the eccentric behavior characteristic of the condition recedes. However, the longer that appropriate placement is delayed, the less likely it is that the child will catch up.

Prognosis & Course of Illness

The prognosis is poor, unless adequate, surrogate parental care is provided. Short stature, delayed puberty, stunted intellectual development, and conduct problems are likely to result from untreated psychosocial dwarfism.

Benoit D: Phenomenology and treatment of failure to thrive. Child Adolesc Psychiatr Clin N Am 1993;2:61.

Benoit D: Failure to thrive and feeding disorders. Pages 317–331 in Zeanah C (editor): *Handbook of Infant Mental Health.* Guilford Press, 1993.

Lucas AR: Anorexia and bulimia nervosa. Pages 586–592 in Lewis M (editor): *Child and Adolescent Psychiatry: A Comprehensive Textbook,* 2nd ed. Williams & Wilkins, 1996.

Mayes LC, Volkmar FR: Nosology of eating and growth disorders in early childhood. Child Adolesc Psychiatr Clin N Am 1993;2:15.

Minde K: The effect of disordered parenting on the development of children. In: Lewis M (editor): *Child and Adolescent Psychiatry: A Comprehensive Textbook,* 2nd ed. Williams & Wilkins, 1996.

Ramsey M: Feeding disorders and failure to thrive. Child Adolesc Psychiatr Clin N Am 1995;4:605.

ELIMINATION DISORDERS

ENCOPRESIS

DSM-IV Diagnostic Criteria

A. Repeated passage of feces into inappropriate places (eg, clothing or floor) whether involuntary or intentional.

B. At least one such event a month for at least 3 months.

C. Chronological age is at least 4 years (or equivalent developmental level).

D. The behavior is not due exclusively to the direct physiological effects of a substance (eg, laxatives) or a general medical condition except through a mechanism involving constipation.

General Considerations

A. Major Etiologic Theories: The etiology of encopresis is multifactorial. Normal continence and voiding requires the following sequence of neuromuscular events: (1) sensitivity to rectal fullness; (2) constriction of the external anal sphincter, puborectalis, and internal anal sphincter; (3) rectal contraction waves; (4) increase of intra-abdominal pressure following contraction of the diaphragm and abdominal muscles; and (5) relaxation of the sphincters.

Children with encopresis exhibit abnormal anorectal dynamics, such as a weak internal sphincter, or a failure of the external sphincter to relax in concert with rectal contraction waves and abdominal straining. There are two types of encopresis: (1) with constipation and overflow incontinence and (2) without constipation and overflow incontinence.

Toilet training involves the learning of the appropriate place and time for defecation; sensitivity to rectal fullness; and the sequential coordination of withholding, finding the right place, adopting the appropriate posture, relaxing the sphincters, and increasing intra-abdominal pressure. Most children are capable of learning the sequence by 18–24 months of age; however, learning may be interrupted by several antecedent conditions or concurrent events. Particularly important are the parent's attunement to the infant's signals and the parent's capacity to introduce the child to the toilet calmly; offer praise and encouragement for a favorable result; and avoid discouragement, coercion, or punishment for failures.

A significant number of children who experience fecal retention were constipated in the first year of life. In other children, physiologic constipation has followed an attack of diarrhea. The preliminary constipation causes painful defecation, in some cases with anal fissure, which precipitates withholding. A pattern of withholding, fecal retention, and involuntary overflow may be created if withholding coincides with faulty toilet training (eg, with coercion, harsh criticism, or physical punishment) or if the parent is emotionally unavailable or poorly attuned to the child (eg, as a result of depression). Thus an initially physiologic condition disrupts the mother-child relationship, and psychogenic retention culminates in abnormal anorectal dynamics, megacolon, rectal insensitivity, and leakage or involuntary voiding.

A small number of children with severe behavioral disturbance, often from neglectful or rejecting homes, exhibit no retention and constipation but deliberately defecate in closets or other inappropriate places. Two other nonretentive groups of encopretics are associated with (1) an apparent insensitivity to rectal fullness and the involuntary passage of feces or (2) the passage of (often liquid) feces when emotionally aroused by anxiety, fear, or laughter.

The degree to which encopresis is associated with psychopathology in the parent or child is disputed. Enuresis, oppositional-defiant behavior, tantrums, school refusal, fire setting, and developmental immaturities have been described as concomitants, although the degree to which these symptoms are primary or secondary to the encopresis is uncertain.

B. Epidemiology: A Scandinavian population study revealed a prevalence of 1.5% among children aged 7–8 years. The sex ratio was 3.4:1 in favor of boys. A British study found a prevalence of about 1.5% among children aged 10–11 years, with a sex ratio of 4.3:1 in favor of boys.

Clinical Findings

Some younger children who deliberately soil in inappropriate places do so at a time of stress or family change, for example after the birth of a sibling. Others, as described earlier in this chapter, do so in reaction to severe neglect or rejection, as in psychosocial dwarfism. A second group appears to lose sphincter control when emotionally aroused. These are often highly strung children exposed to emotional stress, for example, after a change of school.

The most serious cases are associated with constipation, retention, megarectum, megacolon, and the involuntary passage of small amounts of stool, together with liquefaction, fecal leakage, and virtually constant soiling, or the intermittent involuntary passage of large stools. Children with extreme megacolon can become disabled with abdominal distension, anorexia, and loss of weight.

Differential Diagnosis

The following causes of incontinence or constipation should be distinguished from encopresis: Hirschsprung's disease, anal stenosis, and endocrine disorder. However, the combination of soiling; constipation; a ballooned, loaded rectum; and a loaded colon occurs only in encopresis.

The clinician should evaluate the child for other developmental problems or psychiatric disorders (eg, mental retardation, learning problems, disruptive behavior disorder, anxiety disorder).

Treatment

If the child has a loaded colon and rectum, it is likely that his or her rectum is insensitive to distension. Thus the colon should be washed out and laxatives and stool softeners used until fecal masses can no longer be palpated and the child is passing regular stools of normal consistency. In severe cases, hospitalization is required.

Parents should be educated to administer a behavioral program. Coercion, punishment, and criticism should be avoided. It is ill-advised, for example, to punish the child by making him or her clean soiled clothes. The child should be asked to sit briefly on the toilet at the same time twice per day: after breakfast and after school. All tension should be removed from the toileting experience. The child may be read to or may read to himself or herself. The parent should make no comment if no bowel movement is passed; in contrast, the parent should praise and offer individualized reward to the child if toileting is successful. Star charts are useful both as a record and for reinforcement (see "Treatment" discussion in the "Enuresis" section).

Depressed or compulsive parents often find it difficult to institute a consistent, gentle program of this type and may need treatment in their own right. Fathers should be involved in order to provide support and to cooperate in instituting the behavioral program. Marital problems may need attention.

The child may require individual psychotherapy for associated anxiety disorders, disruptive behavior disorders, or other psychopathology. Because the possibility of relapse is high, treatment is often needed for one or more years, with a combination of laxatives, stool softeners, a high-fiber diet, parental education, parental behavior management, individual psychotherapy, and when necessary, psychiatric help for the parents. The results of this regimen are good, particularly in younger children. Success rates of 50–90% have been reported. Imipramine has been prescribed to treat encopresis, but no controlled studies of its effectiveness are available.

Prognosis & Course of Illness

Most cases of encopresis resolve by adolescence. A small minority of encopretic individuals remain incontinent as adults.

Hersov L: Encopresis. Pages 520–528 in Rutter M, Taylor E, Hersov L (editors): *Child and Adolescent Psychiatry,* 3rd ed. Blackwell Scientific, 1994.

Mikkelson EJ: Modern approaches to enuresis and encopresis. Pages 590–601 in Lewis M (editor): *Child and Adolescent Psychiatry: A Comprehensive Textbook,* 2nd ed. Williams & Wilkins, 1996.

ENURESIS (NOT DUE TO A GENERAL MEDICAL CONDITION)

DSM-IV Diagnostic Criteria

A. Repeated voiding of urine into bed or clothes (whether involuntary or intentional).

B. The behavior is clinically significant as manifested by either a frequency of twice a week for at least 3 consecutive months or the presence of clinically significant distress or impairment in social, academic (occupational), or other important areas of functioning.

C. Chronological age is at least 5 years (or equivalent developmental level).

D. The behavior is not due exclusively to the direct

physiological effect of a substance (eg, a diuretic) or a general medical condition (eg, diabetes, spina bifida, a seizure disorder).

Reprinted, with permission, from *Diagnostic and Statistical Manual of Mental Disorders,* 4th ed. Copyright 1994 American Psychiatric Association.

General Considerations

A. Major Etiologic Theories: The cause of enuresis is unknown. One study has found an abnormality in circadian rhythms: Enuretics did not reduce the output of urine at night as do normal children over 12 months of age. Enuretics have low functional bladder volume, a finding that correlates with behavioral disturbance, suggesting a common etiologic factor. Indeed, enuresis correlates with other maturational delays, particularly in language, speech, motor skills, and social development. An association has been noted between the tendency to sleep for long periods each day, between 1 and 2 years of age, and later enuresis, but the significance of this finding is uncertain. Bedwetting occurs at any stage of sleep, and no abnormalities of sleep architecture have been identified.

Primary enuresis refers to enuresis without a period of continence. **Secondary enuresis** is enuresis after a period of normal bladder control. Two general population studies found that if toilet training is delayed until after 18 months, the prevalence of enuresis increases. Secondary enuresis, but not primary enuresis, is associated with psychosocial stressors. Secondary enuresis is more likely to be associated with behavioral disturbance. About 50% of enuretic children between 7 and 12 years of age have had a previous period of continence.

B. Epidemiology: The sex ratio is equal until 5 years of age, after which males predominate (2:1 at 11 years of age). Boys are more likely to develop secondary enuresis. Scandinavian and New Zealand population studies have found the prevalence of enuresis at 7 and 8 years of age to be 9.8% and 7.4%, respectively. In the United States bedwetting is more common in African Americans and Asian immigrants than among other populations. Most enuretic children achieve continence by puberty. Approximately 3% of childhood enuretics are still incontinent at 20 years of age.

C. Genetics: A genetic factor may be involved in enuresis. Bedwetting runs in families and is significantly more common in monozygotic than dizygotic twins.

Differential Diagnosis

Urinalysis, microurine, and urine culture should be ordered routinely. If daytime enuresis is present, if the patient has a history of urinary tract infections or other urinary symptoms (eg, dysuria, urinary frequency, dribbling), or if the patient's urine grows bacteria, further urologic examinations are required in order to rule out urinary tract infection, bladder neck obstruction, urethral valves, or other structural abnormalities. Epilepsy, diabetes mellitus, diabetes insipidus, and spina bifida should be excluded by history, physical examination, and urinalysis.

Treatment

A. Star Charts: The child is given a star to add to a calendar for each dry night. The star chart alone results in a cure for a minority of enuretic children. It also provides useful records of baseline and the child's progress.

B. Surgical Treatment & Retention Control Training: The efficacy of radical surgical treatments such as urethral dilatation, bladder neck repair, cystoplasty, or division of the sacral nerves has not been demonstrated. Bladder training, which involves the retention of urine for longer and longer periods of time, is no longer used.

C. Medication: Heterocyclic antidepressants reduce the frequency of bedwetting in about 80% of patients and suppress it entirely in about 30%. However, most patients will relapse within about 3 months of withdrawal from the drug. The effective nighttime dosage is usually 1–2.5 mg/kg and occasionally as much as 3.5 mg/kg. This treatment essentially aims to suppress wetting while waiting for maturation in bladder control. The drug should be tapered and discontinued every 3 months and titrated back to a therapeutic level if enuresis recurs. The neuropharmacologic basis of the antienuretic effect is unknown.

The synthetic antidiuretic desmopressin acetate (desamine-D-arginine vasopressin, DDAVP) is an antienuretic. It may be administered intranasally or orally. DDAVP may operate by reducing urine volume below that which triggers bladder contraction. As with antidepressant therapy, relapse is common following withdrawal.

Sympathomimetic (eg, ephedrine) and anticholinergic (eg, belladonna) drugs are ineffective in treating enuresis.

D. Behavioral Treatment: The alarm-and-pad technique (in which an alarm is triggered when the first drop of urine onto a pad closes an electrical circuit) has a 75–80% rate of cure and a 30% relapse rate. It is the most effective treatment available for both primary and secondary enuresis. Children with daytime enuresis, behavioral problems, and a lack of motivation may be resistant to behavioral treatment. Optimal improvement requires at least 6–8 weeks of treatment. For maximum benefit, the alarm-and-pad technique may be combined with antidepressant or antidiuretic medication and a star chart.

If behavioral treatment is clearly the most effective method, why is it not the standard? Probably because it is cumbersome, lengthy, embarrassing, and requires good motivation. It is reasonable to begin treating enuresis with drugs and to move to behavioral treatment if medication is ineffective.

Prognosis & Course of Illness

Most cases of enuresis remit between 5 and 7 years of age or 12 and 15 years of age. A minority of cases continue into adulthood.

Mikkelson EJ: Modern approaches to enuresis and encopresis. Pages 590–601 in Lewis M (editor): *Child and Adolescent Psychiatry: A Comprehensive Textbook,* 2nd ed. Williams & Wilkins, 1996.

SLEEP DISORDERS

Sleep problems often commence before 2 years of age. Sleep disorders are described more fully in Chapter 30. This section deals with the sleep disorders of infancy and early childhood. Four types of sleep problems affect this age group: (1) dyssomnia (nightwaking); (2) hypersomnia (sleep apnea); (3) parasomnia (somnambulism, night terrors, nightmares, head banging, body rocking); and (4) circadian rhythm disorder (irregular sleep habits). The first three disorders are discussed in the sections that follow.

NIGHTWAKING

General Considerations

Nightwaking is most likely to be associated with psychosocial stress, maternal depression, inconsistent limits, and anxiety. It also occurs in association with sedative medication, Tourette's syndrome, attention-deficit/hyperactivity disorder (ADHD), mental retardation, autism, and Rett's syndrome.

Different parents have different tolerances for nightwaking. Thus prevalence is a relative matter. Breast-fed infants wake more often than those who are bottle-fed. Waking is not associated with parity or sex; however, it is associated with perinatal adversity other than prematurity.

Clinical Findings

Nightwaking is sometimes associated with colic, a condition in which the child flexes the legs and cries paroxysmically as though in pain. The cause of colic is unknown. The condition seldom lasts beyond 4 months of age.

Treatment

Minde has proposed a treatment approach that starts with several preliminary steps (Table 37–2). Treatment should aim to help the child regulate his or her own sleep without disturbing the parents (Table 37–3). The treatment of marital problems, if any, should be reserved until a later date. Minde claims an 85% success rate with this regimen. Failures are most likely if the parents cannot establish daytime and nighttime routines, or if the father is not involved.

Table 37–2. Preliminary steps in the treatment of nightwaking.

1. Involve both parents in diagnosis and treatment.
2. Obtain full information about the details of the sleep disorder: its antecedents, nature, consequences, and previous treatment.
3. Inquire about other problem behaviors and about any disruptions in the child's typical day.
4. Obtain information about the parents, including their backgrounds, health, personalities, and marital relationship.
5. Have the parents keep a detailed daily record, for 2 weeks, of the child's sleep habits (eg, bedtime, time of falling asleep, number of times awake) and daily routine (eg, mealtimes, naptime).
6. Observe the parent-child interaction during free play; observe the parent-infant interaction during feeding.

SLEEP APNEA

General Considerations

Sleep apnea is peripheral or central in origin. Peripheral apnea is caused by oropharyngeal obstruction (eg, by enlarged tonsilloadenoid tissue). Central apnea occurs in the sudden infant death syndrome. It may be associated with sleeping prone and excessive environmental temperature.

Clinical Findings

In obstructive sleep apnea, the sleeping child's breathing stops intermittently and is then followed by snoring respirations. Chronic apnea can be associated with failure to thrive, cognitive impairment, daytime drowsiness, and chronic headache.

Treatment

Prone sleeping and excessive bedding (eg, blankets and comforters) should be avoided. Tonsillectomy and adenoidectomy may be necessary.

Table 37–3. Treatment of nightwaking.

1. Help the parents establish regular daytime and nighttime routines.
2. Ask the father to handle the nighttime routine and waking.
3. If the child is waking at night, have the father check on the child every 5–10 minutes; if the child is awake, have the father soothe the child with words but without picking up the child.
4. If the child must be weaned from the parental bed, shaping can be used. The child is moved to his or her own bed, and the mother sits on the bed soothing the child to sleep. After 2–3 nights, she sits beside the bed. Gradually, she moves the chair further and further away, unitl she is outside the room.
5. Ask the parents to keep a daily journal, monitoring the progress of the sleep disturbance.
6. Schedule return visits every 2 weeks for about 8 weeks.

PARASOMNIA

General Considerations

Somnambulism and night terrors are probably of inherited origin. Nightmares are more prevalent in association with anxiety, particularly posttraumatic stress disorder. The etiology of head banging and body rocking is unknown.

Somnambulism and night terrors occur in 2.5–9% of children. Head banging and body rocking occur in 30–40% of children at 9–12 months. Their prevalence drops to about 3% after age 3 years.

Clinical Findings

Nightmares should be distinguished from night terrors. In nightmares the child wakens and recounts a frightening, realistic dream but is consolable. In night terrors the apparently terrified child sits up screaming, sometimes moving about the bedroom, but is not truly awake. When the child is laid down again, he or she returns to sleep. In somnambulism the child walks about the house, unresponsive and blank-faced.

In head banging, the child rhythmically hits his or her head against the crib, sometimes vigorously. In body rocking, the child moves his or her torso rhythmically, sometimes with accompanying vocalizations. These sleep problems affect parents and in extreme cases may so disrupt the parents' sleep that they become exhausted, begin to despair, or are set at odds with one another.

Differential Diagnosis

Somnambulism must be distinguished from nocturnal complex seizures. Complex seizures are usually associated with violent thrashing about and stereotyped movements.

Treatment

A. Nightmares: If nightmares are associated with posttraumatic stress disorder, anxiety disorder, or environmental stress, the cause of the sleep disturbance should be treated or addressed.

B. Night Terrors & Somnambulism: The clinician should reassure the parents that the condition is probably a variant of normal development. The child should not be woken but rather should be laid down or led back to bed to sleep. Extraneous sources of stress should be addressed.

C. Head Banging & Body Rocking: Isolated case reports have described the use of behavioral techniques (eg, extinction, reinforcement of nonrocking behavior) to treat these conditions.

Handford HA, Mattison RE, Kales A: Sleep disturbances and disorders. Pages 716–726 in Lewis M (editor): *Child and Adolescent Psychiatry.* Williams & Wilkins, 1991.
Minde K: Sleep disorders in infants and toddlers. Child Adolesc Psychiatr Clin N Am 1995;4:589.

II. MENTAL RETARDATION

Mark L. Wolraich, MD

DSM-IV Diagnostic Criteria

A. Significantly subaverage intellectual functioning: an IQ of approximately 70 or below on an individually administered IQ test (for infants, a clinical judgment of significantly subaverage intellectual functioning).

B. Concurrent deficits or impairments in present adaptive functioning (ie, the person's effectiveness in meeting the standards expected for his or her age by his or her cultural group) in at least two of the following areas: communication, self-care, home living, social/interpersonal skills, use of community resources, self-direction, functional academic skills, work, leisure, health, and safety.

C. The onset is before age 18 years.

Reprinted, with permission, from *Diagnostic and Statistical Manual of Mental Disorders,* 4th ed. Copyright 1994 American Psychiatric Association.

General Considerations

A. Major Etiologic Theories: Mental retardation is diagnosed if an individual is significantly below average in intellectual abilities and impaired in adaptive behaviors. It is not a homogeneous condition. Although an assessment of general intellectual abilities can be represented by an intelligence quotient (IQ), it is misleading to conceptualize intelligence as a single trait. Intelligence entails a number of different areas such as memory, vocabulary, conceptual thinking, computation, perception of patterns, and the association of concepts. Recent changes in the definition provided by the American Association on Mental Retardation have further emphasized the importance of impairment in adaptive skills as a key diagnostic criterion.

Mental retardation, in the majority of affected individuals, has no known cause or is attributed to sociocultural causes. However, in a considerable number of individuals with mental retardation, particularly those with more severe mental retardation, a cause can be identified (Table 37–4).

B. Epidemiology: The prevalence rates of mental retardation vary from 1% to 3%. Rates vary depending on the definitions used, methods of ascertainment, and populations studied.

C. Genetics: Mental retardation with no underlying etiology is usually related to a combination of polygenic and environmental factors. Often it is impossible to determine the relative contribution of each factor. For those cases of mental retardation with specific etiologies, the genetic pattern follows the genetic pattern of the underlying disorder, for example, sex-

Table 37–4. Major causes of mental retardation.

Cause	Examples
Chromosomal	XXY syndrome (Klinefelter's syndrome) Trisomy 21 (Down syndrome) Trisomy 18 Trisomy 13 Fragile X syndrome
Mendelian	Acrocephalosyndactyly (Apert syndrome); dominant Neurofibromatosis (von Recklinghausen's disease); dominant Tuberous sclerosis (characterized by adenoma sebaceum); dominant Mucopolysaccharidosis type I (Hurler's syndrome); autosomal recessive Mucopolysaccharidosis type II (Hunter's syndrome); X-linked recessive
Prenatal exposure	Fetal alcohol syndrome Fetal hydantoin syndrome Rubella
Postnatal exposure	Shaken baby syndrome Kernicterus Meningitis

linked in fragile X syndrome or autosomal recessive in Hurler's syndrome.

Clinical Findings

A. Signs & Symptoms: The initial presentation of mental retardation varies greatly depending on the severity of the retardation. Children with severe mental retardation may present at birth or within the first year of life, with delay in expected developmental landmarks such as sitting, walking, and talking. Children with moderate mental retardation may not exhibit delay until 2–4 years of age, and children with mild mental retardation may not be identified until they are in a school setting and are unable to attain the skills expected for children their age. Early developmental landmarks tend to involve motor skills, which often correlate poorly with general cognitive abilities. Thus the less severe forms of mental retardation can be difficult to detect in children under 2 years of age. In some cases, the underlying cause of the mental retardation provides the initial symptomatology. For example, an abnormally appearing face (eg, due to Down syndrome or fetal alcohol syndrome) may alert the clinician to the possibility of mental retardation before developmental delays are noted. It is important to take seriously parental concerns about delays and to have such children evaluated appropriately.

B. Psychological Testing: The current system, used in *Diagnostic and Statistical Manual of Mental Disorders,* 4th edition (DSM-IV), determines diagnosis and severity according to psychometric measures of general intellectual ability. The most commonly used tests have been the Wechsler Scales (Wechsler Preschool and Primary Scale of Intelligence, Wechsler Intelligence Scale for Children, and Wechsler Adult Intelligence Scale) and the Stanford-Binet Scales. Both of these scales have verbal and performance sections. The Kaufman Assessment Battery for Children, a newer test, has had less extensive use. Other intellectual assessment measures that depend less on verbal abilities and are useful for hearing impaired, language impaired, or culturally different children, include the Leiter International Performance Scale and the Hiskey-Nebraska Test of Learning Aptitude.

All tests convert their results to IQs based on a mean of 100. The deviations appropriate for the levels of severity are presented in Table 37–5. A recent recommendation by the American Association on Mental Retardation is to use the IQ (70–75 or below) as a diagnostic requirement but to include the degree of impairment of adaptive skills both for diagnosis and consideration of severity. The domains of adaptive skills suggested include communication, self-care, home living, social/interpersonal skills, use of com-

Table 37–5. Severity of impairment of intellectual function.

Degree of Impairment	Standard Deviation (SD) Scores	Wechsler Scales (SD = 15)	Stanford-Binet Scales (SD = 16)
Mild	–3.00 to –2.01	55 to 69	52 to 67
Moderate	–4.00 to –3.01	40 to 54	36 to 51
Severe	–5.00 to –4.01	25 to 39	20 to 35
Profound	Below –5.00	Under 25	Under 20

munity resources, self-direction, functional academic skills, work, leisure, health, and safety. Some of these adaptive domains can be measured with the Vineland Social Maturity Scale, but the assessment of social maturity has not revealed the same precision as that of general cognitive abilities.

Luckasson R, Coulter DL, Polloway EA, et al: *Mental Retardation: Definition, Classification, and Systems of Support.* American Association on Mental Retardation, 1992.

C. Laboratory Findings & Imaging: The aim of laboratory testing should be to identify an underlying etiology, as directed by the history and physical findings. The three main areas to address are metabolic/endocrinologic, chromosomal, and brain imaging.

Newborn nurseries now screen for metabolic/endocrinologic conditions that would often go undetected at birth, such as phenylketonuria, hypothyroidism, and galactosemia. Even if screenings are negative, if the history and physical findings suggest a particular condition, repeat testing is required to eliminate the occasional false negative. Patients with severe to profound mental retardation should be screened for other inborn errors of metabolism.

Chromosomal analysis is indicated in patients who have minor or major anomalies as well as in those with strong family histories of mental retardation. One of the more common causes of mental retardation is fragile X syndrome. This condition occurs most frequently in males, but it can occur in females and should be suspected if many family members are retarded. Specific karyotyping with folate-deficient medium and identification of DNA sequencing is required.

Brain imaging is indicated only if history or neurologic examination suggests central nervous system (CNS) malformation or brain injury.

Duitch D, Bernstein NR: Inpatient management of mental retardation. Pages 220–224 in Jellinek MS, Herzog DB (editors): *Psychiatric Aspects of General Hospital Pediatrics.* Yearbook Medical Publishers, 1990.

McMillan DL, Gresham FM, Siperstein GN: Conceptual and psychometric concerns about the 1992 AAMR definitions of mental retardation. Am J Ment Retard 1993;98:325.

Differential Diagnosis

Four kinds of condition can cause children to be delayed in development yet not be mentally retarded: adverse environment, sensory impairment, motor impairment, and psychiatric disorder.

A. Adverse Environment: Children raised in severely deprived situations with neglect and abuse may be delayed in development and score badly on intellectual assessment. Such children frequently improve if they are placed, without excessive delay, in a more stimulating and nurturing environment.

B. Sensory Impairment: Children with auditory or visual impairment may exhibit developmental delays. Accurate assessment requires compensation for sensory deficit. However, because many children with mental retardation also have sensory impairment, it is essential to test the sight and hearing of all children suspected to have mental retardation.

C. Motor Impairment: Children with motor impairments may also exhibit developmental delays. If there is oral involvement, as in children with athetotic cerebral palsy, speech can also be delayed. Assessment by clinicians experienced in working with individuals with motor impairments is essential to ensure that a true estimate of intellectual capability is obtained.

D. Psychiatric Disorder: In young children, pervasive developmental disorders often present as developmental delay (discussed later in this chapter). Although many of these children are also mentally retarded, this is not true for all cases, and even those with some intellectual impairment require intervention oriented to the primary diagnosis (ie, the pervasive developmental disorder).

Comorbidity

Most of the important comorbid conditions have already been described in the preceding section: sensory and motor impairments and pervasive developmental disorders. In addition, individuals with mental retardation can have other psychiatric conditions including depressive disorders, ADHD, and anxiety disorders. Because the patient's behavioral repertoire may be limited, these disorders may not appear with the full or typical symptomatic features. Common manifestations are self-injury, stereotypies, rumination, and aggressive behavior.

Treatment

Treatment should aim to maximize the potential of those with mental retardation, with a particular focus on adaptive skills. Treatment generally includes special educational instruction with educational mainstreaming of children in the regular school environment, whenever possible. Families may need help with behavior management. Psychopharmacologic management and behavioral management may be required for those with severe behavior problems.

Prognosis & Course of Illness

Mental retardation generally does not resolve or progress. The course, in fact, will be determined by the underlying etiology. Severity or degree of impairment may not be clear at the time of diagnosis, but it usually emerges as a child becomes older and is expected to acquire more complex skills. The ultimate course is determined by the extent to which adaptive skills are acquired and depends on the interactions between innate ability and the quality of home, school, and community.

In the past, society has tended to be overly pessimistic about the capabilities of mentally retarded individuals. Low expectation resulted in the institutionalization of many people. Institutionalization restricted development, limiting outcome and thus fulfilling the expectation of limited performance. With the advent of better educational programs in public schools and because most children with mental retardation today grow up with their families, the expectation and outcome of these individuals have greatly improved. Guidelines for the capabilities of individuals with mental retardation are provided in Table 37–6. These guidelines are general; individual attainment varies widely. Furthermore, the guidelines are based on current experience; more intensive and better developed programming, together with societal alternatives, may prove that these guidelines are still conservative.

Wolraich ML, Siperstein GN, Reed D: The prognostications of physicians about mentally retarded individuals. Pages 109–129 in Wolraich ML, Routh DK (editors): *Advances in Developmental and Behavioral Pediatrics.* Vol 10. Kingsley, 1992.

III. PERVASIVE DEVELOPMENTAL DISORDERS

Barry Nurcombe, MD, & Wendy Stone, PhD

The pervasive developmental disorders include several conditions characterized by different degrees of impairment and deviance in intellectual development, language development, communication skills, and social competence, together with stereotyped behavior and interests. These conditions are autistic disorder, Rett's disorder, childhood disintegrative disorder, Asperger's disorder, and pervasive developmental disorder not otherwise specified (NOS).

Table 37–6. Guidelines for capabilities for individuals with mental retardation.[1]

Capability	Mild	Moderate	Severe
Find own way in unfamiliar surroundings	+	+	
Make change for a dollar	+		
Use public transportation independently	+		
Follow national news events	+		
Dress and toilet independently	+	+	+
Drink from a cup unassisted	+	+	+
Eat with utensils	+	+	+
Carry on a simple conversation	+	+	+
Follow one-stage commands	+	+	+
Address two people by name	+	+	+
Use lock and key	+	+	
Choose appropriate clothing	+	+	+
Sustain friendships	+	+	+
Indicate symptoms verbally	+	+	
Recognize traffic signs	+	+	+
Schedule daily activities	+	+	
Act appropriately toward strangers	+	+	+
Anticipate hazards	+	+	
Tell time	+	+	
Cook meals unsupervised	+		
Use pay phone	+	+	
Do own laundry	+	+	
Employment	Competitive environment	Sheltered workshop or competitive environment	Sheltered workshop

[1] + indicates that this skill is likely to occur in a majority of individuals.

AUTISTIC DISORDER

DSM-IV Diagnostic Criteria

A. A total of six (or more) items from (1), (2), and (3), with at least two from (1), and one each from (2) and (3):

    (1) qualitative impairment in social interaction, as manifested by at least two of the following:

        (a) marked impairment in the use of multiple nonverbal behaviors such as eye-to-eye gaze, facial expression, body postures, and gestures to regulate social interaction

        (b) failure to develop peer relationships appropriate to developmental level

        (c) a lack of spontaneous seeking to share enjoyment, interests, or achievements with other people (eg, by a lack of showing, bringing, or pointing out objects of interest)

        (d) lack of social or emotional reciprocity

    (2) qualitative impairments in communication as manifested by at least one of the following:

        (a) delay in, or total lack of, the development of spoken language (not accompanied by an attempt to compensate through alternative modes of communication such as gesture or mime)

        (b) in individuals with adequate speech, marked impairment in the ability to initiate or sustain a conversation with others

        (c) stereotyped and repetitive use of language or idiosyncratic language

        (d) lack of varied, spontaneous make-believe play or social imitative play appropriate to developmental level

    (3) restricted repetitive and stereotyped patterns of behavior, interests, and activities, as manifested by at least one of the following:

        (a) encompassing preoccupation with one or more stereotyped and restricted patterns of interest that is abnormal either in intensity or focus

        (b) apparently inflexible adherence to specific, nonfunctional routines or rituals

        (c) stereotyped and repetitive motor mannerisms (eg, hand or finger flapping or twisting, or complex whole-body movements)

        (d) persistent preoccupation with parts of objects

B. Delays or abnormal functioning in at least one of the following areas, with onset prior to age 3 years: (1) social interaction, (2) language as used in social communication, or (3) symbolic or imaginative play.

C. The disturbance is not better accounted for by Rett's disorder or childhood disintegrative disorder.

Reprinted, with permission, from *Diagnostic and Statistical Manual of Mental Disorders,* 4th ed. Copyright 1994 American Psychiatric Association.

General Considerations

A. Major Etiologic Theories: Early views of autistic disorder suggested a psychogenic cause. Autistic disorder was thought to result from early environmental stress or trauma, deficient parent-child interaction, or parental psychopathology. Research over the past several decades has failed to support these views. Currently, autistic disorder is conceptualized as a biological disorder with diverse etiology. Advances in diagnostic techniques have yielded evidence of brain dysfunction and an association with neurologic conditions. Organic conditions have been reported in 28–49% of individuals with autistic disorder (see Table 37–7 for a summary of neurobiological conditions associated with autistic disorder). Seizure disorders have been found in 11–42% of autistic individuals, with increased prevalence in individuals functioning at lower cognitive levels. Several studies have found an increased frequency of prenatal and perinatal complications in the birth histories of children with autistic disorder, lending further support to an organic etiology.

Psychological theories have emphasized the importance of cognitive factors in the development of many of the characteristic features of autistic disorder. The basic deficit in individuals with autistic disorder has been described as an inability to recognize and understand that other people have mental states (eg, thoughts, beliefs) and to modify one's own behavior accordingly. This defect, thought to be unique to autistic disorder, is referred to as an "impaired theory of mind." Numerous studies have found that high-functioning, verbal individuals with autistic disorder perform more poorly than do control subjects on a variety of social cognitive tasks. Although the impaired-theory-of-mind hypothesis has been of considerable heuristic value, the extent to which it applies to lower-functioning autistic patients is unclear.

B. Epidemiology: Autistic disorder is estimated to occur in about 1 out of 1000 children. It is distributed equally among all socioeconomic levels, with a male-to-female sex ratio of about 3:1. Although fe-

Table 37–7. Major neurobiological conditions associated with autistic disorder.

Congenital rubella
Cytomegalovirus
Epilepsy
Fragile X syndrome
Herpes encephalitis
Möbius' syndrome
Neurofibromatosis
Phenylketonuria
Tuberous sclerosis

males are affected less frequently, they tend to be affected more severely, functioning at lower intellectual levels with greater evidence of neurologic impairment.

C. Genetics: There is strong evidence that genetic factors are involved in the etiology of autistic disorder. The evidence derives from family pedigree and twin studies as well as from the association of autistic disorder with disorders of known genetic etiology. First, the prevalence of autistic disorder in siblings of autistic children is 2–3%, about 50 times greater than chance. Second, concordance rates for autistic disorder are higher for monozygotic twins (36–96%) than for dizygotic twins (0–24%). Third, an increased prevalence of cognitive, language, and social impairments has been found in the families of individuals with autistic disorder. Finally, autistic disorder appears to be associated with several known genetic disorders, particularly fragile X syndrome, phenylketonuria, tuberous sclerosis, and neurofibromatosis. Although several hypothetical models of genetic transmission have been proposed, none has received conclusive support.

Clinical Findings

A. Signs & Symptoms: The accurate diagnosis of autistic disorder is complicated by the variability of the symptomatology. The overall severity of autistic disorder, as well as the specific behavioral manifestations of each characteristic, can vary as a function of age and developmental level. For example, very young children are unlikely to demonstrate the language abnormalities or repetitive rituals and routines that characterize older children.

1. Social deficits—Deficits in social relating and reciprocity are currently viewed as the core characteristics of autistic disorder. Social difficulties are usually first apparent in the child's interaction with parents. Peer problems (ie, lack of interest, inability to play cooperatively, failure to make friends) become evident in the preschool years. A number of social behaviors have been investigated in an attempt to elucidate the somewhat elusive construct of reciprocity: eye-to-eye gaze, imitation, attachment, affect, and social cognition or social perspective-taking.

One of the earliest social deficits is in motor imitation. Young children with autistic disorder have been consistently found to have more difficulty imitating body movements and the use of objects than do developmentally matched control subjects. Although these skills tend to improve with age, subtle deficits in the imitation of body movements have been found even in high-functioning autistic adolescents. Deficits in eye-to-eye gaze represent another early-developing social behavior associated with autistic disorder. Recent research suggests that children with autistic disorder differ from control subjects not in the absolute amount of eye contact, but rather in the ways it is used, particularly for social or communicative purposes, such as sharing enjoyment or directing another person's attention.

A variety of deficits in the recognition and use of affect are associated with autistic disorder. Young autistic children, compared to control subjects, display less positive affect, more neutral affect, and more incongruent combinations of affect. Positive affect occurs more often during solitary activities than during social interaction. Children with autistic disorder smile less often in response to their mothers' smiles and pay less attention to an adult simulating distress. Unusual affective expressions and difficulty with affective understanding and empathy have also been noted in older, high-functioning individuals with autistic disorder.

In contrast to the social deficits described here, research on attachment behavior suggests that children with autistic disorder, compared to other children of the same mental age, seek attachment security. For example, autistic children demonstrate increased proximity-seeking upon reunion with their mothers and more proximity-seeking toward their mothers than toward strangers. However, their behavioral and affective expressions of attachment may be qualitatively different from those of other children; for example, they may exhibit affective changes without seeking physical contact.

2. Language & communication impairment—Individuals with autistic disorder exhibit extensive language and communication difficulties. About 50% of autistic individuals fail to develop functional spoken language. Those who do acquire spoken language often exhibit delayed milestones and a deviant pattern of development. A number of unusual language features may be present, including immediate and delayed echolalia, pronoun reversal, repetitive language, idiosyncratic use of words and phrases, and abnormal prosody (ie, eccentric pitch, stress, rate, and rhythm). Deficits in the pragmatic aspects of language (ie, the ability to use speech and gesture in a communicative and socially appropriate manner) are also common (eg, pedantic speech, one-sided rather than reciprocal conversation, difficulty using and understanding facial expressions or gestures, and a tendency to perseverate on particular topics). In contrast, the semantic aspects of language, such as syntax and grammar, are relatively unimpaired.

Communication deficits are also present in autistic children who have not yet acquired speech. At young ages, one salient aspect of abnormal communication in autistic disorder is the failure to develop the capacity for joint attention, such as showing a toy to another person, pointing toward an object of interest, or alternating gaze between a person and an object. The impairment of joint attention with another person is considered by some to represent an early example of impaired theory of mind.

3. Restricted activities & interests—Stereotyped movements, sensory abnormalities, and an insistence on complex routines impose some degree of regularity or invariance on a perceptually confusing or unstable environment. The most common motor stereotypies are arm, hand, or finger flapping; head or body rocking; and spinning. Sensory abnormalities include hyporeactivity, heightened awareness, and heightened sensitivity in one or more modalities. Restricted and repetitive forms of play are common in younger children with autistic disorder. Young autistic children demonstrate less diverse, less functional, and more sensory-based play (eg, spinning, shaking, or twirling toys) than do control children. They also exhibit less play with dolls and less pretend play.

The particular repetitive activities exhibited by children with autistic disorder are related to developmental level. For example, low-functioning children are more likely to demonstrate stereotyped movements, whereas high-functioning individuals are more likely to engage in complex routines and to exhibit perseverative interests. Young children are less likely than older children to exhibit unusual habits or routines.

B. Psychological Testing: Between 70% and 80% of children with autistic disorder have mental retardation. Many demonstrate an uneven pattern of cognitive abilities, with relative strength in visual-motor skills and auditory memory and relative weaknesses in language and abstract thinking. In view of the cognitive and behavioral deficits of children with autistic disorder, specialized assessment techniques (eg, nonverbal tests) may be required for the best estimate of cognitive functioning and learning potential. Under appropriate testing conditions, the IQ scores obtained for children with autistic disorder are as valid and stable as those for nonautistic children.

A number of specialized instruments have been developed for the purpose of gathering diagnostic information. Examples of observational measures are the Childhood Autism Rating Scale and the Autism Diagnostic Observation Schedule. Parental report instruments include the Parent Interview for Autism and the Autism Diagnostic Interview.

C. Laboratory Findings & Imaging: No single neurobiological factor has been uniquely and universally associated with autistic disorder. Rather, a variety of organic conditions may contribute to the development of autistic disorder. Specific structural abnormalities found in autistic individuals include ventricular enlargement (especially in the left temporal horn); cerebellar abnormalities (ie, loss of Purkinje cells and hypoplasia of vermal lobules); decreased brain stem size, especially of the pons; and forebrain abnormalities. Neurophysiologic studies have revealed dysfunction at cortical and subcortical levels. Abnormal electroencephalograms (EEGs) have been reported in 32–43% of autistic children, and atypical patterns of hemispheric lateralization have also been found. The P300 component of event-related potentials (ie, the component associated with detection of novel, unpredictable stimuli) may be reduced in am-

plitude. Evidence for subcortical dysfunction has been found in a subgroup of autistic individuals and includes abnormal vestibular and autonomic responses as well as prolonged brain stem transmission times.

The most consistent finding from neurochemical studies has been increased levels of serotonin; however, the implications of this finding are unclear, as hyperserotonemia is found in only about one third of autistic patients, and elevated serotonin levels are also common in nonautistic patients with mental retardation. Abnormal levels of endogenous opioids (eg, β-endorphin) have also been reported. Neuropsychological studies have implicated frontal lobe dysfunction. Autistic individuals have consistently been found to perform more poorly than control subjects on executive function tasks measuring frontal lobe functions such as cognitive flexibility and response inhibition.

Lord C, Rutter M, LeCouteur A: Autism Diagnostic Interview—Revised: a revised version of a diagnostic interview for caregivers of individuals with possible pervasive developmental disorders. J Autism Dev Disord 1994; 24:659.

Lord C et al: Autism Diagnostic Observation Schedule: a standardized observation of communicative and social behavior. J Autism Dev Disord 1989;19:185.

Schopler E, Reichler RJ, Renner BR: *The Childhood Autism Rating Scale*. Western Psychological, 1988.

Stone WL, Hogan KL: A structured parent interview for identifying young children with autism. J Autism Dev Disord 1993;23:639.

Differential Diagnosis

Autistic disorder can be differentiated from other pervasive developmental disorders on the basis of severity, age at onset, and progression of symptomatology. Table 37–8 illustrates the similarities and differences between autistic disorder and other pervasive developmental disorders.

Autistic disorder can be differentiated from other developmental and psychiatric disorders by the characteristic triad of clinical features; delay and deviation in the development of social skills; communication, and language; and a restricted behavioral repertoire. Children with mixed receptive-expressive language disorder do not demonstrate the qualitative impairments in social reciprocity or the restricted and repetitive activities associated with autistic disorder. Moreover, children with language disorders usually do not exhibit impairments in nonverbal communication to the extent observed in autistic disorder. The majority of children with autistic disorder function within the range of mental retardation; however, children with mental retardation are less likely to demonstrate an uneven profile of cognitive skills, and they do not exhibit the impairments in social behavior and communication and the restricted activities and interests associated with autistic disorder. Children with autistic disorder may exhibit social isolation and abnormal af-

Table 37–8. Major diagnostic features of DSM-IV pervasive developmental disorders.

Feature	Autistic Disorder	Asperger's Disorder	Childhood Disintegrative Disorder	Rett's Disorder	Pervasive Developmental Disorder NOS
Social impairment	+	+	+[1]	+	+[2]
Language or communication disorder	+		+[1]	+	+[2]
Repetitive interests and activities	+	+	+	+	+[2]
Onset prior to 36 months	+			+	
Average intelligence		+			
Period of normal development			+	+	
Loss of skills in several areas			+	+	

[1] At least two of the three features must be present.
[2] At least one of the three features must be present.

fective responses similar to those observed in childhood-onset schizophrenia; however, schizophrenia is associated with a later age at onset, a clearer family history of schizophrenia, and less-impaired intellectual functioning relative to autistic disorder. Although repetitive activities and behavior are associated with obsessive-compulsive disorder, children with obsessive-compulsive disorder have a more normal course of development otherwise, and do not exhibit impairment in social interaction or communication.

Comorbidity

Comorbid conditions include ADHD, mood disorders, and anxiety disorders. The diagnosis of other psychiatric disorders is hampered by the difficulties that autistic individuals have communicating and describing feelings; diagnosis may have to rely on observation rather than self-report. Poor concentration, hyperactivity, and impulsivity are commonly observed in individuals with autistic disorder, particularly in the preschool and school-age years. Depression appears to be the most common affective disorder, although mania has also been reported. Affective disorders have been reported in high-functioning individuals and in those with moderate to severe levels of mental retardation. High levels of generalized anxiety have been described primarily in high-functioning individuals with autistic disorder.

Treatment

There is no cure for autistic disorder. The primary goals of treatment are to promote social, communicative, and adaptive living skills; to reduce the frequency and intensity of maladaptive behavior such as rigidity and stereotypies; and to alleviate family stress. The best-established treatments for children with autistic disorder use educational and behavioral interventions. Early intervention programs appear to be beneficial. The following are effective in promoting learning and development, especially if begun early: a structured learning environment; specialized, individualized, and developmentally based programming; the use of nondisabled peers as intervention agents; the use of behavioral techniques for the acquisition and generalization of new skills; and the involvement of parents in their child's treatment.

Pharmacotherapy is not a routine component of treatment, although in some cases it can be a useful adjunct. Haloperidol has been used to alleviate agitation, hyperactivity, aggression, and stereotyped behavior; however, it is associated with side effects such as tardive dyskinesia. Fenfluramine received a flurry of attention after initial reports of improvements in IQ, hyperactivity, withdrawal, and stereotypies; however, these results have not been replicated. Less well-studied medications include the following: naltrexone for self-injurious behavior, stereotypies, aggression, and social withdrawal; clomipramine for compulsive and repetitive behavior; and psychostimulants for inattention and hyperactivity in higher-functioning individuals.

Prognosis & Course of Illness

Although the average age at diagnosis has been reported to be about 4 years, many parents become concerned about their children at 18 months or younger. Parental concerns at this age are usually related to delayed speech development and lack of responsiveness to sounds rather than to other behavior typical of autistic disorder. The behavioral manifestations of autistic disorder change as a function of age and maturation, although the characteristic triad of clinical features is typically present throughout life. The preschool years have been described as the most problematic, because behavior and skill development often improve during the school years. During adolescence, improvements in social behavior, language, and self-help skills continue, and hyperactivity tends to decrease. However, aggression and self-injurious behavior intensify in a small subgroup of autistic adolescents, and a second peak of seizure onset also occurs.

The prognosis is variable. Some autistic individuals require high levels of supervision and care. A few others obtain educational degrees and attain competitive employment. The best predictors of outcome are IQ level and the presence of functional speech by age 5 years. Over the years, the proportion of children achieving a favorable outcome has increased, a positive trend that most likely reflects advances in educational and community-based services. Recent follow-up studies of autistic individuals with a wide variation of cognitive impairment have revealed a good outcome for 4–32% and a poor outcome for 20–48%. The outcome for high-functioning individuals with autistic disorder is more promising: Recent studies have revealed that 9–31% were living independently, 27–38% were in competitive employment, and 11–50% had at least some tertiary education.

Lord C, Rutter M: Autism and pervasive developmental disorders. Pages 569–593 in Rutter M, Taylor E, Hersov L (editors): *Child and Adolescent Psychiatry: Modern Approaches,* 3rd ed. Blackwell Scientific, 1994.

RETT'S DISORDER

DSM-IV Diagnostic Criteria

A. All of the following:
   (1) apparently normal prenatal and perinatal development
   (2) apparently normal psychomotor development through the first 5 months after birth
   (3) normal head circumference at birth
B. Onset of all of the following after a period of normal development:
   (1) deceleration of head growth between ages 5 and 48 months
   (2) loss of previously acquired purposeful hand skills between ages 5 and 30 months with the subsequent development of stereotyped hand movements (eg, hand-wringing or hand washing)
   (3) loss of social engagement early in the course (although often social interaction develops later)
   (4) appearance of poorly coordinated gait or trunk movements
   (5) severely impaired expressive and receptive language development with severe psychomotor retardation

General Considerations

A. Major Etiologic Theories: The brains of patients with Rett's disorder exhibit low weight without evidence of dysgenesis or abnormal intraneuronal storage. On microscopic examination, limited dendritic branching of small densely packed cortical neurons has been observed. This is thought to be consistent with an arrest of brain development between 1 and 3 months postnatally, causing a "neuronal disconnection failure."

Seventy percent of patients with Rett's disorder have an abnormal plasma glycosphingolipid absent from normal control subjects but found in 10% of patients with other brain disorders. One study has noted a reduction in GD1a and GD1b gangliosides in the cerebrum and cerebellum.

B. Epidemiology: Prevalence is thought to be 1 in 10,000–12,000 girls. There have been no confirmed cases in boys. All ethnic groups and social classes are affected. Among severely retarded girls, Rett's disorder may be third in prevalence to Down syndrome and fragile X syndrome.

C. Genetics: Most cases of Rett's disorder are sporadic. Familial cases are fewer than 1%; nevertheless, cooccurrence is greater than would be expected by chance. In several case reports the concordance in monozygotic twins has been recorded as 100%, whereas the concordance in dizygotic twins was 0%. An autosomal dominant or X-linked mutation, lethal in males, has been postulated. In one case, balanced translocation has been found between the short arm of the X chromosome (p22.11) and the long arm of chromosome 3. In another case, a translocation has been discovered between Xp11.22 and Xp22.11.

Clinical Findings

A. Signs & Symptoms: Although the diagnosis of Rett's disorder is considered tentative until 2–5 years of age, deviant development is apparent by 24 months in all cases. Many patients have been regarded as behaviorally "very good" in the first 6 months of life. The following stages have been described: (1) normal development (0–6 months); (2) stagnation (6–18 months); (3) deterioration (1–3 years); (4) plateau (5–20 years); and (5) further deterioration (beyond 20 years).

The first signs of Rett's disorder are hypotonia, reduced mobility, repetitive movements, and lack of involvement in play. Between 6 and 18 months the child may be sociable and content, but head growth decelerates, hypotonia increases, and the child loses all interest in play. Between 1 and 3 years, there is a rapid developmental regression, together with the appearance of autistic features (eg, lack of social interest, stereotypic responses). Episodes of crying, screaming, rage, and chaotic hyperactivity may occur. At about 5 years of age, the condition appears to plateau, the child often remaining in a pseudo-stationary phase for years. During preadolescence or adolescence there is often a sudden or gradual regression with loss of manipulative movements. Pincer grasp is lost early. Hand stereotypies appear along with so-called fractured gestures (jerky movements of the face, mouth, trunk, and limbs).

The loss of social interest and apparent social withdrawal often cause the child to be referred for assessment between 2 and 3 years of age. Communicative intent and joint referencing are usually retained at this stage. With increasing age, the child exhibits breathing problems characterized by hyperventilation and apneic spells, with bruxism (teeth grinding) and an increase of hand movements. Breathing appears to be normal when the child is asleep. Aerophagia and abdominal distension are sometimes noted. In 50% of patients, seizures appear at an average age at onset of 4 years. Virtually all patients have an abnormal EEG. Grand mal, focal, generalized, myoclonic, and atonic seizures have been reported. Abnormalities of the sleep-wake cycle are common, with increased daytime sleeping, nighttime waking, and early waking. Spasticity, muscle wasting, scoliosis, and limb deformities occur late in the disease.

B. Psychological Testing & Laboratory Findings: The general psychological and medical evaluation of children with Rett's disorder is similar to that described for autistic disorder. Medical examination should exclude the following conditions: intrauterine growth retardation, organomegaly associated with storage disease, retinopathy or optic atrophy, microcephaly, perinatally acquired brain damage, identifiable metabolic or progressive neurologic disease, and acquired neurologic disorder. To aid in the differential diagnosis (see next section), the clinician should screen for the following: aminoacidopathies, organic acidopathies, polysaccharidoses and oligosaccharidoses, brain dysfunction or abnormality (using EEG and computed tomography [CT] scan), and abnormal chromosomes.

Differential Diagnosis

Rett's disorder is most likely to be confused with the following conditions: autistic disorder, childhood disintegrative disorder (in which there is no neurologic dysfunction), infantile neuronal ceroid lipofuscinosis (in which there are transient drop spells, loss of head control, and irregular myoclonus), mucopolysaccharidoses, and infantile spasms.

Rett's disorder differs from autistic disorder in that the former is associated with the following characteristics: normal social development and social reciprocity for up to 12 months; deceleration of head growth; loss of pincer grip and manipulative skills; slow movements, hypoactivity, and stereotypic hand movements; hyperventilation and bruxism; abnormal gait; language normal early but lost by 18 months without

recovery; profound mental retardation with neurologic impairment; seizures in 50% of patients from early childhood.

Treatment

Treatment is symptomatic and supportive. The episodes of anxiety and weeping associated with the stage of rapid deterioration may be alleviated by hydrotherapy, massage, and music therapy. Behavior modification is ineffective in alleviating emotional distress, hand movements, and abnormal breathing. Physical and occupational therapy are indicated for ataxia, scoliosis, and spasticity. Arm splints may be applied to decrease stereotypic hand movements. Bromocryptine has been used to alleviate chaotic behavior. Carbamazepine appears to be the most effective medication for complex partial seizures. Parent education and support groups are indicated.

Prognosis & Course of Illness

The prognosis of Rett's disorder is poor; however, many patients survive into the fourth decade of life. Sudden death (possibly from respiratory arrest) is not uncommon.

Gillberg C: Rett syndrome. Pages 235–243 in Gilberg C: *Clinical Child Neuropsychiatry.* Cambridge University Press, 1995.
Harris JC: Rett's disorder. Pages 228–238 in Harris JC (editor): *Developmental Neuropsychiatry.* Vol 2. Oxford University Press, 1995.
Tsai LY: Rett syndrome. Child Adolesc Psychiatr Clin N Am 1994;3:105.

CHILDHOOD DISINTEGRATIVE DISORDER

DSM-IV Diagnostic Criteria

A. Apparently normal development for at least the first 2 years after birth as manifested by the presence of age-appropriate verbal and nonverbal communication, social relationships, play, and adaptive behavior.
B. Clinically significant loss of previously acquired skills (before age 10 years) in at least two of the following areas:
  (1) expressive or receptive language
  (2) social skills or adaptive behavior
  (3) bowel or bladder control
  (4) play
  (5) motor skills
C. Abnormalities of functioning in at least two of the following areas:
  (1) qualitative impairment in social interaction (eg, impairment in nonverbal behaviors, failure to develop peer relationships, lack of social or emotional reciprocity)

(2) qualitative impairments in communication (eg, delay or lack of spoken language, inability to initiate or sustain a conversation, stereotyped and repetitive use of language, lack of varied make-believe play)

(3) restricted, repetitive, and stereotyped patterns of behavior, interests, and activities, including motor stereotypies and mannerisms

D. The disturbance is not better accounted for by another specific pervasive developmental disorder or by schizophrenia.

Reprinted, with permission, from *Diagnostic and Statistical Manual of Mental Disorders,* 4th ed. Copyright 1994 American Psychiatric Association.

General Considerations

Child disintegrative disorder has been included in DSM-IV and *International Classification of Disease,* 9th edition (ICD-9) because no clear neurologic cause has been determined. The diagnostic criteria for this condition are essentially those described by Heller in 1930. The essential features are as follows: apparently normal development for at least 2 years, followed by deterioration and deviance of communication and the emergence of autistic behavior.

This condition is very rare: Slightly more than 100 clear-cut cases of childhood disintegrative disorder have been described. The incidence is thought to be 11 in 1,000,000 children born. The male-to-female ratio is 8:1. The mean age at onset is 3.4 years with a range of 1–9 years.

Clinical Findings

A. Signs & Symptoms: The onset of childhood disintegrative disorder may be insidious or abrupt. A premonitory phase of agitation has been noted in some patients. Seventy-five percent of patients deteriorate to a plateau of development. A few patients exhibit a partial recovery. One small subgroup of patients progresses downhill to an early death. In a recent survey of known patients, 42% were mute, 38% used single words or phrases, and 19% used sentences. Seizure disorder occurs in approximately 70% of patients.

B. Psychological Testing & Laboratory Findings: The assessment of patients who have childhood disintegrative disorder is the same as that for autistic disorder.

Treatment

Treatment is supportive and symptomatic.

Gillberg C: Childhood disintegrative disorder (Heller dementia infantilis). Pages 88–90 in Gilberg C: *Clinical Child Neuropsychiatry.* Cambridge University Press, 1995.

Harris JC: Childhood disintegrative disorder. Pages 239–243 in Harris JC (editor): *Developmental Neuropsychiatry.* Vol 2. Oxford University Press, 1995.

Volkmar FR: Childhood disintegrative disorder. Child Adolesc Psychiatr Clin N Am 1994;3:119.

Volkmar FR et al: "Nonautistic" pervasive developmental disorders. Pages 429–448 in Coffey CE, Brumback RA (editors): *Textbook of Pediatric Neuropsychiatry.* American Psychiatric Press, 1998.

ASPERGER'S DISORDER

DSM-IV Diagnostic Criteria

A. Qualitative impairment in social interaction, as manifested by at least two of the following:
(1) marked impairment in the use of multiple nonverbal behaviors such as eye-to-eye gaze, facial expression, body postures, and gestures to regulate social interaction
(2) failure to develop peer relationships appropriate to developmental level
(3) a lack of spontaneous seeking to share enjoyment, interests, or achievements with other people (eg, by a lack of showing, bringing, or pointing out objects of interest to other people)
(4) lack of social or emotional reciprocity

B. Restricted repetitive and stereotyped patterns of behavior, interests, and activities, as manifested by at least one of the following:
(1) encompassing preoccupation with one or more stereotyped or restricted patterns of interest that is abnormal either in intensity or focus
(2) apparently inflexible adherence to specific, nonfunctional routines or rituals
(3) stereotyped and repetitive motor mannerisms (eg, hand or finger flapping or twisting, or complex whole-body movements)
(4) persistent preoccupation with parts of objects

C. The disturbance causes clinically significant impairment in social, occupational, or other important areas of functioning.

Reprinted, with permission, from *Diagnostic and Statistical Manual of Mental Disorders,* 4th ed. Copyright 1994 American Psychiatric Association.

General Considerations

Asperger's disorder was first described in 1944 by Hans Asperger, who was unaware of Kanner's description of infantile autistic disorder 2 years earlier. Asperger applied the term "autistic psychopathy" to the condition, relating it to a difficulty in personal relationships and a failure to comprehend other peoples' emotional expression. There has been a continuing debate as to whether Asperger's disorder is on a continuum with autistic disorder or whether it is distinct.

Furthermore, the distinction between Asperger's disorder, schizoid personality disorder, and nonverbal learning disabilities syndrome is unclear. Nonverbal learning disabilities syndrome is characterized by deficits in visuospatial, social, and communicative functioning but well-developed rote memory and verbal skills. Nonverbal learning disabilities syndrome is also associated with difficulty adapting to new situations, defective pragmatic speech, and impaired social skills. It is unclear whether Asperger's disorder and nonverbal learning disabilities syndrome overlap, whether Asperger's disorder is a subset of the syndrome, or whether the two conditions are distinct.

The lack of social reciprocity associated with Asperger's disorder is evident in the child's socially inappropriate behavior, egocentrism, failure to appreciate social cues, and apparent difficulty in sensing other peoples' feelings. The patient with Asperger's disorder may express a great interest in making friends, but the patient's desire to do so is frustrated by his or her one-sided insensitivity and gaucherie. The patient with Asperger's disorder may have a theoretical understanding that other people have feelings, but he or she is characteristically unable to respond appropriately. As a result, patients tend to rely on rigid, formal rules of behavior in order to negotiate social situations.

The restricted patterns of interest that are characteristic of this condition tend to emphasize rote memory rather than conceptualization, with the amassing of information about a highly specific topic (eg, the navies of the world). The topic of interest may change over time.

Although there is no delay in language development, early pragmatic-semantic language deviance has been described. Communication tends to be formal, pedantic, long-winded, tangential, circumstantial, and verbose. It is difficult for the listener to change the speaker's topic of conversation. Prosody is eccentric, with a restricted range of intonation. Intonation patterns are poorly matched to the content of conversation. Peculiar voice characteristics, idiosyncratic use of words, misinterpretation of metaphors, and absence of humor are characteristic of this condition.

The motor clumsiness often noted in individuals with Asperger's disorder is characterized by awkward movements, rigid gait, and odd, eccentric postures.

A. Major Etiologic Theories: Family concentrations have been reported among the first-degree relatives of probands with Asperger's disorder, apparently more so than in autistic disorder. Asperger's disorder has been reported in association with aminoaciduria, Tourette's syndrome, tuberous sclerosis, and ligamentous laxity. In one third of cases, CT scan and EEG are abnormal.

B. Epidemiology: Because of uncertainties about the boundaries of the condition, the prevalence of Asperger's disorder is unclear. Asperger's disorder is more common in boys than girls (10:1). It is not associated with socioeconomic status or parental education. In one survey, the prevalence was thought to be 0.6–4 per 10,000. A Swedish survey has estimated the prevalence of Asperger's disorder as 10–26 per 10,000, suggesting that Asperger's disorder is more prevalent than autistic disorder.

Clinical Findings

A. Signs & Symptoms: Parents are not usually concerned about the development of a child with Asperger's disorder until the child reaches 2–4 years of age. It is then noted that the child either has no need for playmates or has great difficulty relating to other children. By the time the child reaches elementary school, he or she is regarded as eccentric because of his or her peculiar interests, pedantic speech, and lack of emotional reciprocity. However, the child is usually of normal or above normal intelligence. Most individuals with the disorder are never referred for psychiatric evaluation.

B. Psychological Testing & Laboratory Findings: Case assessment involves history taking; a review of mental health, medical, and educational records; mental status examination, and pediatric examination. Full psychological testing is required with regard to intelligence, style of learning, adaptive functioning, academic achievement, neuropsychological functioning, and personality.

Differential Diagnosis

Asperger's disorder is distinguished from autistic disorder by the following characteristics: (1) Asperger's disorder is associated with normal intellectual and language development, (2) the social defect in Asperger's disorder is less severe than that in autistic disorder, (3) Asperger's disorder is more likely to be associated with motor clumsiness, (4) Asperger's disorder is associated with a higher Similarity score on the Wechsler Intelligence Scale for Children—Revised, (5) patients with Asperger's disorder have a less severe impairment of metarepresentation (ie, theory of mind), and (6) associated defects or handicaps (eg, epilepsy) are less common in Asperger's disorder.

Treatment

The treatment of Asperger's disorder is similar to the psychoeducational management of nonverbal learning disabilities syndrome. The social-emotional and metarepresentational impairment are best treated by a speech and language pathologist, using a social-cognitive approach that addresses the following issues: (1) social problem solving (ie, use of language, logical reasoning, goal-setting, considering alternative solutions, choosing a solution and monitoring the outcome); (2) self-control (stopping and thinking before responding); (3) affective understanding (learning the vocabulary of emotions for oneself and others); (4) pragmatic skills (appropriate nonverbal behavior, the capacity to decode other peoples' nonverbal behavior, and the capacity to take the perspective of other people); and (5) the enhancement of self-esteem.

Patients with Asperger's disorder adapt best to occupations that do not make heavy social demands.

Prognosis & Course of Illness

Most patients with Asperger's disorder appear to cope with adult life; however, they are often frustrated by their difficulty in making friends. Some become depressed and suicidal. Alcoholism, schizophrenia, and paranoid disorder have been recorded. Criminality is unlikely, but the patient's extreme egocentrism may cause him or her to be ridiculed or socially rejected, with consequent aggressiveness.

Gillberg C: Asperger syndrome. Pages 90–97 in Gilberg C: *Clinical Child Neuropsychiatry.* Cambridge University Press, 1995.

Harris JC: Asperger's disorder. Pages 221–228 in Harris JC (editor): *Developmental Neuropsychiatry.* Vol 2. Oxford University Press, 1995.

Volkmar FR, Lord C: Diagnosis and definition of autism and other pervasive disorders. Pages 1–31 in Volkmar FR (editor): *Autism and Pervasive Developmental Disorders.* Cambridge University Press, 1998.

PERVASIVE DEVELOPMENTAL DISORDER NOS

General Considerations

This residual category lacks clear defining features. It includes a heterogeneous group of patients who have some but not all of the criteria required to diagnose a specific pervasive developmental disorder. These patients meet the criteria for pervasive developmental disorder in at least one area but not all three areas of impairment (ie, social competence; communicative competence; and restricted, repetitive behavior). The condition is diagnosed more often among children who are too profoundly retarded to be socially interactive. This residual category has also been known as atypical autistic disorder or autistic-like or atypical pervasive developmental disorder. An associated term, multiplex complex developmental disorder, refers to a group of patients characterized by impaired social relatedness, affective dysregulation, and disorganized thinking. The differentiation of pervasive developmental disorder NOS from schizotypal personality disorder is unclear.

A. Major Etiologic Theories: Because the definition of this condition is still unclear, and because it is probably heterogeneous, the etiology has not been studied.

B. Epidemiology: Different studies have estimated the prevalence of pervasive developmental disorder NOS as between 2 and 16 per 10,000. It appears to be at least as common as autistic disorder.

C. Genetics: The genetics of this condition have not been studied.

Clinical Findings

A. Signs & Symptoms: Multivariate cluster analytic studies have yielded inconsistent results. Using the Rimland Diagnostic Checklist on children with pervasive developmental disorder, Prior found two classes: (1) with early onset and core symptoms of social isolation and communication defect and (2) with later onset and impairments in socialization and communication and less stereotypic behavior. Siegel identified the following clusters: (1) autistic, (2) mentally retarded, and (3) schizoid. Szatmari performed a cluster analysis on children with pervasive developmental disorder and a normal IQ, using dimensional scores of socialization, communication, and imaginative activity. He found three clusters: (1) autistic, (2) Asperger's syndrome, and (3) an atypical group with less impaired socialization but impaired language and defective imagination. Volkmar first distinguished children who had autistic disorder, atypical pervasive developmental disorder, or schizophreniform disorder and then compared them on associated features. The children with atypical pervasive developmental disorder group had a later age at onset and higher IQ, were less impaired in social competence and communication, exhibited less stereotyped behavior, and manifested more affective disturbance.

It has been suggested that there are two subgroups of atypical pervasive developmental disorder: (1) a low-functioning group, containing more females, with a higher degree of organicity and a less favorable outcome; and (2) a high-functioning group, with more males, less organicity, and better outcome.

B. Psychological & Medical Evaluation: The assessment of patients who have pervasive developmental disorder NOS is the same as that for autistic disorder.

Differential Diagnosis

The chief differential diagnoses are autistic disorder, mental retardation, semantic-pragmatic language disorder, and multiplex complex developmental disorder.

Treatment

The treatment of this condition is similar to that for autistic disorder.

Prognosis & Course of Illness

The prognosis of this condition has not been studied separately from that of autistic disorder.

Volkmar FR et al: "Nonautistic" pervasive developmental disorders. Pages 429–448 in Coffey CE, Brumback RA (editors): *Textbook of Pediatric Neuropsychiatry.* American Psychiatric Press, 1998.

IV. MOTOR SKILLS DISORDER & COMMUNICATION DISORDERS

Michael Tramontana, PhD,
& Barry Nurcombe, MD

MOTOR SKILLS DISORDER (DEVELOPMENTAL COORDINATION DISORDER)

DSM-IV Diagnostic Criteria

A. Performance in daily activities that require motor coordination is substantially below that expected given the person's chronological age and measured intelligence. This may be manifested by marked delays in achieving motor milestones (eg, walking, crawling, sitting), dropping things, "clumsiness," poor performance in sports, or poor handwriting.

B. The disturbance in Criterion A significantly interferes with academic achievement or activities of daily living.

C. The disturbance is not due to a general medical condition (eg, cerebral palsy, hemiplegia, or muscular dystrophy) and does not meet criteria for a pervasive developmental disorder.

D. If mental retardation is present, the motor difficulties are in excess of those usually associated with it.

Reprinted, with permission, from *Diagnostic and Statistical Manual of Mental Disorders,* 4th ed. Copyright 1994 American Psychiatric Association.

General Considerations

Recent research suggests that developmental coordination disorder can be divided into several subcategories (Table 37–9).

A. Major Etiologic Theories: Motor development involves the gradual acquisition of central control over reflex movement. There is controversy over whether this acquisition involves the suppression of reflex and spontaneous cyclic movements of early infancy or whether infantile movements are incorporated into the elements that become voluntary motor skills.

Skilled movement requires a program of action with a specified objective or set goal. The program is composed of a sequence of hierarchically organized subroutines under executive control. Once acquired, motor skills are flexible. For example, the child who has learned to walk can do so on smooth, rugged, soft, or hard surfaces. The adaptation to different situations of the programmed subroutines requires accurate per-

Table 37–9. Subcategories of developmental coordination disorder.

Clumsiness: inefficiency in the performance of fine motor movements
Adventitious movements: synkinesis, chorea, tremor, or tics
Dyspraxia: inability to learn or perform serial voluntary movements to complete skilled acts
Material-specific dyspraxia: motor execution below expected for age with regard to writing (dysgraphia), drawing (constructional dyspraxia), or speech (verbal dyspraxia)
Neurologic soft signs: nonnormative performance on motor or sensory neurologic tests in the absence of localizable neurologic disease or defect
Pathologic handedness: left-handedness associated with left-hemispheric defect and paresis of the right hand

ception, central processing, executive control, and progressive feedback. Feedback monitors the approximation of the program to the set goal and modifies the timing, speed, force, and direction of movement until the desired endpoint is achieved. Initially, feedback produces jerky movements, as the child struggles to master the skill. Eventually, the skill is regulated centrally and the subroutines automated. A variety of skills can be built up from a limited number of practiced subroutines deployed in accordance with combinatorial rules. The combinatorial rules act as a kind of grammar, organizing the subroutines in hierarchical fashion. Skilled performance can be delayed or disrupted if basic reflexes are not suppressed or incorporated into the program, or if the following functions are delayed, defective, or disrupted: perception, central processing and programming, motor function, or feedback.

The hypothesis of minimal brain damage or minimal brain dysfunction was formerly invoked to explain minor sensorimotor abnormalities or immaturities; however, there is no way to prove this hypothesis. It is unclear whether the defects or delays occur in the peripheral or in the central apparatus or, if so, how they relate to developmental coordination disorder.

B. Epidemiology: It is estimated that 6% of schoolchildren have developmental coordination disorder. Children with perceptual motor defects have a high incidence of educational problems and psychological maladjustment.

Clinical Findings

A. Signs & Symptoms:

1. Clumsiness—The clumsy child is slow, jerky, and inefficient in fine-motor performance. Agonist and antagonist muscles are poorly coordinated. Motor milestones are delayed. The child drops things, tends to lose his or her balance, and is poor at activities requiring hand-eye coordination. Clumsiness can affect a particular set of muscles (eg, orofacial, hand and finger, shoulder girdle), several sets, or the entire body musculature. The child's social development is likely to be affected, particularly if clumsiness is associated with learning problems.

2. Adventitious movements—These movements involve one or more of the following unwilled movements during a purposeful motor activity: synkinesis, chorea, tremor, or tic.

Synkinesis refers to movement in a set of muscles other than that in which the primary motor action takes place. It may be homologous (ie, symmetrical) or heterologous (ie, asymmetrical). For example, while drawing with the right hand, the child with synkinesis moves his or her left hand (homologous) or tongue (heterologous). **Chorea** refers to repetitive abrupt movements of the limbs or face. **Tremor** refers to rhythmic oscillations of a body part. A **tic** is an abrupt, involuntary, repetitive movement of a particular set of muscles, usually in the face, mouth, head, neck, or diaphragm.

3. Dyspraxia—Despite normal strength, coordination, and perception, the dyspraxic child is unable to learn or perform motor skills. Dyspraxia may involve all effector muscles or may affect mainly the orofacial musculature, hand, or trunk and lower limb. The components of the motor skill are intact, but they are combined in an incoherent manner. A clumsy child will slowly get the job done. The dyspraxic child will not get the job done at all.

4. Material-specific dyspraxia—Children with material-specific dyspraxia exhibit defective motor performance in regard to specific tasks such as handwriting (specific dysgraphia), drawing and construction (constructional dyspraxia), or the articulation of words (verbal dyspraxia).

5. Neurologic soft signs—Found normally in younger children, neurologic soft signs represent a heterogeneous group of phenomena that disappear with normal development. Soft signs are regarded as abnormal if detected beyond a normative cut-off age (8–10 years). They are usually found incidentally unless tested for specifically. Their reliability, validity, and significance are disputed. A number of studies have suggested an association with cognitive dysfunction, learning problems, and psychiatric disturbance. In some cases soft signs may be related to mild brain damage; in other cases they may be related to a genetically determined factor that also correlates with a nonspecific vulnerability to psychiatric disturbance.

6. Pathologic handedness—Pathologic left-handedness occurs following damage during early development to the left hemisphere, causing a shift from right- to left-handedness. Right-sided hypoplasia, impaired visuospatial functioning, and language impairment are often found in association with this condition.

B. Assessment Procedures: After taking a developmental history, processing questions directed at elucidating motor performance, and administering a neurologic examination, the clinician can apply the specific assessment procedures described in the following sections:

1. Clumsiness—Gubbay's standardized test battery for the assessment of clumsy children, Denckla's Finger Tapping Test, and Rapin et al's Peg-Moving Procedures Test for Clumsiness are useful screening instruments.

2. Adventitious movements—The Fog Test and Wolff et al's procedure screen for synkinesis are useful. In order to elicit choreiform movements, Wolff and Hurwitz had children stand with their eyes closed; arm, wrists, and fingers extended; and wrists pronated.

3. Dyspraxia—The Lincoln-Oseretsky Test includes a subtest for dyspraxia. Dyspraxia can be tested by having the child imitate hand postures, pantomime manual activities, and use actual objects (eg, pen, cup) in an appropriate way.

4. Material-specific dyspraxia—Dysgraphia is tested by observing handwriting. Constructional dyspraxia is tested by having the child copy drawings (eg, the Bender-Gestalt Test) or block designs. Verbal dyspraxia is screened for using the Reynell Developmental Language Scales.

5. Neurologic soft signs—Neurologic soft signs can be screened for with the Physical and Neurological Examination for Soft Signs (PANESS) or the Examination for Minor Neurological Signs in Children (EXAMINS). The EXAMINS tests the following: digit span, visual tracking, speech, nystagmus, eye symmetry, hand dominance, crossed dominance of arm and leg, right-left self-identification, right-left identification on examiner, bilateral hand stimulation, face-hand apposition, finger localization, graphesthesia, stereognosis, synkinesis, finger-to-nose apposition, diadochokinesis, and passive head turning.

Pincus JH: The neurological meaning of soft signs. Pages 479–484 in Lewis M (editor): *Child and Adolescent Psychiatry: A Comprehensive Textbook,* 2nd ed. Williams & Wilkins, 1996.

Shafer SO et al: Hard thoughts on neurological "soft signs." Pages 113–143 in Rutter M (editor): *Developmental Neuropsychiatry.* Guilford Press, 1983.

Shaffer D et al: Neurological "soft signs": their origins and significance for behavior. Pages 144–163 in Rutter M (editor): *Developmental Neuropsychiatry.* Guilford Press, 1983.

Differential Diagnosis

Clumsiness is observed in chronic intoxication with neuroleptic and anticonvulsant drugs, in neuromuscular disorders (eg, Charcot-Marie-Tooth disease, Duchenne's disease), and in upper motor neuron disorders (eg, cerebral palsy, degenerative disorders). Children with Down syndrome, autism, Asperger's syndrome, specific dyslexia, and ADHD are sometimes more clumsy than is appropriate for their mental age.

Synkinesis is associated with agenesis of the corpus callosum, Klippel-Feil syndrome, hypogonadism, midline facial defects, and a rare familial syndrome. It may be associated with ADHD and conduct disorder. Chorea is observed in Sydenham's chorea (antistreptolysin titer and electrocardiogram should be ordered to test for rheumatic fever), hyperthyroidism, benign familial chorea, CNS degenerations (eg, Wilson's disease, Hallervorden-Spatz disease, homocystinuria, Huntington's disease), and tardive dyskinesia. Tremor is associated with posterior fossa tumors; neuroleptic, lithium, or phenytoin toxicity; hyperthyroidism; and benign familial tremor. Simple motor tics should be distinguished from Tourette's syndrome.

Dyspraxia is associated with subacute sclerosing panencephalitis, HIV encephalopathy, Rett's disorder, and degenerative disorders of the CNS, whether inborn or acquired. Dyspraxia can be associated with learning disorders and possibly ADHD and autism. Dysgraphia and oral-motor dyspraxia may be associated with neurofibromatosis, congenital heart disease, and homocystinuria. Constructional dyspraxia is observed in William's disease. Verbal dyspraxia has been described in galactosemia and fragile X syndrome.

Treatment

A number of treatment methods have been proposed, but it is not clear whether any of them is effective. Ayres designed a motor training program based on the theory that motor skills disorders are caused by a failure to inhibit primitive reflexes. Kephart's motor training targets posture, balance, locomotion, manipulation, catching, and propulsion. Bobath and Connolly have designed physiotherapy and occupational therapy techniques for the remediation of motor handicaps.

Connolly K: Motor development and motor disability. Pages 138–153 in Rutter M (editor): *Developmental Psychiatry.* University Park, 1981.

Deuel RK: Motor skills disorders. Pages 239–281 in Hooper SR, Hynd GW, Mattison RE (editors): *Developmental Disorders: Diagnostic Criteria and Clinical Assessment.* Lawrence Erlbaum Associates, 1992.

Greenhill LL: The physical examination in child psychiatry. Pages 409–431 in Shaffer D, Ehrhardt AA, Greenhill LL (editors): *The Clinical Guide to Child Psychiatry.* Free Press, 1985.

Voeller KKS: Nonverbal learning disabilities and motor skills disorders. Pages 719–768 in Coffey CE, Brumback RA (editors): *Textbook of Pediatric Neuropsychiatry.* American Psychiatric Press, 1998.

COMMUNICATION DISORDERS

Diagnostic Criteria

DSM-IV identifies the following categories of communication disorder:

- **Expressive language disorder:** a disturbance manifested by symptoms such as markedly limited vocabulary, errors in grammatical relationships, or difficulties with word recall or sentence production

- **Mixed receptive-expressive language disorder:** a disturbance that includes the symptoms of an expressive language disorder together with deficits involving the processing or understanding of spoken words and sentences

- **Phonological disorder:** a disturbance, formerly known as a developmental articulation disorder, manifested by developmentally inappropriate production, use, representation, or organization of speech sounds, such as sound substitutions or sound omissions

- **Stuttering:** a disturbance in the normal fluency and temporal patterning of speech characterized by one or more of the following: sound and syllable repetitions, whole-word repetitions, prolongations, interjections, broken words, blocking, circumlocutions, and excess tension in word production

In each disorder, the problem must be severe enough to interfere with the patient's school or occupational achievement or with social communication. The problem also must exceed what would be expected based on the patient's age, intelligence, or dialect and on the presence of environmental deprivation or speech-motor or sensory deficits (if a sensory, speech-motor, or known neurologic deficit is present, it should be coded as an Axis III disorder). In addition, the diagnosis of either an expressive language disorder or mixed receptive-expressive language disorder requires that the criteria for a pervasive developmental disorder are not met.

The DSM-IV category communication disorder not otherwise specified refers to any disturbance in communication that does not meet the criteria for a specific disorder of communication as noted in this section. Such disorders include voice disorders, cluttering (in which excessive wordiness interferes with idea expression), and so on. Although not specifically mentioned in DSM-IV, deficits in pragmatic language abilities are included in this category. The term "pragmatics" refers to the use of language in a social context, with respect to either the understanding or expression of intended meanings. "Getting the message" entails more than simply a literal decoding and processing of words according to syntactic rules. It relies on the incorporation of a broader range of features, many of them nonverbal, such as prosodic and gestural cues. The interpretation of indirect meaning, humor, or sarcasm often depends heavily on these features. The same is true with respect to effective expression within a social context, which from a psychiatric standpoint is an especially important dimension of language functioning, as it often may relate to problems with interpersonal relationships and social skills development.

General Considerations

DSM-IV criteria reflect a number of advancements in the conceptualization and definition of communication disorders in childhood. Many discussions on the topic make a distinction between acquired and developmental language disorders. An **acquired language disorder,** or acquired aphasia in childhood, is a syndrome involving impairment in one or more language abilities after the normal onset of speech. It usually has an identifiable neurologic basis and in general can be classified using the same terms used to classify adult aphasias. By contrast, a **developmental language disorder** (sometimes referred to as congenital aphasia) impedes the normal acquisition of language. It has no obvious point of onset, and although a neurologic basis may be suspected, it may not be verifiable. Earlier versions of DSM criteria specifically referred to developmental speech and language disorders. This distinction was dropped in DSM-IV, where the criteria are treated purely on functional grounds without implicit reference to type of onset.

Another improvement was the elimination of a category of communication disorders in childhood referring solely to receptive language impairment. The possibility of a specific disorder of receptive language, similar to Wernicke's aphasia, cannot exist in a child who has never learned to speak. Any disorder affecting receptive language, which would interfere with a child's ability to process and understand spoken input, will necessarily impede the child's ability to produce spoken language. Thus language disorders in children generally are either global or primarily expressive in nature.

A. Major Etiologic Theories: Speech and language disorder have multiple etiologies, some genetic, some congenital, and some arising from perinatal trauma such as prematurity and anoxia. Some form of underlying brain dysfunction has generally been assumed, even in disorders of the so-called developmental variety, although evidence to support this assumption may be lacking. Many studies examining children with language disorders—especially earlier studies—failed to document the presence of any CNS abnormalities.

New and important insights have begun to unfold, especially with recent technological advances in the study of brain function. For example, electrophysiologic features in the newborn—specifically involving auditory evoked responses over the left hemisphere—are predictive of language skills at 3 years of age. Such findings support a general presumption of left-hemispheric dysfunction in many speech and language disorders. Pragmatic language functions, and their dependence on various nonverbal abilities, are thought to be influenced strongly by right-hemispheric processes.

B. Epidemiology: Prevalence rates for childhood speech and language deficits vary according to the classification criteria and cutoff points used in defining abnormality. Such deficits can be defined strictly on statistical grounds, as when impaired performance is defined as falling below a particular score on a standardized test. For example, if the cutoff is set at two standard deviations (SDs) below the mean, then by definition, 2% of the reference group would fall in the impaired range; this impairment rate would rise to roughly 7% if the cutoff were set at 1.5 SDs, and so forth. Shrinkage in the estimates would result if exclusionary criteria were considered.

Language disorders occur more frequently in families with a history of language or learning problems than in the general population and are about four times more likely in boys than girls. There also appears to be an elevated rate of comorbidity with childhood psychopathology. For example, in one study 60% of children with language disorders met diagnostic criteria for ADHD.

Clinical Findings

Several key issues must be addressed in the diagnosis and evaluation of communication disorders. First, a child's speech or language functioning must be assessed through the use of standardized, individually administered tests. Basing the diagnosis on clinical observations alone is generally insufficient, except when the nature or severity of the disorder prevents formal testing. Table 37–10 describes sample measures and instruments.

Second, cutoff points should be set in determining abnormality or impairment on specific measures. In other words, what constitutes a significant deficit? This is somewhat arbitrary, although the cutoff is typically set at about 2 SDs below the mean on any particular measure, at or below which the obtained score would be considered to reflect impairment. A slightly higher cutoff may be used (eg, −1 to −1.5 SDs) if the goal pertains more to initial screening than to formal diagnosis. A more liberal cutoff may also be used when it reflects a level of performance that is clearly discrepant with the child's more general functioning. Thus a score of 85 on a standardized language measure—which technically falls in a low average range—could be viewed as reflecting a significant problem in a child with an intelligence quotient of 115 or more.

Finally, how is an unbiased estimate of a child's global abilities obtained, against which his or her language performance can be compared? DSM-IV requires that this estimate be based specifically on a nonverbal measure of intellectual capacity. This is because many intelligence measures depend heavily on verbal abilities; thus their results would be unduly lowered when a specific language impairment is involved. Measures of nonverbal intelligence include the Test of Nonverbal Intelligence, the Leiter Interna-

Table 37–10. Assessments for specific speech and language capabilities.

Capabilities Measured	Tests
Word comprehension	Peabody Picture Vocabulary Test—Revised
Expressive vocabulary, or naming abilities	Expressive One-Word Picture Vocabulary Test—Revised
Listening comprehension for spoken instructions of increasing length and complexity	Token Test for Children
Multifaceted measures of language	Clinical Evaluation of Language Fundamentals—Revised Test of Language Development—Revised
Speech articulation	Goldman-Fristoe Test of Articulation
Pragmatic language functions	No standardized tests; Wigg has developed a series of checklists for evaluating pragmatics behaviorally in children 3 years of age and up

tional Performance Scale, and the Performance section of the Wechsler Intelligence Scales.

Differential Diagnosis

The valid diagnosis of a communication disorder requires that it be differentiated from other factors that could interfere with effective communication. Language acquisition can be impeded by environmental deprivation, although such deprivation rarely would constitute the primary cause of a language disorder. Hearing-impaired children and children with neuromotor dysfunction may exhibit slow oral language growth. However, a specific language impairment may also be inferred if the degree of impairment exceeds what would be expected due to the sensory or sensorimotor deficit(s) alone. The same is true with respect to mental retardation, if present.

It is especially difficult to distinguish language disorders from autism or other pervasive developmental disorders. A communication impairment of one kind or another is a defining characteristic in various forms of pervasive developmental disorders. Important differences that may distinguish pervasive developmental disorders include the idiosyncratic use of words, aprosodic features, deviant eye contact, and an apparent disinterest in communication as reflected in the absence of a gestural language system or other nonverbal means of communication. Also, unlike the poor auditory memory often observed in language-impaired children, many children with pervasive developmental disorders exhibit superior memory.

It is also difficult sometimes to distinguish language impairment and ADHD. In both disorders, the child may have difficulties following spoken language or in expressing ideas in a focused and goal-directed manner. In ADHD, however, the problems with efficient focusing would not be limited to verbal areas. Both disorders may coexist (indeed the comorbidity rate appears fairly high), in which case the attention deficits may be especially pronounced when verbal processing is involved.

Many forms of learning disabilities can be viewed as the extension of language processing problems into the school-age period, especially when skills such as reading, spelling, and writing are involved. These problems can be considered language-based forms of learning disorders, particularly if accompanied by broader problems with language comprehension or production. The range of learning disabilities is varied, however, in that nonverbal types of learning disabilities also exist.

Treatment

Therapeutic services in the area of communication disorders are provided by appropriately certified speech and language pathologists. Services may focus on speech impediments, including problems with voice quality, oral-motor control, and phonologic and fluency weaknesses. Receptive and expressive language processing problems may also be addressed, with exercises aimed at improving word comprehension, naming abilities, syntactic awareness, and higher-order listening comprehension and formulation skills.

Depending on the therapist's qualifications, services may be directed toward facilitating pragmatic language abilities such as interpreting indirect meanings, utilizing nonverbal cues, and applying associated skills necessary for effective social communication (eg, taking turns, maintaining eye contact). Treating pragmatic deficits is a more specialized aspect of language intervention that is related closely to behaviorally oriented treatment approaches focusing on social skills development. Such approaches are not necessarily emphasized in the training and experience of all speech and language pathologists; thus it must be considered specifically when exploring potential referral options. The same is true with respect to identifying speech and language pathologists who are suited for remedial work in areas such as mnemonics and language-based learning disabilities.

Arthur G: *Arthur Adaptation of the Leiter International Performance Scale.* Psychological Services Center, 1952

Brown L, Sherbenou RJ, Dollar SJ: *Test of Nonverbal Intelligence.* Pro-ed, 1982.

Cohen DJ, Paul R, Volkmar FR: Issues in the classification of pervasive and other developmental disorders: toward DSM-IV. J Am Acad Child Psychiatry 1986;25:213.

Crary MA, Voeller KKS, Haak NJ: Questions of developmental neurolinguistic assessment. Pages 249–279 in Tramontana MG, Hooper SR (editors): *Assessment Issues in Child Neuropsychology.* Plenum Publishing, 1988.

DiSimoni F: *The Token Test for Children.* Teaching Resources, 1978.

Dunn LM, Dunn LM: *Peabody Picture Vocabulary Test—Revised.* American Guidance Service, 1981.

Gardner MF: *Expressive One-Word Picture Vocabulary Test—Revised.* Academic Therapy Publications, 1990.

Goldman R, Fristoe M: *Goldman-Fristoe Test of Articulation.* American Guidance Service, 1969.

Hammil DD, Newcomer PL: *Test of Language Development.* Pro-ed, 1988.

Molfese DL: The use of auditory evoked responses recorded from newborn infants to predict language skills. Pages 1–23 in Tramontana MG, Hooper SR (editors): *Advances in Child Neuropsychology.* Vol 1. Springer-Verlag, 1992.

Paul R, Cohen DJ, Caparulo BK: A longitudinal study of patients with severe developmental disorders of language learning. J Am Acad Child Psychiatry 1983;22:525.

Semel E, Wiig EH, Secord W: *Clinical Evaluations of Language Fundamentals—Revised.* The Psychological Corporation, 1987.

Wechsler D: *Wechsler Intelligence Scale for Children,* 3rd ed. Psychological Corporation, 1991.

Wigg EH: *Let's Talk: Developing Prosocial Communication Skills.* Merrill, 1982.

38

Disorders Usually Presenting in Middle Childhood (6–11 years) or Adolescence (12–18 years)

Barry Nurcombe, MD, Michael G. Tramontana, PhD, Mark L. Wolraich, MD, Anna Baumgaertel, MD, William Bernet, MD, & Roy Q. Sanders, MD

I. LEARNING DISORDERS

Michael G. Tramontana, PhD

Diagnostic Criteria

Diagnostic and Statistical Manual of Mental Disorders, 4th edition (DSM-IV) identifies three types of learning disorders: (1) reading disorder, (2) mathematics disorder, and (3) disorder of written expression. In each disorder, the diagnosis depends on documentation that

- Achievement in the area, as assessed on an individually administered standardized test, falls substantially below expectations based on the person's age, measured intelligence, and education
- The deficiency significantly interferes with academic achievement or daily activities requiring the particular skill
- The skill deficiency exceeds what usually would be associated with any sensory deficit, if present

Inherent in these criteria are considerations pertaining to the severity, extent, and specificity of the observed deficit—whether it be in reading, mathematics, or written expression. The deficit must be nontrivial or substantial, although this is not defined further by DSM-IV. It must affect relevant aspects of daily functioning. It also must be specific and not simply reflective of intellectual, sensory, or educational limitations.

The diagnostic category of learning disorder not otherwise specified refers to deficiencies in reading, mathematics, or written expression that interfere with academic achievement but do not meet criteria for a specific learning disorder. This is an ambiguous category that probably should not be viewed as representing a disorder. At best, it implies that a learning disorder is suspected but cannot be documented through ordinary means.

General Considerations

A. Definition Issues: Terms such as learning disorder and learning disability often are used interchangeably, although the latter term is used more commonly. A major stride in the definition of learning disabilities came from The National Joint Committee for Learning Disabilities (NJCLD). NJCLD defined a learning disability as

> a generic term that refers to a heterogeneous group of disorders manifested by significant difficulties in the acquisition and use of listening, speaking, reading, writing, reasoning or mathematical abilities. These disorders are intrinsic to the individual and presumed to be due to central nervous system dysfunction. Even though a learning disability may occur concomitantly with other handicapping conditions (e.g., sensory impairment, mental retardation, social and emotional disturbance) or environmental influences (e.g., cultural differences, insufficient/inappropriate instruction, psychogenic factors), it is not the direct result of those conditions or influences (Hammill et al 1981, p. 336).

This definition went further than the earlier one contained in the Education for All Handicapped Children Act of 1975 (P.L. 94-142) by stipulating specifically that a learning disability must be presumed to be due to central nervous system (CNS) dysfunction. Although this was implied in previous definitions, never before was it made explicit. Accordingly, the newer definition helps to resolve a good deal of confusion and ambiguity involving identification and differential diagnosis. Deficiencies in academic achievement can arise from a variety of factors, operating alone or in combination. To say that there is a learning disability, however, means that there must be a basis for inferring that some form of brain dysfunction is involved.

B. Major Etiologic Theories: The issue of etiology is addressed, at least in broad terms, by the NJCLD definition of learning disabilities. In one form or another, brain dysfunction is the source of a learning-disabled individual's deficit(s) in reading, mathematics, or written expression. The dysfunction may stem from genetic or congenital factors, arising especially during middle to later stages of fetal brain development. Neuropathologic studies suggest the presence of relatively subtle irregularities (eg, focal dysplasia, abnormal cortical layering, polymicrogyria), often clustering in the left perisylvian region, although the precise pattern will vary with the type of learning disabilities involved. This observation accounts for the specific nature of learning disabilities, in that earlier or more widespread abnormalities in brain development typically would give rise to more generalized disorders such as mental retardation. Insults occurring after birth may be a factor, provided that they affect the acquisition rather than loss of a particular skill. Although similar deficits may arise, the convention is to regard a learning disability as a neurodevelopmental disorder rather than as an acquired brain injury.

There have been a number of misconceptions regarding the cause of learning disabilities. One misconception has suggested that children with disabilities are not disordered but rather delayed on certain developmental dimensions, their difficulties presumably reflecting a slower rate of maturation of an otherwise normal brain. This would explain why a fairly severe disability can exist in the absence of documented brain impairment, at least when gross indices are used. However, current research does not support such a hypothesis. There is no evidence that the brains of learning-disabled individuals are immature, or unfinished, in some way. Rather, newer and more detailed investigations have documented specific structural abnormalities. Nor is there any indication that the disabled learner's performance resembles that of a normal younger child or that the disability is eventually outgrown. The child with learning disabilities is not merely delayed but rather deviant in the performance of processes necessary for normal reading, math, or writing. The disability may be "silent" in earlier years, giving the false impression of normal brain development, only to become evident when the child enters school.

C. Epidemiology: Estimates have varied, but about 2–8% of all school-aged children in the United States are thought to have a learning disability. The estimates are arbitrary to some extent, as they are based on the adoption of an agreed-upon cutoff in a continuous distribution. These estimates are influenced not only by debates over what the objective criteria for identification should be (see below) but also by public policy considerations having to do with the allocation of special services.

Galaburda AM, Kemper TL: Cytoarchitectonic abnormalities in developmental dyslexia: a case study. Ann Neurol 1979;6:94.

Hammill DD et al: A new definition of learning disabilities. Learning Disability Quarterly 1981;4:336.

Clinical Findings

A. Psychometric Criteria: Clear operational criteria are needed in order to identify learning disabilities. For example, how does one decide whether an individual's achievement falls "substantially below expectations" (a DSM-IV diagnostic criterion)? This determination is usually based on some type of discrepancy criterion that stipulates the minimum difference that must exist between scores obtained on standardized tests of the individual's intelligence quotient (IQ) and scores obtained on one or more areas of an achievement test.

In what is probably the most commonly used form of evaluation, IQ-achievement comparisons are made using standard scores. Different school systems set their own cutoffs, although the minimum discrepancy is typically one to two standard deviations (SDs), or 15 to 30 points for standard scores with a mean of 100 and a SD of 15. For example, for an individual with a measured IQ of 105, an achievement test score of 90 or less would be needed to meet discrepancy criteria at 1 SD, 75 or less at 2 SDs, and so forth. The problem with this method is that it does not correct for the correlation between IQ and achievement test scores. IQ and achievement test scores usually correlate moderately, so that a high score on one test will often be accompanied by a less extreme (lower) score on the other because of regression to the mean. As a result, high-IQ individuals tend to be over-identified, and low-IQ individuals under-identified, as having a learning disability.

A better approach utilizes regression-based criteria that adjust the standard test score comparisons for the correlation between IQ and achievement. A regression equation is derived for each achievement measure based on its obtained correlation with IQ (this correlation is usually available in the published test manual). This approach allows for an examination of any discrepancy between actual achievement and expected achievement predicted by the IQ measure. A cutoff between 1 and 2 standard errors of prediction (SE_{pred}) typically would be used in determining whether the discrepancy is significant.

B. Subtypes: Learning disabilities occur singly or in combination. Obviously, the underlying pattern of cognitive deficits will vary depending on how many types of learning disability are involved.

Each type of learning disability also can be further differentiated or subtyped based on the pattern of underlying deficits. To date, much of the research has focused mainly on reading and has identified two especially robust patterns of reading disability, or dyslexia: an auditory-linguistic subtype and a visual-spatial subtype. For example, the problem with letter reversals and other perceptual distortions that are commonly thought to characterize dyslexia are associated with the visual-spatial subtype of reading disability. However, the auditory-linguistic subtype of reading disability is the more prevalent subtype. A common feature of most poor readers (and spellers) is a weakness in phonologic processing, which makes it difficult for the reader to phonemically segment spoken or printed words. Poor fluency in extracting words from printed material (and vice versa) is the result.

C. Assessment Procedures: The most commonly used measure of general intelligence for school-aged children is the Wechsler Intelligence Scale for Children, 3rd edition (WISC-III). For measuring academic achievement, numerous individually administered standardized measures are available. Comprehensive or broad-band batteries include the Wechsler Individual Achievement Test and the Woodcock-Johnson Psycho-Educational Battery—Revised. Both of these tests include specific subtests that assess skills in reading, mathematics, and written expression.

Hynd GW, Connor RT, Nieves N: Learning disabilities subtypes: perspectives and methodological issues in clinical assessment. Pages 281–312 in Tramontana MG, Hooper SR (editors): *Assessment Issues in Child Neuropsychology.* Plenum Publishing, 1988.
Psychological Corporation: *Wechsler Individual Achievement Test.* Harcourt, Brace, & Jovanovich, 1992.
Shankweiler DP, Crain S: Language mechanisms and reading disorder: a modular approach. Cognition 1986;24:139.
Wechsler D: *Wechsler Intelligence Scale for Children: Third Edition.* Psychological Corporation, 1991.
Woodcock RW, Johnson MB: *Woodcock-Johnson Tests of Achievement.* DLM Teaching Resources, 1989.

Differential Diagnosis

A key issue to consider is whether an individual's poor achievement in one or more areas is merely the result of low intelligence. That is, a child's reading skills may be poor not because of a specific processing disorder but because of generally low aptitude or learning ability. Although similar underlying deficits (eg, poor phonology) may be involved in both mentally retarded and nonretarded disabled readers, the requirement for specificity would not be met in the case of mental retardation. By definition, discrepancy-based criteria for learning disabilities would help to make this differentiation.

Similarly, other exclusionary criteria pertaining to the diagnosis of learning disabilities (eg, sensory impairment, cultural differences, inadequate instruction) must be considered. If such factors are present, it must be assumed that, whether operating alone or in combination, they cannot fully account for deficits exhibited by a particular child.

One of the more common differentiations to be made is between learning disabilities and attention-deficit/hyperactivity disorder (ADHD). In both disorders, poor school achievement is likely, although the underlying mechanisms differ. In ADHD, the problems have to do more with the disruptive effects of inattention and poor task persistence that result in poor learning or skill acquisition. The child's performance is generally more variable in ADHD than in learning disabilities, and close observation often will reveal that the child is capable of processing the material but becomes unfocused or distracted at times. In learning disabilities, the processing deficits persist even when attention is optimal. Of course, some children have both conditions: estimates of comorbidity are at about 25%.

Emotional factors also must be distinguished from learning disabilities. School functioning can become impaired by a significant emotional disturbance, which makes it essential for the clinician to gather a careful history of the onset of academic symptoms. Emotional factors tend to exert a generalized or nonspecific effect, usually by impeding concentration or motivation. Although not the direct cause of specific disabilities, emotional factors may often worsen or compound the disabilities. In some cases, phobic reactions may occur to certain types of material, causing significant avoidance and further decreases in achievement. Careful evaluation will almost always document an underlying pattern of relatively lower aptitude upon which specific anxiety reactions become superimposed.

Barkley RA: Attention deficit disorder with hyperactivity. Pages 66–104 in Mash EJ, Terdal LG (editors): *Behavioral Assessment of Childhood Disorders,* 2nd ed. Guilford Press, 1988.

Treatment

Generally speaking, there are three types of treatment or intervention for learning disabilities: remedial approaches, compensatory approaches, and interventions for secondary social-emotional problems.

A. Remedial Approaches: Remedial approaches are aimed directly at improving specific skills. For example, a child with poor phonologic processing may receive intensive instruction and practice with phoneme-grapheme correspondence to improve word-attack skills in reading. Although there is no age cutoff per se, remedial interventions tend to have more of an impact earlier on, usually before the child reaches about 10 years of age. Effectiveness also depends on whether the interventions appropriately target the child's particular pattern of underlying deficits. A child with dyslexia may receive intensive help with visual tracking, even though visual problems may have nothing to do with why he or she is unable to read fluently (as would be true in the vast majority of cases). There has been a proliferation of therapies for learning disabilities, many of which lack empirical validation of their effectiveness.

B. Compensatory Approaches: Compensatory approaches help the individual to compensate, or work around, a particular deficit rather than to change it directly. These approaches are usually deferred until after an adequate course of remediation has been tried and the deficit persists. The individual should be assisted in developing strategies for containing the problem and managing to go on despite it. For example, the person with poor phonology may be taught to rely more on whole word recognition to improve reading fluency. In more severe cases, the individual may have to learn how to adapt without being a proficient reader—concentrating efforts instead on developing minimal "survival skills" (eg, recognizing common phrases, reading a menu) while emphasizing other areas.

C. Interventions for Secondary Social-Emotional Problems: Children with learning disabilities are at increased risk for problems with frustration, performance anxiety, negative peer interactions, school avoidance, and low self-esteem. Services may include education of parents on how to manage common emotional reactions, school-based interventions that teach positive coping skills, and individual psychotherapy for patients in whom more significant emotional problems have emerged. Pharmacotherapy should be considered when more pronounced or persistent anxiety or depressive symptoms are present and when ADHD is also present.

Prognosis & Course of Illness

Children generally do not outgrow learning disabilities. As noted earlier in this chapter, one of the common misconceptions regarding learning disabilities was that they merely reflect a delay—the implication being that the child will catch up eventually and exhibit normal functioning. Children with learning disabilities do improve, but except in the mildest cases, a relative weakness in the affected skill will persist. Children may even improve to roughly average levels, although this achievement would still fall below the expectations for an otherwise bright individual.

Reviews of research on adult outcomes suggest that, as a group, individuals with learning disabilities attain lower educational and occupational levels. Outcomes are poorer in patients with more severe learning disabilities, lower IQ, frank neurologic impairment, and lower socioeconomic status. Evidence regarding the long-term benefits of early educational intervention is inconclusive.

Spreen O: Prognosis of learning disability. J Consult Clin Psychol 1988;56:836.

II. DISRUPTIVE BEHAVIOR DISORDERS

Barry Nurcombe, MD, Anna Baumgaertel, MD, & Mark L. Wolraich, MD

OPPOSITIONAL DEFIANT DISORDER

DSM-IV Diagnostic Criteria

A. A pattern of negative, hostile, and defiant behavior lasting at least 6 months, during which four (or more) of the following are present:
   (1) often loses temper
   (2) often argues with adults
   (3) often actively defies or refuses to comply with adults' requests or rules
   (4) often deliberately annoys people
   (5) often blames others for his or her mistakes or misbehavior
   (6) is often touchy or easily annoyed by others
   (7) is often angry or resentful
   (8) is often spiteful or vindictive

   Note: Consider a criterion met only if the behavior occurs more frequently than is typically observed in individuals of comparable age and developmental level.

B. The disturbance in behavior causes clinically significant impairment in social, academic, or occupational functioning.

C. The behaviors do not occur exclusively during the course of psychotic or mood disorder.

D. Criteria are not met for conduct disorder, and, if the individual is age 18 years or older, criteria are not met for antisocial personality disorder.

Reprinted, with permission, from *Diagnostic and Statistical Manual of Mental Disorders*, 4th ed. Copyright 1994 American Psychiatric Association.

General Considerations

As with conduct disorder and ADHD (described later in this chapter), with which it is often entangled, it is uncertain whether oppositional defiant disorder is a truly distinctive nosological category. Specifically, it is unclear whether oppositional behavior is better considered to be on a continuum between normal developmental limit-testing on the one hand and pathologically disruptive behavior on the other. The distinction between categorical disorders and dimensional psychopathology is more than a theoretical quibble. Valid categories delimit disorders that are likely to have a significantly biological (eg, neurochemical) basis. Dimensional sets of behavior masquerading as categories may, in fact, obscure true categories that nest within their fictitious boundaries.

Oppositional defiant disorder, as defined in DSM-IV, is manifest as age-inappropriate, persistent, intemperate, argumentative, defiant, deliberately annoying, irritable, resentful, vindictive behavior associated with the tendency of the subject to blame others for his or her own transgressions or omissions. The aggression of the oppositional child or adolescent is predominantly verbal rather than physical. The aggression tends to be reactive (eg, in response to an unwelcome imposition of rules) rather than proactive (eg, bullying), and overt (eg, shouting) rather than covert (eg, spreading malicious rumors).

A. Major Etiologic Theories: The genesis of oppositional defiant disorder has not been studied separately from that of conduct disorder. Because conduct disorder often evolves from earlier oppositional behavior, and because the two disorders have similar risk factors, oppositional defiant disorder and conduct disorder are often discussed together.

Many young children who exhibit oppositional defiant behavior were, as infants, already temperamentally hyperreactive, irritable, difficult to soothe, and slow to adapt to new circumstances. Infants who exhibit disorganized attachment behavior are at risk of oppositional, disruptive behavior in middle childhood. Often the families of these children are highly stressed, as a result, for example, of marital discord, single parenthood, parental psychopathology, or socioeconomic disadvantage. Maternal depression may be particularly common. Preoccupied with their own problems, parents fail to provide these children with adequate praise and attention. When parents seek to set limits, they do so harshly and inconsistently. The children react defiantly, testing the limits, and the stage is set for repetitive cycles of escalating coerciveness, with shouting and mutual accusations, often terminated by harsh physical punishment or by the capitulation of one or other of the antagonists. Children's aggressiveness is associated with how aggressive their parents were at the same age. Often parents respond to their children in the manner (and even in the same words) that their parents responded to them. In summary, a lack of positive reinforcement for acceptable behavior is associated with increasing negative attention for oppositional behavior and with inconsistent, unpredictable, harsh punishment. Table 38–1 lists the characteristics of a coercive interaction. These factors can be targeted for therapeutic intervention (see "Treatment" section later in this chapter).

B. Epidemiology: The prevalence of oppositional defiant disorder is uncertain, but it has been estimated at 5.7–9.9%. The average age at onset is 6 years. Oppositional defiant disorder is regarded by many researchers as a milder, precocious form of conduct disorder. The male-to-female sex ratio in childhood conduct disorder is 4:1. There is a clinical impression that childhood oppositional defiant disorder is more common among preadolescent males than females; however, the relative prevalence in females appears to rise in adolescence.

C. Genetics: The genetics of oppositional defiant disorder has not been studied apart from that of

Table 38–1. The characteristics of coercive parent-child/adolescent interactions.

Characteristic	Example
Unclear communication	Failure to address the child directly, lack of eye contact, hard-to-follow instructions
Lack of sincerity or conviction in communication	Poor eye contact; incongruity between words, gesture, and body language
Harsh, sarcastic tone of communication	"You'll do what you're told, young lady, or . . ."
Accusatory, denigrating, shaming statements	"You'll never amount to anything, you slut."
Empty threats	"If you do that once more, I'll . . ."
Bringing up the past	"I'll never forgive you for the time when you . . ."
Rigid, overgeneralized, black-and-white, "catastrophizing"	"People who smoke die young."
Preaching, moralizing, "psychologizing"	"When I was young, kids did what they were told . . ."
Failure to listen to the other person	Interrupting, changing the topic, discounting the other person's opinion ("How would you know . . .?"), monopolizing the conversation
Capitulation, impotence, hopelessness, despair	"What's the use of talking to you? It never does any good."
Failure to praise the child's or adolescent's achievements	
Failure to follow through and monitor the child's behavior	
Inconsistent, unpredictable, excessively harsh punishment	

conduct disorder. Behavioral genetic studies of aggressive behavior in children have yielded inconsistent estimates of its heritability, probably because of variations in the measurement instruments used. Most studies suggest that the trait of aggressiveness has low heritability.

Caspi A, Moffitt TE: The continuity of maladaptive behavior: from description to understanding in the study of antisocial behavior. Pages 472–511 in Cicchetti D, Cohen DJ (editors): *Developmental Psychopathology.* Vol 2: *Risk, Disorder, and Adaptation.* John Wiley & Sons, 1995.

Hinshaw SP, Anderson CA: Conduct and oppositional defiant disorders. Pages 113–152 in Mash EJ, Barkley RA (editors): *Child Psychopathology.* Guilford Press, 1996.

Clinical Findings

A. Signs & Symptoms: The persistent, recurrent aggressive and defiant behavior associated with oppositional defiant disorder may be restricted to the home or may be generalized as an antiauthoritarian attitude, for example, to teachers and other adults outside the home. It is usually evident before 8 years of age but may emerge for the first time in adolescence. Oppositional, hostile, limit-testing behavior disrupts family relationships and can interfere with learning. At school, oppositional children or adolescents may be moody, irritable, lacking in self-esteem, and often in conflict with teachers and peers. As a result, the oppositional child or adolescent often appears to have a "chip on his or her shoulder." Oppositional adolescents may be solitary or inclined to gravitate to the company of others who regard themselves as outlaws. Precocious tobacco use is likely, as is alcohol and substance abuse.

B. Psychological Testing: Aside from questionnaires that are useful for assessing aggressive behavior (eg, the Child Behavior Checklist and the Eyberg Child Behavior Inventory), a number of behavioral observation rating scales and questionnaires have been developed for the assessment of conflictual parent-child or family behavior (Table 38–2). These tests may be useful as monitors of the progress and effectiveness of treatment, in accordance with treatment goals and objectives.

Differential Diagnosis & Comorbidity

Oppositional defiant disorder should be differentiated from normal developmental limit-testing in toddlers and preschool children, and from the challenging confrontations that occur between parents and normal adolescents who are seeking to be more independent. Developmental oppositional behavior is transitory and causes no significant impairment.

Oppositional defiant disorder should be discriminated from ADHD, with which it frequently coexists, and from conduct disorder, which often succeeds it. An underlying mood disorder may be manifest, to the superficial observer, as sullen defiance. Premorbid schizophrenia or early schizophrenia is sometimes associated with negativism and marked contrasuggestibility. A comprehensive history and mental status examination will differentiate these two disorders.

Children with mental retardation, hearing loss, or impaired language comprehension are sometimes oppositional and defiant at school. Selective mutism often has oppositional features.

Oppositional defiant behavior often coexists with the following situations or conditions: parental conflict, parental psychopathology (especially depression), physical or sexual abuse, conduct disorder, ADHD, and adolescent substance use disorder. In re-

Table 38–2. Behavioral observation scales and questionnaires useful for assessing parent-child or family interaction.

Assessment Tools	Reference
The Dyadic Parent-Child Interaction Coding System	Eyberg & Robinson 1983
The Family Interaction Coding System	Reid 1978
The Marital Interaction Coding System	Robin 1988
The Interaction Behavior Code	Robin & Koepke 1985
Wahler's Standardized Observation Codes	Wahler et al 1976
The Family Process Code	Dishion et al 1976
The Parent Daily Report	Chamberlain & Reid 1987
The Parenting Stress Index	Loyd & Abidin 1985
The Issues Checklist	Robin & Foster 1989
The Conflict Behavior Questionnaire	Robin & Foster 1989
The Parent-Adolescent Relationship Questionnaire	Robin et al 1986
The Family Beliefs Inventory	Vincent et al 1986
The Family Environment Scale	Moos & Moos 1983
The Family Adaptability and Cohesion Evaluation Scales—II	Olsen & Portner 1983

gard to the comorbidity of oppositional defiant disorder with ADHD and conduct disorder, it is unclear whether these disorders have mixed symptoms, whether they share risk factors, whether oppositional defiant disorder is a risk factor for other disorders, or whether it is an early manifestation of conduct disorder.

Treatment

A. Children: With children under 12 years of age, treatment is provided primarily through the parents. Whether as single parents, as parental dyads, or in parental groups, parents are educated concerning the origin and meaning of oppositional defiant behavior and are trained to replace coercive discipline with more effective child-rearing techniques. Table 38–3 describes the essentials of effective parenting.

The Positive Parenting Program (Triple P) contains all these elements and has been designed as a population-based intervention strategy. Triple P is a parenting and family support program that can be delivered in five levels: Level 1 targets common, everyday behavior problems; level 2 targets oppositional defiant disorder; and levels 3–5 target severe behavior problems complicated by severe family psychopathology. The program can be delivered through parent information nights; through videotapes; by information and skills training delivered through individual, self-directed, and group programs; and through three levels of intensive family therapy (requiring specific training for the clinicians who implement the therapy). Table 38–4 lists the principles and objectives of the Triple P program.

B. Adolescents: In adolescent oppositional defiant disorder, a family therapy approach has had the most success. In the Problem Solving Communication Training (PSCT) program, the family is first assessed with regard to the issues described in Table 38–5. These issues can be described as molecular (ie, fam-

Table 38–3. The essentials of effective parenting with oppositional defiant children.[1]

Provide positive attention with praise and reinforcement of desirable behavior.
Ignore inappropriate behavior unless it is serious.
Give clear, brief commands, reduce task complexity, and eliminate competing influences (eg, television).
Establish a token economy at home with tokens or points awarded for compliance (to be "cashed in," weekly). Do not remove points for noncompliance, at first. Maintain the token economy for at least 6–8 weeks.
When the token economy is established, use response cost (removal of tokens) or time out, contingent on noncompliance, applied soon after the noncompliance (1–2 minutes time out per year of age). Do not release the child from time out until he or she is quiet and agrees to obey.
Extend time out to noncompliance in public places.

[1] Adapted, with permission, from Barkley RA: *Defiant Children: A Clinician's Manual for Parent Training.* Guilford Press, 1987.

Table 38–4. The principles and objectives of the Triple P program.[1]

Principles
Children need a safe environment that provides opportunities for exploration and play.
Parents should respond constructively to help children solve their own problems.
Assertive discipline is more effective than coercive discipline.
Parents should take care of themselves by communicating better with each other, understanding their own emotional states, and coping with their own disruptive emotions.

Objectives
The promotion in parents of better self-regulation and problem solving.
The enhancement of child competencies that protect against adverse mental health outcomes (eg, social skills, affect regulation, problem solving).
The reduction of family conflict.
The reduction of parental distress and the promotion of parental competence.
The provision of social support.

[1] Adapted, with permission, from Sanders MR: *Healthy Families, Healthy Nation: Strategies for Promoting Family Mental Health in Australia.* Australian Academic Press, 1995.

ily communication problems and poor problem solving) or molar (ie, family structural and functional problems). Molecular issues provide the specific goals and objectives of therapy, whereas molar issues inform its strategy and tactics.

The treatment objectives of PSCT are also listed in Table 38–5. Family communication and problem solving are addressed by eliciting the common causes of family disagreement and then ranking them in order of seriousness or difficulty. The family is directed to address one cause of dispute per session, starting with the least acrimonious, by using a formula for problem solution (Table 38–6). As the family addresses these problems, family communication pathology can be remediated with the use of feedback, instruction, modeling, and behavioral rehearsal. Sometimes the family's communication patterns are so adverse that they must be addressed before PSCT can begin.

In the course of treatment, the family's rigid, biased beliefs will be revealed and targeted for cognitive restructuring (Table 38–7). In cognitive restructuring, the therapist challenges each dysfunctional belief, suggests a more reasonable alternative, and helps the family to conduct an "experiment" that will disconfirm the belief.

In a complex family system, PSCT and cognitive restructuring are unlikely to be effective unless the family's functional and structural pathology can also be addressed. PCST can be undermined by family members who are not involved in therapy or by outside agencies that oppose it. Severe psychopathology in a family member (eg, maternal depression, paternal alcoholism, adolescent substance abuse) may need treatment before PSCT can proceed. A minimal level

Table 38–5. Problem-Solving Communication Training: assessment and treatment.[1]

Assessment
What are the specific issues that provoke discord in the family?
How effective are the family's communication patterns?
Is the family involved in coercive interactions (see Table 38–1)?
Do the parents model and convey effective problem-solving techniques?
Does the family endorse negatively biased, inflexible beliefs about each other (eg, "catastrophizing," perfectionism) (see Table 38–7)?
Are structural problems evident in the family (eg, misalignments, coalitions, triangulation, disengagement, enmeshment, conflict, "detouring")?
What functional purpose does the adolescent's behavior serve (eg, to distract parents who would otherwise quarrel, or to drive parents apart, or to attract attention away from a sibling regarded as more favored)?

Treatment objectives
Promote better family communication and more effective problem solving.
Help the family generalize their skills to the home.
Reverse or neutralize structural and functional problems.

[1] Adapted, with permission, from Foster SL, Robin AL: Parent-adolescent conflict. Pages 493–528 in Mash EJ, Barkley RA (editors): *Treatment of Childhood Disorders.* Guilford Press, 1989.

of verbal ability in family members is required for PSCT to be successful. PSCT by itself is unlikely to be effective if the adolescent patient has conduct disorder.

Foster SL, Robin AL: Parent-adolescent conflict. Pages 493–528 in Mash EJ, Barkley RA (editors): *Treatment of Childhood Disorders.* Guilford Press, 1989.
Sanders MR: *Healthy Families, Healthy Nation: Strategies for Promoting Family Mental Health in Australia.* Australian Academic Press, 1995.
Sanders MR: New directions in behavioral family intervention with children. Pages 283–330 in Ollendick TH, Prinz RJ (editors): *Advances in Clinical Child Psychology.* Vol 18. Plenum Publishing, 1996.

Prognosis & Course of Illness

Oppositional defiant disorder is predicted by the same risk factors as is conduct disorder (eg, marital discord, socioeconomic stress, maternal depression) but to a lesser degree. Although about 90% of children and adolescents with conduct disorder have previously met (and still meet) criteria for oppositional defiant disorder, only about 25% of children with oppositional defiant disorder go on to exhibit conduct disorder. About 50% continue to exhibit oppositional defiant disorder in late childhood and adolescence; and the remaining 25%, when assessed later, cease to meet criteria for either oppositional defiant disorder or conduct disorder.

The significance of these findings has been debated. Should oppositional defiant disorder be regarded as a precocious (albeit milder) form of conduct disorder? Or is it an extreme form of (and continuous with) normal oppositional behavior? What determines the developmental trajectory of the individual child? It has been postulated that one developmental trajectory proceeds from early oppositional-defiant behavior, along an authority conflict pathway, to serious conflict with adults during adolescence. This pathway is likely to intersect with the covert or overt antisocial trajectories described in the next section.

Oppositional behavior is common during adolescence. As described earlier in this chapter, when such behavior is severe, it is usually a manifestation of family dysfunction. The association between childhood oppositional defiant disorder and adolescent oppositional defiant disorder is unknown.

Table 38–7. Dysfunctional beliefs.[1]

Parents
If my adolescent is given freedom, he or she will be ruined.
My adolescent should always obey me.
My adolescent should always make the right decision.
My adolescent is out to upset and hurt his or her parents.
If my adolescent does wrong, I must be to blame.

Adolescents
Rules are unfair.
Rules will ruin my life.
I should be allowed complete freedom.
People should always be fair to each other.
If my parents loved me, they would always trust me.
I should never upset my parents.

[1] Adapted, with permission, from Foster SL, Robin AL: Parent-adolescent conflict. Pages 493–528 in Mash EJ, Barkley RA (editors): *Treatment of Childhood Disorders.* Guilford Press, 1989.

Table 38–6. The steps of problem solving for families.[1]

1. Define the problem. Each family member tells the others what the problem is and why it is a problem. The other family members paraphrase the statement to check their understanding of it.
2. Generate alternative solutions, taking turns.
3. Take turns to evaluate each proposed solution. The solution with the greatest number of positive ratings wins.
4. Implement the solution and check its effectiveness.

[1] Adapted, with permission, from Foster SL, Robin AL: Parent-adolescent conflict. Pages 493–528 in EJ Mash, RA Barkley (editors): *Treatment of Childhood Disorders.* Guilford Press, 1989.

Lahey BB et al: Oppositional defiant and conduct disorders: issues to be resolved for DSM-IV. J Am Acad Child Adolesc Psychiatry 1992;31:539.

Loeber R et al: Developmental pathways in disruptive child behavior. Dev Psychopathol 1993;5:103.

CONDUCT DISORDER

DSM-IV Diagnostic Criteria

A. A repetitive and persistent pattern of behavior in which the basic rights of others or major age-appropriate societal norms or rules are violated, as manifested by the presence of three (or more) of the following criteria in the past 12 months, with at least one criterion present in the past 6 months:

Aggression to people and animals

(1) often bullies, threatens, or intimidates others

(2) often initiates physical fights

(3) has used a weapon that can cause serious physical harm to others

(4) has been physically cruel to people

(5) has been physically cruel to animals

(6) has stolen while confronting a victim

(7) has forced someone into sexual activity

Destruction of property

(8) has deliberately engaged in fire setting with the intention of causing serious damage

(9) has deliberately destroyed others' property (other than by fire setting)

Deceitfulness or theft

(10) has broken into someone else's house, building, or car

(11) often lies to obtain goods or favors or to avoid obligations

(12) has stolen items of nontrivial value without confronting a victim

Serious violations of rules

(13) often stays out at night despite parental prohibitions, beginning before 13 years of age

(14) has run away from home overnight at least twice while living in parental or parental surrogate home (or once without returning for a lengthy period)

(15) often truant from school, beginning before age 13 years

B. The disturbance in behavior causes clinically significant impairment in social, academic, or occupational functioning.

C. If the individual is age 18 years or older, criteria are not met for antisocial personality disorder.

Specify type based on age at onset: *childhood-onset type* or *adolescent-onset type.*

Specify severity: *mild, moderate, severe.*

General Considerations

As described in DSM-IV, the diagnostic features of conduct disorder have evolved from earlier multivariate factor analytic studies of child and adolescent clinical populations. A former division of delinquency syndromes into undersocialized aggression and socialized aggression has been dropped in favor of the atheoretical subcategories of childhood-onset and adolescent-onset types, either of which may be mild, moderate, or severe.

It has been difficult to disentangle the taxon of conduct disorder from several other behavior disorders with which it is frequently associated (eg, oppositional defiant disorder, ADHD, and substance use disorder). Although conduct disorder is formally described as though it were categorically distinct, it almost certainly comprises a number of associated continua.

Conduct disorder must be distinguished from transient antisocial behavior that reflects the risk-taking and group contagion that are part of normal adolescence. Antisocial behavior is common in adolescence; in most cases it requires no psychiatric attention. Conduct disorder, in contrast, represents severe, persistent, and pervasive dysfunction.

Two types of aggression have been described, variously designated as reactive/proactive, overt/covert, affective/predatory, defensive/offensive, socialized/undersocialized, impulsive/controlled, or hostile/instrumental. Reactive, affective, impulsive aggression is likely to be associated with child maltreatment.

A. Major Etiologic Theories:

1. Psychosis, epilepsy, & brain dysfunction— Careful history taking, mental status examination, neuropsychological testing, and electroencephalography (EEG) of violent juvenile offenders often reveal hallucinatory experiences, mental absences, episodes of illogical thinking, lapses of concentration, memory gaps, suspiciousness, explosive aggression, and nonspecific EEG abnormalities. These findings, along with the history of physical abuse and neglect often encountered among violent delinquents, have suggested that some antisocial youths could be experiencing covert psychosis or subclinical epilepsy caused by brain injury. An alternative explanation is that a high proportion of explosively aggressive youths harbor overt or residual posttraumatic stress disorder secondary to physical or sexual abuse and that their absences, hallucinations, lapses in concentration, and explosiveness represent dissociation stemming from unresolved trauma.

2. Psychophysiologic theories— Childhood-onset, aggressive conduct disorder (in contrast to adolescent-onset, nonaggressive conduct disorder) is associated with low tonic psychophysiologic arousal, low autonomic reactivity, and rapid habituation. These characteristics may be associated with an impairment of avoidance conditioning to social stimuli, a failure to respond to punishment, and deficient behavioral inhibition. An imbalance between central reward and inhibition systems has been postulated. It is unclear whether these psychophysiologic phenomena are inherent, whether they are secondary to disruptive experiences in early childhood, or whether they are the result of an unstable lifestyle.

3. Neuroendocrine & biochemical theories— Research into the relationship between testosterone and aggressive crime has yielded inconsistent results. Several studies have found an association between low levels of 3-methoxy-4-hydroxyphenylglycol in cerebrospinal fluid and impulsive behavior in older youths. Other abnormalities in the dopaminergic and noradrenergic systems have been described, although only in very small population samples. Low levels of cerebrospinal 5-hydroxyindoleacetic acid, a serotonin metabolite, are associated with psychopathy, aggression, and suicide; and one study correlated defiance and aggression with low levels of whole blood 5-hydroxytryptamine. Another study has suggested a relationship between disruptive behavior disorder (ie, conduct disorder and oppositional defiant disorder) and lower concentrations of cerebrospinal fluid somatostatin. These studies must be interpreted with caution because of the following limitations: (1) They have small sample sizes, (2) they gathered data from areas (ie, cerebrospinal fluid) that are far "downstream" from the areas in question (ie, central neurotransmitter synapses), and (3) their cross-sectional correlative nature makes it difficult to determine the direction and timing of causal sequences. Many of the children in these studies experienced severe maltreatment; moreover, conduct disorder itself may generate traumatic experiences that could affect the neurochemical systems in question.

4. Neuropsychological & neurodevelopmental theories—Associations have been found among severe and extended child maltreatment, dissociative symptoms, chronic posttraumatic stress disorder, memory defects, and reduction in hippocampal size. Low circulating cortisol has been associated with emotional numbing in chronic posttraumatic stress disorder, and high cortisol levels have been associated with flashbacks.

Delinquent populations subjected to cognitive testing have consistently exhibited IQs about eight points below those of nondelinquent populations, a difference that persists when socioeconomic status is statistically controlled. This discrepancy is primarily the result of deficits in word knowledge, verbally coded information, verbal reasoning, verbally mediated response regulation, and metalinguistic skills. The most impulsive, aggressive subjects exhibit the widest discrepancy between verbal and performance IQs. These

deficits probably antedate school entry and are associated with learning problems.

Research into time-orientation, impulsivity, sensation seeking, and locus of control in youths with conduct disorder has not yielded consistent results, possibly because juvenile delinquency is not homogeneous. In terms of moral reasoning, unsocialized aggressive delinquents operate at a preconventional level and have deficient role-taking abilities. The characteristic egocentrism, hedonism, unreflectiveness, and denial of responsibility of offenders have been associated with developmental immaturity of the frontal lobe and left hemisphere.

5. Psychoanalytic & attachment theory— Early psychoanalytic theories postulated a relationship between crime and unconscious guilt. Later studies described the deficient ego and superego functioning of adult criminals, with impairment in reality testing, judgment, affect regulation, object relations, adaptive regression, and synthetic functioning. A connection has been postulated between parental psychopathology and the parent's unconscious fostering of deviant behavior in the child.

The observation that early neglect and bond disruption were prevalent in delinquents who exhibited so-called affectionless psychopathy led attachment theorists to examine the contributions of emotional neglect, attachment disruption, separation, and object loss to sociopathy. Disruptive behavior patterns are postulated to stem from three complementary processes: disorganized attachment patterns, distorted affective-cognitive structures, and the motivational consequences of insecure attachment. Disruptive behavior patterns are thought to arise ultimately from a combination of neurobiological risk factors, attachment disturbance, inappropriate parenting practices, and adverse family ecology.

6. Child maltreatment & adverse parenting practices—Maternal depression has been linked, via disorganized attachment, to disruptive behavior in middle childhood. Marital conflict, domestic violence, parental neglect, and child maltreatment are also associated with later antisocial behavior. The effect of divorce on child behavior is likely to be mediated mainly by exposure to marital discord before, during, and after parental separation. Physical abuse is related to later aggressive behavior and can be transferred from one generation to the next. The prevalence of sexual abuse among girls with conduct disorder is very high. According to a recent study of delinquent girls placed in therapeutic foster care, the girls first engaged in sexual activity at age 6 years, on average.

The following adverse parenting practices convey a risk for antisocial behavior: low parental involvement in child-rearing; poor supervision; and harsh, punitive discipline. Characteristic parent-child interactions involve unclear communication; lax and inconsistent monitoring; lack of follow-through; unpredictable, explosive, coercive, harsh, and overpunitive verbal or physical discipline; and a failure to provide verbal reinforcement for desirable behavior. Parents tend to back down from their child's increasingly coercive demands until, unable to tolerate them further, they lash out angrily. At such times, the parents are likely to berate the child in terms of the same undesirable characteristics that their own parents ascribed to them. Thus parents unwittingly reinforce negative behavior, fail to model and reinforce desirable behavior, and at the same time distort the child's attributional style: The child is primed to view himself or herself as bad and to expect other people, particularly authority figures, to be hostile and uncaring.

The combination of aggressive, antiauthoritarian behavior and verbal reasoning impairment causes the child to fail at school, to perceive himself or herself as rejected by teachers and peers, and to gravitate toward like-minded companions. Aggregations of high-risk youths incite and perpetuate antisocial behavior, providing a training ground for criminality and drug abuse. The parents of disruptive children are likely to have difficulty in preventing their children from mixing with rogue companions who promote delinquent behavior.

7. Attributional style—Children who are prone to conduct disorder develop a characteristic interpersonal style that reflects a complex interplay among the following factors: biological predisposition, adverse environment, distorted information processing, and the influence of peers. Aggressive children have been found to underutilize social cues, to interpret neutral or ambiguous cues as hostile, to generate few assertive solutions to social problems, and to expect that aggressive behavior will be rewarded. This is particularly likely in those children who, early in development, exhibit aggressive, hyperactive, impulsive behavior. Presumably their impulsivity limits their capacity to scan the environment for cues.

8. Sociologic theories—The following sociologic factors are related to antisocial behavior: severe family adversity; multiple family transitions; unemployment; socioeconomic disadvantage; disorganized, crime-ridden neighborhoods; and the prevalence of juvenile gangs. Family adversity, family transitions, and low socioeconomic status are particularly likely to be associated with childhood-onset, aggressive conduct disorder. However, the effect of low socioeconomic status is nullified when the effect of adverse parenting practices is statistically controlled. Adverse family circumstances appear to affect the child via adverse parenting.

Sociologic research has generated five main theories concerning the roots of antisocial behavior: (1) social segregation theory, (2) culture conflict theory, (3) criminogenic social organization theory, (4) blocked-opportunity theory, and (5) theories to do with differential justice and labeling.

Social segregation theory postulates that disadvantaged social or ethnic groups, particularly recent immigrants, become relegated to decaying neighborhoods ringing the inner city. Socially disorganized slums become battlegrounds for competing ethnic groups and spawn criminogenic cultural organizations such as juvenile gangs. Economically blocked from mainstream culture, many residents seek a criminal solution whereas others tolerate or adapt to the local criminal tradition.

Culture conflict theory relates the antisocial behavior of the children of socially disadvantaged immigrants to the confusion and disempowerment of immigrant parents, leading to a conflict between traditional parental control and the influence of the new society. Criminogenic social organization theorists have studied the informal organization of street gangs and their focal concerns with masculinity, toughness, status, the capacity to outwit others, a hunger for excitement, and the belief that life is dictated by fate rather than planning. Blocked-opportunity theorists have emphasized the function of the gang as an illegitimate means to acquire desirable amenities in a materialistic society that accords high status to affluence.

Alternative views suggest that differential delinquency rates are related to variations in the activity of police and juvenile justice authorities: The chances for apprehension are higher in areas where there is greater police surveillance. Labeling theorists suggest that delinquency is caused by designating a juvenile as "delinquent." Evidence indicates that delinquent attitudes can be hardened by legal processing, but this is a contributory rather than a root cause of antisocial behavior.

B. Epidemiology: Definitive conclusions about the prevalence of conduct disorder are difficult to reach because studies have differed in the geographic areas and age ranges studied and in the methods of assessment. However, it is evident that conduct disorder is one of the most common problems in childhood and adolescence. Overall prevalence rates for conduct disorder have varied from 0.9% (Germany) to 8.7% (Missouri). Prevalence rates in adolescents have varied from 9% to 10% in boys and from 3% to 4% in girls. The prevalence of antisocial personality disorder in adults is estimated to be 2.6%. Two studies found that African-American youths were more likely to be assigned the diagnosis of conduct disorder; however, comparative studies are few.

Prospective studies have identified the following individual variables as associated with later adjudications for delinquency: drug use, stealing, aggression, general problem behavior, truancy, poor educational achievement, and lying. The following environmental variables predict delinquency: poor parental supervision, lack of parental involvement, poor discipline, parental absence, poor parental health, low socioeconomic status, and association with deviant peers. The following factors are protective: high IQ, easy temperament, good social skills, good school achievement, and a good relationship with at least one adult.

Composite behavioral indices have greater predictive power than do single variables, supporting a cumulative risk model. One model of transmission postulates a genetic propensity that is triggered if the subject is exposed to parental risk factors and is subsequently expressed fully in an adverse social environment. It has not been demonstrated whether genetic propensity or adverse parenting alone can generate conduct disorder. However, a Danish study found that birth complications and maternal rejection predicted antisocial violence in late adolescence.

Gender differences in prevalence and trajectory have been identified. Whereas males predominate in disruptive behavior disorders prior to adolescence, prevalence rates among the two sexes are closer by age 15 years, due to an increase in covert, nonaggressive delinquent behavior among girls. Girls are more likely to follow the nonaggressive pathway with late onset, covert offenses, and a greater likelihood of recovery. Because of the emphasis on aggressive behavior in formal diagnostic schedules for conduct disorder, it is possible that the behavioral precursors and adult outcome of female conduct disorder have been obscured. Indirect aggression (eg, spreading malicious rumors) is more common in girls.

C. Genetics: Studies have examined the concordance for adult criminality between monozygotic (MZ) and dizygotic (DZ) twins (determining heritability), the concordance for criminality between MZ twins reared apart (correcting for shared environment), and the prevalence of criminality in adopted-away offspring of adult criminals (separating environmental and genetic influences). In 10 twin comparison studies, the concordance rates for adult criminality have been up to 50% for MZ twins and 20% for DZ twins. In contrast, seven studies of adolescent antisocial behavior have demonstrated a high but equivalent concordance in MZ and DZ twins, suggesting a preponderant environmental effect. Studies of the adopted-away offspring of adult criminals suggest an additive effect, for adult property crime, between biological predisposition and criminogenic environment. Interestingly, this effect does not appear to apply to aggressive crime.

Improvements in the subtyping of conduct disorder will likely lead to advances in genetic research. For example, recent studies found evidence for the heritability of an aggression trait, whereas little evidence was found for a genetic factor in adolescent-onset, nonpersisting delinquent behavior. Research into the genetics of adolescent antisocial behavior has been impeded by the tendency to regard conduct disorder as a homogeneous, categorically distinct disorder rather than as a loosely assorted conglomerate of dimensional types exhibiting multifactorial etiology (multiple causal factors), heterotypic continuity (the tendency for behavioral patterns to change over time), and equifinality (the tendency for different causal factors to result in a common phenotype).

Pedigree studies suggest an association between adult antisocial personality disorder (in men), alcoholism (in men), and hysteria (in women). Recent research suggests that antisocial personality disorder and alcoholism have separate modes of inheritance.

In summary, it appears likely that polygenic factors have a moderate influence on adult criminality, particularly in regard to recidivism for property offenses, and that adverse genetic and environmental influences interact. At this point, definitive studies have not been conducted with adolescents. Future research into the genetics of juvenile delinquency should examine subtypes of juvenile antisocial and aggressive behavior.

Three chromosomal abnormalities have been associated with antisocial behavior: 47XXY, 47XYY, and an abnormally long Y chromosome. These conditions are so uncommon as to be of little practical import. In developmentally retarded groups, the XXY anomaly may be associated with antisocial behavior. The XYY anomaly is characterized by tallness, hypotonia, hyperactivity, delayed language development, tantrums, EEG abnormality, recidivism for minor property offenses, and (in one study) a sadistic sexual orientation. The long Y anomaly may also be associated with recidivism.

Bauermeister JJ, Canino G, Bird H: Epidemiology of disruptive behavior disorders. Child Adolesc Psychiatr Clin N Am 1994;3:177.

Lahey BB et al: Psychobiology. Chapter 2, pages 27–44 in Sholevar GP (editor): *Conduct Disorders in Children and Adolescents.* American Psychiatric Press, 1995.

Rogeness GA: Biologic findings in conduct disorder. Child Adolesc Psychiatr Clin N Am 1994;3:271.

Clinical Findings

A. Signs & Symptoms: Children with conduct disorder are usually referred for evaluation during childhood or adolescence—by parents; caregivers; pediatricians; or educational, child welfare, or juvenile justice authorities—because their behavior has become intolerably disruptive or dangerous at home, in school, or in the community. Often the referral occurs in response to threatened or actual suspension from school.

The overlap among conduct disorder, oppositional defiant disorder, and ADHD has raised questions concerning the distinctiveness of each disorder. Furthermore, the many associated problems exhibited by these children dictate the need to gather diagnostic data from a number of informants (eg, parents, the patient, teachers). Categorical diagnosis alone is almost useless for treatment planning. A comprehensive biopsychosocial evaluation is required with an assessment of the patient's perceptual-motor, cognitive, linguistic, academic, and social competencies; an analysis of family functioning; and an examination of the child's behavior in school, with peers, and in relation to the community. Clinical interviewing of the patient and the family allows the clinician to explore different areas in response to diagnostic hypotheses. Structured clinical interviews may be more reliable than semistructured interviews, but their rigidity and cumbersome nature virtually restrict them to research purposes.

B. Psychological Testing: Cognitive, educational achievement, and neuropsychological testing, while not helpful in categorical diagnosis, can provide important information concerning the patient's perceptual-motor, cognitive, and linguistic functioning and educational performance—data that are important in the design of a comprehensive treatment plan. Table 38–8 lists rating scales that are useful in diagnosis and, possibly, in the monitoring of treatment.

Differential Diagnosis & Comorbidity

Conduct disorder is likely to coexist with oppositional defiant disorder and ADHD, and with substance use disorder, learning disorder, depression, posttraumatic stress disorder, and other anxiety disorders. In longitudinal studies, the prevalence of ADHD declines with age, whereas the prevalence of conduct disorder rises. Oppositional defiant disorder and conduct disorder are temporally continuous (see "Prognosis & Course of Illness" discussion later in this section), whereas conduct disorder and ADHD often coexist. The coexistence of conduct disorder and ADHD significantly complicates treatment and conveys a worse prognosis than the diagnosis of ADHD or conduct disorder alone.

Many youths with conduct disorder have specific developmental disorders, particularly reading disabil-ity and verbal and metalinguistic deficits. Conduct disorder is also associated with early-onset substance use and with a rapid progression to serious substance abuse. Childhood-onset conduct disorder is more likely to be associated with comorbidity than is adolescent-onset conduct disorder.

Dysthymia, major depressive disorder, and anxiety disorders have been described as comorbid with conduct disorder. Conduct problems may precede depression or become apparent after its onset. Completed or attempted suicide has often been associated with conduct problems, particularly explosive aggression. A high proportion of incarcerated delinquents have posttraumatic stress disorder, in full or subclinical form. Of patients with combined Tourette's syndrome and ADHD, 30% also have conduct disorder. Conduct disorder should be differentiated from mania, which is often associated with irritable, belligerent, and rule-breaking behavior.

Loeber R, Keenan K: Interaction between conduct disorder and its comorbid conditions. Clin Psychol Rev 1994; 14:497.

Prevention & Treatment

Conduct disorder is too complex a group of problems to be treated by a single method. Individually tailored combinations of biological, psychosocial, and ecological interventions will likely be most effective. The task is to find the most effective treatment combinations for different groups of children and adolescents with conduct problems. The following sections discuss the most common approaches to prevention and treatment.

Table 38–8. Psychological testing for conduct disorder.

Scale	Comments
Achenbach-Conners-Quay Questionnaire (ACQ)	An expansion of the authors' respective scales, the ACQ yields two aggression factors: aggressive behavior and delinquent behavior.
Child Behavior Checklist (CBCL)	Has parent, youth, teacher, and observer versions. A multidimensional, omnibus scale analyzed separately for boys and girls age 2–3 and 4–18 years. Total behavior problem scores are broken down into externalizing and internalizing band factors and further still into aggressive and delinquent factor scores.
Conners Parent Rating Scale (CPRS) and Conners Teacher Rating Scale (CTRS)	Particularly helpful in the assessment of hyperactivity and conduct problems. All versions of the CPRS have a conduct problem or aggression factor. An abbreviated form of the scale, the Conners Abbreviated Symptom Questionnaire (CASQ), combines items relevant to conduct disorder and hyperactivity and may be useful in the monitoring of treatment in comorbid cases.
Eyberg Child Behavior Inventory (ECBI)	Designed specifically to rate aggressive behavior on a unidimensional scale. It is particularly useful as a treatment monitor.
Jessness Inventory, Carlson Psychological Survey, and Hare Psychopathy Checklist	Assess conduct-disordered behavior in adolescents.
Preschool Behavior Checklist (PBCL) and Burks Preschool and Kindergarten Behavior Rating Scale	Designed to assess behavior in younger children.
Quay's Revised Behavior Problem Checklist	Yields two factorized subscales that reflect aggressive behavior: conduct disorder and socialized aggression.

A. Early Intervention Programs: Early intervention programs such as Head Start may have a preventative function. Head Start programs attend to the child's physical health and provide an early education program that prepares the child for elementary school. They also educate parents about child development and offer support in times of crisis. Early mental health intervention programs, such as Triple P and Fast Track, identify aggressive children and provide intensive parent education to counteract the poor communication, inconsistency, lack of follow-through, coercive discipline, and failure to model or reward prosocial behavior that so frequently accompany nascent conduct disorder. Both Triple P and Fast Track have demonstrated promising short-term effects; however, their long-term benefits are unclear.

B. Treatment Programs for School-Aged Children: Behavioral programs targeting parental effectiveness and the child's social problem-solving capacity, social skills, prosocial behavior, and academic functioning are more effective in the short term than are nonspecific treatment methods.

C. Treatment Programs for Adolescents: During the 1980s, a number of meta-analyses confirmed generally pessimistic impressions of the effectiveness of community and institutional interventions. During the past decade, however, several therapeutic approaches have had promising results.

The Adolescent Transition Program combines initial assessment with feedback and motivational enhancement, followed by a menu of interventions including family-focused training, family therapy, and comprehensive case management.

Evidence is accumulating that it is ineffective to treat youths who have conduct disorder in community or institutional groups. The contagious reinforcement of antisocial behavior generated by antisocial youth groups likely counteracts any benefit derived from group-oriented therapeutic programs. For that reason, therapeutic foster homes have been developed. Youths who would otherwise have been incarcerated are placed with specially trained foster parents who provide daily structure and support; institute an individualized point program; and ensure close supervision of peer associations, consistent nonphysical discipline, and social-skill-building activities supplemented by weekly individual psychotherapy. When treatment foster care was compared with group care, a significant reduction of offending was demonstrated in the 12 months following discharge. The most significant differences between treatment foster care and group care were in the capacity of treatment foster care to prevent the adolescent from associating with deviant peers and in the quality of discipline provided.

Multisystemic therapy provides home-based community treatment for violent antisocial and substance-abusing youths. Based on social ecological and family systems theory, and applying family preservation principles, multisystemic therapy aims to empower parents with parenting skills and to enable youths to cope with family, peer, school, and neighborhood problems. Multisystemic interventions target specific problems, particularly adverse sequences of behavior within and between ecological systems (eg, between child, family, and school), and are continually evaluated from a number of perspectives. Interventions are designed to promote the generalization and long-term maintenance of therapeutic change. Strategic and structural family therapy, behavioral parent training, cognitive-behavioral therapy, and community consultation are combined in accordance with individualized treatment plans. Deviant peer contact is monitored, discouraged, and counteracted. Parent-teacher communication is promoted. Several controlled evaluation studies have demonstrated the efficacy of multisystemic therapy compared to juvenile correctional placement, conventional individual psychotherapy, and no specific treatment.

D. Medication: Until recently, conduct disorder was thought to be resistant to drug treatment. Medication was thought to be useful for treating comorbid problems, for example, ADHD (using stimulants, tricyclic antidepressants, buspirone, or serotonin reuptake inhibitors), anxiety (using propranolol or bupropion), and explosive aggression (using propranolol, carbamazepine, trazodone, or neuroleptics). The rationale for medication was based primarily on hypothetical reasoning and clinical impressions. Three controlled studies have now been completed. One study has demonstrated the efficacy of methylphenidate in reducing defiance, oppositionalism, aggression, and mood changes in outpatients age 5–8 years who were diagnosed as having conduct disorder, with or without ADHD. Another controlled study has demonstrated the effectiveness of divalproex, an "antikindling" agent, in reducing hyperarousal, anger, and aggressiveness in incarcerated adolescents. Divalproex appears to be particularly effective for those adolescents whose explosive aggression is related to posttraumatic stress disorder. A third controlled study has demonstrated the effectiveness of lithium in reducing aggressiveness in inpatient adolescents with conduct disorder. In three previous controlled studies of the effectiveness of lithium in conduct disorder, two demonstrated efficacy and one did not.

Kazdin A et al: Cognitive-behavioral therapy and relationship therapy in the treatment of children referred for antisocial behavior. J Consult Clin Psychol 1989;57:522.

Steiner H: Practice parameters for the assessment and treatment of children and adolescents with conduct disorder. J Am Acad Child Adolesc Psychiatry 1997;36:122S.

Zavodnick JM: Pharmacotherapy. Chapter 14, pages 269–298 in Sholevar GP (editor): *Conduct Disorders in Children and Adolescents.* American Psychiatric Press, 1995.

Prognosis & Course of Illness

The developmental trajectories of the disruptive behavior disorders illustrate the principle of heterotypic continuity (the tendency of behavior patterns to evolve and change with development). For example, temperamental impulsiveness and oppositional defiant behavior in infancy and the preschool period evolve to antiauthoritarian behavior and stealing during middle childhood; to assault, breaking and entering, sexual misbehavior, and substance abuse in adolescence; and to criminality in adulthood. Such a developmental pathway is the result of a complex interplay among biological, environmental, and ecological factors.

A recent meta-analysis of factor analyses of disruptive child behavior has yielded a two-factor solution: an overt/covert factor and an orthogonal destructive/nondestructive factor, with four quadrants: property violations (eg, fire setting, stealing, vandalism); aggression (eg, spitefulness, bullying, assault); oppositional behavior (eg, anger, argumentativeness, stubbornness, defiance); and status violations (eg, truancy, rule-breaking, substance use).

Oppositional defiant disorder usually precedes conduct disorder; and conduct disorder incorporates oppositionalism; however, only about 25% of preschoolers with oppositional defiant disorder progress to conduct disorder. In view of the similar pattern of risk factors between the two disorders, it has been contended that oppositional defiant disorder and conduct disorder do not merit a separate diagnostic status. Similarly, whereas by definition all adults with antisocial personality disorder have manifested conduct disorder in adolescence, only 25–40% of adolescents with conduct disorder progress to antisocial personality disorder. Conduct disorder in adolescent girls predicts internalizing disorders (eg, depression, somatoform disorder) and antisocial behavior.

Aside from the oppositional defiant disorder–conduct disorder–antisocial personality disorder pathway, other developmental trajectories have been identified: an exclusive substance abuse pathway; a covert, nonaggressive pathway; and an aggressive, versatile pathway. The exclusive substance abuse pathway involves a progression from less serious to more dangerous illicit drugs, without aggressive or nonaggressive delinquency. The covert, nonaggressive pathway proceeds from minor theft to serious property violations. The aggressive, versatile path has an early onset, is associated with early hyperactivity and impulsivity, and involves increasingly violent behavior (eg, from frequent fighting to assaultive behavior). A fourth pathway, authority conflict, is described as progressing from oppositionalism to serious antiauthoritarianism. Many youths with conduct disorder cross over from one trajectory to another.

ATTENTION-DEFICIT/ HYPERACTIVITY DISORDER

DSM-IV Diagnostic Criteria

A. Either (1) or (2):

(1) six (or more) of the following symptoms of inattention have persisted for at least 6 months to a degree that is maladaptive and inconsistent with developmental level:

Inattention

(a) often makes careless mistakes
(b) often has difficulty sustaining attention
(c) often does not listen
(d) often fails to follow through on instructions or to finish tasks
(e) often has difficulty organizing tasks and activities
(f) often avoids tasks requiring sustained attention
(g) often loses things
(h) often is easily distracted
(i) often is forgetful

(2) six (or more) of the following symptoms of hyperactivity-impulsivity have persisted for at least 6 months to a degree that is maladaptive and inconsistent with developmental level:

Hyperactivity

(a) often fidgets or squirms
(b) often leaves seat
(c) often moves excessively (may feel restless)
(d) often has difficulty playing or engaging in leisure activities quietly
(e) is often "on the go"
(f) often talks excessively

Impulsivity

(g) often blurts out answers
(h) often has difficulty awaiting turn
(i) often interrupts or intrudes on others

B. Some hyperactive-impulsive or inattention symptoms that caused impairment were present before age 7 years.

C. Some impairment from the symptoms is present in two or more settings.

D. There must be clear evidence of clinically significant impairment in social, academic, or occupational functioning.

E. The symptoms do not occur exclusively during the course of a pervasive developmental disorder, schizophrenia, or other psychotic disorder and are not better accounted for by another mental disorder.

There are three subtypes of ADHD: (1) predominantly inattentive, (2) predominantly hyperactive-impulsive, and (3) combined. If symptom criteria are not met fully, clinical judgment may confer the diagnosis of ADHD not otherwise specified (NOS).

Adapted, with permission, from *Diagnostic and Statistical Manual of Mental Disorders,* 4th ed. Copyright 1994 American Psychiatric Association.

General Considerations

A. Major Etiologic Theories: ADHD symptoms are the result of multiple, as yet largely inferred, etiologies rooted in the interaction of CNS dysfunction with environmental factors. Gestational adversity and postnatal insults to the developing brain—such as prenatal exposure to CNS toxins and infections, complications of prematurity, postnatal malnutrition, and some systemic and genetic diseases—are associated with ADHD but are not usually found in the history of persons diagnosed with the disorder.

There is a high incidence of first-degree relatives with ADHD, implying a genetic, familial etiology. Specific aspects of early caregiver-child interaction and other less well-delineated environmental characteristics may affect the development of attention and of impulsive and hyperactive behavior. The central pathophysiologic mechanisms appear to consist of dysfunction of dopaminergic pathways involving the connections among basal ganglia, the limbic system, and the frontal and prefrontal cortexes.

B. Epidemiology: ADHD is the single most common chronic behavior disorder in preadolescent children. Reported rates range widely from 5% to 12% depending on study methodology and population. Much higher rates are found in inner-city populations in the United States. ADHD is more common in boys than in girls, with male-to-female sex ratios ranging from 5:1 for the predominantly hyperactive-impulsive type to 2:1 for the predominantly inattentive type.

C. Genetics: Familial, including genetic factors, play a dominant role in the etiology of ADHD. The incidence of ADHD reported in first-degree relatives of persons diagnosed with ADHD is 30–50%. Specific inheritance patterns have not been established except for those cases in which ADHD occurs in the context of a defined genetic disorder such as in fragile X syndrome or neurofibromatosis. In addition to ADHD, clustering of specific neuropsychopathology—such as anxiety disorders, learning and language disorders, major depression, and antisocial personality disorders—clusters among relatives of children with ADHD.

Lou H, Henriksen I, Bruhn P: Focal cerebral hypoperfusion in children with dysphasia and/or attention deficit disorder. Arch Neurol 1984;41:825.

Wolraich ML et al: Comparison of diagnostic criteria for attention deficit hyperactivity disorder in a county-wide sample. J Child Adolesc Psychiatry 1996;35:319.

Zametkin AJ et al: Cerebral glucose metabolism in adults with hyperactivity of childhood onset. New Engl J Med 1990;323:1361.

Clinical Findings

A. Signs & Symptoms: Because ADHD is a developmental disorder, symptom manifestations are highly individualistic and core symptoms may shift with age. Hyperactivity and impulsivity tend to become less apparent as children get older and attentional and cognitive problems move into the foreground. Secondary symptoms such as perceptual and emotional immaturity, poor social skills, and motor coordination problems may be observed. Academic underachievement is often further enhanced by commonly comorbid language and learning disorders. Disruptive and impulsive behaviors often lead to peer rejection and low self-esteem, and emotional and social complications frequently are the dominating features by adolescence, whether or not the core symptoms persist.

B. Psychological & Medical Evaluation: In the school-aged child, it is important to obtain the child's educational history and records of academic achievement. A current psychoeducational evaluation should be obtained to exclude learning and language disorders as causing or contributing to the ADHD symptoms. This should include complete intelligence and achievement testing. Neuropsychological testing may be necessary when ADHD is associated with complex CNS dysfunction, such as in seizure disorders or systemic disease. The medical history should consider familial, prenatal, developmental, and social risk factors as well as possible underlying medical conditions and medications contributing to ADHD symptoms. Distinguishing inattention from absence seizures is a further consideration in the differential diagnosis, as is identifying possible behavioral effects of medications the child is taking regularly.

A detailed social history is salient because parents of children with ADHD have an increased rate of psychopathology and marital discord. A large percentage of mothers of children diagnosed with ADHD have been found to be depressed, whereas fathers show increased problems with antisocial behavior and job instability when compared to control subjects. This information is important because of its implications related to cause, but also because it can affect the choice of interventions. Information about family functioning, including behavioral or academic problems in siblings, is important. Children with ADHD frequently place a great deal of stress on the family, and family dynamics themselves may improve when specific interventions for ADHD are implemented.

Barkley R: Nature and diagnosis. In: *Attention Deficit Hyperactivity Disorder: A Handbook for Diagnosis and Treatment.* Guilford Press, 1990.

Biederman J et al: Further evidence for family genetic risk factors in attention deficit hyperactivity disorder. Patterns of comorbidity in probands and relatives psychiatrically and pediatrically referred samples. Arch Gen Psychiatry 1992;49:728.

Schacha R et al: Changes in family functioning and relationships in children who respond to methylphenidate. J Am Acad Child Adolesc Psychiatry 1987;26:728.

Differential Diagnosis, Comorbidity, & Etiologically Linked Disorders

Table 38–9 lists conditions in which the patient may exhibit hyperactive, impulsive, and inattentive behaviors and conditions that sometimes look like or may be comorbid with ADHD.

Treatment

Documented efficacious interventions for children with ADHD fall into three broad categories of treatment approaches that can, and often should be, used together: stimulant medication, behavior modification, and educational modifications. Undocumented treatments have also been proposed.

A. Stimulant Medication: The most extensively prescribed and studied medications prescribed to treat ADHD are CNS stimulants and, to a much lesser degree, tricyclic antidepressants and α-adrenergic agonists (primarily clonidine). Antipsychotic drugs were used in the past but have fallen into disuse because of their significant potential for serious side effects. Psychostimulants are the most popular form of psychotropic medication prescribed for children in the United States and are by far the drugs of choice for ADHD. Methylphenidate is the most popular and extensively researched stimulant; dextroamphetamine and pemoline are used much less frequently. The properties and appropriate dosages of the psychostimulants are presented in Tables 38–10 and 38–11.

B. Behavioral Modification: Behavioral interventions may be likened to pharmacologic interventions in that their effects are essentially symptomatic and effective only as long as they are being applied. The programs generally consist of targeting appropriate behaviors for increase and inappropriate behaviors for decrease or extinction. The appropriate behaviors are rewarded with praise as well as points or tokens as part of a reward system. Inappropriate behaviors cause loss of points or tokens or result in a punishment such as "time out." Social skills training, preferably in peer groups and within the school setting, is important because most children with ADHD have weak social skills.

C. Educational Modification: Modifications of the classroom environment and academic tasks and goals are significant aspects of the treatment plan. Since the implementation of P.L. 101-476, the effect of ADHD on academic and cognitive performance has been acknowledged and necessary classroom modifications must be specified in an Individualized Educational Plan for children certified as having ADHD and educational impairment.

D. Undocumented Treatments: In response to observations that some children show hyperactive behavior associated with certain foods, especially sugar, chocolate, food dyes, and other additives, various restriction diets have been used with variable clinical success. The best known of these diets is the Feingold diet. Several methodologically stringent (ie, double-blind placebo-controlled) studies failed to support dietary effects of sugar and food additives on behavior except in possibly a very small percentage of children. However, recent studies have demonstrated behavioral responses to hypoallergenic restriction diets and challenge with foods indicated by parents to produce disruptive behavior in their children. Currently these studies are few in number and need replication. Megavitamin therapy is considered to be ineffective and potentially dangerous because of possible toxicity. More recently, biofeedback training has been pro-

Table 38–9. Differential diagnoses, comorbid conditions, and etiologically linked diagnoses.

Differential Diagnoses	Comorbid Conditions	Etiologically Linked Diagnoses
Mental retardation or advanced skills with inappropriate school placement Abuse, family adversity, poor temperamental "fit" in family or in school Learning disabilities Language disorders Asperger's syndrome Autistic disorder Obsessive-compulsive disorder Major affective disorders, including bipolar disorder Anxiety disorders Absence seizure disorder Sleep disorders	Learning disabilities Oppositional defiant disorder or conduct disorder Anxiety or mood disorder Language and communication disorders Developmental coordination disorder (dyspraxia) Tourette's syndrome or chronic tic disorder Personality disorders (in adolescence)	Posttraumatic encephalopathy Fetal alcohol syndrome Fragile X syndrome Chronic lead poisoning Untreated phenylketonuria Postinfectious encephalopathy Cerebral palsy Neurocutaneous syndromes Generalized unresponsiveness to thyroid hormone

Table 38–10. Pharmacologic management of ADHD: short-acting psychostimulants.

Psychostimulant	Onset	Maximum Effect	Duration	Half-life	Standard Dosage (average)	Dosage (mg/kg)
Methylphenidate	20–30 min	1–2 hours	3–5 hours	2–3 hours	2.5–25 mg (10 mg twice or three times daily)	0.2–1.0
Dextroamphetamine	20–60 min	1–2 hours	4–5 hours	4–6 hours	1.25–10 mg (5 mg twice or three times daily)	0.1–0.5

moted by a small group of therapists as improving ADHD symptoms.

Wender EH: The food additive–free diet in the treatment of behavior disorders: a review. J Dev Behav Pediatr 1986;7:35.
Wolraich ML, Wilson DB, White JW: The effect of sugar on behavior or cognition in children: a meta-analysis. J Am Med Assoc 1995;274:1617.

Prognosis & Course of Illness

The outcome of ADHD depends on continuation of ADHD symptomatology, type and degree of comorbidity, intelligence, and psychosocial factors such as parental psychopathology. The period of formal schooling is usually the most difficult life phase for persons with ADHD. At later stages, these individuals often find occupational or educational niches that accommodate their behavioral and cognitive idiosyncrasies. Social outcomes are often threatened by persisting cognitive disorganization, poor impulse control, and perceptual dysfunction.

About 50% of children with ADHD continue to manifest dysfunctional symptoms into adulthood. Longitudinal studies show relatively poorer occupational and educational outcomes regardless of current psychiatric status, greater psychiatric comorbidity than in control subjects, and significantly higher rates of socialization disorders and substance use disorders in adults in whom ADHD symptoms per-

sist. Much of what is known related to ADHD in children is not necessarily transferable directly to adults, which makes diagnosing the disorder in adults a challenge. Caution must be taken when treating ADHD in adults because the primary recommended treatment, stimulant medication, has a greater risk for abuse in adults.

III. ANXIETY DISORDERS & PHOBIAS

Barry Nurcombe, MD

SEPARATION ANXIETY DISORDER

Diagnostic Features

A. Developmentally inappropriate and excessive anxiety concerning separation from home or from those to whom the individual is attached, as evidenced by three (or more) of the following:
   (1) recurrent excessive distress when separation from home or major attachment figures occurs or is anticipated
   (2) persistent and excessive worry about losing, or about possible harm befalling, major attachment figures

Table 38–11. Pharmacologic management of ADHD: long-acting psychostimulants.

Psychostimulant	Onset	Maximum Effect	Duration	Half-life	Average Dosage (daily, occasionally, or twice daily)	Response
Methylphenidate SR	1–3 hours	2 hours	8 hours	2–6 hours	20 mg	Very variable
Dextroamphetamine SR	1+ hours	2+ hours	9+ hours	6+ hours	10 mg	Variable
Pemoline	2 hours (after achieving maintenance)	2+ hours	7+ hours	7–8 hours	56.25 mg (18.5–112.5 mg)	Good with adequate dosage

(3) persistent and excessive worry that an untoward event will lead to separation from a major attachment figure (eg, getting lost or being kidnapped)

(4) persistent reluctance or refusal to go to school or elsewhere because of fear of separation

(5) persistently and excessively fearful or reluctant to be alone or without major attachment figures at home or without significant adults in other settings

(6) persistent reluctance or refusal to go to sleep without being near a major attachment figure or to sleep away from home

(7) repeated nightmares involving the theme of separation

(8) repeated complaints of physical symptoms (such as headaches, stomachaches, nausea, or vomiting) when separation from major attachment figures occurs or is anticipated

B. The duration of the disturbance is at least 4 weeks.

C. The onset is before age 18 years.

D. The disturbance causes clinically significant distress or impairment in social, academic (occupation), or other important areas of functioning.

E. The disturbance does not occur exclusively during the course of a pervasive developmental disorder, schizophrenia, or other psychotic disorder and, in adolescents and adults, is not better accounted for by panic disorder with agoraphobia.

Specify if:
Early onset: if onset occurs before age 6 years.

Reprinted, with permission, from *Diagnostic and Statistical Manual of Mental Disorders,* 4th ed. Copyright 1994 American Psychiatric Association.

General Considerations

A. Major Etiologic Theories: Separation anxiety disorder is linked to insecure attachment (see Chapter 37). It may be precipitated by loss, separation, or the threat of either. Parental anxiety and an enmeshed mother-child relationship is commonly associated with this condition. The combination of parental anxiety and depression is an additional risk factor. The prevalence of anxiety disorders in other family members might indicate a genetic factor.

A psychodynamic theory concerning the etiology of separation anxiety disorder postulates the following: (1) The mother has a hostile-dependent relationship with her own mother; (2) the mother is lonely and unsatisfied in her marriage; (3) following a threat to security, the child responds to an overly dependent relationship with the mother; (4) the mother is gratified by the child's overdependence; (5) the mother and child develop a mutually ambivalent hostile-dependent relationship; (6) the child responds to the normal stresses of school with fear and avoidance; (7) the mother is pleased by having the child at home, while at the same time annoyed by it; and (8) both mother and child focus on the somatic symptoms of anxiety and become convinced that the child has a physical disorder.

B. Epidemiology: Separation anxiety disorder occurs in 2–4% of children and adolescents. It represents about 50% of all referrals for evaluation of anxiety disorder at this age. Separation anxiety disorder may be slightly more prevalent in girls and in families of lower socioeconomic status. School refusal is equally common in all socioeconomic groups. Its incidence is 1–2% in school-aged children, and it may be more common in boys.

Clinical Findings

The average age at onset is 8–9 years. Children with separation anxiety disorder exhibit severe distress when separated or threatened with separation from their parent, usually the mother. Fearing that harm will befall the attachment figure or themselves, they typically want to sleep in the parental bed, refuse to be alone, plead not to go to school, have nightmares about separation, and exhibit numerous somatic symptoms when threatened with separation. For example, when it is time to go to school these children complain of abdominal pain, nausea, vomiting, diarrhea, urinary frequency, and palpitations. Sometimes they have to be forced to leave the house. They may run away and hide near the home.

Differential Diagnosis, Treatment, Comorbidity, & Prognosis

See end of section.

Black B: Separation anxiety disorder and panic disorder. Pages 212–234 in March J (editor): *Anxiety Disorders in Children and Adolescents.* Guilford Press, 1995.

GENERALIZED ANXIETY DISORDER

Diagnostic Features

Generalized anxiety disorder (GAD) involves excessive anxiety and worry about a number of events or activities (eg, school performance, social relations, clothes), causing significant impairment or distress, manifested by somatic symptoms, self-consciousness, and social inhibition. See Chapter 22 for diagnostic criteria.

General Considerations

A. Major Etiologic Theories: As with separation anxiety disorder, GAD is associated with a familial concentration of anxiety disorders. Parents of children with GAD have been described as anxious and hypercritical, with high expectations for their children's performance. Children with GAD are more likely to have exhibited behavioral inhibition when younger, a temperamental trait that involves shyness and withdrawal from unfamiliar situations. Behavioral inhibition is probably genetically determined.

B. Epidemiology: GAD occurs in about 3% of children and in 6–7% of adolescents. The sex ratio is equal. GAD is more prevalent among children of higher socioeconomic status.

Clinical Findings

The average age at onset of GAD is 10 years. Children with GAD worry about their clothes, schoolwork, social relationships, and sporting performance—past, present, and future. They are exceedingly self-conscious, have low self-esteem, and complain of many somatic symptoms (particularly abdominal pain and headaches).

Differential Diagnosis, Treatment, Comorbidity, & Prognosis

See end of section.

Silverman WK, Ginsberg G: Specific phobias and generalized anxiety disorder. Pages 151–180 in March J (editor): *Anxiety Disorders in Children and Adolescents.* Guilford Press, 1995.

AVOIDANT PERSONALITY DISORDER & SOCIAL PHOBIA

DSM-IV Diagnostic Criteria

A. Avoidant Personality Disorder: In general, avoidant personality disorder involves pervasive social inhibition, a sense of inadequacy, and hypersensitivity to criticism, which leads to avoidance of academic and social involvement, preoccupation with being rejected, and low self-esteem. See Chapter 33 for diagnostic criteria.

B. Social Phobia: In general, social phobia involves marked, persistent fear of social or performance situations that involve potential scrutiny by other people. The fear is sufficiently severe to interfere with normal social and academic functioning. See Chapter 22 for diagnostic criteria.

General Considerations

A. Major Etiologic Theories: Adults with social phobia often report that the phobia was precipitated by a traumatic event. Compared to patients with ADHD and to normal control groups, anxiety disorders are more common among first-degree relatives of children with anxiety disorders (including avoidant personality disorder and social phobia), but there is no tendency for children with avoidant personality disorder or social phobia to have parents with the same anxiety disorder. In contrast to the development of GAD, behaviorally inhibited children show no greater tendency than do normal children to develop avoidant

personality disorder or social phobia. However, the parents of behaviorally inhibited children are more likely to have, or to have had, social phobia, avoidant personality disorder, or GAD. There may be a familial predisposition to the development of fear. Social phobia has been associated with the predisposition of some children to assume a low status position in the social dominance hierarchy of their peers.

B. Epidemiology: The prevalence of social phobia among children and adolescents is 0.9–1.1%. Girls predominate over boys in a ratio of about 7:3. The prevalence of social phobia has been estimated at 0.08% and 0.7% in 7-year-old and 5-year-old children, respectively. Among children in these two age groups, girls predominate over boys in a ratio of about 2:1.

Clinical Findings

Children with avoidant personality disorder or social phobia experience anxiety in the company of other people or when expected to perform in some way. For example, when unfamiliar visitors arrive, they hide; they prefer single playmates; they avoid sports events and parties; and they detest taking examinations, reading aloud in class, eating in front of others, using public toilets, answering telephones, or speaking up to people in authority. Most of these children are afraid of two or more situations. When threatened, they experience the somatic concomitants of anxiety (eg, rapid breathing, palpitations, shakiness, chills, sweating, nausea).

Differential Diagnosis, Treatment, Comorbidity, & Prognosis

See end of section.

Beidel DC, Morris TL: Social phobia. Pages 181–211 in March J (editor): *Anxiety Disorders in Children and Adolescents.* Guilford Press, 1995.

PANIC DISORDER

Diagnostic Features

In general, panic disorder involves recurrent, unexpected panic attacks, with fear of future attacks, with or without agoraphobia (a fear of being in places from which escape might be difficult such as in a crowd, on a bridge, or while traveling). The disorder is manifested as acute anxiety with autonomic concomitants (eg, racing heart; dilated pupils; rapid breathing; cold, sweaty palms), and it may present as hyperventilation, with tetany. See Chapter 22 for diagnostic criteria.

General Considerations

A. Major Etiologic Theories: In adults with panic disorder, lactate infusion provokes panic symptoms, a phenomenon not found in other anxiety disorders. Agoraphobia is probably a secondary phenomenon, produced by conditioning, when the individual is apprehensive between attacks about the next panic attack. Despite plausible hypotheses, no evidence has been found for an early history of loss or traumatic separation in adults with panic disorder, and childhood separation anxiety disorder is related to adult anxiety disorders generally, not to panic disorder specifically. It is not clear whether childhood separation anxiety disorder predisposes to adult agoraphobia; however, childhood separation anxiety disorder is statistically associated with the early onset of adult panic disorder.

B. Epidemiology: Panic disorder appears to be equally prevalent in both sexes. Its base-rate prevalence is not known.

Clinical Findings

Panic disorder can begin as early as the preschool years, but the peak age at onset is 15–19 years. About 25% of patients report an onset prior to 15 years of age. The condition has probably been underdiagnosed and confused with separation anxiety disorder. Typical symptoms are episodes of hyperventilation, trembling, palpitations, shortness of breath, sweating, numbness, depersonalization, chest pain, choking, fear of dying, dizziness, and fainting.

Differential Diagnosis, Treatment, Comorbidity, & Prognosis

See end of section.

Black B: Separation anxiety disorder and panic disorder. Pages 212–234 in March J (editor): *Anxiety Disorders in Children and Adolescents*. Guilford Press, 1995.

SELECTIVE MUTISM

DSM-IV Diagnostic Criteria

A. Consistent failure to speak in specific social situations (in which there is an expectation of speaking, eg, at school) despite speaking in other situations.

B. The disturbance interferes with educational or occupational achievement or with other social communication.

C. The duration of the disturbance is at least 1 month (not limited to the first month of school).

D. The failure to speak is not due to a lack of knowledge of, or comfort with, the spoken language required in the social situation.

E. The disturbance is not better accounted for by a communication disorder (eg, stuttering) and does not occur exclusively during the course of a pervasive developmental disorder, schizophrenia, or other psychotic disorder.

General Considerations

A. Major Etiologic Theories: The cause of selective mutism is probably multifactorial. Four types of the disorder have been postulated. In symbiotic mutism, the child manipulates the environment, using shyness and clinging to avoid separation. In passive-aggressive mutism, a child scapegoated by his or her peers trenchantly refuses to speak when called on to do so. Reactive mutism is precipitated by a stressor such as illness, separation, or abuse. In speech phobic mutism, the child is afraid to hear his or her own voice.

Shyness and selective mutism run in families. Selective mutism may be a form of social anxiety. One study found a high incidence of social phobia, avoidant personality disorder, and simple phobia in this condition, along with a familial aggregation of social phobia and selective mutism. No clear relationship has been found between trauma and selective mutism.

B. Epidemiology: Selective mutism is more common in girls than boys. Prevalence estimates have varied from 0.08% to 0.7%.

Clinical Findings

The age at onset of selective mutism is 1–5 years (average, 2.7 years). Children with selective mutism are most reluctant to speak at school, away from home, to adults, and to unfamiliar people. They are more likely to speak to peers than to teachers. One study found that 13% of children with selective mutism had a learning disorder and 10% had a history of delayed language development, but all had normal speech and language by 5 years of age. No clear association has been found between trauma and the onset of selective mutism, nor has the often-reported association with oppositional behavior been corroborated. Selective mutism may be regarded more appropriately as a symptom of social anxiety, akin to the "freezing" that some adults with social phobia experience when called on to speak in public.

Differential Diagnosis, Treatment, Comorbidity, & Prognosis

See remainder of this section.

Black B, Uhde TW: Psychiatric characteristics of children with selective mutism. J Am Acad Child Adolesc Psychiatry 1995;34:847.

Differential Diagnosis

Separation anxiety disorder and school refusal are most likely to be confused with physical disorders when they have salient somatic anxiety equivalents.

Thus gastrointestinal symptoms can be confused with peptic ulcer, esophageal reflux, abdominal emergency, or disorders associated with bowel hurry. Separation anxiety disorder with school refusal can also masquerade as chronic fatigue syndrome, chronic muscular pain, and prolonged convalescence from infectious mononucleosis. In panic disorder, mitral valve prolapse should be investigated only if auscultation indicates the need to do so.

Selective mutism should be differentiated from deafness, mental retardation, developmental language disorder, aphonia, and the lack of understanding of English by recent immigrants. Panic disorder should be distinguished from substance-induced anxiety disorder (eg, caffeinism), posttraumatic stress disorder, and medical disorders that cause anxiety (eg, pheochromocytoma).

See Table 38–12 for the general and specific standard interviews and questionnaires useful in screening for and diagnosing anxiety disorders and phobias and in monitoring the treatment outcome of these disorders.

Treatment

Obsessive-compulsive disorder is the only anxiety disorder for which a best treatment can be recommended (see Chapter 24). With other anxiety disorders and phobias, it is reasonable to start with behavioral treatments and to try medication only if such treatments are unsuccessful. Family therapy, individual psychotherapy for unresolved conflict, and liaison with the patient's school are also commonly required.

The behavioral techniques most often used are systematic desensitization and exposure, operant conditioning, modeling, and cognitive-behavioral therapy (see Chapter 2). High-potency benzodiazepines (eg, alprazolam, clonazepam) and tricyclic antidepressants hold some promise in the treatment of anxiety disorders, and fluoxetine has been recommended for the treatment of social phobia. Four placebo-controlled studies have examined the effectiveness of tricyclic antidepressants in the treatment of separation anxiety disorder. In only one of these studies was the experimental drug more effective than placebo. One controlled study of the effectiveness of clonazepam in treating separation anxiety disorder showed no superiority over placebo. Controlled trials of clonazepam in treating GAD and social phobia showed no superiority over placebo. There are no controlled studies of the effectiveness of medication in the treatment of panic disorder. β-Blockers have shown promise in the alleviation of examination performance anxiety in undergraduate students.

Allen JA, Leonard H, Swedo S: Current knowledge of medications for the treatment of childhood anxiety disorders. J Am Acad Child Adolesc Psychiatry 1995;34:976.

Leonard H, Dow S: Selective mutism. Pages 235–250 in March J (editor): *Anxiety Disorders in Children and Adolescents.* Guilford Press, 1995.

Comorbidity

Anxiety disorders (particularly separation anxiety disorder) and depressive disorders frequently coincide. Anxiety disorders are also often encountered in children who have ADHD. Many children with one type of anxiety disorder have at least one other anxiety disorder (eg, separation anxiety disorder with panic disorder, GAD, or avoidant personality disorder). The high degree of comorbidity may be explained on the basis of a risk hypothesis, on the basis of a hypothesis that there is a single underlying pathogenesis, or on the assumption that the symptoms of anxiety and depression overlap in a dimensional, noncategorical manner.

Curry JF, Murphy LB: Comorbidity of anxiety disorders. Pages 301–320 in March J (editor): *Anxiety Disorders in Children and Adolescents.* Guilford Press, 1995.

Prognosis & Course of Illness

The onset of separation anxiety disorder may be acute and precipitated by stress, or it may be gradual, without apparent precipitant. The prognosis is variable. Some children recover completely; others experience chronic or recurrent separation anxiety. These children are likely to relapse when their attachment relationships are threatened, even into maturity. Children with separation anxiety disorder are likely to develop panic disorder, agoraphobia, or depressive disorders in adolescence or adulthood.

The natural history of GAD is not understood. One study has shown that 65% of children diagnosed as having GAD or phobic disorder no longer carry the diagnosis after 2 years. Social phobia in childhood may become associated with alcohol abuse in adolescence. Most children with selective mutism "outgrow" it within a year of onset, although there may be residual shyness. In a minority of cases, mutism continues into late childhood or adolescence.

Table 38–12. Psychological testing for anxiety disorders.

Standardized interviews

Schedule for Affective Disorders and Schizophrenia in School-Aged Children (K-SADS) (Puig-Antich & Chambers 1978)

Anxiety Disorders Interview for Children (ADIS-C) (Silverman & Nellis 1988)

Diagnostic Interview Schedule for Children (DISC) (Costello et al 1985)

Questionnaires

Revised Children's Manifest Anxiety Scale (RCMAS) (Reynolds & Richman 1978)

Revised Fear Survey Schedule for Children (FSSC-R) (Ollendick 1983)

Multidimensional Anxiety Scale for Children (MASC) (March et al 1994)

IV. GENDER IDENTITY DISORDER

Roy Q. Sanders, MD, & William Bernet, MD

DSM-IV Diagnostic Criteria

A. A strong and persistent cross-gender identification (not merely a desire for any perceived cultural advantages of being the other sex).

In children, the disturbance is manifested by four (or more) of the following:

(1) repeatedly stated desire to be, or insistence that he or she is, the other sex

(2) in boys, preference for cross-dressing or simulating feminine attire; in girls, insistence on wearing only stereotypical masculine clothing

(3) strong and persistent preferences for cross-sex roles in make-believe play or persistent fantasies of being the other sex

(4) intense desire to participate in the stereotypical games and pastimes of the other sex

(5) strong preferences for playmates of the other sex

In adolescents and adults, the disturbance is manifested by symptoms such as a stated desire to be the other sex, frequent passing as the other sex, desire to live or be treated as the other sex, or the conviction that he or she has the typical feelings and reaction of the other sex.

B. Persistent discomfort with his or her sex or sense of the inappropriateness in the gender role of that sex.

In children, the disturbance is manifested by any of the following: in boys, assertion that his penis or testes are disgusting or will disappear or assertion that it would be better not have a penis, or aversion toward rough-and-tumble play and rejection of male stereotypical toys, games, and activities; in girls, rejection of urinating in a sitting position, assertion that she has or will grow a penis, or assertion that she does not want to grow breasts or menstruate, or marked aversion towards normative feminine clothing.

In adolescents and adults, the disturbance is manifested by symptoms such as preoccupation with getting rid of primary and secondary sex characteristics (eg, request for hormones, surgery, or other procedures to physically alter sexual characteristics in such a way as to simulate the other sex) or belief that he or she was born the wrong sex.

C. The disturbance is not concurrent with a physical intersex condition.

D. The disturbance causes clinically significant distress or impairment in social, occupational or other important areas of functioning.

General Considerations

Gender identity disorder (GID) is not simply a child's nonconformity to stereotypic sex roles but a significant and pervasive disturbance in the child's view of himself or herself. The disturbance is generally severe enough to disrupt both familial and social interactions.

A. Major Etiologic Theories: The etiology of gender identity disorder is probably multifactorial. Overall, much more attention has been paid to the etiology and treatment of the disorder in boys, most likely owing to the greater social stigma attached to gender-atypical behavior in boys. However, recent studies have examined gender-atypical behaviors in girls as compared with boys.

The disorder is located at the extreme of a continuum that begins with mild gender-atypical behavior through gender dysphoria and on to gender identity disturbance. As with most psychiatric disorders, the etiology is probably best comprehended by a biopsychosocial approach.

Research on the biological issues involved in this disorder have not yielded clear conclusions. Animal models suggest that intra- and extrauterine hormonal influences play a significant role in gender-specific behavior. Many psychosocial theories have been proposed. Researchers have suggested a window of psychological vulnerability between age 2½ years, when the child establishes a self-gender identification, and ages 5 or 6 years when he or she recognizes that gender assignment is stable over time. Researchers continue to examine the family dynamics for clues concerning the development of this disorder. Some authors suggest that particular children are especially vulnerable to the development of GID in response to trauma. Other children would possibly never exhibit gender-atypical behavior and certainly not GID, regardless of trauma or the family dynamics.

Intersex patients (individuals who manifest physical characteristics of both sexes, caused by a flaw in embryonic development) present a different set of issues, although they often exhibit many of the features mentioned in this discussion. Nonetheless, these individuals' gender identity difficulties have separate and distinct characteristics, including prevalence, age at onset, and relative occurrence in males and females.

B. Epidemiology: GID appears to be rare, and there are no good epidemiologic data for children. Boys are referred for treatment of the disorder six to eight times as frequently as girls. Only a very small number of the children referred for GID of childhood will have symptoms that persist as GID of adolescence or adulthood. In Western countries the prevalence of transsexualism or adolescent/adult GID has been estimated as 1 in 30,000 in men and 1 in 110,000 in women.

C. Genetics:

Although it is likely that some children are predisposed to develop GID because of inborn constitutional factors, no genetic pattern or marker has been identified.

Coates S, Wolfe S: Gender identity disorder in boys: the interface of constitution and early experience. Psychoanalytic Inquiry 1995;15:6.

Meyer-Bahlburg HFL: Intersexuality and the diagnosis of gender identity disorder. Arch Sex Behav 1994;23:21.

Sandberg DE et al: The prevalence of gender-atypical behavior in elementary school children. J Am Acad Child Adolesc Psychiatry 1993;32:306.

Clinical Findings

The clinical findings of GID are for the most part outlined in the DSM-IV diagnostic criteria. Some researchers are working to develop instruments to diagnose the disorder earlier and more precisely. Efforts have shifted to look more intently at the disorder and the continuum of difficulties in girls as well as in boys. Because the disorder usually presents at a very early age in nonintersexed patients, diagnostic workup should include interviews with all available caregivers. Reports should be limited to directly observable behavioral characteristics and not to presumed inner states or self-concepts.

Differential Diagnosis

The differential diagnosis of GID depends on the age of the individual presenting for evaluation. In children, the overriding concern is the significance of the behaviors leading to referral and the presence of impairment in social or other important areas of function. Special consideration should be paid to the parents' expectations and concerns. In all ages it is important to determine whether any intersex condition exists as this precludes a diagnosis of GID. Individuals with intersex difficulties usually present with problems of gender identity disturbance during adolescence and not in early childhood.

During adolescence, the differential diagnosis can be expanded to include a struggle, internally or externally, with homosexual impulses that may or may not be related to gender-atypical behaviors. Careful consideration should be given to the development of transvestic fetishism with a heterosexual orientation. Gender disturbance with this paraphilia generally presents in adult middle age (see Chapter 28).

Treatment

Treatment of GID should address, primarily, problems with social ostracism and conflict. Treatment also should be directed at any contributing or comorbid psychopathology. Some therapists have attempted to prevent transsexualism or homosexuality. As mentioned earlier, the development of heterosexual orientation is probably preferred by most parents, but there is no strong evidence that shows the effectiveness of treatment on sexual orientation. In adolescents and adults the prevailing opinion is that treatment goals should foster the integration of a homosexual orientation. Most therapists work with the primary short-term goal of reducing gender identity conflict.

Treatment modalities have included behavioral therapy, psychotherapy, parental counseling, group therapy, and eclectic combinations of these approaches. There have been no comprehensive studies to show the comparative efficacy of these treatment approaches; however, all have been beneficial to a degree.

Blanchard R, Steiner BW (editors): *Clinical Management of Gender Identity Disorders in Children and Adults.* American Psychiatric Press, 1990.

Bradley SJ, Zucker KJ: Gender identity disorder: a review of the past 10 years. J Am Acad Child Adolesc Psychiatry 1997;36:872.

Comorbidity

Comorbidity of GID has been studied with patient and teacher report measures, such as the Child Behavior Checklist. Boys with GID are significantly more disturbed than sibling control subjects but are comparable to clinical control subjects. There is a predominance of internalizing psychopathology. Many boys with GID have separation anxiety disorder.

Zucker KJ, Bradley SJ: *Gender Identity Disorder and Psychosexual Problems in Children and Adolescents.* Guilford Press, 1995.

Complications

The major complication in GID is the disruption of social and familial relationships and, subsequently, a potential derailment of associated developmental opportunities. A common concern of parents and other caregivers who bring children for evaluation and treatment is the development of homosexuality. Although many boys with GID do become homosexual as adults, GID is rare and is not experienced by most homosexual men. According to self-reports, homosexual men exhibited a greater degree of gender-atypical behavior and nonconformity in childhood. These behaviors are usually not within the clinical range. Many parents seek treatment for their gender-identity–disturbed sons solely to prevent homosexuality. Therapeutic neutrality about this subject is as important as it is in other attempts to have the clinician act as a narcissistic extension of the parents.

Of course, a potential complication is the continuation of the disorder into adolescence and adulthood. In these age groups, treatment options are limited; and good outcomes, meaning a patient with resolved conflict—whether through sex reassignment or other accommodation—are few.

Prognosis & Course of Illness

As mentioned earlier, most children with GID outgrow the disorder. However, if the disorder persists into adolescence, treatment will have limited success in eliminating the conflict. The best results occur when treatment is undertaken early in a supportive, nonjudgmental but directive frame. Persistent conflicts from childhood seem much more likely to occur in children whose primary caregivers either passively or actively encourage the atypical behaviors. Parents and therapists should be noncritical but clearly supportive of more conventional gender roles. There is evidence that a high percentage of the males with this disturbance in childhood grow up with a homosexual orientation, and there is no clear evidence that intervention in childhood averts the development of a homosexual orientation. No studies have been done with regard to the outcome in females. There is no evidence that early intervention will change sexual orientation; however, early intervention may reduce subsequent gender dysphoria and transsexualism. Interventions in adolescence are much less successful and to achieve a good outcome should probably be geared toward integration and increased self-esteem in gender role and sexual orientation.

Other Conditions Occurring in Childhood or Adolescence

39

William Bernet, MD, & Barry Nurcombe, MD

I. PSYCHOLOGICAL REACTIONS TO ACUTE & CHRONIC SYSTEMIC ILLNESS

Barry Nurcombe, MD

PSYCHOLOGICAL REACTIONS TO ACUTE PHYSICAL ILLNESS OR TRAUMA

Regression is a normal reaction to acute physical illness. Physically ill children become more dependent, clinging, and demanding. Younger children may revert to bedwetting and immature speech. Preschool children may interpret the illness as a punishment for something they have done.

Younger children react to hospitalization with protest, if they are separated from, and perceive they have been abandoned by, their parents. Depression and detachment occur subsequently. These serious sequelae can be averted if a parent can stay with the child and help with daily care. Because all modern pediatric hospitals encourage parents to do so, the long-term effects of traumatic separation are seldom seen today.

Adolescents are most affected by acute illness if they see it as shameful, if they are immobilized, or if they have fantastic ideas about the cause or nature of the illness (eg, that it was caused by masturbation).

Pain complicates adaptation to acute illness. A child's coping can be enhanced if a familiar person is present during a painful procedure; if the procedure is explained ahead of time (eg, in play); if the medical attendant is truthful, calm, and efficient; and if appropriate reassurance and praise is offered by the physician and the parents after the procedure. If the child does break down emotionally during the procedure, the medical attendant or team must studiously avoid showing irritation or provoking guilt.

Younger children sometimes react to acute burn trauma with dissociation, and delirium may occur as a result of associated fever or tissue breakdown. Badly burned children are subsequently immobilized and exposed to repeated painful procedures (eg, changes of dressing) and to plastic surgery, which may be required for years. The effect of disfigurement on self-esteem is discussed later in this chapter.

DELIRIUM

Delirium is an acute or subacute, fluctuating, reversible derangement of cerebral metabolism, characterized by (1) impairment of attention, thinking, awareness, orientation, and memory; (2) illusions and hallucinations; and (3) reversal of the sleep-wake cycle. In children, delirium is most often encountered in infectious illness (particularly with fever); trauma (particularly in relation to burns or after cardiotomy); hypoxia; metabolic disturbance (eg, acidosis, hepatic failure, renal failure); endocrinopathy (eg, hypoglycemia); or intoxication (eg, with drugs, pesticides, or heavy metals). In adolescents, withdrawal from illicit drugs or alcohol must be considered.

The full diagnostic evaluation of delirium requires physical and neurologic examination; a mental status examination; screening investigations (eg, blood chemistry, blood count, urinalysis, toxicology screen, blood gases, electrocardiogram, chest x-ray); and discretionary investigations (eg, electroencephalogram, computed tomography scan, lumbar puncture, specialized blood chemistries) directed by the clinician's diagnostic hypotheses. See Chapter 17 for a more detailed discussion of delirium.

Treatment

The treatment of delirium is directed at the cause. The child psychiatrist is likely to be called on to diagnose it, especially when the cognitive impairment is subtle and delirium has been mistaken for functional psychosis. Agitation can be alleviated with oral or intramuscular haloperidol, with the addition of small doses of lorazepam, if required. Good nursing and the presence of a parent can help to calm the patient.

PSYCHOLOGICAL REACTIONS TO CHRONIC PHYSICAL ILLNESS

The factors that affect a child's response to chronic illness can be classified as follows: (1) factors in the child, (2) factors in the family, (3) factors related to chronic disease in general, and (4) factors related to specific diseases.

Factors in the Child

The child's age at the onset of a disease affects his or her psychological reaction. Preschool children are affected by hospitalization if they are separated from their parents. School-aged children are affected by being cut off from their peers and education and by forced immobility. Adolescents are particularly affected if the disease affects their body image or their capacity to relate to peers, particularly if heterosexual relationships are interrupted or precluded.

The child's beliefs about the cause, nature, or prognosis of the illness may be inaccurate and interfere with coping. Children with oppositional defiant disorder may transfer their behavior to the medical condition, becoming noncompliant with treatment—a serious problem, for example, in juvenile diabetes, hemophilia, or epilepsy. Other preexisting psychiatric disorders can interfere with coping. Illness can aggravate psychiatric disorders such as anxiety, depression, or disruptive disorders.

Factors in the Family

Parents should receive a full explanation of the cause, nature, treatment, and prognosis of the disease. They may have a false, unhelpful sense of responsibility for the illness, particularly if they are carriers of what proves to be a genetic disease. Some parents react initially with denial. Others react by becoming overprotective, by having unrealistic expectations for improvement, by withdrawing, or by rejecting and abandoning the child. Latent tensions between the parents can be aggravated and, at times, separation or divorce precipitated.

Parents with preexisting psychiatric illness, particularly affective disorder, borderline personality disorder, or substance abuse, are likely to have particular difficulty and to need special support. Significant is the quality of the attachment experiences the parents have been able to provide for the child as an infant, before the onset of the disease. If, because of parental inadequacy or extremes of infant temperament or both, the child experienced insecure or disorganized attachment, his or her adaptation to illness may be compromised.

The psychological health of siblings may be overlooked as a result of parental preoccupation with the physically ill child. Siblings may experience deprivation of attention, causing sadness and withdrawal or resentment and acting-out.

Factors Related to Chronic Disease in General

Parents find it particularly difficult to cope when the diagnosis is unclear. Similarly, a disease with a hopeless prognosis, such as metastatic osteosarcoma, puts severe stress on the family system. Some chronic diseases (eg, sickle cell anemia) have intermittent episodes, causing the child and parents to be hypervigilant. Diseases that affect the child's physical appearance or for which the treatment is disfiguring (eg, the cushingoid appearance caused by corticosteroid treatment) are particularly problematic for adolescents who may become noncompliant with treatment. Diseases that cause severe pain or require invasive treatment (eg, intravenous chemotherapy for cancer) are also likely to produce adverse psychological reactions. Some treatments can have adverse neurocognitive effects (eg, cranial irradiation for leukemia).

Specific Diseases or Conditions

A. Asthma: Attacks of asthma can be triggered by a variety of allergic, infectious, physiologic, or psychological factors. Severely asthmatic children are at markedly increased risk of psychological disorder, particularly depression. Affective disorder and family dysfunction increase the risk of a fatal asthmatic attack. The use of corticosteroids and the limitations on activity caused by chronic asthma can impede academic and social functioning.

B. Cystic Fibrosis: Individuals with cystic fibrosis, a chronic genetic disease, are now surviving into their 30s. Almost all the males are sterile. Pregnancy in women with cystic fibrosis carries a severe risk. One study identified one third of the children with this disease as emotionally disturbed. Eating disorders are more common in adolescents with cystic fibrosis. Family dysfunction and disease severity increase the risk of psychological disorder.

C. Juvenile-Onset Diabetes Mellitus: Family dysfunction predicts poor diabetic control. About 18% of diabetic adults exhibit emotional disturbance, usually depression or anxiety; and about 50% of severely diabetic adults are so affected. About 36% of children with diabetes are depressed or otherwise disturbed. Fear of hypoglycemia or ketosis, resistance to dietary restrictions, tampering with insulin dosage, and even suicide attempts by insulin overdose have been reported. Poor diabetic control is associated with reading problems and with psychiatric disorder in the child or parent.

D. Leukemia: Despite improved survival statistics, many children with leukemia exhibit the "Damocles" syndrome, the sense of living on borrowed time, not knowing when a fatal relapse will occur. Bone marrow biopsies, repeated hospitalizations, and chemotherapy can be frightening experiences. Cranial irradiation and intrathecal methotrexate can cause neurocognitive deficits.

E. HIV Encephalopathy: In HIV encephalopathy, the neurologic disease progresses in parallel with the immunodeficiency. The disease follows one of three courses: subacute progressive, plateau type, or static. Subacute encephalopathy is associated with gradual deterioration and loss of function including motor impairment, apathy, loss of facial expression, emotional lability, and loss of concentration. In some patients the disease plateaus for months before the patient finally deteriorates. Other patients exhibit neurocognitive defects that do not progress.

HIV infection acquired from the mother is usually associated with an environment of social deprivation. Parental guilt is a common accompaniment. Infection caused by contaminated transfusions (eg, in hemophilia) often provokes parental rage against the source of the contamination. The psychiatrist's task is to keep the child in the mainstream as long as possible, help the family deal with guilt and anger, and prepare the child for the required hospitalization and medical procedures.

F. Sensory Impairment: When parents are apprised that their child is blind or deaf, they often experience grief. If they become depressed, the child may be affected by relative deprivation of attention. Both blind and deaf children are affected by the difficulty their parents have in establishing joint reference and shared attention (ie, for parent and child to focus their attention, together, on an object). The prelinguistic games characteristic of normal children and their parents may be replaced by manual gestures.

Hearing adults and children have difficulty making social contact with deaf children. Blind children tend to be even more socially isolated. Although deaf children have been described as egocentric and impulsive, and blind children as introverted and dependent, it is not clear that these generalities are valid.

Blind children exhibit delayed acquisition of classification and conservation skills. Deaf children are slow to conserve; however, many deaf adolescents are capable of formal operations. Reading and writing are delayed in both groups. There is fierce controversy over whether oral methods or sign language should be used in teaching the deaf, whether oral language should be combined with signing, and whether deaf children should be mainstreamed into schools. The prevalence of psychiatric disorder among the deaf has been estimated as 2.5–3 times that of those with normal hearing. Increased rates of psychiatric disorder have been found among students who attend residential schools for the deaf. Hearing-impaired children are at risk of physical and sexual abuse. The prevalence of psychiatric disorder among the visually impaired is less certain. One study estimated a prevalence rate of 45% (including 18.6% with mental retardation). There may be an association between retrolental fibroplasia and autism.

G. Cerebral Palsy: Most children with cerebral palsy have three or more disabilities (eg, cognitive defect, epilepsy, communication disorders, sensory impairment, orthopedic disorders, psychiatric disorder). Between 50% and 75% are mentally retarded. The prevalence of psychiatric disorder is 3–5 times as high as in control groups, but there is no typical psychiatric disorder. Children with organic brain dysfunction are more likely to develop psychiatric disorder. By the age of 4 years, children with cerebral palsy become aware that they are different from their peers, and they become increasingly aware of social rejection and limited prospects. Only 10% marry. By adolescence, their difficulties in forming social relationships and attaining independence are likely to have caused depression, anxiety, lack of confidence, low self-esteem, and in some adolescents, attacks of rage.

H. Epilepsy: Epilepsy carries an increased risk of psychiatric disorder (eg, depression, anxiety, conduct disorder, suicide). The risk is increased if other neurologic abnormalities are present. Epileptic adolescents are particularly affected by the stigma attached to seizures in public. Phenytoin and phenobarbitone, which are used as anticonvulsants, can dull intellectual performance. There is controversy over the assertion that epilepsy is associated with violent behavior. One study showed that patients with temporal lobe epilepsy had an 85% prevalence of psychiatric disorder, particularly catastrophic rage and hyperkinesis. Another study suggested that the rate of psychiatric disorder in patients with temporal lobe epilepsy is no higher than in patients with other forms of epilepsy. About 10% of children with temporal lobe epilepsy develop a psychotic illness in adolescence or adulthood.

Fritz GK: Common clinical problems in pediatric consultation. Pages 47–66 in Fritz GK et al (editors): *Child and Adolescent Mental Health Consultation in Hospitals, Schools, and Courts.* American Psychiatric Press, 1993.

Goodman R: Brain disorders. Pages 172–190 in Rutter M, Taylor E, Hersov L (editors): *Child and Adolescent Psychiatry,* 3rd ed. Blackwell Scientific, 1994.

Hindley P, Brown RMA: Psychiatric aspects of specific sensory impairments. Pages 720–736 in Rutter M, Taylor E, Hersov L (editors): *Child and Adolescent Psychiatry,* 3rd ed. Blackwell Scientific, 1994.

Mrazek D: Psychiatric aspects of somatic disease and disorders. Pages 697–710 in Rutter M, Taylor E, Hersov L (editors): *Child and Adolescent Psychiatry,* 3rd ed. Blackwell Scientific, 1994.

Ryan RM, Sundheim STPV, Voeller KKS: Medical diseases. Pages 1223–1274 in Coffey CE, Brumback RA (editors): *Textbook of Pediatric Neuropsychiatry.* American Psychiatric Press, 1998.

Thompson C, Westwell P, Viney D: Psychiatric aspects of human immunodeficiency virus in childhood and adolescence. Pages 711–719 in Rutter M, Taylor E, Hersov L (editors): *Child and Adolescent Psychiatry,* 3rd ed. Blackwell Scientific, 1994.

Williams DT, Pleak RR, Hanesian H: Neurological disorders. Pages 636–649 in Lewis M (editor): *Child and Adolescent Psychiatry.* Williams & Wilkins, 1996.

II. CHILD MALTREATMENT

William Bernet, MD

General Considerations

Practitioners in private practice, as well as those employed by courts or other agencies, see children who may have been mentally, physically, or sexually abused. As a clinician, the practitioner may provide assessments and treatment for abused children and their families in both outpatient and inpatient settings. As a forensic investigator, the practitioner may work with an interdisciplinary team at a pediatric medical center and assist the court in determining what happened to the child.

A. Definitions: The legal definitions regarding child maltreatment vary from state to state. In general, **neglect** is the failure to provide adequate care and protection for children. It may involve failure to feed the child adequately, failure to provide medical care, or failure to protect the child from danger. **Physical abuse** is the infliction of injury by a caretaker. It may take the form of beating, punching, kicking, biting, or other methods. The abuse can result in injuries such as broken bones, internal hemorrhages, bruises, burns, and poisoning. Cultural factors should be considered in assessing whether the discipline of a child is abusive or normative. **Sexual abuse** of children refers to sexual behavior between a child and an adult or be-

tween two children when one of them is significantly older or more dominant. The sexual behaviors include the following: touching breasts, buttocks, and genitals, whether the victim is dressed or undressed; exhibitionism; fellatio; cunnilingus; penetration of the vagina or anus with sexual organs or with objects; and pornographic photography. **Emotional abuse** occurs when a caretaker causes serious psychological injury by repeatedly terrorizing or berating a child. When it is serious, it is often accompanied by neglect, physical abuse, or sexual abuse.

B. Epidemiology: Each year about 3 million alleged incidents of child maltreatment are reported to protective services. Of those reports, about 1 million are substantiated. Of the substantiated cases, about 55% involve neglect; about 23% involve physical abuse; about 10% involve sexual abuse; about 4% involve emotional abuse; and the rest are unspecified. About 1300 children die each year as the result of maltreatment.

Briere JN et al: *The APSAC Handbook on Child Maltreatment.* Sage Publications, 1996.

Nurcombe B, Partlett DJ: *Child Mental Health and the Law.* Free Press, 1994.

Schmitt B: The child with nonaccidental trauma. Pages 178–196 in Helfer RE, Kempe CH (editors): *The Battered Child,* 4th ed. University of Chicago Press, 1987.

Clinical Findings

Children who have been abused manifest pleomorphic symptoms in a variety of emotional, behavioral, and psychosomatic reactions. As a general rule, children who have been physically abused are likely to become aggressive, and children who have been sexually abused are likely to display inappropriate sexual behavior. Table 39–1 lists symptoms that are associated with child abuse, but they are not specific or pathognomonic; the same symptoms may occur without a history of abuse.

The parents of physically abused children have certain characteristics. Typically, they have delayed seeking help for the child's injuries. The history given by

Table 39–1. Symptoms associated with child abuse.

Type of Abuse	Associated Symptoms
Any abuse	Psychological symptoms related to emotional distress, such as fear, anxiety, nightmares, phobias, depression, low self-esteem, anger, and hostility More serious psychological problems such as suicidal behavior; posttraumatic stress disorder; and dissociative reactions, with periods of amnesia, trance-like states, and, in some cases, dissociative identity disorder Physical symptoms (eg, somatic complaints, encopresis, eating disorders) Somatoform symptoms (eg, pseudoseizures)
Sexual abuse	Abnormal sexual behavior: Sexual hyperarousal (eg, open masturbation, excessive sexual curiosity, talking excessively about sexual acts, masturbating with an object, imitating intercourse, inserting objects into the vagina or anus) Sexually aggressive behavior (eg, frequent exposure of the genitals, trying to undress other people, rubbing against other people, sexual perpetration) Avoidance of sexual stimuli through phobias and inhibitions In adolescents: sexual acting-out with promiscuity and, possibly, homosexual contact

the parents is implausible or incompatible with the physical findings. There may be evidence of repeated suspicious injuries. The parents may blame a sibling or claim the child injured himself or herself.

In cases of intrafamilial sexual abuse and other sexual abuse that occurs over a period of time, there is a typical sequence of events: (1) engagement, when the perpetrator induces the child into a special relationship; (2) sexual interaction, in which the sexual behavior progresses from less intimate to more intimate forms of abuse; (3) the secrecy phase; (4) disclosure, when the abuse is discovered; and (5) suppression, when the family pressures the child to retract his or her statements.

The child sexual abuse accommodation syndrome is sometimes seen when children are sexually abused over a period of time. This syndrome has five characteristics: (1) secrecy; (2) helplessness; (3) entrapment and accommodation; (4) delayed, conflicted, and unconvincing disclosure; and (5) retraction. The process of accommodation occurs as the child learns that he or she must be available without complaint to the parent's demands. The child often finds ways to accommodate: by maintaining secrecy in order to keep the family together, by turning to imaginary companions, and by employing altered states of consciousness. Other children become aggressive, demanding, and hyperactive.

It is possible to distinguish the psychological sequelae of children who have experienced single-event and repeated-event trauma. The following four characteristics occur after both types of trauma: (1) visualized or repeatedly perceived memories of the event; (2) repetitive behavior; (3) fears specifically related to the trauma; and (4) changed attitudes about people, life, and the future. Children who sustain single-event traumas manifest full, detailed memories of the event; an interest in "omens," such as looking retrospectively for reasons why the event occurred; and misperceptions, including visual hallucinations and time distortion. In contrast, many children who have experienced severe, chronic trauma (eg, repeated sexual abuse) manifest massive denial and psychic numbing, self-hypnosis and dissociation, and rage.

Cicchetti D, Toth SL: A developmental psychopathology perspective on child abuse and neglect. J Am Acad Child Adolesc Psychiatry 1995;34:541.

Kendall-Tacket KA, Williams LM, Finkelor D: Impact of sexual abuse on children: a review and synthesis of recent empirical studies. Psychol Bull 1993;113:164.

Summit RC: The child sexual abuse accommodation syndrome. Child Abuse and Neglect 1983;7:177.

Terr LC: Childhood traumas: an outline and overview. Am J Psychiatry 1991;148.

Clinical Evaluation

The professional who evaluates children who may have been abused has several important tasks: finding out what happened; evaluating the child for emotional disorder; considering other possible explanations for any disorder; being aware of developmental issues, avoiding biasing the outcome with his or her preconceptions; pursuing these objectives in a sensitive manner so as not to retraumatize the child; being supportive to family members; and keeping an accurate record because it may be subpoenaed for future court proceedings.

It is important to be familiar with normative sexual behavior of children for two reasons. First, normal sexual play activities between children should not be taken to be sexual abuse. In assessing this issue, the evaluator should consider the age difference between the children; the developmental level of the children; whether one child was dominating or coercing the other child; and whether the act itself was intrusive, forceful, or dangerous. Second, sexually abused children manifest more sexual behavior than do normal children.

A. Patient Interview: The clinical interview may need some modification when evaluating a child who may have been abused. The following sections describe the components of an interview that is particularly suited for forensic evaluations:

1. Build rapport and make informal observations of the child's behavior, social skills, and cognitive abilities.

2. Ask the child to describe two specific past events, in order to assess the child's memory and to model the form of the interview for the child by asking nonleading, open-ended questions, a pattern that will hold through the rest of the interview.

3. Establish the need to tell the truth. Reach an agreement that in this interview only the truth will be discussed, not "pretend" or imagination.

4. Introduce the topic of concern. Start with more general questions, such as, "Do you know why you are talking with me today?" Proceed, if necessary, to more specific questions, such as, "Has anything happened to you?" or "Has anyone done something to you?" Drawings may be helpful in initiating disclosure. For example, either the child or the interviewer draws an outline of a person. Then the child is asked to add and name each body part and describe its function. If sexual abuse is suspected, the interviewer could ask, when the genitals are described, if the child has seen that part on another person and who has seen or touched that part on the child. If physical abuse is suspected, the interviewer could ask if particular parts have been hurt in some way.

5. Elicit a free narrative. Once the topic of abuse has been introduced, the interviewer encourages the child to describe each event from the beginning without leaving out any details. The child is allowed to proceed at his or her pace, without correction or interruption. If abuse has occurred over a period of time, the interviewer may ask for a description of the general pattern and then for an account of particular episodes.

6. Pose general questions. The interviewer may ask general questions in order to elicit further details. These questions should not be leading and should be phrased in such a way that an inability to recall or lack of knowledge is acceptable.

7. Pose specific questions, if necessary. It may be helpful to obtain clarification by asking specific questions. For example, the interviewer may follow up on inconsistencies in a gentle, nonthreatening manner. Avoid repetitive questions and the appearance of rewarding particular answers in any way.

8. Use interview aids, if necessary. Anatomically correct dolls may be useful in understanding exactly what sort of abusive activity occurred. The dolls are not used to diagnose child abuse, only to clarify what happened.

9. Conclude the interview. Toward the end of the interview, the interviewer may ask a few leading questions about irrelevant issues (eg, "You came here by taxi, didn't you?"). If the child demonstrates a susceptibility to the suggestions, the interviewer would need to verify that the information obtained earlier did not come about through contamination. Finally, the interviewer thanks the child for participating, regardless of the outcome of the interview. The interviewer should not make promises that cannot be kept.

B. Parent Interview: In order to evaluate a child who may have been abused, it is necessary to do more than simply interview the child and ask him or her what happened. It is also important to interview the parents and perhaps obtain information from outside sources. The parents should be able to provide information regarding the child's experiences with particular people; the duration and evolution of the child's symptoms; the child's developmental and medical history; and factors in the child's life, other than abuse, that might explain the symptoms. It may also be important to assess the parents' motivations and psychological strengths and weaknesses. For instance, some parents (who perpetrated the abuse or allowed another individual to do so) may be motivated to deny or minimize the possibility that the child was abused. Other parents (who are vengeful or overly suspicious of another person) may be motivated to exaggerate the possibility that the child was abused or may even fabricate symptoms of abuse.

C. Psychological Testing: Although psychological testing cannot diagnose child abuse, it may be a useful part of the evaluation.

American Academy of Child and Adolescent Psychiatry: Practice parameters for the forensic evaluation of children and adolescents who may have been physically or sexually abused. J Am Acad Child Adolesc Psychiatry 1997;36:423.

Benedek EP, Schetky DH: Problems in validating allegations of sexual abuse. Part 2: clinical evaluation. J Am Acad Child Adolesc Psychiatry 1987;26:916.

Everson MD, Boat BW: Putting the anatomical doll controversy in perspective: an examination of the major uses and criticisms of the dolls in child sexual abuse evaluations. Child Abuse and Neglect 1994;18:113.

Friedrich WN et al: Normative sexual behavior in children. Pediatrics 1991;88:456.

Yuille JC et al: Interviewing children in sexual abuse cases. Pages 95–115 in Goodman GS, Bottoms BL (editors): *Child Victims, Child Witnesses: Understanding and Improving Testimony.* Guilford Press, 1993.

Differential Diagnosis

Children may make false statements in psychiatric evaluations. Sometimes they falsely deny abuse; sometimes they make false allegations. A number of mental processes, both conscious and unconscious, can result in false allegations. For example, a delusional mother, who believed that her ex-husband had been molesting their daughter, induced the girl to state that the father had rubbed against her in bed. By repeatedly asking leading or suggestive questions, inept interviewers have induced children to make false allegations of abuse. Some children manifest pathologic lying in making false allegations. Young children may tell tall tales, making innocent statements that evolve or are molded into false allegations of abuse. Older children may lie about abuse for revenge or personal advantage. In some cases, multiple allegations of abuse have been generated through group contagion or have been spread by parental panic or overzealous clinical investigation.

Bernet W: False statements and the differential diagnosis of abuse allegations. J Am Acad Child Adolesc Psychiatry 1993;32:903.

Assessing the Child's Credibility

Credibility refers to the child's truthfulness and accuracy, which sometimes is an issue in assessing children who allege abuse. The following factors seem to indicate the child is credible: The child uses his or her own vocabulary rather than adult terms and tells the story from his or her own point of view; the child reenacts the trauma in spontaneous play; sexual themes are present in play and drawings; the child's affect is consonant with the accusations; the child's behavior is seductive, precocious, or regressive; the child has good recall of details, including sensory motor and idiosyncratic details; and the child has a history of telling the truth.

The following factors seem to indicate the child is making unreliable or fictitious allegations: The child's statements become increasingly inconsistent over time; the child's statements are dramatic or implausible, for example, involving the presence of multiple perpetrators or situations in which the perpetrator has not taken ordinary steps against discovery; and the child's account progresses from relatively innocuous behavior to increasingly intrusive, abusive, and aggressive activities.

Rogers ML: Coping with alleged false sexual molestation: Examination and statement analysis procedures. Issues in Child Abuse Accusations 1990;2:57.

III. SUICIDAL BEHAVIOR

Barry Nurcombe, MD

General Considerations

Suicide is intentional self-destruction. In **attempted suicide,** the individual harms himself or herself, in some cases with the intent to die, in other cases for a purpose or purposes other than self-destruction. **Suicidal ideation** refers to a preoccupation with committing suicide that could vary from occasional and transient to frequent, persistent, and compelling. The term **parasuicide** refers to suicidal attempts or gestures. Suicidal behavior includes completed suicide, parasuicide, suicidal ideation, and suicidal communications.

Suicidal behavior should be distinguished from deliberate self-injury that is not suicidal in intent. The latter involves wrist, arm, body or thigh cutting; head banging; or wall punching apparently in an attempt to express intense emotion, alleviate distress, or counteract depersonalization.

A. Major Etiologic Theories:

1. Sociologic factors—The relevance of Durkheim's theories concerning altruistic, egoistic, and anomic forms of suicide is unclear. His concept of anomie has some parallel to Erikson's concept of **identity diffusion**—the sense of rootlessness, confusion, lack of connectedness, and hopelessness that precedes some cases of suicide. Anomie may relate particularly to the high prevalence of impulsive suicide among indigenous groups in North America and Australia that have been dispossessed of their land and culture and exposed, as children, to domestic violence and parental alcoholism.

Recent studies have pointed to an increase in the number of adolescent suicides after television "docudramas" about suicide or after publicity concerning the suicides of well-known entertainers, perhaps because their suicides are depicted or perceived as romantic or heroic gestures. Several so-called epidemics of suicide have been reported, usually among males (not all of whom have been closely associated) in small communities. Though dramatic, such occurrences are relatively uncommon.

2. Genetic factors—The genetics of suicide are probably linked with the genetics of affective disorders. However, because not all completed or attempted suicides are associated with affective disorders, and because affective disorders are not heterogeneous, it is little wonder that genetic research in this area is rudimentary. Nevertheless, there is an increased risk of suicide in the relatives of probands who have had major depressive disorder or who committed suicide and in the biological relatives of adoptees who committed suicide. The likelihood of suicide is increased in families with a history of bipolar disorder.

3. Neuroendocrine & neurochemical factors—Major depression in childhood has been associated with the following: abnormal hypothalamo-pituitary-adrenocortical functioning, growth hormone hyposecretion following the insulin tolerance test, hypersecretion of growth hormone during sleep, lower levels of urinary secretion of 3-methoxy-4-hydroxy-phenylglycol, and abnormality of central serotonin metabolism. Impulsive behavior, including suicide, has been associated with low levels of cerebrospinal fluid 5-hydroxy-indoleacetic acid, a serotonin metabolite.

4. Psychiatric disorders—Studies of adolescents who have attempted suicide and retrospective psychological autopsy studies of adolescents who have committed suicide indicate a high prevalence of psychiatric disorder. The following diagnoses are the most frequently encountered, alone or in combination: major depressive disorder; dysthymic disorder; bipolar disorder; conduct disorder; substance use disorder; borderline personality disorder; complex, abuse-related posttraumatic stress disorder; intermittent explosive disorder; and schizophrenia or schizoaffective disorder.

5. Transactional diathesis-stress model—The transactional diathesis-stress model proposes that predisposing psychological factors (eg, exposure to domestic violence, abuse, neglect, rejection, parental psychopathology, parental separation, and conflictual divorce), together with a genetic predisposition to affective disorder or impulsivity, lay the foundation for a vulnerable personality. By adolescence, personality vulnerability is manifested by low self-esteem and high interpersonal neediness, combined with heightened sensitivity to criticism, rejection, or humiliation. Vulnerable individuals have difficulty regulating affect by identifying and expressing emotion in words, if they seek help, or by using their imagination to work out their own solutions to life problems. As a result, they brood fruitlessly and drift into a state of hopelessness. Vulnerable individuals are prone to perceive desirable events as a matter of chance or luck. They see misfortune as their due. Because they do not perceive themselves as in control of their fate, they are chronically pessimistic. In terms of ego defense, these individuals lack the capacity for a realistic appraisal of situations and events and are impaired in the capacity for self-reflection, emotional expression, and impulse control. When things go wrong, their pessimistic expectations are fulfilled and they blame themselves. Rather than seeking help and tackling their problems, these individuals rely on displacement or introjection. In summary, an adverse early environment, acting in some cases in concert with a genetic predisposition to affective disorder, produces a vulnerable personality characterized by low self-esteem, pessimism, fatalism, and an impaired capacity to regulate affect and impulse when stressed.

In early adolescence, the vulnerable individual struggles with normal developmental issues of autonomy and efficacy, sexual identity, peer relations, and a sense of identity. In late adolescence and early adulthood, issues of identity, emancipation, the capacity for intimacy, love relationships, and career choice become important.

Against this backdrop the vulnerable individual is confronted by a stressful situation. The stressor might be something that emotionally stronger individuals would take in stride; however, the vulnerable person is plunged into a downward spiral of self-blame, despair, and hopelessness, or into an impulsive explosion of self-directed aggression. Impulsive suicide is often associated with alcohol or substance abuse and may occur while the subject is intoxicated or in withdrawal.

Typical stressors involve conflict, separation, loss, rejection, failure, or humiliation. Examples include conflict with a parent; separation from or death of a loved parent, sibling, relative, friend, or pet; rejection by a desired romantic partner; academic failure; suspension from school; unemployment or loss of employment; humiliation by peers or family; or police involvement. In Asian adolescents, shame at having dishonored the family can lead to suicide. Some researchers report an association between suicide and conflict over homosexuality, or persecution by peers on account of gender identity issues. Many adolescents have experienced the suicide of relatives or friends. All have been exposed to media accounts of the subject (eg, news reports on the demise of popular entertainers). Eventually, suicide is perceived as a reasonable, honorable, even romantic, solution to life's problems.

Table 39–2 describes common motivations for the suicidal act. Sometimes, the suicidal act is a response to command hallucinations or delusions (eg, in schizophrenia, schizoaffective disorder, or dissociative hallucinosis).

B. Epidemiology:

1. Incidence—International data on deaths by suicide must be interpreted with care, because methods of ascertainment differ. The suicide rate has increased in many countries but has decreased in others.

Table 39–2. Common motivations for the suicidal act.

Motivation	Example
Atonement	I will punish myself for what I have done.
Control	I am unfraid of death.
Escape	I want to be free of my body and my life.
Rebirth	After I die, I can start again.
Reunion	I'll join my mother in heaven.
Revenge	They'll be sorry when I've gone.
Self-sacrifice	My death will bring them together.

The reasons for these differences are not known. According to recent statistical data on the incidence of suicide in male youths, the United States has the 6th highest rate out of 14 Western industrialized countries (Table 39–3). Prepubertal suicide is rare and has not increased in incidence (0.7 per 100,000 in 1993). In contrast, the rate of suicide in the 15- to 19-year-old age group has increased steadily from 1960 (3.6 per 100,000) to 1990 (11.1 per 100,000) and is now, after accidents, the second most common cause of death in this age group.

In the United States, as in Canada and Australia, a cohort effect is evident: Since 1960, at successive 5-year intervals, each 5-year period has begun with a higher suicide rate, in the 15- to 24-year-old age group. The incidence of attempted suicide has also risen. Suicide is attempted about 50 times more often than it is completed. Suicidal ideation is highly prevalent: 40% of rural adolescents have entertained thoughts of suicide, compared to the 9% who have attempted it. The increase in suicide rate is due mainly to an increase in the frequency of suicide among 15- to 24-year-old white males (21.7 per 100,000) compared to that of nonwhite males (11.8 per 100,000) or to that of females of all races. Adolescents with a history of psychiatric hospitalization are nine times more likely to commit suicide than are those with no such history.

Among U.S. male adolescents, the two most common methods of completed suicide are firearms and hanging. Among females the most common methods are firearms and jumping from a height.

2. Risk factors—The following events are associated with suicide: family conflict, family problems, personal loss, problems with the opposite sex, recent rejection or humiliation by family or peers, problems at school, suspension from school, problems at work, and loss of a job.

Compared to individuals who attempt suicide, those who succeed are more likely to have experienced the suicide of a parent, relative, or friend; to have been exposed to parental conflict, absence, or psychopathology; to have been maltreated; to have communicated suicidal ideation or attempted suicide in the past; to have used alcohol or drugs; to have been socially inhibited; to have exhibited antisocial behavior; or to have had a history of psychiatric treatment.

The reasons for the cohort effect described in the preceding section are unknown but are thought to be related to profound changes in Western society over the past 50 years. Such changes include increased social mobility, divorce, prevalence of single-parent families, and parental absence due to work obligations; weakened religious ties; and an increase of alcohol and drug abuse among youth.

Among prepubertal children who exhibit suicidal behavior, high rates of physical and sexual abuse have been found, together with an accumulation of stress-

Table 39–3. Changing suicide rates (per 100,000 of population) among males age 15–24 years, from selected industrial countries, 1981–1993.[1,2]

Country	1981–1982	1984–1985	1987–1988	1991–1993
New Zealand	17.5	19.6	35.7	39.9
Norway	20.2	21.9	26.6	28.2
Switzerland	38.2	34.1	26.3	25.0
Canada	NA	25.2	26.9	24.7
Australia	19.3	24.0	27.8	24.6
United States	19.8	20.5	21.9	21.9
France	15.7	17.0	14.7	14.0
Denmark	17.1	17.0	16.5	13.4
Germany	21.2	19.4	15.8	13.0
United Kingdom	7.0	8.2	12.3	12.2
Japan	14.7	14.1	10.4	10.1
Netherlands	5.3	10.6	9.2	9.1
Spain	5.0	5.3	8.4	7.1
Italy	5.3	NA	5.1	5.7

[1] From World Health Organization: *World Health Statistics Manual,* 1983, 1985, 1987, 1989–1994.
[2] Rates for each column refer to one of the two or three years specified, according to available data (NA, not available). The last column represents the latest data available.

ful life events in the year prior to psychiatric treatment.

Emergency Evaluation & Management

A. Identification & Assessment: If a primary care clinician suspects that an adolescent is harboring suicidal ideation, he or she should ask the adolescent one of the following questions: "Have you ever thought of harming yourself?" or "Do you ever get so low that you think of suicide?" There is no evidence that either question will suggest the possibility of suicide to somebody who is not already thinking about it.

Table 39–4. Issues to address in evaluating suicidal patients.

Is the suicidal ideation insistent and persistent?
Does the adolescent sincerely want to die?
Does the adolescent have a plan for how he or she will commit suicide?
Is the plan potentially lethal (in terms of means and likelihood of discovery)?
Does the adolescent have a history of suicide attempts, impulsive violence, or risk taking?
Does the adolescent have a history of physical or sexual abuse?
Is the adolescent intoxicated or subject to alcohol or drug abuse?
Has the adolescent experienced recent serious loss, separation, rejection, humiliation, or disappointment?
Is there evidence of major depression or psychotic thought disorder (eg, command hallucinations)?

Indeed, many adolescents are relieved to be able to speak about suicidal thoughts. Table 39–4 lists the issues that an evaluation should address in order to weigh the degree of risk against protective factors.

If the adolescent has attempted suicide, the following additional issue should be addressed: Was the suicide attempt potentially lethal, or did the adolescent think it was? Table 39–5 lists protective factors that should be assessed, regardless of whether the patient has attempted suicide or has suicidal thoughts.

B. Hospitalization: If the clinician considers that the immediate risk outweighs the protective factors, the patient should be referred for emergency evaluation with regard to psychiatric hospitalization, preferably in an adolescent unit. The aims of hospitalization are as follows: (1) protection, (2) comprehensive diagnostic evaluation, (3) goal-directed treatment planning,

Table 39–5. Protective factors to consider in evaluating suicidal risk.

Does the adolescent have a protective, cohesive family that is aware of the seriousness of the situation, willing to secure all potentially lethal means of suicide in the home, and able to monitor the patient adequately?
Does the adolescent have supportive friends?
Does the adolescent have strong religious adherence?
Does the adolescent have any insight into the seriousness of the suicidal behavior and its causation?
Does the adolescent have a good relationship with a therapist, or is he or she capable of forming one?
Is the adolescent prepared to enter into a suicide contract?

(4) stabilization, and (5) coordination with community clinicians or agencies for postdischarge treatment. During hospitalization, the individualized stabilization plan is likely to involve brief individual psychotherapy, group therapy, family therapy, and, if appropriate, suitable medication.

In-home 24-hour nursing observation is a less-expensive alternative to hospitalization. However, imminently suicidal, disruptive, or psychotic patients cannot be managed safely in this manner, and the diagnostic evaluation in the home is likely to be less comprehensive, particularly in regard to associated physical disorder.

Outpatient Treatment

An individualized goal-directed treatment plan should be implemented before the patient is discharged from the hospital or immediately if the patient is not hospitalized. In some cases, brief supportive psychotherapy with crisis-oriented family therapy is sufficient. If the patient's psychopathology is more complex and severe, extended individual psychotherapy, cognitive-behavioral therapy, family therapy, or a combination of these therapies will be required, together with targeted pharmacotherapy, if appropriate.

During treatment, the therapist must monitor the patient's progressive risk of suicide and take appropriate precautions. Countertransference issues (eg, strong dislike, need to rescue, feelings of hurt at being rejected, panic, or feelings of isolation and helplessness) indicate the need for consultation with a colleague.

Postvention

Abundant evidence indicates that families and friends are often devastated by the suicide of a child or peer. Families are likely to feel guilt, remorse, shame, and anger. Family counseling can facilitate the resolution of these feelings and promote a reintegration of the surviving family. Surviving peers and teachers can also be helped by means of group counseling aimed at the sharing of feelings and their resolution. It is also possible for the counselor to identify those family or group members who need more extended, individualized treatment.

Prevention

The increasing incidence of attempted and completed suicide has stimulated many communities to consider preventative action. The following interventions have been proposed: population-based strategies, early identification strategies, high-risk strategies, and educational and community awareness strategies.

A. Population-Based Strategies: Population-based strategies aim to limit the availability of lethal means to suicide. These strategies include limiting the availability of firearms; reducing the pack-size of nonprescription analgesics (eg, acetaminophen); us-ing catalytic converters on cars to reduce carbon monoxide emissions; positioning automobile exhaust pipes in such a way as to deter hose attachment; and prescribing safer antidepressants (ie, selective serotonin reuptake inhibitors instead of tricyclic antidepressants) and anxiolytics.

A reduction in unemployment and improved measures to prevent or treat domestic violence, child maltreatment, and conflictual divorce could also have a beneficial effect in the long term. Furthermore, measures to raise community awareness of youth problems and to provide recreational and protective facilities for youths could also be helpful. Unfortunately, economic policies associated with unemployment may not be influenced by health concerns, and the will of the community to unite to help youths has scarcely been tested.

B. Early Identification & Treatment: Adolescents who commit suicide generally fall into one of two groups: those with a depressive disorder or those with an impulse-control disorder (often complicated by alcohol or drug abuse). Both groups can be identified in early adolescence, or before, by school counselors or teachers. Depressed adolescents manifest sadness, social withdrawal, deteriorating school performance, and allusions to suicide in letters or essays. Impulsive adolescents manifest impulsive, oppositional, and aggressive behavior. All children suspended from school should be evaluated by a child mental health clinician. Treatment could be provided in mental health clinics or preferably in satellite clinics located in schools. Many adolescents who are contemplating suicide visit their family practitioner in the month before the attempt. Family practitioners should be trained in the identification and assessment of suicide risk and in appropriate referral techniques.

C. High-Risk Strategies: Adolescents who were recently discharged from the hospital or who were evaluated in an emergency room after a suicide attempt are at increased risk of further self-harm. Effective evaluation, referral, and service coordination should ensure that those who need treatment are linked with a community clinician or mental health clinic as soon as possible and that those who do not appear for scheduled appointments are contacted.

Community education and treatment services should be provided for high-risk groups such as Native Americans and Australian Aborigines, particularly for those in juvenile correctional institutions.

Community hotline services provide telephone assessment, counseling, and when possible, referral for children and adolescents in emotional crisis. About 10% of calls to these services are suicide related. Although these services are used by youths when they are well publicized, it is not clear that those who are at greatest risk (usually males) are inclined to do so.

D. Educational Strategies: School-based suicide prevention curricula aim to raise students' awareness of suicide, to encourage those with problems to seek help, and to encourage other students to recognize, refer, or report their friends who need help. Evaluations of these programs have not supported their efficacy. These programs have ignored or alienated adolescents who are most in need, and other adolescents who originally had unfavorable views of suicide were inclined to view it as a rational alternative after these programs concluded.

E. Summary: The measures likely to convey the greatest benefit are the population-based and high-risk strategies, particularly those limiting the availability of lethal means, reducing unemployment, and providing effective treatment for adolescents who have attempted suicide. Early identification, assessment, and referral by teachers, school counselors, and family practitioners is promising but as yet untested. Community hotline services probably fail to reach those who are most at risk. School-based suicide prevention curricula are of doubtful effectiveness and may even be deleterious. Aside from the population-based strategies, the interventions described in this section presuppose the availability of child and adolescent mental health facilities that provide effective treatment services. Few communities have treatment resources that are adequate for this task.

de Wilde EJ et al: The relationship between adolescent suicidal behavior and life events in childhood and adolescence. Am J Psychiatry 1992;149:45.

Gould MS et al: Pages 180–196 in the clinical prediction of adolescent suicide. In: Maris RW, Berman AL, Maltsburger JT (editors): *Assessment and Prediction of Suicide.* Guilford Press, 1992.

Group for the Advancement of Psychiatry, Committee on Adolescence: *Adolescent Suicide,* Report No. 140. American Psychiatric Press, 1996.

Hendin H: Psychodynamics of suicide, with particular reference to the young. Am J Psychiatry 1991;148:1150.

Lewis G, Hawton K, Jones P: Strategies for preventing suicide. Br J Psychiatry 1997;171:351.

Pfeffer CR: Suicidal behavior in children and adolescents: causes and management. Chapter 61, pages 661–673 in Lewis M (editor): *Child and Adolescent Psychiatry: A Comprehensive Textbook,* 2nd ed. Williams & Wilkins, 1996.

Shaffer D: Suicide: risk factors and the public health. Am J Public Health 1993;83:171.

NOTE: Page numbers in bold face type indicate a major discussion. A *t* following a page number indicates tabular material and an *f* following a page number indicates a figure. Drugs are listed under their generic names. When a drug trade name is listed, the reader is referred to the generic name.